CW01424995

MEDICINE

engelsk-svensk-engelsk

P. H. Collin

MEDICINE

engelsk-svensk-engelsk

Norstedts Akademiska Förlag

Översättning
Margit Bönnemark Myrman

Granskning
Jan Fohlman

Redaktion
Inger Hesslin Rider
Mona Wiman

ISBN 978-91-7227-049-7

Första upplagan, sjunde tryckningen

First published in Great Britain
by Peter Collin Publishing Ltd with the title
ENGLISH MEDICAL DICTIONARY

Norstedts Akademiska Förlag ingår i
Norstedt Förlagsgrupp AB, grundad 1823

www.norstedtsakademiska.se

Tryckt hos NordBook, Norge 2008

Förord

Norstedts fackordböcker har som grund en serie engelska fackordböcker utgivna av Peter Collin Publishing Ltd. Tidigare utgivna engelsk-svensk-engelska titlar är Business, Computing/Information Technology och Law. Nu fogas ytterligare en titel till serien: Medicine, som omfattar ett brittiskt-amerikanskt ordförråd om ca 12 000 ord och fraser från det medicinska området.

I den tvåspråkiga versionen har uppslagsord och definierade fraser försetts med översättningar. Definitionerna av uppslagsord och fraser på enkel engelska har behållits. Förutom de översatta fraserna innehåller ordboken ett rikt urval autentiska språkexempel som visar i vilket sammanhang uppslagsordet vanligen används. Användaren får också hjälp med enklare grammatik, t ex konstruktion eller oregelbunden böjning, eller olikheter mellan brittisk och amerikansk engelska.

För att ytterligare anpassa serien till den svenska användarens behov anges uttal för engelska uppslagsord. Vidare finns ett antal svenska uppslagsord insorterade i bokstavsordning bland de engelska. De fungerar som ingångsord tillbaka till engelskan:

Ex. blodgivare ⇒ blood

I artikeln *blood* hittar man så *blood donor* med översättningen blodgivare. Man måste alltså slå upp artikeln för att finna översättningen.

Medicine innehåller dessutom ett antal bilder på organ m m, vilka försetts med både engelsk och svensk text. Det finns också ett supplement med tabeller och termer med anknytning till det medicinska området.

Norstedts Akademiska Förlag

Ordboken innehåller ett antal ord som har sitt ursprung i varumärken. Detta får inte feltolkas så, att ordens förekomst här och sättet att förklara dem skulle ändra varumärkenas karaktär av skyddade kännetecken eller kunna anföras som giltigt skäl att beröva innehavarna deras skyddade ensamrätt till de ifrågavarande beteckningarna.

Aa

Vitamin A [ˌvɪtəmɪn ˈeɪ] *or* **retinol** [ˈretɪˌnɒl] *subst.* vitamin which is soluble in fat and can be formed in the body from precursors but is mainly found in food, such as liver, vegetables, eggs and cod liver oil. *A-vitamin, retinol*

> COMMENT: lack of Vitamin A affects the body's growth and resistance to disease and can cause night blindness or xerophthalmia. Carotene (the yellow substance in carrots) is a precursor of Vitamin A, which accounts for the saying that eating carrots helps you to see in the dark

A band [ˈeɪˌbænd] *subst.* part of the pattern in muscle tissue, seen through a microscope as a dark band *A-band, det mörka bandet i tvärstrimmig muskulatur*

abdomen [ˈæbdəmən, æbˈdəʊmen] *subst.* space in front of the body below the diaphragm and above the pelvis, containing the stomach, intestines, liver and other vital organs *abdomen, buken, bukhålan;* **acute abdomen** = any serious condition of the abdomen which requires surgery *akut buk*

> COMMENT: the abdomen is divided for medical purposes into nine regions: at the top, the right and left hypochondriac regions with the epigastrium between them; in the centre, the right and left lumbar regions with the umbilical between them; and at the bottom, the right and left iliac regions with the hypogastric between them

abdomin- [æbˈdɒmɪn, -ˌ--] *prefix* referring to the abdomen *abdomin(o)-, bukhåle-, buk-*

abdominal [æbˈdɒmɪn(ə)l] *adj.* referring to the abdomen *abdominal, abdominell, buk-, bukhåle-;* **abdominal aorta** *see* AORTA; **abdominal cavity** = space in the body below the chest *cavum abdominis, bukhålan;* **abdominal distension** = condition where the abdomen is stretched (because of gas *or* fluid) *utspänd buk;* **abdominal pain** = pain in the abdomen caused by indigestion or more serious disorders *buksmärta;* **abdominal viscera** = organs contained in the abdomen (such as the stomach, liver, etc.) *inälvorna;* **abdominal wall** = muscular tissue which surrounds the abdomen *bukväggen*

abdominell ➪ **abdominal**

abdominoperineal excision [æbˌdɒmɪnəʊˌperɪˈniːəl ɪkˈsɪʒ(ə)n] *subst.* cutting out of tissue in both the abdomen and the perineum *operativt avlägsnande av vävnad både i buk och bäckenbotten*

abdominoscopy [æbˌdɒmɪˈnɒskəpi] *subst.* internal examination of the abdomen, usually with an endoscope *laparoskopi*

abdominothoracic [æbˌdɒmɪnəʊθɔːˈræsɪk] *adj.* referring to the abdomen and thorax *som avser el. hör till både buken och bröstkorgen* NOTE: for other terms referring to the abdomen, see words beginning with **coeli-**

abducens [æbˈdjuːsənz] *or* **abducent nerve** [æbˈdjuːsənt ˌnɜːv] *subst.* sixth cranial nerve, which controls the muscle which makes the eyeball turn outwards *(nervus) abducens, 6:e kranialnerven*

abducera ➪ **abduct**

abduct [æbˈdʌkt] *vb.* to pull away from the centre line of the body *abducera;* **vocal folds abducted** = normal condition of the vocal cords in quiet breathing *abducerade stämband, stämband i respirationsställning*

abduction [æbˈdʌkʃ(ə)n] *subst.* movement where part of the body moves away from the midline or from a neighbouring part *abduktion*

abductor (muscle) [æbˈdʌktə ˌmʌs(ə)l] *subst.* muscle which pulls a part of the body away from the midline of the body or from a neighbouring part *abduktor, abducerande (isärförande) muskel*
NOTE: the opposite is **adducted, adduction, adductor**

abduktion ➪ **abduction**

abduktor ➪ **abductor (muscle)**

aberrant [æˈber(ə)nt] *adj.* not normal *aberrant, avvikande, onormal*

aberration [ˌæbəˈreɪʃ(ə)n] *subst.* action *or* growth which is not normal *aberration, avvikelse;* **mental aberration** = slight forgetfulness *or* slightly abnormal mental process *sinnesförvirring*

ability [ə'bɪləti] *subst.* being able to do something *förmåga, färdighet*

ablation [æb'leɪʃ(ə)n] *subst.* removal of an organ *or* of part of the body by surgery *ablation, avlägsnande;* **segmental ablation** = surgical removal of part of a nail, as treatment for an ingrowing toenail *Königs operation*

able ['eɪb(ə)l] *adj.* **after the injection he was able to breathe more easily** = he could breathe more easily *efter injektionen kunde han andas lättare*
NOTE: opposite is **unable.** Note also that **able** is used with **to** and a verb

abnorm ➪ **abnormal, anomalous**

abnormal [æb'nɔːm(ə)l] *adj.* not normal *abnorm, onormal, avvikande;* **abnormal behaviour** = conduct which is different from the way normal people behave *onormalt (avvikande) beteende;* **abnormal motion** *or* **abnormal stool** = faeces which are different in colour *or* which are very liquid *onormal avföring*

> QUOTE the synovium produces an excess of synovial fluid, which is abnormal and becomes thickened. This causes pain, swelling and immobility of the affected joint
> **Nursing Times**

abnormality [,æbnɔː'mæləti] *subst.* form *or* action which is not normal *abnormitet, avvikelse*

> QUOTE Even children with the milder forms of sickle-cell disease (SCD) have an increased frequency of pneumococcal infection. The reason for this susceptibility is a profound abnormality of the immune system in children with SCD
> **Lancet**

abnormally [æb'nɔːm(ə)li] *adv.* in a way which is not normal *abnormt, onormalt, på ett avvikande sätt;* **he had an abnormally fast pulse; her periods were abnormally frequent** NOTE: for other terms referring to abnormality, see words beginning with **terat-**

abnormitet ➪ **abnormality**

abnormt ➪ **abnormally**

abort [ə'bɔːt] *vb.* (i) to eject the embryo *or* fetus and so end a pregnancy before the fetus is fully developed *abortera, få missfall, framkalla abort;* (ii) to have an abortion *göra (genomgå) abort;* **the doctors decided to abort the fetus; the tissue will be aborted spontaneously**

abort ➪ **abortion, termination**

abortera ➪ **abort**

abortframkallande ➪ **abortifacient, -facient**

abortifacient [ə,bɔːtɪ'feɪʃ(ə)nt] *subst.* drug *or* surgical instrument which provokes an abortion *abortframkallande*

abortion [ə'bɔːʃ(ə)n] *subst.* situation where an unborn baby leaves the womb before the end of pregnancy, especially during the first twenty-eight weeks of pregnancy when it is not likely to survive birth *abort, missfall;* **the girl asked the clinic if she could have an abortion; she had two abortions before her first child was born; to have an abortion** = to have an operation to make a fetus leave the womb during the first period of pregnancy *göra (genomgå) abort;* **complete abortion** = abortion where the whole contents of the uterus are expelled *abortus completus, fullständig abort;* **criminal abortion** *or* **illegal abortion** = abortion which is carried out illegally *abortus criminalis (illegalis), illegal abort;* **habitual abortion** *or* **recurrent abortion** = condition where a woman has several abortions with successive pregnancies *abortus habitualis, habituell abort;* **incomplete abortion** = abortion where part of the contents of the uterus is not expelled *abortus incompletus, ofullständig abort;* **induced abortion** = abortion which is produced by drugs *or* by surgery *abortus provocatus, framkallad abort;* **legal abortion** = abortion which is carried out legally *abortus legalis, legal abort;* **spontaneous abortion** = MISCARRIAGE; **therapeutic abortion** = abortion which is carried out because the health of the mother is in danger *abort pga att havandeskapet medför allvarlig fara för moderns liv eller hälsa;* **threatened abortion** = possible abortion in the early stages of pregnancy, indicated by bleeding *abortus imminens, hotande abort*

> COMMENT: in the UK an abortion can be carried out legally if two doctors agree that the mother's life is in danger or that the fetus is likely to be born with severe handicaps. *I Sverige krävs ej längre s.k. tvåläkarintyg (övers. anm.)*

abortionist [ə'bɔːʃ(ə)nɪst] *subst.* person who makes a woman abort, usually a person who performs an illegal abortion *abortör*

abortive [ə'bɔːtɪv] *adj.* which does not succeed *abortiv, förkrympt, ofullgången, hämmad (i sin utveckling);* **abortive poliomyelitis** = mild form of polio which only affects the throat and intestines *abortiv poliomyelit*

abort, spontan ⇨ **miscarriage**

abortus fever [ə'bɔːtəs ˌfiːvə] *or* **brucellosis** [ˌbruːsɪ'ləʊsɪs] *subst.* disease which can be caught from cattle, or from drinking infected milk, spread by a species of the bacterium Brucella *brucellos, febris undulans, undulantfeber*

> COMMENT: symptoms include tiredness, arthritis, headaches, sweating and swelling of the spleen

abortör ⇨ **abortionist**

ABO system [ˌeɪbiː'əʊ ˌsɪstəm] *subst.* system of classifying blood groups *ABO-systemet; see note at* BLOOD GROUP

above [ə'bʌv] *adv. & prep.* higher than *över, högre än;* **his temperature was above 100 degrees; her pulse rate was far above normal**

abrasio ⇨ **dilatation**

abrasion [ə'breɪʒ(ə)n] *subst.* condition where the surface of the skin has been rubbed off by a rough surface and bleeds *abrasion, skrubbsår*

> COMMENT: even minor abrasions can allow infection to enter the body, and should be cleaned and treated with an antiseptic

abreaction [ˌæbrɪ'ækʃ(ə)n] *subst. (in psychology)* treatment of a neurotic patient by making him think again about past bad experiences *avreagering*

abscess ['æbses] *subst.* swollen area where pus forms, and which is painful, and often accompanied by high temperature *abscess, varhärd, böld;* **he had an abscess under a tooth; the doctor decided to lance the abscess; acute abscess** = abscess which develops rapidly *akut abscess (böld);* **chronic abscess** = abscess which develops slowly over a period of time *kronisk abscess (böld)* NOTE: plural is **abscesses**

> COMMENT: an acute abscess can be dealt with by opening and draining when it has reached the stage where sufficient pus has been formed; a chronic abscess is treated with drugs

abscesshåla ⇨ **vomica**

absence ['æbs(ə)ns] *subst.* not being here *or* there *frånvaro, brist, avsaknad;* **in the absence of any other symptoms** = because no other symptoms were present *i brist (avsaknad) på andra symtom*

absent ['æbs(ə)nt] *adj.* not here *or* not there *frånvarande, obefintlig;* **normal symptoms of malaria are absent in this form of the disease; three children are absent because they are ill**

absolutely ['æbsəluːtli] *adv.* really *or* completely *absolut, fullständigt, helt;* **he's still not absolutely fit after his operation; the patient must remain absolutely still while the scan is taking place**

absolutist ⇨ **abstainer**

absorb [əb'sɔːb] *vb.* to take in (a liquid) *absorbera, suga upp;* **cotton wads are used to absorb the discharge from the wound**

absorbent [əb'sɔːb(ə)nt] *adj.* which absorbs *absorberande;* **absorbent cotton** = soft white stuff used as a dressing to put on wounds *kompress*

absorbera ⇨ **absorb**

absorberande ⇨ **absorbent**

absorption [əb'sɔːpʃ(ə)n] *subst.* (i) action of taking a liquid into a solid *absorption, uppsugning;* (ii) taking substances into the body, such as proteins *or* fats which have been digested from food, and are taken into the bloodstream from the bowels *absorption, uppsugning, upptag(ning);* **absorption rate** = rate at which a liquid is absorbed by a solid *absorptionshastighet;* **percutaneous absorption** = absorbing a substance through the skin *perkutan absorption, upptag genom huden*
NOTE: the spellings: **absorb** but **absorption**

absorptionsförband ⇨ **lint**

absorptionshastighet ⇨ **absorption**

abstain [əb'steɪn] *vb.* not to do something voluntarily *avstå, avhålla sig, vara avhållsam;* **he abstained from taking any drugs for two months; they decided to abstain from sexual intercourse**

abstainer [əb'steɪnə] *subst.* person who does not drink alcohol *absolutist, helnykterist*

abstinence ['æbstɪnəns] *subst.* not doing something voluntarily *abstinens, avhållsamhet, nykterhet;* **the clinic recommended total abstinence from alcohol** *or* **from drugs**

abstinens ⇨ **abstinence, withdrawal**

abstinenssymtom ⇨ **withdrawal**

abulia [ə'bu:liə] *subst.* lack of will power *abuli, viljesvaghet, viljeförlamning*

abuse [ə'bju:s; ə'bju:z] **1** *subst.* **(a)** using something wrongly *abusus, missbruk;* **alcohol abuse** *or* **amphetamine abuse** *or* **drug abuse** = being mentally and physically dependent on taking alcohol *or* a drug regularly *alkoholmissbruk, spritmissbruk, amfetaminmissbruk, narkotikamissbruk, drogmissbruk* **(b)** bad treatment of a person *misshandel, (sexuellt) utnyttjande;* **child abuse or sexual abuse of children** NOTE: no plural **2** *vb.* **(a)** to use something wrongly *missbruka;* **heroin and cocaine are commonly abused drugs; to abuse one's authority** = to use one's powers in an illegal or harmful way *missbruka sin makt eller ställning* **(b)** to treat someone badly *misshandla, utnyttja (sexuellt);* **he had sexually abused small children**

a.c. [ˌeɪ'si:] *abbreviation of* "ante cibum": meaning "before food" (used on prescriptions) *ante cibum, före måltid*

acanthosis [ˌækən'θəʊsɪs] *subst.* disease of the prickle cell layer of thew skin, where warts appear on the skin or inside the mouth *akantos*

acaricide [ə'kærəsaɪd] *subst.* substance which kills mites *medel som dödar kvalster*

acatalasia ['ækætə'leɪziə] *subst.* inherited condition which results in a defect of catalase in all tissue *akatalasemi*

accelerate [ək'seləreɪt] *vb.* to go faster *accelerera, öka hastigheten (takten)*

acceleration [əkˌselə'reɪʃ(ə)n] *subst.* going more quickly *acceleration, tilltagande (ökande) hastighet;* **the nurse noticed an acceleration in the patient's pulse rate**

accelerera ➪ **accelerate**

accepteras ➪ **take**

accessorisk ➪ **accessory**

accessory [ək'ses(ə)rɪ] *adj.* (thing) which helps, without being most important *accessorisk, bidragande, extra, hjälp-;* **accessory nerve** = eleventh cranial nerve, which supplies the muscles in the neck and shoulders *nervus accessorius, 11:e kranialnerven;* **accessory organ** = organ which has a function which is controlled by another organ *accessoriskt organ*

accident ['æksɪd(ə)nt] *subst.* **(a)** something which happens by chance *tillfällighet, slump;* **I met her by accident at the bus stop** **(b)** unpleasant event which happens suddenly and harms someone's health *olycka, olyckshändelse, olycksfall;* **she had an accident in the kitchen and had to go to hospital; three people were killed in the accident on the motorway; accident and emergency department (A & E)** = department of a hospital which deals with accidents and emergency cases *akutklinik, akutmottagning, olycksfallsavdelning, klinik för vård av akut- och olycksfall;* **accident prevention** = taking steps to prevent accidents from happening *olycksförebyggande åtgärder;* **accident ward** = ward in a hospital for victims of accidents *akutmottagning, olycksfallsavdelning*

accidentally [ˌæksɪ'dent(ə)li] *adv.* **(a)** by chance *av en händelse (slump, tillfällighet);* **I found the missing watch accidentally** **(b)** in an accident *i en olycka (olyckshändelse);* **he was killed accidentally**

accident-prone ['æksɪd(ə)ntprəʊn] *adj.* (person) who has awkward movements and frequently has minor accidents *or* who frequently causes minor accidents *som lätt (ofta) råkar ut för olyckor*

accommodation [əˌkɒmə'deɪʃ(ə)n] *subst. (of the lens of the eye)* being able to focus on objects at different distances, using the ciliary muscle *ackommodation(sförmåga)*

accommodative squint [əˌkɒmədeɪtɪv 'skwɪnt] *subst.* squint when the eye is trying to focus on an object which is very close *kisande för att få föremål i fokus*

accompany [ə'kʌmp(ə)ni] *vb.* to go with *beledsaga, åtfölja, göra sällskap med;* **he accompanied his wife to hospital; the pain was accompanied by high temperature**

according to [ə'kɔ:dɪŋ tʊ] *adv.* as someone says or writes *enligt, efter;* **according to the dosage on the bottle, the medicine can be given to very young children**

accretion [ə'kri:ʃ(ə)n] *subst.* growth of a substance which sticks to an object *ackretion, avlagring;* **an accretion of calcium round the joint**

accumulate [ə'kju:mjəleɪt] *vb.* to grow together in a group *ackumulera, ansamla, upplagra;* **large quantities of fat accumulated in the arteries**

accumulation [əˌkju:mjə'leɪʃ(ə)n] *subst.* (i) act of accumulating *ackumulation, ansamling, upplagring;* (ii) material which has accumulated *anhopning, ansamling;* **the drug**

aims at clearing the accumulation of fatty deposits in the arteries

accurate ['ækjərət] *adj.* very correct *exakt, riktig, noggrann;* **the sphygmomanometer does not seem to be giving an accurate reading; the scan helped to give an accurate location for the operation site; the results of the lab tests should help the consultant make an accurate diagnosis**

accurately ['ækjərətli] *adv.* very correctly *exakt, riktigt, noggrant;* **the GP accurately diagnosed a tumour in the liver**

acefal ⇨ **acephalus**

acephalus [ˌeɪ'sef(ə)ləs] *subst.* fetus born without a head *acefal, acranius, foster utan huvud*

acetabularplastik ⇨ **acetabuloplasty**

acetabuloplasty [ˌæsɪ'tæbjʊlə(ʊ)ˌplæsti] *subst.* surgical operation to repair *or* rebuild the acetabulum *acetabularplastik, höftledsplastik*

acetabulum [ˌæsɪ'tæbjʊləm] *or* **cotyloid cavity** ['kɒtiˌlɔɪd ˌkævəti] *subst.* part of the pelvic bone, shaped like a cup, into which the head of the femur fits to form the hip joint *acetabulum, höftledspannan*
NOTE: plural is **acetabula**

acetic acid [əˌsiːtɪk 'æsɪd] *subst.* acid which turns wine into vinegar *ättiksyra, metylkarbonsyra*

> COMMENT: a weak solution of acetic acid can be used to cool the body in hot weather; a strong solution can be used to burn away warts

aceton ⇨ **acetone**

acetone ['æsətəʊn] *subst.* substance, smelling like nail varnish, formed in the body after vomiting or during diabetes *aceton*

acetonuria [ˌæsɪtə'njʊəriə] *subst.* presence of acetone in the urine, giving off a sweet smell *acetonuri*

acetylcholine [ˌæsɪˌtaɪ(ə)l'kəʊliːn] *subst.* substance released from nerve endings, which allows nerve impulses to move from one nerve to another, or from a nerve to the organ it controls *acetylcholin, acetylkolin*

acetylkolin ⇨ **acetylcholine**

acetylsalicylic acid [ˌæsɪˌtaɪ(ə)lˌsælə'sɪlɪk 'æsɪd] *subst. see* ASPIRIN

acetylsalicylsyra ⇨ **aspirin**

achalasia [ˌækə'leɪziə] *subst.* being unable to relax the muscles *achalasi, akalasi;* **cardiac achalasia** *or* **achalasia cardia** = being unable to relax the cardia *or* the muscle at the entrance to the stomach, with the result that food cannot enter the stomach *kardiospasm; see also* HELLER'S OPERATION

ache [eɪk] **1** *subst.* pain which goes on for a time, but is not very acute *värk;* **he complained of various aches and pains; she said she had an ache in one of her front teeth** *used with other words to show where the pain is situated: see* BACKACHE, HEADACHE, STOMACH ACHE, TOOTHACHE **2** *vb.* to have a pain in part of the body *värka, göra ont;* **reading in bad light can make the eyes ache; his tooth ached so much he went to the dentist**

Achilles tendon [əˌkɪliːz 'tendən] *subst.* tendon at the back of the ankle which connects the calf muscles to the heel, and which acts to pull up the heel when the calf muscle is tense *tendo calcaneus (Achillis), akillessenan*

achillorrhaphy [ˌækɪ'lɔːrəfi] *subst.* surgical operation to stitch a torn Achilles tendon *akillorrafi, suturering av akillessenan*

achillotomy [ˌækɪ'lɒtəmi] *subst.* act of dividing the Achilles tendon *akillotomi*

aching ['eɪkɪŋ] *adj.* with a continuous pain *värkande*

achlorhydria [ˌeɪklɔː'haɪdriə] *subst.* condition where the gastric juices do not contain hydrochloric acid, a symptom of stomach cancer or pernicious anaemia *aklorhydri, akyli*

acholia [ə'kəʊliə] *subst.* absence of bile *acholi, akoli, gallbrist*

acholuria [ˌækə'lʊəriə] *subst.* absence of bile colouring in the urine *acholuri, akoluri*

acholuric jaundice [ˌækə'lʊərɪk ˌdʒɔːndɪs] *subst.* hereditary spherocytosis *or* disease where abnormally round red blood cells form, leading to anaemia, enlarged spleen and the formation of gallstones *akolurisk ikterus, gulsot*

achondroplasia [ˌeɪˌkɒndrə(ʊ)'pleɪziə] *subst.* hereditary condition where the long bones in the arms and legs do not grow fully, while the rest of the bones in the body do so, producing dwarfism *achondroplasi, akondroplasi*

acid ['æsɪd] *subst.* **(a)** chemical compound containing hydrogen, which reacts with an alkali to form a salt and water *syra;* **hydrochloric acid is secreted in the stomach and forms part of the gastric juices; bile acids** = acids (such as cholic acid) found in the bile *gallsyror;* **inorganic acids** = acids which come from minerals, used in dilute form to help indigestion *oorganiska syror;* **organic acids** = acids which come from plants, taken to stimulate the production of urine *organiska syror* **(b)** any bitter juice *surt ämne*

aciditet ⇨ **acidity**

acidity [ə'sɪdəti] *subst.* **(a)** level of acid in a liquid *aciditet, surhet(sgrad);* **the alkaline solution may help to reduce acidity (b)** acid stomach *or* form of indigestion where the patient has a burning feeling in his stomach caused by too much acid forming in the stomach *sur mage*

acidos ⇨ **acidosis**

acidosis [ˌæsɪ'dəʊsɪs] *subst.* (i) condition when there are more acid waste products (such as urea) than normal in the blood because of a lack of alkali *acidos;* (ii) acid stomach *sur mage*

acinus ['æsɪnəs] *subst.* (i) tiny alveolus which forms part of a gland *acinus, druvklaseliknande del av körtel;* (ii) part of a lobule in the lung *acinus, grupp lungblåsor i bronkiol* NOTE: plural is **acini**

ackommodation(sförmåga) ⇨ **accommodation**

ackommodationsreflex ⇨ **reflex**

ackretion ⇨ **accretion**

ackumulera ⇨ **accumulate**

acne ['ækni] *or* **acne vulgaris** [ˌækni vʌl'geərɪs] *subst.* inflammation of the sebaceous glands during puberty, which makes blackheads appear on the skin, usually on the face, neck and shoulders, and these then become infected *acne (vulgaris, simplex), akne, finnar;* **he suffers from acne; she is using a cream to clear up her acne**

acoustic [ə'ku:stɪk] *adj.* referring to sound *or* hearing *akustisk, ljud-, hörsel-;* **acoustic nerve** *see* NERVE; **acoustic neurofibroma** *or* **acoustic neuroma** = tumour in the sheath of the auditory nerve, causing deafness *tumör som utgår från hörselnervens skida*

acquired [ə'kwaɪəd] *adj.* (condition) which is neither congenital nor hereditary, and which a person develops after birth in reaction to his environment *förvärvad;* **acquired immunity** = immunity which a body acquires and which is not congenital *förvärvad immunitet;* **acquired immunodeficiency syndrome** = AIDS *see also* CONGENITAL, HEREDITARY

acranius ⇨ **acephalus**

acro- ['ækrə(ʊ), ˌ--] *prefix* referring to a point *or* tip *akro-*

acrocyanosis [ˌækrə(ʊ)sa(ɪ)ə'nəʊsɪs] *subst.* blue colour of the extremities (fingers, toes, ears and nose) due to bad circulation *akrocyanos*

acrodynia [ˌækrə(ʊ)'dɪniə] *or* **pink disease** ['pɪnk dɪˌzi:z] *subst.* children's disease where the child's hands, feet and face swell and become pink, with a fever and loss of appetite, caused by allergy to mercury *akrodyni, pink disease, erythroedema*

acromegaly [ˌækrə(ʊ)'megəli] *subst.* disease caused by excessive quantities of growth hormone produced by the pituitary gland, causing a slow enlargement of the hands, feet and jaws in adults *akromegali*

acromial [ə'krəʊmiəl] *adj.* referring to the acromion *akromial;* **coraco-acromial =** referring to both the coracoid process and the acromion *coraco-acromialis, som avser el. hör till både det korpnäbblika utskottet från skulderbladet och akromion (skulderhöjden)*

acromion [ə'krəʊmiən] *subst.* pointed top of the scapula, which forms the tip of the shoulder ⇨ *illustration* SHOULDER, SKELETON *akromion, skulderhöjden*

acronyx ['ækrə(ʊ)nɪks] *subst. (of a nail)* growing into the flesh *akronyx, inväxt nagel*

acroparaesthesia [ˌækrə(ʊ)ˌpæri:s'θi:ziə] *subst.* condition where the patient suffers sharp pains in the arms and numbness in the fingers after sleep *akroparestesi*

acrophobia [ˌækrə(ʊ)'fəʊbiə] *subst.* fear of heights *akrofobi, höjdskräck*

acrosclerosis [ˌækrə(ʊ)sklə'rəʊsɪs] *subst.* sclerosis which affects the extremities *akroskleros, sklerodaktyli*

act [ækt] *vb.* to do something *or* to have the effect of *handla, fungera, tjänstgöra, verka;* **the connecting tissue acts as a supporting framework; he had to act quickly to save his sister**

ACTH [ˌeɪsiːtiːˈeɪtʃ, ækə] = ADRENOCORTICOTROPHIC HORMONE

actin [ˈæktɪn] *subst.* protein which, with myosin, forms the contractile tissue of muscle *aktin*

actinomycosis [ˌæktɪnəmaɪˈkəʊsɪs] *subst.* disease transmitted by cattle, where the patient is infected with fungus which forms abscesses in the mouth and lungs (pulmonary actinomycosis) or in the ileum (intestinal actinomycosis) *aktinomykos, strålsvampsjuka*

action [ˈækʃ(ə)n] *subst.* thing which is done *or* effect *handling, verkan, effekt;* **the injection will speed up the action of the antibiotic**

activate [ˈæktɪveɪt] *vb.* to make something start to work *aktivera, göra aktiv (verksam, effektiv);* **the muscle activates the heart; hormones from the pituitary gland activate other glands**

active [ˈæktɪv] *adj.* lively *or* energetic *or* doing something *aktiv, verksam;* **although he is over eighty he is still very active; active ingredient** = main medicinal ingredient of an ointment *or* lotion (as opposed to the base) *aktiv (verksam) substans;* **active movement** = movement made by a patient using his own willpower and muscles *aktiv rörelse;* **active principle** = main medicinal ingredient of a drug which makes it have the required effect on a patient *aktiv beståndsdel*

activity [ækˈtɪvəti] *subst.* what something does *aktivitet, verksamhet, effekt;* **the drug's activity did not last more than a few hours**

actomyosin [ˌæktəʊˈmaɪəsɪn] *subst.* combination of actin and myosin, which forms the contractile tissue of muscle *aktomyosin*

act on [ˈækt ˌɒn] *or* **upon** [əˈpɒn] *vb.* **(a)** to do something as the result of something which has been said *handla enligt (efter);* **he acted upon your suggestion (b)** to have an effect on *inverka (verka, göra verkan) på, ha effekt på;* **the antibiotic acted quickly on the infection**

actual [ˈæktʃ(u)əl] *adj.* real *faktisk, verklig;* **what are the actual figures for the number of children in school?**

actually [ˈæktʃ(u)əli] *adv.* really *faktiskt, verkligen;* **is he actually going to discharge himself from the hospital?**

acuity [əˈkjuːəti] *subst.* sharpness *skärpa;* **visual acuity** = being able to see objects clearly *visus, synskärpa*

acupuncture [ˈækjupʌŋktʃə] *subst.* treatment originating in China, where needles are inserted through the skin into nerve centres to relieve pain *akupunktur*

acupuncturist [ˈækjuˌpʌŋktʃ(ə)rɪst] *subst.* person who practises acupuncture *akupunktör*

acute [əˈkjuːt] *adj.* (i) (disease) which comes on rapidly and can be dangerous *akut, brådskande, plötslig;* (ii) (pain) which is sharp and intense *akut, häftig, skarp;* **she had an acute attack of shingles; he felt acute chest pains; after the acute stage of the illness had passed, he felt very weak; acute abdomen** = any serious condition of the abdomen which may require surgery *akut buk; compare* CHRONIC

> QUOTE twenty-seven adult patients admitted to hospital with acute abdominal pains were referred for study
>
> **Lancet**

> QUOTE the survey shows a reduction in acute beds in the last six years. The bed losses forced one hospital to send acutely ill patients to hospitals up to sixteen miles away
>
> **Nursing Times**

acute yellow atrophy [əˈkjuːt ˌjeləʊ ˈætrəfi] *see* YELLOW

acystia [əˈsɪstiə] *subst.* congenital defect, where a baby is born without a bladder *acysti*

Adam's apple [ˌædəmz ˈæp(ə)l] *subst.* piece of the thyroid cartilage surrounding the voice box, which projects from the neck below the chin in a man, and moves up and down when he speaks *prominentia laryngea, pomum Adami, adamsäpplet*

Adams-Stokes syndrom ⇨ **Stokes-Adams syndrome**

adamsäpplet ⇨ **Adam's apple, laryngeal, prominence**

adapt [əˈdæpt] *vb.* to change to fit a new situation *adaptera, anpassa (sig);* **she has adapted very well to her new job in the children's hospital; the brace has to be adapted to fit the patient**

adaptation [ˌædæpˈteɪʃ(ə)n] *subst.* (i) changing something so that it fits a new situation *adap(ta)tion, anpassning;* (ii) process by which sensory receptors become accustomed to a sensation which is repeated *adap(ta)tion;* **dark adaptation** *or* **light adaptation** = changes in the eye in response to changes in light conditions *mörkeradap(ta)tion, ljusadap(ta)tion*

adaptera ➪ **adapt**

addict [ˈædɪkt] *subst.* **drug addict** = person who is physically and mentally dependent on taking drugs regularly *missbrukare, narkotikamissbrukare, narkoman;* **a heroin addict; a morphine addict**

addicted [əˈdɪktɪd] *adj.* **addicted to alcohol** *or* **drugs** = being unable to live without taking alcohol *or* drugs regularly *hemfallen åt alkoholmissbruk (narkotikamissbruk)*

addiction [əˈdɪkʃ(ə)n] *subst. missbruk;* **drug addiction** *or* **drug dependence** = being mentally and physically dependent on taking a drug regularly *narkomani, narkotikamissbruk, läkemedelsmissbruk, drogmissbruk, narkotikaberoende, läkemedelsberoende, drogberoende*

> QUOTE three quarters of patients aged 35-64 on GPs' lists have at least one major risk factor: high cholesterol, high blood pressure or addiction to tobacco
>
> **Health Services Journal**

addictive [əˈdɪktɪv] *adj.* (drug) which is habit-forming *or* which people can become addicted to *vanebildande, beroendeframkallande;* **certain narcotic drugs are addictive**

Addisonanemi ➪ **anaemia**

Addison's anaemia [ˈædɪs(ə)nz əˌniːmiːə] = PERNICIOUS ANAEMIA

Addison's disease [ˈædɪs(ə)nz dɪˌziːz] *subst.* disease of the adrenal glands, resulting in general weakness, anaemia, low blood pressure and wasting away *Addisons sjukdom*

> COMMENT: the most noticeable symptom of the disease is the change in skin colour to yellow and then to dark brown. Treatment consists of corticosteroid injections

additive [ˈædətɪv] *subst.* chemical substance which is added, especially to food to improve its appearance or to prevent it going bad *tillsats;* **the tin of beans contains a number of additives; asthmatic and allergic reactions to additives are frequently found in workers in food processing factories**

adducerad ➪ **adducted**

adducted [əˈdʌktɪd] *adj.* brought towards the middle of the body *adducerad;* **vocal folds adducted** = position of the vocal cords for speaking *adducerade stämband, stämband i fonationsställning*

adduction [əˈdʌkʃ(ə)n] *subst.* movement of a limb towards the midline of the body *adduktion*

adductor (muscle) [əˈdʌktə ˌmʌs(ə)l] *subst.* muscle which pulls a part of the body towards the midline of the body *(musculus) adductor*
NOTE: the opposite is **abducted, abduction, abductor**

adduktion ➪ **adduction**

aden- [ˌædən, ˌædɪn] *or* **adeno-** [ˌædɪnəʊ, ˌædɪˈnəʊ, ˌædɪˈnɒ] *prefix* referring to glands *aden(o)-, körtel-*

adenectomy [ˌædəˈnektəmi] *subst.* surgical removal of a gland *adenektomi*

adenektomi ➪ **adenectomy**

adenitis [ˌædəˈnaɪtɪs] *subst.* inflammation of the lymph glands *adenit, körtelinflammation*

adenocarcinoma [ˌædɪnəʊˌkɑːsɪˈnəʊmə] *subst.* malignant tumour of a gland *adenocarcinom, adenokarcinom*

adenohypofysen ➪ **adenohypophysis**

adenohypophysis [ˌædɪnəʊhaɪˈpɒfɪsɪs] *subst.* front lobe of the pituitary gland which secretes several hormones which themselves stimulate the adrenal and thyroid glands, or which stimulate the production of sex hormones, melanin and milk *adenohypofysen, främre hypofysloben*

adenoid [ˈædɪnɔɪd] *adj.* like a gland *adenoid, körtelliknande, polyp-*

adenoidal [ˌædɪˈnɔɪd(ə)l] *adj.* referring to adenoids *körtel-;* **adenoidal expression** = common symptom of child suffering from adenoids, where his mouth is always open, the nose is narrow and the top teeth appear to project forward *symtom hos barn med polyper bakom näsan;* **adenoidal tissue** *or* **pharyngeal tonsils** = glands at the back of the throat where the passages from the nose join the throat *tonsilla pharyngea, farynxtonsillen, polyp (bakom näsan)*

adenoidectomy [ˌædɪnɔɪ'dektəmi] *subst.* surgical removal of the adenoids *adenoidektomi, adenoidotomi, borttagande av polyp*

adenoidektomi ⇨ **adenoidectomy**

adenoidism ['ædɪnɔɪdɪz(ə)m] *subst.* condition of a person with adenoids *adenoidism;* **the little boy suffers from adenoidism**

adenoidotomi ⇨ **adenoidectomy**

adenoids ['ædɪnɔɪdz] *subst pl.* condition where growths form on the glands at the back of the throat where the passages from the nose join the throat, which prevent the patient breathing through the nose *polyper (bakom näsan);* **enlargement of the adenoids** *or* **adenoid vegetation** = condition in children where the adenoidal tissue is covered with growths and can block the nasal passages or the Eustachian tubes *adenoida vegetationer;* **removal of the adenoids is sometimes indicated**

adenokarcinom ⇨ **adenocarcinoma**

adenoma [ˌædɪ'nəʊmə] *subst.* benign tumour of a gland *adenom, körtelsvulst*

adenomyoma [ˌædɪnəʊmaɪ'əʊmə] *subst.* benign tumour made up of glands and muscle *adenomyom*

adenopathy [ˌædɪ'nɒpəθi] *subst.* disease of a gland *adenopati, körtelsjukdom*

adenopati ⇨ **adenopathy, adenosis**

adenosclerosis [ˌædɪnəʊsklə'rəʊsɪs] *subst.* hardening of a gland *adenoskleros*

adenosine triphosphate (ATP) [ə'denə(ʊ)si:n ˌtraɪ'fɒsfeɪt (ˌeɪti:'pi:)] *subst.* chemical which occurs in all cells, but mainly in muscle, where it forms the energy reserve *adenosintrifosfat, ATP*

adenosintrifosfat ⇨ **adenosine triphosphate (ATP)**

adenosis [ˌædɪ'nəʊsɪs] *subst.* any disease *or* disorder of the glands *adenopati, körtelsjukdom*

adenoskleros ⇨ **adenosclerosis**

adenovirus [ˌædɪnəʊ'vaɪ(ə)rəs] *subst.* virus which produces upper respiratory infections and sore throats, and can cause fatal pneumonia in infants *adenovirus*

adequate ['ædɪkwət] *adj.* enough *tillräcklig;* **the brain must have an adequate supply of blood; does the children's diet provide them with an adequate quantity of iron?**

adermin ⇨ **Vitamin B**

ADH [ˌeɪdi:'eɪtʃ] = ANTIDIURETIC HORMONE

adhesion [əd'hi:ʒ(ə)n] *subst.* abnormal connection between two surfaces in the body which should not be connected *adhesion, sammanväxning*

adhesive [əd'hi:sɪv] *adj.* which sticks *häft-, självhäftande;* **adhesive dressing** *or* **adhesive plaster** = dressing with a sticky substance on the back, so that it can stick to the skin *häftplåster, plåster, häfta;* **adhesive strapping** = overlapping strips of adhesive plaster, used to protect a lesion *häftförband*

adipose ['ædɪpəʊs] *adj.* containing fat *or* made of fat *adipös, fet, fettrik, fett-;* **adipose tissue** = body fat *or* tissue where the cells contain fat *fettväv(nad), kroppsfett;* **adipose degeneration** *see* DEGENERATION

> COMMENT: normal fibrous tissue is replaced by adipose tissue when more food is eaten than is necessary

adiposis dolorosa [ˌædɪ'pəʊsɪs ˌdɒlə'rəʊsə] *or* **Dercum's disease** ['dɜ:kəmz dɪˌzi:z] *subst.* disease of middle-aged women where painful lumps of fatty substance form in the body *adipositas dolorosa, (neuro)lipomatosis dolorosa, Dercums sjukdom*

adipositet ⇨ **obesity**

adiposogenitalis [ˌædɪˌpəʊsəʊˌdʒenɪ'teɪlɪs] *see* DYSTROPHIA

adiposuria [ˌædɪpəs'jʊəriə] *subst.* fat in the urine *adiposuri*

adiposus [ˌædɪ'pəʊsəs] *see* PANNICULUS

adipös ⇨ **adipose, obese**

aditus ['ædɪtəs] *subst.* opening *or* entrance to a passage *aditus, öppning, mynning*

administer [əd'mɪnɪstə] *vb.* to give (a medicine) to a patient *administrera, ge,* *tillföra;* **to administer orally** = to give a medicine by the mouth *ge peroralt, tillföra genom munnen*

administration [əd,mɪnɪs'treɪʃ(ə)n] *subst.* **(a)** giving of a drug *administrering, "läkemedelsdelning", "delning";* **administration of drugs must be supervised by a qualified doctor or nurse (b)** management *or* running of a hospital, service, etc. *administration, förvaltning;* **medical administration** = the running of hospitals and other health services *administration (förvaltning) av hälso- och sjukvård;* **she has started her career in medical administration**

administrations- ⇨ **administrative**

administrative [əd'mɪnɪstrətɪv] *adj.* referring to administration *administrativ, administrations-, förvaltnings-;* **most of the GP's spare time is taken up with administrative work**

administrator [əd'mɪnɪstreɪtə] *subst.* person who runs (a hospital *or* district health authority, etc.) *administratör*

administratör ⇨ **administrator**

administrera ⇨ **administer**

administrering ⇨ **administration**

admission [əd'mɪʃ(ə)n] *subst.* being allowed into a place *tillträde, inläggning, intagning;* **admission to the hospital** = official registering of a patient in a hospital *inläggning (intagning) på sjukhus*

admit [əd'mɪt] *vb.* to allow (someone) to go in *släppa in, ge tillträde;* to register a patient in a hospital *ta (lägga) in;* **children are admitted free; he was admitted (to hospital) this morning**

> QUOTE 80% of elderly patients admitted to geriatric units are on medication
> **Nursing Times**

> QUOTE ten patients were admitted to the ICU before operation, the main indications being the need for evaluation of patients with a history of severe heart disease
> **Southern Medical Journal**

adnexa [æd'neksə] *subst pl.* structures attached to an organ *adnexa, bihang*

adolescence [,ædə'les(ə)ns] *subst.* period of life when a child is developing into an adult *adolescens, ungdomstiden*

adolescens ⇨ **adolescence**

adolescent [,ædə'les(ə)nt] *subst. & adj.* (person) who is at the stage of life when he is developing into an adult *adolescent, ungdom, tonåring*

adopt [ə'dɒpt] *vb.* to become the legal parent of a child who was born to other parents *adoptera*

> COMMENT: if a child's parents are divorced, or if one parent dies, the child may be adopted by a step-father or step-mother

adoptera ⇨ **adopt**

adoption [ə'dɒpʃ(ə)n] *subst.* act of becoming the legal parent of a child which is not your own *adoption;* **adoption order** = order by a court which legally transfers the rights of the natural parents to the adoptive parents *adoptionsbevis;* **adoption proceedings** = court action to adopt someone *adoptionsförfarande*

adoptionsbevis ⇨ **adoption**

adoptionsförfarande ⇨ **adoption**

adoptivbarn ⇨ **adoptive**

adoptive [ə'dɒptɪv] *adj.* **adoptive child** = child who has been adopted *adoptivbarn;* **adoptive parent** = person who has adopted a child *adoptivförälder*

adrenal [ə'dri:n(ə)l] *adj.* situated near the kidney *adrenal, binjure-;* **adrenal body** = an adrenal gland *glandula suprarenalis, binjure;* **adrenal cortex** = firm outside layer of an adrenal gland, which secretes a series of hormones affecting the metabolism of carbohydrates and water *cortex suprarenis, binjurebarken;* **adrenal glands** *or* **suprarenal glands** *or US* **the adrenals** = two endocrine glands at the top of the kidneys, which secrete cortisone, adrenaline and other hormones *glandulae suprarenales, binjurarna;* **adrenal medulla** = soft inner part of the adrenal gland which secretes adrenaline and noradrenaline ⇨ *illustration* KIDNEY *medulla glandulae suprarenalis, binjuremärgen*

adrenalectomy [ə,dri:nə'lektəmi] *subst.* surgical removal of one of the adrenal glands *adrenalektomi;* **bilateral adrenalectomy** = surgical removal of both adrenal glands *bilateral adrenalektomi*

adrenalektomi ⇨ **adrenalectomy**

adrenalin ⇨ **adrenaline, epinephrine**

adrenaline [ə'dren(ə)lɪn] *subst.* hormone secreted by the medulla of the adrenal glands which has an effect similar to stimulation of the sympathetic nervous system *adrenalin*
NOTE: US English is **epinephrine**

> COMMENT: adrenaline is produced when a person is experiencing surprise *or* shock *or* fear *or* excitement, and speeds up the heart beat and blood pressure

adrenergic receptors [ˌædrə'nɜːdʒɪk rɪ'septəz] *subst pl.* nerves which are stimulated by adrenaline *adrenerga receptorer*

> COMMENT: three types of adrenergic receptor act in different ways when stimulated by adrenaline. Alpha receptors constrict the bronchi; beta 1 receptors speed up the heartbeat, and beta 2 receptors dilate the bronchi. See also BETA BLOCKER

adrenocortical [əˌdriːnəʊ'kɔːtɪk(ə)l] *adj.* referring to the cortex of the adrenal glands *adrenokortikal, binjurebark-*

adrenocorticotrophic hormone (ACTH) [əˌdriːnəʊˌkɔːtəkəʊ'trɒfɪk 'hɔːməʊn] *or* **corticotrophin** [ˌkɔːtɪkəʊ'trəʊfɪn] *subst.* hormone secreted by the pituitary gland and which makes the cortex of the adrenal glands produce corticosteroids *adrenokortikotropt hormon, ACTH, kortikotropin*

adrenocorticotrophin [əˌdriːnəʊˌkɔːtəkəʊ'trəʊfɪn] *subst.* adrenaline extracted from animals' adrenal glands and used to prevent haemorrhages or to help asthmatic conditions *adrenokortikotropin*

adrenogenital syndrome [əˌdriːnəʊ'dʒenit(ə)l 'sɪndrəʊm] *subst.* condition caused by overproduction of male sex hormones, where boys show rapid sexual development and females show virilization *adrenogenitalt syndrom*

adrenokortikal ⇨ **adrenocortical**

adrenokortikotropin ⇨ **adrenocorticotrophin**

adrenolytic [əˌdriːnəʊ'lɪtɪk] *adj.* acting against the secretion of adrenaline *som motverkar adrenalinutsöndring*

adsorbent [æd'sɔːbənt] *adj.* (solid) which attracts gas to its surface *adsorberande*

adsorberande ⇨ **adsorbent**

adsorption [æd'sɔːpʃ(ə)n] *subst.* attraction of gas *or* liquid to the surface of a solid *adsorption*

adstringerande ⇨ **astringent**

adstringerande (medel) ⇨ **styptic**

adult ['ædʌlt, ə'dʌlt] *subst. & adj.* grown-up (person *or* animal) *vuxen;* **adolescents reach the adult stage about the age of eighteen or twenty**

advanced [əd'vɑːnst] *adj.* which has developed *avancerad, långt framskriden;* **the advanced stages of a disease; he is suffering from advanced syphilis**

adventitia [ˌædven'tɪʃ(i)ə] *subst.* **(tunica) adventitia** = outer layer of the wall of an artery *or* vein *(tunica) adventitia*

adventitious [ˌædv(ə)n'tɪʃəs] *adj.* which is on the outside *utifrån kommande, främmande;* **adventitious bursa** *see* BURSA

advice [əd'vaɪs] *subst.* suggestion about what should be done *råd;* **he went to the psychiatrist for advice on how to cope with his problem; she would not listen to my advice; the doctor's advice was that he should take a long holiday; the doctor's advice was to stay in bed; he took the doctor's advice and went to bed**
NOTE: no plural: **some advice** or **a piece of advice**

advise [əd'vaɪz] *vb.* to suggest what should be done *råda;* **the doctor advised him to stay in bed; she advised me to have a checkup; I would advise you not to drink alcohol**

advise against [əd'vaɪz əˌgeɪnst] *vb.* to suggest that something should not be done *avråda från;* **he wanted to leave hospital but the consultant advised against it; the doctor advised against going to bed late**

adynamic ileus [ˌædɪ'næmɪk 'ɪliəs] *subst.* obstruction in the ileum caused by paralysis of the muscles of the intestine *paralytisk ileus*

A & E [ˌeɪənd'iː] = ACCIDENT AND EMERGENCY **an A & E ward; A & E nurses**

aegophony [iː'gɒfəni] *subst.* high sound of the voice heard through a stethoscope, where there is fluid in the pleural cavity *(a)egofoni, tragofoni*

aerob ⇨ **aerobic**

aeroba [eə'rəʊbə] *or* **aerobe** ['eərəʊb] *subst.* tiny organism which needs oxygen to survive *aerob (syrekrävande) organism*

aerobic [eə'rəʊbɪk] *adj.* needing oxygen to live *aerob;* **aerobic respiration** = process where the oxygen which is breathed in is used to conserve energy *or* ATP *aerob andning*

aerobics [eə'rəʊbɪks] *subst pl.* exercises which aim to increase the amount of oxygen taken into the body *aerobics, slags syrekrävande gymnastik*

aeroembolism ⇨ **caisson disease**

aerofagi ⇨ **aerophagy**

aerogenous [eə'rɒdʒənəs] *adj.* (bacterium) which produces gas *aerogen, gasbildande, gasproducerande*

aerophagy [eə'rɒfədʒi] *or* **aerophagia** [ˌeərə'feɪdʒiə] *subst.* habit of swallowing air when suffering from indigestion, so making the stomach pains worse *aerofagi, luftslukande*

aerosol ['eərə(ʊ)sɒl] *subst.* liquid and gas under pressure, which is used to spray sterilizing liquid *or* medicinal liquid in the form of tiny drops *aerosol, spray, sprej*

aetiological agent [ˌiːtiə'lɒdʒik(ə)l 'eɪdʒ(ə)nt] *subst.* agent which causes a disease *etiologiskt agens, sjukdomsframkallare (bakterie el. likn.)*

aetiology [ˌiːti'ɒlədʒi] *or US* **etiology** [ˌiːti'ɒlədʒi] *subst.* (study of) the cause *or* origin of a disease *etiologi, sjukdomsorsak*

> QUOTE a wide variety of organs or tissues may be infected by the Salmonella group of organisms, presenting symptoms which are not immediately recognised as being of Salmonella aetiology
> **Indian Journal of Medical Sciences**

afagi ⇨ **aphagia**

afaki ⇨ **aphakia**

afasi ⇨ **aphasia**

afebrile [æ'fiːbraɪl] *adj.* with no fever *afebril, feberfri*

affect [ə'fekt] *vb.* to make something change *påverka, angripa, drabba;* **some organs are rapidly affected if the patient lacks oxygen for even a short time**

affection [ə'fekʃ(ə)n] *or* **affect** [ə'fekt] *subst.* type of feeling; general state of a person's emotions *affekt, känsla, sinnesrörelse*

affective disorder [ə'fektɪv dɪs'ɔːdə] *subst.* disorder which makes the patient depressed *or* excited *affektiv psykos*

affekt ⇨ **affection**

affektiv psykos ⇨ **affective disorder**

afferent ['æf(ə)rənt] *adj.* which conducts liquid *or* impulses towards the inside *afferent, inåtledande* NOTE: opposite is **efferent**

affinitet ⇨ **affinity**

affinity [ə'fɪnəti] *subst.* attraction between two substances *affinitet*

afford [ə'fɔːd] *vb.* to have enough money to pay for something *ha råd;* **I can't afford to go to hospital; how can you afford this expensive treatment?**

afoni ⇨ **aphonia**

afrikansk sömnsjuka ⇨ **sleeping sickness**

afrodisiakum ⇨ **aphrodisiac, philtrum**

afte ⇨ **aphthae**

after- ['ɑːftə] *prefix* which comes later *or* which take place later *efter-*

afterbirth ['ɑːftəbɜːə] *subst.* tissues (including the placenta and umbilical cord) which are present in the uterus during pregnancy and are expelled after the birth of the baby *efterbörd; see also* PLACENTA

aftercare ['ɑːftəkeə] *subst.* care of a person who has had an operation *or* care of a mother who has just given birth *eftervård, efterbehandling;* **aftercare treatment involves changing dressings and helping the patient to look after himself again**

after-effects ['ɑːftərɪˌfekts] *subst pl.* changes which appear only some time after the cause *efterverkningar, sviter, men;* **the operation had some unpleasant after-effects**

after-image ['ɑːftərˌɪmɪdʒ] *subst.* image of an object which remains in a person's sight after the object itself has gone *efterbild*

afterpains ['ɑ:ftəpeɪnz] *subst pl.* regular pains in the uterus which are sometimes experienced after childbirth *eftervärkar*

aftertaste ['ɑ:ftəteɪst] *subst.* taste which remains in the mouth after the substance which caused it has been removed *eftersmak;* **the linctus leaves an unpleasant aftertaste**

aftöst sår ⇨ **ulcer**

Ag *chemical symbol for* silver *Ag, silver*

agalactia [ˌægə'lækʃ(i)ə] *subst. (of mother after childbirth)* being unable to produce milk *agalakti, agalorré*

agalakti ⇨ **agalactia**

agalorré ⇨ **agalactia**

agammaglobulinaemia [æˌgæməˌglɒbjʊlɪ'ni:miə] *subst.* deficiency *or* absence of gamma globulin in the blood, which results in a reduced ability to provide immune responses *agammaglobulinemi*

agar ['eɪgə] *or* **agar agar** [ˌeɪgər'eɪgə] *subst.* jelly made from seaweed, used to cultivate bacterial cultures in laboratories, and also as a laxative *agar, agarsubstrat*

agarsubstrat ⇨ **agar**

age [eɪdʒ] **1** *subst.* number of years which a person has lived *ålder;* **what's your age on your next birthday? he was sixty years of age; she looks younger than her age; the size varies according to age; mental age =** age of a person's mental state, measured by intelligence tests (usually compared to that of a normal person of the same chronological age) *intelligensålder, mental ålder;* **old age =** period when a person is old (usually taken to be after the age of sixty-five) *ålderdom(en)* **2** *vb.* to grow old *åldras*

COMMENT: changes take place in almost every part of the body as the person ages. Bones become more brittle, skin is less elastic. The most important changes affect the blood vessels which are less elastic, making thrombosis more likely. This also reduces the supply of blood to the brain, which in turn reduces the mental faculties

aged [eɪdʒd, 'eɪdʒɪd] *adj.* **(a)** with a certain age *i en ålder av, ...gammal;* **a boy aged twelve; he died last year, aged 64 (b)** very old *mycket gammal, ålderstigen;* **an aged man**

ageing ['eɪdʒɪŋ] *subst.* growing old *åldrande;* **the ageing process =** the physical changes which take place in a person as he grows older *åldrandet*

agency ['eɪdʒ(ə)nsi] *subst.* **(a)** action of causing something to happen *inverkan, förmedling;* **the disease develops through the agency of certain bacteria present in the bloodstream (b)** office *or* organization which provides nurses for temporary work in hospitals *or* clinics *or* in private houses *kontor, byrå, förmedling*

QUOTE the cost of employing agency nurses should be no higher than the equivalent full-time staff
Nursing Times

QUOTE growing numbers of nurses are choosing agency careers, which pay more and provide more flexible schedules than hospitals
American Journal of Nursing

agenesi ⇨ **aplasia**

agens ⇨ **agent**

agent ['eɪdʒ(ə)nt] *subst.* **(a)** person who acts for another, usually in another country *agent, ombud, representant;* **he is the agent for an American pharmaceutical firm (b)** chemical substance which makes another substance react *agens, medel;* substance *or* organism which causes a disease *or* condition *orsak, medel*

agglutinate [ə'glu:tɪneɪt] *vb.* to form into groups *agglutineras(s), klibba ihop (sig)*

agglutination [əˌglu:tɪ'neɪʃ(ə)n] *subst.* action of grouping together of cells (as of bacteria cells in the presence of serum *or* blood cells when blood of different types is mixed) *agglutinering, agglutination, hopklibbning;* **agglutination tests =** (i) tests to identify bacteria *agglutinationsprov;* (ii) tests to identify if a woman is pregnant *slags graviditetstest*

agglutinationsprov ⇨ **agglutination**

agglutinering ⇨ **agglutination**

agglutinin [ə'glu:tɪnɪn] *subst.* factor in a serum which makes cells group together *agglutinin*

agglutinogen [ˌæglu'tɪnədʒən] *subst.* factor in red blood cells which reacts with a specific agglutinin in serum *agglutinogen; see also* PAUL-BUNNELL, WEIL-FELIX, WIDAL

aggravate ['ægrəveɪt] *vb.* to make worse *förvärra, försämra, försvåra;* **playing football**

only aggravates his knee injury; the treatment seems to aggravate the disease

aggression [ə'greʃ(ə)n] *subst.* state of feeling violently angry towards someone *or* something *aggression*

agitans ['ædʒɪt(ə)ns] *see* PARALYSIS

agitated ['ædʒɪteɪtɪd] *adj.* moving about *or* twitching nervously (because of worry or other psychological state) *rastlös, upprörd, upphetsad;* **the patient became agitated and had to be given a sedative**

aglutition ⇨ **aphagia**

agnosia [æg'nəʊziə] *subst.* brain disorder where the patient cannot understand what his senses tell him and so fails to recognise places *or* people *or* tastes *or* smells which he used to know well *agnosi*

agoni ⇨ **agony**

agony ['æg(ə)nɪ] *subst.* very severe pain *agoni, svår smärta (plåga);* **he lay in agony on the floor; she suffered agonies until her condition was diagnosed**

agorafobi ⇨ **agoraphobia**

agorafobiker ⇨ **agoraphobic**

agoraphobia [ˌæg(ə)rə'fəʊbiə] *subst.* fear of being in open spaces *agorafobi, torgskräck*

agoraphobic [ˌæg(ə)rə'fəʊbɪk] *subst. & adj.* (person) suffering from agoraphobia *agorafobiker, som lider av agorafobi*
NOTE: the opposite is **claustrophobia**

agraff ⇨ **clamp, clip**

agrafi ⇨ **agraphia**

agranulocytosis [əˌgrænjʊləʊsaɪ'təʊsɪs] *subst.* usually fatal disease where the number of granulocytes (white blood cells) falls sharply because of a defect in the bone marrow *agranulocytos*

agraphia [eɪ'græfiə] *subst.* being unable to put ideas in writing *agrafi*

agreement [ə'gri:mənt] *subst.* action of agreeing *enighet, överensstämmelse;* **they are in agreement with our plan** = they agree with it *de samtycker till (går med på) planen*

agree with [ə'gri: ˌwið] *vb.* **(a)** to say that you think the same way as someone; to say yes *samtycka till, gå med på, vara enig (överens) med;* **the consultant agreed with the GP's diagnosis (b)** to be easily digested *vara lättsmält;* **this rich food does not agree with me**

AHF ⇨ **antihaemophilic factor**

AHG ⇨ **antihaemophilic factor**

AID [ˌeɪaɪ'di:] = ARTIFICIAL INSEMINATION BY DONOR

aid [eɪd] **1** *subst.* **(a)** help *hjälp, bistånd;* **medical aid** = treatment of someone who is ill *or* injured, given by a doctor *läkarvård; see also* FIRST **(b)** machine *or* tool *or* drug which helps someone do something *hjälpmedel;* **he uses a walking frame as an aid to exercising his legs 2** *vb.* to help *hjälpa, bistå, underlätta;* **the reason for the procedure is to aid repair of tissues after surgery**

aider ['eɪdə] *subst.* person who helps *person som ger hjälp (vård);* **first aider** = person who offers first aid to someone who is suddenly ill *or* injured *person som ger första hjälpen*

AIDS [eɪdz] *or* **Aids** [eɪdz] *subst.* acquired immunodeficiency syndrome *or* viral infection which breaks down the body's immune system *AIDS, förvärvat immunbristsyndrom*

> COMMENT: AIDS is a virus disease, spread by the HIV virus. It is spread mostly by sexual intercourse, and although at first associated with male homosexuals, it is now known to affect anyone. It is also transmitted through infected blood and plasma transfusions, through using unsterilized needles for injections, and can be passed from a mother to a fetus. The disease takes a long time, even years, to show symptoms, so there are many carriers. It causes a breakdown of the body's immune system, making the patient susceptible to any infection and often results in the development of rare skin cancers. It is not curable

AIH [ˌeɪaɪ'eɪtʃ] = ARTIFICIAL INSEMINATION BY HUSBAND

ailing ['eɪlɪŋ] *adj.* not well for a period of time *sjuk, krasslig, opasslig;* **he stayed at home to look after his ailing parents**

ailment ['eɪlmənt] *subst.* illness, though not generally a very serious one *krämpa, sjukdom;* **measles is one of the common childhood ailments**

ailurophobia [aɪˌlʊərəʊ'fəʊbiə] *subst.* fear of cats *kattfobi*

aim [eɪm] *vb.* **(a)** to point at *måtta på, sikta (rikta) mot;* **the X-ray beam is aimed at the patient's jaw (b)** to intend to do something *ämna, tänka, ha för avsikt;* **we aim to eradicate tuberculosis by the end of the century**

air [eə] *subst.* mixture of gases (mainly oxygen and nitrogen) which cannot be seen, but which exists all around us and which is breathed *luft;* **the air in the mountains felt cold; he breathed the polluted air into his lungs; air bed** = mattress which is filled with air, used to prevent the formation of bedsores *luftmadrass; see also* CONDUCTION; **air embolism** = interference with blood flow caused by air bubbles *luftemboli;* **air hunger** = condition where the patient needs air because of lack of oxygen in the tissues *lufthunger;* **air passages** = tubes, formed of the nose, pharynx, larynx, trachea and bronchi, which take air to the lungs *luftvägarna;* **air sac** *or* **alveolus** = small sac in the lungs which contains air *alveol, lungblåsa*

airsick ['eəsɪk] *adj.* being ill because of the movement of an aircraft *luftsjuk, flygsjuk*

airsickness ['eəsɪknəs] *subst.* feeling sick because of the movement of an aircraft *luftsjuka, flygsjuka*

airway ['eəweɪ] *subst.* passage through which air passes, especially the trachea *luftväg;* **airway clearing** = making sure that the airways in a newborn baby are free of any obstruction *rensugning av luftvägarna (hos nyfödd);* **airway obstruction** = something which blocks the air passages *luftvägshinder*

akademiker ⇨ **graduate**

akalasi ⇨ **achalasia**

akantos ⇨ **acanthosis**

akatalasemi ⇨ **acatalasia**

akillessenan ⇨ **Achilles tendon, calcaneal, tendo calcaneus**

akilles(sene)reflex ⇨ **ankle**

akillorrafi ⇨ **achillorrhaphy**

akillotomi ⇨ **achillotomy**

akinesia [ˌækɪ'niːziə] *subst.* lack of voluntary movement (as in Parkinson's disease) *akines(i), orörlighet, stelhet*

akinetic [ˌækɪ'netik] *adj.* without movement *akinetisk*

aklorhydri ⇨ **achlorhydria**

akne ⇨ **acne**

akoli ⇨ **acholia**

akoluri ⇨ **acholuria**

akondroplasi ⇨ **achondroplasia**

akrocyanos ⇨ **acrocyanosis**

akrodyni ⇨ **pink**

akrofobi ⇨ **acrophobia**

akromegali ⇨ **acromegaly**

akromial ⇨ **acromial**

akromion ⇨ **acromion**

akronyx ⇨ **acronyx**

akroparestesi ⇨ **acroparaesthesia**

akroskleros ⇨ **acrosclerosis**

aktin ⇨ **actin**

aktinomykos ⇨ **actinomycosis**

aktiv ⇨ **active**

aktivera ⇨ **activate**

aktivitet ⇨ **activity**

aktomyosin ⇨ **actomyosin**

aktuell ⇨ **date, present**

akupunktur ⇨ **acupuncture**

akupunktör ⇨ **acupuncturist**

akustisk ⇨ **acoustic**

akut ⇨ **acute, out of hours**

akutklinik ⇨ **accident**

akutmottagning ⇨ **accident, casualty, emergency**

akyli ⇨ **achlorhydria**

alactasia [ˌælæk'teɪziə] *subst.* condition where there is a deficiency of lactase in the intestine, making the patient incapable of digesting milk sugar (lactose) *tillstånd som medför laktosintolerans, laktasbrist*

alanine ['ælәniːn] *subst.* amino acid in protein *alanin*

alar cartilage ['eɪlә ˌkɑːt(ә)lɪdʒ] *subst.* cartilage in the outer wings of the nose *cartilago alaris (major och minores), delar av näsbrosket*

alba ['ælbә] *see* LINEA

Albee's operation ['ɔːlbiːz ˌɒpә'reɪʃ(ә)n] *subst.* (i) surgical operation to fuse two or more vertebrae *operation för att förena två el. flera ryggkotor;* (ii) surgical operation to fuse the femur to the pelvis *operation för att förena lårbenet med bäckenet*

albicans ['ælbɪkænz] *see* CANDIDA ALBICANS, CORPUS ALBICANS

albinism ['ælbɪnɪz(ә)m] *subst.* condition where the patient lacks melanin, and so has pink skin and eyes and white hair *albinism; see also* VITILIGO

> COMMENT: albinism is hereditary, and cannot be treated

albino [æl'biːnәʊ] *subst.* person who is deficient in melanin, with little or no pigmentation in skin, hair or eyes *albino*

albuginea [ˌælbju'dʒɪniә] *subst.* layer of white tissue covering a part of the body *tunica albuginea;* **albuginea oculi** = sclera *or* white outer covering of the eyeball *tunica albuginea oculi, sclera, sklera, senhinnan, ögonvitan*

albumin ['ælbjʊmɪn] *subst.* common protein, soluble in water and found in plant and animal tissue, and digested in the intestine *albumin;* **serum albumin** = protein in blood plasma *serumalbumin*

albuminometer [ælˌbjuːmɪ'nɒmɪtә] *subst.* instrument for measuring the level of albumin in the urine *instrument för att mäta mängden albumin (äggvita) i urinen*

albuminuria [ælˌbjuːmɪ'njʊәriә] *subst.* condition where albumin is found in the urine, usually a sign of kidney disease, but also sometimes of heart failure *albuminuri*

albumose ['ælbjʊmәʊs] *subst.* intermediate product in the digestion of protein *albumos*

alcohol ['ælkәhɒl] *subst.* pure colourless liquid, which forms part of drinks such as wine *or* whisky, and which is formed by the action of yeast on sugar solutions *alkohol, sprit;* **alcohol abuse** *or* **alcohol addiction** = condition where a patient is addicted to drinking alcohol, and cannot stop *alkoholmissbruk, spritmissbruk;* **alcohol poisoning** = poisoning and disease caused by excessive drinking of alcohol *alkoholförgiftning;* **ethyl alcohol** *or* **ethanol** = colourless liquid, which is the basis of drinking alcohols (whisky *or* gin *or* vodka, etc.) and also used in medicines and as a disinfectant *etylalkohol, etanol;* **denatured alcohol** = ethyl alcohol with an additive (usually methyl alcohol) to make it unpleasant to drink (such as methylated spirit, rubbing alcohol *or* surgical spirit) *denaturerad sprit;* **methyl alcohol** = wood alcohol (poisonous alcohol used for heating) *metylalkohol, metanol, träsprit;* **alcohol rub** = rubbing a bedridden patient with alcohol to help protect against bedsores and as a tonic *spritavtvättning*

> COMMENT: alcohol is used medicinally to dry wounds or harden the skin. When drunk, alcohol is rapidly absorbed into the bloodstream. It is a source of energy, so any carbohydrates taken at the same time are not used by the body and are stored as fat. Alcohol is a depressant, not a stimulant, and affects the mental faculties

alcohol-fast ['ælkәhɒlˌfɑːst] *adj.* (organ stained for testing) which is not discoloured by alcohol *som inte avfärgas av alkohol*

alcoholic [ˌælkә'hɒlɪk] **1** *adj.* (i) containing alcohol *alkohol-, sprit-;* (ii) caused by alcoholism *orsakad av alkoholism;* **children should not be encouraged to take alcoholic drinks; alcoholic cirrhosis** = cirrhosis of the liver caused by alcoholism *levercirros orsakad av alkoholism* **2** *subst.* person who is addicted to drinking alcohol and shows changes in behaviour and personality *alkoholist*

Alcoholics Anonymous [ˌælkәˌhɒlɪks ә'nɒnɪmәs] *subst.* organization of former alcoholics which helps sufferers from alcoholism to overcome their dependence on alcohol by encouraging them to talk about their problems in group therapy *Anonyma Alkoholister*

alcoholicum [ˌælkә'hɒlɪkәm] *see* DELIRIUM

alcoholism ['ælkәhɒlɪz(ә)m] *subst.* excessive drinking of alcohol which becomes addictive *alkoholism*

alcoholuria [ˌælkәhɒ'ljʊәriә] *subst.* condition where alcohol is present in the urine (the level of alcohol in the urine is used as a test for drunken drivers) *alkohol i urinen*

aldosterone [æl'dɒstәrәʊn] *subst.* hormone secreted by the cortex of the adrenal gland, and which regulates the balance of sodium and potassium in the body and the amount of body fluid *aldosteron*

aleppoböld ➪ **Baghdad boil**

alert [ə'lɜ:t] *adj.* (person) who takes an intelligent interest in his surroundings *vaken, pigg, uppmärksam;* **the patient is still alert, though in great pain**

aleukaemic [ˌælu'ki:mɪk] *adj.* (i) (state) where leukaemia is not present *aleukemisk;* (ii) state where leucocytes are not normal *aleukemisk*

aleukemisk ➪ **aleukaemic**

alexia [ə'leksiə] *or* **word blindness** ['wɜ:d ˌblaɪndnəs] *subst.* condition where the patient cannot understand printed words *alexi, ordblindhet, förlust av läsförmågan*

alfacell ➪ **cell**

alfafetoprotein ➪ **alpha-fetoprotein**

algae ['ældʒi:] *subst pl.* class of lower plants, many of which are seaweeds *alger, tång*

alger ➪ **algae**

algesimeter [ˌældʒɪ'sɪmɪtə] *subst.* instrument to measure the sensitivity of the skin to pain *instrument för att mäta hudens smärtkänslighet*

algid ['ældʒɪd] *adj.* cold *or* (stage in an attack of cholera or malaria) where the body becomes cold *kall, med frossbrytningar*

alimentary canal [ˌælɪ'ment(ə)ri kə'næl] *subst.* digestive tract *canalis alimentarius, digestionskanalen, magtarmkanalen*

alimentation [ˌælɪmen'teɪʃ(ə)n] *subst.* feeding *or* taking in food *näring, näringsintag*

alive [ə'laɪv] *adj.* living *or* not dead *levande;* **the patient was still alive, even though he had been in the sea for two days**
NOTE: **alive** cannot be used in front of a noun: **the patient is alive** but **a living patient** Note also that **live** can be used in front of a noun: **the patient was injected with live vaccine**

alkalaemia [ˌælkə'li:miə] *subst.* excess of alkali in the blood *alkalemi*

alkalemi ➪ **alkalaemia**

alkali ['ælkəlaɪ] *subst.* one of many substances which neutralize acids and form salts *alkali*

alkaliliknande ➪ **alkaloid**

alkaline ['ælkəlaɪn] *adj.* containing more alkali than acid *alkalisk*

COMMENT: alkaline solutions are used to counteract the effects of acid poisoning, and also of bee stings. If strong alkali (such as ammonia) is swallowed, the patient should drink water and an acid such as orange juice

alkalinitet ➪ **alkalinity**

alkalinity [ˌælkə'lɪnəti] *subst.* level of alkali in a body *alkalinitet;* **hyperventilation causes fluctuating carbon dioxide levels in the blood, resulting in an increase of blood alkalinity**

alkalisk ➪ **alkaline**

alkaloid ['ælkəlɔɪd] **1** *adj.* similar to an alkali *alkaliliknande* **2** *subst.* one of many poisonous substances found in plants, used as medicines (such as atropine *or* morphine *or* quinine) *alkaloid*

alkalosis [ˌælkə'ləʊsɪs] *subst.* condition where the alkali level in the body tissue is high, producing cramps *alkalos*

alkaptonuria [ælˌkæptə'njʊəriə] *subst.* hereditary condition where dark pigment is present in the urine *alkaptonuri*

alkohol ➪ **alcohol, spirit**

alkohol- ➪ **alcoholic**

alkoholförgiftning ➪ **alcohol**

alkoholism ➪ **alcoholism**

alkoholist ➪ **alcoholic**

alkoholmissbruk ➪ **alcohol**

alkoholproblem ➪ **problem**

allantoin [ə'læntəʊɪn] *subst.* powder from a herb (comfrey), used to treat skin disorders *allantoin*

allantois [ə'læntəʊɪs] *subst.* one of the membranes in the embryo, shaped like a sac, which grows out of the embryonic hindgut *allantois, navelblåsan*

allergen ['ælədʒen] *subst.* substance which produces hypersensitivity *allergen*

> COMMENT: allergens are usually proteins, and include foods, dust, hair of animals, as well as pollen from flowers. Allergic reaction to serum is known as anaphylaxis. Treatment of allergies depends on correctly identifying the allergen to which the patient is sensitive. This is done by patch tests, in which drops of different allergens are placed on scratches in the skin. Food allergens discovered in this way can be avoided, but other allergens (such as dust and pollen) can hardly be avoided, and have to be treated by a course of desensitizing injections

allergen ⇨ **allergenic**

allergenic [ˌælə'dʒenɪk] *adj.* which produces an allergy *allergen, allergiframkallande*

allergi ⇨ **allergy, hypersensitivity**

allergic [ə'lɜːdʒɪk] *adj.* suffering from an allergy *allergisk;* **she is allergic to cats; I'm allergic to penicillin; he showed an allergic reaction to chocolate; allergic person =** person who has an allergy to something *allergiker; see also* ALVEOLITIS NOTE: you have an allergy or you are allergic **to** something

allergiframkallande ⇨ **allergenic**

allergiker ⇨ **allergic**

allergisk ⇨ **allergic**

allergist ['ælədʒɪst] *subst.* doctor who specializes in the treatment of allergies *specialist på allergiska sjukdomar*

allergy ['ælədʒɪ] *subst.* being sensitive to certain substances (such as pollen *or* dust) which cause a physical reaction *allergi;* **drug allergy =** reaction to a certain drug *läkemedelsallergi;* **he has a penicillin allergy** *see also* FOOD

alleviate [ə'liːvɪeɪt] *vb.* to make (a pain) lighter *or* to relieve (a pain) *lätta, lindra, mildra;* **he was given injections to alleviate the pain; the nurses tried to alleviate the suffering of the injured**

allmän ⇨ **common, general, generalized, widespread**

allmänpraktiker ⇨ **general practitioner (GP)**

allmänprevention ⇨ **secondary**

allmän(t förekommande) ⇨ **prevalent**

allmäntjänstgöring ⇨ **internship**

allmänt sjukhus ⇨ **hospital**

allo- ['ælə(ʊ)] *prefix* different *allo-*

allograft ['ælə(ʊ)grɑːft] *or* **homograft** ['hɒməgrɑːft] *subst.* graft of an organ *or* tissue from one person to another *allograft, homograft, allogent (homologt) transplantat; compare* AUTOGRAFT

allopathy [ə'lɒpəθɪ] *subst.* treatment of a condition using drugs which produce opposite symptoms to those of the condition *allopati; compare* HOMEOPATHY

allopati ⇨ **allopathy**

all or none law [ˌɔːl ɔː nʌn lɔː] *subst.* rule that the heart muscle either contracts fully or does not contract at all *lagen (principen) om allt eller intet, allt-eller-intet-principen*

all over [ˌɔːl'əʊvə] **(a)** everywhere *överallt, över hela;* **there were red marks all over the child's body; she poured water all over the patient's head (b)** finished *över, slut;* **when it was all over we went home**

allow [ə'laʊ] *vb.* to say that someone can do something *tillåta, låta;* **the consultant allowed him to watch the operation; patients are not allowed to go outside the hospital; he is allowed to eat certain types of food**

all right [ˌɔːl'raɪt] *adj.* well *or* not ill *all right, bra;* **he's feeling very sick at the moment, but he will be all right in a few hours; my mother had flu but she is all right now; his hearing is all right, but his sight is failing**

allt-eller-intet-principen ⇨ **all or none law**

allvarlig ⇨ **bad, major, profound, serious, severe**

allvarligt ⇨ **seriously, severely**

almoner ['ɑːmənə, 'ælm-] *subst.* formerly a person working in a hospital, looking after the welfare of patients and the families of patients (now called medical social worker) *tidigare kurator, sjukhuskurator*

alopeci ⇨ **baldness**

alopecia [ˌælə'piːʃ(ɪ)ə] *subst.* baldness *alopeci, håravfall, skallighet;* **alopecia areata**

= condition where the hair falls out in patches *alopecia areata (circumscripta)*

COMMENT: baldness in men is hereditary; it can also occur in men and women as a reaction to an illness or to a drug

alpha ['ælfə] *subst.* first letter of the Greek alphabet *alfa*

alpha cells ['ælfə,selz] *subst pl.* one of the types of cells in glands (such as the pancreas) which have more than one type of cell *alfaceller*

alpha-fetoprotein [,ælfə,fi:təʊ'prəʊti:n] *subst.* protein found in the amniotic fluid when the fetus has an open neurological deficiency such as meningomyelocele *alfafetoprotein*

ALS [,eɪel'es] = ANTILYMPHOCYTIC SERUM

ALS ⇨ **amyotrophic lateral sclerosis**

alster ⇨ **product**

alstra ⇨ **produce**

alternativmedicin ⇨ **naturopathy**

alternativodlad ⇨ **organic**

altitude sickness ['æltɪtju:d ,sɪknəs] = MOUNTAIN SICKNESS

aluminiumhydroxid ⇨ **aluminium hydroxide**

aluminium hydroxide [,ælə'mɪniəm haɪ'drɒksaɪd] *subst.* chemical substance used as an antacid to treat indigestion *aluminiumhydroxid* NOTE: chemical symbol is **$Al(OH)_3$**

alveol ⇨ **air, alveolus**

alveolar [,ælvɪ'əʊlə, æl'vi:ələ] *adj.* referring to alveoli *alveolar, alveolär;* **alveolar bone** = part of the jawbone to which the teeth are attached *käkben med håligheter för tändernas rötter*

alveolarpyorré ⇨ **pyorrhoea**

alveolitis [,ælviə'laɪtɪs] *subst.* inflammation of an alveolus in the lungs or the socket of a tooth *alveolit;* **extrinsic allergic alveolitis** = condition where the lungs are allergic to fungus and other allergens *inflammation i lungalveolerna på grund av allergi*

alveolus [,ælvɪ'əʊləs, æl'vi:ələs] *subst.* small cavity, such as one of the air sacs in the lungs or the socket into which a tooth fits *alveol, lungblåsa* NOTE: plural is **alveoli**

alveolär ⇨ **alveolar**

Alzheimer's disease ['æltshaɪməz dɪ,zi:z] *subst.* condition where a patient suffers from presenile dementia in middle age, caused when areas of the brain atrophy, making the ventricles expand *Alzheimers sjukdom*

COMMENT: no cause has been identified for the disease, although it is more prevalent in certain families than in others

amalgam [ə'mælgəm] *subst.* mixture of metals (based on mercury and tin) used by dentists to fill holes in teeth *amalgam*

amaurosis [,æmɔ:'rəʊsɪs] *subst.* blindness where there is no visible defect in the eye, caused by a defect in the optic nerves *amauros, svart starr;* **amaurosis fugax** = temporary blindness on one eye, caused by problems of circulation *amaurosis partialis fugax, flimmerskotom*

amaurotic familial idiocy [,æmɔ:'rɒtɪk fə,mɪliəl 'ɪdiəsi] = TAY-SACHS DISEASE

ambi- ['æmbi, ,--] *prefix* meaning both *ambi-, bi-*

ambidextrous [,æmbi'dekstrəs] *adj.* (person) who can use both hands equally well, and who is not right- or left-handed *ambidexter*

ambisexual [,æmbi'sekʃuəl] *or* **bisexual** ['baɪ'sekʃu(ə)l] *adj.* (person) who is sexually attracted to both males and females *bisexuell*

amblyopia [,æmbli'əʊpiə] *subst.* partial blindness, leading to blindness, for which no cause seems to exist, although it may be caused by the cyanide in tobacco smoke or by drinking methylated spirits (toxic amblyopia) *amblyopi*

amblyopic [,æmbli'ɒpɪk] *adj.* suffering from amblyopia *amblyop*

amblyoscope ['æmbliəʊskəʊp] *subst.* surgical instrument for training an amblyopic eye *amblyoskop*

ambulance ['æmbjələns] *subst.* van for taking sick *or* injured people to hospital *ambulans;* **the injured man was taken away in an ambulance; the telephone number of**

the local ambulance service is in the telephone book

ambulanceman ['æmbjələnsmæn] *subst.* man who drives or assists in an ambulance *ambulansman, ambulansförare* NOTE: plural is **ambulancemen**

ambulans ⇨ **ambulance**

ambulansförare ⇨ **ambulanceman**

ambulant ⇨ **ambulatory**

ambulation [ˌæmbju'leɪʃ(ə)n] *subst.* walking *ambulerande, uppegående;* **early ambulation is recommended** = patients should try to get out of bed and walk about as soon as possible after the operation *patienter bör upp och gå så snart som möjligt* NOTE: no plural

ambulatory ['æmbjulət(ə)ri] *adj.* (patient) who is able to walk *ambulant, inte sängbunden, uppegående;* **ambulatory fever** = mild fever (such as the early stages of typhoid fever) where the patient can walk about, and can therefore act as a carrier *mild feber som kommer och går*

> QUOTE ambulatory patients with essential hypertension were evaluated and followed up at the hypertension clinic
> **British Medical Journal**

ambulerande ⇨ **ambulation**

ambustio ⇨ **burn**

ameba [ə'miːbə] *US* = AMOEBA

amelia [ə'miːliə] *subst.* congenital absence of a limb *or* condition where a limb is congenitally short *ameli*

amelioration [əˌmiːliə'reɪʃ(ə)n] *subst.* improvement *or* getting better *amelioration, förbättring*

ameloblastoma [əˌmelə(ʊ)blæ'stəʊmə] *subst.* tumour in the jaw, usually in the lower jaw *ameloblastom, adamantin(oblast)om, emaljsvulst*

amenity bed [ə'miːnəti ˌbed] *subst.* bed (usually in a separate room) in an NHS hospital, for which the patient pays extra *sängplats som patienten betalar extra för*

amenorré ⇨ **amenorrhoea**

amenorré, falsk ⇨ **cryptomenorrhoea**

amenorrhoea [ˌeɪˌmenə'riːə] *subst.* absence of one or more menstrual periods, normal during pregnancy and after the menopause, but otherwise abnormal in adult women *amenorré;* **primary amenorrhoea** = condition where a woman has never had menstrual periods *primär amenorré;* **secondary amenorrhoea** = situation where a woman's menstrual periods have stopped *sekundär amenorré*

amens ⇨ **amentia**

amentia [eɪ'menʃ(i)ə] *subst.* being mentally subnormal *amens, amentia*

ametropia [ˌæmɪ'trəʊpiə] *subst.* condition where the eye cannot focus light correctly on to the retina, as in astigmatism, myopia and hypermetropia *ametropi, refraktionsanomali; compare* EMMETROPIA

amfetamin ⇨ **amphetamine**

amfetaminmissbruk ⇨ **amphetamine**

amfiartros ⇨ **amphiarthrosis**

amfotericin ⇨ **amphotericin**

amino acid [əˌmiːnəʊ 'æsɪd] *subst.* chemical compound which is broken down from proteins in the digestive system and then used by the body to form its own protein *aminosyra;* **proteins are first broken down into amino acids; essential amino acids** = eight amino acids which are essential for growth, but which cannot be synthesized and so must be obtained from food or medicinal substances *essentiella aminosyror*

> COMMENT: amino acids all contain carbon, hydrogen, nitrogen and oxygen, as well as other elements. Some amino acids are produced in the body itself, but others have to be absorbed from food. The eight essential amino acids are: isoleucine, leucine, lysine, methionine, phenylalanine, threopine, tryptophan and valine

aminobutyric acid [əˌmiːnəʊbjuˌtɪrik 'æsɪd] *see* GAMMA

aminosyra ⇨ **amino acid**

aminotransferas ⇨ **transaminase**

amitosis [ˌæmɪ'təʊsɪs] *subst.* multiplication of a cell by splitting the nucleus *amitos*

amma ⇨ **nurse**

ammande moder ⇨ **nursing**

ammonia [ə'məʊniə] *subst.* gas with a strong smell, one of the normal products of human metabolism *ammoniak* NOTE: chemical symbol is **NH_3**

ammonshornet ⇨ **hippocampal formation**

amnesia [æm'ni:ziə] *subst.* loss of memory *amnesi, minnesförlust;* **general amnesia** = loss of all memory *or* a state where a person does not even remember who he is *generell (total, allmän) minnesförlust;* **partial amnesia** = being unable to remember certain facts, such as names of people *partiell (ofullständig) minnesförlust*

amning ⇨ **breast, lactation**

amningsperiod ⇨ **lactation**

amniocentesis [ˌæmniəʊsen'ti:sɪs] *subst.* taking a test sample of the amniotic fluid during pregnancy using a hollow needle and syringe *amniocentes*

> COMMENT: amniocentesis and amnioscopy are the examination and testing of the amniotic fluid, giving information about possible congenital abnormalities in the fetus, and also the sex of the unborn baby

amnion ['æmniən] *subst.* thin sac (containing the amniotic fluid) which covers an unborn baby in the womb *amnion*

amnion- ⇨ **amniotic**

amnionsäcken ⇨ **amniotic, bag**

amnionvatten ⇨ **amniotic, water**

amnionvätska ⇨ **amniotic, water**

amnioscopy [ˌæmni'ɒskəpi] *subst.* examination of the amniotic fluid during pregnancy *amnioskopi*

amniotic [ˌæmni'ɒtɪk] *adj.* referring to the amnion *amnion-, fostervatten-;* **amniotic fluid** = fluid contained in the amnion, which surrounds an unborn baby *liquor amnii, amnionvätska, amnionvatten, fostervatten;* **amniotic sac** = thin sac which covers an unborn baby in the womb, containing the amniotic fluid *amnionsäcken*

amniotomy [ˌæmni'ɒtəmi] *subst.* puncture of the amnion to help induce labour *amniotomi*

amoeba [ə'mi:bə] *subst.* form of animal life, made up of a single cell *amöba* NOTE: plural is **amoebae.** Note also the US spelling **ameba**

amoebiasis [ˌæmɪ'baɪəsɪs] *subst.* infection caused by amoeba, which can result in amoebic dysentery in the large intestine (intestinal amoebiasis) and can sometimes infect the lungs (pulmonary amoebiasis) *amoebiasis, amöbainfektion*

amoebic [ə'mi:bɪk] *adj.* referring to an amoeba *amöba-;* **amoebic dysentery** = mainly tropical form of dysentery which is caused by **Entamoeba histolytica** which enters the body through contaminated water or unwashed food *amöbadysenteri*

amoebicide [ə'mi:bɪsaɪd] *subst.* substance which kills amoebae *amöbadödande ämne*

amorf ⇨ **amorphous**

amorphous [ə'mɔ:fəs] *adj.* with no regular shape *amorf, formlös*

amount [ə'maʊnt] **1** *subst.* quantity *mängd;* **he is not allowed to drink a large amount of water; she should not eat large amounts of fried food 2** *vb.* to add up (to) *belöpa sig till, uppgå till;* **the bill for surgery amounted to £1,000**

amphetamine [æm'fetəmi:n] *or* **pep pill** ['pepˌpɪl] *subst.* addictive drug, similar to adrenaline, used to give a feeling of well-being and wakefulness *amfetamin;* **amphetamine abuse** = repeated addictive use of amphetamines which in the end affects the mental faculties *amfetaminmissbruk*

amphiarthrosis [ˌæmfiɑ:'θrəʊsɪs] *subst.* joint which only has limited movement (such as the joints in the spine) *amfiartros, dubbelartros, stram led*

amphotericin [ˌæmfəʊ'terɪsɪn] *subst.* antifungal agent, used against Candida *amfotericin*

ampicillin [ˌæmpɪ'sɪlɪn] *subst.* type of penicillin, used as an antibiotic *ampicillin*

ampoule ['æmpu:l] *or* **ampule** ['æmpju:l] *subst.* small glass container, closed at the neck, used to contain sterile drugs for use in injections *ampull*

ampull ⇨ **ampoule, ampulla**

ampulla [æm'pʊlə] *subst.* swelling of a canal *or* duct, shaped like a bottle *ampull, ampulla*

NOTE: plural is **ampullae**

amputate [æmpjʊteɪt] *vb.* to remove a limb *or* part of a limb in a surgical operation *amputera;* **a patient whose leg needs to be amputated; after gangrene set in, surgeons had to amputate her toes**

amputation [ˌæmpjʊ'teɪʃ(ə)n] *subst.* surgical removal of a limb *amputation*

amputationsstump ⇨ **stump**

amputee [ˌæmpju'tiː] *subst.* patient who has lost a limb through amputation *person som genomgått amputation*

amputera ⇨ **amputate**

amuse [ə'mjuːz] *vb.* to make someone happy *roa, underhålla;* **the nurses amused the children at Christmas**

amusement [ə'mjuːzmənt] *subst.* being made happy *nöje, förströelse, munterhet;* **Father Christmas gave out presents to the great amusement of the children in the ward**

amusing [ə'mjuːzɪŋ] *adj.* which makes you happy *roande, lustig*

amygdala [ə'mɪgdələ] *or* **amygdaloid body** [ə'mɪgdəlɔɪd ˌbɒdi] *subst.* almond-shaped body in the brain, at the end of the caudate nucleus of the thalamus *corpus amygdaloideum, mandelkärnan*

amyl- ['æm(ə)l, ˌ--] *prefix* starch *amyl(o)-*

amylas ⇨ **amylase, diastase**

amylase ['æmɪleɪz] *subst.* enzyme which converts starch into maltose *amylas*

amyloid disease ['æmɪlɔɪd dɪˌziːz] *or* **amyloidosis** [ˌæmɪlɔɪ'dəʊsɪs] *subst.* disease of the kidneys and liver, where the tissues are filled with amyloid, a wax-like protein *amyloidos*

amyloidos ⇨ **amyloid disease**

amylopsin [ˌæmɪ'lɒpsiːn] *subst.* enzyme which converts starch into maltose *amylopsin*

amylose ['æmɪləʊz] *subst.* carbohydrate of starch *amylos*

amyotonia [ˌeɪmaɪə'təʊniə] *subst.* lack of muscle tone *amyotoni;* **amyotonia congenita** *or* **floppy baby syndrome** = congenital disease of children, where the muscles lack tone *myatonia congenita*

amyotrofi ⇨ **amyotrophia**

amyotrophia [əˌmaɪə'trəʊfiə] *subst.* wasting away of a muscle *amyotrofi, muskelatrofi*

amyotrophic lateral sclerosis [ˌeɪmaɪə'trɒfɪk 'læt(ə)r(ə)l sklə'rəʊsɪs] *or* **Gehrig's disease** ['geɪrɪgz dɪˌziːz] *subst.* a motor neurone disease, similar to muscular sclerosis, where the limbs twitch and the muscles gradually waste away *amyotrofisk lateralskleros, ALS*

amöba ⇨ **amoeba**

amöba- ⇨ **amoebic**

amöbadysenteri ⇨ **amoebic**

amöbainfektion ⇨ **amoebiasis**

an- ['æn, ˌ-] *prefix* without *or* lacking *an-*

anabolic [ˌænə'bɒlɪk] *adj.* (substance) which synthesizes protein *anabol(isk);* **anabolic steroids** = drugs which encourage the synthesis of new living tissue from nutrients *anabola steroider*

> QUOTE insulin, secreted by the islets of Langerhans, is the body's major anabolic hormone, regulating the metabolism of all body fuels and substrates
>
> **Nursing Times**

anabol(isk) ⇨ **anabolic**

anabolism [ə'næbəlɪz(ə)m] *subst.* process of building up complex chemical substances on the basis of simpler ones *anaboli(sm)*

anae- [ə'niː, ˌænɪ]
NOTE: words beginning with **anae-** are spelt **ane-** in US English

anaemia [ə'niːmiə] *or US* **anemia** [ə'niːmiə] *subst.* condition where the level of red blood cells is less than normal, or where the haemoglobin is less, making it more difficult for the blood to carry oxygen *anemi, blodbrist;* **haemolytic anaemia** = anaemia caused by the destruction of red blood cells *hemolytisk anemi;* **iron-deficiency anaemia** = anaemia caused by lack of iron in red blood cells *sideropeni, serumjärnbrist, järnbristanemi;* **pernicious anaemia** *or* **Addison's anaemia** = disease where a lack of vitamin B_{12} prevents the absorption of red blood cells and damages the spinal cord *perniciös anemi, Addisonanemi;* **splenic anaemia** = type of anaemia where the patient has an enlarged spleen caused by cirrhosis of the liver *hepatolienal fibros, Bantis sjukdom (syndrom); see also* APLASTIC, SICKLE-CELL

> COMMENT: symptoms of anaemia are tiredness and pale colour, especially pale lips, nails and the inside of the eyelids. The condition can be fatal if not treated

anaemic [ə'ni:mɪk] *adj.* suffering from anaemia *anemisk, blodfattig*

> COMMENT: symptoms of anaemia are tiredness and pale colour, especially pale lips, nails and the inside of the eyelids. The condition can be fatal if not treated

anaerobe [æn'eərəʊb] *subst.* microorganism (such as the tetanus bacillus) which lives without oxygen *anaerob (icke syrekrävande) organism*

anaerobic respiration [ˌænə'rəʊbɪk ˌrespə'reɪʃ(ə)n] *subst.* biochemical processes which lead to the formation of ATP without oxygen *anaerob respiration*

anaesthesia [ˌænəs'θi:ziə] *or US* **anesthesia** [ˌænəs'θi:ziə] *subst.* loss of the feeling of pain *anestesi, bedövning, okänslighet;* **general anaesthesia** = loss of feeling and loss of consciousness *narkos, sövning;* **local anaesthesia** = loss of feeling in a part of the body *lokalanestesi, lokalbedövning*

anaesthesiologist [ˌænəsˌθi:zi'ɒlədʒɪst] *subst.* specialist in the study of anaesthetics *anestesiolog, narkosläkare*

anaesthesiology [ˌænəsˌθi:zi'ɒlədʒi] *subst.* study of anaesthetics *anestesiologi*

anaesthetic [ˌænəs'θetɪk] **1** *adj.* which produces loss of feeling *anestetisk, narkos-, bedövnings-;* **anaesthetic risk** = risk that a drug may cause unwanted serious side-effects *anestetisk risk, risk vid bedövning (narkos);* **anaesthetic induction** = methods of inducing anaesthesia in a patient *narkosinledning, induktion vid narkos (sövning)* **2** *subst.* substance given to a patient to remove feeling, so that he can undergo an operation without feeling pain *anestetikum, narkosmedel, bedövningsmedel;* **caudal anaesthetic** = anaesthetic often used in childbirth, where the drug is injected into the base of the spine to remove feeling in the lower part of the trunk *epiduralanestesi, epiduralbedövning;* **general anaesthetic** = substance given to make a patient lose consciousness so that a major surgical operation can be carried out *narkosmedel;* **local anaesthetic** = substance which removes the feeling in a certain part of the body only *lokalanestetikum, lokalbedövningsmedel;* **spinal anaesthetic** = anaesthetic given by injection into the spine, which results in large parts of the body losing the sense of feeling *spinalanestesi, spinalbedövning*

anaesthetist [ə'ni:sθətɪst] *subst.* specialist who administers anaesthetics *anestesiolog, narkosläkare*

anaesthetize [ə'ni:sθətaɪz] *vb.* to produce a loss of feeling in a patient *or* in part of the body *bedöva, söva (ned);* **the patient was anaesthetized before the operation**

anafas ⇨ **anaphase**

anafylaktisk chock ⇨ **anaphylactic shock**

anafylaxi ⇨ **anaphylaxis**

anal ['eɪn(ə)l] *adj.* referring to the anus *anal;* **anal canal** = passage leading from the rectum to the anus *canalis analis, analkanalen;* **anal fissure** = crack in the mucous membrane of the wall of the anal canal *fissura ani, analfissur, rektalfissur;* **anal fistula** *or* **fistula in ano** = fistula which develops between the rectum and the outside of the body after an abscess near the anus *fistula in ano, analfistel;* **anal sphincter** = strong ring of muscle which closes the anus *(musculus) sphincter ani, analsfinktern;* **anal triangle** *or* **rectal triangle** = posterior part of the perineum *bakre delen av bäckenbotten*

analeptic [ˌænə'leptɪk] *subst.* drug used to make someone regain consciousness *or* to stimulate a patient *analeptikum, uppiggande medel*

analeptikum ⇨ **analeptic**

analfissur ⇨ **fissure**

analfistel ⇨ **fistula**

analgesia [ˌæn(ə)l'dʒi:ziə] *subst.* reduction of the feeling of pain without loss of consciousness *analgesi, smärtfrihet;* **caudal analgesia** = technique often used in childbirth, where an analgesic is injected into the extradural space at the base of the spine to remove feeling in the lower part of the trunk *epiduralanestesi, epiduralbedövning*

analgesic [ˌæn(ə)l'dʒi:zɪk] **1** *adj.* referring to analgesia *analgetisk, smärtstillande* **2** *subst.* pain-killing drug which produces analgesia *analgetikum, smärtstillande medel;* analgesics are commonly used as local anaesthetics, for example in dentistry

analgetikum ⇨ **analgesic, pain killer**

analgetisk ⇨ **analgesic**

analkanalen ⇨ **anal**

anally ['eɪn(ə)li] *adv.* through the anus *analt;* **the patient is not able to pass faeces anally**

analpekten ⇨ **pecten**

analsfinktern ⇨ **anal**

analt ⇨ **anally**

analys ⇨ **analysis**

analyse ['ænəlaɪz] *vb.* to examine something in detail *analysera, undersöka noga;* **the laboratory is analysing the blood samples; when the food was analysed it was found to contain traces of bacteria**

analyser ['ænəlaɪzə] *subst.* machine which analyses blood *or* tissue samples automatically *apparat för analys av blod el. vävnadsprov, autoanalyser, multianalyser*

analysera ⇨ **analyse**

analysis [ə'næləsɪs] *subst.* examination of a substance to find out what it is made of *analys, noggrann undersökning*
NOTE: plural is **analyses**

analyst ['ænəlɪst] *subst.* person who examines samples of substances *or* tissue, to find out what they are made of *laboratorieassistent, kemist; see also* PSYCHOANALYSIS, PSYCHOANALYST

analöppning ⇨ **anus**

anamnes ⇨ **past**

anaphase ['ænəfeɪz] *subst.* stage in cell division, after the metaphase and before the telophase *anafas*

anaphylactic shock [,ænəfɪ'læktɪk 'ʃɒk] *subst.* sudden allergic reaction to an allergen such as an injection, which can be fatal *anafylaktisk chock*

anaphylaxis [,ænəfɪ'læksɪs] *subst.* reaction, similar to an allergic reaction, to an injection *or* to a bee sting *anafylaxi*

anaplasia [,ænə'pleɪsiə] *subst.* loss of a cell's characteristics, caused by cancer *anaplasi*

anaplastic [,ænə'plæstɪk] *adj.* referring to anaplasia *anaplastisk;* **anaplastic neoplasm** = cancer where the cells are not similar to those of the tissue from which they come *anaplastisk cancer*

anaplastisk ⇨ **anaplastic**

anasarca [,ænə'sɑːkə] *subst.* dropsy *or* presence of fluid in the body tissues *anasarka, utbrett ödem*

anasarka ⇨ **anasarca**

anastomos ⇨ **anastomosis**

anastomose [ə'næstəməʊz] *vb.* to attach two arteries *or* tubes together *göra en anastomos*

anastomosis [ə,næstə'məʊsɪs] *subst.* connection made between two vessels *or* two tubes, either naturally or by surgery *anastomos*

anatom ⇨ **anatomist**

anatomi ⇨ **anatomy**

anatomical [,ænə'tɒmɪk(ə)l] *adj.* referring to anatomy *anatomisk;* **the anatomical features of a fetus**

anatomisk ⇨ **anatomical**

anatomist [ə'nætəmɪst] *subst.* scientist who specializes in the study of the anatomy *anatom*

anatomy [ə'nætəmi] *subst.* (i) structure of the body *anatomi, kroppens byggnad (struktur);* (ii) study of the structure of the body *anatomi;* **he is studying anatomy; she failed her anatomy examination; human anatomy** = structure, shape and functions of the human body *människans anatomi;* **the anatomy of a bone** = description of the structure and shape of a bone *ett bens anatomi (uppbyggnad)*

anatoxin ⇨ **toxoid**

anbringa ⇨ **apply, fix**

ancestor ['ænsestə] *subst.* person from whom someone is descended, usually a person who lived a long time ago *förfader*

ancillary staff [æn'sɪləri ,stɑːf] *subst.* staff in a hospital who are not administrators, doctors or nurses (such as cleaners, porters, kitchen staff, etc.) *hjälppersonal (såsom städare, vaktmästare o.dyl.)*

anconeus [æŋ'kəʊniəs] *subst.* small triangular muscle at the back of the elbow *musculus anconaeus, armbågsmuskeln*

Ancylostoma [ˌænsɪ'lɒstəmə] *or* **Ankylostoma** [ˌæŋkɪ'lɒstəmə] *or* **hookworm** ['hʊkwɜːm] *subst.* parasitic worm in the intestine, with holds onto the wall of the intestine with its teeth and lives on the blood and protein of the carrier *Ancylostoma duodenale, hakmask*

ancylostomiasis [ˌænsɪˌlɒstə'maɪəsɪs] *or* **hookworm disease** ['hʊkwɜːm dɪˌziːz] *subst.* disease caused by a hookworm which lives on the blood of the host, where the patient suffers weakness and anaemia *ancylostomiasis, ankylostomiasis; see also* NECATOR

ancylostomiasis ⇨ **ankylostomiasis, necatoriasis**

andas ⇨ **breathe**

andetag ⇨ **breath**

andfådd ⇨ **breathless, wheezy**

andfåddhet ⇨ **breathlessness, orthopnoea, shortness of breath**

andning ⇨ **breath, breathing, respiration, ventilation**

-andning ⇨ **-pnea, -pnoea**

andning, paradox ⇨ **paradoxical breathing**

andningsapparaten ⇨ **respiratory**

andningscentrum ⇨ **respiratory**

andningsfrekvens ⇨ **breathing, respiration**

andningsinsufficiens ⇨ **respiratory, ventilatory failure**

andningsljud ⇨ **breath**

andningsmask ⇨ **respirator**

andningsstillestånd ⇨ **apnoea**

andnöd ⇨ **dyspnoea**

andra ⇨ **second, secondary**

andra gradens brännskada ⇨ **burn**

andra ordningens neuron ⇨ **neurone**

androgen ['ændrədʒ(ə)n] *subst.* male sex hormone *or* hormone which increases the male characteristics of the body *androgen, manligt könshormon*

androgen ⇨ **androgen, androgenic**

androgenic [ˌændrə'dʒenɪk] *adj.* which produces male characteristics *androgen*

androsterone [æn'drɒstərəʊn] *subst.* one of the male sex hormones *androsteron*

anemi ⇨ **anaemia, erythropenia, hyphaemia**

anemia [ə'niːmiə] *US* = ANAEMIA

anemisk ⇨ **anaemic**

anencefali ⇨ **anencephaly**

anencephalous [ˌænen'kef(ə)li] *adj.* with no brain *utan hjärna*

anencephaly [ˌænen'kefələs] *subst.* absence of a brain, which causes a fetus to die a few hours after birth *anencefali*

anergi ⇨ **anergy**

anergy ['ænədʒi] *subst.* (i) being weak *or* lacking energy *anergi, utan ork (energi);* (ii) lack of immunity *anergi, avsaknad av immunologisk reaktion på antigen*

anestesi ⇨ **anaesthesia**

anestesiolog ⇨ **anaesthesiologist, anaesthetist**

anestesiologi ⇨ **anaesthesiology**

anestetikum ⇨ **anaesthetic**

anestetisk ⇨ **anaesthetic**

aneurin ⇨ **aneurine, Vitamin B**

aneurine [ə'njʊərɪn] *subst.* thiamine *or* vitamin B_1 *aneurin, thiamin, vitamin* B_1

aneurysm ['ænjəˌrɪz(ə)m] *subst.* swelling caused by the weakening of a wall of a blood vessel *aneurysm, artärbråck, pulsåderbråck;* **congenital aneurysm** = weakening of the arteries at the base of the brain, occurring in a baby from birth *medfött aneurysm*

COMMENT: aneurysm usually occurs in the wall of the aorta, and is often due to atheroma and sometimes to syphilis

anfall ⇨ **attack, bout, fit, seizure, spell, turn**

ange ⇨ **indicate**

angelägen ⇨ **anxious, urgent**

angiectasis [ˌændʒi'ektəsɪs] *subst.* swelling of the blood vessels *angiektasi, kärlutvidgning*

angiektasi ⇨ **angiectasis**

angiitis [ˌændʒi'aɪtɪs] *subst.* inflammation of a blood vessel *angit, kärlinflammation*

anginal [æn'dʒaɪn(ə)l] *adj.* referring to angina *anginös;* **he suffered anginal pains**

angina (pectoris) [æn'dʒaɪnə (ˌpekt(ə)rɪs)] *subst.* pain in the chest caused by inadequate supply of blood to the heart muscles, following exercise or eating, because of narrowing of the arteries *angina (pectoris), kärlkramp;* **stable angina** = angina which has not changed for a long time *stabil angina (pectoris);* **unstable angina** = angina which has suddenly become worse *instabil angina (pectoris)*

anginös ⇨ **anginal**

angio- ['ændʒiə(ʊ), ˌ---] *prefix* referring to a blood vessel *angio-, kärl-*

angiocardiography [ˌændʒiəʊˌkɑːdi'ɒgrəfi] *subst.* X-ray examination of the cardiac system after injecting it with an opaque dye so that the organs appear clearly on the film *angiokardiografi, angiografi*

angiografi ⇨ **angiocardiography, angiography**

angiogram ['ændʒiəʊgræm] *subst.* X-ray picture of blood vessels *angiogram*

angiography [ˌændʒi'ɒgrəfi] *subst.* X-ray examination of blood vessels after injection with an opaque dye so that they show up in an X-ray *angiografi*

angiokardiografi ⇨ **angiocardiography**

angioma [ˌændʒi'əʊmə] *subst.* benign tumour (such as a naevus) formed in blood vessels *angiom*

angioneurotic oedema [ˌændʒiəʊnju(ə)'rɒtɪk ɪ'diːmə] *subst.* sudden accumulation of liquid under the skin, similar to nettlerash *angioneurotiskt ödem, Quinckeödem*

angioplastik ⇨ **angioplasty**

angioplasty ['ændʒiə(ʊ)plæsti] *subst.* plastic surgery to repair a blood vessel, such as a narrowed coronary artery *angioplastik, kärlplastik;* **percutaneous angioplasty** = repair of a narrowed artery by passing a balloon into the artery through a catheter, and then inflating it *perkutan kärlplastik*

angiosarcoma [ˌændʒiəʊsɑː'kəʊmə] *subst.* malignant tumour in the blood vessels *angiosarkom*

angiosarkom ⇨ **angiosarcoma**

angiospasm ['ændʒiə(ʊ)spæz(ə)m] *subst.* spasm which constricts blood vessels *angiospasm, vasospasm, kärlspasm*

angiotensin ['ændʒiə(ʊ)ˌtensiːn] *subst.* one of the factors responsible for high blood pressure *angiotensin, angiotonin, hypertensin*

angiotonin ⇨ **angiotensin**

angit ⇨ **angiitis**

angle ['æŋg(ə)l] *subst.* bend *or* corner *vinkel, hörn; see also* STERNOCLAVICULAR

angrepp ⇨ **onset**

angripa ⇨ **affect**

angripen ⇨ **diseased**

angular vein ['æŋgjʊlə ˌveɪn] *subst.* vein which continues the facial vein at the side of the nose *vena angularis*

anhidrosis [ˌænhɪ'drəʊsɪs] *subst.* condition where the amount of sweat is reduced or there is no sweat at all *anhidros*

anhidrotic [ˌænhɪ'drɒtɪk] *adj.* drug which reduces sweating *anhidrotisk*

anhopning ⇨ **accumulation, cluster, cumulative**

anhydraemia [ˌænhaɪ'driːmiə] *subst.* lack of sufficient fluid in the blood *anhydremi*

anhydremi ⇨ **anhydraemia**

anhörig ⇨ **kin**

anidrosis [ˌænɪ'drəʊsɪs] *subst.* = ANHIDROSIS

animal ['ænim(ə)l] *subst.* living and moving thing *djur;* **dogs and cats are animals, and man is also an animal; animal bite =** bite from an animal *djurbett*

COMMENT: bites from animals should be cleaned immediately. The main danger from animal bites is the possibility of catching rabies

aniridia [ˌænɪ'rɪdiə] *subst.* congenital absence of the iris *aniridi, irideremi*

anisometropia [ænˌaɪsəʊmə'trəʊpiə] *subst.* state where the refraction in the two eyes is different *anisometropi*

ankelbenen ➪ **tarsal**

ankeln ➪ **ankle, tarsus**

ankle ['æŋk(ə)l] *subst.* part of the body where the foot is connected to the leg *fotleden, vristen, ankeln;* **he twisted his ankle** *or* **he sprained his ankle** = he hurt it by stretching it *or* bending it *han vrickade (stukade) foten;* **ankle bone** *or* **talus =** bone which is part of the tarsus, and links the bones of the lower leg to the calcaneus *talus, språngbenet;* **ankle fracture =** break in any of the bones in the ankle *fotledsfraktur;* **ankle joint =** joint which connects the bones of the lower leg (the tibia and fibula) to the talus *fotleden;* **ankle jerk =** sudden jerk as a reflex action of the foot when the back of the ankle is tapped *akilles(sene)reflex*

ankyloblepharon [ˌæŋkɪləʊ'blef(ə)rɒn] *subst.* state where the edges of the eyelids are stuck together *ankyloblefaron, sammanvuxna ögonlock*

ankylos ➪ **ankylosis**

ankylose ['æŋkɪləʊz] *vb. (of bones)* to fuse together *ankylosera, växa samman, bli orörlig (stel); see also* SPONDYLITIS

ankylosis [ˌæŋkɪ'ləʊsɪs] *subst.* condition where the bones of a joint fuse together *ankylos*

Ankylostoma [ˌæŋkɪ'lɒstəmə] *or* **Ancylostoma** [ˌæŋkɪ'lɒstəmə] *or* **hookworm** ['hʊkwɜːm] *subst.* parasitic worm in the intestine, with holds on to the wall of the intestine with its teeth and lives on the blood and protein of the carrier *Ancylostoma duodenale, hakmask*

ankylostomiasis [ˌæŋkɪˌlɒstə'maɪəsɪs] *or* **hookworm disease** ['hʊkwɜːm dɪˌziːz] *subst.* disease caused by the hookworm, where the patient suffers weakness and anaemia, and can in severe cases die *ancylostomiasis, ankylostomiasis*

ankylostomiasis ➪ **ancylostomiasis**

anlag ➪ **diathesis, predisposition, tendency**

anlagsbärare ➪ **carrier**

anledning ➪ **reason**

anläggning ➪ **complex**

anmäla ➪ **notify, report**

anmälan ➪ **report**

anmälningspliktig sjukdom ➪ **notifiable disease**

anmärkning ➪ **complaint**

annular ['ænjʊlə] *adj.* shaped like a ring *annular, annulär, ringformad*

annulus ['ænjʊləs] *subst.* ring *or* structure shaped like a ring *annulus, ring*

annulär ➪ **annular**

anococcygeal [ˌænəˌkɒksɪ'dʒiːəl] *adj.* referring to both the anus and coccyx *som avser el. hör till både ändtarmsmynningen och svansbenet*

anomal ➪ **anomalous**

anomali ➪ **anomaly**

anomalous [ə'nɒm(ə)ləs] *adj.* different from what is usual *anomal, abnorm, onormal;* **anomalous pulmonary venous drainage =** condition where oxygenated blood from the lungs drains into the right atrium instead of the left *onormalt venöst avflöde från lungorna*

anomaly [ə'nɒm(ə)lɪ] *subst.* something which is different from the usual *anomali*

anonychia [ˌænə(ʊ)'nɪkiə] *subst.* congenital absence of one or more nails *anonyki*

anonyki ➪ **anonychia**

Anopheles [ə'nɒfəliːz] *subst.* mosquito which carries the malaria parasite *Anopheles mygga*

anorchism [æn'ɔ:kɪz(ə)m] *subst.* congenital absence of testicles *anorki(dism)*

anordning ➪ **device, facilities**

anorectal [ˌænə'rekt(ə)l] *adj.* referring to both the anus and rectum *anorektal*

anorektal ➪ **anorectal**

anoretisk ➪ **anorexic**

anorexia [ˌænə'reksiə] *subst.* loss of appetite *anorexi, aptitlöshet;* **anorexia nervosa** = psychological condition (usually found in girls) where the patient refuses to eat because of a fear of becoming fat *anorexia nervosa*

anorexic [ˌænə'reksɪk] *adj.* referring to anorexia *anoretisk;* **the school has developed a programme of counselling for anorexic students**

anosmia [æn'ɒzmiə] *subst.* lack of the sense of smell *anosmi*

anovular bleeding [æn'ɒvjʊlə ˌbli:dɪŋ] *subst.* bleeding from the uterus when ovulation has not taken place *anovulvatorisk blödning, menstruationsblödning utan ägglossning*

anoxaemia [ˌænɒk'si:miə] *subst.* reduction of the amount of oxygen in the blood *anox(i)emi*

anoxia [æn'ɒksiə] *subst.* lack of oxygen in body tissue *anoxi*

anoxic [æn'ɒksɪk] *subst.* referring to anoxia *anoxisk*

anpassa ➪ **fit, vary**

anpassning ➪ **adaptation**

ansamla ➪ **accumulate**

ansamling ➪ **accumulation**

anse ➪ **feel**

anserina ['ænseraɪn] *see* CUTIS

ansiktet ➪ **face**

ansiktsartären ➪ **facial**

ansiktsbjudning ➪ **delivery, face**

ansiktsbrand, fuktig ➪ **noma**

ansiktsdrag ➪ **features**

ansiktsfärg ➪ **complexion**

ansiktslyftning ➪ **face**

ansiktsnerven ➪ **facial**

anslagstavla ➪ **noticeboard**

ansluta ➪ **connect**

anslutning ➪ **connection**

anstränga ➪ **strain**

ansträngande ➪ **strenuous**

ansträngning ➪ **effort, exertion, strain**

anställa ➪ **employ, recruit**

ansvarig ➪ **responsible**

ansvarsnämnd, medicinsk ➪ **professional**

ansvällning ➪ **bulb**

answer ['ɑ:nsə] **1** *subst.* reply *or* words spoken or written when someone has spoken to you or asked you a question *svar;* **he phoned the laboratory but there was no answer; have the tests provided an answer to the problem? 2** *vb.* to reply *or* to speak or write words after someone has spoken to you or asked you a question *svara, besvara;* **when asked if the patient would survive the consultant did not answer; to answer an emergency call** = to go to the place where the call came from to bring help *göra en akut utryckning*

ansöka ➪ **apply**

ansökan ➪ **application**

antacid [ænt'æsɪd] *subst.* medicinal substance (tablet *or* liquid) which counteracts acidity in the stomach *antacidum, medel mot magsyra*

antagonist ➪ **blocker**

antagonistisk ➪ **incompatible**

ante- ['ænti, ˌ--] *prefix* meaning before *ante-, före, framåt-*

ante cibum [ˌænti 'saɪbəm] *Latin phrase meaning* "before food" (used in prescriptions) *ante cibum, före måltid*

antefixation ➪ **ventrofixation, ventrosuspension**

anteflexion [ˌæntiˈflekʃ(ə)n] *subst.* abnormal bending forward, especially of the uterus *anteflexion, framåtböjning*

antemortem [ˌæntiˈmɔːtəm] *subst.* period before death *period före döden*

antenatal [ˌæntiˈneɪt(ə)l] *adj.* during the period between conception and childbirth *antenatal, prenatal, foster-;* **antenatal diagnosis** *or* **prenatal diagnosis** = medical examination of a pregnant woman to see if the fetus is developing normally *prenataldiagnostik, fosterdiagnostik; see also* CLINIC

antenatal ⇨ **prenatal**

antepartum [ˌæntiˈpɑːtəm] *subst. & adj.* period of three months before childbirth *tredje trimestern, de tre månaderna före nedkomsten*

anterior [ænˈtɪəriə] *adj.* in front *anterior, främre;* **anterior superior iliac spine** = projection at the front end of the iliac crest of the pelvis *spina iliaca anterior superior;* **anterior jugular** = small jugular vein in the neck *vena jugularis anterior, främre halsvenen;* **anterior synechia** = condition of the eye, where the iris sticks to the cornea *främre syneki* NOTE: opposite is **posterior**

anteversion [ˌæntiˈvɜːʃ(ə)n] *subst.* leaning forward of an organ, especially of the uterus *anteversion, framåtvridning*

anthelmintic [ˌænθelˈmɪntɪk] *subst. & adj.* (drug) which removes worms from the intestine *ant(i)helmintikum, medel mot inälvsmask, maskmedel*

anthracosis [ˌænθrəˈkəʊsɪs] *subst.* lung disease from breathing coal dust *antrakos, kolsjuka*

anthrax [ˈænθræks] *subst.* disease of cattle and sheep which can be transmitted to humans *anthrax, mjältbrand*

COMMENT: caused by *Bacillus anthracis,* anthrax can be transmitted by touching infected skin, meat or other parts of an animal (including bone meal used as a fertilizer). It causes pustules on the skin or in the lungs (woolsorter's disease)

anti- [ˈænti, ˌ--] *prefix* meaning against *anti-, mot-*

antibacterial [ˌæntibækˈtɪəriəl] *adj.* which destroys bacteria *antibakteriell*

antibakteriell ⇨ **antibacterial**

antibiotic [ˌæntibaiˈɒtɪk] **1** *adj.* which stops the spread of bacteria *antibiotisk* **2** *subst.* drug (such as penicillin) which is developed from living substances and which stops the spread of microorganisms *antibiotikum;* **he was given a course of antibiotics; antibiotics have no use against virus diseases; broad spectrum antibiotics** = antibiotics which are used to control many types of bacteria *bredspektrumantibiotika*

antibiotikum ⇨ **antibiotic**

antibody [ˈæntiˌbɒdi] *subst.* substance which is naturally present in the body and which attacks foreign substances (such as bacteria) *antikropp;* **tests showed that he was antibody positive**

anti-cancer drug [ˌæntiˈkænsə ˌdrʌg] *subst.* drug which can control *or* destroy cancer cells *cytostatikum*

anticoagulant [ˌæntikəʊˈægjʊlənt] *subst. & adj.* (drug) which slows down or stops blood clotting *antikoagulans*

anti-convulsant [ˌæntikənˈvʌls(ə)nt] *subst. & adj.* (drug) used to control convulsions, as in the treatment of epilepsy *antiepileptikum, antikonvulsivt medel*

antidepressant [ˈæntidɪˈpres(ə)nt] *subst. & adj.* (drug) used to treat depression *antidepressivt medel*

anti-D-globulin ⇨ **anti D immunoglobulin**

anti D immunoglobulin [ˌænti ˌdiː ˌɪmjunəʊˈglɒbjʊlɪn] *subst.* immunoglobulin administered to Rh-negative mothers after the birth of a Rh-positive baby, to prevent haemolytic disease of the newborn in the next pregnancy *anti-D-globulin*

antidiuretic [ˌæntiˌdaɪju(ə)ˈretɪk] *adj.* which stops the production of excessive amounts of urine *antidiuretisk;* **hormones which have an antidiuretic effect on the kidneys; antidiuretic hormone (ADH)** *or* **vasopressin** = hormone secreted by the pituitary gland which acts on the kidneys to regulate the quantity of salt in body fluids and the amount of urine excreted by the kidneys *vasopressin, antidiuretiskt hormon, ADH*

antidot ⇨ **antidote**

antidote [ˈæntidəʊt] *subst.* substance which counteracts the effect of a poison *antidot, motgift;* **there is no satisfactory antidote to cyanide**

antiemetic [ˌæntiɪ'metik] *subst. & adj.* (drug) which prevents sickness *or* vomiting *antiemetisk(t medel), ant(i)emetikum*

antiepileptikum ➪ **anti-convulsant**

antifungal [ˌænti'fʌŋg(ə)l] *adj.* (substance) which kills *or* controls fungi *antimykotisk*

antigen ['æntidʒ(ə)n] *subst.* substance (such as a virus *or* germ) in the body which makes the body produce antibodies to attack it *antigen*

antigenic [ˌænti'dʒenɪk] *adj.* (substance) which stimulates the formation of antibodies *som stimulerar till antikroppsbildning*

antigen, inkomplett ➪ **hapten**

antihaemophilic factor [ˌæntiˌhiːmə'fɪlɪk 'fæktə] *subst.* factor VIII (used to encourage clotting in haemophiliacs) *(koagulations)faktor VIII, antihemofilifaktor A, AHF, AHG*

antihistamine (drug) [ˌænti'hɪstəmiːn (ˌdrʌg)] *subst.* drug used to control the effects of an allergy which releases histamine *antihistamin*

antihypertensive [ˌæntiˌhaɪpə'tensɪv] *adj. & subst.* (drug) used to reduce high blood pressure *antihypertensiv(t medel), blodtryckssänkande (medel)*

antikoagulans ➪ **anticoagulant**

antikropp ➪ **antibody**

antilymfocytserum ➪ **antilymphocytic serum (ALS)**

antilymphocytic serum (ALS) [ˌæntiˌlɪmfəʊ'sɪtɪk 'sɪərəm (ˌeɪel'es)] *subst.* serum used to produce immunosuppression in transplants *antilymfocytserum*

antimalarial [ˌæntimə'leəriəl] *adj. & subst.* (drug) used to treat malaria *antimalaria-, malaria(medel)*

antimetabolite [ˌæntimə'tæbəlaɪt] *subst.* substance which can replace a cell metabolism, but which is not active *antimetabolit*

antimitotic [ˌæntimaɪ'tɒtɪk] *adj.* which prevents the division of a cell by mitosis *mitoshämmare, som förhindrar celldelning genom mitos*

antimycotic [ˌæntimaɪ'kɒtɪk] *adj.* which destroys fungi *antimykotisk*

antimykotisk ➪ **antifungal, antimycotic**

antiperistalsis [ˌæntiˌperɪ'stælsɪs] *subst.* movement in the oesophagus *or* intestine where the contents are moved in the opposite direction to normal peristalsis, so leading to vomiting *antiperistaltik*

antiperistaltik ➪ **antiperistalsis**

antiperspirant [ˌænti'pɜːsp(ə)rənt] *subst.* substance which prevents sweating *antitranspirationsmedel, deodorant*

antipruritic [ˌæntipru'rɪtɪk] *subst. & adj.* (substance) which prevents itching *klådstillande (medel)*

antipyretic [ˌæntipaɪ(ə)'retɪk] *subst. & adj.* (drug) which helps to reduce a fever *antipyretikum, antipyretisk(t medel), febernedsättande (medel)*

antipyretikum ➪ **antipyretic, febrifuge**

anti Rh body [ˌænti 'ɑːrˌeɪtʃ 'bɒdi] *subst.* antibody formed in the mother's blood in reaction to a Rhesus antigen in the blood of the fetus *antikropp mot Rh-positivt antigen*

antisepsis [ˌænti'sepsɪs] *subst.* preventing sepsis *antiseptik*

antiseptic [ˌænti'septɪk] **1** *adj.* which prevents germs spreading *antiseptisk;* **she gargled with an antiseptic mouthwash** **2** *subst.* substance which prevents germs growing or spreading *antiseptikum, bakteriedödande medel;* **the nurse painted the wound with antiseptic**

antiseptisk ➪ **antiseptic**

antiserum [ˌænti'sɪərəm] *subst.* serum taken from an animal which has developed antibodies to bacteria, used to give temporary immunity to a disease *antiserum* NOTE: plural is **antisera**

antiserum ➪ **antitoxic serum, antivenene**

antisocial [ˌænti'səʊʃ(ə)l] *adj.* (behaviour) which is dangerous to other people *samhällsfarlig;* **antisocial hours** = hours of work (such as night duty) which can disrupt the worker's family life *tider som kan medföra sociala problem*

antispasmodic [ˌæntispæz'mɒdɪk] *subst.* drug used to prevent spasms *antispasmodikum, krampstillande medel*

antitetanus serum (ATS) [ˌænti'tet(ə)nəs ˌsɪərəm (ˌeɪti:'es)] *subst.* serum which protects a patient against tetanus *tetanusserum*

antithrombin [ˌænti'θrɒmbɪn] *subst.* substance present in the blood which prevents clotting *antitrombin*

antitoxic serum [ˌænti'tɒksɪk ˌsɪərəm] *subst.* immunizing agent, formed of serum taken from an animal which has developed antibodies to a disease, used to protect a person from that disease *antiserum*

antitoxin [ˌænti'tɒksɪn] *subst.* antibody produced by the body, which counteracts a poison in the body *antitoxin*

antitragus [æn'tɪtrəgəs] *subst.* small projection on the outer ear opposite the tragus *antitragus*

antitranspirationsmedel ➪ **antiperspirant**

antitrombin ➪ **antithrombin**

antituberculous drug [ˌæntitju'bɜ:kjʊləs ˌdrʌg] *subst.* drug used to treat tuberculosis *tuberkulosmedel*

antitussive [ˌænti'tʌsɪv] *subst.* drug used to reduce coughing *antitussivum, hostdämpande medel, hostmedicin*

antivenene [ˌæntivə'ni:n] *or* **antivenom (serum)** [ˌænti'venəm (ˌsɪərəm)] *subst.* serum which is used to counteract the poison from bites of snakes *or* insects *antiserum, ormserum*

antiviral drug [ˌænti'vaɪ(ə)r(ə)l ˌdrʌg] *subst.* drug which is effective against a virus *antiviralt medel*

antivärdreaktion ➪ **graft**

antrakos ➪ **anthracosis**

antral ['æntrəl] *adj.* referring to an antrum *som avser el. hör till håla;* **antral puncture** = making a hole in the wall of the maxillary sinus to remove fluid *punktering av överkäkshålan för bihålespolning*

antrectomy [æn'trektəmi] *subst.* surgical removal of an antrum in the stomach to prevent gastrin being formed *antrektomi, antrumextirpation*

antrektomi ➪ **antrectomy**

antrostomy [æn'trɒstəmi] *subst.* surgical operation to make an opening in the maxillary sinus *antrotomi*

antrotomi ➪ **antrostomy**

antrum ['æntrəm] *subst.* any cavity inside the body, especially one in bone *antrum, håla, hålrum;* **antrum of Highmore** = maxillary air sinus *antrum Highmori, sinus maxillaris, överkäkshålan;* **mastoid antrum** = cavity linking the air cells of the mastoid process with the middle ear *antrum mastoideum;* **pyloric antrum** = space at the bottom of the stomach, before the pyloric sphincter *antrum pyloricum (ventriculi)*

antrumextirpation ➪ **antrectomy**

antyda ➪ **suggest**

anures ➪ **anuria**

anuria [æn'jʊəriə] *subst.* condition where the patient does not make urine, either because of a deficiency in the kidneys or because the urinary tract is blocked *anuri, anures*

anus ['eɪnəs] *subst.* opening at the end of the rectum, leading outside the body between the buttocks, through which the faeces are passed ➪ *illustration* DIGESTIVE SYSTEM, UROGENITAL SYSTEM *anus, analöppning*
NOTE: for terms referring to the anus, see also **anal** and words beginning with **ano-**

anvil ['ænvɪl] *or* **incus** ['ɪŋkəs] *subst.* one of the three ossicles in the middle ear *incus, städet*

använda ➪ **employ, exert**

anxiety [æŋ'zaɪəti] *subst.* state of being very worried and afraid *oro, ängslan, ångest;* **anxiety disorders** = various mental disorders where the patient is worried and afraid (including the phobias) *ångestneuroser*

anxious ['æŋ(k)ʃəs] *adj.* **(a)** worried and afraid *orolig, ängslig;* **my sister is ill - I am anxious about her (b)** eager *ivrig, angelägen;* **she was anxious to get home; I was anxious to see the doctor**

aorta [eɪ'ɔ:tə] *subst.* large artery which takes blood away from the left side of the heart, and takes it to other arteries ➪ *illustration* HEART *aorta, stora kroppspulsådern;* **abdominal aorta** = the part of the aorta between the diaphragm and the point where it divides into the iliac arteries

➪ *illustration* KIDNEY *aorta abdominalis, bukaorta;* **ascending aorta** *or* **descending aorta**= first two sections of the aorta as it leaves the heart, first rising and then turning downwards *aorta ascendens, aorta descendens;* **thoracic aorta** = the part of the aorta which crosses the thorax *aorta thoracica, bröstaorta*

> COMMENT: the aorta is about 45 centimetres long. It leaves the left ventricle, rises (where the carotid arteries branch off) then goes downwards through the abdomen and divides into the two iliac arteries. The aorta is the blood vessel which carries all arterial blood from the heart

aortabågen ➪ **aortic**

aortagapet ➪ **aortic**

aortainflammation ➪ **aortitis**

aortainsufficiens ➪ **incompetence, regurgitation**

aortaklaffen ➪ **aortic**

aortakoarktation ➪ **coarctation**

aortastenos ➪ **aortic**

aortic [eɪ'ɔːtɪk] *adj.* referring to the aorta *aorta-;* **aortic arch** = bend in the aorta which links the ascending aorta to the descending *arcus aortae, aortabågen;* **aortic hiatus** = opening in the diaphragm through which the aorta passes *hiatus aorticus, aortagapet;* **aortic incompetence** = defective aortic valve, causing regurgitation *aortainsufficiens;* **aortic regurgitation** = backwards flow of blood caused by a defective aortic valve *återflöde i aorta beroende på aortainsufficiens;* **aortic sinuses** = swellings in the aorta from which the coronary arteries lead back into the heart itself *sinus aortae;* **aortic stenosis** = condition where the aortic valve is narrow, caused by rheumatic fever *stenosis aortae, aortastenos;* **aortic valve** = valve with three flaps at the opening into the aorta *valva aortae, aortaklaffen*

aortitis [ˌeɪɔː'taɪtɪs] *subst.* inflammation of the aorta *aortit, aortainflammation*

aortography [ˌeɪɔː'tɒgrəfi] *subst.* X-ray examination of the aorta after an opaque substance has been injected into it *aortografi*

apathetic [ˌæpə'θetɪk] *adj.* (patient) who takes no interest in anything *apatisk*

apatisk ➪ **apathetic, listless**

apelsinhud ➪ **peau d'orange**

aperient [ə'pɪəriənt] *subst. & adj.* (substance, such as a laxative *or* purgative) which helps make bowel movements *(svagt) laxerande (medel), (svagt) avförande (medel)*

aperistalsis [ˌæperɪ'stælsis] *subst.* lack of the peristaltic movement in the bowel *avsaknad av peristaltik*

apertura ➪ **aperture, inlet**

aperture ['æpətʃə] *subst.* hole *apertura, öppning*

apex ['eɪpeks] *subst.* top of the heart *or* lung *apex cordis, hjärtspetsen, apex pulmonis, lungspetsen;* end of the root of a tooth *apex radicis dentis, tandrotsspets;* **apex beat** = heartbeat which can be felt if the hand is placed on the heart *ictus cordis, hjärtspetsstöten*

Apgar score ['æpgɑː ˌskɔː] *subst.* method of judging the condition of a newborn baby *Apgarpoäng, Apgarscore*

> COMMENT: the baby is given a maximum of two points on each of five criteria: colour of the skin, heartbeat, breathing, muscle tone and reaction to stimuli

> QUOTE in this study, babies having an Apgar score of four or less had 100% mortality. The lower the Apgar score, the poorer the chance of survival
> **Indian Journal of Medical Sciences**

aphagia [ə'feɪdʒiə] *subst.* being unable to swallow *afagi, aglutition*

aphakia [ə'feɪkiə] *subst.* absence of a crystalline lens of the eye *afaki*

aphasia [ə'feɪziə] *subst.* being unable to speak or write *or* to understand speech or writing, caused by damage to the brain centres which control speech *afasi*

aphonia [eɪ'fəʊniə] *subst.* being unable to make sounds *afoni*

aphrodisiac [ˌæfrə'dɪziæk] *subst. & adj.* (substance) which increases sexual urges *afrodisiakum, könsdriftshöjande (medel)*

aphthae ['æfθiː] *or* **aphthous ulcers** ['æfθəs ˌʌlsəz] *subst pl.* ulcers in the mouth *aftösa sår, afte*

apical abscess ['æpɪk(ə)l ˌæbses] *subst.* abscess in the socket around the root of a tooth *abscess i tandrotsspets*

apicectomy [ˌæpɪ'sektəmi] *subst.* surgical removal of the root of a tooth *apikoektomi*

apikoektomi ⇨ **apicectomy**

aplasia [ə'pleɪziə] *subst.* lack of growth of tissue *aplasi, agenesi, utebliven organbildning*

aplastic anaemia [eɪˌplæstɪk ə'ni:miə] *subst.* anaemia caused by bone marrow failure which stops the formation of red blood cells *aplastisk anemi*

apné ⇨ **apnoea**

apnoea [æp'ni:ə] *subst.* stopping of breathing *apné, andningsstillestånd*

apnoeic [æp'ni:ɪk] *adj.* where breathing has stopped *apnoisk*

apnoisk ⇨ **apnoeic**

apocrine glands ['æpəkraɪn ˌglændz] *subst.* glands, such as the sweat glands which produce body odour, where part of gland's cells break off with the secretions *apokrina körtlar*

apofys ⇨ **apophysis**

apofysit ⇨ **apophysitis**

aponeurosis [ˌæpəʊnju(ə)'rəʊsɪs] *subst.* band of tissue which attaches muscles to each other *aponeuros, senhinna*

apophyseal [ˌæpə'fɪziəl] *adj.* referring to apophysis *som avser el. hör till apofys*

apophysis [ə'pɒfəsɪs] *subst.* growth of bone, not at a joint *apofys*

apophysitis [ˌæpəfɪ'saɪtɪs] *subst.* inflammation of an apophysis *apofysit*

apoplectic [ˌæpə'plektɪk] *adj.* (person) suffering from apoplexy *or* likely to have a stroke *apoplektisk*

apoplektisk ⇨ **apoplectic**

apoplexy ['æpəpleksi] *subst.* stroke *or* sudden loss of consciousness caused by a cerebral haemorrhage or blood clot in the brain *apoplexi, slag, slaganfall, stroke*

apotek ⇨ **chemist, dispensary, pharmacy**

apotekare ⇨ **chemist, pharmacist**

apoteksburk ⇨ **gallipot**

apparat ⇨ **apparatus, device; tract**

apparatus [ˌæpə'reɪtəs] *subst.* equipment used in a laboratory *or* hospital *apparat, instrument;* **the hospital has installed new apparatus in the physiotherapy department; the blood sample was tested in a special piece of apparatus**
NOTE: no plural: **a piece of apparatus; some new apparatus**

appear [ə'pɪə] *vb.* **(a)** to start being seen *bli (vara) synlig, visa sig, uppträda;* **a rash suddenly appeared on the upper part of the body (b)** to seem *synas, förefalla, verka;* **he appears to be seriously ill**

appearance [ə'pɪər(ə)ns] *subst.* how a person or thing looks *utseende, yttre;* **you could tell from her appearance that she was suffering from anaemia**

appendage [ə'pendɪdʒ] *subst.* part of the body *or* piece of tissue which hangs down from another part *appendix, bihang*

appendektomi ⇨ **appendicectomy**

appendiceal [ˌæpən'dɪsiəl] *adj.* referring to the appendix *som avser el. hör till appendix ("blindtarmen");* **there is a risk of appendiceal infection**

appendicectomy [əˌpendɪ'sektəmi] *subst.* surgical removal of an appendix *appendektomi, vanligen "blindtarmsoperation"*

appendicit ⇨ **appendicitis**

appendicitis [əˌpendə'saɪtɪs] *subst.* inflammation of the vermiform appendix *appendicit, blindtarmsinflammation*

> COMMENT: appendicitis takes several forms, the main ones being: acute appendicitis, which is a sudden attack of violent pain in the right lower part of the abdomen, accompanied by a fever. Acute appendicitis normally requires urgent surgery. A second form is chronic appendicitis, where the appendix is continually slightly inflamed, giving a permanent dull pain or a feeling of indigestion

appendicular skeleton [ˌæpən'dɪkjʊlə ˌskelətən] *subst.* part of the skeleton formed of the arms and legs, together with the shoulder bones and pelvis which are attached to the spine *de (hängande) delar av skelettet som fäster vid ryggraden; compare* AXIAL SKELETON

appendix [ə'pend ɪks] *subst.* **(a)** any small tube *or* sac hanging from an organ *appendix, bihang* **(b)** **(vermiform) appendix** = small tube shaped like a worm, attached to the caecum, which serves no function but can become infected *appendix vermiformis, blindtarmens maskformiga bihang, "blindtarmen"*; **grumbling appendix** = chronic appendicitis *kronisk (recidiverande) appendicit (blindtarmsinflammation)* NOTE: plural is **appendices** ➪ *illustration* DIGESTIVE SYSTEM

appendix ➪ **appendage, appendix**

appetite ['æpɪtaɪt] *subst.* wanting food *aptit;* **loss of appetite** = lack of interest in eating food *aptitförlust, nedsatt aptit*

appliance [ə'plaɪəns] *subst.* piece of apparatus used on the body *hjälpmedel;* **he wore a surgical appliance to support his neck**

application [ˌæplɪ'keɪʃ(ə)n] *subst.* **(a)** asking for a job (usually in writing) *ansökan;* **if you are applying for the job, you must fill in an application form** **(b)** putting a substance on *applicering;* **two applications of the lotion should be made each day**

applicator ['æplɪkeɪtə] *subst.* instrument for applying a remedy *applikator, påstrykare*

applicera ➪ **apply**

applicering ➪ **application**

applikator ➪ **applicator**

apply [ə'plaɪ] *vb.* **(a)** to ask for a job *ansöka;* **she applied for a job in a teaching hospital** **(b)** to refer to *gälla, tillämpas;* **this order applies to all medical staff; the rule applies to visitors only** **(c)** to put (a substance) on *applicera, anbringa, lägga (sätta, stryka)på;* **the ointment should not be applied to the face**

appoint [ə'pɔɪnt] *vb.* to give someone a job *utnämna, förordna, tillsätta;* **she was appointed night sister**

appointment [ə'pɔɪntmənt] *subst.* **(a)** giving someone a job *utnämning;* **on his appointment as head of the clinical department** = when he was made head of the clinical department *när han blev utnämnd till klinikchef* **(b)** arrangement to see someone at a particular time *(avtalat) möte, (tid för ett) sammanträffande (samtal);* **I have an appointment with the doctor** *or* **to see the doctor on Tuesday** *or* **I have a doctor's appointment on Tuesday; can I make an appointment to see Dr Jones? I'm very busy - I've got appointments all day**

appreciate [ə'priːʃɪeɪt] *vb.* to notice how good something is *uppskatta, sätta värde på;* **the patients always appreciate a talk with the ward sister**

approach [ə'prəʊtʃ] *vb.* to go *or* come nearer *närma sig, nalkas;* **as the consultant approached, all the patients looked at him**

approve [ə'pruːv] *vb.* **to approve of something** = to think that something is good *godkänna, godta, tillstyrka;* **I don't approve of patients staying in bed; the Medical Council does not approve of this new treatment; the drug has been approved by the Department of Health**

apraxia [eɪ'præksiə] *subst.* being unable to make proper movements *apraxi, handlingsoförmåga*

apron ['eɪpr(ə)n] *subst.* cloth or plastic cover which you wear in front of your clothes to stop them getting dirty *förkläde;* **the surgeon was wearing a green apron**

aptit ➪ **appetite**

aptitbefordrande medel ➪ **stomachic**

aptitförlust ➪ **appetite**

aptitlöshet ➪ **anorexia**

aptitretande medel ➪ **stomachic**

apyrexia [ˌæpaɪ(ə)'reksiə] *subst.* absence of fever *apyrexi, feberfrihet*

aqua ['ækwə] *subst.* water *aqua, vatten*

aquaeductus ➪ **aqueduct**

aqueduct ['ækwɪdʌkt] *subst.* canal *or* tube which carries fluid from one part of the body to another *aquaeductus, vätskeförande gång (kanal);* **cerebral aqueduct** *or* **aqueduct of Silvius** = canal connecting the third and fourth ventricles in the brain *aquaeductus cerebri (Sylvii)*

aqueous ['eɪkwiəs, 'æk-] *adj.* (solution) made with water *aquosus, vatten-*

aqueous (humour) ['eɪkwiəs (ˌhjuːmə)] *subst.* fluid in the eye between the lens and the cornea *humor aqueus, ögonkammarvatten* NOTE: usually referred to as "the aqueous"

aquiline nose ['ækwɪlaɪn ˌnəʊz] *subst.* nose which is large and strongly curved *örnnäsa*

aquosus ⇨ **aqueous**

arachidonic acid [ˌærəkə'dɒnɪk 'æsɪd] *subst.* essential fatty acid *arachidonsyra*

arachidonsyra ⇨ **arachidonic acid**

arachnidism [ə'ræknɪdɪz(ə)m] *subst.* poisoning by the bite of a spider *förgiftning pga spindelbett*

arachnodactyly [ə'ræknə'dæktɪli] *subst.* one of the conditions of Marfan's syndrome, a congenital condition where the fingers and toes are long and thin *araknodaktyli, spindelfingrar*

arachnoidea ⇨ **arachnoid mater**

arachnoiditis [əˈræknɔɪ'daɪtɪs] *subst.* inflammation of the arachnoid membrane *araknoidit, araknit*

arachnoid mater [ə'ræknɔɪd ˌmeɪtə] *or* **arachnoid membrane** [ə'ræknɔɪd ˌmembreɪn] *subst.* middle membrane covering the brain *arachnoidea, meninx serosa, spindelvävshinnan*

araknit ⇨ **arachnoiditis**

araknodaktyli ⇨ **arachnodactyly**

araknoidit ⇨ **arachnoiditis**

arbetarskyddslag ⇨ **health**

arbetssjukdom ⇨ **industrial, occupational**

arbetsterapeut ⇨ **occupational**

arbetsterapi ⇨ **occupational**

arborisation ⇨ **arborization**

arborization [ˌɑːbəraɪ'zeɪʃ(ə)n] *subst.* (i) branching ends of some nerve fibres or of a motor nerve in muscle fibre *nervändslut;* (ii) normal tree-like appearance of venules, capillaries and arterioles *arborisation, förgrening;* (iii) branching of capillaries when inflamed *kapillärernas förgrening vid inflammation*

arbor vitae ['ɑːbə 'vaɪtiː] *subst.* structure of the cerebellum *or* of the womb which looks like a tree *arbor vitae, livsträdet*

arbovirus [ˌɑːbə'vaɪ(ə)rəs] *subst.* virus transmitted by blood-sucking insects *arbovirus*

arc [ɑːk] *subst.* (i) nerve pathway *nervbana;* (ii) part of a curved structure in the body *båge, valv;* **arc eye** *or* **snow blindness** = temporary painful blindness caused by ultraviolet rays, especially in arc welding or from sunlight shining on snow *ophthalmia nivalis, snöblindhet;* **reflex arcs** = nerve pathways of a reflex action *reflexbågar*

arch [ɑːtʃ] *subst.* curved part of the body, especially under the foot *båge, valv, hålfoten;* **aortic arch** = curved part of the aorta which joins the ascending aorta to the descending *arcus aortae, aortabågen;* **deep plantar arch** = curved artery crossing the sole of the foot *arcus plantaris, hålfotsbågen;* **palmar arch** = one of two arches formed by arteries in the palm of the hand *arcus palmaris profundis, djupa hålhandsbågen;* **longitudinal arch** *or* **plantar arch** = curved part of the sole of the foot running along the length of the foot *hålfoten, fotvalvet;* **metatarsal arch** *or* **transverse arch** = arch across the sole of the foot from side to side *fotvalvet, hålfoten;* **zygomatic arch** = ridge of bone across the temporal bone between the ear and the bottom of the eye socket *arcus zygomaticus, okbågen, kindbågen;* **fallen arches** = condition where the arches in the sole of the foot are not high *sänkta fotvalv, plattfot*

arcuate ['ɑːkjuɪt] *adj.* arched *böjd, bågformig;* **medial arcuate ligament** = fibrous arch to which the diaphragm is attached *psoasarkaden, ligamentum arcuatum mediale; see also* ARTERY

arcus ['ɑːkəs] *subst.* arch *arcus, båge;* **arcus senilis** = grey ring round the cornea, found in old people *arcus senilis, gerontoxon, åldringsbåge*

area ['eəriə] *subst.* **(a)** measurement of the space occupied by something *area, yta, ytinnehåll;* **to measure the area of a room you must multiply the length by the width; the area of the ward is 250 square metres** **(b)** space occupied by something *område, centrum;* **there is a small area of affected tissue in the right lung; treat the infected area with antiseptic; visual area** = part of the cerebral cortex which is concerned with sight *syncentrum;* **bare area of liver** = large triangular part of the liver not covered with peritoneum *facies diaphragmatica, den del av levern som inte täcks av bukhinnan*

areata [ˌæri'eɪtə] *see* ALOPECIA

areola [ə'riːələ] *subst.* (i) coloured part round the nipple *areola mammae, vårtgården, bröstvårtgården;* (ii) part of the iris closest to the pupil *den del av regnbågshinnan som ligger närmast pupillen*

areolar tissue [ə'ri:ələ ˌtɪʃu:] *subst.* type of connective tissue *slags stödjevävnad*

arginine ['ɑ:dʒɪni:n] *subst.* amino acid which helps the liver form urea *arginin*

Argyll Robertson pupil [ɑ:ˌgaɪ(ə)l 'rɒbəts(ə)n ˌpju:p(ə)l] *subst.* condition of the eye, where the lens is able to focus, but the pupil does not react to light *Argyll Robertsons tecken (pupiller)*

COMMENT: a symptom of general paralysis of the insane, or of locomotor ataxia

arise [ə'raɪz] *vb.* (i) to begin in *or* to come from (a place) *härröra;* (ii) to start to happen *uppstå, uppkomma, framträda;* **a muscle arising in the scapula; two problems have arisen concerning the removal of the geriatric patients to the other hospital** NOTE: **arising - arose - has arisen**

QUOTE the target cells for adult myeloid leukaemia are located in the bone marrow, and there is now evidence that a substantial proportion of childhood leukaemias also arise in the bone marrow
British Medical Journal

QUOTE one issue has consistently arisen - the amount of time and effort which nurses need to put into the writing of detailed care plans
Nursing Times

arm [ɑ:m] *subst.* one of the limbs *or* part of the body which goes from the shoulder to the hand, formed of the upper arm, the elbow and the forearm *brachium, armen;* **she broke her arm skiing; lift your arms up above your head; arm bones** = the humerus, the ulna and the radius *armens ben;* **arm sling** = sling made of cloth attached round the neck, used to support an injured arm *mitella*

armartären ⇨ **brachial**

armavledning ⇨ **limb**

armband ⇨ **bracelet**

armbågen ⇨ **elbow**

armbågs- ⇨ **cubital**

armbågsbenet ⇨ **ulna**

armbågsmuskeln ⇨ **anconeus**

armbågsutskottet ⇨ **olecranon (process)**

armböjaren ⇨ **brachialis muscle**

armen ⇨ **arm, brachium, limb**

armflätan ⇨ **brachial**

armhålan ⇨ **armpit, axilla**

armhåle- ⇨ **axillary**

armpit ['ɑ:mpɪt] *or* **axilla** [æk'sɪlə] *subst.* hollow under the shoulder, between the arm and the body, where the upper arm joins the shoulder *axilla, armhålan, axelhålan*
NOTE: for other terms referring to the arm see words beginning with **brachi-**

armplexus ⇨ **brachial**

armsträckaren ⇨ **triceps**

Arnold-Chiari malformation [ˌɑ:nɒldki'eəriz ˌmælfɔ:'meɪʃ(ə)n] *subst.* congenital condition where the base of the skull is malformed, allowing parts of the cerebellum into the spinal canal *Arnold-Chiaris syndrom*

arrange [ə'reɪn(d)ʒ] *vb.* **(a)** to put in order *arrangera, ordna, göra (ställa) i ordning;* **the beds are arranged in rows; the patients' records are arranged in alphabetical order** **(b)** to organize *arrangera, ordna med, planera, avtala;* **he arranged the appointment for 6 o'clock**

arrangemang ⇨ **arrangement**

arrangement [ə'reɪn(d)ʒmənt] *subst.* way in which something is put in order *arrangemang, ordnande;* way in which something is organized *arrangemang, ordning*

arrangera ⇨ **arrange, fix**

arrector pili muscle [əˌrektə 'paɪlaɪ ˌmʌs(ə)l] *subst.* small muscle which is attached to a hair follicle and makes the hair stand upright, and also forms goose pimples ⇨ *illustration* SKIN, SENSORY RECEPTOR **arrector pili muscles** ***(musculi) arrectores pilorum***

arrest [ə'rest] *subst.* stopping of a bodily function *stillestånd; see also* CARDIAC

arrhythmia [ə'riðmiə] *subst.* variation in the rhythm of the heartbeat *arrytmi, oregelbundenhet*

arrytmi ⇨ **arrhythmia**

arsenic ['ɑ:snɪk] *subst.* poison which was once used in some medicines *arsenik* NOTE: the chemical symbol is **As**

arsenik ⇨ **arsenic**

art ⇨ **species**

artefact ['ɑ:tɪfækt] *subst.* something which is made *or* introduced artificially *artefakt, konstprodukt; see also* DERMATITIS

artefakt ⇨ **artefact**

arterial [ɑ:'tɪəriəl] *adj.* referring to arteries *arteriell, artär-, pulsåder-;* **arterial bleeding** = bleeding from an artery *artärblödning;* **arterial block** = blocking of an artery by a blood clot *stopp i artär, blodpropp;* **arterial blood** = oxygenated blood *or* bright red blood in an artery which has received oxygen in the lungs and is being taken to the tissues *arteriellt (syrsatt) blod;* **arterial supply to the brain** = supply of blood to the brain by the internal carotid arteries and the vertebral arteries *hjärnans blodförsörjning*

arteriectomy [ɑ:ˌtɪəri'ektəmi] *subst.* surgical removal of an artery *or* part of an artery *arteriektomi*

arteriektomi ⇨ **arteriectomy**

arteriell ⇨ **arterial**

arterio- [ɑ:'tɪəriəʊ, -ˌ---] *prefix* referring to arteries *arteri(o)-, artär-, pulsåder-*

arteriografi ⇨ **arteriography**

arteriogram [ɑ:'tɪəriəʊgræm] *subst.* X-ray photograph of an artery, taken after it has been injected with opaque dye *arteriogram*

arteriography [ɑ:ˌtɪəri'ɒgrəfi] *subst.* taking of X-ray photographs of arteries after injecting an opaque dye *arteriografi*

arteriole [ɑ:'tɪəriəʊl] *subst.* very small artery *arteriol*

arteriopathy [ɑ:ˌtɪəri'ɒpəθi] *subst.* disease of an artery *artärsjukdom*

arterioplasty [ɑ:'tɪəriəʊplæsti] *subst.* plastic surgery to make good a damaged *or* blocked artery *artärplastik*

arteriorrhaphy [ɑ:ˌtɪəri'ɔ:rəfi] *subst.* stitching of an artery *artärrafi*

arteriosclerosis [ɑ:ˌtɪəriəʊsklə'rəʊsɪs] *subst.* hardening of the arteries *or* condition where the walls of arteries become thick and more rigid, making it more difficult for the blood to pass, and so causing high blood pressure, stroke and coronary thrombosis *arterioskleros, åderförkalkning*

arterioskleros ⇨ **arteriosclerosis, artery**

arteriosus [ɑ:ˌtɪəri'əʊsəs] *see* DUCTUS

arteriotomy [ˌɑ:tɪəri'ɒtəmi] *subst.* puncture made into the wall of an artery *arteriotomi*

arteriovenous [ɑ:ˌtɪəriəʊ'vi:nəs] *adj.* referring to both an artery and a vein *arteriovenös*

arteriovenös ⇨ **arteriovenous**

arteritis [ˌɑ:tə'raɪtɪs] *subst.* inflammation of the walls of an artery *arterit, artärinflammation;* **giant-cell arteritis** = disease of old people, which often affects the arteries in the scalp *arteritis temporalis, polyarteritis senilis, Hortons sjukdom, jättecellsarterit, temporalisarterit*

artery ['ɑ:t(ə)ri] *subst.* blood vessel taking blood from the heart to the tissues of the body *artär, pulsåder;* **arcuate artery** = curved artery in the foot *or* kidney *arteria arcuata, fotryggens bågartär, artär i njuren;* **axillary artery** = artery leading from the subclavian artery at the armpit *arteria axillaris, stora armhåleartären;* **basilar artery** = artery which lies at the base of the brain *arteria basilaris, hjärnans basala artär;* **brachial artery** = artery running down the arm from the axillary artery to the elbow, where it divides into the radial and ulnar arteries *arteria brachialis, armartären;* **cerebral arteries** = main arteries taking blood into the brain *arteriae cerebrali, hjärnartärerna;* **common carotid artery** = main artery leading up each side of the lower part of the neck *arteria carotis communis, gemensamma halsartären;* **communicating arteries** = arteries which connect the blood supply from each side of the brain, forming part of the circle of Willis *arteria communicans anterior resp. posterior;* **coronary arteries** = arteries which supply blood to the heart muscle *arteria coronaria dexter resp. sinistra, hjärtats kransartärer, kranskärlen, koronarkärlen;* **femoral artery** = continuation of the external iliac artery, which runs down the front of the thigh and then crosses to the back *arteria femoralis, lårbensartären;* **hardened arteries** *or* **hardening of the arteries** = arteriosclerosis *or* condition (mainly found in old people) where the walls of arteries become thicker because of deposits of fats and minerals, making it more difficult for the blood to pass, and so causing high blood pressure *arterioskleros, åderförkalkning;* **hepatic artery** = artery which takes blood to the liver *arteria hepatica (communis);* **common iliac artery** = one of two arteries which branch from the aorta in the abdomen and divide into the internal and external iliac arteries *arteria iliaca communis, stora höftpulsådern;* **ileocolic artery** = branch of the superior mesenteric artery *arteria ileocolica;* **innominate artery** = largest branch from the aortic arch, which continues as the right common carotid and right subclavian arteries *arteria brachiocephalica, "namnlösa artären"*; **interlobar artery** = artery running towards the cortex on each side of a renal pyramid *arteria interlobaris renis;* **interlobular arteries** = arteries running to the glomeruli of the kidneys *arteriae interlobulares renis;* **lingual artery** = artery which supplies the tongue *arteria lingualis, tungartären;* **lumbar artery** = one of four arteries which supply the back muscles and skin *arteria lumbalis;* **popliteal artery** = artery which branches from the femoral artery at the knee and leads into the tibial arteries *arteria poplitea, knävecksartären;* **pulmonary arteries** = arteries which take deoxygenated blood from the heart to the lungs to be oxygenated *arteria pulmonalis dextra resp. sinistra, pulmonalisartärerna, lungpulsådrorna;* **radial artery** = artery which branches from the brachial artery, starting at the elbow and ending in the palm of the hand *arteria radialis, radialartären;* **renal arteries** = pair of arteries running from the abdominal aorta to the kidneys *arteriae renales, njurartärerna;* **subclavian artery** = artery running from the aorta to the axillary artery in each arm *arteria subclavia, nyckelbensartären;* **tibial arteries** = two arteries which run down the front and back of the lower leg *arteria tibialis, skenbensartären;* **ulnar artery** = artery which branches from the brachial artery at the elbow and joins the radial artery in the palm of the hand *arteria ulnaris; compare* VEIN

COMMENT: In most arteries, the blood has been oxygenated in the lungs and is bright red in colour. In the pulmonary artery, the blood is deoxygenated and so is darker. The arterial system begins with the aorta, which leaves the heart and from which all the arteries branch

arthr- [ɑːθr] *prefix* referring to a joint *artr(o)-, led-, ledgångs-*

arthralgia [ɑːˈθrældʒə] *subst.* pain in the joints *artralgi, artrodymi, ledsmärta*

arthrectomy [ɑːˈθrektəmi] *subst.* surgical removal of a joint *artrektomi, ledresektion*

arthritic [ɑːˈθrɪtɪk] **1** *adj.* referring to arthritis *artritisk;* **he has an arthritic hip 2** *subst.* person suffering from arthritis *person som lider av ledgångsinflammation*

arthritis [ɑːˈθraɪtɪs] *subst.* painful inflammation of a joint *artrit, ledgångsinflammation;* **rheumatoid arthritis** = general painful disabling disease affecting any joint, but usually the hands, feet, and hips *reumatoid artrit, RA, kronisk ledgångsreumatism; see also* OSTEOARTHRITIS

arthroclasia [ˌɑːθrəʊˈkleɪʒə] *subst.* removal of ankylosis in a joint *artroklasi*

arthrodesis [ˌɑːθrəʊˈdiːsɪs] *subst.* surgical operation where a joint is fused in a certain position so preventing pain from movement *artrodes, steloperation av led*

arthrodynia [ˌɑːθrəˈdɪniə] *subst.* pain in a joint *artrodyni, ledsmärta*

arthrography [ɑːˈθrɒgrəfi] *subst.* X-ray photography of a joint *artrografi*

arthropathy [ɑːˈθrɒpəθi] *subst.* disease in a joint *artropati, ledsjukdom, ledgångssjukdom*

arthroplasty [ˈɑːθrəʊplæsti] *subst.* surgical operation to repair a joint *or* to replace a joint *artroplastik*

arthroscope [ˈɑːθrəʊskəʊp] *subst.* instrument which is inserted into the cavity of a joint to inspect it *artroskop*

arthroscopy [ɑːˈθrɒskəpi] *subst.* examining the inside of a joint by means of an arthroscope *artroskopi*

arthrosis [ɑːˈθrəʊsɪs] *subst.* degeneration of a joint *artros*

arthrotomy [ɑːˈθrɒtəmi] *subst.* cutting into a joint to drain pus *artrotomi*

articular [ɑːˈtɪkjʊlə] *adj.* referring to joints *artikulär, led-;* **articular cartilage** = layer of cartilage at the end of a bone where it forms a joint with another bone ⇨ *illustration* BONE STRUCTURE *cartilago articularis, ledbrosk;* **articular facet of a rib** = point at which a rib articulates with the spine *revbens ledyta*

articulate [ɑːˈtɪkjʊleɪt] *vb.* to be linked with another bone in a joint *leda mot;* **articulating bones** = bones which form a joint *ben som ledar mot varanda;* **articulating process** = piece of bone which sticks out from a vertebra and links with the next vertebra *processus articularis, ledutskott*

articulation [ɑːˌtɪkjʊˈleɪʃ(ə)n] *subst.* joint *or* series of joints *artikulation, led, ledgång*

artificial [ˌɑːtɪˈfɪʃ(ə)l] *adj.* which is made by man *or* which is not a natural part of the body *artificiell, konstgjord;* **artificial cartilage; artificial kidney; artificial lung; artificial leg; artificial insemination** = introduction of semen into a woman's womb by artificial means *artificiell insemination, konstgjord befruktning; see also* AID, AIH; **artificial respiration** = way of reviving someone who has stopped breathing (as by mouth-to-mouth resuscitation) *artificiell respiration, konstgjord andning;* **artificial ventilation** = breathing which is assisted *or* controlled by a machine *artificiell ventilation, konstgjord andning (med hjälp av respirator)*

artificially [ˌɑːtɪˈfɪʃ(ə)li] *adv.* in an artificial way *artificiellt, på konstgjord väg*

artificiell ➪ **artificial, synthetic**

artificiellt ➪ **artificially, synthetically**

artikulation ➪ **articulation**

artikulär ➪ **articular**

artralgi ➪ **arthralgia**

artrektomi ➪ **arthrectomy**

artrit ➪ **arthritis**

artritisk ➪ **arthritic**

artrodymi ➪ **arthralgia**

artrodyni ➪ **arthrodynia**

artrofyt ➪ **osteophyte**

artrografi ➪ **arthrography**

artroklasi ➪ **arthroclasia**

artros ➪ **arthrosis, osteoarthritis**

artroskopi ➪ **arthroscopy**

artrotomi ➪ **arthrotomy**

artär ➪ **artery**

artär- ➪ **arterial, arterio-**

artärblödning ➪ **arterial, haemorrhage**

artärbråck ➪ **aneurysm**

artärinflammation ➪ **arteritis**

artärplastik ➪ **arterioplasty**

artärrafi ➪ **arteriorrhaphy**

artärsjukdom ➪ **arteriopathy**

artärstammen ➪ **truncus**

arvsanlag ➪ **gene**

arytenoid [ˌærɪˈtiːnɔɪd] *adj.* (cartilage) at the back of the larynx *arytenoid, kannformig*

As *chemical symbol for* arsenic *As, arsenik*

asbestosis [ˌæsbeˈstəʊsɪs] *subst.* disease of the lungs caused by inhaling asbestos dust *asbestos*

ascariasis [ˌæskəˈraɪəsɪs] *subst.* disease of the intestine and sometimes the lungs, caused by infestation with Ascaris lumbricoides *ascariasis, askaridos, spolmaskinfektion*

Ascaris lumbricoides [ˈæskərɪs ˌlʌmbrɪˈkɔɪdiːz] *subst.* type of large roundworm which is a parasite in the human intestine *Ascaris lumbricoiden, vanliga spolmasken*

ascending [əˈsedɪŋ] *adj.* going upwards *uppåtstigande, uppåtgående;* **ascending aorta** = first part of the aorta which goes up from the heart until it turns at the aortic arch *aorta ascendens;* **ascending colon** = first part of the colon which goes up the right side of the body from the caecum ➪ *illustration* DIGESTIVE SYSTEM *colon ascendens, uppåtstigande delen av tjocktarmen*

Aschoff nodules [ˈæʃɒf ˌnɒdjuːlz] *subst pl.* nodules which are formed mainly in or near the heart in rheumatic fever *Aschoffs knutor*

ascites [əˈsaɪtiːz] *subst.* abnormal accumulation of liquid from the blood in the peritoneal cavity, occurring in dropsy *ascites, askites, vatten i bukhålan*

ascorbic acid [əˌskɔːbɪk ˈæsɪd] *subst.* vitamin C *askorbinsyra, C-vitamin*

> COMMENT: ascorbic acid is found in fresh fruit (especially oranges and lemons) and in vegetables. Lack of Vitamin C can cause anaemia and scurvy

-ase [eɪz, eɪs] *suffix* meaning an enzyme *-as*

asepsis [eɪˈsepsɪs] *subst.* state of being sterilized *or* with no infection *asepsis*

aseptic [eɪˈseptɪk] *adj.* referring to asepsis *aseptisk;* **it is important that aseptic techniques should be used in**

microbiological experiments; aseptic meningitis = relatively mild form of viral meningitis *aseptisk meningit (hjärnhinneinflammation);* **aseptic surgery** = surgery using sterilized equipment, rather than relying on killing germs with antiseptic drugs *aseptisk kirurgi; compare* ANTISEPTIC

aseptisk ⇨ **aseptic**

asexual *adj.* not involving sex *asexuell, könlös;* **asexual reproduction** = reproduction of a cell by cloning *asexuell reprodukion, könlös förökning (fortplantning)*

asexuell ⇨ **asexual**

asfyxi ⇨ **asphyxia**

Asian flu ['eɪʃ(ə)n 'flu:] *see* FLU

askaridos ⇨ **ascariasis**

askites ⇨ **ascites**

askorbinsyra ⇨ **ascorbic acid**

asleep [ə'sli:p] *adj.* sleeping *sovande;* **the patient is asleep and must not be disturbed; she fell asleep** = she began to sleep *hon somnade (in);* **fast asleep** = sleeping deeply *i djup sömn;* **the babies are all fast asleep**
NOTE: **asleep** cannot be used in front of a noun **the patient is asleep** but **a sleeping patient**

asparagine and aspartic acid [ə'spærədʒi:n ənd ə'spɑ:tɪk 'æsɪd] *subst.* two amino acids in protein *asparagin och asparaginsyra*

aspergillos ⇨ **aspergillosis**

aspergillosis [æˌspɜ:dʒɪ'ləʊsɪs] *subst.* infection of the lungs with **Aspergillus,** a type of fungus *aspergillos*

aspermi ⇨ **aspermia**

aspermia [ə'spɜ:miə] *subst.* absence of sperm in semen *aspermi*

asphyxia [æs'fɪksiə] *subst.* suffocation *or* condition where someone is prevented from breathing and therefore cannot take oxygen into the bloodstream *asfyxi, kvävning;* **asphyxia neonatorum** = failure to breathe in a newborn baby *asphyxia neonatorum*

COMMENT: asphyxia can be caused by strangulation *or* by breathing poisonous gas *or* by having the head in a plastic bag, etc.

asphyxiate [æs'fɪksieɪt] *vb.* to stop someone from breathing *kväva;* **the baby caught his head in a plastic bag and was asphyxiated; an unconscious patient may become asphyxiated if left lying on his back**

asphyxiation [æsˌfɪksi'eɪʃ(ə)n] *subst.* state of being asphyxiated *kvävning*

aspiration [ˌæspə'reɪʃ(ə)n] *subst.* removing fluid from a cavity in the body (often using a hollow needle) *aspiration, utsugning, tömning;* **aspiration pneumonia** = form of pneumonia where infected matter is inhaled from the bronchi or oesophagus *aspirationspneumoni*

aspiration ⇨ **Mendelson's syndrome; suction**

aspirationspneumoni ⇨ **aspiration**

aspirator ['æspəreɪtə] *subst.* instrument to suck fluid out of a cavity, out of the mouth in dentistry, from an operation site *sug*

aspirin ['æsprɪn] *subst.* (i) common pain-killing drug *or* acetylsalicylic acid *acetylsalicylsyra;* (ii) tablet of this drug *huvudvärkstablett;* **he took two aspirin tablets** *or* **two aspirins before going to bed**

COMMENT: aspirin can have an irritating effect on the lining of the stomach, and even causes bleeding

assimilate [ə'sɪməleɪt] *vb.* to take substances which have been absorbed into the blood from digested food, into the body's tissues *assimilera*

assimilation [əˌsɪmə'leɪʃ(ə)n] *subst.* action of assimilating food *assimilation*

assimilera ⇨ **assimilate**

assist [ə'sɪst] *vb.* to help *assistera, hjälpa, bistå;* **assisted respiration** = breathing helped by a machine *assisterad andning (ventilation)*

assistance [ə'sɪst(ə)ns] *subst.* help *hjälp, vård;* **medical assistance** = help provided by a nurse *or* by a member of the Red Cross, etc. *medicinsk vård*

assistant [ə'sɪst(ə)nt] *subst.* person who helps *assistent, medhjälpare;* **six assistants helped the consultant**

assistent ⇨ **assistant, auxiliary**

assistera ⇨ **assist**

associate [ə'səʊʃieɪt, -eɪt] *vb.* to be related to *or* to be connected with *associera, ha samband (med), vara förknippad med* *(relaterad till);* **the condition is often associated with diabetes; side-effects which may be associated with the drug**

association [əˌsəʊsiˈeɪʃ(ə)n] *subst.* **(a)** relating one thing to another in the mind *association, förknippning;* **association area** = area of the cortex of the brain which is concerned with relating stimuli coming from different sources *associationsområde, associationscentrum;* **association neurone** = neurone which links an association area to the main parts of the cortex *associationsnervcell;* **association tracts** = tracts which link areas of the cortex in the same cerebral hemisphere *associationsbanor* **(b)** group of people in the same profession *or* with the same interests *sammanslutning, förening, förbund; see also* BRITISH MEDICAL ASSOCIATION

associationscentrum ⇨ **association**

associera ⇨ **associate**

asteni ⇨ **asthenia**

astenisk ⇨ **asthenic**

astenopi ⇨ **asthenopia, eyestrain**

aster [ˈæstə] *subst.* structure shaped like a star, seen around the centrosome in cell division *aster*

asthenia [æsˈθiːniə] *subst.* being weak *or* not having any strength *asteni, kraftlöshet*

asthenic [æsˈθenɪk] *adj.* (general condition) where the patient has no strength and no interest in things *astenisk, kraftlös*

asthenopia [ˌæsθɪˈnəʊpiə] *subst.* eyestrain *astenopi, överansträngning av ögonen*

asthma [ˈæsmə] *subst.* narrowing of the bronchial tubes where the muscles go into spasm and the patient has difficulty in breathing *astma;* **cardiac asthma** = difficulty in breathing caused by heart failure *asthma cardiale, hjärtastma*

asthmatic [æsˈmætɪk] **1** *adj.* referring to asthma *astmatisk;* **he has an asthmatic attack every spring; asthmatic bronchitis** = asthma associated with bronchitis *asthma bronchiale, luftrörsastma* **2** *subst.* person suffering from asthma *astmatiker*

asthmaticus [æsˈmætɪkəs] *see* STATUS

astigmatic [ˌæstɪgˈmætɪk] *adj.* referring to astigmatism *astigmatisk;* **he is astigmatic** = he suffers from astigmatism *han är astigmatiker (lider av astigmatism)*

astigmatisk ⇨ **astigmatic**

astigmatism [əsˈtɪgməˌtɪz(ə)m] *subst.* defect in the eye, which prevents the eye from focusing correctly *astigmatism*

astigmatoskop ⇨ **keratoscope**

astma ⇨ **asthma**

astmatiker ⇨ **asthmatic**

astmatisk ⇨ **asthmatic**

astonish [əˈstɒnɪʃ] *vb.* to surprise *förvåna, överraska;* **I was astonished to hear that she had recovered**

astonishing [əˈstɒnɪʃɪŋ] *adj.* which surprises *förvånande, överraskande;* **it's astonishing how many people catch flu in the winter**

astonishment [əˈstɒnɪʃmənt] *subst.* great surprise *förvåning;* **to the doctor's great astonishment, she suddenly started to walk**

astragalus [əˈstræg(ə)ləs] *subst.* old name for talus *or* the ankle bone *astragalus, talus, språngbenet*

astringent [əˈstrɪn(d)ʒ(ə)nt] *subst. & adj.* (substance) which stops bleeding and makes the skin tissues contract and harden *adstringerande, kärlsammandragande*

astrocyt ⇨ **astrocyte**

astrocyte [ˈæstrə(ʊ)saɪt] *subst.* star-shaped brain cell *astrocyt, stjärnformad gliacell*

astrocytom ⇨ **astrocytoma**

astrocytoma [ˌæstrə(ʊ)saɪˈtəʊmə] *subst.* type of brain tumour, consisting of star-shaped cells which develop slowly in the brain and spinal cord *astrocytom*

asymmetri ⇨ **asymmetry**

asymmetry [æˈsɪmətrɪ] *subst.* state where the two sides of the body are not closely similar to each other *asymmetri*

asymptomatic [æˌsɪmptəˈmætɪk] *adj.* which does not show any symptoms of disease *asymtomatisk, symtomfri*

asymtomatisk ⇨ **asymptomatic**

asynclitism [æ'sɪnklɪtɪz(ə)m] *subst.* situation at childbirth, where the head of the baby enters the vagina at an angle *hjässbensinställning (främre el. bakre)*

asynergia [ˌæsɪ'nɜːdʒə] *or* **dyssynergia** [ˌdɪsɪ'nɜːdʒə] *subst.* awkward movements and bad coordination, caused by a disorder of the cerebellum *asynergi, dyssynergi*

asystole [ə'sɪstəli] *subst.* state where the heart has stopped beating *asystoli, hjärtstillestånd*

asystoli ⇨ **asystole**

ataktisk ⇨ **ataxic**

ataractic [ˌætə'ræktɪk] *or* **ataraxic** [ˌætə'ræksɪk] *adj.* (drug) which calms a patient *ataraktisk, lugnande*

ataraktisk ⇨ **ataractic**

ataraxi ⇨ **ataraxia**

ataraxia [ˌætə'ræksiə] *subst.* being calm *or* not worrying *ataraxi, sinneslugn, oberördhet*

atavism ['ætəvɪz(ə)m] *subst.* situation where a patient suffers from a condition which an ancestor was known to have suffered from, but not his immediate parents *atavism*

ataxia [ə'tæksiə] *subst.* lack of control of movements due to defects in the nervous system *ataxi;* **cerebellar ataxia** = disorder where the patient staggers and cannot speak clearly *ataxia cerebellaris, cerebellar ataxi;* **locomotor ataxia** = TABES DORSALIS

ataxic [ə'tæksɪk] *adj.* referring to ataxia *ataktisk, okoordinerad; see also* GAIT

atelectasis [ˌætə'lektəsɪs] *subst.* collapse of a lung, where lung fails to expand properly *atelektas*

atelektas ⇨ **atelectasis**

aterogen ⇨ **atherogenic**

aterom ⇨ **cyst, steatoma**

ateroskleros ⇨ **atherosclerosis**

aterosklerotisk ⇨ **atherosclerotic**

atetos ⇨ **athetosis**

atherogenic [ˌæθərəʊ'dʒenɪk] *adj.* which may produce atheroma *aterogen, som ger åderförkalkning*

atheroma [ˌæθə'rəʊmə] *subst.* thickening of the walls of an artery by deposits of fatty substance such as cholesterol *(fett)avlagringar i artärvägg*

atherosclerosis [ˌæθərəʊsklə'rəʊsɪs] *subst.* condition where deposits of fats and minerals form on the walls of an artery (especially the aorta, the coronary arteries and the cerebral arteries) and prevent blood from flowing easily *ateroskleros, åderförkalkning*

atherosclerotic [ˌæθərəʊsklə'rɒtɪk] *adj.* referring to atherosclerosis *aterosklerotisk, åderförkalknings-;* **atherosclerotic plaque** = deposit on the walls of an artery *aterosklerotiskt plack*

athetosis [ˌæθə'təʊsɪs] *subst.* repeated slow movements of the limbs, caused by a brain disorder such as cerebral palsy *CP, atetos*

athlete's foot [ˌæθliːts 'fʊt] = TINEA PEDIS

atlas ['ætləs] *subst.* top vertebra in the spine, which supports the skull and pivots on the axis *or* second vertebra ⇨ *illustration* VERTEBRAL COLUMN *atlas, atlaskotan*

atlaskotan ⇨ **atlas**

AT-läkare ⇨ **intern**

atmospheric pressure [ˌætməs'ferɪk 'preʃə] *subst.* normal pressure in the air *lufttryck*

> COMMENT: disorders due to atmospheric pressure include altitude sickness and caisson diseases

atomizer ['ætəmaɪzə] *or* **nebulizer** ['nebjʊlaɪzə] *subst.* instrument which sprays liquid in the form of tiny drops *nebulisator, sprej(flaska), spray(flaska)*

atoni ⇨ **atony**

atony ['æt(ə)ni] *subst.* lack of tone *or* tension in the muscles *atoni, minskad muskeltonus el. muskelspänning*

atopen ['ætəpen] *subst.* allergen which causes an atopy *allergen som orsakar atopi*

atopi ⇨ **atopy**

atopic eczema [ə'tɒpɪk ˌeksɪmə] *or* **atopic dermatitis** [ə'tɒpɪk ˌdɜːmə'taɪtɪs] *subst.* eczema caused by a hereditary allergy *atopiskt eksem, atopisk dermatit*

atopy ['ætəpi] *subst.* hereditary allergic reaction *atopi*

ATP [ˌeɪtiː'piː] = ADENOSINE TRIPHOSPHATE

ATP ⇨ **adenosine triphosphate (ATP)**

atresia [ə'triːziə] *subst.* abnormal closing *or* absence of a tube in the body *atresi*

atretic [ə'tretɪk] *adj.* referring to atresia *atretisk;* **atretic follicle** = scarred remains of an ovarian follicle *folliculus atreticus, atretisk follikel (äggstocksblåsa)*

atretisk ⇨ **atretic**

atrial ['eɪtriəl] *adj.* referring to the heart *atrial, förmaks-;* **atrial fibrillation** = rapid uncoordinated fluttering of the atria of the heart, causing an irregular heartbeat *fibrillatio atrii cordis, förmaksflimmer*

atrioventricular [ˌætriəʊven'trɪkjʊlə] *adj.* referring to the atria and ventricles *atrioventrikular(-), atrioventrikulär;* **atrioventricular bundle** *or* **AV bundle** *or* **bundle of His** = bundle of fibres which conduct impulses and which pass from the atrioventricular node to the septum and then divide to connect with the two ventricles *atrioventrikulära muskelknippet, His bunt (knippe, knut), Hisska bunten (knippet, knutan);* **atrioventricular groove** = groove round the outside of the heart, showing the division between the atria and ventricles *AV-fåra, fåra på hjärtats utsida som visar gränsen mellan förmaken och kamrarna;* **atrioventricular node** *or* **AV node** = mass of conducting tissue in the right atrium, which continues as the bundle of His and passes impulses from the atria to the ventricles *atrioventrikularknutan, atrioventrikulärknutan, AV-knutan, AV-noden*

atrioventrikular ⇨ **atrioventricular**

atrioventrikularklaffen ⇨ **tricuspid valve**

atrioventrikularknutan ⇨ **atrioventricular**

atrioventrikulär ⇨ **atrioventricular**

atrium ['eɪtriəm] *subst.* (i) one of the two upper chambers in the heart *atrium (cordis), förmak;* (ii) cavity in the ear behind the eardrum ⇨ *illustration* HEART *cavum tympani, trumhålan* NOTE: plural is **atria**

atrofi ⇨ **atrophy**

atrofiera ⇨ **atrophy**

atrophy ['ætrəfɪ] **1** *subst.* wasting of an organ *or* part of the body *atrofi, förtvining* **2** *vb. (of part of the body)* to waste away *or* to become smaller *atrofiera, förtvina*

atropine ['ætrəpiːn] *subst.* alkaloid substance derived from belladonna, a poisonous plant, used, among other things, to enlarge the pupil of the eye *atropin*

ATS [ˌeɪtiː'es] = ANTITETANUS SERUM

attach [ə'tætʃ] *vb.* to fix *or* to fasten *fästa, häfta vid;* **the stomach is attached to the other organs by the greater and lesser omenta**

attachment [ə'tætʃmənt] *subst.* (i) something which is attached *tillsats, bihang;* (ii) arrangement where a home nurse is attached to a particular general practice *slags arrangemang med sjuksköterska som ger vård i hemmet*

attack [ə'tæk] *subst.* sudden illness *anfall, attack;* **he had an attack of fever; she had two attacks of laryngitis during the winter; heart attack** = state where the heart suffers from defective blood supply because one of the arteries becomes blocked by a blood clot (coronary thrombosis) *hjärtattack*

attack ⇨ **attack, fit, seizure, spell, turn**

attempt [ə'tem(p)t] **1** *subst.* try *försök;* **they made an attempt to treat the disease with antibiotics 2** *vb.* to try *försöka;* **the surgeons attempted to sew the finger back on**

attend [ə'tend] *vb.* **(a)** to be present at *närvara, delta;* **will you attend the meeting tomorrow? seventeen patients are attending the antenatal clinic (b)** to look after (a patient) *vårda, sköta, behandla;* **he was attended by two doctors; attending physician** = doctor who is looking after a certain patient *behandlande läkare;* **he was referred to the hypertension unit by his attending physician**

attend to [ə'tend tʊ] *vb.* to deal with *vårda, sköta, behandla;* **the doctor is attending to his patients**

attention [ə'tenʃ(ə)n] *subst.* care in looking after a patient *omsorg, vård;* **he has had the best medical attention; she needs urgent medical attention**

attest ⇨ **certificate**

attract [ə'trækt] *vb.* to make something come nearer *attrahera, dra till sig;* **the solid attracts the gas to its surface; the patient is sexually attracted to both males and females**

attraction [ə'trækʃ(ə)n] *subst.* act of attracting *attraktion, dragning(skraft);* **sexual attraction** = feeling of wanting to have sexual intercourse with someone *sexuell attraktion (dragningskraft)*

attrahera ⇨ **attract**

attraktion ⇨ **attraction**

Au *chemical symbol for* gold *Au, guld*

audi- [ˌɔ:də, ˌɔ:di] *prefix* referring to hearing *or* sound *audi(o)-, hör(sel)-*

audible ['ɔ:dəb(ə)l] *adj.* which can be heard *hörbar;* **audible limits** = upper and lower limits of sound frequencies which can be heard by humans *gränser för hörbara ljudfrekvenser*

audiogram ['ɔ:diəʊgræm] *subst.* graph drawn by an audiometer *audiogram*

audiometer [ˌɔ:di'ɒmɪtə] *subst.* apparatus for testing hearing *audiometer, hörselmätare*

audiometry [ˌɔ:di'ɒmətri] *subst.* science of testing hearing *audiometri*

audit ['ɔ:dɪt] *subst.* (i) analysis of the accounts of a hospital *or* doctor's practice, to see if they are correct *revision, räkenskapsgranskning;* (ii) analysis of statistics relating to a doctor's practice (as numbers of patients *or* incidence of disease *or* numbers of patients referred to specialists, etc.) for research purposes *analys av patientstatistik etc.*

auditiv ⇨ **auditory**

auditory ['ɔ:dɪt(ə)ri] *adj.* referring to hearing *auditiv, hörsel-;* **external auditory canal** *or* **meatus** = tube leading from the outer ear to the eardrum *meatus acusticus externus, yttre hörselgången;* **internal auditory meatus** = channel which takes the auditory nerve through the temporal bone *meatus acusticus internus, inre hörselgången;* **auditory nerve** *or* **vestibulocochlear nerve** = eighth cranial nerve which governs hearing and balance ⇨ *illustration* EAR *nervus vestibulo-cochlearis, hörsel- och balansnerven, 8:e kranialnerven*

Auerbach's plexus ['auərbɑ:ks ˌpleksəs] *subst.* group of nerve fibres in the intestine wall *plexus myentericus, Auerbachs plexus*

aura ['ɔ:rə] *subst.* warning sensation of varying kinds which is experienced before an attack of epilepsy *or* migraine *or* asthma *aura (epileptica), föraning, förebud*

aural ['ɔ:r(ə)l] *adj.* (i) referring to the ear *aurikular, aurikulär, öron-;* (ii) like an aura *auraliknande;* **aural polyp** = polyp in the middle ear *polyp i mellanörat;* **aural surgery** = surgery on the ear *öronkirurgi*

auraliknande ⇨ **aural**

auricle ['ɔ:rɪk(ə)l] *subst.* tip of each atrium in the heart *auricula (cordis, atrii), hjärtörat*

auriculae [ɔ:'rɪkjʊli:] *subst. pl. see* CONCHA

auricular [ɔ:'rɪkjʊlə] *adj.* (i) referring to the ear *aurikular, aurikulär, öron-;* (ii) referring to an auricle *som avser el. hör till öronmussla;* **auricular veins** = veins which lead into the posterior facial vein *venae auriculares*

aurikular ⇨ **aural, auricular**

aurikulär ⇨ **aural, auricular**

auriscope ['ɔ:rəskəʊp] *or* **otoscope** ['əʊtəskəʊp] *subst.* instrument for examining the ear and eardrum *auriskop, otoskop*

auriskop ⇨ **auriscope**

auscultation [ˌɔ:sk(ə)l'teɪʃ(ə)n] *subst.* listening to the sounds of the body using a stethoscope *auskultation*

auscultatory [ɔ:'skʌltət(ə)rɪ] *adj.* referring to auscultation *som avser el. hör till auskultation*

auskultation ⇨ **auscultation**

australiensiskt lyft ⇨ **shoulder**

authority [ɔ:'θɒrəti] *subst.* **(a)** power to act *makt;* **to abuse one's authority** = to use powers in an illegal *or* harmful way *missbruka sin makt, utöva maktmissbruk* **(b)** official body which controls an area *myndighet, styrelse; see also* DISTRICT, REGIONAL

autism ['ɔ:tɪz(ə)m] *subst.* condition of children and adolescents, where the patient is completely absorbed in himself, pays no attention to others and does not communicate with anyone *autism*

autistic [ɔːˈtɪstɪk] *adj.* referring to autism *autistisk;* **autistic child** = child suffering from autism *autistiskt barn*

autistisk ⇨ **autistic**

auto- [ˈɔːtəʊ, ˌ--] *prefix* meaning oneself *auto-, egen-, själv-*

autoallergisk ⇨ **autoimmune**

autoanalyser ⇨ **analyser**

autoantibody [ˌɔːtəʊˈæntɪˌbɒdi] *subst.* antibody formed to attack the body's own cells *autoantikropp*

autoantikropp ⇨ **autoantibody**

autoclave [ˈɔːtəʊkleɪv] **1** *subst.* equipment for sterilizing surgical instruments using heat under high pressure *autoklav* **2** *vb.* to sterilize using heat under high pressure *autoklavera;* **autoclaving is the best method of sterilization; waste should be put into autoclavable plastic bags**

autodigestion ⇨ **autolysis**

autograft [ˈɔːtəgrɑːft] *subst.* graft *or* transplant made using parts of the patient's own body *autotransplantat, autogent (autologt) transplantat*

autoimmune [ˌɔːtəʊɪˈmjuːn] *adj.* referring to an immune reaction in a person to antigens in his own tissue *autoimmun, autoallergisk;* **autoimmune disease** = disease where the patient's own cells are attacked by autoantibodies *autoimmun sjukdom;* **rheumatoid arthritis is thought to be an autoimmune disease**

autoimmunity [ˌɔːtəʊɪˈmjuːnəti] *subst.* state where an organism produces autoantibodies to attack its own cells *autoimmunitet*

autoinfection [ˌɔːtəʊɪnˈfekʃ(ə)n] *subst.* infection by a germ already in the body *reaktivering (av infektion);* infection of one part of the body by another *autoinfektion, självinfektion*

autoinfektion ⇨ **autoinfection**

autointoxication [ˌɔːtəʊɪnˌtɒksɪˈkeɪʃ(ə)n] *subst.* poisoning of the body by toxins produced in the body itself *autointoxikation, autotoxikos*

autointoxikation ⇨ **autointoxication**

autoklav ⇨ **autoclave**

autolys ⇨ **autolysis**

autolysis [ɔːˈtɒlɪsɪs] *subst.* action of destroying cells by their own enzymes *autolys, autodigestion*

automatic [ˌɔːtəˈmætɪk] *adj.* which works by itself, with no one making it work *automatisk*

automatically [ˌɔːtəˈmætɪk(ə)li] *adv.* working without a person giving instructions *automatiskt;* **the heart beats automatically**

automatisk ⇨ **automatic**

automatiskt ⇨ **automatically**

automatism [ɔːˈtɒmətɪz(ə)m] *subst.* state where a person acts without consciously knowing that he is acting *automati(sm)*

> COMMENT: automatic acts can take place after concussion or epileptic fits. In law, automatism can be a defence to a criminal charge when the accused states that he acted without knowing what he was doing

autonom ⇨ **autonomic**

autonomi ⇨ **autonomy**

autonomic [ˌɔːtəˈnɒmɪk] *adj.* which governs itself independently *autonom, självständig, självstyrande;* **autonomic nervous system** = nervous system formed of ganglia linked to the spinal column, which regulates the automatic functioning of the main organs of the body, such as the heart and lungs, and which works when a person is asleep or even unconscious *autonoma nervsystemet; see also* PARASYMPATHETIC SYSTEM, SYMPATHETIC SYSTEM

autonom reflex ⇨ **reflex**

autonomy [ɔːˈtɒnəmi] *subst.* being free to act as one wishes *autonomi, självständighet*

autopsy [ˈɔːtɒpsi] *or* **post mortem** [ˌpəʊst ˈmɔːtəm] *subst.* examination of a dead body by a pathologist, to find out the cause of death *obduktion*

autosome [ˈɔːtəʊˌsəʊm] *subst.* one of a pair of similar chromosomes *autosom*

autotoxikos ⇨ **autointoxication**

autotransfusion [ˌɔːtəʊtrænsˈfjuːʒ(ə)n] *subst.* infusion into a patient of his own blood *autotransfusion*

autotransplantat ⇨ **autograft**

auxiliary [ɔːgˈzɪliəri] **1** *adj.* which helps *hjälp-, reserv-;* **the hospital has an auxiliary power supply in case the electricity supply breaks down 2** *subst.* assistant *assistent, medhjälpare;* **nursing auxiliary** = helper who does general work in a hospital *or* clinic *ung. sjukvårdsbiträde*

available [əˈveɪləb(ə)l] *adj.* which can be got *tillgänglig, till buds (stående), till hands;* **the drug is available only on prescription; all available ambulances were rushed to the scene of the accident**

avancerad ⇨ **advanced**

avascular [əˈvæskjʊlə] *adj.* with no blood vessels *or* with a deficient blood supply *avaskulär;* **avascular necrosis** = condition where tissue cells die because their supply of blood has been cut *avaskulär nekros*

avaskulär ⇨ **avascular**

avbrott ⇨ **stoppage**

avbrutet samlag ⇨ **coitus**

avbryta ⇨ **discontinue**

AV bundle [ˌeɪˈviːˌbʌnd(ə)l] *or* **AV node** [ˌeɪˈviːˌnəʊd] = ATRIOVENTRICULAR

avdelning ⇨ **unit, ward**

avdelningsföreståndare ⇨ **sister**

avdelningsläkare ⇨ **registrar**

avdunsta ⇨ **vaporize**

avdunstning ⇨ **evaporation**

aversion ⇨ **aversion to, dislike**

aversionsterapi ⇨ **therapy**

aversion to [əˈvɜːʃ(ə)n tʊ] *subst.* great dislike of something *aversion, motvilja, avsmak;* **aversion therapy** = treatment where the patient is cured of a type of behaviour by making him develop a great dislike for it *aversionsterapi*

avfallsprodukt ⇨ **detritus, waste**

AV-fåra ⇨ **atrioventricular**

avfärgning ⇨ **counterstain**

avförande ⇨ **aperient, cathartic, efferent, laxative, purgative**

avföring ⇨ **defaecation, excrement, excretion, faecal, faeces, motion, passage**

avföringsinkontinens ⇨ **encopresis, incontinence**

avföringsmedel ⇨ **evacuant, laxative, purgative**

avgiftning ⇨ **detoxication**

avgångsbetyg ⇨ **diploma**

avgöra ⇨ **determine**

avhållsamhet ⇨ **abstinence**

A-vitamin ⇨ **retinol, Vitamin A**

avitaminosis [æˌvɪtəmɪnˈəʊsɪs] *subst.* disorder caused by lack of vitamins *avitaminos*

avkok ⇨ **infusion**

avkoppling ⇨ **relaxation**

avkylning ⇨ **refrigeration**

avlagring ⇨ **accretion, deposit, sediment, sedimentation**

avledande ⇨ **deferent**

avledning, unipolär ⇨ **unipolar**

avlida ⇨ **die**

avlossning ⇨ **separation**

avlägsna ⇨ **remove**

avlägsna (kirurgiskt) ⇨ **resect**

avlägsnande ⇨ **ablation, removal**

avläsning ⇨ **reading**

avmagrad ⇨ **emaciated**

avmagring ⇨ **emaciation, wasting**

avnötning ⇨ **detrition**

avoid [əˈvɔɪd] *vb.* to try not to do something; to try not to hit something *undvika, avhålla sig från;* **you must try to avoid over exerting yourself; the patient on a diet should avoid alcohol**

avpassa ⇨ **fit**

avreagering ⇨ **abreaction**

avråda från ⇨ **advise against**

avsaknad ⇨ **absence**

avsikt ⇨ **intention**

avskilja ⇨ **detach, sever**

avskiljande av vätska ⇨ **syneresis**

avslag ⇨ **lochia**

avslappande ⇨ **relaxant**

avslappning ⇨ **relaxation**

avslappningsterapi ⇨ **relaxation**

avslutas ⇨ **end**

avslutning ⇨ **ending, termination**

avslöja ⇨ **expose, reveal**

avsmak ⇨ **aversion to**

avsmakning ⇨ **gustation**

avsnitt ⇨ **section**

avstå ⇨ **abstain, give up**

avstöta ⇨ **shed; reject**

avstötning ⇨ **rejection**

avsvällande medel ⇨ **decongestant**

avsätta ⇨ **deposit**

avsöndra ⇨ **discharge, eliminate, excrete, secrete**

avsöndring ⇨ **discharge, elimination, excretion, secretion**

avsöndring, tunn ⇨ **gleet**

avta ⇨ **fall off, subside, wear off**

avtala ⇨ **arrange**

avtrubbning ⇨ **hebetude, obtusion**

avtryck ⇨ **die, impression**

avulsion [ə'vʌlʃ(ə)n] *subst.* pulling away tissue by force *avulsio, bortslitande;* **nail avulsion** = pulling away an ingrowing toenail *evulsio;* **phrenic avulsion** = surgical removal of part of the phrenic nerve in order to paralyse the diaphragm *avulsio*

avvara ⇨ **spare**

avvikande ⇨ **aberrant, abnormal**

avvikelse ⇨ **aberration, abnormality, deviation**

avvisa ⇨ **turn away**

avvänja ⇨ **wean**

awake [ə'weɪk] **1** *vb.* **(a)** to wake somebody up *väcka (upp);* **he was awoken by pains in his chest (b)** to wake up *vakna (upp);* **after the accident he awoke to find himself in hospital** NOTE: **awakes - awaking - awoke - has awoken 2** *adj.* not asleep *vaken;* **he was still awake at 2 o'clock in the morning; the patients were kept awake by shouts in the next ward; the baby is wide awake** = very awake *barnet är klarvaket* NOTE: **awake** cannot be used in front of a noun

awaken [ə'weɪk(ə)n] *vb.* to wake someone *väcka (upp);* to stimulate someone's senses *väcka*

awareness [ə'weənəs] *subst.* being aware (especially of a problem) *medvetenhet*

> QUOTE doctors should use the increased public awareness of whooping cough during epidemics to encourage parents to vaccinate children
> **Health Visitor**

aware of [ə'weər əv] *adj.* knowing *or* conscious enough to know what is happening *medveten om, uppmärksam på;* **she is not aware of what is happening around her; the surgeon became aware of a problem with the heart-lung machine**

awkward ['ɔːkwəd] *adj.* difficult to reach *or* find *or* to deal with *besvärlig, obekväm;* **the tumour is in a very awkward position for surgery**

awkwardly ['ɔːkwədli] *adv.* in a difficult way *besvärligt, obekvämt;* **the tumour is awkwardly placed and not easy to reach**

axel ⇨ **axis, shoulder**

axel- ⇨ **axial**

axelhålan ⇨ **armpit, axilla**

axelleden ⇨ **glenohumeral, shoulder**

axial ['æksiəl] *adj.* referring to an axis *axial, axiell, axel-;* **axial skeleton** = main part of the skeleton, formed of the skull, backbone and ribs *de delar av skelettet som består av skallen, ryggraden och revbenen; compare* APPENDICULAR SKELETON; **computerized axial tomography** (CAT) = X-ray examination using a computer to build up a picture of a section of the body *datortomografi, DT, skiktröntgen*

axiell ⇨ **axial**

axilla [æk'sɪlə] *subst.* armpit *or* hollow under the shoulder between the upper arm and the body, where the arm joins the shoulder *axilla, armhålan, axelhålan* NOTE: plural is **axillae**

COMMENT: the armpit contains several important blood vessels, lymph nodes and sweat glands

axillar ⇨ **axillary**

axillarknutorna ⇨ **axillary**

axillary [æk'sɪləri] *adj.* referring to the armpit *axillar, axillär, armhåle-;* **axillary artery** = artery which branches from the subclavian artery in the armpit *arteria axillaris, stora armhåleartären;* **axillary nodes** = part of the lymphatic system in the arm *axillarknutorna*

axillär ⇨ **axillary**

axis ['æksɪs] *subst.* **(a)** imaginary line through the centre of the body *axel* **(b)** central vessel, which divides into other vessels *centralt blodkärl som delar upp sig i andra kärl* **(c)** second vertebra, on which the atlas sits ⇨ *illustration* VERTEBRAL COLUMN *axis, andra cervikalkotan (halskotan)*
NOTE: plural is **axes**

axodendrite [ˌæksəʊ'dendraɪt] *subst.* appendage like a fibril on the axon of a nerve *utskott på nervaxon*

axon ['æksɒn] *subst.* nerve fibre which sends impulses from one neurone to another, linking with the dendrites of the other neurone *axon;* **axon covering** = myelin sheath which covers a nerve *myelinskida;* **postsynaptic axon** *or* **presynaptic axon** = nerves on either side of a synapse ⇨ *illustration* NEURONE *postsynaptiskt (presynaptiskt) axon*

azoospermia [eɪˌzəʊə'spɜːmiə] *subst.* absence of sperm *azoospermi*

azotaemia [ˌæzəʊ'tiːmiə] *subst.* presence of urea or other nitrogen compounds in the blood *azotemi, uremi*

azotemi ⇨ **azotaemia**

azoturia [ˌæzəʊ'tjʊəriə] *subst.* presence of urea or other nitrogen compounds in the urine, caused by kidney disease *azoturi*

azygos ['æzɪgəs] *adj.* single *or* not one of a pair *oparig;* **azygos vein** = vein which brings blood back into the vena cava from the abdomen *vena azygos, opariga venen*

Bb

Vitamin B [ˌvɪtəmɪn 'biː] *subst.* **Vitamin B complex** = group of vitamins which are soluble in water, including folic acid, pyridoxine, riboflavine and many others *B-vitamin;* **Vitamin B_1** *or* **thiamine** = vitamin found in yeast, liver, cereals and pork *vitamin B_1, tiamin, aneurin;* **Vitamin B_2** *or* **riboflavine** = vitamin found in eggs, liver, green vegetables, milk and yeast *vitamin B_2, riboflavin;* **Vitamin B_6** *or* **pyridoxine** = vitamin found in meat, cereals and molasses *vitamin B_6, adermin, pyridoxin;* **Vitamin B_{12}** *or* **cyanocobalamin** = vitamin found in liver and kidney, but not present in vegetables *vitamin B_{12}, cykobemin, kobalamin, cyanokobalamin, extrinsic factor*

COMMENT: lack of vitamins from the B complex can have different results: lack of thiamine causes beriberi; lack of riboflavine affects a child's growth, and can cause anaemia and inflammation of the tongue and mouth; lack of pyridoxine causes convulsions and vomiting in babies; lack of vitamin B_{12} causes anaemia

Ba *chemical symbol for* barium *Ba, barium*

Babinski reflex [bə'bɪnskɪ ˌriːfleks] *or* **Babinski test** [bə'bɪnskɪ ˌtest] *subst.* abnormal response of the toes to running a finger lightly across the sole of the foot *Babinskis reflex (fenomen), plantarreflex; see* PLANTAR REFLEX

COMMENT: the normal response is for all the toes to turn down, but in the case of the Babinski reflex, the big toe turns up, while the others turn down and spread out, a sign of hemiplegia and pyramidal tract disease

baby ['beɪbi] *subst.* very young child *baby, spädbarn;* **babies start to walk when they are about 12 months old; baby care** = looking after babies *spädbarnsvård;* **baby clinic** =

special clinic which deals with babies *spädbarnsklinik*
NOTE: if you do not know the sex of a baby you can refer to it as **it: "the baby was sucking its thumb"**

bacill ▷ **bacillus**

bacillaemia [ˌbæsɪ'liːmiə] *subst.* infection of the blood by bacilli *bakteriemi*

bacillary [bə'sɪləri] *adj.* referring to bacillus *bacillär;* **bacillary dysentery =** dysentery caused by the bacillus **Shigella** in contaminated food *bacillär dysenteri*

bacille Calmette-Guérin (BCG) [ba'sɪl kalˌmet ge'rʃ) (ˌbiːsiː'dʒiː)] *subst.* vaccine which immunizes against tuberculosis *Calmette-Guérins bacill, BCG*

bacilluria [ˌbæsɪ'ljʊəriə] *subst.* presence of bacilli in the urine *bakteriuri*

bacillus [bə'sɪləs] *subst.* bacterium shaped like a rod *bacill* NOTE: plural is **bacilli**

bacillär ▷ **bacillary**

back [bæk] *subst.* **(a)** dorsum *or* part of the body from the neck downwards to the waist, which is made of the spine, and the bones attached to it *dorsum, ryggen;* **he complained of a pain in the back; he hurt his back lifting the piece of wood; she strained her back working in the garden; back muscles =** strong muscles in the back which help hold the body upright *ryggmusklerna;* **back pain =** pain in the back *ryggvärk, smärtor (ont) i ryggen (jfr lumbago);* **back strain =** condition where the muscles *or* ligaments in the back have been strained *sträckning i ryggen* **(b)** other side to the front *baksida;* **she has a swelling on the back of her hand; the calf muscles are at the back of the lower leg**

backache ['bækeɪk] *subst.* pain in the back *ryggvärk, smärtor (ont) i ryggen*

> COMMENT: backache can result from bad posture or a soft bed, or by straining a muscle, but it can also be caused by rheumatism (lumbago), fevers such as typhoid fever, and osteoarthritis. Pains in the back can also be referred pains, from gallstones or kidney disease

backbone ['bækbəʊn] *or* **rachis** ['reɪkɪs] *subst.* spine *or* series of bones (the vertebrae) linked together to form a flexible column running from the pelvis to the skull *columna vertebralis, ryggraden; see also* SPINE, SPINAL COLUMN, VERTEBRAL COLUMN

NOTE: for other terms referring to the back, see words beginning with **dors-**

baclofen ['bækləʊfen] *subst.* drug which is a muscle relaxant *slags muskelavslappande medel*

bacteraemia [ˌbæktə'riːmiə] *subst.* blood poisoning *or* having bacteria in the blood *bakteriemi, blodförgiftning*

bacteria [bæk'tɪəriə] *subst pl.* tiny organisms, some of which are permanently present in the gut and can break down tissue; many of them can cause disease *bakterier*
NOTE: the singular is **bacterium**

> COMMENT: bacteria can be shaped like rods (bacilli), like balls (cocci) or have a spiral form (such as spirochaetes). Bacteria, especially bacilli and spirochaetes, can move and reproduce very rapidly

bacterial [bæk'tɪəriəl] *adj.* referring to bacteria *or* caused by bacteria *bakteriell;* **children with sickle-cell anaemia are susceptible to bacterial infection; (subacute) bacterial endocarditis =** infection of the endocardium (the membrane covering the inner surfaces of the heart) by bacteria *(subakut) bakteriell endokardit*

bactericidal [bækˌtɪərɪ'saɪd(ə)l] *adj.* which kills bacteria *bakteri(o)cid, bakteriedödande*

bactericide [bæk'tɪərɪsaɪd] *subst.* substance which kills bacteria *bakteri(o)cid, bakteriedödande ämne*

bacteriological [bækˌtɪəriə'lɒdʒɪk(ə)l] *adj.* referring to bacteriology *bakteriologisk*

bacteriologist [bækˌtɪəri'ɒlədʒɪst] *subst.* doctor who specializes in the study of bacteria *bakteriolog*

bacteriology [bækˌtɪəri'ɒlədʒɪ] *subst.* study of bacteria *bakteriologi*

bacteriolysin [bækˌtɪəri'ɒlɪsiːn] *subst.* protein, usually an immunoglobulin, which destroys bacterial cells *bakteriolysin*

bacteriolysis [bækˌtɪəri'ɒlɪsɪs] *subst.* destruction of bacterial cells *bakteriolys*

bacteriophage [bæk'tɪəriə(ʊ)feɪdʒ] *subst.* virus which infects bacteria *bakteriofag*

bacteriostasis [bækˌtɪəriəʊ'steɪsɪs] *subst.* action of stopping bacteria from multiplying *bakteriostas*

bacteriostatic [bæk,tɪəriəʊ'stætɪk] *adj.* (substance) which does not kill bacteria but stops them from multiplying *bakteriostatisk*

bacterium [bæk'tɪəriəm] *subst. see* BACTERIA

bacteriuria [bæk,tɪəri'jʊəriə] *subst.* having bacteria in the urine *bakteriuri*

bad [bæd] *adj.* **(a)** not good *or* not well *dålig, sjuk;* **he has a bad leg and can't walk fast; eating too much fat is bad for you** = it will make you ill *det är inte bra att äta alltför mycket fett;* **bad breath** = halitosis *or* condition where a person's breath has an unpleasant smell *halitosis, dålig andedräkt;* **bad tooth** = tooth which has caries *dålig (kariesangripen) tand* **(b)** unpleasant *or* quite serious *allvarlig, svår;* **she has got a bad cold; he had a bad attack of bronchitis**
NOTE: **bad - worse - worst**

bad ⇨ **bath**

bada ⇨ **bath**

badda ⇨ **bathe, dab**

badkar ⇨ **bath**

bag [bæg] *subst.* something made of paper *or* cloth *or* tissue which can contain things *påse, säck, blåsa;* **a bag of potatoes; he put the apples in a paper bag; colostomy bag** *or* **ileostomy bag** = bags attached to the openings made by a colostomy *or* ileostomy to collect faeces as they are passed out of the body *kolostomipåse, ileostomipåse;* **sleeping bag** = comfortable warm bag for sleeping in *sovsäck;* **bag of waters** = part of the amnion which covers an unborn baby in the womb and contains the amniotic fluid *amnionsäcken*

bagareksem ⇨ **baker's itch**

Baghdad boil ['bægdæd ,bɔɪl] *or* **Baghdad sore** ['bægdæd ,sɔː] *or* **Leishmaniasis** [,liːʃmə'naɪəsɪs] *or* **oriental sore** [,ɔːri'ent(ə)l ,sɔː] *subst.* skin disease of tropical countries caused by the parasite Leishmania *leishmaniasis cutanae, orientböld, aleppoböld*

Baker's cyst ['beɪkəz ,sɪst] *subst.* swelling filled with synovial fluid, at the back of the knee, caused by weakness of the joint membrane *Bakercysta*

baker's itch ['beɪkəz ,ɪtʃ] *or* **baker's dermatitis** [,beɪkəz ,dɜːmə'taɪtɪs] *subst.* irritation of the skin caused by handling yeast *bagareksem*

bakgrund ⇨ **history**

bakhjärnan ⇨ **hindbrain, rhombencephalon**

bakhuvudet ⇨ **occiput**

bakre ⇨ **post-, posterior**

bakre gombågen ⇨ **palatopharyngeal arch**

baksida ⇨ **back**

baksmälla ⇨ **hangover**

baktarmen ⇨ **hindgut**

bakterie ⇨ **bacteria, germ**

bakterie- ⇨ **germinal**

bakteriedödande ⇨ **bactericidal**

bakteriedödande medel ⇨ **antiseptic**

bakterieflora ⇨ **flora**

bakteriell ⇨ **bacterial, infective**

bakteriell lunginflammation ⇨ **pneumonia**

bakteriemi ⇨ **bacillaemia, bacteraemia**

bakteriespektrum ⇨ **spectrum**

bakteriestam, resistent ⇨ **resistant**

bakteriofag ⇨ **bacteriophage**

bakteriologi ⇨ **bacteriology**

bakteriologisk ⇨ **bacteriological**

bakteriolys ⇨ **bacteriolysis**

bakteriuri ⇨ **bacilluria, bacteriuria**

bakåtböjning ⇨ **retroflexion**

bakåtgående ⇨ **retrograde**

bakåtlutad livmoder ⇨ **tipped womb**

bakåtlutning ⇨ **retroversion**

bakåtvridning ⇨ **retroversion**

BAL [,biːeɪ'el] = BRITISH ANTI-LEWISITE

balance ['bæləns] **1** *subst.* **(a)** device for weighing, made with springs or weights *våg;* **he weighed the powder in a spring balance** **(b)** staying upright *or* not falling *balans;* **sense of balance** = feeling that keeps someone upright, governed by the fluid in the inner ear balance mechanism *balanssinnet;* **he stood on top of the fence and kept his balance** = he did not fall off *han stod uppe på staketet och höll balansen* **(c) balance of mind** = good mental state *mental jämvikt (balans), sinneslugn;* **disturbed balance of mind** = state of mind when someone is for a time incapable of reasoned action (because of illness *or* depression) *störd mental jämvikt (balans)* **2** *vb.* to stand on something narrow without falling *balansera;* **he was balancing on top of the fence; how long can you balance on one foot?**

balanitis [ˌbælə'naɪtɪs] *subst.* inflammation of the glans of the penis *balanit*

balanoposthitis [ˌbælənəupɒs'θaɪtɪs] *subst.* inflammation of the foreskin and the end of the penis *balanopostit*

balans ⇨ **balance, equilibrium**

balanserad kost (diet) ⇨ **diet**

balanssinnet ⇨ **balance**

balantidiasis [ˌbæləntɪ'daɪəsɪs] *subst.* infestation of the large intestine by a parasite **Balantidium coli,** which causes ulceration of the wall of the intestine, giving diarrhoea and finally dysentery *balantidiasis*

balanus ['bælənəs] *subst.* glans *or* the round end of the penis *glans (penis), ollonet*

bald [bɔːld] *adj.* with no hair *or* (man) who has lost his hair *skallig, flintskallig;* **he is going bald** *or* **he is becoming bald** = he is beginning to lose his hair *han börjar bli flintskallig;* **he went bald when he was still young; after the operation she became quite bald**

balding ['bɔːldɪŋ] *adj.* (man) who is going bald *som börjar bli flintskallig*

baldness ['bɔːldnəs] *or* **alopecia** [ˌælə'piːʃiə] *subst.* state of not having any hair *alopeci, håravfall, skallighet*

baljfrukter ⇨ **pulse**

Balkan frame [ˌbɔːlk(ə)n 'freɪm] *or* **Balkan beam** [ˌbɔːlk(ə)n 'biːm] *subst.* frame fitted above a bed to which a leg in plaster can be attached *slags ställning för upphängning av gipsat ben*

ball [bɔːl] *subst.* (i) round object *boll;* (ii) soft part of the hand below the thumb *or* soft part of the foot below the big toe *thenar, tumvalken, tåvalken*

ball and socket joint [ˌbɔːl ənd 'sɒkɪt ˌdʒɔɪnt] *subst.* joint where the round end of a long bone is attached to a cup-shaped hollow in another bone in such a way that the long bone can move in almost any direction *articulatio sphaeroidea (cotylica), enartros, kulled*

ballong ⇨ **balloon**

balloon [bə'luːn] *subst.* bag of light material inflated with air or a gas (used to unblock arteries) *ballong; see also* ANGIOPLASTY

ballottement [bə'lɒtmənt] *subst.* method of examining the body by tapping or moving a part, especially during pregnancy *balott(e)mang*

balneoterapi ⇨ **balneotherapy**

balneotherapy [ˌbælniəu'θerəpi] *subst.* treatment of diseases by bathing in hot water *or* water containing certain chemicals *balneoterapi*

balsam ['bɔːls(ə)m] *subst.* mixture of resin and oil, used to rub on sore joints or to put in hot water and use as an inhalant *balsam; see also* FRIARS' BALSAM

balsamera ⇨ **embalm**

ban [bæn] *vb.* to forbid *or* to say that something should not be done *förbjuda;* **alcohol has been banned by his doctor** *or* **he has been banned alcohol by his doctor; smoking is banned in most restaurants**

bana ⇨ **pathway, tract**

band [bænd] *subst.* thin piece of material for tying things together *band, snöre;* **the papers were held together with a rubber band**

band ⇨ **cord, vinculum; tape**

bandage ['bændɪdʒ] **1** *subst.* piece of cloth which is wrapped around a wound *bandage, förband, binda;* **his head was covered with bandages; put a bandage round your knee; elastic bandage** = stretch bandage used to support a weak joint, or for treatment of a varicose vein *elastiskt förband;* **rolled** *or* **roller bandage** = bandage which is a long strip of cloth, which can be kept rolled up when not in use *gasbinda;* **spiral bandage** = bandage which is wrapped round a limb, each turn overlapping the one before *förband med överlappande turer;* **T bandage** = bandage shaped like the letter T, used for bandaging the area between the legs *T-binda, T-format förband;* **triangular bandage** = bandage made of a triangle of cloth, used to make a sling for an arm *mitella;* **tubular bandage** = bandage made of a tube of elastic cloth *(förband av) tubgas (tubigrip); see also* ESMARCH'S **2** *vb.* to wrap a piece of cloth around a wound *bandagera, förbinda, sätta på förband;* **she bandaged his leg; his arm is bandaged up**

bandagera ➪ **bandage**

Bandl's ring [ˌbændlz 'rɪŋ] = RETRACTION RING

bandmask ➪ **cestode, taenia, tapeworm**

bank [bæŋk] *subst.* place where blood *or* organs from donors can be stored until needed *bank; see also* BLOOD BANK, EYE BANK, SPERM BANK

banka ➪ **throb**

Bankhart's operation ['bæŋkhɑ:ts ˌɒpə'reɪʃ(ə)n] *subst.* operation to repair a recurrent dislocation of the shoulder *Bankarts operation*

banta ➪ **diet, slim**

Banti's syndrome ['bæntɪz ˌsɪndrəʊm] *or* **disease** [dɪ'zi:z] *or* **splenic anaemia** [ˌsplenɪk ə'ni:miə] *subst.* type of anaemia where the patient has an enlarged spleen, haemorrhages, portal hypertension and cirrhosis of the liver *hepatolienal fibros, Bantis sjukdom (syndrom)*

bantning ➪ **dieting**

bantningsdiet ➪ **slim**

bar ➪ **bare**

Barbados leg [bɑ:'beɪdɒs ˌleg] *subst.* form of elephantiasis *or* large swelling due to a Filaria worm *slags elefantiasis*

barber's itch ['bɑ:bəz ˌɪtʃ] *or* **barber's rash** ['bɑ:bəz ˌræʃ] = SYCOSIS

barbitalism ➪ **barbiturism**

barbitone ['bɑ:bitəʊn] *subst.* type of barbiturate *slags barbiturat*

barbiturate [bɑ:'bɪtʃʊrət] *subst.* sleeping pill *or* drug which is used to make people sleep, and which may become addictive if taken frequently *barbiturat;* **barbiturate abuse** = repeated addictive use of barbiturates which in the end affects the brain *barbituratmissbruk;* **barbiturate dependence** = being dependent on regularly taking barbiturate tablets *barbituratberoende;* **barbiturate poisoning** = poisoning caused by an overdose of barbiturates *barbituratförgiftning*

barbituratförgiftning ➪ **barbiturate**

barbituratmissbruk ➪ **barbiturate**

barbiturism [bɑ:'bɪtʃʊrɪz(ə)m] *subst.* addiction to barbiturates *barbiturism, barbitalism*

barbotage [ˌbɑ:bə'tɑ:ʒ] *subst.* method of spinal analgesia, where cerebrospinal fluid is injected into the spinal cord and then removed, used as a treatment for cancer *slags spinalbedövning*

bare [beə] *adj.* **(a)** not covered by clothes *bar, naken;* **the children had bare feet; her dress left her arms bare (b) bare area of the liver** = large triangular part of the liver not covered with peritoneum *den del av levern som inte är täckt av bukhinnan*

barium ['beəriəm] *subst.* chemical element used as a contrast in X-ray examinations *barium;* **barium enema** = enema made of barium sulphate which is put into the rectum so that an X-ray can be taken of the lower intestine *kolonröntgen;* **barium meal** *or* **barium solution** = liquid solution containing barium sulphate which a patient drinks so that an X-ray can be taken of his alimentary tract *bariumgröt, bariumsulfat; see also* SULPHATE NOTE: chemical symbol is **Ba**

bariumgröt ➪ **barium**

bariumsulfat ➪ **barium**

bark ➪ **cortex**

Barlow's disease ['bɑ:ləʊz dɪˌzi:z] *subst.* scurvy in children, caused by lack of vitamin C *Barlows sjukdom*

barmhärtighetsmord ➪ **mercy killing**

barn ➪ **child**

barn- ➪ **infantile, paed-, ped-**

barnafödande ➪ **childbearing**

barnaföderska ⇨ **puerpera**

barnavård ⇨ **child care**

barnavårdscentral ⇨ **child health clinic (CHC)**

barnbeck ⇨ **meconium**

barnbördsavdelning ⇨ **maternity**

barndom ⇨ **childhood**

barnförlamning ⇨ **polioencephalitis**

barnförlamning, epidemisk ⇨ **poliomyelitis**

barnhem ⇨ **home**

barnläkare ⇨ **paediatrician, pediatrician**

barnmisshandel ⇨ **child**

barnmisshandelssyndrom ⇨ **battered baby**

barnmorska ⇨ **midwife, visitor**

barnmorska, legitimerad ⇨ **register**

barnmorska vid sjukhus ⇨ **staff**

barnmorskeutbildning ⇨ **midwifery**

barnsbörd ⇨ **childbirth, parturition**

barnsbörds- ⇨ **puerperal**

barnsjukdomar ⇨ **childhood**

barnsjukhus ⇨ **child**

barnsäker ⇨ **child-proof**

barnsängsfeber ⇨ **puerperal**

barnsängstiden ⇨ **puerperium**

barntandläkare ⇨ **pediodontist**

baroreceptor ['bærəʊrɪˌseptə] *subst.* one of a group of nerves near the carotid artery and aortic arch, which sense changes in blood pressure *baroreceptor*

barotrauma [ˌbærəʊ'trɔːmə] *subst.* injury caused by a sharp increase in pressure *barotrauma, slags tryckskada*

Barr body ['bɑː ˌbɒdi] *see* CHROMATIN

barrier ['bæriə] *subst.* thing which prevents contact *barriär, hinder, spärr, skydd;* **barrier cream** = cream put on the skin to prevent the skin coming into contact with irritating substances *skyddskräm;* **barrier nursing** = nursing of a patient suffering from an infectious disease, while keeping him away from other patients and making sure that faeces and soiled bedclothes do not carry the infection to other patients *ung. smittskyddsvård*

> QUOTE those affected by salmonella poisoning are being nursed in five isolation wards and about forty suspected sufferers are being barrier nursed in other wards
>
> **Nursing Times**

barriär ⇨ **barrier**

bartholinit ⇨ **bartholinitis**

bartholinitis [ˌbɑːθɒlɪ'naɪtɪs] *subst.* inflammation of Bartholin's glands *bartholinit*

Bartholin's glands ['bɑːθ(ə)lɪnz ˌglændz] *or* **greater vestibular glands** [ˌgreɪtə ve'stɪbjʊlə ˌglændz] *subst pl.* two glands at the side of the entrance to the vagina which secrete a lubricating substance *glandulae vestibularis majores, Bartholins körtlar*

Bartholins körtel ⇨ **vestibular**

bas ⇨ **base, basis**

bas- ⇨ **basic, basilar**

basal ['beɪs(ə)l] *adj.* extremely important *or* which affects a base *basal(-), grund-;* **basal cell carcinoma** = RODENT ULCER; **basal ganglia** = masses of grey matter in the cerebrum *basala ganglierna;* **basal metabolism** *or* **basal metabolic rate (BMR)** = amount of energy which a person uses in exchanging oxygen and carbon dioxide when at rest *basalmetabolism, basalomsättning, BMB;* **basal narcosis** = making a patient unconscious by administering a narcotic before giving a general anaesthetic *narkosinledning, nedsövning;* **basal nuclei** = mass of grey matter at the bottom of each cerebral hemisphere *basala ganglierna*

basal ⇨ **basal**

basalcellscancer ⇨ **rodent ulcer**

basale [bə'seɪli] *see* STRATUM

basaliom ⇨ **rodent ulcer**

basalis [bə'seɪlɪs] *see* DECIDUA

basalmembran ⇨ **basement membrane**

basalmetabolism ⇨ **basal**

basalomsättning ⇨ **basal**

base [beɪs] **1** *subst.* **(a)** bottom part *bas;* **the base of the spine; base of the brain** = bottom surface of the cerebrum *hjärnstammen* **(b)** main ingredient of an ointment, as opposed to the active ingredient *bas, grundbeståndsdel* **(c)** substance which reacts with an acid to form a salt *bas* **2** *vb.* to make, using a substance as a main ingredient *basera;* **cream based on zinc oxide** = cream which uses zinc oxide as a base *krämen har zinkoxid som bas (är baserad på zinkoxid)*

Basedow's disease ['beɪzɪdəʊz dɪˌziːz] = THYROTOXICOSIS

basement membrane ['beɪsmənt ˌmembreɪn] *subst.* membrane at the base of an epithelium *basalmembran*

basera ⇨ **base**

basic ['beɪsɪk] *adj.* very simple *or* which everything else comes from *bas-, grund-, grundläggande;* **you should know basic maths if you want to work in a shop; basic structure of the skin** = the two layers of skin (the inner dermis and the outer epidermis) *hudens grundläggande struktur*

basilar ['bæzɪlə] *adj.* referring to a base *basilar(-), basal(-), bas-, grund-;* **basilar artery** = artery which lies at the base of the brain *arteria basilaris, hjärnans basala artär;* **basilar membrane** = membrane in the cochlea which transmits nerve impulses from sound vibrations to the auditory nerve *basilarmembran*

basilarmembran ⇨ **basilar**

basilic [bə'sɪlɪk] *adj.* important *or* prominent *viktig, framstående;* **basilic vein** = vein in the arm, running from the elbow along the inside of the upper arm *vena basilica*

basin ['beɪs(ə)n] *subst.* large bowl *fat, skål;* **wash basin** = bowl in a kitchen or bathroom where you can wash your hands *handfat*

basis ['beɪsɪs] *subst.* **(a)** main part of which something is formed *bas, grundbeståndsdel;* **water forms the basis of the solution; the basis of the treatment is quiet and rest** **(b)** main reason for deciding *grundval, utgångspunkt;* **the basis for the diagnosis is the result of the test for the patient's blood sugar**

basofili ⇨ **basophilia**

basophil ['beɪsə(ʊ)fɪl] *or* **basophilic granulocyte** [ˌbeɪsə(ʊ)'fɪlɪk ˌgrænjʊləsaɪt] *subst.* type of white blood cell which contains granules *basofil granulocyt;* **basophil leucocyte** = blood cell which carries histamines *basofil leukocyt*

basophilia [ˌbeɪsə(ʊ)'fɪliə] *subst.* increase in the number of basophils in the blood *basofili*

bastard ⇨ **hybrid**

Batchelor plaster [ˌbætʃ(ə)lə 'plɑːstə] *subst.* plaster cast which keeps both legs apart *gipsförband som håller isär benen*

bath [bɑːθ] **1** *subst.* **(a)** large container for water, in which you can wash your whole body *badkar;* **there's a shower and a bath in the bathroom; eye bath** = small dish into which a solution can be put for bathing the eye *ögonbad* **(b)** washing your whole body *bad;* **the patient was given a hot bath; he believes that a cold bath every morning is good for you; medicinal bath** = treatment where the patient lies in a bath of hot water with special chemicals in it *or* hot mud or other substances *medicinskt bad;* **sponge bath** = washing a patient in bed, using a sponge *helavtvättning;* **the nurse gave her a sponge bath** **2** *vb.* to wash with a lot of liquid *bada;* **he's bathing the baby**

bathe [beɪð] *vb.* to wash (a wound) *badda, tvätta;* **he bathed his knee with boiled water**

bathroom ['bɑːθruːm] *subst.* small room with a bath or shower and usually a toilet *badrum*

battered baby [ˌbætəd 'beɪbi] *or* **battered child syndrome** [ˌbætəd 'tʃaɪld ˌsɪndrəʊm] *subst.* condition where a baby *or* small child is frequently beaten by one or both of its parents, usually with multiple fractures and other injuries *misshandlat barn, barnmisshandelssyndrom, spädbarnsmisshandelssyndrom*

battledore placenta ['bæt(ə)lˌdɔː plə'sentə] *subst.* placenta where the umbilical cord is attached to the edge and not the centre *placenta där navelsträngen utgår från kanten och inte från mitten*

Bauhins klaff ⇨ **valve**

Bazin's disease ['beɪzɪnz dɪˌzi:z] = ERYTHEMA INDURATUM

BB ⇨ **maternity**

BC [ˌbi:'si:] *see* BONE CONDUCTION

BCG [ˌbi:si:'dʒi:] = BACILLE CALMETTE-GUERIN **the baby had a BCG vaccination**

BCG ⇨ **bacille Calmette-Guérin (BCG)**

BCh [ˌbi:si:'eɪtʃ] = BACHELOR OF SURGERY

BDA [ˌbi:di:'eɪ] = BRITISH DENTAL ASSOCIATION

Be *chemical symbol for* beryllium *Be, beryllium*

beam [bi:m] *subst.* line of light *or* rays *stråle, ljusstråle, strålknippe;* **the X-ray beam is directed at the patient's jaw**

bearing down [ˌbeərɪŋ 'daʊn] *subst. (of a woman giving birth)* stage in childbirth when the woman starts to push out the baby from the uterus *utdrivningsskiftet*

beat [bi:t] **1** *subst.* regular sound which forms a rhythm *slag;* **the patient's heart had an irregular beat 2** *vb.* **(a)** to hit *slå;* **beat joint (beat elbow** *or* **beat knee) =** inflammation of a joint (such as the elbow *or* knee) caused by frequent sharp blows or other pressure *s.k. studentarmbåge el. skurgummeknä* **(b)** to make a regular sound *slå (regelbundet);* **his heart was beating fast**
NOTE: **beats - beating - beat - has beaten**

Bechterews sjukdom ⇨ **spondylitis**

becquerel ['bek(ə)r(ə)l] *subst.* unit of measurement of radiation *becquerel; see also* RAD
NOTE: written **bq** with figures: **200bq**

bed [bed] *subst.* **(a)** piece of furniture for sleeping on *bädd, säng;* **lie down on the bed if you're tired; she always goes to bed at 9 o'clock; he was sitting up in bed drinking a cup of coffee; she's in bed with a cold (b) hospital bed =** special type of bed used in hospitals *sjukhussäng;* **ward with twenty beds; a 250-bed hospital; bed occupancy rate =** number of beds occupied in a hospital shown as a percentage of all the beds in the hospital *beläggningsgrad*

bedbug ['bedbʌg] *subst.* small insect which lives in dirty bedclothes and sucks blood *cimex lectularius, vägglus*

bedclothes ['bedkləʊðz] *subst pl.* sheets and blankets which cover a bed *sängkläder*

bedpan ['bedpæn] *subst.* dish into which a patient can urinate or defecate without getting out of bed *bäcken*

bedridden ['bedˌrɪd(ə)n] *adj.* (patient) who cannot get out of bed *sängbunden, sängliggande;* **he is bedridden and has to be looked after by a nurse; she stayed at home to look after her bedridden mother**

bedroom ['bedru:m] *subst.* room where you sleep *sovrum*

bedside manner [ˌbedsaɪd 'mænə] *subst.* way in which a doctor behaves towards a patient in bed *uppträdande (sätt) mot patienten;* **doctor with a good bedside manner =** doctor who comforts and reassures patients when he examines them in hospital *läkare med ett förtroendeingivande sätt mot patienter*

bedsore ['bedsɔ:] *or* **decubitus ulcer** [dɪ'kju:bɪtəs ˌʌlsə] *subst.* inflamed patch of skin on a bony part of the body, which develops into an ulcer, caused by pressure of the part on the mattress after lying for some time in one position *dekubitalsår, trycksår, liggsår*

> COMMENT: special types of mattresses can be used to try to prevent the formation of bedsores. See AIR BED, RIPPLE BED, WATER BED

bedtime ['bedtaɪm] *subst.* time when you usually go to bed *sängdags, läggdags;* **9 o'clock is the patients' bedtime; go to bed - it's past your bedtime**

bedwetting ['bedˌwetɪŋ] *or* **nocturnal enuresis** [nɒk'tɜ:n(ə)l ˌenjʊ(ə)'ri:sɪs] *subst.* passing urine in bed at night (especially used of children) *enuresis nocturna, sängvätning, nattvätning*

bedöma ⇨ **evaluate**

bedömning ⇨ **evaluation**

bedöva ⇨ **anaesthetize**

bedövning ⇨ **anaesthesia**

bedövnings- ⇨ **anaesthetic, narco-, narcotic**

bedövningsmedel ⇨ **anaesthetic**

Beer's knife ['bɪəz ˌnaɪf] *subst.* knife with a triangular blade, used in eye operations *kniv med triangulärt blad som används vid ögonoperationer*

bee sting ['biː stɪŋ] *subst.* sting by a bee *bistick*

COMMENT: because a bee injects acid into the body, relief can be obtained by dabbing an alkaline solution onto a sting

befolkning ⇨ **population**

befolkningsstatistik ⇨ **vital**

befrukta ⇨ **fertilize, impregnate**

befruktning ⇨ **conception, fertilization, impregnation, insemination**

befrämja ⇨ **promote**

begrava ⇨ **bury**

begränsa ⇨ **limit, restrict**

begränsad ⇨ **confined, localized**

begränsad syn(förmåga) ⇨ **partial**

begynnande ⇨ **incipient**

begär ⇨ **desire, urge**

begära ⇨ **require**

behandla ⇨ **attend, treat**

behandling ⇨ **cure, intervention, management, procedure, therapy, treatment**

behandlingskur ⇨ **course**

behandlingsmetod ⇨ **procedure**

behandlingsserie ⇨ **programme**

behandling(stillfälle) ⇨ **session**

behave [bɪ'heɪv] *vb.* to do things (usually well) *bete (uppföra) sig;* **the children all behaved (themselves) very well when the doctor visited the ward; after she was ill she started to behave in a very strange way**

behaviorism ⇨ **behaviourism**

behaviour *or US* **behavior** [bɪ'heɪvjə] *subst.* way of doing things *beteende, uppträdande;* **his behaviour was very strange; the behaviour of the patients in the mental ward is causing concern; behaviour therapy** = psychiatric treatment where the patient learns to improve his condition *beteendeterapi*

behavioural [bɪ'heɪvjər(ə)l] *adj.* referring to behaviour *beteende-*

behaviourism [bɪ'heɪvjərɪz(ə)m] *subst.* psychological theory that only the patient's behaviour should be studied to discover his psychological problems *behaviorism*

behaviourist [bɪ'heɪvjərɪst] *subst.* psychologist who follows behaviourism *behaviorist*

Behçet's syndrome ['beɪsets ˌsɪndrəʊm] *subst.* condition with no known cause, in which the patient has mouth ulcers and inflamed eyes accompanied by polyarthritis *Behçets sjukdom*

behov ⇨ **requirement**

behålla ⇨ **keep, keep down, retain**

behörighet ⇨ **qualification**

bejel ['bedʒ(ə)l] *or* **endemic syphilis** [ɪn'demɪk 'sɪfəlɪs] *subst.* non venereal form of syphilis which is endemic among children in some areas of the Middle East *endemisk syfilis*

beklädnad, invändig ⇨ **lining**

bekräfta ⇨ **confirm**

bekämpa ⇨ **combat**

belagd ⇨ **fur**

belasta ⇨ **strain**

belastning ⇨ **strain**

belch [beltʃ] **1** *subst.* eructation *or* allowing air in the stomach to come up through the mouth *eruktation, rap(ning)* **2** *vb.* to make air in the stomach come up through the mouth *rapa*
NOTE: with babies use the word **burp**

beledsaga ⇨ **accompany**

belladonna [ˌbelə'dɒnə] *or* **deadly nightshade** [ˌdedli 'naɪtʃeɪd] *subst.* poisonous plant which produces atropine *(Aropa) belladonna*

belle indifférence [ˌbel ɛ̃ˌdɪfe'rɑ̃s] *subst.* excessively calm state of a patient, when normally he should show emotion *belle indifférence*

Bellocq's cannula [be'lɒks ˌkænjʊlə] *or* **sound** [saʊnd] *subst.* instrument used to control a nosebleed *instrument som används för att stoppa näsblödning*

Bell's mania ['belz ˌmeɪnɪə] *subst.* form of acute mania with delirium *slags akut mani med delirium*

Bell's palsy ['belz ˌpɔːlzi] *or* **facial paralysis** [ˌfeɪʃ(ə)l pə'ræləsɪs] *subst.* paralysis of one side of the face, preventing the patient from closing one eye, caused by a defect in the facial nerve *Bells pares (förlamning), facialispares*

belly ['beli] *subst.* **(a)** abdomen *or* space in the front of the body below the diaphragm and above the pelvis, containing the stomach *buken, magen* **(b)** fatter central part of a muscle *venter, buk*

bellyache ['belieɪk] *subst.* pain in the abdomen *or* stomach *buksmärtor, ont i magen*

belly button ['beli ˌbʌt(ə)n] *subst. (used mainly by children)* navel *naveln*

belt [belt] *subst.* long piece of leather *or* plastic which goes around the waist to keep trousers up or to attach a coat *bälte, skärp;* **seat belt** = belt in a car *or* in a plane which holds you safely in your seat *säkerhetsbälte, bilbälte;* **surgical belt** = fitted covering, worn to support parts of the chest *or* abdomen *korsett*

belysning ➪ **light, lighting**

belägen ➪ **situated**

beläggning ➪ **coating**

beläggningsgrad ➪ **bed, occupancy rate**

ben ➪ **bone, os; leg, limb**

ben- ➪ **bony, osseous, ost-**

benavledning ➪ **limb**

benbildning ➪ **ossification, osteogenesis**

ben-brosktumör ➪ **osteochondroma**

benbrott ➪ **break, fracture**

Bence Jones protein [ˌbens 'dʒəʊnz ˌprəʊtiːn] *subst.* protein found in the urine of patients suffering from myelomatosis, lymphoma, leukaemia and some other cancers *Bence-Jones protein (äggvita)*

bend [bend] **1** *subst.* curved shape *böj(ning), krök(ning);* **the pipe under the wash basin has two bends in it; the bends** = CAISSON DISEASE **2** *vb.* **(a)** to make something curved *or* to be curved *böja, kröka;* **he bent the pipe into the shape of an S (b)** to lean towards the ground *böja sig;* **he bent down to tie up his shoe; she was bending over the table**
NOTE:
NOTE: **bends - bending - bent - has bent**

Benedict's solution ['beɪdɪkts sə'luːʃ(ə)n] *subst.* solution used to carry out Benedict's test *slags lösning för att undersöka socker i urinen*

Benedict's test ['benɪdɪkts ˌtest] *subst.* test to see if sugar is present in the urine *slags prov för att undersöka socker i urinen*

benelevatorium ➪ **levator**

benfog ➪ **suture**

benförhårdning ➪ **osteosclerosis**

benförtätning ➪ **osteosclerosis**

benhinnan ➪ **periosteum**

benhinneinflammation ➪ **periostitis**

benhölje ➪ **involucrum**

benig ➪ **bony**

benign [bɪ'naɪn] *adj.* generally harmless *benign, godartad;* **benign tumour** *or* **benign growth** = tumour which will not grow again *or* spread to other parts of the body if it is removed surgically, but which can be fatal if not treated *benign (godartad) tumör*
NOTE: opposite is **malignant**

beninflammation ➪ **osteitis**

benlabyrinten ➪ **labyrinth**

benledning ➪ **conduction**

benlära ➪ **osteology**

benmärg ➪ **bone marrow, medulla**

benmärgs- ➪ **myel-, myeloid**

benmärgsinflammation ➪ **myelitis, osteomyelitis**

benmärgssvulst ➪ **myeloma**

benmärgstransplantat ➪ **bone marrow**

Bennett's fracture ['benɪts ˌfræktʃə] *subst.* fracture of the first metacarpal *or* the bone between the thumb and the wrist *Bennetts fraktur*

benorylate [be'nɔrɪleɪt] *subst.* drug used as a pain killer in treatment of arthritis *slags smärtstillande medel*

benröta ➪ **caries, osteomyelitis**

bensammansmältning ➪ **synostosis**

bensjukdom ➪ **osteopathy**

benskada ➪ **damage**

benskörhet ➪ **fragilitas, osteoporosis**

bensoe(harts) ➪ **benzoin**

bensporre ➪ **exostosis**

benstomme ➪ **skeleton**

benstruktur ➪ **bone**

bensylpenicillin ➪ **benzyl penicillin**

bensår ➪ **ulcer**

bensöm ➪ **suture**

bentagg ➪ **spicule**

bentransplantat ➪ **bone**

benutskott, godartat ➪ **osteophyte**

benutväxt ➪ **exostosis**

benvävsförtunning ➪ **rarefaction**

benvävssvulst ➪ **osteoma**

benvävsuppmjukning ➪ **osteomalacia**

benzoin ['benzəʊɪn] *subst.* resin used to make friars' balsam *bensoe(harts)*

benzyl penicillin ['benzɪl ˌpenə'sɪlɪn] *subst.* penicillin G *bensylpenicillin, penicillin G*

benägenhet ➪ **tendency**

bereda ➪ **prepare**

bergsjuka ➪ **mountain sickness**

beriberi [ˌberi'beri] *subst.* disease of the nervous system caused by lack of vitamin B_1 *polyneuritis epidemica perniciosa, beriberi;* **dry beriberi** = beriberi where the patient suffers loss of feeling and paralysis *beriberi med känselförlust och förlamning;* **wet beriberi** = beriberi where the patient's body swells with oedema *beriberi med ödem*

> COMMENT: beriberi is prevalent in tropical countries where the diet is mainly formed of white rice which is deficient in thiamine

beroende ➪ **addiction, dependence**

-beroende ➪ **-related**

beroendeframkallande ➪ **addictive**

beroende, fysiskt ➪ **physical**

beroende, psykologiskt ➪ **habituation**

berusa ➪ **intoxicate**

berusad ➪ **drunk, drunken**

berusning ➪ **inebriation, intoxication**

berusningsmedel ➪ **intoxicant**

berylliosis [bə'rɪli'əʊsɪs] *subst.* poisoning caused by breathing in particles of beryllium oxide *beryll(i)os*

beryllium [bə'rɪliəm] *subst.* chemical element *beryllium, Be* NOTE: chemical symbol is **Be**

beröring ➪ **contact, touch**

besegra ➪ **overcome**

besiktning ➪ **inspection**

besk ➪ **bitter**

beskaffenhet ➪ **nature**

beskriva ➪ **describe**

beskrivning ➪ **description**

beslöjad ➪ **husky**

Besnier's prurigo [beni'eɪz prʊ(ə)ˌraɪgəʊ] *see* PRURIGO

bespruta ⇨ **spray**

bestrålning ⇨ **radiation**

bestå ⇨ **persist**

bestående ⇨ **permanent, persistent**

beståndsdel ⇨ **component, constituent, ingredient**

beståndsdel, aktiv ⇨ **principle**

bestämma ⇨ **determine**

besvara ⇨ **answer**

besvär ⇨ **bother, complaint, condition, problem, trouble, upset**

besvärande hårväxt ⇨ **hair**

besvärlig ⇨ **awkward, difficult**

besök ⇨ **call, session, visit**

besöka ⇨ **call, visit**

besökare ⇨ **visitor**

besökstider ⇨ **visit**

besökstid, obegränsad ⇨ **open**

beta ['bi:tə] *subst.* second letter of the Greek alphabet *beta;* **beta blocker** = drug which blocks the beta-adrenergic receptors and so reduces the activity of the heart *betablockerare, beta(receptor)blockare;* **beta cell** = cell which produces insulin *betacell*

betablockerare ⇨ **blocker**

betacell ⇨ **cell**

betametason ⇨ **betamethasone**

betamethasone [ˌbi:tə'meθəsəʊn] *subst.* very strong corticosteroid drug *betametason*

beteende ⇨ **behavior, manner**

beteende- ⇨ **behavioural**

beteendeterapi ⇨ **behaviour**

betingad reflex ⇨ **conditioned reflex**

bett ⇨ **bite, sting**

better ['betə] *adj. & adv.* healthy again *or* not as ill as before *bättre;* **I had a cold last week but now I'm better; I hope you're better soon; she had flu but now she's feeling better; vegetables are better for you than sweets** = vegetables make you healthier *grönsaker är bättre för en (hälsan) än sötsaker*

bevara ⇨ **conserve**

bevis ⇨ **certificate**

B-glukosnivå ⇨ **glucose, sugar**

Bi *chemical symbol for* bismuth *Bi, vismut*

bi- ['baɪ, ˌbaɪ] *prefix* two *or* twice *bi-, två-, dubbel-*

bi- ⇨ **ambi-, bi-, para-**

bicarbonate of soda [baɪˌkɑ:b(ə)nət əv 'səʊdə] *subst.* sodium salt used to treat acidity in the stomach *bikarbonat, natriumbikarbonat* NOTE: chemical symbol is **$NaHCO_3$**

bicellular [baɪ'seljʊlə] *adj.* which has two cells *bicellulär*

biceps ['baɪseps] *subst.* any muscle formed of two parts joined to form one tendon, especially the muscles in the front of the upper arm and the back of the thigh *biceps, tvåhövdad muskel;* **biceps femoris** = extensor muscle in the back of the thigh *musculus biceps femoris, tvåhövdade lårmuskeln; compare* TRICEPS NOTE: plural is **biceps**

bicipital [baɪ'sɪpɪt(ə)l] *adj.* (i) referring to a biceps muscle *som avser el. hör till tvåhövdad muskel;* (ii) with two parts *tvådelad, tudelad*

biconcave [baɪ'kɒŋkeɪv] *adj.* (lens) which is concave on both sides *bikonkav*

biconvex [baɪ'kɒnveks] *adj.* (lens) which is convex on both sides *bikonvex*

bicornuate [baɪ'kɔ:njuit] *adj.* which is divided into two parts (sometimes applied to a malformation of the uterus) *tvådelad, tudelad*

bicuspid [ˌbaɪ'kʌspɪd] *subst. & adj.* with two points, such as a premolar tooth *tvåfliktig, tvåspetsig;* **bicuspid (mitral) valve** = valve in the heart which allows blood to flow from the left atrium to the left ventricle but not in the opposite direction ⇨ *illustration* HEART *valvula mitralis (bicuspidalis), bikuspidalklaffen, mitralisklaffen*

b.i.d. [ˌbi:aɪ'di:] *or* **bis in die** [ˌbɪs ɪn 'di:e] Latin phrase meaning twice daily *bis in die, två gånger dagligen*

bidragande ⇨ **accessory**

bifid ['baɪfɪd] *adj.* in two parts *bifidus, tvådelad, tudelad*

bifida ['bɪfɪdə] *see* SPINA BIFIDA

bifidus ⇨ **bifid**

bifocal lenses [ˌbaɪ'fəʊk(ə)l ˌlenzɪz] *or* **bifocals** [ˌbaɪ'fəʊk(ə)lz] *subst pl.* type of glasses, where two lenses are combined in the same piece of glass, the top lens being for seeing at a distance and the lower lens for reading *bifokala linser, bifokalglasögon; see also* TRIFOCAL

bifokalglasögon ⇨ **bifocal lenses**

bifurcation [ˌbaɪfə'keɪʃ(ə)n] *subst.* place where something divides into two parts *bifurkation, förgrening, klyvning*

bifurkation ⇨ **bifurcation**

bigeminy [baɪ'dʒemɪni] *or* **pulsus bigeminus** ['pʌlsəs baɪˌdʒemɪnəs] *subst.* condition where double heartbeats can be felt at the pulse *pulsus bigeminus, tvåslagspuls*

big toe ['bɪg təʊ] *subst.* largest of the five toes, in the inside of the foot *hallux, stortån*

bihang ⇨ **adnexa, appendage, appendix, attachment**

bihåla ⇨ **sinus**

bihåleinflammation ⇨ **sinusitis**

bikarbonat ⇨ **bicarbonate of soda**

bikonkav ⇨ **biconcave**

bikonvex ⇨ **biconvex**

bikuspidalklaffen ⇨ **bicuspid**

bilateral [baɪ'læt(ə)r(ə)l] *adj.* which affects both sides *bilateral, dubbelsidig;* **bilateral pneumonia** = pneumonia affecting both lungs *bilateral pneumoni, dubbelsidig lunginflammation;* **bilateral vasectomy** = surgical operation to cut both vasa deferentia and so make the patient sterile *bilateral vasektomi*

bilbälte ⇨ **belt, safety**

bild ⇨ **image**

bilda ⇨ **produce**

bildanalys ⇨ **imaging**

bildning ⇨ **formation**

bildskärm ⇨ **monitor**

bile [baɪl] *subst.* thick bitter brownish yellow fluid produced by the liver, stored in the gall bladder and used to digest fatty substances and to neutralize acids *galla;* **bile acids** = acids (such as cholic acid) found in bile *gallsyror;* **bile duct** = tube which links the cystic duct and the hepatic duct to the duodenum *gallgång;* **bile pigment** = colouring matter in bile *gallfärgämne;* **bile salts** = sodium salts of bile acids *gallsalter*
NOTE: for other terms referring to bile see words beginning with **chol-**

> COMMENT: in jaundice, excess bile pigments flow into the blood and cause the skin to turn yellow

Bilharzia [bɪl'hɑːziə] *or* **Schistosoma** [ˌʃɪstə'səʊmə] *subst.* fluke which enters the patient's bloodstream and causes bilharziasis *bilharzia*

bilharzia ⇨ **Bilharzia, bilharziasis**

bilharziasis [ˌbɪlhɑː'zaɪəsɪs] *or* **schistosomiasis** [ˌʃɪstəsəʊ'maɪəsɪs] *subst.* tropical disease caused by flukes in the intestine or bladder *bilharzia, bilharzios*
NOTE: although strictly speaking, **Bilharzia** is the name of the fluke, it is also generally used for the name of the disease: **bilharzia patients; six cases of bilharzia**

> COMMENT: the larvae of the fluke enter the skin through the feet and lodge in the walls of the intestine or bladder. They are passed out of the body in stools or urine and return to water, where they lodge and develop in the water snail, the secondary host, before going back into humans. Patients suffer from fever and anaemia

bilharzios ⇨ **bilharziasis**

biliary ['bɪliərɪ] *adj.* referring to bile *biliär, gall-;* **biliary colic** = pain in the abdomen caused by gallstones in the bile duct *or* by inflammation of the gall bladder *colica hepatica, gallstenskolik;* **primary biliary cirrhosis** = cirrhosis of the liver caused by autoimmune disease *primär biliär cirros;* **secondary biliary cirrhosis** = cirrhosis of the liver caused by an obstruction of the bile ducts *sekundär biliär cirros;* **biliary fistula** = opening which discharges bile on to the surface of the skin from the gall bladder, bile duct or liver *gallfistel*

bilious ['bɪliəs] *adj.* (condition) caused by bile *or* where bile is brought up into the mouth *gall-, gallsjuk;* (any condition) where the patient suffers nausea *med illamående;* **he had a bilious attack** = he had indigestion together with nausea *han hade ont i magen och mådde illa (pga. gallstensanfall)*

biliousness ['bɪliəsnəs] *subst.* feeling of indigestion and nausea *känsla av illamående och magont*

bilirubin [ˌbɪli'ruːbɪn] *subst.* red pigment in bile *bilirubin;* **serum bilirubin** = bilirubin in serum, converted from haemoglobin as red blood cells are destroyed *serumbilirubin*

bilirubinaemia [ˌbɪliˌruːbɪ'niːmiə] *subst.* excess of bilirubin in the blood *bilirubinemi*

bilirubinemi ⇨ **bilirubinaemia**

biliuria [ˌbɪli'jʊəriə] *subst.* presence of bile in the urine *biliuri; see* CHOLURIA

biliverdin [ˌbɪli'vɜːdɪn] *subst.* green pigment in bile, produced by oxidation of bilirubin *biliverdin*
NOTE: for other terms referring to bile, see words beginning with **chol-**

biliär ⇨ **biliary**

biljud ⇨ **bruit**

Billroth's operations ['bɪlrɒθs ˌɒpə'reiʃ(ə)nz] *subst. pl.* surgical operations where the lower part of the stomach is removed and the part which is left is linked to the duodenum or jejunum *Billroths operation*

bilobate [baɪ'ləʊbeɪt] *adj.* with two lobes *med två lober*

"bilringar" ⇨ **flab**

bimanual [baɪ'mænjʊ(ə)l] *adj.* done with two hands *or* needing both hands to be done *bimanuell*

bimanuell ⇨ **bimanual**

binary ['baɪn(ə)ri] *adj.* (i) made of two parts *binär;* (ii) (compound) made of two elements *binär, dubbel-;* **binary fission** = splitting into two parts (in some types of cell division) *tudelning*

binaural [baɪn'ɔːr(ə)l] *adj.* referring to both ears *binaural;* using both ears *binaural*

bind [baɪnd] *vb.* to tie *binda, förbinda;* to fasten *fästa, binda fast;* **the burglars bound his hands and feet with string** NOTE: **binds - binding - bound - has bound**

binda ⇨ **bandage, bind**

binder ['baɪndə] *subst.* bandage which is wrapped round an organ for support *stödförband*

bindhinnan ⇨ **conjunctiva**

bindhinne- ⇨ **conjunctival**

bindhinneinflammation ⇨ **conjunctivitis**

bindning ⇨ **bonding**

bindväv ⇨ **connective tissue, stroma**

bindväv, lucker ⇨ **cellular**

bindvävs- ⇨ **collagenous, fibroid, fibrous, syndesm-**

bindvävsbrosk ⇨ **fibrocartilage**

bindvävsfog ⇨ **fibrous, syndesmosis**

bindvävshinna ⇨ **fascia**

bindvävsinflammation ⇨ **fibrositis**

bindvävssjukdom ⇨ **collagen**

bindvävssträng ⇨ **retinaculum**

bindvävssvulst ⇨ **fibroma**

bindvävsvandling ⇨ **fibroid**

Binet's test ['bɪneɪz ˌtest] *subst.* intelligence test for children *slags intelligenstest för barn*

binjurarna ⇨ **adrenal**

binjurebark- ⇨ **adrenocortical**

binjurebarken ⇨ **cortex**

binjurebarkhormon ⇨ **cortical, corticosteroid**

binjuremärgen ⇨ **adrenal**

binnikemask ⇨ **tapeworm**

binocular [bɪ'nɒkjʊlə] *adj.* referring to the two eyes *binokular, binokulär;* **binocular vision** = ability to see with both eyes at the same time, which gives a stereoscopic effect and allows a person to judge distances *binokulärt seende; compare* MONOCULAR

binokular ⇨ **binocular**

binokulär ⇨ **binocular**

binovular [bɪ'nɒvjʊlə] *adj.* (twins) which come from two different ova *tvåäggs-*

binucleate [baɪ'nju:kliеɪt] *adj.* with two nuclei *tvåkärnig*

binär ⇨ **binary**

bio- ['baɪə(ʊ), ˌ--] *prefix* referring to living organisms *bio-*

bioassay [ˌbaɪəʊə'seɪ] *subst.* test of the strength of drugs *or* hormones *or* vitamins *or* sera, by noting their effects on living animals *or* tissue *bioassay*

biochemical [ˌbaɪə(ʊ)'kemɪk(ə)l] *adj.* referring to biochemistry *biokemisk*

biochemist [ˌbaɪəʊ'kemɪst] *subst.* scientist who specializes in biochemistry *biokemist*

biochemistry [ˌbaɪə(ʊ)'kemɪstri] *subst.* chemistry of living tissues *biokemi*

bioengineering [ˌbaɪəʊˌendʒɪ'nɪərɪŋ] *subst.* science of manipulating and combining different genetic material to produce living organisms with particular characteristics *DNA-manipulering, genetisk ingenjörskonst*

biofeedback [ˌbaɪəʊ'fi:dbæk] *subst.* control of the autonomic nervous system by the patient's conscious thought (as he sees the results of tests *or* scans) *biofeedback*

biogenesis [ˌbaɪə(ʊ)'dʒenəsɪs] *subst.* theory that living organisms can only develop from other living organisms *biogenes*

biokemi ⇨ **biochemistry**

biokemisk ⇨ **biochemical**

biokemist ⇨ **biochemist**

biolog ⇨ **biologist**

biologi ⇨ **biology**

biological [ˌbaɪə'lɒdʒɪk(ə)l] *adj.* referring to biology *biologisk;* **biological clock** *or* **circadian rhythm** = rhythm of physiological functions (eating *or* defecating *or* sleeping, etc.) which is repeated every twenty-four hours *biologisk klocka*

biologisk ⇨ **biological**

biologisk klocka ⇨ **biological**

biologist [baɪ'ɒlədʒɪst] *subst.* scientist who specializes in biology *biolog*

biology [baɪ'ɒlədʒi] *subst.* study of living organisms *biologi*

bionics [baɪ'ɒnɪks] *subst.* applying knowledge of biological systems to mechanical and electronic devices *bioteknik, bionik*

bionik ⇨ **bionics**

biopsi ⇨ **biopsy**

biopsy ['baɪɒpsi] *subst.* taking a small piece of living tissue for examination and diagnosis *biopsi;* **the biopsy of the tissue from the growth showed that it was benign**

biorhythms ['baɪə(ʊ)ˌrɪð(ə)mz] *subst pl.* recurring cycles of different lengths which some people believe affect a person's sensitivity and intelligence *biorytm*

biorytm ⇨ **biorhythms**

biostatistics [ˌbaɪəʊstə'tɪstɪks] *subst pl.* statistics used in medicine and the study of disease *medicinsk statistik*

bioteknik ⇨ **bionics**

biotin ['baɪətɪn] *subst.* type of vitamin B, found in egg yolks, liver and yeast *biotin*

bipara [baɪ'peərə] *subst.* woman who has been pregnant twice and each time has given birth normally *bipara*

biparietal [ˌbaɪpə'raɪət(ə)l] *adj.* referring to the two parietal bones *biparietal, hjässbens-*

biparous ['bɪpərəs] *adj.* which produces twins *som ger tvillingar*

bipennat ⇨ **bipennate**

bipennate [baɪ'peneɪt] *adj.* (muscle) with fibres which rise from either side of the tendon *bipennat*

bipolar [ˌbaɪ'pəʊlə] *adj.* with two poles *bipolar, bipolär;* **bipolar disorder** = mental disorder where the patient moves from mania to depression *bipolär psykos (affektiv sjukdom);* **bipolar neurone** = nerve cell with two processes, a dendrite and an axon ⇨ *illustration* NEURONE *bipolart (bipolärt) neuron, bipolar (bipolär) nervcell*

bipolär ⇨ **bipolar**

birth [bɜ:θ] *subst.* being born *födelse;* **date of birth** = date when a person was born *födelsedatum;* **to give birth** = to have a baby *föda;* **she gave birth to twins; breech birth** = birth where the baby's buttocks appear first *sätesförlossning;* **birth canal** = uterus, vagina and vulva *förlossningskanalen;* **birth certificate** = official document giving details of a person's date and place of birth *födelseattest;* **birth control** = using contraceptive devices to regulate births *födelsekontroll;* **birth defect** = congenital defect *or* defect which exists in a person from birth *medfödd missbildning (defekt);* **birth injury** = injury (such as brain damage) which is done to a baby during a difficult childbirth *förlossningsskada;* **birth rate** = number of births per year, per thousand of population *nativitet, födelsetal;* **premature birth** = birth of a baby earlier than nine months from conception *partus praematurus, för tidig födelse (förlossning), förtidsbörd*

birthing chair ['bɜːθɪŋ ˌtʃeə] *subst.* special chair in which a mother sits to give birth *förlossningsstol*

birthmark ['bɜːθmɑːk] *or* **naevus** ['niːvəs] *subst.* mark on the skin which a baby has from birth *naevus, födelsemärke*

bisexual [ˌbaɪ'sekʃʊ(ə)l] *adj.* (person) who feels sexual attraction to both males and females *bisexuell*

bisexuality [ˌbaɪˌsekʃu'æləti] *subst.* having both male and female physical characteristics *bisexualitet; compare* AMBISEXUAL, HETEROSEXUAL, HOMOSEXUAL

bisexuell ⇨ **ambisexual, bisexual**

bisköldkörtel ⇨ **parathyroid (gland)**

bisköldkörtelhormon ⇨ **parathormone, parathyroid (gland)**

bismuth ['bɪzməθ] *subst.* chemical element *vismut, Bi;* **bismuth salts** = salts used to treat acid stomach, and formerly used in the treatment of syphilis *vismutsalter* NOTE: chemical symbol is **Bi**

bistick ⇨ **bee sting**

bistoury ['bɪstəri] *subst.* sharp, thin surgical knife *bist(o)uri, slags operationskniv*

bistå ⇨ **aid, assist**

bistånd ⇨ **aid, help**

bite [baɪt] **1** *vb.* to cut into something with the teeth *bita(s);* **the dog bit the postman; he bit a piece out of the apple; she was bitten by an insect; to bite on something** = to hold onto something with the teeth *bita i (på);* **the dentist told him to bite on the bite wing** NOTE: **bites - biting - bit - has bitten** **2** *subst.* action of being bitten *bett, stick, sting;* place where someone has been bitten *bett;* **animal bite** *or* **insect bite** *or* **snake bite; her arm was covered with bites**

bitestikel ⇨ **epididymis**

bite wing ['baɪt wɪŋ] *subst.* holder for dental X-ray film, which the patient holds between the teeth, so allowing an X-ray of both upper and lower teeth to be taken *bitewing*

Bitot's spots ['bitəʊz ˌspɒts] *subst pl.* small white spots on the conjunctiva, caused by vitamin A deficiency *Bitots fläckar*

biträdande överläkare ⇨ **registrar**

biträde ⇨ **helper**

bitter ['bɪtə] *adj.* one of the four tastes, not sweet, sour or salt *bitter, besk;* **quinine is bitter but oranges are sweet** ⇨ *illustration* TONGUE

bitter ⇨ **bitter**

bivalve ['baɪvælv] *subst.* (organ) which has two valves *organ med två klaffar*

biverkning ⇨ **side-effect**

bjuda sig ⇨ **present**

bjudning ⇨ **presentation**

black [blæk] *adj. & subst.* of the darkest colour which is the opposite of white *svart;* **the surgeon was wearing a black coat; black coffee** = coffee with no milk in it *svart kaffe;* **black death** = severe form of bubonic plague *svarta döden, digerdöden;* **black eye** = bruising and swelling of the tissues round an eye, caused by a blow *blått öga;* **he got a black eye in the fight** NOTE: **black - blacker - blackest**

blackhead ['blækhed] *or* **comedo** ['kɒmɪdəʊ] *subst.* point of dark, hard matter in a sebaceous follicle, often found associated with acne on the skin of adolescents *comedo, komedon, pormask; see* ACNE

blackout ['blækaʊt] *subst.* fainting fit *or* sudden loss of consciousness *blackout, tillfällig medvetslöshet;* **he must have had a blackout while driving**

black out [ˌblæk ˈaʊt] *vb.* to have a sudden fainting fit *tillfälligt förlora medvetandet;* **I suddenly blacked out and I can't remember anything more**

blackwater fever [ˈblækˌwɔːtə ˌfiːvə] *subst.* tropical disease, a form of malaria, where haemoglobin from red blood cells is released into plasma and makes the urine dark *malaria perniciosa haemoglobinurica, svartvattenfeber*

blad ⇨ **blade, lamella**

bladder [ˈblædə] *subst.* any sac in the body, especially the sac where the urine collects before being passed out of the body *blåsa, urinblåsan;* **he is suffering from bladder trouble; she is taking antibiotics for a bladder infection; gall bladder** = sac in which bile produced by the liver is stored ⇨ *illustration* DIGESTIVE SYSTEM *gallblåsan;* **neurogenic bladder** = any disturbance of the bladder function caused by lesions in the nerve supply to the bladder *neurogen blåsa;* **urinary bladder** = sac where urine collects before being passed out of the body ⇨ *illustration* UROGENITAL SYSTEM *vesica urinaria, urinblåsan*

bladder worm [ˈblædə ˌwɜːm] *or* **cysticercus** [ˌsɪstɪˈsɜːkəs] *subst.* larva of a tapeworm which grows in a cyst *cysticerk, dynt, blåsmask*
NOTE: for other terms referring to the bladder, see words beginning with **cyst-, vesico-**

blade [bleɪd] *subst.* flat piece of metal *blad;* **this bistoury has a very sharp blade**

Blalock's operation [ˈbleɪlɒks ˌɒpəˈreɪʃ(ə)n] *or* **Blalock-Taussig operation** [ˌbleɪlɒkˈtɔːsɪg ˌɒpəˌreɪʃ(ə)n] *subst.* surgical operation to connect the pulmonary artery to the subclavian artery, to increase blood flow to the lungs in patients suffering from tetralogy of Fallot *Blalock-Taussig-anastomos*

Blalock-Taussig-anastomos ⇨ **Blalock's operation**

bland [blænd] *adj.* (food) which is not spicy *or* not irritating *or* not acid *mild, skonsam;* **bland diet** = diet in which the patient eats mainly milk-based foods, boiled vegetables and white meat, as a treatment for peptic ulcers *skonkost*

blandbarhet ⇨ **compatibility**

blandbar, inte ⇨ **immiscible**

blank [blæŋk] *adj.* (paper) with nothing written on it *blank, ren, oskriven;* **the doctor took out a blank prescription form**

blanket [ˈblæŋkɪt] *subst.* thick woollen cover which is put over a person to keep him warm in bed *filt;* **he woke up when his blankets fell off**

blankett ⇨ **form**

blast [blɑːst] *subst.* **(a)** immature form of a cell before definite characteristics develop *blast* **(b)** wave of air pressure from an explosion, which can cause concussion *tryckvåg, explosion;* **blast injury** = severe injury to the chest following a blast *explosionsskada*

blast ⇨ **blast**

-blast [blæst] *suffix* referring to a very early stage in the development of a cell *-blast*

blasto- [ˈblæstəʊ, ˌ--] *prefix* referring to a germ cell *blasto-, grodd-*

blastocoele [ˈblæstəʊsiːl] *subst.* cavity filled with fluid in a morula *blastoc(o)ele*

blastocyst [ˈblæstəʊsist] *subst.* early stage in the development of an embryo *blastocyt, groddcell*

Blastomyces [ˌblæstə(ʊ)ˈmaɪsiːz] *subst.* type of parasitic fungus which affects the skin *Blastomyces*

blastomycosis [ˌblæstəʊmaɪˈkəʊsɪs] *subst.* infection caused by Blastomyces *blastomykos, sackaromykos*

blastomykos ⇨ **blastomycosis**

blastula [ˈblæstjʊlə] *subst.* first stage of the development of an embryo in animals *blastula*

bleb [bleb] *subst.* small blister *liten blåsa, blemma; compare* BULLA

bled [bled] *see* bleed

bleed [bliːd] *vb.* to lose blood *blöda;* **his knee was bleeding; his nose began to bleed; when she cut her finger it bled; he was bleeding from a cut on the head** NOTE: **bleeds - bleeding - bled - has bled**

bleeder [ˈbliːdə] *subst.* person who suffers from haemophilia *blödarsjuk (person)*

bleeding [ˈbliːdɪŋ] *subst.* abnormal loss of blood from the body through the skin or internally *blödning;* **bleeding point** *or* **bleeding site** = place in the body where bleeding is taking place *blödningskälla;* **bleeding time** = test of clotting of a patient's blood, by timing the length of time it takes for the blood to congeal *blödningstid;* **control of bleeding** = ways of stopping bleeding by applying pressure to blood vessels *blödningskontroll;* **internal bleeding** = loss of blood inside the body (as from a wound in the intestine) *inre blödning*

> COMMENT: blood lost through bleeding from an artery is bright red, and can rush out because it is under pressure. Blood from a vein is darker red and flows more slowly

blefarit ⇨ **blepharitis**

blefaroptos ⇨ **blepharoptosis**

blefarospasm ⇨ **blepharospasm**

bleforrafi ⇨ **tarsorrhaphy**

blek ⇨ **pale**

blekfet ⇨ **flabby**

blekhet ⇨ **paleness, pallor**

blekna ⇨ **pale**

blemma ⇨ **bleb, papule, pimple**

blenno- ['blenəʊ, ˌ--] *prefix* referring to mucus *blenn(o)-, slem-*

blennorrhagia [ˌblenəʊ'reɪdʒ(i)ə] *subst.* (i) discharge of mucus *blenorragi;* (ii) gonorrhoea *gonorré*

blennorrhoea [ˌblenə'rɪə] *subst.* (i) discharge of watery mucus *blenorré;* (ii) gonorrhoea *gonorré*

blenorragi ⇨ **blennorrhagia**

blenorré ⇨ **blennorrhoea**

blephar- ['blefə, ˌ--] *prefix* referring to the eyelids *blefar(o)-, ögonlocks-*

blepharitis [ˌblefə'raɪtɪs] *subst.* inflammation of the eyelid *blefarit, ögonlocksinflammation*

blepharon ['blefərɒn] *subst.* eyelid *blepharon, ögonlocket*

blepharon ⇨ **eyelid**

blepharoptosis [ˌblefərəʊ'təʊsɪs] *subst.* condition where the upper eyelid is half closed because of paralysis of the muscle or nerve *blefaroptos*

blepharospasm ['blefərəʊˌspæz(ə)m] *subst.* sudden contraction of the eyelid, as when a tiny piece of dust gets in the eye *blefarospasm, ögonlockskramp*

blind [blaɪnd] **1** *adj.* not able to see *blind;* **a blind man with a white stick; after her illness she became blind; colour blind** = not able to tell the difference between certain colours, especially red and green *färgblind;* **blind spot** = point in the retina where the optic nerve joins it, which does not register light *blinda fläcken;* **blind loop syndrome** *see* LOOP **2** *subst.* **the blind** = people who are blind *de blinda;* **blind register** = official list of blind people *officiellt register över blinda i Storbritannien* **3** *vb.* to make someone blind *blända, göra blind;* **he was blinded in the accident**

blind ⇨ **blind**

blinda fläcken ⇨ **blind**

blindhet ⇨ **blindness**

blindness ['blaɪndnəs] *subst.* not being able to see *blindhet;* **colour blindness** = not being able to tell the difference between certain colours *färgblindhet;* **day blindness** *or* **hemeralopia** = being able to see better in poor light than in ordinary daylight *hemeralopi, dagblindhet;* **night blindness** *or* **nyctalopia** = being unable to see in bad light *nyktalopi, nattblindhet;* **snow blindness** = temporary blindness caused by bright sunlight shining on snow *ophthalmia nivalis, snöblindhet;* **sun blindness** *or* **photoretinitis** = damage done to the retina by looking at the sun *solblindhet*

blindskrift ⇨ **Braille**

blindtablett ⇨ **placebo**

blindtarmen ⇨ **caecum**

"blindtarmen" ⇨ **appendix, vermiform, vermix**

blindtarmsinflammation ⇨ **appendicitis**

blindtarmsinflammation, egentlig ⇨ **typhlitis**

blindtarmsoperation ⇨ **-ectomy**

blink [blɪŋk] *vb.* to close and open the eyelids rapidly *or* to make the eyelids move rapidly to cover the eye once *blinka;* **he blinked in the bright light**

blinka ⇨ **blink, wink**

blinkning ⇨ **nictation**

blister ['blɪstə] **1** *subst.* (i) swelling on the skin containing serous liquid *blåsa;* (ii) substance which acts as a counterirritant *ämne som ger upphov till ytlig irritation, vilken verkar smärtlindrande* **2** *vb.* to have blisters *få (ha) blåsor;* **after the fire his hands and face were badly blistered**

COMMENT: blisters contain serum, or watery liquid from the blood. They can be caused by rubbing, burning or by a disease such as chickenpox. Blood blisters contain blood which has passed from broken blood vessels under the skin. Water blisters contain lymph

blivande mor ⇨ **expectant mother**

block [blɒk] **1** *subst.* **(a)** stopping of a function *block(ad), hinder, stopp;* **caudal block** = local analgesia of the cauda equina nerves in the lower spine *kaudalblockad;* **epidural block** = analgesia produced by injecting an analgesic solution into the space between the vertebral canal and the dura mater *epiduralblockad, epiduralanestesi, epiduralbedövning;* **heart block** = slowing of the action of the heart because of damage to the conducting system which takes impulses from the SA node to the ventricle *hjärtblock;* **mental block** = temporary inability to remember something due to nervous effect on the mental processes *mental blockering (hämning);* **nerve block** = stopping the function of a nerve by injection of an anaesthetic *nervblockad;* **speech block** = temporary inability to speak, caused by a nervous effect on mental processes *talblockering, talhämning;* **spinal block** = reduction of pain by injection of the spinal cord with an anaesthetic *spinalblockad* **(b)** large piece *block, kloss;* **a block of wood fell on his foot (c)** one of the different buildings forming a section of a hospital *byggnad(skomplex), kvarter;* **the patient is in Ward 7, Block 2; she is having treatment in the physiotherapy block 2** *vb.* to stop something moving *blockera, spärra (stänga) av, täppa till, hindra;* **the artery was blocked by a clot; he swallowed a piece of plastic which blocked his oesophagus**

block ⇨ **pulley**

blockad ⇨ **block**

blockage ['blɒkɪdʒ] *subst.* thing which blocks *hinder, stopp;* being blocked *blockering;* **there is a blockage in the rectum**

blocker ['blɒkə] *subst.* substance which blocks *block(er)are, antagonist;* **beta blocker** = drug which blocks the beta-adrenergic receptors and so reduces the activity of the heart *betablockerare, beta(receptor)blockare*

blockera ⇨ **block, obstruct**

blockering ⇨ **blockage, blocking, inhibition, occlusion**

blocking ['blɒkɪŋ] *subst.* psychiatric disorder, where the patient suddenly stops one train of thought and switches to another *blockering*

blod ⇨ **blood**

blod- ⇨ **haem-, sanguineous**

blodbank ⇨ **blood**

blodbildande ⇨ **haematogenous**

blodbildning ⇨ **blood, haemopoiesis**

blodbrist ⇨ **anaemia, erythropenia, hyphaemia**

blodbrist, lokal ⇨ **ischaemia**

blodbråck ⇨ **haematocoele**

blodcirkulationen ⇨ **circulation (of the blood)**

blodcylindrar ⇨ **blood**

blodfattig ⇨ **anaemic**

blodfull ⇨ **plethoric, sanguineous**

blodförgiftning ⇨ **bacteraemia, blood, sepsis, toxaemia**

blodförgiftning, allmän ⇨ **pyaemia**

blodförlust ⇨ **blood**

blodförsörjning ⇨ **arterial**

blodgivare ⇨ **blood**

blodgrupp ⇨ **blood group**

blodgruppering ⇨ **group**

blodgruppsbestämning ⇨ **group**

blod-hjärnbarriären ⇨ **blood-brain barrier**

blodig ⇨ **bloodstained**

blodigel ⇨ **leech**

blodkoagulation ⇨ **blood**

blodkoagulationstid ⇨ **clotting**

blodkropp ⇨ **blood**

blodkroppsräkning ⇨ **blood**

blodkräkning ⇨ **haematemesis**

blodkärl ⇨ **blood**

blodkärls- ⇨ **vas-, vascular, vaso-**

blodlever ⇨ **clot, coagulum**

blodlever- ⇨ **thrombo-**

blododling ⇨ **blood**

blodomloppet ⇨ **circulation (of the blood)**

blodparasit ⇨ **haematozoon**

blodplasma ⇨ **blood**

blodplatta ⇨ **blood, platelet**

blodplätt ⇨ **blood, platelet**

blodpropp ⇨ **arterial, clot, embolus, thrombus, thrombosis**

blodproppsupplösande ⇨ **thrombolytic**

blodprov ⇨ **blood**

blodsband ⇨ **consanguinity**

blodserum ⇨ **blood**

blodsinus ⇨ **sinus**

blodsockernivå ⇨ **glucose, sugar**

blodsockernivå, normal ⇨ **glycaemia**

blodspottning ⇨ **haemoptysis**

blodstatus ⇨ **blood, chemistry**

blodstillande (medel) ⇨ **styptic**

blodstillning ⇨ **haemostasis**

blodstockning ⇨ **congestion, engorgement, haemostasis, stasis**

blodström ⇨ **bloodstream**

blodsänkningsreaktion ⇨ **erythrocyte, sedimentation**

blodtappning ⇨ **exsanguination**

blodtillblandad ⇨ **bloodstained**

blodtransfusion ⇨ **blood**

blodtryck ⇨ **blood pressure**

blodtryck, normalt ⇨ **normotension**

blodtrycksmanschett ⇨ **cuff**

blodtrycksmätare ⇨ **sphygmomanometer**

blodtryckssänkande (medel) ⇨ **antihypertensive**

blodupphostning ⇨ **haemoptysis**

blodvallning ⇨ **flush**

blodvolym ⇨ **volume**

blodåder ⇨ **vein**

blodåder- ⇨ **vene-, venous**

blodöverfyllnad ⇨ **congestion, engorgement**

blomkålsöra ⇨ **cauliflower ear**

blond ⇨ **fair, light**

blood [blʌd] *subst.* red liquid in the body *blod;* **the police followed the spots of blood to find the wounded man; blood was pouring from the cut in his hand; he suffered serious loss of blood** *or* **blood loss in the accident; blood bank** = section of a hospital where blood given by donors is stored for use in transfusions *blodbank;* **blood casts** = pieces of blood cells which are secreted by the kidneys in kidney disease *blodcylindrar, rester av blodkroppar som utsöndras av njurarna vid njursjukdom;* **blood cell** *or* **blood corpuscle** = cell (red blood cell *or* white blood cell) which is one of the parts of blood *blodkropp;* **blood chemistry** = substances which make up blood, which can be analysed in blood tests, the results of which are useful in diagnosing disease *blodstatus;* **blood clot** *or* **thrombus** = mass of coagulated blood in a vein or artery *tromb, blodpropp;* **blood**

clotting *or* **blood coagulation** = process where the blood changes from being liquid to being solid and so stops bleeding *blodkoagulation;* **blood count** = test to count the number of different blood cells in a certain quantity of blood *blodkroppsräkning, blodstatus;* **blood culture** = putting a sample of blood into a culture medium to see if foreign organisms in it grow *blododling;* **blood donor** = person who gives blood which is then used in transfusions to other patients *blodgivare;* **blood formation** *or* **haemopoiesis** = the continual production of new blood cells *hemopo(i)es, hematopo(i)es, blodbildning;* **blood letting** *or* **venesection** = opening of an artery *or* vein to take away blood *venesektion, flebotomi, åderlåtning;* **blood loss** = loss of blood from the body by bleeding *blodförlust;* **blood plasma** = watery liquid which forms the greatest part of blood *blodplasma;* **blood platelet** = small blood cell which releases thromboplastin and which multiplies rapidly after an injury *trombocyt, blodplätt, blodplatta;* **blood poisoning** *or* **septicaemia** = condition where bacteria are present in blood and cause illness *septikemi, sepsis, blodförgiftning;* **blood serum** = watery liquid which separates from coagulated blood *blodserum, serum;* **blood sugar level** = amount of glucose in the blood *blodsockernivå, B-glukosnivå;* **blood test** = laboratory test to find the chemical composition of a patient's blood *blodprov;* **blood transfusion** = giving a patient blood from another person *blodtransfusion;* **blood type** = BLOOD GROUP; **blood urea** = urea present in the blood (a high level occurs following heart failure or kidney disease *urea i blodet;* **blood vessel** = any tube (artery *or* vein *or* capillary) which carries blood round the body *blodkärl* NOTE: for other terms referring to blood vessels, see words beginning with **anglo-** NOTE: for other terms referring to blood, see words beginning with **haem-, haemato-**

COMMENT: blood is formed of red and white corpuscles, platelets and plasma. It circulates round the body, going from the heart and lungs along arteries and returns to the heart through the veins. As it moves round the body it takes oxygen to the tissues and removes waste material which is cleaned out through the kidneys or exhaled through the lungs. It also carries hormones produced by glands to the various organs which need them. Each adult person has about six litres or ten pints of blood in his body.

blood-brain barrier ['blʌdbreɪn ˌbæriə] *subst.* process by which certain substances are held back by the endothelium of cerebral capillaries (where in other parts of the body the same substances will diffuse from capillaries) so preventing these substances from getting into contact with the fluids round the brain *blod-hjärnbarriären*

blood group ['blʌd gru:p] *subst.* one of the different types of blood by which groups of people are identified *blodgrupp*

COMMENT: blood is classified in various ways. The most common classifications are by the agglutinogens in red blood corpuscles (factors A and B) and by the Rhesus factor. Blood can therefore have either factor (Group A and Group B), or both factors (Group AB) or neither (Group O), and each of these groups can be Rhesus negative or positive

blood pressure ['blʌd ˌpreʃə] *subst.* pressures (measured in millimetres of mercury) at which the blood is pumped round the body by the heart *blodtryck*

COMMENT: blood pressure is measured using a sphygmomanometer, where a rubber tube is wrapped round the patient's arm and blown up. Two readings of blood pressure are taken: the systolic pressure, when the heart is contracting and so pumping out, and the diastolic pressure (which is always a lower figure) when the heart relaxes

QUOTE raised blood pressure may account for as many as 70% of all strokes. The risk of stroke rises with both systolic and diastolic blood pressure in the normotensive and hypertensive ranges. Blood pressure control reduces the incidence of first stroke and aspirin appears to reduce the risk of stroke after TIAs

British Journal of Hospital Medicine

bloodstained ['blʌdsteɪnd] *adj.* stained with traces of blood *blodig, blodtillblandad, blodfläckad;* **he coughed up bloodstained sputum; the nurses took away the bloodstained sheets**

bloodstream ['blʌdstri:m] *subst.* blood flowing round the body *blodström;* **the antibiotics are injected into the bloodstream; hormones are secreted by the glands into the bloodstream**

blossande ⇨ **flushed**

blot [blɒt] *see* RORSCHACH

blotta ⇨ **expose**

blue [blu:] *adj. & subst.* a colour like the colour of the sky in the daytime *blå;* **the sister was dressed in a blue uniform; blue baby** = baby suffering from congenital cyanosis, born either with a congenital heart defect or with atelectasis (a collapsed lung), which prevents

an adequate supply of oxygen reaching the tissues, giving the baby's skin a bluish colour *blue baby*
NOTE: **blue - bluer - bluest**

Blue Cross [ˌbluː 'krɒs] *or* **Blue Shield** [ˌbluː 'ʃiːld] *subst. US* systems of private medical insurance *slags sjukförsäkringssystem i USA*

blueness ['bluːnəs] *or* **blue disease** [ˌbluː dɪ'ziːz] *or* **cyanosis** [ˌsaɪə'nəʊsɪs] *subst.* blue colour of the skin, a symptom of lack of oxygen in the blood *cyanos*

blunt [blʌnt] *adj.* not sharp *or* which does not cut well *slö, trubbig;* **he hurt his hand with a blunt knife; the surgeon's instruments must not be blunt**
NOTE: **blunt - blunter - bluntest**

blurred [blɜːd] *adj.* not clear *oskarp, suddig;* **blurred vision** = condition where the patient does not see objects clearly *suddig (oskarp) syn*

blurring of vision [ˌblɜːrɪŋ əv 'vɪʒ(ə)n] *subst.* condition where a patient does not see clearly, caused by loss of blood or sometimes by inadequate diet *suddig (oskarp) syn, oskärpa*

blush [blʌʃ] **1** *subst.* rush of red colour to the skin of the face (caused by emotion) *rodnad* **2** *vb.* to go red in the face because of emotion *rodna*

bly ⇨ **lead**

blyfri ⇨ **lead-free**

blyförgiftning ⇨ **lead poisoning, plumbism, saturnism**

blygd- ⇨ **pubic, pudendal**

blygdbenet ⇨ **pubic, pubis**

blygdbensfogen ⇨ **interpubic joint**

blygdbenskammen ⇨ **pecten**

blygden ⇨ **pubes, pudendum, vulva**

blygdhår ⇨ **public**

blygdläpp ⇨ **labium**

blykolik ⇨ **painter's colic**

blysöm ⇨ **lead**

blå ⇨ **blue, livid**

blå- ⇨ **cyano-**

blåblindhet ⇨ **tritanopia**

blåmärke ⇨ **bruise, contusion, ecchymosis, haematoma**

blåsa ⇨ **bag, bladder, blister, bulla**

blåsa, liten ⇨ **phlyctenule, vesicle**

blåsbildning ⇨ **vesiculation**

blåsdermatos ⇨ **pompholyx**

blåsdragande medel ⇨ **vesicant**

blåshalskörtelinflammation ⇨ **prostatitis**

blåshalskörteln ⇨ **prostate (gland)**

blåskatarr ⇨ **cystitis**

blåsljud ⇨ **bruit, heart, souffle**

blåsmask ⇨ **bladder worm**

blåsmasksjuka ⇨ **echinococciasis**

blåsmola ⇨ **hydatidiform mole**

blåsyra ⇨ **cyanide, hydrocyanic acid**

blått öga ⇨ **black**

blända ⇨ **blind**

blöda ⇨ **bleed**

blödarsjuk ⇨ **haemophiliac**

blödning ⇨ **bleeding**

blödning, kraftig ⇨ **haemorrhage**

blödning, ockult ⇨ **occult**

blödningskontroll ⇨ **bleeding**

blödningskälla ⇨ **bleeding**

blödningstid ⇨ **bleeding**

blöja ⇨ **diaper, napkin, nappy**

blöjdermatit ⇨ **rash**

blöjeksem ⇨ **rash**

blöt ⇨ **wet**

blöta ⇨ **soak**

BM [ˌbiːˈem] = BACHELOR OF MEDICINE

BMA [ˌbiːemˈeɪ] = BRITISH MEDICAL ASSOCIATION

BMB ⇨ **basal**

BMR [ˌbiːemˈɑː] = BASAL METABOLIC RATE; **BMR test** = test of thyroid function *basalmetabolism, BMB*

BO [ˌbiːˈəʊ] = BODY ODOUR

bodily [ˈbɒdɪli] *adj.* referring to the body *kroppslig, kropps-, fysisk;* **the main bodily functions are controlled by the sympathetic nervous system; he suffered from several minor bodily disorders**

body [ˈbɒdi] *subst.* **(a)** the trunk *or* main part of a person, not including the head and arms and legs *bålen* **(b)** all of a person (as opposed to the mind) *kropp;* **the dead man's body was found several days later; body fat** = adipose tissue *or* tissue where the cells contain fat, which replaces normal fibrous tissue when too much food is eaten *fettväv(nad), kroppsfett;* **body fluids** = liquid in the body, including mainly water and blood *kroppsvätskor;* **body image** *or* **body schema** = the mental image which a person has of his own body *kroppsbild;* **body odour** = smell caused by perspiration *kroppslukt, kroppsodör;* **body scan** = X-ray examination of a patient's body *(hel)kroppscint(igrafi);* **body temperature** = internal temperature of the human body (normally about 37°C) *kroppstemperatur* **(c)** mass *or* piece of material (of any size) *kropp;* **pineal body** *or* **pineal gland** = small cone-shaped gland on the third ventricle of the brain, believed to have a connection with the development of the sex glands *corpus pineale, tallkottkörteln;* **cell body** = part of a nerve cell which surrounds the nucleus and from which the axon and dendrites leave *cellkropp;* **ciliary body** = part of the eye which connects the iris to the choroid *corpus ciliare, ciliarkroppen;* **inclusion bodies** = minute particles in cells infected by a virus *inklusionskroppar, lysomer;* **Nissl bodies** *or* **Nissl granules** = granules surrounding the nucleus of nerve cells *Nisslpartiklar, Nisslsubstans* **(d)** main part of something *huvuddel, viktigaste del, stomme;* **body of sternum** = main central part of the breastbone *corpus sterni;* **body of vertebra** = main part of a vertebra which supports the weight of the body *corpus vertebrae;* **body of the stomach** = main part of the stomach between the fundus and the pylorus ⇨ *illustration* STOMACH *corpus ventriculi* **(e) foreign body** = piece of material which is not part of the surrounding tissue and should not be there *främmande kropp;* **the X-ray showed the presence of a foreign body; swallowed foreign bodies** = anything (a pin *or* coin *or* button) which should not have been swallowed *nedsvalda främmande kroppar (föremål)*

Boeck's disease [ˈbeks dɪˈziːz] *or* **Boeck's sarcoid** [ˈbeks ˌsɑːkɔɪd] = SARCOIDOSIS

Bohn's nodules [ˈbɔːnz ˌnɒdjuːlz] *or* **Bohn's epithelial pearls** [ˈbɔːnz ˌepɪˈθiːliəl ˈpɜːlz] *subst pl.* tiny cysts found in the mouths of healthy infants *slags små cystor som uppträder i munnen på friska spädbarn*

boil [bɔɪl] **1** *subst.* furuncle *or* tender raised mass of infected tissue and skin, usually caused by staphylococcal infection of a hair follicle *furunkel, böld* **2** *vb.* to heat water (or another liquid) until it changes into gas *koka; (of water, etc.)* to change into a gas because of heating *koka;* **can you boil some water so we can sterilize the instruments?**

boll ⇨ **ball, bolus**

bolus [ˈbəʊləs] *subst.* food which has been chewed and is ready to be swallowed *or* mass of food passing along the intestine *bolus, boll*

bomull ⇨ **cotton**

bomullstopp ⇨ **swab**

bonding [ˈbɒndɪŋ] *subst.* making a psychological link between the baby and its mother *bindning;* **in autistic children bonding is difficult**

bone [bəʊn] *subst.* **(a)** one of the calcified pieces of connective tissue which make the skeleton *ben;* **he fell over and broke a bone in his ankle; there are several small bones in the human ear; cranial bones** = bones of the skull ⇨ *illustration* SKULL *skallbenen;* **metacarpal bones** = bones of the hand ⇨ *illustration* HAND *ossa metacarpalia, metakarpalbenen, mellanhandsbenen* **(b)** hard substance which forms a bone *ben(vävnad);* **compact bone** *or* **dense bone** = type of bone tissue which forms the hard outer layer of a bone ⇨ *illustration* BONE STRUCTURE *pars compacta, kompakt ben(vävnad);* **spongy bone** *or* **cancellous bone** = bone tissue which forms the inner part of a bone, containing the marrow ⇨ *illustration* BONE STRUCTURE *pars spongiosa, porös benvävnad, spongiöst ben;* **bone conduction** *see* CONDUCTION; **bone graft** = piece of bone taken from one part of the body to repair a defect in another bone *bentransplantat;* **bone structure** = (i) system of jointed bones as it forms the body *skelettet;* (ii) the arrangement of the various components of a bone *benstruktur*

COMMENT: bones are formed of a hard outer layer (compact bone) which is made up of a series of layers of tissue (Haversian systems) and a softer inner part (cancellous *or* spongy bone) which contains bone marrow

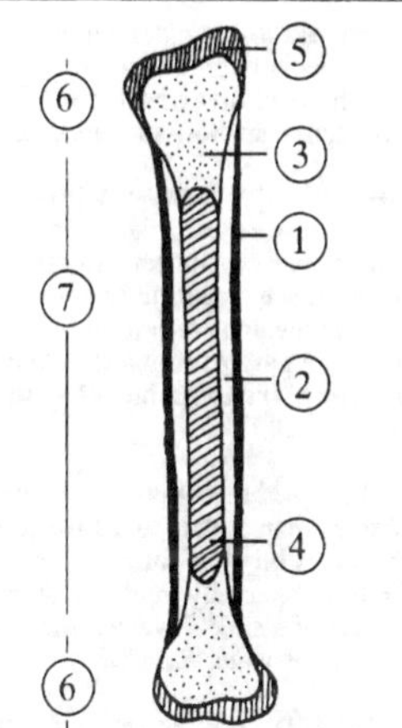

BONE STRUCTURE	BENSTRUKTUR
1. periosteum	1. periost, (yttre) benhinnan
2. compact bone	2. kompakt ben
3. cancellous (spongy) bone (red marrow)	3. poröst (spongiöst) ben (röd benmärg)
4. medullary cavity (yellow marrow)	4. märghåla (gul benmärg)
5. articular cartilage	5. ledbrosk
6. epiphysis	6. epifys, ändstycke
7. diaphysis	7. diafys, skaft

bone marrow ['bəʊn ˌmærəʊ] *subst.* soft tissue in cancellous bone *benmärg, märg;* **bone marrow transplant** = transplant of marrow from a donor to a recipient *benmärgstransplantat*

COMMENT: two types of bone marrow are to be found: red bone marrow *or* myeloid tissue, which forms red blood cells and is found in cancellous bone; as a person gets older, fatty yellow bone marrow develops in the central cavity of long bones

NOTE: for other terms referring to bone marrow, see words beginning with **myel-, myelo-**

Bonney's blue ['bɒnɪz ˌbluː] *subst.* blue dye used as a disinfectant *slags blått desinfektionsmedel*

bony ['bəʊni] *adj.* (i) referring to bones *ben-;* (ii) part of the body which shows the structure of the bones underneath *benig, knotig;* **she has long bony hands; bony labyrinth** = hard part of the temporal bone surrounding the inner ear *labyrinthus osseus, benlabyrinten*

NOTE: for other terms referring to bone, see words beginning with **ost-, osteo-**

boosterdos ▷ **booster (injection)**

booster (injection) ['buːstə(rɪnˌdʒekʃ(ə)n)] *subst.* repeat injection of vaccine given some time after the first injection so as to keep the immunizing effect *boosterdos*

boot [buːt] *subst.* strong shoe which goes above the ankle *känga, stövel;* **surgical boot** = specially made boot for a person who has a deformed foot *ortopedisk känga*

boracic acid [bəˌræsɪk 'æsɪd] *or* **boric acid** [ˌbɔːrɪk 'æsɪd] *subst.* soluble white powder, which is used as a general disinfectant *borsyra*

borax ['bɔːræks] *subst.* white powder used as a household cleanser and disinfectant *borax*

borborygmus [ˌbɔːbə'rɪgməs] *subst.* rumbling noise in the the abdomen, caused by gas in the intestine *borborygmi (jfr meteorism), kurr i magen*

NOTE: plural is **borborygmi**

border ['bɔːdə] *subst.* edge *kant, rand;* **vermilion border** = external red parts of the lips *rubor labii, läppsömmen*

Bordetella [ˌbɔːdə'telə] *subst.* bacteria of the family Brucellaceae (**Bordetella pertussis** causes whooping cough) *Bordetella, kikhostebakterie*

boric acid [ˌbɔːrɪk 'æsɪd] *see* BORACIC ACID

born [bɔːn] *vb.* **to be born** = to begin to live outside the mother's womb *född;* **he was born in Germany; she was born in 1963**

NOTE: **born** is usually only used with **was** or **were**

Bornholm disease ['bɔːnhəʊm dɪˌziːz] *or* **epidemic pleurodynia** [ˌepɪ'demɪk ˌplʊərəʊ'daɪniə] *see* PLEURODYNIA

bornholmssjuka ▷ **pleurodynia**

borr ▷ **burr, drill**

borra ▷ **drill**

borrkropp ▷ **Trypanosoma**

borsta ⇨ **brush, clean**

borsyra ⇨ **boracic acid**

bortförande ⇨ **deferent, efferent**

bortskärning ⇨ **excision, resection**

bortslitande ⇨ **avulsion**

bortstötning ⇨ **rejection**

borttagande ⇨ **extirpation, removal, withdrawal**

bortträngning ⇨ **repression**

borttynande ⇨ **cadaveric, wasting**

bostad ⇨ **domicile**

bota ⇨ **cure**

botande ⇨ **curative, remedial**

botemedel ⇨ **corrective, cure, remedy**

bother ['bɒðə] **1** *subst.* thing which is annoying or worrying *besvär, bråk;* **the new government instructions have caused a lot of bother 2** *vb.* (i) to take trouble to do something *göra sig besvär, bry sig;* (ii) to worry about something *oroa sig, plåga, besvära;* **she didn't bother to send a telegram; don't bother about cleaning the room; smoke bothers him because he has asthma**

botten ⇨ **bottom, fundus**

bottensats ⇨ **sediment**

bottle ['bɒt(ə)l] *subst.* glass container for liquids *flaska;* **he drinks a bottle of milk a day; open another bottle of orange juice; baby's (feeding) bottle** = special bottle with a rubber teat, used for giving milk (or other liquids) to babies *nappflaska;* **bottle feeding** = giving a baby milk from a bottle, as opposed to the mother's breast *flaskuppfödning; compare* BREAST FEEDING

bottom ['bɒtəm] *subst.* **(a)** lowest part *botten, underdel;* **there was some jam left in the bottom of the jar (b)** part of your body on which you sit *stjärten, sätet; see also* BUTTOCKS

botulism ['bɒtjuˌlɪz(ə)m] *subst.* type of food poisoning, caused by a toxin of **Clostridium botulinum** in badly canned or preserved food *botulism*

> COMMENT: the symptoms include paralysis of the muscles, vomiting and hallucinations. Botulism is often fatal

bougie ['bu:ʒi:] *subst.* thin tube which can be inserted into passages in the body (such as the oesophagus *or* rectum) either to allow liquid to be introduced, or simply to dilate the passage *bougie*

bout [baʊt] *subst.* sudden attack of a disease, especially one which recurs *anfall, "släng";* **he is recovering from a bout of flu; she has recurrent bouts of malarial fever**

bowel ['baʊəl] *or* **bowels** ['baʊəlz] *subst.* the intestine, especially the large intestine *tarmen, tarmarna;* **bowel movement** = defecation *or* evacuation of solid waste matter from the anus *tarmtömning, defekation, avföring;* **the patient had a bowel movement this morning; irritable bowel syndrome** = MUCOUS COLITIS

bowl [bəʊl] *subst.* **(a)** wide container with higher sides than a plate, used for semi-liquids *skål, bunke;* **a bowl of soup** *or* **of cream; soup bowl** = bowl specially made for soup *soppskål* **(b)** the part of a sink *or* wash basin *or* toilet which contains water *handfat*

bow-legged ['bəʊleg(ɪ)d] *adj.* with bow legs *hjulbent*

bow legs ['bəʊ legz] *or* **genu varum** [ˌdʒenju: 'veərəm] *subst.* condition where the ankles touch and the knees are apart when a person is standing straight *genu varum, hjulbenthet, O-benthet*

Bowman's capsule ['bəʊmənz ˌkæpsju:l] *or* **Malpighian glomerulus** [mælˌpɪgiən gləʊ'meruləs] *subst.* expanded end of a renal tubule, surrounding a glomerular tuft *Bowmans kapsel*

boxaröra ⇨ **cauliflower ear**

boy [bɔɪ] *subst.* male child *pojke;* **they have three children - two boys and a girl; the boys were playing in the field**

BP [ˌbi:'pi:] = BLOOD PRESSURE, BRITISH PHARMACOPOEIA

bq [ˌbi:'kju:] *abbreviation for* becquerel, a measurement of radiation *Bq, becquerel*

Br *chemical symbol for* bromine *Br, brom*

bra ⇨ **all right, fine, well**

brace [breɪs] *subst.* any type of splint *or* appliance worn for support, such as a metal support used on children's legs to make the bones straight *or* on teeth which are forming badly *stöd, spjäla, skena, korsett, tandställning;* **she wore a brace on her front teeth**

bracelet ['breɪslət] *subst.* chain *or* band which is worn around the wrist *armband;* **identity bracelet** = label attached to the wrist of a newborn baby *or* patient in hospital, so that he can be identified *identitetsband, ID-band*

brachi- ['breɪki, ,--] *prefix* referring to the arm *brachi-, braki-, arm-*

brachial ['breɪkiəl] *adj.* referring to the arm, especially the upper arm *brakial, arm-;* **brachial artery** = artery running from the axillary artery to the elbow, where it divides into the radial and ulnar arteries *arteria brachialis, armartären;* **brachial plexus** = group of nerves at the armpit which lead to the nerves in the arms and hands (injury to the brachial plexus at birth leads to Erb's palsy) *plexus brachialis, armplexus, armflätan;* **brachial pressure point** = point on the arm where pressure will stop bleeding from the brachial artery *ställe på armen där tryck får blödning från armartären att upphöra;* **brachial veins** = veins accompanying the brachial artery, draining into the axillary vein *venae brachiales*

brachialis muscle [breɪ'kaɪəlɪs ,mʌs(ə)l] *subst.* flexor of the elbow *musculus brachialis, armböjaren*

brachiocephalic artery [,breɪkiəʊsə'fælɪk ,ɑːt(ə)ri] *subst.* largest branch of the arch of the aorta, which continues as the right common carotid and the right subclavian arteries *arteria brachiocephalica, "namnlösa artären"*

brachiocephalic veins [,breɪkiəʊsə'fælɪk ,veɪnz] *subst.* innominate veins *or* veins which continue the subclavian and jugular veins to the superior vena cava *vena brachiocephalica dextra resp. sinistra*

brachium ['breɪkiəm] *subst.* arm, especially the upper arm between the elbow and the shoulder *brachium, armen, överarmen*
NOTE: plural is **brachia**

brachy- ['bræki, ,--] *prefix* short *brachy-, braky-, kort-*

brachycephaly [,bræki'sefəli] *subst.* condition where the skull is shorter than normal *brakycefali(sm), kortskallighet*

Bradford's frame ['brædfədz ,freɪm] *subst.* frame of metal and cloth, used to support a patient *slags lift*

brady- ['brædi, ,--] *prefix* slow *brady-, långsam*

bradycardia [,brædi'kɑːdiə] *subst.* slow rate of heart contraction, shown by a slow pulse rate (less than 70 per minute) *bradykardi*

bradykardi ⇨ **bradycardia**

bradykinesia [,brædikə'niːziə] *subst.* walking slowly *or* making slow movements (because of disease) *bradykinesi*

bradypné ⇨ **bradypnoea**

bradypnoea [,brædi'niə] *subst.* abnormally slow breathing *bradypné*

Braille [breɪ(ə)l] *subst.* system of writing using raised dots on the paper to indicate letters, which allows a blind person to read by passing his fingers over the paper *Braille(s alfabet), blindskrift;* **she was reading a Braille book; the book has been published in Braille**

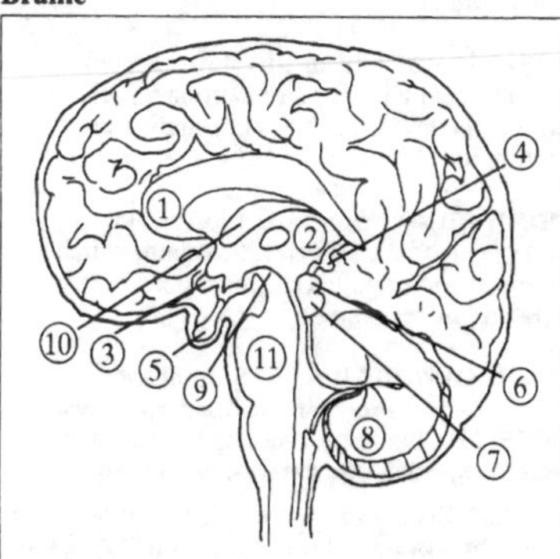

BRAIN	HJÄRNAN
1. corpus callosum	1. hjärnbalken
2. thalamus	2. talamus
3. hypothalamus	3. hypotalamus
4. pineal body	4. epifysen, tallkottkörteln
5. pituitary gland	5. hypofysen
6. superior colliculi	6. collicus superior, övre kullen
7. inferior colliculi	7. collicus inferior, nedre kullen
8. cerebellum	8. lillhjärnan
9. cerebral peduncle	9. hjärnskänklarna, hjärnstjälkarna
10. fornix	10. hjärnvalvet
11. pons	11. hjärnbryggan

brain [breɪn] *or* **encephalon** [en'kefəlɒn] *subst.* cranial part of the central nervous system, situated inside the skull *encefalon, hjärnan;* **brain death** = condition where the nerves in the brain stem have died, and the patient can be certified as dead, although the heart may not have stopped beating *hjärndöd;* **brain haemorrhage** = bleeding inside the brain from a burst blood vessel *hemorrhagia cerebri, hjärnblödning; see also* FOREBRAIN, HINDBRAIN, MIDBRAIN

COMMENT: the main part of the brain is the cerebrum, formed of two sections or hemispheres, which relate to thought and to sensations from either side of the body; at the back of the head and beneath the cerebrum is the cerebellum which coordinates muscle reaction and balance. Also in the brain are the hypothalamus which governs body temperature, hunger, thirst and sexual urges, and the tiny pituitary gland which is the most important endocrine gland in the body

brain damage ['breɪn ˌdæmɪdʒ] *subst.* damage caused to the brain in an accident *hjärnskada;* **he suffered brain damage in the car crash**

brain-damaged ['breɪnˌdæmɪdʒd] *adj.* (person) who has suffered brain damage *hjärnskadad*

brain fever ['breɪn ˌfiːvə] *subst.* non-medical term for an infection which affects the brain (such as encephalitis or meningitis) *hjärnfeber*

brain stem ['breɪn ˌstem] *subst.* lower part of the brain, shaped like a stem, which connects the brain to the spinal cord *truncus cerebri, hjärnstammen*

brain tumour ['breɪn ˌtjuːmə] *subst.* tumour which grows in the brain *hjärntumör*
NOTE: for other terms referring to brain, see words beginning with **cerebr-, encephal-**

COMMENT: tumours may grow in any part of the brain. The symptoms of brain tumour are usually headaches and dizziness, and as the tumour grows it may affect the senses or mental faculties. Operations to remove brain tumours can be very successful

brakial ⇨ **brachial**

branch [brɑːn(t)ʃ] **1** *subst.* (i) part of a tree growing out of the main trunk *gren;* (ii) any part which grows out of a main part *gren, förgrening* **2** *vb.* to split out into smaller parts *(för)grena sig;* **the radial artery branches from the brachial artery at the elbow**

branchial cyst ['bræŋkiəl ˌsist] *or* **branchial fistula** ['bræŋkiəl ˌfɪstjʊlə] *subst.* cyst on the side of the neck of an embryo *gälgångscysta, gälgångsfistel*

branchial pouch ['bræŋkiəl ˌpaʊtʃ] *subst.* pouch on the side of the neck of an embryo *gälspringan*

brand ⇨ **gangrene**

brandskorpa ⇨ **eschar**

Braun's frame ['braʊnz ˌfreɪm] *or* **splint** [splɪnt] *subst.* metal splint and frame to which pulleys are attached, used for holding up a fractured leg while a patient is lying in bed *slags beställning för sängliggande patient*

bread [bred] *subst.* food made by baking flour and yeast *bröd*

break [breɪk] **1** *subst.* point at which a bone has broken *fraktur, brott, benbrott;* **a clean break** = break in a bone which is not complicated *or* where the two parts will join again easily *okomplicerat (ben)brott* **2** *vb.* to make something go to pieces *bryta (av, sönder);* to go to pieces *brytas (av), gå sönder;* **she fell off the wall and broke her leg; he can't play football with a broken leg** NOTE: **breaks - breaking - broke - has broken**

breakbone fever ['breɪkbəʊn ˌfiːvə] = DENGUE

breakdown ['breɪkdaʊn] *subst.* **(a) (nervous) breakdown** = non-medical term for a sudden illness where a patient becomes so depressed *or* worried that he is incapable of doing anything *nervsammanbrott* **(b) breakdown product** = substance which is produced when a compound is broken down into its parts *nedbrytningsprodukt, slaggprodukt*

break down [ˌbreɪk 'daʊn] *vb.* **(a)** to reduce a compound to its parts *bryta ned, dela (spalta, lösa) upp* **(b)** to collapse in a nervous state *bryta samman, falla ihop, kollapsa;* **she broke down and cried as she described the symptoms to the doctor**

breakfast ['brekfəst] *subst.* first meal of the day *frukost;* **the patient had a boiled egg for breakfast; she didn't have any breakfast because she was due to have surgery later in the day; we have breakfast at 7.30 every day**

breast [brest] *or* **mamma** [mə'mɑː, 'mɑːmə, 'mæmə] *subst.* one of two glands in a woman which secrete milk *mamma, bröstet, bröstkörteln;* **breast cancer** = malignant tumour in the breast *bröstcancer;* **breast**

feeding = feeding a baby from the mother's breast as opposed to from a bottle *amning; see also* BOTTLE FEEDING

breastbone ['brestbəʊn] *or* **sternum** ['stɜ:nəm] *subst.* bone which is in the centre of the front of the thorax *sternum, bröstbenet*

breastfed ['brestfed] *adj.* (baby) which is fed from the mother's breast *ammad, uppfödd på bröstmjölk;* **she was breastfed for the first two months**
NOTE: for other terms referring to breast, see words beginning with **mamm-, mast-**

breath [breθ] *subst.* air which goes in and out of your body when you breathe *andan, andning, andetag, andedrag;* **he ran so fast he was out of breath; stop for a moment to get your breath back; she took a deep breath and dived into the water; to hold your breath** = to stop breathing out, after having inhaled deeply *hålla andan;* **breath sounds** = sounds heard through a stethoscope placed on a patient's chest, used in diagnosis *andningsljud;* **bad breath** = HALITOSIS

breathe [bri:ð] *vb.* to inhale or exhale *or* to take air in and out of your body through your nose or mouth *andas;* **he could not breathe under water; he breathed in the smoke from the fire and it made him cough; the patient has begun to breathe normally; the doctor told him to take a deep breath and breathe out slowly**

COMMENT: children breathe about 20 to 30 times per minute, men 16-18 per minute, and women slightly faster. The breathing rate increases if the person is taking exercise or has a fever. Some babies hold their breath and go blue in the face, especially when crying or during a temper tantrum

breathing ['bri:ðɪŋ] *subst.* respiration *or* taking air into the lungs and pushing it out again through the mouth or nose *respiration, andning;* **if breathing is difficult or has stopped, begin artificial ventilation immediately; breathing rate** = number of times a person breathes in and out *andningsfrekvens* NOTE: for other terms referring to breathing, see words beginning with **pneumo-**

breathless ['breθləs] *adj.* (patient) who finds it difficult to breathe enough air *andfådd, som tappat andan;* **after running upstairs she became breathless and had to sit down**

breathlessness ['breθləsnəs] *subst.* difficulty in breathing enough air *andfåddhet*

QUOTE 26 patients were selected from the outpatient department on grounds of disabling breathlessness present for at least five years
Lancet

breda ryggmuskeln ⇨ **latissimus dorsi**

bredspektrumantibiotika ⇨ **antibiotic**

breech [bri:tʃ] *subst.* buttocks *nates, klinkorna, sätet;* **breech birth** *or* **breech delivery** = birth where the baby's buttocks appear first *sätesförlossning;* **breech presentation** = position of a baby in the womb with the buttocks about to appear first *sätesbjudning*

breed [bri:d] *vb.* to reproduce and spread *föröka (sig), fortplanta (sig);* **the bacteria breed in dirty water**

bregma ['bregmə] *subst.* point at the top of the head where the soft gap between the bones of a baby's skull (the anterior fontanelle) hardens *bregma, hjässan*

Brickerblåsa ⇨ **ileal**

bridge [brɪdʒ] *subst.* **(a)** top part of the nose, where it joins the forehead *näsryggen* **(b)** *(for teeth)* artificial tooth (or teeth) which is joined to natural teeth which hold it in place *tandbrygga, tandbro*

Bright's disease ['braɪts dɪˌzi:z] *or* **(glomerulo)nephritis** [(gləʊˌmɜ:juləʊ)nɪ'fraɪtɪs] *subst.* inflammation of the kidney *glomerulonefrit*

brim [brɪm] *subst.* edge *brädd, kant;* **pelvic brim** = line on the ilium which separates the false pelvis from the true pelvis *linea terminalis*

bring up [ˌbrɪŋ 'ʌp] *vb.* **(a)** to look after and educate a child *uppfostra, föda upp;* **he was brought up by his uncle in Scotland; I was brought up in the country (b)** (i) to vomit *or* to force material from the stomach back into the mouth *kräkas, kasta upp;* (ii) to cough up material such as mucus from the lungs *or* throat *hosta upp;* **he was bringing up mucus**

brist ⇨ **absence, defect, deficiency, lack**

-brist ⇨ **-penia**

brista ⇨ **burst, perforate, rupture**

bristfällig ⇨ **defective**

bristning ⇨ **rupture**

-bristning ⇨ **-rrhexis**

bristsjukdom ⇨ **deficiency**

British ['brɪtɪʃ] *adj.* referring to Great Britain *brittisk, engelsk*

British anti-lewisite (BAL) ['brɪtɪʃ ˌæntɪ'luːɪsaɪt (ˌbiːeɪ'el)] *subst.* antidote for blister gases, but also used to treat cases of poisoning, such as mercury poisoning *antidot (motgift) mot bl.a. kvicksilver*

British Dental Association (BDA) ['brɪtɪʃ 'dent(ə)l əˌsəʊsɪ'eɪʃ(ə)n (ˌbiːdiː'eɪ)] *subst.* professional association of dentists *brittiska tandläkarförbundet*

British Medical Association (BMA) ['brɪtɪʃ 'medɪk(ə)l əˌsəʊsɪ'eɪʃ(ə)n (ˌbiːem'eɪ)] *subst.* professional association of doctors *brittiska läkarförbundet*

British Pharmacopoeia (BP) ['brɪtɪʃ ˌfɑːməkə'piːə (ˌbiː'piː)] *subst.* book listing approved drugs and their dosages *slags Fass, brittiskt register över godkända läkemedel och deras dosering*

> COMMENT: drugs listed in the British Pharmacopoeia have the letters BP written after them on labels

brits ⇨ **couch**

brittle ['brɪtl] *adj.* which breaks easily *spröd, skör, bräcklig;* **the bones of old people become brittle** *see also* DUCTILE, OSTEOGENESIS

bro ⇨ **pons**

broad [brɔːd] *adj.* wide in relation to length *bred;* **broad ligament** = peritoneal folds supporting the uterus on either side *ligamentum latum uteri, breda livmoderbanden;* **broad spectrum antibiotics** = antibiotics which are used to control many types of bacteria *bredspektrumantibiotika*
NOTE: opposite is **narrow**

Broadbent's sign ['brɔːdbents ˌsaɪn] *subst.* movement of a patient's left side near the lower ribs at each beat of the heart, indicating adhesion between the diaphragm and pericardium in cases of pericarditis *slags rörelse hos bröstkorgen vid perikardit (hjärtsäcksinflammation)*

Broca's aphasia ['brəʊkəz əˌfeɪziə] *subst.* being unable to speak or write, caused by damage to Broca's area *afasi pga skada i Brocas centrum*

Broca's area ['brəʊkəz ˌeəriə] *subst.* area on the left side of the brain which governs the motor aspects of speaking *Brocas centrum*

Brodie's abscess ['brəʊdiz ˌæbses] *subst.* abscess of a bone, caused by staphylococcal osteomyelitis *Brodies benabscess*

brom ⇨ **bromine**

bromhidrosis [ˌbrɒmhɪ'drəʊsɪs] *subst.* condition where the perspiration has an unpleasant smell *bromidros, osmidros*

bromides ['brəʊmaɪdz] *subst pl.* bromine salts, formerly used as depressants or sedatives *bromider*

bromidros ⇨ **bromhidrosis**

bromine ['brəʊmiːn] *subst.* chemical element *brom, Br*
NOTE: the chemical symbol is **Br**

bromism ['brəʊmɪz(ə)m] *or* **bromide poisoning** ['brəʊmaɪd ˌpɔɪz(ə)nɪŋ] *subst.* chronic ill health caused by excessive use of bromides *bromi(ni)sm*

bronch- ['brɒŋk, ˌ-] *prefix* referring to the windpipe *bronch-, bronk-, luftrörs-*

bronchi ['brɒŋkaɪ] *subst pl.* air passages leading from the trachea into the lungs *bronkerna, luftrören;* **lobar bronchi** *or* **secondary bronchi** = air passages leading to a lobe of the lung *lobbronkerna;* **main** *or* **primary bronchi** = two main bronchi which branch from the trachea outside the lung *bronchi principalis, huvudbronkerna;* **segmental bronchi** *or* **tertiary bronchi** = air passages supplying a segment of the lung ⇨ *illustration* LUNGS *bronchi segmentali, segmentbronkerna* NOTE: singular is **bronchus**

bronchial ['brɒŋkiəl] *adj.* referring to the bronchi *bronkial(-), bronko-;* **bronchial asthma** = type of asthma mainly caused by an allergen *or* exertion *bronkialastma;* **bronchial breath sounds** = distinctive breath sounds from the lungs which help diagnosis *bronkiellt andningsljud;* **bronchial pneumonia** = inflammation of the bronchioles, which may lead to general infection of the lungs *bronkopneumoni;* **bronchial tree** = system of tubes (bronchi and bronchioles) which take the air from the trachea into the lungs *bronkialträdet;* **bronchial tubes** = bronchi *or* air tubes leading from the windpipe into the lungs *bronkerna, luftrören*

> QUOTE 19 children with mild to moderately severe perennial bronchial asthma were selected. These children gave a typical history of exercise-induced asthma and their symptoms were controlled with oral or aerosol bronchodilators
>
> **Lancet**

bronchiectasis [ˌbrɒŋki'ektəsɪs] *subst.* disorder of the bronchi, which become wide, infected and filled with pus, and can lead to pneumonia *bronkiektasi, bronkutvidgning*

bronchiolar [ˌbrɒŋki'əʊlə] *adj.* referring to the bronchioles *som avser el. hör till bronkiolerna*

bronchiole ['brɒŋkiəʊl] *subst.* very small air tube in the lungs leading from a bronchus to the alveoli ⇨ *illustration* LUNGS *bronkiol*

bronchiolitis [ˌbrɒŋkiəʊ'laɪtɪs] *subst.* inflammation of the bronchioles *bronkiolit*

bronchitic [brɒŋ'kɪtɪk] *adj.* (i) referring to bronchitis *som avser el. hör till bronkit (luftrörskatarr);* (ii) (patient) suffering from bronchitis *som lider av bronkit (luftrörskatarr)*

bronchitis [brɒŋ'kaɪtɪs] *subst.* inflammation of the mucous membrane of the bronchi *bronkit, luftrörskatarr;* **acute bronchitis** = attack of bronchitis caused by a virus *or* exposure to cold and wet *akut bronkit (luftrörskatarr);* **chronic bronchitis** = long-lasting form of bronchial inflammation *kronisk bronkit (luftrörskatarr)*

bronchoconstrictor [ˌbrɒŋkəʊkən'strɪktə] *subst.* drug which narrows the bronchi *medel som orsakar bronkokonstriktion*

bronchodilator [ˌbrɒŋkəʊdaɪ'leɪtə] *subst.* drug which makes the bronchi wider *medel som orsakar bronkodilatation*

bronchogram ['brɒŋkəʊgræm] *subst.* X-ray picture of the bronchial tubes after an opaque substance has been injected into them *bronkogram*

bronchography [brɒŋ'kɒgrəfi] *subst.* X-ray examination of the lungs, after an opaque substance has been put into the bronchi *bronkografi*

bronchomediastinal trunk [ˌbrɒŋkəʊˌmiːdiə'staɪn(ə)l ˌtrʌŋk] *subst.* lymph nodes draining part of the chest *truncus bronchomediastinalis, lymfkärl som dränerar en del av bröstet*

bronchomycosis [ˌbrɒŋkəʊmaɪ'kəʊsɪs] *subst.* infection of the bronchi by a fungus *svampinfektion i luftrören*

bronchophony [brɒŋ'kɒfəni] *subst.* vibrations of the voice heard when the consolidation of the lungs produces a loud sound *bronkofoni*

bronchopleural [ˌbrɒŋkəʊ'plʊər(ə)l] *adj.* referring to a bronchus and pleura *som avser el. hör till både bronkerna och lungsäckarna*

bronchopneumonia [ˌbrɒŋkəʊnju'məʊniə] *subst.* infectious inflammation of the bronchioles, which may lead to general infection of the lungs *bronkopneumoni*

bronchopulmonary [ˌbrɒŋkəʊ'pʌlmən(ə)ri] *adj.* referring to the bronchi and the lungs *som avser el. hör till både bronkerna och lungorna*

bronchoscope ['brɒŋkəʊskəʊp] *subst.* instrument which is passed down the trachea into the lungs, which a doctor can use to inspect the inside passages of the lungs *bronkoskop*

bronchoscopy [brɒŋ'kɒskəpi] *subst.* examination of a patient's bronchi using a bronchoscope *bronkoskopi*

bronchospasm ['brɒŋkəʊˌspæz(ə)m] *subst.* tightening of the bronchial muscles which causes the tubes to contract *bronkospasm*

bronchospirometer [ˌbrɒŋkəʊspaɪ(ə)'rɒmɪtə] *subst.* instrument for measuring the volume of the lungs *(bronko)spirometer*

bronchospirometry [ˌbrɒŋkəʊspaɪ(ə)'rɒmɪtri] *subst.* measuring the volume of the lungs *bronkospirometri*

bronchostenosis [ˌbrɒŋkəʊste'nəʊsɪs] *subst.* abnormal constriction of the bronchial tubes *bronkostenos*

bronchotracheal [ˌbrɒŋkəʊtrə'kiːəl] *adj.* referring to the bronchi and the trachea *som avser el. hör till både bronkerna och luftstrupen*

bronchus ['brɒŋkəs] *subst.* air passage from the trachea to the lungs, where it splits into many bronchioles *bronk, luftrör*
NOTE: plural is **bronchi**

bronkerna ⇨ **bronchi, bronchial**

bronkial ⇨ **bronchial**

bronkialastma ⇨ **bronchial**

bronkialträdet ⇨ **bronchial**

bronkiektasi ⇨ **bronchiectasis**

bronkiol ⇨ **bronchiole**

bronkiolit ⇨ **bronchiolitis**

bronkit ⇨ **bronchitis**

bronko- ⇨ **bronchial**

bronkofoni ⇨ **bronchophony**

bronkografi ⇨ **bronchography**

bronkogram ⇨ **bronchogram**

bronkopneumoni ⇨ **bronchial, bronchopneumonia**

bronkoskop ⇨ **bronchoscope**

bronkoskopi ⇨ **bronchoscopy**

bronkospasm ⇨ **bronchospasm**

bronkospirometri ⇨ **bronchospirometry**

bronkostenos ⇨ **bronchostenosis**

bronkutvidgning ⇨ **bronchiectasis**

bronsdiabetes ⇨ **haemochromatosis**

bronze diabetes ['brɒnz ˌda(i)ə'biːtiːz] = HAEMOCHROMATOSIS

bror ⇨ **brother**

brosk ⇨ **cartilage, gristle**

brosk- ⇨ **cartilaginous, chondr-**

broskbildningscell ⇨ **chondroblast**

broskfog ⇨ **cartilaginous**

broskförkalkning ⇨ **chondrocalcinosis**

broskhinna ⇨ **perichondrium**

broskinflammation ⇨ **chondritis**

brosksvulst ⇨ **chondroma, ecchondroma**

broskuppmjukning ⇨ **chondromalacia**

broth [brɒθ] *subst.* (i) light soup made from meat *buljong;* (ii) medium in which bacteria can be cultivated *näringssubstrat*

brother ['brʌðə] *adj. & subst.* male who has the same mother and father as another child *bror;* **he's my brother; that girl has three brothers; his brother's a doctor**

brott ⇨ **break, fracture**

brow [braʊ] *subst.* (i) forehead *or* part of the face above the eyes *pannan;* (ii) eyebrow *or* line of hair above the eye *ögonbryn*

brown [braʊn] *adj. & subst.* of a colour like the colour of earth or wood *brun;* **he has brown hair and blue eyes; you're very brown - you must have been sitting in the sun; brown bread** = bread made with flour which has not been refined *mörkt bröd, limpa;* **brown bread is better for you than white; brown fat** = animal fat which can easily be converted to energy, and is believed to offset the effects of ordinary white fat *brunt fett*
NOTE: **brown - browner - brownest**

Brown-Séquard syndrome [ˌbraʊn'seɪkɑː ˌsɪndrəʊm] *subst.* condition of a patient where the spinal cord has been partly severed or compressed, with the result that the lower half of the body is paralysed on one side and loses feeling in the other side *Brown-Séquards förlamning*

Brucella [bru'selə] *subst.* type of rod-shaped bacterium *Brucella*

brucellos ⇨ **abortus fever, brucellosis**

brucellosis [ˌbruːsɪ'ləʊsɪs] *or* **undulant fever** ['ʌndjʊlənt ˌfiːvə] *or* **Malta fever** ['mɔːltə ˌfiːvə] *or* **mountain fever** ['maʊntɪn ˌfiːvə] *subst.* disease which can be caught from cattle or goats or from drinking infected milk, spread by a species of the bacterium Brucella *brucellos, febris undulans, undulantfeber*

> COMMENT: symptoms include tiredness, arthritis, headache, sweating, irritability and swelling of the spleen

bruise [bruːz] **1** *subst.* contusion *or* dark painful area on the skin, where blood has escaped under the skin following a blow *ekkymom, blåmärke, utgjutning; see also* BLACK EYE **2** *vb.* to make a bruise *ge blåmärke (utgjutning);* **she bruised her knee on the corner of the table; the nurse put a**

compress on his bruised leg; she bruises easily = even a soft blow will give her a bruise *hon får lätt blåmärken*

bruising ['bru:zɪŋ] *subst.* area of bruises *område med blåmärken (utgjutningar);* **the baby has bruising on the back and legs**

bruit [bru:t] *subst.* abnormal noise heard through a stethoscope *blåsljud, biljud*

brun ⇨ **brown**

Brunner's glands ['brʊnəz ˌglændz] *subst.* glands in the duodenum and jejunum *Brunners körtlar*

brush [brʌʃ] **1** *subst.* stiff hairs *or* wire set in a hard base, used for cleaning *borste;* **you need a stiff brush to remove the dandruff from the scalp 2** *vb.* to clean with a brush *borsta;* **have you brushed your hair? remember to brush your teeth after a meal**

brygga ⇨ **pons**

bryta ⇨ **refract**

bryta ut ⇨ **erupt**

brytningsmätare ⇨ **refractometer**

bråck ⇨ **hernia, rupture**

bråckband ⇨ **truss**

bråckbildning ⇨ **herniation**

bråckoperation ⇨ **herniotomy**

bråcksäck ⇨ **hernial**

brådmogen ⇨ **precocious**

brådskande ⇨ **acute, urgent**

bräcklig ⇨ **brittle, fragile, frail**

bräcklighet ⇨ **fragilitas**

brädd ⇨ **brim**

bränna ⇨ **cauterize**

bränning ⇨ **cauterization**

brännjärn ⇨ **cautery**

brännpunkt ⇨ **focus**

brännskada ⇨ **burn**

brännskadeavdelning ⇨ **burn**

brännvidd ⇨ **focal**

brässen ⇨ **gland, thymus (gland)**

bröst- ⇨ **mammary, mast-, pectoral, precordial, thoracic**

bröstaorta ⇨ **aorta**

bröstbenet ⇨ **breastbone, sternum**

bröstbens- ⇨ **sternal**

bröstböld ⇨ **mastitis**

bröstcancer ⇨ **breast**

bröstet ⇨ **breast, chest, mamma, pectus**

brösthålan ⇨ **chest, thoracic**

bröstkorgen ⇨ **chest, pectus, rib, thorax**

bröstkotorna ⇨ **dorsal, thoracic**

bröstkörtel ⇨ **breast, mamma, mammary**

bröstmuskel ⇨ **chest, pectoral, pectoralis**

bröstpalpation ⇨ **palpation**

bröstsmärtor ⇨ **pain**

bröstttermografi ⇨ **mammothermography**

bröstvårta ⇨ **nipple, mamilla**

bröstvårteliknande ⇨ **mastoid**

bröstvårtgård ⇨ **areola**

bubble ['bʌbl] *subst.* small amount of air *or* gas surrounded by a liquid *bubbla;* **air bubbles formed in the blood vessel, causing embolism**

bubo ['bju:bəʊ] *subst.* swelling of a lymph node in the groin or armpit *bubon, lymfkörtelinflammation (särskilt vid pest)*

bubon ⇨ **bubo**

bubonic plague [bjuˌbɒnɪk 'pleɪg] *subst.* fatal disease caused by bacteria transmitted to humans by fleas from rats *pestis bubonica, bubonpest, böldpest, digerdöden*

COMMENT: bubonic plague was the Black Death of the Middle Ages. Symptoms are fever, delirium, vomiting and swellings of the lymph nodes

bubonpest ⇨ **bubonic plague**

buccal ['bʌk(ə)l] *adj.* referring to the cheek *buckal, kind-;* **buccal cavity** = the mouth *cavum oris, munhålan;* **buccal fat** = pad of fat separating the buccinator muscle from the masseter *fett som ligger mellan kindmuskeln och tuggmuskeln*

buccinator ['bʌksɪneɪtə] *subst.* cheek muscle which helps the jaw to chew *musculus buccinator, kindmuskeln*

buckal ⇨ **buccal**

bud [bʌd] *subst.* small appendage *knopp, litet bihang;* **taste buds** = tiny sensory receptors in the vallate and fungiform papillae of the tongue and in part of the back of the mouth *caliculi gustatorii, smaklökarna*

budbärar-RNA ⇨ **messenger**

Budd-Chiari syndrome [ˌbʌdkɪ'eəri ˌsɪndrəʊm] *subst.* disease of the liver, where thrombosis has occurred in the hepatic veins *Budd-Chiaris syndrom*

Buerger's disease ['bɜːgəz dɪˌziːz] = THROMBO-ANGIITIS OBLITERANS

buffer ['bʌfə] *subst.* solution where the pH factor is not changed by adding acid or alkali *buffert*

buffert ⇨ **buffer**

bug [bʌg] *subst. informal* infectious disease *slang för infektionssjukdom;* **he caught a bug on holiday; half the staff are sick with a stomach bug**

build [bɪld] *subst.* general size of a person's body *kroppsbyggnad;* **he has a heavy** *or* **strong build for his height; the girl has a slight build, but she can run very fast**

build up [ˌbɪld 'ʌp] *vb.* to form by accumulation *bygga upp*

build-up ['bɪldʌp] *subst.* gradual accumulation *gradvis uppbyggnad;* **a build-up of fatty deposits on the walls of the arteries**

-built [bɪlt] *suffix* referring to the general size of a person's body *-byggd;* **a heavily-built man; she's slightly-built**

buk- ⇨ **abdomin-, abdominal, coeli-, coeliac, laparo-, ventro-**

bukaorta ⇨ **aorta**

bukbäckenet ⇨ **pelvis**

bukduk ⇨ **tampon**

buken ⇨ **abdomen, belly, stomach**

bukhinnan ⇨ **peritoneum**

bukhinnans yttre blad ⇨ **peritoneum**

bukhinne- ⇨ **peritoneal**

bukhinneinflammation ⇨ **peritonitis**

bukhinnenätet ⇨ **omentum**

bukhålan ⇨ **abdomen, abdominal, cavity, enterocoele**

bukinälvsartären ⇨ **coeliac**

bukmuskeln, raka ⇨ **rectus**

buksmärtor ⇨ **abdominal, bellyache, stomach, tormina**

bukspott ⇨ **pancreatic**

bukspottkörtelinflammation ⇨ **pancreatitis**

bukspottkörteln ⇨ **pancreas**

bukta ut ⇨ **bulge**

bukväggen ⇨ **abdominal**

bula ⇨ **bump, lump, swelling**

bulb [bʌlb] *subst.* round part at the end of an organ *or* bone *knöl, ansvällning;* **olfactory bulb** = end of the olfactory tract, where the processes of the sensory cells in the nose are linked to the fibres of the olfactory nerve *bulbus olfactorius, luktloben;* **bulb of the penis** *or* **glans penis** = round end of the penis *bulbus penis, glans (penis), ollonet*

bulbar ['bʌlbə] *adj.* referring to a bulb *or* to the medulla oblongata *bulbär(-), som avser el. hör till medulla oblongata;* **bulbar paralysis** *or* **palsy** = motor neurone disease which affects the muscles of the mouth, jaw and throat *paralysis bulbaris, bulbärparalys;* **bulbar poliomyelitis** = type of polio affecting the brain stem, which makes it difficult for a patient to swallow or breathe *bulbär paralys*

bulbospongiosus muscle [ˌbʌlbəʊˌspʌndʒi'əʊsəs ˌmʌs(ə)l] *subst.*

muscle in the perineum behind the penis *musculus bulbocavernosum*

bulbourethral glands [ˌbʌlbəʊjʊ(ə)'riːər(ə)l ˌglændz] *or* **Cowper's glands** ['kuːpəz ˌglændz] *see* GLAND

bulbärparalys ⇨ **bulbar**

bulge [bʌldʒ] *vb.* to swell out *or* to push out *bukta ut, svälla ut;* **the wall of the stomach becomes weak and part of the intestine bulges through**

bulimia (nervosa) [bju'lɪmiə (nəˌvəʊsa)] *subst.* psychological condition where the patient eats too much and is incapable of controlling his eating *bulimi, hetshunger*

> COMMENT: although the patient eats a large quantity of food, this is followed by vomiting which is induced by the patient himself, so that the patient does not in fact become overweight

bulla ['bʊlə] *subst.* large blister *bulla, blåsa*
NOTE: plural is **bullae**

bulna ⇨ **fester**

bulnad ⇨ **lump**

bulta ⇨ **throb**

bump [bʌmp] **1** *subst.* **(a)** slight knock against something *stöt, duns;* **the plane landed with a bump (b)** slightly swollen part on the skin, caused by a blow *or* sting, etc. *bula, svulst, knöl;* **she has a bump on the back of her head where the door hit her; the vaccination has left a little bump on her left arm 2** *vb.* to knock slightly *stöta, dunsa;* **she bumped her head on the door**

bumper fracture ['bʌmpə ˌfræktʃə] *subst.* fracture of the upper part of the tibia (so called, because it can be caused by a blow from the bumper of a car) *slags brott på tibia (skenbenet)*

bunden till ⇨ **confined**

bundle ['bʌnd(ə)l] *subst.* (i) collection of things roughly fastened together *knippe, bunt;* (ii) group of nerves running in the same direction *fascikel, nervstråk;* **bundle branch block** = defect in the heart's conduction tissue *grenblock;* **bundle of His** *or* **atrioventricular bundle** = bundle of fibres which run from the atrioventricular node to the septum, and then divide to connect with the two ventricles *atrioventrikulära muskelknippet, His bunt (knippe, knut), Hisska bunten (knippet, knutan)*

bunion ['bʌnjən] *subst.* inflammation and swelling of the big toe, caused by tight shoes which force the toe sideways with a callus developing over the joint between the toe and the metatarsal *bunio, pseudobursa*

bunt ⇨ **bundle, fasciculus**

buphthalmos [bʌf'θælməs] *subst.* type of congenital glaucoma occurring in infants *slags medfödd starr hos spädbarn*

burk ⇨ **jar**

Burkitt's tumour ['bɜːkɪts ˌtjuːmə] *or* **lymphoma** [lɪm'fəʊmə] *subst.* malignant tumour, usually on the maxilla *Burkitts tumör (lymfom)*

> COMMENT: Burkitt's tumour is found especially in children in Africa

burn [bɜːn] **1** *subst.* injury to skin and tissue caused by light *or* heat *or* radiation *or* electricity *or* chemicals *combustio, ambustio, brännskada;* **cold burn** = injury to the skin caused by touching very cold surfaces *congelatio, frostskada;* **dry burn** = injury to the skin caused by touching very hot dry surfaces *brännskada orsakad av beröring med het, torr yta;* **wet burn** *or* **scald** = injury to the skin caused by touching very hot wet substances *skållskada;* **deep burn** = burn which is so severe that a graft will be necessary to repair the skin damage *djup brännskada;* **superficial burn** = burn which leaves enough tissue for the skin to grow again *ytlig brännskada;* **first degree burn** = burn where the skin turns red because the epidermis has been affected *combustio erythematosa, första gradens brännskada;* **second degree burn** = burn where the skin becomes very red and blisters *combustio bullosa, andra gradens brännskada;* **third degree burn** = burn where both the epidermis and dermis are destroyed, and a skin graft will be required to repair the damage *necrosis, tredje gradens brännskada;* **fourth degree burn** = burn where the tissue becomes black *carbonizio, brännskada där vävnaden är förkolnad;* **burns unit** = special department in a hospital which deals with burns *brännskadeavdelning* **2** *vb.* to destroy by fire *(för)bränna, sveda;* **she burnt her hand on the hot frying pan; most of his hair** *or* **his skin was burnt off** NOTE: **burns - burning - burnt/burned - has burnt/burned**

> COMMENT: burns were formerly classified by degrees, and are still often referred to in this way. The modern classification is into two categories: deep and superficial

burp [bɜːp] **1** *subst.* allowing air in the stomach to come up into the mouth *rap(ning)* **2** *vb.* to allow the air in the stomach to come up into the mouth *rapa;* **to burp a baby** = to pat a baby on the back until it burps *rapa ett barn, få ett barn att rapa* NOTE: used particularly of babies. For adults use **belch**

burr [bɜː] *subst.* bit used with a drill to make holes in a bone (as in the cranium) or a tooth *borr*

bursa ['bɜːsə] *subst.* sac containing fluid, which is normally present at joints where frequent pressure or rubbing is experienced (especially found at the knee *or* the elbow) *bursa, slemsäck;* **adventitious bursa** = abnormal bursa which develops as a result of continued pressure *bursa som utvecklas pga långvarigt tryck* NOTE: plural is **bursae**

bursitis [bɜː'saɪtɪs] *subst.* inflammation of a bursa, especially in the shoulder *bursit, slemsäcksinflammation;* **prepatellar bursitis** *or* **housemaid's knee** = condition where the bursa in the knee becomes inflamed, caused by kneeling on hard surfaces *bursitis prepatellaris, skurgummeknä*

burst [bɜːst] *vb. (of a sac or blister)* to break open *brista, spricka;* **never use a needle to burst a blister; he was rushed to hospital with a burst appendix**
NOTE: **bursts - bursting - burst - has burst**

bury ['beri] *vb.* to put a dead person's body into the ground *begrava;* **he died on Monday and was buried on Friday**

butter ['bʌtə] *subst.* solid yellow edible fat made from cream *smör;* **he was spreading butter on a piece of bread; fry the onions in butter** NOTE: no plural

buttocks ['bʌtəks] *or* **nates** ['neɪtiːz] *subst pl.* two fleshy parts below the back on which a person sits, made up mainly of the gluteal muscles *nates, klinkorna, sätet;* **he had a boil on his right buttock**

B-vitamin ➪ **Vitamin B**

bypass ['baɪpɑːs] *subst.* act of going round an obstruction *bypass, shunt;* **cardiopulmonary bypass** = method of artificially circulating the patient's blood during open heart surgery, where the heart and lungs are cut off from the circulation and replaced by a pump *(användning av) hjärtlungmaskin, hjärtlungbypass, shuntning av blod vid öppen hjärtkirurgi;* **heart bypass operation** *or* **coronary bypass surgery** = surgical operation to treat angina by grafting pieces of vein to go around the diseased part of a coronary artery *bypassoperation i hjärtats kranskärl*

byssinosis [ˌbɪsɪ'nəʊsɪs] *subst.* lung disease (a form of pneumoconiosis) caused by inhaling cotton dust *byssinos*

byte ➪ **change**

båge ➪ **arc, arch, arcus**

bågformig ➪ **arcuate**

båggångarna ➪ **semicircular**

bålen ➪ **body, torso, trunk**

bår ➪ **stretcher**

bårbärare ➪ **stretcher**

bår(vagn) ➪ **trolley**

båtbenet ➪ **navicular bone**

båtben, handlovens ➪ **scaphoid (bone)**

båtskallighet ➪ **scaphocephaly**

bäcken ➪ **bedpan; pelvis**

bäckenbotten ➪ **pelvic, perineum**

bäckenbotten- ➪ **perineal**

bäckenbottenmuskulaturen ➪ **perineal**

bäckenet ➪ **pelvis**

bäckenfraktur ➪ **pelvic**

bäckenförträngning ➪ **cephalopelvic**

bäckengördeln ➪ **girdle**

bäckenhålan ➪ **pelvic**

bäckenhögläge ➪ **Trendelenburg's position**

bäckenmätning ➪ **pelvimetry**

bäckenringen ➪ **girdle**

bäckenträngsel ➪ **cephalopelvic**

bäckenvidd ➪ **conjugate**

bädd ➪ **bed**

bädd(plats) ➪ **hospital**

bägarcell ⇨ **goblet cell**

bältros ⇨ **herpes**

bärare ⇨ **vector**

"bärare" ⇨ **orderly, porter**

bärbar ⇨ **portable**

bättre ⇨ **better**

bättring ⇨ **recovery**

bättringsvägen, vara på ⇨ **convalesce**

böja ⇨ **bend, curve, flex**

böjare ⇨ **flexor**

böjd ⇨ **arcuate, circumflex, curved**

böjlig ⇨ **ductile, flexible, pliable**

böjning ⇨ **flexion, flexure**

böld ⇨ **abscess, boil, carbuncle, furuncle**

böldpest ⇨ **bubonic plague**

Cc

C [siː] **1** *abbreviation for* Celsius *C, Celsius* **2** *chemical symbol for* carbon *C, kol* **3** *subst.* **vitamin C** *or* **ascorbic acid** = vitamin which is soluble in water, and is found in fresh fruit (especially oranges and lemons) and in raw vegetables, liver and milk *C-vitamin, askorbinsyra*

COMMENT: lack of vitamin C can cause anaemia and scurvy

Ca *chemical symbol for* calcium *Ca, kalcium, kalk*

CABG [ˌsiːeɪbiːˈdʒiː] = CORONARY ARTERY BYPASS GRAFT

cabinet [ˈkæbɪnət] *subst.* cupboard *skåp;* **the drugs cabinet must be kept locked at all times**

cachet [ˈkæʃeɪ] *subst.* quantity of a drug wrapped in paper, to be swallowed *kapsel*

cachexia [kæˈkeksiə] *subst.* state of ill health with wasting and general weakness *kakexi*

cadaver [kəˈdævə] *subst.* dead body, especially one used for dissection *kadaver, lik*

cadaveric [kəˈdæv(ə)rɪk] *or* **cadaverous** [kəˈdæv(ə)rəs] *adj.* (person who is) thin *or* wasting away *mycker mager, borttynande*

cadmium [ˈkædmiəm] *subst.* metallic element, which if present in soil can make plants poisonous *kadmium, Cd*
NOTE: chemical symbol is **Cd**

caecalporten ⇨ **orifice**

caecostomy [siːˈkɒstəmi] *subst.* surgical operation to make an opening between the caecum and the abdominal wall to allow faeces to be passed without going through the rectum and anus *cekostomi*

caecum [ˈsiːkəm] *subst.* wider part of the large intestine in the lower right-hand side of the abdomen at the point where the small intestine joins it and which has the appendix attached to it ⇨ *illustration* DIGESTIVE SYSTEM *(intestinum) caecum, blindtarmen*

Caesarean section [sɪˌzeəriən ˈsekʃ(ə)n] *or* **caesarean** [sɪˈzeəriən] *subst.* surgical operation to deliver a baby by cutting through the abdominal wall into the uterus *tomotoki, sectio caesarea, kejsarsnitt*
NOTE: the operation is correctly called **Caesarean section** but informally most people use **caesarean: "she had her baby by Caesarean section** *or* **she had a caesarean"**

COMMENT: Caesarean section is performed only when it appears that normal childbirth is impossible, or might endanger mother or child, and only after the 28th week of gestation

caesium [ˈsiːziəm] *subst.* radioactive element, used in treatment by radiation *cesium, Cs*
NOTE: chemical symbol is **Cs**

caffeine [ˈkæfiːn] *subst.* alkaloid found in coffee and tea, which acts as a stimulant *koffein*

COMMENT: apart from acting as a stimulant, caffeine also helps in the production of urine. It can be addictive, and exists in both tea and coffee in about the same percentages as well as in chocolate and other drinks

caisson disease ['keɪs(ə)n dɪ,zi:z] *or* **decompression sickness** [,di:kəm'preʃ(ə)n ,sɪknəs] *or* **compressed air sickness** [kəm'prest 'eə ,sɪknəs] *or* **the bends** [ðə 'bendz] *subst.* condition where the patient suffers pains in the joints and stomach, and dizziness caused by nitrogen in the blood *caissonsjuka, aeroembolism, dykarsjuka*

COMMENT: found when a person has moved rapidly from high atmospheric pressure to a lower pressure area, especially in divers who come back to the surface too quickly after a deep dive. The first symptoms of pains in the joints are known as "the bends". The disease can be fatal

caissonsjuka ⇨ **caisson disease**

Cal [,si:eɪ'el] *abbreviation for* kilocalorie *kcal, kilokalori*

calamine (lotion) ['kæləmaɪn (,ləʊʃ(ə)n)] *subst.* lotion, based on zinc oxide, which helps relieve skin irritation (such as that caused by sunburn *or* chickenpox) *slags zinkliniment*

calc- [kælk] *or* **calci-** ['kælsɪ, ,--] *prefix* referring to calcium *kalci-, kalk-*

calcaemia [kæl'si:miə] *subst.* condition where the blood contains an abnormally large amount of calcium *kalcemi, hyperkalcemi*

calcaneal [kæl'keiniəl] *adj.* referring to the calcaneus *som avser el. hör till calcaneus (hälbenet);* **calcaneal tendon** *or* **Achilles tendon** = tendon at the back of the ankle which connects the calf muscles to the heel and pulls the heel upwards when the calf muscles are tense *tendo calcaneus (Achillis), akillessenan*

calcaneus [kæl'keɪniəs] *subst.* heel bone, situated underneath the talus ⇨ *illustration* FOOT *calcaneus, hälbenet*

calcareous degeneration [kæl'keəriəs dɪ,dʒenə'reɪʃ(ə)n] *subst.* formation of calcium on bones *or* at joints in old age *förkalkning, kalkinlagring*

calciferol [kæl'sɪfərɒl] *subst.* vitamin D_2 *calciferol, kalciferol, vitamin* D_2

calcification [,kælsɪfɪ'keɪʃ(ə)n] *subst.* hardening by forming deposits of calcium salts *kalcifikation, förkalkning, kalkinlagring; see also* PELLEGRINI-STIEDA'S DISEASE

COMMENT: calcification can be normal in the formation of bones, but can occur abnormally in joints, muscles and organs, where it is known as calcinosis

calcified ['kælsɪfaɪd] *adj.* made hard *förkalkad;* **bone is calcified connective tissue**

calcitonin [,kælsɪ'təʊnɪn] *or* **thyrocalcitonin** [,θaɪ(ə)rəʊ,kælsɪ'təʊnɪn] *subst.* hormone, produced by the thyroid gland, which is believed to regulate the level of calcium in the blood *kalcitonin, tyrokalcitonin*

calcium ['kælsɪəm] *subst.* metallic chemical element which makes up a large part of the bones and teeth, and which is essential for various bodily processes such as blood clotting *kalcium, kalk, Ca* NOTE: chemical symbol is **Ca**

COMMENT: calcium is an important element in correct diet. Milk, cheese, eggs and certain vegetables are its main sources. Calcium deficiency can be treated by injections of calcium salts

calculosis [,kælkjʊ'ləʊsɪs] *subst.* condition where calculi exist in an organ *tillstånd med konkrement (stenar) i ett organ*

calculus ['kælkjʊləs] *or* **stone** [stəʊn] *subst.* hard mass like a little stone, which forms in an organ *calculus, konkrement, sten;* **renal calculus** = kidney stone *calculus renalis, njursten* NOTE: plural is **calculi**

COMMENT: calculi are formed of cholesterol and various inorganic substances, and are commonly found in the bladder, the gall bladder (gallstones), and various parts of the kidney

Caldwell-Luc operation [,kɔ:ldwel'lʌk ,ɒpə,reɪʃ(ə)n] *subst.* surgical operation to drain the maxillary sinus by making an incision above the canine tooth *Caldwell-Lucs operation*

calf [kɑ:f] *subst.* muscular fleshy part at the back of the lower leg, formed by the gastrocnemius muscles *vaden*
NOTE: plural is **calves**

calibrate ['kælɪbreɪt] *vb.* **(a)** to measure the inside diameter of a tube or passage *mäta innermått på kanal, gång etc.* **(b)** *(in surgery)* to measure the sizes of two parts of the body to be joined together *inom kirurgin: mäta storleken på två kroppsdelar som skall förenas*

calibrator ['kæləbreɪtə] *subst.* (i) instrument used to enlarge a passage *instrument för att vidga gång, kanal etc.;* (ii) instrument for measuring the diameter of passages *instrument för att mäta innermått på gång, kanal etc.*

caliper ['kælɪpə] *subst.* **(a)** instrument with two legs, used for measuring the width of the pelvic cavity *tång, instrument för att mäta bäckenmått* **(b)** instrument with two sharp points which are put into a fractured bone, and weights attached to cause traction *frakturinstrument* **(c)** metal splints made of a pair of rods attached to a thigh and to a special boot to support an injured leg *skena, spjäla*

call [kɔ:l] **1** *subst.* **(a)** speaking by telephone *telefonsamtal;* **I want to make a (phone) call to Canada; there were three calls for you while you were out; on call** = ready to be called for duty *jourhavande;* **three nurses are on call during the night (b)** visit *besök;* **the district nurse makes a regular call every Thursday 2** *vb.* **(a)** to telephone *telefonera, ringa;* **if he comes, tell him I'll call him when I'm at the surgery; Mr Smith is out - shall I ask him to call you back? (b)** to visit *besöka, göra hembesök;* **the district nurse called at the house, but there was no one there; she called on the patient for the last time on Tuesday**

calliper ['kælɪpə] = CALIPER

callosity [kə'lɒsəti] *or* **callus** ['kæləs] *subst.* hard patch on the skin resulting from frequent pressure or rubbing (such as a corn) *callus, förhårdnad, valk*

callosum [kə'ləusəm] *see* CORPUS

callus ['kæləs] *subst.* **(a)** = CALLOSITY **(b)** tissue which forms round a broken bone as it starts to mend, leading to consolidation *callus, valk;* **callus formation is more rapid in children and young adults than in elderly patients**

calm [kɑ:m] *adj.* quiet *or* not upset *lugn;* **the patient was delirious but became calm after the injection**

calm down [ˌkɑ:m 'daun] *vb.* to become calm *or* to make someone calm *lugna (ner) sig;* **he was soon calmed down** *or* **he soon calmed down when the nurse gave him an injection**

Calmette-Guérins bacill ⇨ **bacille Calmette-Guérin (BCG)**

calomel ['kæləmel] *subst.* drug based on mercury, used to treat pinworms in the intestine *kalomel*

calor ['kælə] *subst.* heat *calor, hetta, värme*

Calorie ['kæl(ə)ri] *or* **large calorie** ['lɑ:dʒ ˌkæl(ə)ri] *subst.* kilocalorie *or* 1,000 calories *kilokalori* NOTE: written **cal** after figures: **250cal**

> COMMENT: one calorie is the amount of heat needed to raise the temperature of one gram of water by one degree Celsius. A Calorie or kilocalorie is the amount of heat needed to raise the temperature of a kilogram of water by one degree Celsius. The Calorie is also used as a measurement of the energy content of food, and to show the amount of energy needed by an average person. The average adult in an office job, requires about 3000 Calories per day, supplied by carbohydrates and fats to give energy and proteins to replace tissue; more strenuous physical work needs more Calories. If a person eats more than the number of Calories needed by his energy output or for his growth, the extra Calories are stored in the body as fat.

calorie ['kæl(ə)ri] *or* **small calorie** ['smɔ:l ˌkæl(ə)ri] *subst.* unit of measurement of heat *or* energy *kalori*

calorific value [ˌkælə'rɪfɪk ˌvælju:] *subst.* heat value of food *or* number of Calories which a certain amount of a certain food contains *kalorivärde;* **the tin of beans has 250 calories** *or* **has a calorific value of 250 calories**

calvaria [kæl'veəriə] *or* **calvarium** [kæl'veəriəm] *subst.* top part of the skull *calvaria, kalvariet, skalltaket*

calyx ['keɪlɪks] *subst.* part of the body shaped like a cup especially the tube leading to a renal pyramid *kalk, calyx renalis, njurkalk* NOTE: the plural is **calyces** ⇨ *illustration* KIDNEY

> COMMENT: the renal pelvis is formed of three major calyces, which themselves are formed of several smaller minor calyces

camphor ['kæmfə] *subst.* white crystals with a strong smell, made from a tropical tree, used to keep insects away *or* as a liniment *kamfer;* **camphor oil** *or* **camphorated oil** = mixture of 20% camphor and oil, used as a rub *kamferolja*

canal [kə'næl] *subst.* tube along which something flows *kanal, gång;* **alimentary canal** = passage from the mouth to the rectum, along which food passes and is digested *canalis alimentarius, digestionskanalen, matspjälkningskanalen;* **anal canal** = passage leading from the rectum to the anus *analkanalen;* **auditory canals** = external and internal passages of the ear *meatus acusticus* *externus resp. internus, yttre resp. inre hörselgången;* **bile canal** = bile duct *gallgång;* **central canal** = thin tube in the centre of the spinal cord containing cerebrospinal fluid *canalis centralis, ryggradens centralkanal;* **cervical canal** *or* **cervicouterine canal** = tube running through the cervix from the point where the uterus joins the vagina to the entrance of the uterine cavity *cervikalkanalen;* **Eustachian canal** = passage through the porous bone forming the outside part of the Eustachian tube *tuba auditiva, otosalpinx, eustachiska röret, örontrumpeten;* **femoral canal** = inner tube of the femoral sheath which surrounds the femoral artery and femoral vein *canalis femoralis, femoralkanalen, kruralkanalen;* **Haversian canals** = canals which run vertically through Haversian systems in compact bone, containing blood vessels, and lymph ducts *canales nutricius (ossis), Havers kanaler, haver(si)ska kanalerna;* **inguinal canal** = passage in the lower abdominal wall, carrying the spermatic cord in the male and the round ligament of the uterus in the female *canalis inguinalis, inguinalkanalen, ljumskkanalen;* **root canal** = canal in the root of a tooth which carries nerves and blood vessels *rotkanal;* **Schlemm's canal** = circular canal in the sclera of the eye, which drains the aqueous humour *sinus venosus sclerae, Schlemms kanal;* **semicircular canals** = three canals in the inner ear partly filled with fluid and which regulate the sense of balance ⇨ *illustration* EAR *canales semicirculares, båggångarna;* **vertebral canal** = hole in the centre of each vertebra, through which the spinal cord passes *canalis vertebralis, spinalkanalen, vertebralkanalen, ryggradskanalen;* **Volkmann's canal** = canal running horizontally through compact bone, carrying blood to the Haversian systems *Volkmanns (volkmannsk) kanal*

canaliculotomy [ˌkænəˌlɪkjʊˈlɒtəmi] *subst.* surgical operation to open up a little canal *operativt ingrepp för att öppna liten kanal*

canaliculus [ˌkænəˈlɪkjʊləs] *subst.* little canal, such as a canal leading to the Haversian systems in compact bone, or a canal leading to the lacrimal duct *canaliculus, liten kanal* NOTE: plural is **canaliculi**

cancellous bone [ˈkænsɪləs ˌbəʊn] *subst.* light spongy bone tissue which forms the inner core of a bone (where it contains the red bone marrow) and also the ends of long bones ⇨ *illustration* BONE STRUCTURE *pars spongiosa, porös benvävnad, spongiöst ben*

cancer [ˈkænsə] *subst.* malignant growth *or* tumour, which develops in tissue and destroys it, which can spread by metastasis to other parts of the body and cannot be controlled by the body itself *cancer, kräfta;* **cancer cells developed in the lymph; he has been diagnosed as having lung cancer** *or* **as having cancer of the lung** NOTE: used with **the** or **a** to indicate one particular tumour, and without **the** or **a** to indicate the disease: **doctors removed a cancer from her breast; she has breast cancer.** NOTE: for other terms referring to cancer see words beginning with **carcin-**

> COMMENT: cancers can be divided into cancers of the skin (carcinomas) or cancers of connective tissue, such as bone or muscle (sarcomas). Cancer can be caused by tobacco, radiation and many other factors. Many cancers are curable by surgery, by chemotherapy or by radiation, especially if they are detected early

cancer ⇨ **cancer, neoplasm**

cancer- ⇨ **cancerous, carcin-**

cancerframkallande ⇨ **carcinogenesis, carcinogenic**

cancer-in-situ ⇨ **carcinoma**

cancerofobi ⇨ **cancerophobia**

cancerophobia [ˌkænsərəʊˈfəʊbiə] *subst.* fear of cancer *cancerofobi, cancerskräck*

cancerous [ˈkæns(ə)rəs] *adj.* referring to cancer *cancerös, cancer-;* **the X-ray revealed a cancerous growth in the breast**

cancerskräck ⇨ **cancerophobia**

cancerös ⇨ **cancerous**

cancrum oris [ˈkænkrəm ˈɔːrɪs] *or* **noma** [ˈnəʊmə] *subst.* severe ulcers in the mouth, leading to gangrene *cancrum oris, noma*

Candida [ˈkændɪdə] *or* **Monilia** [məˈnɪliə] *subst.* type of fungus which causes mycosis *Candida;* **Candida albicans** = one type of Candida which is normally present in the mouth and throat without causing any illness, but which can cause thrush *Candida albicans*

> COMMENT: when the infection occurs in the vagina or mouth it is known as "thrush". Thrush in the mouth usually affects small children

> QUOTE It is incorrect to say that oral candida is an infection. Candida is easily isolated from the mouths of up to 50% of healthy adults and is a normal commensal
>
> **Nursing Times**

candidainfektion ⇨ **candidiasis, perleche**

candidate ['kændɪdeɪt] *subst.* (i) person who is applying for a job *or* for a promotion *kandidat, sökande;* (ii) patient who could have an operation *kandidat (för operation);* **the board is interviewing the candidates for the post of administrator; these types of patients may be candidates for embolization; candidate vaccine** = vaccine which is being tested for use in immunization *vaccin under utprövning*

candidiasis [ˌkændɪ'da(ɪ)əsɪs] *or* **candidosis** [ˌkændɪ'dəʊsɪs] *or* **moniliasis** [məˌnɪlɪ'eɪsɪs] *subst.* infection with Candida *moniliasis, muntorsk, torsk, candidainfektion*

canicola fever [kə'nɪkələ ˌfiːvə] *subst.* form of leptospirosis, giving high fever and jaundice *slags leptospiros med hög feber och gulsot, slags hundsmitta*

canine (tooth) ['kænaɪn (ˌtuːθ)] *or* **eye tooth** ['aɪ ˌtuːθ] *subst.* pointed tooth next to an incisor ⇨ *illustration* TEETH *dens cuspidatus (caninus), hörntand*

> COMMENT: there are four canines in all, two in the upper jaw and two in the lower; those in the upper jaw are referred to as the "eye teeth"

canities [kə'nɪʃiiːz] *subst.* loss of pigments, which makes the hair turn white *canities, gråhårighet*

canker ['kæŋkə] *subst.* lesion of the skin *kräftsår*

cannabis ['kænəbɪs] *or* **hemp** [hemp] *or* **marijuana** [ˌmæri'wɑːnə] *subst.* addictive drug made from the leaves *or* flowers of the Indian hemp plant *cannabis, hampa, marijuana, marihuana*

cannula ['kænjʊlə] *subst.* tube with a trocar *or* blunt needle inside, inserted into the body to drain off or introduce fluid *kanyl*

canthal ['kænθəl] *adj.* referring to the corner of the eye *som avser el. hör till ögonvinkeln (ögonvrån)*

canthus ['kænθəs] *subst.* corner of the eye *canthus, ögonvinkeln, ögonvrån*

cap [kæp] *subst.* **(a)** type of hat which fits tightly on the head *mössa;* **the surgeons were wearing white caps (b)** top which covers something *lock, kapsyl;* **screw the cap back on the bottle; child-proof cap** = special cap on a bottle of a drug, which is made so that a young child cannot open it *barnsäkert lock* **(c)** covering which protects something *lock, skydd;* **Dutch cap** = diaphragm *or* contraceptive device similar to a condom, which is placed in the woman's vagina before sexual intercourse *pessar* **(d)** artificial hard covering for a damaged or broken tooth *jacketkrona*

capable ['keɪpəb(ə)l] *adj.* which can do something *kunnig, mottaglig;* **the disease is capable of treatment**

capacity [kə'pæsəti] *subst. (of a person)* ability to do something *kapacitet, förmåga; (of an organ)* ability to contain *or* absorb a substance *rymd, volym*

capillary [kə'pɪl(ə)ri] *subst.* (i) tiny blood vessel, between the arterioles and the venules, which carries blood and nutrients into the tissues *vas capillare, kapillär;* (ii) any tiny tube carrying a liquid in the body *hårfint kärl, hårrörskärl;* **capillary bleeding** = bleeding where blood oozes out from small blood vessels *kapillärblödning*

capitate (bone) ['kæpɪteɪt (ˌbəʊn)] *subst.* largest of the eight small carpal bones in the wrist ⇨ *illustration* HAND *(os) capitatum*

capitis [kə'paɪtɪs] *see* CORONA

capitulum [kə'pɪtjʊləm] *subst.* round end of a bone, such as the distal end of the humerus, which articulates with another bone *capitulum*

capsula ⇨ **capsule**

capsular ['kæpsjʊlə] *adj.* referring to a capsule *kapsulär*

capsularis [ˌkæpsjʊ'leərɪs] *see* DECIDUA

capsule ['kæpsjuːl] *subst.* **(a)** membrane round an organ *or* joint *capsula, kapsel;* **fibrous capsule** *or* **renal capsule** = fibrous tissue surrounding the kidney *capsula fibrosa, njurkapseln, njurens bindvävskapsel;* **joint capsule** = white fibrous tissue which surrounds and holds a joint together *capsula articularis, ledkapsel;* **Tenon's capsule** = tissue which lines the orbit of the eye *vagina bulbi, Tenons kapsel* **(b) internal capsule** = bundle of fibres linking the cerebral cortex and other parts of the brain *capsula interna* **(c)**

small hollow digestible case, filled with a drug to be swallowed by the patient *kapsel;* **she swallowed three capsules of pain killer; the doctor prescribed the drug in capsule form**

capsulectomy [ˌkæpsjʊˈlektəmi] *subst.* surgical removal of the capsule round a joint *kapsulektomi*

capsulitis [ˌkæpsjʊˈlaɪtɪs] *subst.* inflammation of a capsule *kapsulit*

caput [ˈkeɪpət, ˈkæpət] *subst.* (i) the head *caput, huvudet;* (ii) top of part of the body *caput, huvud*
NOTE: plural is **capita**

carbohydrates [ˌkɑːbə(ʊ)ˈhaɪdreɪts] *subst.* organic compounds which derive from sugar and which are the main ingredients of many types of food *kolhydrater*

> COMMENT: carbohydrates are compounds of carbon, hydrogen and oxygen. They are found in particular in sugar and starch, and provide the body with energy

carbolic acid [kɑːˌbɒlɪk ˈæsɪd] = PHENOL

carbon [ˈkɑːb(ə)n] *subst.* one of the common non-metallic elements, an essential component of living matter and organic chemical compounds *kol*

carbonated [ˈkɑːb(ə)neɪtɪd] *adj.* (drink) with bubbles in it, because carbon dioxide has been added *kolsyrad*

carbon dioxide [ˌkɑːb(ə)n daɪˈɒksaɪd] *subst.* gas produced by the body's metabolism as the tissues burn carbon, and breathed out by the lungs as waste *koldioxid, kolsyra*

carbonizio ⇨ **burn**

carbon monoxide [ˌkɑːb(ə)n məˈnɒksaɪd] *subst.* poisonous gas found in fumes from car engines, from burning gas and cigarette smoke *koloxid;* **carbon monoxide poisoning** = being poisoned by breathing carbon monoxide *koloxidförgiftning* NOTE: the chemical symbols for carbon, carbon dioxide and carbon monoxide are **C, CO_2, CO**

> COMMENT: carbon dioxide can be solidified at low temperatures and is known as "dry ice" or "carbon dioxide snow", being used to remove growths on the skin. Carbon monoxide is dangerous because it is easily absorbed into the blood and takes the place of the oxygen in the blood. Carbon monoxide has no smell, and people do not realize that they are being poisoned by it until they become unconscious. The treatment for carbon monoxide poisoning is very rapid inhalation of fresh air together with carbon dioxide if this can be provided

carbuncle [ˈkɑːbʌŋk(ə)l] *subst.* localized staphylococcal infection, which goes deep into the tissue *karbunkel, böld*

carcin- [ˈkɑːsɪn, ˌ--] *prefix* referring to carcinoma *or* cancer *carcin(o)-, karcin(o)-, cancer-, kräft-*

carcinogen [kɑːˈsɪnədʒ(ə)n] *subst.* substance which produces carcinoma *carcinogent (karcinogent, cancerframkallande) ämne*

carcinogen ⇨ **carcinogenic**

carcinogenesis [ˌkɑːsɪnəˈdʒenəsɪs] *subst.* process of forming carcinoma in tissue *cancerframkallande*

carcinogenic [ˌkɑːsɪnəˈdʒenɪk] *adj.* which produces carcinoma *carcinogen, karcinogen, cancerframkallande*

carcinoid ⇨ **carcinoid (tumour)**

carcinoidsyndrom ⇨ **carcinoid (tumour)**

carcinoid (tumour) [ˈkɑːsɪnɔɪd (ˌtjuːmə)] *subst.* type of intestinal tumour (especially in the appendix), which causes diarrhoea *carcinoid, karcinoid;* **carcinoid syndrome** = group of symptoms which are associated with a carcinoid tumour *carcinoidsyndrom*

carcinom ⇨ **carcinoma**

carcinoma [ˌkɑːsɪˈnəʊmə] *subst.* cancer of the epithelium or glands *carcinom, karcinom, kräftsvulst;* **carcinoma-in-situ** = first stage in the development of a cancer, where the epithelial cells begin to change *cancer-in-situ, noninvasiv cancer, stadium 0 av cancer*

carcinomatos ⇨ **carcinomatosis**

carcinomatosis [ˌkɑsɪˌnəʊməˈtəʊsɪs] *subst.* carcinoma which has spread to many sites in the body *carcinomatos*

carcinomatous [ˌkɑːsɪˈnɒmətəs] *adj.* referring to carcinoma *som avser el. hör till carcinom*

card [kɑːd] *subst.* stiff piece of paper which can carry information on it for reference *kort;* **filing card** = card with information written on it, used to classify information in correct order *registerkort;* **index card** = card used to make a card index *kartotekskort;* **punched card** = card with holes punched in it which a computer can read *hålkort*

cardi- ['kɑːdi, ˌ--] *or* **cardio-** ['kɑːdiə(ʊ), ˌ--] *prefix* referring to the heart *cardi(o)-, kardi(o)-, hjärt-*

cardia ['kɑːdɪə] *subst.* (i) opening at the top of the stomach which joins it to the gullet *cardia, kardia, övre magmunnen;* (ii) the heart ➪ *illustration* STOMACH *hjärtat*

cardiac ['kɑːdɪæk] *adj.* (i) referring to the heart *hjärt-;* (ii) referring to the cardia *som avser el. hör till övre magmunnen;* **cardiac achalasia** *see* ACHALASIA; **cardiac arrest** = stopping of the heart *or* condition where the heart muscle stops beating *hjärtstillestånd;* **cardiac asthma** = difficulty in breathing caused by heart failure *asthma cardiale, hjärtastma;* **cardiac catheterization** = passing a catheter into the heart to take samples of tissue *or* to check blood pressure *hjärtkatetrisering;* **cardiac cirrhosis** = cirrhosis of the liver caused by heart disease *cirrhose (biliare) cardiaque;* **cardiac compression** = compression of the heart by fluid in the pericardium *hjärttamponad, hopklämning av hjärtat pga vätska i hjärtsäcken;* **cardiac conducting system** = nerve system in the heart which links an atrium to a ventricle, so that the two beat at the same rate *hjärtats retledningssystem;* **cardiac cycle** = repeated beating of the heart, formed of the diastole and systole *hjärtcykeln;* **cardiac decompression** = removal of a haematoma *or* constriction in the heart *avlägsnande av ngt som orsakar hopklämning av hjärtat;* **cardiac failure** *or* **heart failure** = situation where the heart cannot function in a satisfactory way and is unable to circulate blood normally *hjärtsvikt;* **cardiac impressions** = hollow parts in the surface of the liver and lungs where they are in contact with the pericardium *incisurae cardiacae, hjärtats avtryck på omgivande organ;* **cardiac massage** = treatment to make a heart which has stopped beating start working again, where the first aider presses on the patient's chest *hjärtmassage;* **cardiac monitor** = electrocardiograph *or* instrument which checks the functioning of the heart in an intensive care unit *oscilloskop, övervaknings-TV, EKG-apparat;* **cardiac murmur** = abnormal sound made by the heart, heard through a stethoscope *hjärtblåsljud;* **cardiac muscle** = special muscle which forms the heart *hjärtmuskeln;* **cardiac neurosis** *or* **da Costa's syndrome** = condition where the patient suffers palpitations caused by worry *hjärtneuros;* **cardiac notch** = (i) point in the left lung, where the right inside wall is bent *incisura cardiaca;* (ii) notch at the point where the oesophagus joins the greater curvature of the stomach *incisura angularis, vinkeln mellan matstrupen och magsäckens övre del;* **cardiac orifice** = opening where the oesophagus joins the stomach *ostium cardiacum, öppningen där matstrupen övergår i magsäcken;* **cardiac pacemaker** = electronic device implanted on a patient's heart or worn by the patient attached to his chest, which stimulates and regulates the heartbeat *(konstgjord) pacemaker; see also* PACEMAKER; **cardiac patient** = patient suffering from heart disorder *hjärtpatient;* **cardiac reflex** = reflex which controls the heartbeat automatically *nervimpuls som styr hjärtats kontraktioner;* **cardiac tamponade** = pressure on the heart when the pericardial cavity fills with blood *hjärt(säcks)tamponad;* **cardiac veins** = veins which lead from the myocardium to the right atrium *hjärtats vener*

cardialgia [ˌkɑːdi'ældʒiə] *subst.* heartburn *or* pain in the chest from indigestion *kardialgi, hjärtsmärta*

card index [ˌkɑːd 'ɪndeks] *subst.* series of cards with information written on them, kept in special order so that the information can be found easily *kortregister, kartotek;* **the hospital records used to be kept on a card index, but have been transferred to the computer; card-index file** = information kept on filing cards *information i kortregister*

card-index [ˌkɑːd'ɪndeks] *vb.* to put information onto a card index *föra in information på kort (i register)*

cardiogram ['kɑːdɪə(ʊ)græm] *subst.* graph showing the heartbeat, produced by a cardiograph *elektrokardiogram, EKG, kardiogram*

cardiograph ['kɑːdɪə(ʊ)grɑːf] *subst.* instrument which records the heartbeat *(elektro)kardiograf*

cardiographer [ˌkɑːdi'ɒgrəfə] *subst.* technician who operates a cardiograph *person som tar EKG*

cardiologist [ˌkɑːdɪ'ɒlədʒɪst] *or* **heart specialist** ['hɑːt ˌspeʃəlɪst] *subst.* doctor who specializes in the study of the heart *kardiolog, hjärtspecialist*

cardiology [ˌkɑːdi'ɒlədʒi] *subst.* study of the heart and its diseases and functions *kardiologi*

cardiomegaly [ˌkɑːdiə(ʊ)'megəli] *subst.* enlarged heart *kardiomegali, hjärthypertrofi, hjärtförstoring*

cardiomyopathy [ˌkɑːdiə(ʊ)maɪˈɒpəθi] *subst.* disorder of the heart muscle *kardiomyopati*

cardiomyotomy [ˌkɑːdiə(ʊ)maɪˈɒtəmi] *subst.* Heller's operation *or* operation to treat cardiac achalasia by splitting the ring of muscles where the oesophagus joins the stomach *kardiomyotomi*

cardiopathy [ˌkɑːdiˈɒpəθi] *subst.* any kind of heart disease *kardiopati, hjärtsjukdom*

cardiophone [ˈkɑːdiə(ʊ)fəʊn] *subst.* microphone attached to a patient to record sounds (used to record the heart of an unborn baby) *mikrofon som fångar upp ljud (t.ex. fosterljud)*

cardiopulmonary bypass [ˌkɑːdiə(ʊ)ˈpʌlmənəri ˈbaɪpɑːs] *subst.* machine *or* method for artificially circulating the patient's blood during open heart surgery, where the heart and lungs are cut off from the circulation and replaced by a pump *hjärtlungmaskin, hjärtlungbypass, shuntning av blod vid öppen hjärtkirurgi*

cardiopulmonary resuscitation (CPR) [ˌkɑːdiə(ʊ)ˈpʌlmənəri rɪˌsʌsɪˈteɪʃ(ə)n (ˌsiːpiːˈɑː)] *subst.* method of resuscitation which stimulates both heart and lungs *hjärtlungräddning*

> COMMENT: the first aider applies massage to the patient's heart by pressing on his chest, and from time to time also applies mouth-to-mouth resuscitation

cardioscope [ˈkɑːdiə(ʊ)skəʊp] *subst.* instrument formed of a tube with a light at the end, used to inspect the inside of the heart *kardioskop*

cardiospasm [ˈkɑːdiə(ʊ)spæz(ə)m] *subst.* being unable to relax the cardia (the muscle at the entrance to the stomach), with the result that food cannot enter the stomach *kardiospasm; see also* HELLER'S OPERATION

cardiotocography [ˌkɑːdiə(ʊ)tɒˈkɒgrəfi] *subst.* recording of the heartbeat of a fetus *kardiotokografi*

cardiovascular [ˌkɑːdiə(ʊ)ˈvæskjʊlə] *adj.* referring to the heart and the blood circulation system *kardiovaskulär;* **cardiovascular disease** = any disease (such as hypertension) which affects the circulatory system *kardiovaskulär sjukdom;* **cardiovascular system** = system of blood circulation *kardiovaskulära systemet, hjärt-kärlsystemet, cirkulationsapparaten*

> QUOTE Cardiovascular diseases remain the leading cause of death in the United States
> **Journal of American Medical Association**

cardioversion [ˈkɑːdiə(ʊ)ˌvɜːʃ(ə)n] *or* **defibrillation** [diːˌfɪbrɪˈleɪʃ(ə)n] *subst.* correcting an irregular heartbeat by using an electric impulse *elkonvertering, defibrillering*

carditis [kɑːˈdaɪtɪs] *subst.* inflammation of the connective tissue of the heart *kardit, hjärtinflammation*

care [keə] *subst.* attention *or* general treatment (of a patient) *vård, omsorg, omvårdnad;* **the patient is under the care of a cancer specialist; she is responsible for the care of patients in the outpatients department; coronary care unit** = section of a hospital reserved to treat patients suffering from heart attacks *hjärtintensivavdelning, hjärtinfarktavdelning, HIA;* **a coronary care unit has been opened at a London hospital; intensive care** = constant supervision and treatment of a patient in a special section of a hospital *intensivvård;* **she is in intensive care** *or* **in the intensive care unit**

> QUOTE the experience of the ward sister is the most important factor in the standard of care
> **Nursing Times**

care for [ˈkeə fɔː] *vb.* to look after *vårda, sköta om;* **nurses were caring for the injured people at the scene of the accident; severely handicapped children are cared for in special clinics**

care plan [ˈkeə ˌplæn] *subst.* plan drawn up by the nursing staff for the treatment of an individual patient *vårdplan, omvårdnadsplan*

> QUOTE all relevant sections of the nurses' care plan and nursing process had been left blank
> **Nursing Times**

carer [ˈkeərə] *subst.* someone who looks after a sick person *vårdare*

> QUOTE most research has focused on those caring for older people or for adults with disability and chronic illness. Most studied are the carers of those who might otherwise have to stay in hospital for a long time
> **British Medical Journal**

caries [ˈkeərɪz] *subst.* decay in a tooth *or* bone *karies, tandröta, benröta;* **dental caries** = decay in a tooth *(tand)karies, tandröta*

carina [kəˈriːnə] *subst.* structure shaped like the bottom of a boat, such as the cartilage at the point where the trachea branches into the bronchi *carina*

cariogenic [ˌkeəriəʊˈdʒenɪk] *adj.* (substance) which causes caries *kariogen, kariesframkallande*

carminative [ˈkɑːmɪnətɪv] *adj. & subst.* (substance) which relieves colic *or* indigestion *carminativum, karminativum, medel mot gasbildning*

carminativum ⇨ **carminative**

carotenaemia [ˌkærətɪˈniːmiə] *or* **xanthaemia** [zænˈθiːmiə] *subst.* excessive amount of carotene in the blood as a result of eating mainly too many carrots or tomatoes, which gives the skin a yellow colour *karotinemi, xantemi*

carotene [ˈkærətiːn] *subst.* orange or red pigment in carrots, egg yolk and some natural oils, which is converted by the liver into vitamin A *karotin, karoten*

carotid [kəˈrɒtɪd] *subst.* artery in the neck *carotis, stora halspulsådern;* **common carotid artery** *or* **carotid** = main artery running up each side of the lower part of the neck *arteria carotis communis, gemensamma halsartären;* **carotid body** = tissue in the carotid sinus which is concerned with cardiovascular reflexes *glomus caroticum, vävnad i sinus caroticus som reglerar blodtryck och hjärtfrekvens;* **carotid pulse** = pulse in the carotid artery at the side of the neck *carotispuls;* **carotid sinus** = expanded part attached to the carotid artery, which monitors blood pressure *sinus caroticus, carotissinus*

COMMENT: the common carotid artery is in the lower part of the neck, and branches upwards into the external and internal carotids. The carotid body is situated at the point where the carotid divides

carotis ⇨ **carotid**

carotispuls ⇨ **carotid**

carotissinus ⇨ **carotid**

carp- [kɑːp] *or* **carpo-** [ˈkɑːpə(ʊ), ˌ--] *prefix* referring to the wrist *carp(o)-, karp(o)-, handlovs-*

carpal [ˈkɑːp(ə)l] *adj. & subst.* referring to the wrist *karpal(-), handlovs-;* **carpal bones** *or* **carpals** = the eight bones which make up the carpus *or* wrist ⇨ *illustration* HAND *ossa carpalia (carpi), karpalbenen;* **carpal tunnel syndrome** = condition (usually in women) where the fingers tingle and hurt at night, caused by compression of the median nerve *karpaltunnelsyndrom*

carphology [kɑːˈfɒlədʒi] *or* **floccitation** [ˌflɒksɪˈteɪʃ(ə)n] *subst.* pulling at the bedclothes (a sign of delirium in typhoid and other fevers) *floccilegium*

carpometacarpal joints (CM joints) [ˌkɑːpə(ʊ)ˌmetəˈkɑːp(ə)l ˌdʒɔɪnts (ˌsiːˈemˌdʒɔɪnts)] *subst.* joints between the carpals and metacarpals *articulationes carpometacarpae, karpometakarpallederna, cmc-lederna*

carpopedal spasm [ˌkɑːpə(ʊ)ˈpiːd(ə)l ˌspæz(ə)m] *subst.* spasm in the hands and feet caused by lack of calcium *carpopedalspasm, karpopedalspasm*

carpus [ˈkɑːpəs] *subst.* wrist *or* bones by which the lower arm is connected to the hand *carpus, handloven*

COMMENT: the carpus is formed of eight small bones (the carpals): these are the capitate, hamate, lunate, pisiform, scaphoid, trapezium, trapezoid and triquetral

carrier [ˈkærɪə] *subst.* **(a)** person who carries bacteria of a disease in his body, and who can transmit the disease to others without showing any sign of it himself *smittbärare* **(b)** insect which carries disease and infects humans *vektor, transportör* **(c)** healthy person who carries the chromosome defect of a hereditary disease (such as haemophilia *or* Duchenne muscular dystrophy) *anlagsbärare*

carsick [ˈkɑːsɪk] *adj.* being ill because of the movement of a car *åksjuk*

carsickness [ˈkɑːsɪknəs] *subst.* feeling sick because of the movement of a car *kinetos, åksjuka*

cart [kɑːt] *US* = TROLLEY

cartilage [ˈkɑːtəlɪdʒ] *subst.* gristle *or* thick connective tissue which lines the joints and acts as a cushion, and which forms part of the structure of an organ *cartilago, brosk;* **articular cartilage** = layer of cartilage on the end of a bone where it joins another bone *cartilago articularis, ledbrosk;* **costal cartilage** = cartilage which connects a rib to the breastbone *revbensbrosk;* **cricoid cartilage** = cartilage in the lower part of the larynx *cartilago cricoidea, ringbrosket;* **elastic cartilage** = flexible cartilage in the ear and epiglottis *elastiskt brosk;* **epiphyseal cartilage** = section of cartilage in the bones of children and adolescents which expands and hardens as the bones grow to full size *cartilago epiphysialis, epifysbrosk;* **hyaline cartilage** = type of cartilage in the nose, larynx and joints *hyalint brosk, glasbrosk;* **thyroid cartilage** = large cartilage in the larynx which forms part of the Adam's apple *cartilago thyreoidea, sköldbrosket*

> COMMENT: cartilage in small children is the first stage in the formation of bones

cartilaginous [ˌkɑːtəˈlædʒɪnəs] *adj.* made of cartilage *kartilaginär, brosk-;* **(primary) cartilaginous joint** *or* **synchondrosis** = joint in children before the cartilage has changed to bone *synkondros, broskfog;* **(secondary) cartilaginous joint** *or* **symphysis** = joint where cartilage fixes two bones together so that they cannot move (such as the pubic symphysis) *symfys* NOTE: for other terms referring to cartilage, see words beginning with **chondr-** ⇨ *illustration* BONE STRUCTURE, JOINTS, LUNGS

caruncle [kəˈrʌŋk(ə)l] *subst.* small swelling *karunkel;* **lacrimal caruncle** = red point at the inner corner of each eye *caruncula lacrimalis, tårkarunkeln, ögonkarunkeln*

casantranol ⇨ **cascara (sagrada)**

cascara (sagrada) [kæˈskɑːrə (səˌgrɑːdə)] *subst.* laxative made from the bark of a tropical tree *casantranol, sagrada(extrakt)*

case [keɪs] *subst.* (i) single occurrence of a disease *sjukdomsfall;* (ii) person who has a disease *or* who is undergoing treatment *fall;* **there were two hundred cases of cholera in the recent outbreak; the hospital is only admitting urgent cases; there is an appendicectomy case waiting for the operating theatre; case history** = details of what has happened to a patient who is undergoing treatment *sjukjournal, sjukdomshistoria*

casein [ˈkeɪsiɪn, -siːn] *subst.* protein found in milk *kasein*

> COMMENT: casein is precipitated when milk comes into contact with an acid, and so makes milk form cheese

cast [kɑːst] *subst.* **(a) plaster cast** = hard support, made of bandage soaked in liquid plaster of Paris which is allowed to harden, used to wrap round a fracture to prevent movement while the bone is healing *gips(förband)* **(b)** mass of material formed in a hollow organ *or* tube and excreted in fluid *cylinder;* **blood casts** = pieces of blood cells which are secreted by the kidneys in kidney disease *blodcylindrar*

castor oil [ˈkɑːstərˌɒɪl] *subst.* vegetable oil which acts as a laxative *ricinolja*

castrate [kæsˈtreɪt, ˈ--] *vb.* to remove the testicles *kastrera*

castration [kæsˈtreɪʃ(ə)n] *subst.* surgical removal of the testicles *kastrering*

casualty [ˈkæʒʊ(ə)lti] *subst.* **(a)** person who has suffered an accident *or* who is suddenly ill *offer, olycksfall;* **the fire caused several casualties; the casualties were taken by ambulance to the nearest hospital; casualty department** *or* **hospital** *or* **ward** = department *or* hospital *or* ward which deals with accident victims *akutmottagning, olycksfallsavdelning etc.* **(b)** a casualty department *akutmottagning, olycksfallsavdelning;* **the accident victim was rushed to casualty**

CAT [ˌsiːeɪˈtiː] = COMPUTERIZED AXIAL TOMOGRAPHY; **CAT scan** = scan in which a narrow X-ray beam, guided by a computer to take photographs from various directions, can make a photograph of a thin section of a body *or* organ *datortomografi, DT, CT, skiktröntgen*

cata- [ˈkætə, ˌ--] *prefix* meaning downwards *cata-, kata-*

catabolic [ˌkætəˈbɒlɪk] *adj.* referring to catabolism *katabol(isk)*

catabolism [kəˈtæbəlɪz(ə)m] *subst.* breaking down of complex chemicals into simple chemicals *katabolism*

catalase [ˈkætəleɪs] *subst.* enzyme present in the blood and liver which catalyzes the breakdown of hydrogen peroxide into water and oxygen *katalas*

catalepsy [ˈkætəlepsi] *subst.* condition where a patient becomes incapable of sensation, his body is rigid and he does not move for long periods, especially in schizophrenia *katalepsi*

catalyst [ˈkæt(ə)lɪst] *subst.* substance which produces *or* helps a chemical process but without itself changing *katalysator;* **an enzyme which acts as a catalyst in the digestive process**

catalyze [ˈkætəlaɪz] *vb.* to act as a catalyst *or* to help make a chemical process take place *katalysera*

catamenia [ˌkætəˈmiːniə] *subst.* menstruation *mens(truation), reglering, månadsblödning*

cataplexy [ˈkætəˌpleksi] *subst.* condition where the patient's muscles become suddenly rigid and he falls without losing consciousness, possibly caused by a shock *kataplexi*

cataract ['kætərækt] *subst.* condition where the lens of the eye gradually becomes hard and opaque *katarakt, grå starr;* **diabetic cataract** = cataract which develops in people suffering from diabetes *catarrhacta complicata, grå starr vid diabetes;* **senile cataract** = cataract which occurs in an elderly person *catarrhacta senilis, ålder(dom)sstarr;* **cataract extraction** = surgical removal of an opaque lens from an eye *starroperation*

> COMMENT: cataracts form most often in people after the age of 50. They are sometimes caused by a blow or an electric shock. Cataracts can easily and safely be removed by surgery

catarrh [kə'tɑ:] *subst.* inflammation of mucous membranes in the nose and throat, creating an excessive amount of mucus *katarr, slemhinneinflammation;* **he suffers from catarrh in the winter; is there anything I can take to relieve my catarrh?**

catarrhal [kə'tɑ:r(ə)l] *adj.* referring to catarrh *katarral;* **a catarrhal cough**

catatonia [ˌkætə'təʊniə] *subst.* condition where a psychiatric patient is either motionless *or* shows violent reactions to stimulation *katatoni*

catatonic [ˌkætə'tɒnɪk] *adj.* (behaviour) where the patient is either motionless *or* extremely violent *kataton(isk);* **catatonic schizophrenia** = type of schizophrenia where the patient is alternately apathetic or very active and disturbed *schizophrenia catatonica, kataton schizofreni*

catch [kætʃ] *vb.* to get a disease *få, smittas av, ådra sig;* **he caught a cold after standing in the rain; she caught mumps** NOTE: **catches - catching - caught - has caught**

catching ['kætʃɪŋ] *adj.* infectious *smittsam, smittande;* **is the disease catching?**

catchment area ['kætʃmənt ˌeəriə] *subst.* area around a hospital which is served by that hospital *upptagningsområde*

catecholamines [ˌkætə'kɒləmi:nz] *subst pl.* adrenaline and noradrenaline (hormones released by the adrenal glands) *katekolaminer*

category ['kætəg(ə)rɪ] *subst.* classification *or* way in which things can be classified *kategori, klass;* **his condition is of a non-urgent category**

catgut ['kæ:tgʌt] *subst.* thread made from part of the intestines of sheep, now usually artificially hardened, used to sew up incisions made during surgery *catgut, katgut*

> COMMENT: catgut is slowly dissolved by fluids in the body after the wound has healed and therefore does not need to be removed. Ordinary catgut will dissolve in 5 to 10 days; hardened catgut takes up to three or four weeks

catharsis [kə'θɑ:sɪs] *subst.* purgation of the bowels *katarsis, laxering*

cathartic [kə'θɑ:tɪk] *adj.* laxative *or* purgative *purgerande, laxerande, avförande*

catheter ['kæθɪtə] *subst.* tube passed into the body along one of the passages in the body *kateter;* **cardiac catheter** = catheter passed through a vein into the heart, to take blood samples *or* to record pressure *or* to examine the interior of the heart before surgery *hjärtkateter;* **ureteric catheter** = catheter passed through the ureter to the kidney to inject opaque solution into the kidney before taking an X-ray *uretärkateter;* **urinary** *or* **urethral catheter** = catheter passed up the urethra to allow urine to flow out of the bladder, used to empty the bladder before an abdominal operation *urinkateter, tappningskateter*

catheterization [ˌkæθɪt(ə)raɪ'zeɪʃ(ə)n] *subst.* putting a catheter into a patient's body *katetrisering;* **cardiac catheterization** = passing a catheter into the heart to take samples of tissue *or* to check blood pressure *hjärtkatetrisering*

> QUOTE high rates of disconnection of closed urine drainage systems, lack of hand washing and incorrect positioning of urine drainage bags have been highlighted in a new report on urethral catheterization
>
> **Nursing Times**

> QUOTE the technique used to treat aortic stenosis is similar to that for any cardiac catheterization. A catheter introduced through the femoral vein is placed across the aortic valve and into the left ventricle
>
> **Journal of the American Medical Association**

catheterize ['kæθɪtəraɪz] *vb.* to insert a catheter into a patient *katetrisera*

cat scratch fever ['kæt ˌskrætʃ 'fi:və] *subst.* fever and inflammation of the lymph glands, caught from being scratched by a cat's claws or by other sharp points *feber och lymfkörtelinflammation pga rivsår (av katt)*

cauda equina ['kɔ:də ɪ'kwaɪnə] *subst.* group of nerves which go from the spinal cord to the lumbar region and the coccyx *cauda equina*

caudal ['kɔ:d(ə)l] *adj. (in animals)* referring to the tail *svans-; (in humans)* referring to cauda equina *kaudal, som avser el. hör till cauda equina;* **caudal analgesia** = technique often used in childbirth, where an analgesic is injected into the extradural space at the base of the spine to remove feeling in the lower part of the trunk *epiduralanestesi, epiduralbedövning;* **caudal block** = local analgesia of the cauda equina nerves *kaudalblockad*

caul [kɔ:l] *subst.* **(a)** membrane which sometimes covers a baby's head at childbirth *fosterhinnan* **(b)** = OMENTUM

cauliflower ear [ˌkɒliˌfla(ʊ)ər 'ɪə] *subst.* permanently swollen ear, caused by blows (in boxing) *blomkålsöra, boxaröra*

causalgia [kɔ:'zældʒə] *subst.* burning pain in a limb, caused by a damaged nerve *kausalgi*

cauterization [ˌkɔ:tərai'zeɪʃ(ə)n] *subst.* act of cauterizing *kauterisering, bränning;* **the growth was removed by cauterization**

cauterize ['kɔ:təraɪz] *vb.* to use burning *or* radiation *or* laser beams to remove tissue *or* to stop bleeding *kauterisera, bränna*

cautery ['kɔ:t(ə)rɪ] *subst.* surgical instrument used to cauterize a wound *kauter, brännjärn;* **cold cautery** = removal of a skin growth using carbon dioxide snow *kauterisering med hjälp av kolsyresnö; see also* ELECTROCAUTERY, GALVANOCAUTERY

cava ['keɪvə] *see* VENA CAVA

cavernosa [ˌkævə'nəusə] *see* CORPUS

cavernous ['kæv(ə)nəs] *adj.* hollow *kavernös, ihålig;* **cavernous breathing** *or* **breath sounds** = hollow sounds made by the lungs when heard through a stethoscope *amforisk andning (vid tbc med lungkaverner);* **cavernous haemangioma** = tumour in connective tissue with wide spaces which contain blood *kavernöst hemangiom;* **cavernous sinus** *see* SINUS

cavitation [ˌkævɪ'teɪʃ(ə)n] *subst.* forming of a cavity *bildning av hålrum*

cavity ['kævətɪ] *subst.* (i) hole *or* empty space inside the body *kavitet, hål(a), hålighet;* (ii) hole in a tooth *kavitet, hål;* **abdominal cavity** = space in the body below the chest *cavum abdominis, bukhålan;* **buccal cavity** = mouth *cavum oris, munhålan;* **cerebral cavity** = ventricles in the brain *ventriculi cerebri, hjärnventriklarna;* **chest cavity** = space in the body containing the heart and lungs *cavum thoracis, brösthålan;* **cranial cavity** = space inside the bones of the cranium, inside which the brain fits *hjärnskålen;* **glenoid cavity** = socket in the shoulder joint into which the humerus fits ⇨ *illustration* SHOULDER *cavitas glenoidalis;* **medullary cavity** = hollow centre of a long bone, containing bone marrow ⇨ *illustration* BONE STRUCTURE *cavum medullare, märghåla;* **nasal cavity** = space behind the nose between the skull and the roof of the mouth, divided in two by the nasal septum ⇨ *illustration* THROAT *cavum nasi, näshålan;* **oral cavity** = mouth *cavum oris, munhålan;* **pelvic cavity** = space below the abdominal cavity, above the pelvic bones *cavum pelvis, bäckenhålan;* **peritoneal cavity** = space between the layers of the peritoneum *cavum peritonei (peritoneale), peritonealhålan;* **pleural cavity** = space between the inner and outer pleura of the chest *cavum pleurae, pleurahålan;* **pulp cavity** = centre of a tooth containing soft tissue ⇨ *illustration* TOOTH *cavum dentis, pulpahåla, pulpakammare;* **synovial cavity** = space inside a synovial joint *ledspalt, ledhåla;* **thoracic cavity** = chest cavity, containing the diaphragm, heart and lungs *cavum thoracis, brösthålan*

cavus ['keɪvəs] *see* PES

CBC [ˌsi:bi:'si:] = COMPLETE BLOOD COUNT

cc [ˌsi:'si:] = CUBIC CENTIMETRE

Cd *chemical symbol for* cadmium *Cd, kadmium*

CDH [ˌsi:di:'eɪtʃ] = CONGENITAL DISLOCATION OF THE HIP

cecum ['si:kəm] *subst. US* = CAECUM

cefalalgi ⇨ **cephalalgia**

cefalocele ⇨ **cephalocele**

cefalometri ⇨ **cephalometry**

cekostomi ⇨ **caecostomy**

-cele [si:(ə)l] *suffix* referring to a hollow *-håla*

celiac ['si:lɪæk] *US* = COELIAC

celiaki ⇨ **coeliac**

celioskopi ➪ **coelioscopy**

cell [sel] *subst.* tiny unit of matter which is the base of all plant and animal tissue *cell;* **cell body** = part of a nerve cell which surrounds the nucleus and from which the axon and dendrites begin *cellkropp;* **cell division** = way in which a cell reproduces itself by mitosis *celldelning;* **cell membrane** = membrane enclosing the cytoplasm of a cell *cellmembran, cellvägg;* **alpha cell** *or* **beta cell** = names given to the two types of cell in glands (such as the pancreas) which have two types *alfacell, betacell;* **blood cell** = corpuscle *or* any type of cell found in the blood *blodkropp;* **daughter cell** = one of the cells which develop by mitosis from a single parent cell *dottercell;* **goblet cell** = tube-shaped cell which secretes mucus *bägarcell;* **mast cell** = large cell in connective tissue, which carries histamine and reacts to allergens *mastcell;* **mother cell** *or* **parent cell** = original cell which splits into daughter cells by mitosis *modercell;* **mucous cell** = cell which secretes mucin *muköscell, slemcell;* **parietal cell** *or* **oxyntic cell** = cell in the gastric mucosa which secretes hydrochloric acid *parietalcell;* **receptor cell** = cell which senses a change in the surrounding environment (such as cold *or* heat) and reacts to it by sending an impulse through the nervous system to the brain *receptorcell*

> COMMENT: the cell is a unit which can reproduce itself. It is made up of a jelly-like substance (cytoplasm) which surrounds a nucleus, and contains many other small organisms which are different according to the type of cell. Cells reproduce by division (mitosis), and their process of feeding and removing waste products is metabolism. The division and reproduction of cells is how the human body is formed.

cell- ➪ **cyt-**

celldelning ➪ **cell**

celldelning, indirekt ➪ **mitosis**

cellförband ➪ **syncytium**

cellkropp ➪ **cell**

cellkärna ➪ **nucleus**

cellmembran ➪ **cell**

celloidin ➪ **collodion**

cellskräck ➪ **claustrophobia**

cellstoff ➪ **wadding**

cellular ['seljʊlə] *adj.* **(a)** referring to cells *or* formed of cells *cellular, cellulär* **(b)** made of many similar parts connected together *uppbyggd av celler;* **cellular tissue** = form of connective tissue with large spaces *lucker bindväv* NOTE: for other terms referring to cells, see words beginning with **cyt-**, **cyto-**

cellulit ➪ **cellulitis**

cellulitis [ˌseljʊ'laɪtɪs] *subst.* usually bacterial inflammation of connective tissue *or* of the subcutaneous tissue *cellulit*

cellulosa ➪ **cellulose**

cellulose ['seljʊləʊs] *subst.* carbohydrate which makes up a large percentage of plant matter *cellulosa*

> COMMENT: cellulose is not digestible, and is passed through the digestive system as roughage

cellulär ➪ **cellular**

cellvägg ➪ **cell**

celom ➪ **coelom**

Celsius ['selsiəs] *subst.* scale of temperature where the freezing and boiling points of water are 0° and 100° *Celsius(skala), celsius*
NOTE: used in many countries, except in the USA, where the Fahrenheit system is still preferred. Normally written as a **C** after the number: **52 ° C** (say: 'fifty-two degrees Celsius'). Also called **Centigrade**

celsius ➪ **Celsius, centigrade**

cement [sə'ment] *subst.* **(a)** adhesive used in dentistry to attach a crown to the base of a tooth *cement* **(b)** = CEMENTUM

cementum [sə'mentəm] *subst.* layer of thick hard material which covers the roots of teeth ➪ *illustration* TOOTH *cement, tandcement*

center ➪ **centre, centrum**

centigrade ['sentɪgreɪd] *subst.* scale of temperature where the freezing and boiling points of water are 0° and 100° *Celsius(skala), celsius; see note at* CELSIUS

centimetre ['sentɪˌmiːtə] *or US* **centimeter** ['sentɪˌmiːtə] *subst.* measurement of how long something is (one hundredth of a metre) *centimeter*

NOTE: centimetre is usually written **cm** with figures: **"the appendix is about 6cm (six centimetres) in length"**

central ['sentr(ə)l] *adj.* referring to the centre *central(-), mitt-;* **central canal** = thin tube in the centre of the spinal cord containing cerebrospinal fluid *canalis centralis, ryggradens centralkanal;* **central nervous system (CNS)** = the brain and spinal cord which link together all the nerves *centrala nervsystemet, CNS;* **central sulcus** = one of the grooves which divide a cerebral hemisphere into lobes *sulcus centralis, centralfåran;* **central vein** = vein in the liver *centralven i levern;* **central venous pressure** = blood pressure in the right atrium, which can be measured by means of a catheter *centrala ventrycket, CVP*

centralfåran ➪ **central**

centralgropen ➪ **fovea (centralis)**

centralis [sen'treɪlɪs] *see* FOVEA

centre *or US* **center** ['sentə] *subst.* **(a)** middle point *or* main part *centrum, mitt;* **the aim of the examination is to locate the centre of infection (b)** large building *centrum, center;* **medical centre** = place where several different doctors and specialists practise *medicinskt centrum, ung. läkarhus* **(c)** point where a group of nerves come together *nervcentrum;* **vision centre** = point in the brain where the nerves relating to the eye come together *chiasma opticum, synnervskorsningen*

centrifug ➪ **centrifuge**

centrifugal [ˌsentrɪ'fju:g(ə)l] *adj.* which goes away from the centre *centrifugal*

centrifuge ['sentrɪfju:dʒ] *subst.* device to separate the components of a liquid *centrifug*

centriol ➪ **centriole**

centriole ['sentriəʊl] *subst.* small structure found in the cytoplasm of a cell, which forms asters during cell division *centriol*

centripetal [sen'trɪpɪt(ə)l] *adj.* which goes towards the centre *centripetal, afferent, inåtledande*

centromer ➪ **centromere**

centromere ['sentrə(ʊ)mɪə] *or* **kinetochore** [kaɪ'ni:təkɔ:] *subst.* constricted part of a cell, seen as the cell divides *centromer*

centroplasma ➪ **centrosome**

centrosoma ➪ **centrosome**

centrosome ['sentrə(ʊ)səʊm] *subst.* structure of the cytoplasm in a cell, near the nucleus, and containing the centrioles *centrosoma, centroplasma*

centrum ['sentrəm] *subst.* centre *or* central part of an organ *centrum, center, mitt*
NOTE: the plural is **centra**

centrum ➪ **centrum, centre, area**

cephal- ['sefəl, ˌ--] *prefix* referring to the head *cefal(o)-, huvud-*

cephalalgia [ˌsefə'lældʒə] *subst.* headache *or* pain in the head *cefalalgi, huvudvärk*

cephalhaematoma [ˌsefəˌli:mə'təʊmə] *subst.* swelling found mainly on the head of babies delivered with forceps *kefalhematom*

cephalic [sə'fælɪk] *adj.* referring to the head *kefal-, hjäss-, huvud-, skall-;* **cephalic index** = measurement of the shape of the skull *skallindex;* **cephalic presentation** = normal position of a baby in the womb, where the baby's head appears first *kronbjudning, hjässbjudning, huvudbjudning;* **cephalic version** = turning a wrongly positioned fetus round in the uterus, so that the head will appear first at birth *vändning till huvudläge*

cephalocele ['sef(ə)ləʊsi:l] *subst.* swelling caused by part of the brain passing through a weak point in the bones of the skull *cefalocele, encefalocele, hjärnbråck*

cephalogram ['sef(ə)ləʊgræm] *subst.* X-ray photograph of the bones of the skull *skallröntgen*

cephalometry [ˌsefə'lɒmɪtri] *subst.* measurement of the head *cefalometri, huvudmätning*

cephalopelvic [ˌsef(ə)ləʊ'pelvɪk] *adj.* referring to the head of the fetus and the pelvis of the mother *som avser el. hör till både fostrets huvud och moderns bäcken;* **cephalopelvic disproportion** = condition where the mother's pelvic opening is not large enough for the head of the fetus *bäckenträngsel, bäckenförträngning*

cerat ➪ **salve**

ceratometri ➪ **keratometry**

ceratoskop ➪ **keratoscope**

ceratotom ➪ **keratome**

ceratotomi ▷ **keratotomy**

cerea ['sɪəriə] *see* FLEXIBILITAS

cereal ['sɪəriəl] *subst.* **(a)** plant whose seeds are used for food, especially to make flour *säd(esslag), spannmål;* **the Common Market grows large quantities of cereals** *or* **of cereal crops (b)** food made of seeds of corn, etc. which is usually eaten at breakfast *(frukost)flingor;* **he ate a bowl of cereal; put milk and sugar on your cereal**

cerebellar [ˌserə'belə] *adj.* referring to the cerebellum *cerebellar, cerebellär, lillhjärns-;* **cerebellar ataxia** = disorder where the patient staggers and cannot speak clearly, due to a disease of the cerebellum *ataxia cerebellaris, cerebellar ataxi;* **cerebellar gait** = way of walking where the patient staggers along, caused by a disease of the cerebellum *cerebellär gång;* **cerebellar peduncles** = bands of tissue which support nerve fibres as they enter or leave the cerebellum *pedunculi cerebellares, lillhjärnsskänklarna, lillhjärnsstjälkarna*

cerebellum [ˌserə'beləm] *subst.* section of the hindbrain, located at the back of the head beneath the back part of the cerebrum ▷ *illustration* BRAIN *cerebellum, lillhjärnan;* **tentorium cerebelli** = part of the dura mater which separates the cerebellum from the cerebrum *tentorium cerebelli, lillhjärnstältet*

> COMMENT: the cerebellum is formed of two hemispheres, with the vermis in the centre. Fibres go into or out of the cerebellum through the peduncles. The cerebellum is the part of the brain where voluntary movements are coordinated and is associated with the sense of balance

cerebr- ['serəbr] *or* **cerebro-** [ˌserəbrə(ʊ)] *prefix* referring to the cerebrum *cerebr(o)-, hjärn-*

cerebral ['serəbr(ə)l] *adj.* referring to the cerebrum *or* to the brain in general *cerebral, hjärn-;* **cerebral aqueduct** *or* **aqueduct of Silvius** = canal connecting the 3rd and 4th ventricles in the brain *aquaeductus cerebri (Sylvii);* **cerebral arteries** = main arteries which take blood into the brain *arteriae cerebri, hjärnartärerna;* **cerebral cavity** = ventricles in the brain *ventriculi cerebri, hjärnventriklarna;* **cerebral cortex** = layer of grey matter which covers the cerebrum *cortex cerebri, hjärnbarken, storhjärnsbarken;* **cerebral decompression** = removal of part of the skull to relieve pressure on the brain *avlägsnande av del av skallen för att minska trycket på hjärnan;* **cerebral haemorrhage** = bleeding inside the brain *hemorrhagia cerebri, hjärnblödning;* **cerebral hemisphere** = one of the two halves of the cerebrum *hemisphaerum cerebri, storhjärnshemisfär, hjärnhemisfär;* **cerebral peduncles** = masses of nerve fibres connecting the cerebral hemispheres to the midbrain *pedunculi cerebri, hjärnskänklarna, hjärnstjälkarna;* **cerebral thrombosis** *or* **stroke** = condition where a blood clot enters and blocks a brain artery *cerebral trombos, blodpropp i hjärnan, stroke, slag(anfall)*

cerebral palsy ['serəbr(ə)l ˌpɔːlzi] *subst.* disorder of the brain, mainly due to brain damage occurring before birth, or due to lack of oxygen during birth *cerebral pares, CP*

> COMMENT: cerebral palsy is the disorder affecting spastics. The patient may have bad coordination of muscular movements, impaired speech, hearing and sight, and sometimes mental retardation

cerebration [ˌserə'breɪʃ(ə)n] *subst.* working of the brain *cerebration*

cerebrospinal [ˌserəbrə(ʊ)'spaɪn(ə)l] *adj.* referring to the brain and the spinal cord *cerebrospinal;* **cerebrospinal fever** *or* **meningococcal meningitis** *or* **spotted fever** = infection of the meninges, caused by a bacterium Neisseria meningitidis *meningitis cerebrospinalis (epidemica), epidemisk hjärnhinneinflammation;* **cerebrospinal fluid (CSF)** = fluid which surrounds the brain and the spinal cord *cerebrospinalvätska;* **cerebrospinal tracts** = main motor pathways in the anterior and lateral white columns of the spinal cord *fasciculi cerebrospinales, tractus corticospinales, pyramidbanorna*

> COMMENT: CSF is found in the space between the arachnoid mater and pia mater of the brain, between the ventricles of the brain, and in the central canal of the spinal cord. CSF consists mainly of water, with some sugar and sodium chloride. Its function is to cushion the brain and spinal cord

cerebrospinalvätska ▷ **cerebrospinal**

cerebrovascular [ˌserəbrə(ʊ)'væskjʊlə] *adj.* referring to the blood vessels in the brain *cerebrovaskulär;* **cerebrovascular accident (CVA)** *or* **stroke** = sudden blocking of or bleeding from a blood vessel in the brain resulting in temporary or permanent paralysis or death *stroke, slag(anfall), hjärnblödning;* **cerebrovascular disease** = disease of the blood vessels in the brain *cerebrovaskulär sjukdom*

cerebrovaskulär ⇨ **cerebrovascular**

cerebrum [sə'ri:brəm] *subst.* main part of the brain *cerebrum, hjärnan, storhjärnan;* **falx cerebri** = fold of the dura mater between the two hemispheres of the cerebrum ⇨ *illustration* BRAIN *falx cerebri, stora hjärnskäran*

> COMMENT: the cerebrum is the largest part of the brain, formed of two sections (the cerebral hemispheres) which run along the length of the head. The cerebrum controls the main mental processes, including the memory

certificate [sə'tɪfɪkət] *subst.* official paper which states something *intyg, bevis, attest;* **birth certificate** = paper giving details of a person's date and place of birth and parents *födelseattest;* **death certificate** = paper signed by a doctor, stating that a person has died and giving details of the person *dödsattest, dödsbevis;* **medical certificate** = paper signed by a doctor, giving a patient permission to be away from work *or* not to do certain types of work *läkarintyg, sjukintyg*

certify ['sɜ:tɪfaɪ] *vb.* to make an official statement in writing *intyga, betyga, förklara;* **he was certified dead on arrival at hospital**
NOTE: formerly used to refer to patients sent to a mental hospital

cerumen [sə'ru:men] *subst.* wax in the ear *cerumen, öronvax*

ceruminous glands [sə'ru:mɪnəs ˌglændz] *subst.* glands which secrete earwax ⇨ *illustration* EAR *glandulae ceruminose, öronvaxkörtlarna*

cervic- ['sɜ:vɪk, ˌ--] *or* **cervico-** ['sɜ:vɪkəʊ, ˌ---] *prefix* (i) referring to a neck *cervik(o)-, hals-;* (ii) referring to the cervix of the uterus *cervik(o)-, livmoderhals-*

cervical ['sɜ:vɪk(ə)l] *adj.* (i) referring to any neck *cervikal, hals-;* (ii) referring to the cervix of the uterus *cervikal, cervix-, livmoderhals-;* **cervical canal** = canal running through the cervix between the uterus and the upper vagina *cervikalkanalen;* **cervical cap** = DUTCH CAP; **cervical cancer** = cancer of the cervix of the uterus *cervixcancer;* **cervical collar** *or* **neck collar** = special strong collar to support the head of a patient with a fractured neck *halskrage;* **cervical ganglion** = one of the bundles of nerves in the neck *ganglion cervicale;* **cervical (lymph) node** = lymph node in the neck *cervikalknuta;* **cervical nerves** = spinal nerves in the neck *nervi cervicales, halsnerverna;* **cervical rib** = extra rib sometimes found attached to the vertebrae above the other ribs, and which may cause thoracic inlet syndrome *costa cervicalis, halsrevben;* **cervical smear** = test for cervical cancer, where cells taken from the mucus in the cervix of the uterus are examined *cervixsmear, utstryk från livmoderhalsen;* **cervical vertebrae** = the seven bones which form the neck ⇨ *illustration* VERTEBRAL COLUMN *vertebrae cervicales, halskotorna;* **deep cervical vein** = vein in the neck, which drains into the vertebral vein *vena cervicalis profunda, djupa nackvenen*

cervicectomy [ˌsɜ:vɪ'sektəmi] *subst.* surgical removal of the cervix uteri *konisation, operativt avlägsnande av cervix uteri (livmoderhalsen)*

cervicit ⇨ **cervicitis**

cervicitis [ˌsɜ:vɪ'saɪtɪs] *subst.* inflammation of the cervix uteri *cervicit*

cervicouterine canal [ˌsɜ:vɪkəʊ'ju:tərаɪn kəˌnæl] *subst.* canal running through the cervix between the uterus and the upper vagina *cervikalkanalen*

cervikal ⇨ **cervical**

cervikalkanalen ⇨ **canal, cervicouterine canal**

cervikalknuta ⇨ **cervical**

cervix ['sɜ:vɪks] *subst.* (i) any narrow neck of an organ *cervix, hals;* (ii) neck of the womb *or* narrow lower part of the uterus leading into the vagina *cervix uteri, livmoderhalsen*
NOTE: cervix means "neck", and can refer to any neck; it is most usually used to refer to the narrow part of the uterus, and is then referred to as the **cervix uteri**

cervix- ⇨ **cervical**

cervixcancer ⇨ **cervical**

cervixeversion ⇨ **eversion**

cervixsmear ⇨ **cervical**

cesium ⇨ **caesium**

cestode ['sestəʊd] *subst.* type of tapeworm *cestod, bandmask*

CFT [ˌsi:ef'ti:] = COMPLEMENT FIXATION TEST

chafe [tʃeɪf] *vb.* to rub, especially to rub against the skin *gnida (sönder), skrapa, skrubba, skava;* **the rough cloth of the collar**

chafed the patient's neck; she was experiencing chafing of the thighs

Chagas' disease ['ʃɑːgəs dɪˌziːz] *subst.* type of sleeping sickness found in South America, transmitted by insect bites which pass trypanosomes into the bloodstream *Chagas sjukdom, chagom*

> COMMENT: the first symptom is an inflamed spot at the place of the insect bite, followed later by fever, swelling of the liver and spleen and swelling of tissues in the face. Children are mainly affected, and if untreated the disease can cause fatal heart block in early adult life

chagom ⇨ **Chagas' disease**

chain [tʃeɪn] *subst.* (i) number of metal rings attached together to make a line *kedja;* (ii) number of components linked together *or* number of connected events *kedja, följd;* **chain reaction** = reaction where each stage is started by the one before it *kedjereaktion*

chair [tʃeə] *subst.* piece of furniture for sitting on *stol;* **a badly made chair can affect the posture; dentist's chair** = special chair which can be made to tip backwards, used by dentists when operating on patients' teeth *tandläkarstol; see also* BIRTHING

chalazion [kə'leɪziən] *or* **meibomian cyst** [maɪ'bəʊmiən ˌsɪst] *subst.* swelling of a sebaceous gland in the eyelid *chalazion, chalazium, kronisk vagel*

chalazium ⇨ **chalazion**

chalone ['kæləʊn] *subst.* hormone which stops a secretion, as opposed to those hormones which stimulate secretion *chalon*

chamber ['tʃeɪmbə] *subst.* hollow space (atrium *or* ventricle) in the heart where blood is collected *förmak, kammare, rum;* **anterior** *or* **posterior chambers of the eye** = parts of the aqueous chamber of the eye which are in front of *or* behind the iris *camera anterior resp. posterior bulbi, främre resp. bakre ögonkammaren;* **collection chambers** = sections of the heart where blood collects before being pumped out *atrium (cordis), förmak;* **pumping chambers** = sections of the heart where blood is pumped *(hjärt)ventrikel, kammare*

chancre ['ʃæŋkə] *subst.* sore on the lips *or* penis *or* eyelids which is the first symptom of syphilis *chancre, schanker*

chancroid ['ʃæŋkrɔɪd] *or* **soft chancre** ['sɒft ˌʃæŋkə] *subst.* soft sore on the genitals caused by the bacterium **Haemophilus ducreyi** *ulcus venereum simplex, ulcus molle, mjuk schanker*

change [tʃeɪn(d)ʒ] **1** *subst.* being different *(för)ändring, byte;* **we will try a change of treatment; this patient needs a change of bedclothes; change of life** = MENOPAUSE **2** *vb.* **(a)** to make something different *(för)ändra;* to become different *(för)ändras;* **treatment of tuberculosis has changed a lot in the past few years; he's changed so much since his illness that I hardly recognized him; the doctor decided to change the dosage (b)** to put on different clothes *or* bedclothes *or* bandages *byta (om), lägga om;* **she changed into her uniform before going into the ward; the nurses change the bedclothes every day; make sure the dressing on the wound is changed every morning**

channel ['tʃæn(ə)l] *subst.* tube *or* passage through which fluid flows *kanal, gång*

chaplain ['tʃæplɪn] *subst.* **hospital chaplain** = religious minister attached to a hospital, who visits and comforts patients and their families and gives them the sacraments when necessary *sjukhuspräst*

chapped [tʃæpt] *adj.* cracked (skin) due to cold *sprucken, narig;* **put some cream on your chapped lips**

chapping ['tʃæpɪŋ] *subst.* cracking of the skin, due to cold *sprickning;* **cream will prevent your hands chapping**

character ['kærəktə] *subst.* way in which a person thinks and behaves *karaktär*

characteristic [ˌkærəktə'rɪstɪk] **1** *adj.* typical *or* special *karakteristisk, typisk;* **the inflammation is characteristic of shingles; symptoms characteristic of anaemia 2** *subst.* difference which makes something special *utmärkande egenskap, särdrag;* **cancer destroys the cell's characteristics**

characterize ['kærəktəraɪz] *vb.* to make something different *karakterisera, utmärka, känneteckna;* **the disease is characterized by the development of coarse features**

charcoal ['tʃɑːkəʊl] *subst.* black substance, an impure form of carbon, formed when wood is burnt in the absence of oxygen *träkol, kol*

> COMMENT: charcoal tablets can be used to relieve diarrhoea *or* flatulence

Charcot's joint ['ʃɑːkɒz ˌdʒɔɪnt] *subst.* joint which becomes deformed because the patient cannot feel pain in it when the nerves have been damaged by syphilis *or* diabetes *or* leprosy *Charcots led*

charge nurse ['tʃɑːdʒ ˌnɜːs] *subst.* nurse in charge of a group of patients *ung. avdelningsföreståndare*

chart [tʃɑːt] *subst.* diagram *or* record of information shown as a series of lines *or* points on graph paper *diagram, kurva;* **a chart showing the rise in cases of whooping cough during the first five months of 1987; temperature chart** = chart showing changes in a patient's temperature over a period of time *temperaturkurva, feberkurva*

ChB [ˌsiːeɪtʃ'biː] = BACHELOR OF SURGERY

CHC [ˌsiːeɪtʃ'siː] = CHILD HEALTH CLINIC

CHD [ˌsiːeɪtʃ'diː] = CORONARY HEART DISEASE

checkup ['tʃekʌp] *subst.* test to see if someone is fit *or* general examination by a doctor or dentist *hälsokontroll, undersökning, läkarundersökning;* **he had a heart checkup last week; she has entered hospital for a checkup; he made an appointment with the dentist for a checkup**

cheek [tʃiːk] *subst.* one of two fleshy parts of the face on each side of the nose *kinden;* **a little girl with red cheeks**

cheekbone ['tʃiːkbəʊn] *or* **zygomatic bone** [ˌzaɪgə(ʊ)'mætɪk ˌbəʊn] *subst.* bone in the face beneath the eye socket *os zygomaticum, okbenet, kindknotan; see also* MALAR

chef ▷ **head**

cheil- ['kaɪl, ˌ-] *prefix* referring to lips *cheil(o)-, keil(o)-, läpp-*

cheilitis [kaɪ'laɪtɪs] *subst.* inflammation of the lips *cheilit, keilit, läppinflammation*

cheilosis [kaɪ'ləʊsɪs] *subst.* swelling and cracks on the lips and corners of the mouth caused by lack of vitamin B *cheilos, munvinkelragad*

chelating agent ['kiːleɪtɪŋ ˌeɪdʒ(ə)nt] *subst.* chemical compound which can combine with certain metals, used as a treatment for metal poisoning *kelatkomplexbildare*

cheloid ['kiːlɔɪd] = KELOID

chem- ['kem, ˌ-] *prefix* referring to chemistry *or* chemicals *chem(o)-, kem(o)-, kemisk*

chemical ['kemɪk(ə)l] **1** *adj.* referring to chemistry *kemisk* **2** *subst.* substance produced by a chemical process *or* formed of chemical elements *kemikalie*

> QUOTE The MRI body scanner is able to provide a chemical analysis of tissues without investigative surgery
>
> **Health Services Journal**

chemist ['kemɪst] *subst.* **(a)** scientist who specializes in the study of chemistry *kemist* **(b) dispensing chemist** = pharmacist who prepares and sells drugs according to doctors' prescriptions *apotekare, farmaceut;* **the chemist's** = shop where you can buy medicine, toothpaste, soap, etc. *ung. apotek;* **go to the chemist's to get some cough medicine; the tablets are sold at all chemists'**

chemistry ['kemɪstri] *subst.* study of substances, elements and compounds and their reactions with each other *kemi;* **blood chemistry** *or* **chemistry of the blood** = record of the changes which take place in blood during disease and treatment *blodstatus*

chemo- ['kiːmə(ʊ), ˌ--] *prefix* referring to chemistry *chem(o)-, kem(o)-, kemisk*

chemoreceptor [ˌkiːmə(ʊ)rɪ'septə] *subst.* cell which responds to the presence of a chemical compound by activating a sensory nerve (such as a taste bud reacting to food) *chemoreceptor, kemoreceptor; see also* EXTEROCEPTOR, INTEROCEPTOR, RECEPTOR

chemosis [kiː'məʊsɪs] *subst.* swelling of the conjunctiva *kemos*

chemotaxi ▷ **chemotaxis**

chemotaxis [ˌkiːmə(ʊ)'tæksɪs] *subst.* movement of a cell which is attracted to or repelled by a chemical substance *chemotaxi, kemotaxi, kemotropism*

chemotherapeutic agent [ˌkiːmə(ʊ)ˌθerə'pjuːtɪk ˌeɪdʒ(ə)nt] *subst.* chemical substance used to treat a disease *kemoterapeutikum*

chemotherapy [ˌkiːmə(ʊ)'θerəpi] *subst.* using chemical drugs (such as antibiotics *or* pain killers *or* antiseptic lotions) to fight a disease, especially using toxic chemicals to destroy rapidly developing cancer cells *kemoterapi*

chest [tʃest] *or* **thorax** ['θɔːræks] *subst.* top part of the front of the body above the abdomen, containing the diaphragm, heart and lungs and surrounded by the rib cage *thorax, bröstet, bröstkorgen;* **he placed the stethoscope on the patient's chest** *or* **he listened to the patient's chest; she is suffering from chest pains; after the fight he was rushed to hospital with chest wounds; a day unit set up for disabled chest patients; she has a cold in the chest** = she coughs badly *hon har en svår förkylning (allvarlig hosta);* **chest cavity** = space in the body which contains the heart and lungs *cavum thoracis, brösthålan;* **chest examination** = examination of the patient's chest by percussion, stethoscope or X-rays *undersökning av bröstkorgen (och dess inre organ);* **chest muscle** *or* **pectoral muscle** = one of two muscles which lie across the chest and control movements of the shoulder and arm *musculus pectoralis, bröstmuskeln*
NOTE: for other terms referring to the chest, see words beginning with **pecto-, steth-, thorac-**

chew [tʃuː] *vb.* to masticate *or* to crush food with the teeth *tugga;* **he was chewing a piece of meat; food should be chewed slowly**

> COMMENT: the action of chewing grinds the food into small pieces and mixes it with saliva to start the process of breaking down the food to extract nutrients from it

chewing gum ['tʃuːɪŋ gʌm] *subst.* sweet substance which you can chew for a long time but not swallow *tuggummi*

Cheyne-Stokes respiration [ˌtʃeɪn'stəʊks ˌrespə'reɪʃ(ə)n] *or* **breathing** ['briːðɪŋ] *subst.* condition (usually of unconscious patients) where breathing is irregular, with short breaths gradually increasing to deep breaths, then reducing again, until breathing appears to stop; caused by a disorder of the brain centre which controls breathing *Cheyne-Stokes andning*

chiasm ['kaɪæz(ə)m] *or* **chiasma** [kaɪ'æzmə] *subst.* cross-shaped crossing of fibres *chiasma, korsning;* **optic chiasma** = structure where some of the optic nerves from each eye partially cross each other in the hypothalamus *chiasma opticum, synnervskorsningen*

chiasma ⇨ **chiasm, decussation**

chickenpox ['tʃɪkɪn pɒks] *or* **varicella** [ˌværi'selə] *subst.* infectious disease of children, with fever and red spots which turn into itchy blisters *varicella, vattkoppor, vattenkoppor*

> COMMENT: chickenpox is caused by a herpesvirus. In later life, shingles is usually a re-emergence of a dormant chickenpox virus, and an adult with shingles can infect a child with chickenpox

chigger ['tʃɪgə] *or* **harvest mite larva** ['hɑːvəst ˌmaɪt 'lɑːvə] *subst.* parasite which enters the skin near a hair follicle and travels under the skin causing intense irritation *kvalster av familjen Trombiculidae*

chilblain ['tʃɪlbleɪn] *or* **erythema pernio** [ˌerə θiːmə ˌpɜːniəʊ] *subst.* condition where the skin of the fingers, toes, nose or ears becomes red, swollen and itchy because of exposure to cold *frosterytem, frostskada, kylskada;* **he has chilblains on his toes**

child [tʃaɪ(ə)ld] *subst.* young boy *or* girl *barn;* **here is a photograph of my father as a child; all the children were playing out in the field; when do the children come out of school?; they have six children** = they have six sons or daughters *de har sex barn;* **child abuse** = bad treatment of children, including sexual interference *barnmisshandel, sexuellt utnyttjande av barn;* **children's hospital** = hospital which specializes in treating children *barnsjukhus* NOTE: plural is **children.** Note also that **child** is the legal term for a person under 14 years of age

childbearing ['tʃaɪldˌbeərɪŋ] *subst.* giving birth *barnafödande;* **45 is the upper age limit for childbearing**

childbirth ['tʃaɪldbɜːθ] *or* **parturition** [ˌpɑːtju(ə)'rɪʃ(ə)n] *subst.* act of giving birth *förlossning, barnsbörd;* **natural childbirth** = childbirth where the mother is not given any pain-killing drugs or anaesthetic but is encouraged to give birth after having prepared herself through relaxation and breathing exercises and a new psychological outlook *naturlig förlossning*

child care ['tʃaɪld keə] *subst.* care of young children and study of their special needs *barnavård*

child health clinic (CHC) [ˌtʃaɪld 'helθ ˌklɪnik (ˌsiːeɪtʃ'siː)] *or* **child development clinic** [ˌtʃaɪld dɪ'veləpmənt ˌklɪnik] *subst.* special clinic for checking the health and development of small children under school age *ung. barnavårdscentral (BVC)*

childhood [ˈtʃaɪldhʊd] *subst.* time when a person is a child *barndom;* **he had a happy childhood in the country; she spent her childhood in Canada; childhood illnesses** *or* **disorders** = disorders which mainly affect children and not adults *barnsjukdomar*

child-proof [ˈtʃaɪldpruːf] *adj.* which a child cannot use *barnsäker;* **the pills are sold in bottles with child-proof lids**
NOTE: for terms referring to children see words beginning with **paed-** *or* **ped-**

chill [tʃɪl] *subst.* feeling cold and shivering, usually the sign of the beginning of a fever, of flu or a cold *köldrysning, frossa, frossbrytning;* **he caught a chill on the train**

chin [tʃɪn] *subst.* bottom part of the face, beneath the mouth *hakan;* **she hit him on the chin; he rested his chin on his hand while he was thinking**

Chinese restaurant syndrome [ˌtʃaɪniːz ˈrestərɒnt ˌsɪndrəʊm] *subst.* allergic condition which gives people violent headaches after eating food flavoured with monosodium glutamate *allergi mot glutamat*

chiropodist [kɪˈrɒpədɪst] *subst.* person who specializes in treatment of minor disorders of the feet *fotvårdsspecialist; see also* PODIATRIST, PODIATRY

chiropody [kɪˈrɒpədi] *subst.* study of minor diseases and disorders of the feet *läran om (lindrigare) fotsjukdomar*

chiropractic [ˌkaɪ(ə)rə(ʊ)ˈpræktɪk] *subst.* treatment of disorders by manipulating the bones of the spine *chiropraktik, kiropraktik*

chiropractor [ˈkaɪ(ə)rə(ʊ)ˌpræktə] *subst.* person who practises chiropractic *chiropraktor, kiropraktor*

chiropraktor ▷ **chiropractor**

Chlamydia [kləˈmɪdiə] *subst.* type of parasite, which is transmitted to humans by insects, causing psittacosis and trachoma *Chlamydia*

chloasma [kləʊˈæzmə] *subst.* presence of brown spots on the skin from various causes *chloasma, kloasma, leverfläck*

chloride [ˈklɔːraɪd] *subst.* a salt of hydrochloric acid *klorid;* **sodium chloride** = common salt *natriumklorid, koksalt, NaCl*

chlorination [ˌklɔːrɪˈneɪʃ(ə)n] *subst.* sterilizing water (as in swimming pools) by adding chlorine *klorering*

chlorine [ˈklɔːriːn] *subst.* powerful greenish gas, used to sterilize water *klor(gas), Cl* NOTE: symbol is **Cl**

chlor(o)- [ˈklɔːr(əʊ), ˌ--] *prefix* referring (i) to chlorine *klor(o)-;* (ii) green *grön-*

chloroform [ˈklɒrəfɔːm] *subst.* powerful drug formerly used as an anaesthetic *kloroform*

chloroma [klɔːˈrəʊmə] *subst.* bone tumour associated with acute leukaemia *klorom*

chlorophyll [ˈklɒrəfɪl, ˈklɔːr-] *subst.* green pigment in plants, also used in deodorants and toothpaste *klorofyll*

chloroquine [ˈklɔːrəkwɪn] *subst.* drug used to treat and prevent malaria *klorokin*

chlorosis [klɔːˈrəʊsɪs] *subst.* type of severe anaemia due to iron deficiency, affecting mainly young girls *kloros*

chlorothiazide [ˌklɔːrəʊˈθaɪəzaɪd] *subst.* drug which acts as a diuretic, and also helps reduce high blood pressure *klortiazid*

chlorpromazine [ˌklɔːˈprəʊməziːn] *subst.* tranquillizing drug *klorpromazin*

ChM [ˌsiːeɪtʃˈem] = MASTER OF SURGERY

choana [ˈkəʊənə] *subst.* any opening shaped like a funnel, especially that leading from the nasal cavity to the pharynx *koan, bakre näsöppning*
NOTE: plural is **choanae**

chock ▷ **shock, trauma**

chocka ▷ **shock**

chockartad ▷ **traumatic**

chockbehandling ▷ **shock**

"chockbehandling" ▷ **electric, electroconvulsive therapy (ECT)**

chocklunga ▷ **lung**

chocksyndrom ▷ **shock**

choke [tʃəʊk] *vb.* to stop breathing because the windpipe becomes blocked by a foreign body *or* by inhalation of water *kväva(s);* **to choke on something** = to take something into the windpipe instead of the gullet, so that the breathing is interrupted *sätta ngt i halsen, få ngt i fel strupe;* **he choked on a piece of bread** *or* **a piece of bread made him choke**

choking ['tʃəʊkɪŋ] **1** *subst.* asphyxia *or* condition where someone is prevented from breathing *kvävning* **2** *adj.* (smoke) which makes you choke *kvävande;* **the room filled with choking black smoke**

chol- [kɒl] *prefix* referring to bile *chol-, kol-, gall-*

cholaemia [kə'li:miə] *subst.* presence of abnormal amount of bile in the blood *cholemi*

cholagogue ['kɒləgɒg] *subst.* drug which encourages the production of bile *cholagogum, galldrivande medel*

cholagogum ⇨ **cholagogue**

cholangiografi ⇨ **cholangiography**

cholangiography [kə,lændʒi'ɒgrəfi] *subst.* X-ray examination of the bile ducts and gall bladder *cholangiografi, kolangiografi*

cholangiolitis [kə,lændʒiəʊ'laɪtɪs] *subst.* inflammation of the small bile ducts *inflammation i de små gallgångarna*

cholangit ⇨ **cholangitis**

cholangitis [,kəʊlæn'dʒaɪtɪs] *subst.* inflammation of the bile ducts *cholangit, kolangit, gallvägsinflammation*

chole- [,kɒlɪ, ,kəʊlɪ] *prefix* referring to bile *chole-, kole-, gall-*

cholecystectomy [,kɒlɪsɪ'stektəmi] *subst.* surgical removal of the gall bladder *cholecystektomi, kolecystektomi*

cholecystektomi ⇨ **cholecystectomy**

cholecystit ⇨ **cholecystitis**

cholecystitis [,kɒlɪsɪ'staɪtɪs] *subst.* inflammation of the gall bladder *cholecystit, kolecystit, gallblåseinflammation*

cholecystoduodenostomy [,kɒlɪsɪstə,dju:ədɪ'nɒstəmi] *subst.* surgical operation to join the gall bladder to the duodenum to allow bile to pass into the intestine when the main bile duct is blocked *cholecystoduodenostomi, kolecystoduodenostomi*

cholecystografi ⇨ **cholecystography**

cholecystogram [,kɒlɪ'sɪstəgræm] *subst.* X-ray photograph of the gall bladder *cholecystogram, kolecystogram*

cholecystography [,kɒlɪsɪ'stɒgrəfi] *subst.* X-ray examination of the gall bladder *cholecystografi, kolecystografi*

cholecystostomi ⇨ **cholecystotomy**

cholecystotomy [,kɒlɪsɪ'stɒtəmi] *subst.* surgical operation to make a cut in the gall bladder, usually to remove gallstones *cholecystostomi, kolecystostomi*

choledoch- [kə,ledək] *prefix* referring to the common bile duct *choledoch(o)-, koledoch(o)-, gallgångs-*

choledochostomi ⇨ **choledochotomy**

choledochotomy [kə,ledə'kɒtəmi] *subst.* surgical operation to make a cut in the common bile duct to remove stones *choledochostomi, koledochostomi*

cholelithiasis [,kɒlɪlɪ'θaɪəsɪs] *or* **choledocholithiasis** [kə,ledəkəlɪ'θaɪəsɪs] *subst.* condition where gallstones form in the gall bladder *or* bile ducts *cholelithiasis, gallstenslidande*

cholelithotomy [,kɒlɪlɪ'θɒtəmɪ] *subst.* surgical removal of gallstones by cutting into the gall bladder *cholelitotomi, kolelitotomi*

cholelitotomi ⇨ **cholelithotomy**

cholemi ⇨ **cholaemia**

cholera ['kɒlərə] *subst.* serious bacterial disease spread through food *or* water which has been infected by Vibrio cholerae *kolera;* **he caught cholera while on holiday; a cholera epidemic broke out after the flood**

> COMMENT: the infected person suffers diarrhoea, cramp in the intestines and dehydration. The disease is often fatal, and vaccination is only effective for a relatively short period

choleresis [kə'lɪərəsɪs] *subst.* the production of bile by the liver *gallproduktion*

choleretic [,kɒlɪ'retɪk] *adj.* (substance) which increases the production and flow of bile *som ökar gallproduktionen*

cholestas ⇨ **cholestasis**

cholestasis [,kɒlɪ'steɪsɪs] *subst.* condition where all bile does not pass into the intestine but some remains in the liver and causes jaundice *cholestas, kolestas, gallstas*

cholesteatom ⇨ **cholesteatoma**

cholesteatoma [ˌkɒlɪˌstɪə'təʊmə] *subst.* cyst containing some cholesterol found in the middle ear and also in the brain *cholesteatom, pärlsvulst*

cholesterol [kə'lestərɒl] *subst.* fatty substance found in fats and oils, also produced by the liver, and forming an essential part of all cells *cholesterol, kolesterol*

> COMMENT: cholesterol is found in brain cells, the adrenal glands, liver and bile acids. High levels of cholesterol in the blood are found in diabetes. Cholesterol is formed by the body, and high blood cholesterol levels are associated with diets rich in animal fat (such as butter and fat meat). Excess cholesterol can be deposited in the walls of arteries, causing atherosclerosis

cholesteros ⇨ **cholesterosis**

cholesterosis [kɒˌlestə'rəʊsɪs] *subst.* inflammation of the gall bladder with deposits of cholesterol *cholesteros*

cholic acid [ˌkəʊlɪk 'æsɪd] *subst.* one of the bile acids *cholsyra*

choline ['kəʊli:n] *subst.* essential basic compound which synthesizes acetylcholine *cholin, kolin*

cholinesteras ⇨ **cholinesterase**

cholinesterase [ˌkəʊlɪ'nestəreɪz] *subst.* enzyme which breaks down a choline ester *cholinesteras, kolinesteras*

cholsyra ⇨ **cholic acid**

choluria [kəʊ'ljʊəriə] *subst.* bile in the urine *choluri, koluri*

chondr- ['kɒndr, ˌ--] *prefix* referring to cartilage *chondr(o)-, kondr(o)-, brosk-*

chondritis [kɒn'draɪtɪs] *subst.* inflammation of a cartilage *chondrit, kondrit, broskinflammation*

chondroblast ['kɒndrəʊblæst] *subst.* cell from which cartilage develops in an embryo *chondroblast, kondroblast, broskbildningscell*

chondrocalcinosis [ˌkɒndrəʊˌkælsɪ'nəʊsɪs] *subst.* condition where deposits of calcium phosphate are found in articular cartilage *chondrokalcinos, kondrokalcinos, broskförkalkning*

chondrocyt ⇨ **chondrocyte**

chondrocyte ['kɒndrəʊsaɪt] *subst.* mature cartilage cell *chondrocyt, kondrocyt*

chondrodysplasia [ˌkɒndrəʊdɪs'pleɪziə] *or* **chondrodystrophy** [ˌkɒndrəʊ'dɪstrəʊfi] *subst.* hereditary disorder of cartilage which is linked to dwarfism *chondrodystrofi, kondrodystrofi*

chondrodystrofi ⇨ **chondrodysplasia**

chondrokalcinos ⇨ **chondrocalcinosis**

chondroma [kɒn'drəʊmə] *subst.* tumour formed of cartilaginous tissue *chondrom, kondrom, brosksvulst*

chondromalacia [ˌkɒndrəʊmə'leɪʃ(i)ə] *subst.* degeneration of the cartilage of a joint *chondromalaci, kondromalaci, broskuppmjukning*

chondrosarcoma [ˌkɒndrəʊsɑː'kəʊmə] *subst.* malignant, rapidly growing tumour involving cartilage cells *chondrosarkom, kondrosarkom, elakartad brosktumör*

chondrosarkom ⇨ **chondrosarcoma**

chorda ['kɔːdə] *subst.* cord *or* tendon *chorda, korda, sträng;* **chordae tendineae** = tiny fibrous ligaments in the heart which attach the edges of some of the valves to the walls of the ventricles *chordae tendineae* NOTE: plural is **chordae**

chordee ['kɔːdiː] *subst.* painful condition where the erect penis is curved *induratio penis plastica, smärtsamt tillstånd med böjd erigerad penis*

chorditis [kɔː'daɪtɪs] *subst.* inflammation of the vocal cords *stämbandsinflammation*

chordotomi ⇨ **chordotomy**

chordotomy [kɔː'dɒtəmi] *subst.* surgical operation to cut any cord, such as a nerve pathway in the spinal cord, to relieve intractable pain *chordotomi, kordotomi*

chorea [kɔː'rɪə] *subst.* sudden severe twitching (usually of the face and shoulders), symptom of disease of the nervous system *chorea, korea, danssjuka;* **Huntington's chorea** = progressive hereditary disease which affects adults, where the outer layer of the brain degenerates and the patient makes involuntary jerky movements and develops progressive dementia *Huntingtons chorea (korea);* **Sydenham's chorea** = temporary chorea affecting children, frequently associated with endocarditis and rheumatism *Sydenhams chorea (korea)*

chorion ['kɔːriən] *subst.* membrane covering the fertilized ovum *chorion, korion, fosterhinna*

chorionic [ˌkɔːri'ɒnɪk] *adj.* referring to the chorion *som avser el. hör till fosterhinna;* **human chorionic gonadotrophin (hCG)** = hormone produced by the placenta, which suppresses the mother's normal menstrual cycle during pregnancy; it is found in the urine during pregnancy; it can be given by injection to encourage ovulation and help a woman to become pregnant *(humant) choriongonadotropin, HCG, graviditetshormon*

chorionic villi [ˌkɔːrɪ'ɒnɪk 'vɪlaɪ] *subst.* tiny finger-like folds in the chorion *villi chorii, chorionvilli*

chorionvilli ⇨ **chorionic villi**

choroid ['kɔːrɔɪd] *subst.* middle layer of tissue which forms the eyeball, between the sclera and the retina *chor(i)oidea, kor(i)oidea, åderhinnan;* **choroid plexus** = part of the pia mater, network of small blood vessels in the ventricles of the brain which produce cerebrospinal fluid *plexus chorioideus*

choroiditis [ˌkɔːrɔɪ'daɪtis] *subst.* inflammation of the choroid in the eyeball ⇨ *illustration* EYE *chor(i)oidit, kor(i)oidit*

Christmas disease ['krɪsməs dɪˌziːz] *or* **haemophilia B** [ˌhiːməʊ'fɪliə 'biː] *subst.* clotting disorder of the blood, similar to haemophilia A, but in which the blood coagulates badly due to deficiency of Factor IX *hemofili B*

> COMMENT: haemophilia A is caused by deficiency of Factor VIII

Christmas factor ['krɪsməs ˌfæktə] *subst.* Factor IX *or* one of the coagulating factors in the blood *koagulationsfaktor IX, antihemofilifaktor B*

chrom- ['krəʊm, ˌ-] *prefix* referring to colour *chrom(o)-, krom(o)-*

chromatid ['krəʊmətɪd] *subst.* one of two parallel filaments making up a chromosome *chromatid, kromatid*

chromatin ['krəʊmətɪn] *subst.* network which forms the nucleus of a cell and can be stained with basic dyes *chromatin, kromatin;* **sex chromatin** *or* **Barr body** = chromatin which is only found in female cells, and which can be used to identify the sex of a baby before birth *sexkromatin, könskromatin, kromatinfläck*

chromatofor ⇨ **chromatophore**

chromatografi ⇨ **chromatography**

chromatography [ˌkrəʊmə'tɒgrəfi] *subst.* method of separating chemicals through a porous medium and analysing compounds *chromatografi, kromatografi*

chromatophore ['krəʊmətəˌfɔː] *subst.* any pigment-bearing cell, in the eyes, hair and skin *chromatofor, melanocyt*

chromicized catgut ['krəʊməsaɪzd ˌkætgʌt] *subst.* catgut which is hardened with chromium to make it slower to dissolve in the body *kromcatgut, kromkatgut*

chromium ['krəʊmiəm] *subst.* metallic trace element *krom, Cr*
NOTE: the chemical symbol is **Cr**

chromosomal [ˌkrəʊmə'səʊm(ə)l] *adj.* referring to chromosomes *som avser el. hör till kromosom(er)*

chromosome ['krəʊməsəʊm] *subst.* rod-shaped structure in the nucleus of a cell, formed of DNA which carries the genes *kromosom*

> COMMENT: each human cell has 46 chromosomes, 23 inherited from each parent. The female has one pair of X chromosomes, and the male one pair of XY chromosomes, which are responsible for the sexual difference. Sperm from a male have either an X or a Y chromosome; if a Y chromosome sperm fertilizes the female's ovum the child will be male

chronic ['krɒnɪk] *adj.* (disease *or* condition) which lasts for a long time *kronisk;* **he has a chronic chest complaint; she is a chronic asthma sufferer** *compare* ACUTE

chyle [kaɪ(ə)l] *subst.* fluid in the lymph vessels in the intestine which contains fat, especially after a meal *chylus, kylus, tarmlymfa*

chylomicron [ˌkaɪ(ə)ləʊ'maɪkrən] *subst.* particle of chyle present in the blood *chylomikron*

chylomikron ⇨ **chylomicron**

chyluri ⇨ **chyluria, lipuria**

chyluria [kaɪ'ljʊəriə] *subst.* presence of chyle in the urine *chyluri, lipuri*

chylus ⇨ **chyle**

chyme [kaɪm] *subst.* semi-liquid mass of food and gastric juices which passes from the stomach to the intestine *chymus, kymus*

chymotrypsin [ˌkaɪmə(ʊ)'trɪpsɪn] *subst.* enzyme which digests protein *chymotrypsin, kymotrypsin*

chymus ⇨ **chyme**

Ci [ˌsiː'aɪ] *abbreviation for* curie *Ci, curie*

cicatrix ['sɪkətrɪks] *subst.* scar *or* mark on the skin, left when a wound *or* surgical incision has healed *cicatrix, ärr*

-cide [saɪd] *suffix* referring to killing *-cid, -dödande*

cilia ['sɪliə] *see* CILIUM

ciliarkroppen ⇨ **ciliary**

ciliarmuskeln ⇨ **ciliary**

ciliary ['siliəri] *adj.* (i) referring to cilia *ciliar, ciliär;* (ii) referring to the eyelids *or* eyelashes *som avser el. hör till ögonlock el. ögonfransar;* **ciliary body** = part of the eye which connects the iris to the choroid *corpus ciliare, ciliarkroppen;* **ciliary muscle** = muscle which makes the lens of the eye change its shape to focus on objects at different distances ⇨ *illustration* EYE *musculus ciliaris, ciliarmuskeln;* **ciliary processes** = series of ridges behind the iris to which the lens of the eye is attached *processus ciliares, flikiga utskott på ciliarkroppen*

ciliated epithelium [ˌsɪlieɪtɪd ˌepɪ'θiːliəm] *subst.* simple epithelium where the cells have tiny hairs *or* cilia *flimmerepitel*

cilium ['sɪliəm] *subst.* **(a)** eyelash *cilium, ögonhår, ögonfrans* **(b)** one of many tiny hair-like processes which line cells in passages in the body and by moving backwards and forwards drive particles or fluid along the passage *cilium, flimmerhår*
NOTE: plural is **cilia**

ciliär ⇨ **ciliary**

cinematics [ˌsɪnə'mætɪks] *subst.* science of movement, especially of body movements *kinematik*

cineplasty ['sɪniplæsti] *subst.* amputation where the muscles of the stump of the amputated limb are used to operate an artificial limb *slags amputation där stumpens muskler används för att röra konstgjord lem*

cineradiografi ⇨ **cineradiography**

cineradiography [ˌsɪniˌreɪdi'ɒgrəfi] *subst.* taking a series of X-ray photographs for diagnosis *or* to show how something moves *or* develops in the body *cineradiografi, cineröntgen*

cineröntgen ⇨ **cineradiography**

cinesiology [sɪˌniːsi'ɒlədʒi] *subst.* study of muscle movements, particularly in relation to treatment *undersökning av muskelrörelser*

cingulectomy [ˌsɪŋgju'lektəmi] *subst.* surgical operation to remove the cingulum *cingulektomi, cingulotomi*

cingulektomi ⇨ **cingulectomy**

cingulotomi ⇨ **cingulectomy**

cingulum ['sɪŋgjʊləm] *subst.* long curved bundle of nerve fibres in the cerebrum *cingulum*
NOTE: the plural is **cingula**

circadian rhythm [sɜː'keɪdiən ˌrɪð(ə)m] *subst.* rhythm of daily activities and bodily processes (eating *or* defecating *or* sleeping, etc.) frequently controlled by hormones, which repeats every twenty-four hours *circadisk rytm, biologisk klocka*

circle of Willis [ˌsɜːk(ə)l əv 'wɪlɪs] *subst.* circle of branching arteries at the base of the brain formed by the basilar, anterior and posterior cerebral, anterior and posterior communicating, and internal carotid arteries *circulus arteriosus Willisii, Willis ring*

circular ['sɜːkjʊlə] *adj.* in the form of a circle *cirkulär, (cirkel)rund;* **circular folds** = large transverse folds of mucous membrane in the small intestine *plicae circulares (intestini tenuis)*

circulate ['sɜːkjʊleɪt] *vb. (of fluid)* to move around *cirkulera, gå runt, vara i omlopp;* **blood circulates around the body; bile circulates from the liver to the intestine through the bile ducts**

circulation (of the blood) [ˌsɜːkju'leɪʃ(ə)n (əv ðə ˌblʌd)] *subst.* movement of blood around the body from the heart through the arteries to the capillaries and back to the heart through the veins *blodcirkulationen, blodomloppet;* **she has poor circulation in her legs; rub your hands to get the circulation going; collateral circulation** = enlargement of certain secondary blood vessels, as a response when the main vessels become slowly blocked *kollateralcirkulation;* **pulmonary circulation** *or* **lesser circulation** = circulation of blood from the heart through the pulmonary arteries to the lungs for oxygenation and back to the heart through the pulmonary veins *lungkretsloppet, lilla kretsloppet;* **systemic circulation** *or* **greater circulation**= circulation of blood around all the body (except the lungs) starting with the aorta and returning through the venae cavae *stora kretsloppet*

circulatory [ˌsɜːkjuˈleɪt(ə)ri] *adj.* referring to the circulation of the blood *som avser el. hör till blodcirkulationen;* **circulatory system** = system of arteries and veins, together with the heart, which makes the blood circulate around the body *kardiovaskulära systemet, hjärt-kärlsystemet, cirkulationsapparaten*

> COMMENT: blood circulates around the body, carrying oxygen from the lungs and nutrients from the liver through the arteries and capillaries to the tissues; the capillaries exchange the oxygen for waste matter such as carbon dioxide which is taken back to the lungs to be expelled. At the same time the blood obtains more oxygen in the lungs to be taken to the tissues. The circulation pattern is as follows: blood returns through the veins to the right atrium of the heart; from there it is pumped through the right ventricle into the pulmonary artery, and then into the lungs. From the lungs it returns through the pulmonary veins to the left atrium of the heart, and is pumped from there through the left ventricle into the aorta, and from the aorta into the other arteries

circumcise [ˈsɜːkəmsaɪz] *vb.* to remove the foreskin of the penis *omskära*

circumcision [ˌsɜːkəmˈsɪʒ(ə)n] *subst.* surgical removal of the foreskin of the penis *cirkumcision, omskärelse*

circumduction [ˌsɜːkəmˈdʌkʃ(ə)n] *subst.* moving a part in a circular motion *cirkumduktion*

circumflex [ˈsɜːkəmfleks] *adj.* bent *or* curved *cirkumflex, böjd;* **circumflex arteries** = branches of the femoral artery in the upper thigh *arteria circumflexa;* **circumflex nerve** = sensory and motor nerve in the upper arm *sensorisk och motorisk nerv i överarmen*

circumvallate papillae [ˌsɜːkəmˈvæleɪt pəˌpɪliː] *subst.* large papillae at the base of the tongue, which have taste buds *papillae (circum)vallatae, vallgravspapiller*

cirkel ⇨ **ring**

cirkulationsapparaten ⇨ **cardiovascular, circulatory**

cirkulationssäng ⇨ **ripple bed**

cirkulera ⇨ **circulate**

cirkulär ⇨ **circular**

cirkumcision ⇨ **circumcision**

cirkumduktion ⇨ **circumduction**

cirkumflex ⇨ **circumflex**

cirrhosis of the liver [səˈrəʊsɪs əv ðə ˌlɪvə] *or* **hepatocirrhosis** [ˌhepətəʊsəˈrəʊsɪs] *subst.* condition where some cells of the liver die and are replaced by hard fibrous tissue *cirrhosis hepatis, levercirros, skrumplever*

> COMMENT: cirrhosis can have many causes: the commonest cause is alcoholism (alcoholic cirrhosis *or* Laennec's cirrhosis); it can also be caused by heart disease (cardiac cirrhosis), by viral hepatitis (postnecrotic cirrhosis), by autoimmune disease (primary biliary cirrhosis), or by obstruction or infection of the bile ducts (biliary cirrhosis)

cirrhotic [səˈrɒtɪk] *adj.* referring to cirrhosis *cirrotisk, skrumpen;* **the patient had a cirrhotic liver**

cirros ⇨ **induration, sclerosis**

cirros, postnekrotisk ⇨ **postnecrotic cirrhosis**

cirrotisk ⇨ **cirrhotic**

cirsoid [ˈsɜːsɔɪd] *adj.* dilated (as of a varicose vein) *utvidgad;* **cirsoid aneurysm** = condition where arteries become swollen and twisted *aneurysma cirsoideum (racemosum)*

cistern [ˈsɪst(ə)n] *or* **cisterna** [sɪˈstɜːnə] *subst.* space containing fluid *cistern, reservoar;* **cisterna magna** = large space containing cerebrospinal fluid, situated underneath the cerebellum and behind the medulla oblongata *cisterna cerebellomedullaris,* **lumbar cistern** = subarachnoid space at the base of the spinal cord filled with cerebrospinal fluid *vätskefyllt* *rum under spindelvävshinnan vid ryggmärgens bas*

citric acid [ˌsɪtrɪk ˈæsɪd] *subst.* acid found in fruit such as oranges, lemons and grapefruit *citronsyra*

citric acid cycle [ˌsɪtrɪk ˈæsɪd ˌsaɪk(ə)l] *or* **Krebs cycle** [ˈkrebz ˌsaɪk(ə)l] *subst.* important series of events concerning amino acid metabolism, taking place in the mitochondria *citronsyracykeln, Krebscykeln*

citronsyra ⇨ **citric acid**

citronsyracykeln ⇨ **citric acid cycle**

citrullinaemia [sɪˌtrʊlɪˈniːmiə] *subst.* deficiency of an enzyme which helps break down proteins *citrullinemi*

citrullinemi ⇨ **citrullinaemia**

Cl *chemical symbol for* chlorine *Cl, klor*

clamp [klæmp] **1** *subst.* surgical instrument to hold something tightly (such as a blood vessel during an operation) *klämma, sårklämma, agraff* **2** *vb.* to hold something tightly *klämma ihop*

clap [klæp] *subst. slang* = GONORRHOEA

classic [ˈklæsɪk] *adj.* typically well-known (symptom) *klassisk;* **she showed classic heroin withdrawal symptoms: sweating, fever, sleeplessness and anxiety**

classification [ˌklæsɪfɪˈkeɪʃ(ə)n] *subst.* putting references *or* components into order so that they can be easily identified *klassifikation, klassificering, system;* **the ABO classification of blood**

classify [ˈklæsɪfaɪ] *vb.* **(a)** to put references *or* components into order so as to be able to refer to them again *klassificera, systematisera;* **the medical records are classified under the surname of the patient; blood groups are classified according to the ABO system (b)** to make information secret *hemligstämpla;* **doctors' reports on patients are classified and may not be shown to the patients themselves**

claudicatio ⇨ **claudication**

claudication [ˌklɔːdɪˈkeɪʃ(ə)n] *subst.* limping *or* being lame *claudicatio, hälta, haltande;* **intermittent claudication =** condition caused by impairment of the arteries *claudicatio intermittens, intermittent hälta, fönstertittarsjuka*

> COMMENT: at first, the patient limps after having walked a short distance, then finds walking progressively more difficult and finally impossible. The condition improves after rest

claustrophobia [ˌklɔːstrəˈfəʊbiə] *subst.* being afraid of enclosed spaces *or* crowded rooms *klaustrofobi, cellskräck*

claustrophobic [ˌklɔːstrəˈfəʊbɪk] *adj.* (room) which causes claustrophobia *or* (person) suffering from claustrophobia *klaustrofobisk, klaustrofobiker, som lider av klaustrofobi*
NOTE: opposite is **agoraphobia**

clavicle [ˈklævɪk(ə)l] *or* **collar bone** [ˈkɒlə ˌbəʊn] *subst.* one of two long thin bones which join the shoulder blades to the breastbone ⇨ *illustration* SHOULDER *clavicula, nyckelbenet*

clavicula ⇨ **clavicle**

clavicular [kləˈvɪkjʊlə] *adj.* referring to the clavicle *klavikulär, nyckelbens-*

clavus [ˈkleɪvəs] *subst.* **(a)** corn (on the foot) *clavus, liktorn* **(b)** severe pain in the head, like a nail being driven in *clavus hystericus*

claw foot [ˈklɔː ˌfʊt] *or* **pes cavus** [ˈpes ˈkeɪvəs] *subst.* deformed foot with the toes curved towards the instep and with a very high arch *pes cavus, klofot*

claw hand [ˈklɔː ˌhænd] *subst.* deformed hand, with the fingers (especially the ring finger and little finger) bent towards the palm, caused by paralysis of the muscles *main en griffe, klohand*

clean [kliːn] **1** *adj.* not dirty *ren;* **the beds have clean sheets every morning; these plates aren't clean; the report suggested the hospital kitchens were not as clean as they should have been** NOTE: **clean - cleaner - cleanest** **2** *vb.* to make clean clean, by taking away dirt *rengöra, göra ren, städa, tvätta, borsta;* **the nurses have to make sure the wards are clean before the inspection; have you cleaned your teeth today? she was cleaning the patients' bathroom**

cleanliness [ˈklenlɪnəs] *subst.* state of being clean *renlighet, renhet;* **the report criticized the cleanliness of the hospital kitchen**

cleanse [klenz] *vb.* to make very clean *rengöra*

cleanser ['klenzə] *subst.* powder *or* liquid which cleanses *rengöringsmedel*

clear [klɪə] **1** *adj.* **(a)** easily understood *klar, tydlig;* **the doctor made it clear that he wanted the patient to have a home help; the words on the medicine bottle are not very clear (b)** which is not cloudy and which you can easily see through *klar;* **a clear glass bottle; the urine sample was clear, not cloudy (c) clear of** = free from *fri från;* **the area is now clear of infection**
NOTE: **clear - clearer - clearest 2** *vb.* to take away a blockage *rensa;* **the inhalant will clear your blocked nose; he is on antibiotics to try to clear the congestion in his lungs**

clearance ['klɪər(ə)ns] *subst.* **renal clearance** = measurement of the rate at which kidneys filter impurities from blood *njurclearance*

clearly ['klɪəli] *adv.* plainly *or* obviously *klart, tydligt;* **the swelling is clearly visible on the patient's neck**

clear up [ˌklɪər 'ʌp] *vb.* to clear completely *klarna;* to get better *förbättras, bli bra;* **his infection should clear up within a few days; I hope your cold clears up before the holiday**

cleavage ['kli:vɪdʒ] *subst.* repeated division of cells in an embryo *delning*

cleft palate [ˌkleft 'pælət] *subst.* congenital defect, where there is a fissure in the roof of the mouth, connecting the mouth and nasal cavities *palatum fissum, gomklyvning, gomspalt, kluven gom*

> COMMENT: a cleft palate is usually associated with harelip. Both are due to incomplete fusion of the maxillary processes. Both can be successfully corrected by surgery

client ['klaɪənt] *subst.* person visited by a health visitor *or* social worker *klient*

climacteric [klaɪ'mækt(ə)rɪk] *subst.* **(a)** = MENOPAUSE **(b)** period of diminished sexual activity in a man who reaches middle age *(manligt) klimakterium*

clinic ['klɪnɪk] *subst.* **(a)** small hospital *or* department in a large hospital which deals only with walking patients, or which specializes in the treatment of certain conditions *klinik;* **he is being treated in a private clinic; she was referred to an antenatal clinic; antenatal clinic** *or* **maternity clinic**= clinic where expectant mothers are taught how to look after babies, do exercises and have medical checkups *mödravårdscentral;* **physiotherapy clinic** = clinic where patients can undergo physiotherapy *ung. sjukgymnastikavdelning* **(b)** group of students under a doctor or surgeon who examine patients and discuss their treatment *klinisk undervisningsgrupp*

clinical ['klɪnɪk(ə)l] *adj.* **(a)** (i) referring to a clinic *klinik-;* (ii) referring to a physical examination of patients by doctors (as opposed to a surgical operation *or* a laboratory test *or* experiment) *klinisk;* **clinical medicine** = treatment of patients in a hospital ward *or* in the doctor's surgery (as opposed to the operating theatre *or* laboratory) *klinisk medicin;* **clinical nurse specialist** = nurse who specializes in a particular branch of clinical care *sjuksköterska med specialutbildning inom kliniskt område;* **clinical thermometer** = thermometer for taking a patient's body temperature *febertermometer* **(b)** referring to instruction given to students at the bedside of patients as opposed to class instruction with no patient present *klinisk (som avser undervisning)*

> QUOTE we studied 69 patients who met the clinical and laboratory criteria of definite MS
> **Lancet**

> QUOTE the allocation of students to clinical areas is for their educational needs and not for service requirements
> **Nursing Times**

clinician [klɪ'nɪʃ(ə)n] *subst.* doctor, usually not a surgeon, who has considerable experience in treating patients *kliniker*

clip [klɪp] **1** *subst.* piece of metal with a spring, used to attach things together *klämma, sårklämma, agraff;* **Michel's clips** = clips used to suture a wound *slags sårklämma (agraff)* **2** *vb.* to attach together *fästa (klämma, hålla) ihop;* **the case notes are clipped together with the patient's record card**

clitoris ['klɪt(ə)rɪs] *subst.* small erectile female sex organ *or* structure in females, situated at the anterior angle of the vulva, which can be excited by sexual activity ⇨ *illustration* UROGENITAL SYSTEM (FEMALE) *clitoris, klitoris, kittlaren*

cloaca [kləʊ'eɪkə] *subst.* end part of the hindgut in an embryo *cloaca, kloaken*

clon ⇨ **clone**

clone [kləʊn] *subst.* group of cells derived from a single cell by asexual reproduction and so identical to the first cell *clon, klon*

clonic ['klɒnɪk] *adj.* (i) referring to clonus *klonisk;* (ii) having spasmodic contractions *med kloniska sammandragningar*

cloning ['kləʊnɪŋ] *subst.* method of making an exact copy of a living organism by asexual reproduction *kloning*

clonorchiasis [ˌkləʊnɔ'kaɪəsɪs] *subst.* liver condition, common in the Far East, caused by the fluke **Clonorchis sinensis** *sjukdom orsak av en slags levermask*

clonus ['kləʊnəs] *subst.* rhythmic contraction and relaxation of a muscle (usually a sign of upper motor neurone lesions) *clonus, klonus, klonisk muskelkramp*

Clostridium [klɒ'strɪdiəm] *subst.* type of bacteria *Clostridium*

COMMENT: species of Clostridium cause botulism, tetanus and gas gangrene

clot [klɒt] **1** *subst.* soft mass of blood which has coagulated *tromb, koagel, blodlever, blodpropp;* **the doctor diagnosed a blood clot in the brain; blood clots occur in embolism and thrombosis 2** *vb.* to coagulate *or* to change from liquid to semi-solid *koagulera, levra sig* NOTE: **clotting - clotted**

clothes [kləʊðz] *subst.* things worn to cover the body and keep a person warm *kläder;* **all his clothes had to be destroyed; you ought to put some clean clothes on; bedclothes** = sheets and blankets which cover a bed *sängkläder*

clotting ['klɒtɪŋ] *subst.* action of coagulating *koagulation, koagulering;* **clotting factors** *or* **coagulation factors** = substances (called Factor I, Factor II, and so on) in plasma which act one after the other to make the blood coagulate when a blood vessel is injured *koagulationsfaktorer;* **clotting time** *or* **coagulation time** = time taken for blood to coagulate under normal conditions *koagulationstid, blodkoagulationstid*

COMMENT: deficiency in one or more of the clotting factors results in haemophilia

cloud [klaʊd] *subst.* light white *or* grey mass of vapour floating in the air *or* disturbed sediment in a liquid *moln, grumling;* **I think it is going to rain - look at those grey clouds; clouds of smoke were pouring out of the house**

cloudy ['klaʊdi] *adj.* (i) where the sky is covered with clouds *molnig;* (ii) (liquid) which is not transparent but which has an opaque substance in it *oklar, grumlig;* **the patient is passing cloudy urine**

clubbing ['klʌbɪŋ] *subst.* thickening of the ends of the fingers and toes, a sign of many different diseases *bildning av trumpinnefingrar och trumpinnetår*

club foot ['klʌb ˌfʊt] *or* **talipes** ['tælɪpiːz] *subst.* congenitally deformed foot *talipes, klumpfot*

COMMENT: the most usual form (talipes equinovarus) is where the person walks on the toes, with the foot permanently bent forward; in other forms the foot either turns towards the inside (talipes varus) *or* towards the outside (talipes valgus) *or* upwards (talipes calcaneus) at the ankle so that the patient cannot walk on the sole of the foot

cluster ['klʌstə] *subst.* group of small items which cling together *kluster, anhopning;* **cluster headache** = headache which occurs behind one eye for a short period *clusterhuvudvärk*

clusterhuvudvärk ➪ **cluster**

Clutton's joint ['klʌtənz ˌdʒɔɪnt] *subst.* swollen knee joint occurring in congenital syphilis *svullen knäled pga medfödd syfilis*

cmc-lederna ➪ **carpometacarpal joints (CM joints)**

CMV [ˌsiːem'viː] = CYTOMEGALOVIRUS

CN [ˌsiː'en] = CHARGE NURSE

CNS [ˌsiːen'es] = CENTRAL NERVOUS SYSTEM

Co *symbol for* cobalt *Co, kobolt*

coagulant [kəʊ'ægjulənt] *subst.* substance which can make blood coagulate *ämne som orsakar (blod)koagulering*

coagulase [kəʊ'ægjuleɪz] *subst.* enzyme produced by Staphylococci which makes blood plasma coagulate *enzym som orsakar (blod)koagulering*

coagulate [kəʊ'ægjuleɪt] *vb.* to change from being liquid to semi-solid *koagulera;* **his blood does not coagulate easily**

COMMENT: blood coagulates with the conversion into fibrin of fibrinogen, a protein in the blood, under the influence of the enzyme thromboplastin

coagulation [kəʊˌægju'leɪʃ(ə)n] *subst.* becoming semi-solid (from being liquid) *koagulation, koagulering;* **coagulation**

factors = CLOTTING FACTORS; **coagulation time** = CLOTTING TIME

coagulum [kəʊ'ægjuləm] *subst.* blood clot *or* mass of coagulated blood *koagel, tromb, blodlever*

coarctation [ˌkəʊɑːk'teɪʃ(ə)n] *subst.* narrowing *coar(c)tation, koar(k)tation, striktur, förträngning;* **coarctation of the aorta** = congenital narrowing of the aorta which results in high blood pressure in the upper part of the body and low blood pressure in the lower part *coarctatio aortae, aortakoarktation*

coarse [kɔːs] *adj.* rough *or* not fine *grov;* **coarse hair grows on parts of the body at puberty; disease characterized by coarse features**

coat [kəʊt] **1** *subst.* layer of material covering an organ *or* a cavity *lager, skikt;* **muscle coats** = two layers of muscle forming part of the lining of the intestine *muskellager* **2** to cover *täcka, klä*

coating ['kəʊtɪŋ] *subst.* covering *hinna, dragering, beläggning;* **pill with a sugar coating**

cobalt ['kəʊbɔːlt] *subst.* metallic element *kobolt, Co;* **cobalt 60** = radioactive isotope which is used in radiotherapy to treat cancer *radioaktiv isotop av kobolt*
NOTE: symbol is **Co**

cocaine [kəʊ'keɪn] *subst.* alkaloid from the coca plant, sometimes used as a local anaesthetic but not generally used because its use leads to addiction *kokain*

coccidioidomycosis [kɒkˌsɪdiˌɔɪdəʊmaɪ'kəʊsɪs] *subst.* lung disease, caused by inhaling spores of the fungus Coccidioides immitis *koccidiodomykos, ökenreumatism*

coccus ['kɒkəs] *subst.* bacterium shaped like a ball *coccus, kock* NOTE: plural is **cocci**

> COMMENT: cocci grow together in groups: either in groups (staphylococci) or in long chains (streptococci)

coccy- [ˌkɒksi] *prefix* referring to the coccyx *coccy(g)-, koccy(g)-, svans-, svansbens-*

coccydynia [ˌkɒksi'dɪniə] *or* **coccygodynia** [ˌkɒksigəʊ'dɪniə] *subst.* sharp pain in the coccyx, usually caused by a blow *coccygalgi, coccygodyni*

coccygalgi ⇨ **coccydynia**

coccygeal vertebrae [kɒk'sɪdʒiəl ˌvɜːtɪbreɪ] *subst.* the fused bones in the coccyx *vertebrae coccygeae, svanskotorna*

coccygodyni ⇨ **coccydynia**

coccyx ['kɒksɪks] *subst.* lowest bones in the backbone ⇨ *illustration* VERTEBRAL COLUMN *coccyx, os coccygis, svansbenet*

> COMMENT: the coccyx is a rudimentary tail made of four bones which have fused together into a bone in the shape of a triangle

cochlea ['kɒkliə] *subst.* spiral tube, shaped like a snail shell, inside the inner ear, which is the essential organ of hearing ⇨ *illustration* EAR *cochlea, öronsnäckan*

> COMMENT: sounds are transmitted as vibrations to the cochlea from the ossicles through the oval window. The lymph fluid in the cochlea passes the vibrations to the organ of Corti, which in turn is connected to the auditory nerve

cochlear ['kɒkliə] *adj.* referring to the cochlea *cochlear, koklear, kokleär;* **cochlear duct** = spiral channel in the cochlea *ductus cochlearis;* **cochlear nerve** = division of the auditory nerve *nervus cochlearis, hörselnerven, cochlearisnerven, koklearnerven*

cochlearisnerven ⇨ **cochlear**

code [kəʊd] **1** *subst.* signs which have a hidden meaning *kod;* **genetic code** = characteristics which exist in the DNA of a cell and are passed on when the cell divides, and so are inherited by a child from a parent *genetisk kod* **2** *vb.* to give a meaning *koda;* **genes are sequences of DNA that code for specific proteins**

codeine ['kəʊdiːn] *subst.* alkaloid made from opium, used as a pain killer and to reduce coughing *kodein*

cod liver oil [ˌkɒd lɪvər 'ɒɪ(ə)l] *subst.* oil from the liver of codfish, which is rich in calories and vitamins A and D *torskleverolja, fiskleverolja*

-coele [siː(ə)l] *suffix* referring to a hollow *-håla*

coeli- ['siːli] *prefix* referring to a hollow, usually the abdomen *buk-, bukhåle-* NOTE: words beginning **coeli-** are spelled **celi-** in US English

coeliac ['si:liæk] *adj.* referring to the abdomen *buk-, bukhåle-;* **coeliac artery** *or* **coeliac axis** *or* **coeliac trunk** = main artery in the abdomen leading from the abdominal aorta and dividing into the left gastric, hepatic and splenic arteries *truncus coeliacus, bukinälvsartären;* **coeliac disease** *or* **gluten enteropathy** *or* **malabsorption syndrome** = syndrome mainly affecting children, caused by a reaction to gluten which prevents the small intestine from digesting fat *celiaki, intestinal infantilism, sprue, malabsorption, glutenintolerans;* **adult coeliac disease** = condition where gluten makes the villi of the intestine become smaller, so that the surface available for absorbing is reduced *celiaki, icke-tropisk sprue;* **coeliac plexus** = major plexus of nerves in the abdomen *plexus coeliacus (solaris), solarplexus*

COMMENT: symptoms of coeliac disease include a swollen abdomen, pale diarrhoea, abdominal pains and anaemia

coelioscopy [ˌsi:li'ɒskəpi] *subst.* examining the peritoneal cavity by inflating the abdomen with sterile air and passing an endoscope through the abdominal wall *laparoskopi, celioskopi*

coelom ['si:ləm] *subst.* body cavity in an embryo, which divides to form the thorax and abdomen *celom*

coffee ground vomit [ˌkɒfi graʊnd 'vɒmɪt] *subst.* vomit containing dark pieces of blood, indicating that the patient is bleeding from the stomach or upper intestine *kaffesumpsliknande kräkning, kaffesumpskräkning*

coil [kɔɪl] *subst.* spiral metal wire fitted into a woman's uterus, as a contraceptive *spiral*

coiled [kɔɪld] *adj.* spiral *or* twisted round and round *rulla (ringla) ihop sig;* **a coiled tube at the end of a nephron**

coital ['kəʊɪt(ə)l] *adj.* referring to coitus *som avser el. hör till samlag*

coition [kəʊ'ɪʃ(ə)n] *subst.* sexual intercourse *coitus, samlag, kopulation*

coitus ['kəʊɪtəs] *subst.* sexual intercourse *coitus, samlag, kopulation;* **coitus interruptus** = form of contraception, where the penis is removed from the vagina before ejaculation *coitus interruptus, avbrutet samlag*

COMMENT: this is not a safe method of contraception

coitus ⇨ **coitus, coition, copulation, intercourse, sex**

cold [kəʊld] **1** *adj.* not warm *or* not hot *kall;* **he always has a cold shower in the morning; the weather is colder than last week and they say it will be even colder tomorrow; many old people suffer from hypothermia in cold weather; cold drinks give him colic pains; cold burn** = injury to the skin caused by exposure to extreme cold *congelatio, frostskada;* **cold compress** = cloth pad soaked in cold water, used to relieve a headache *or* bruise *kallt vått omslag;* **cold sore** *or* **herpes simplex** = burning sore, usually on the lips *herpes simplex (labialis)* **2** *subst.* **common cold** *or* **coryza** *or* **cold in the head** = illness, when the patient sneezes and coughs, and has a blocked and running nose *coryza, förkylning, snuva;* **he caught a cold by standing in the rain; she's got a cold so she can't go out; mother's in bed with a cold; don't come near me - I've got a cold and you may catch it**

COMMENT: a cold usually starts with a virus infection which causes inflammation of the mucous membrane in the nose and throat. Symptoms include running nose, cough and loss of taste and smell; there is no cure for a cold at present, though the coronavirus which causes a cold has been identified

colectomy [kə(ʊ)'lektəmi] *subst.* surgical removal of the whole *or* part of the colon *kolektomi*

coli ['kəʊlaɪ] *see* TAENIA

colic ['kɒlɪk] *or* **enteralgia** [ent(ə)r'ældʒd] *subst.* **(a)** pain in any part of the intestinal tract *kolik;* **biliary colic** = pain caused by inflammation of the gall bladder or by stones in the bile duct *colica hepatica, gallstenskolik;* **mucous colic** = inflammation of the colon, with painful spasms in the muscles of the walls of the colon *colica mucosa;* **renal colic** = pain caused by kidney stone or stones in the ureter *colica renalis, njurkolik, ofta njurstensanfall* **(b) right colic** *or* **middle colic** = arteries which lead from the superior mesenteric artery *arteria colica dextra resp. colica media, högra resp. mellersta tjocktarmsartären*

COMMENT: although colic can refer to pain caused by indigestion, it can also be caused by stones in the gall bladder or kidney

colicky ['kɒlɪkɪ] *adj.* referring to colic *som avser el. hör till kolik;* **he had colicky pains in his abdomen**

coliform bacteria ['kəʊlifɔ:m bækˌtɪəriə] *subst.* bacteria which are similar to Bacterium coli *koliform bakterie*

colit ⇨ **colitis**

colitis [kə(ʊ)'laɪtɪs] *subst.* inflammation of the colon *colit, kolit, tjocktarmsinflammation;* **mucous colitis** *or* **irritable bowel syndrome** = inflammation of the mucous membrane in the intestine, where the patient suffers pain caused by spasms in the muscles of the walls of the colon *colica mucosa, colon irritabile, spastisk kolit;* **ulcerative colitis** = severe pain in the colon, together with diarrhoea and ulcers in the rectum, often with a psychosomatic cause *colon ulcerosa, ulcerös kolit*

collagen ['kɒlədʒ(ə)n] *subst.* bundles of protein fibres, which form the connective tissue, bone and cartilage *kollagen;* **collagen disease** = any of several diseases of the connective tissue *kollagenos, bindvävssjukdom;* **collagen fibre** = fibre which is the main component of fasciae, tendons and ligaments, and is essential in bone and cartilage *kollagen fiber (tråd)* NOTE: no plural

COMMENT: collagen diseases include rheumatic fever, rheumatoid arthritis, periarteritis nodosa, scleroderma and dermatomyositis,. Collagen diseases can be treated with cortisone

collagenous [kə'lædʒɪnəs] *adj.* (i) containing collagen *kollagen-, bindvävs-;* (ii) referring to collagen disease *som avser el. hör till kollagenos (bindvävssjukdom)*

collapse [kə'læps] **1** *subst.* condition where a patient is extremely exhausted *or* semi-conscious *kollaps, sammanbrott;* **he was found in a state of collapse 2** *vb.* **(a)** to fall down in a semi-conscious state *kollapsa, klappa ihop, bryta samman;* **after running to catch his train he collapsed (b)** to become flat *or* to lose air *kollabera, falla ihop, sjunka samman;* **collapsed lung** *see* PNEUMOTHORAX

collar ['kɒlə] *subst.* part of a coat, shirt, etc. which goes round the neck *krage;* **my shirt collar's too tight; she turned up her coat collar because of the wind; cervical collar** *or* **neck collar** *or* **surgical collar** = special strong collar to support the head of someone with a fractured neck *halskrage;* **collar bone** *or* **clavicle** = one of two long thin bones which join the shoulder blades to the breastbone *clavicula, nyckelbenet;* **collar bone fracture** = fracture of the collar bone (one of the most frequent fractures in the body) *fractura colli femori, collumfraktur, brott på lårbenshalsen*

collateral [kə'læt(ə)r(ə)l] *adj.* secondary *or* less important *kollateral-;* **collateral circulation** = enlargement of certain secondary blood vessels, as a response when the main vessels become slowly blocked *kollateralcirkulation*

QUOTE embolization of the coeliac axis is an effective treatment for severe bleeding in the stomach or duodenum, localized by endoscopic examination. A good collateral blood supply makes occlusion of a single branch of the coeliac axis safe
British Medical Journal

collect [kə'lekt] *vb.* to bring various things together *samla (ihop, in, upp, på);* to come together *samlas, samla sig;* **fluid collects in the tissues of patients suffering from dropsy**

collecting duct [kə'lektɪŋ ˌdʌkt] *subst.* part of the system by which urine is filtered in the kidney *samlingsrör*

collection [kə'lekʃ(ə)n] *subst.* bringing together of various things *samling;* **the hospital has a collection of historical surgical instruments**

college ['kɒlɪdʒ] *subst.* place of further education where people study after they have left secondary school *college, ung. högskola;* **I'm going to college to study pharmacy**

Colles' fracture [ˌkɒlɪs(ɪz) 'fræktʃə] *see* FRACTURE

colliculus [kə'lɪkjʊləs] *subst.* one of four small projections (the superior and inferior colliculi) in the midbrain ⇨ *illustration* BRAIN *collicus inferior resp. superior, liten upphöjning på fyrhögsplattan*
NOTE: the plural is **colliculi**

collodion [kə'ləʊdiən] *subst.* liquid used to paint on a clean wound, where it dries to form a flexible covering *collodium, kollodium, kollodion, celloidin*

collodium ⇨ **collodion**

collum chirurgicum (humeri) ⇨ **surgical**

collumfraktur ⇨ **collar**

collyrium [kə'lɪriəm] *subst.* solution used to bathe the eyes *collyrium, kollyrium, ögonvatten*

coloboma [ˌkɒləʊ'bəʊmə] *subst.* condition where part of the eye, especially part of the iris, is missing *coloboma, kolobom*

colon ['kəʊlən] *subst.* the large intestine (running from the caecum at the end of the small intestine to the rectum) *colon, kolon, grovtarmen, tjocktarmen;* **ascending colon** = first part of the colon which goes up the right side of the body from the caecum *colon ascendens, uppåtstigande delen av tjocktarmen;* **descending colon** = third section of the colon which goes down the left side of the body *colon descendens, nedåtgående delen av tjocktarmen;* **sigmoid colon** = fourth section of the colon which continues as the rectum *(colon) sigmoideum, sigmaformade delen av tjocktarmen;* **transverse colon** = second section of the colon which crosses the body below the stomach *colon transversum, tvärgående delen av tjocktarmen;* **irritable** *or* **spastic colon** = MUCOUS COLITIS ⇨ *illustration* DIGESTIVE SYSTEM

> COMMENT: the colon is about 1.35 metres in length, and rises from the end of the small intestine up the right side of the body, then crosses beneath the stomach and drops down the left side of the body to end as the rectum. In the colon, water is extracted from the waste material which has passed through the small intestine, leaving only the faeces which are pushed forward by peristaltic movements and passed out of the body through the rectum

colon **⇨ large intestine**

colonic [kəʊ'lɒnɪk] *adj.* referring to the colon *kolisk, kolon-;* **colonic irrigation** = washing out of the large intestine *kolonsköljning, kolonspolning*

colon irritabile **⇨ mucous**

colonoscope [kə'lɒnəskəʊp] *subst.* surgical instrument for examining the interior of the colon *kolo(no)skop*

colonoscopy [ˌkɒlə'nɒskəpi] *subst.* examination of the inside of the colon, using a colonoscope passed through the rectum *kolo(no)skopi*

colony ['kɒləni] *subst.* group *or* culture of microorganisms *koloni*

colostomy [kə'lɒstəmi] *subst.* surgical operation to make an opening (stoma) between the colon and the abdominal wall to allow faeces to be passed out without going through the rectum *kolostomi*

> COMMENT: a colostomy is carried out when the colon or rectum is blocked, or where part of the colon or rectum has had to be removed

colostomy bag [kə'lɒstəmi ˌbæg] *subst.* bag attached to the opening after a colostomy, to collect faeces *kolostomipåse*

colostrum [kə'lɒstrəm] *subst.* fluid secreted by the breasts at the birth of a baby, but before the true milk starts to flow *colostrum, kolostrum, råmjölk*

colour ['kʌlə] *or US* **color** ['kʌlər] **1** *subst.* differing wavelengths of light (red *or* blue *or* yellow, etc.) which are reflected from objects and sensed by the eyes *färg;* **what is the colour of a healthy liver? the diseased parts are shown by the colour red on the chart; he looks unwell, and his face has no colour 2** *vb.* to give colour to *färga;* **the arteries are coloured red on the diagram; bile colours the urine yellow**

colour-blind ['kʌləblaɪnd] *adj.* not able to tell the difference between certain colours *färgblind;* **several of the students are colour-blind**

colour blindness ['kʌləblaɪndnəs] *subst.* being unable to tell the difference between certain colours *färgblindhet*

> COMMENT: colour blindness is a condition which almost never occurs in women. The commonest form is the inability to tell the difference between red and green. The Ishihara test is used to test for colour blindness

colouring (matter) ['kʌlərɪŋ (ˌmætə)] *subst.* substance which colours an organ *färgämne*

colourless ['kʌlələs] *adj.* with no colour *färglös;* **a colourless fluid was discharged from the sore**

colp- ['kɒlp, ˌ-] *prefix* referring to the vagina *colp(o)-, kolp(o)-, vagin(o)-, vaginal-, slid-*

colpocystopexy [ˌkɒlpə'sɪstəpeksi] *subst.* surgical operation to lift and stitch the vagina and bladder to the abdominal wall *slags operation av inkontinens*

colpopexi **⇨ colpopexy**

colpopexy ['kɒlpəpeksi] *subst.* surgical operation to fix a prolapsed vagina to the abdominal wall *colpopexi, kolpopexi*

colpoplasty ['kɒlpəplæsti] *subst.* surgical operation to repair a damaged vagina *vaginalplastik*

colpoptosis [ˌkɒlpə'təʊsɪs] *subst.* prolapse of the walls of the vagina *kolpoptos, vaginalprolaps, framfall av slidan*

colporrhaphy [kɒl'pɒrəfi] *subst.* surgical operation to suture a prolapsed vagina *kolporrafi*

colposcope ['kɒlpəʊskəʊp] *subst.* surgical instrument used to examine the inside of the vagina *kolposkop, vaginoskop*

colposcopy [kɒl'pɒskəpi] *subst.* examination of the inside of the vagina *kolposkopi, vaginoskopi*

colpotomy [kɒl'pɒtəmi] *subst.* any surgical operation to make a cut in the vagina *kolpotomi, vaginotomi, vaginalsnitt*

column ['kɒləm] *subst.* usually circular mass standing upright like a tree *pelare;* **spinal column** *or* **vertebral column** = backbone *or* series of bones and discs which forms a flexible column running from the pelvis to the skull *columna spinalis (vertebralis), kotpelaren, ryggraden*

columnar [kə'lʌmnə] *adj.* shaped like a column *pelarliknande;* **columnar cell** = type of epithelial cell *cylinderepitelcell*

coma ['kəʊmə] *subst.* state of unconsciousness from which a person cannot be awakened by external stimuli *koma, medvetslöshet;* **he went into a coma and never regained consciousness; she has been in a coma for four days; diabetic coma** = unconsciousness caused by untreated diabetes *diabeteskoma*

COMMENT: a coma can have many causes: head injuries, diabetes, stroke, drug overdose. A coma is often fatal, but a patient may continue to live in a coma for a long time, even several months, before dying or regaining consciousness

comatose ['kəʊmətəʊs] *adj.* (i) unconscious *or* in a coma *komatös, medvetslös;* (ii) like a coma *komaliknande*

combat ['kɒmbæt] *vb.* to fight against *bekämpa;* **the medical team is combating an outbreak of diphtheria; what can we do to combat the spread of the disease?**

combination [ˌkɒmbɪ'neɪʃ(ə)n] *subst.* act of joining together *kombination, förening;* **actomyosin is a combination of actin and myosin**

combine [kəm'baɪn] *vb.* to join together *kombinera, förena*

combustio ⇨ **burn**

comedo ['kɒmɪdəʊ] *subst.* blackhead *or* small point of dark, hard matter in a sebaceous follicle, often found in adolescents *comedo, komedon, pormask*
NOTE: plural is **comedones**

comfort ['kʌmfət] *vb.* to make relaxed *or* to help make a patient less miserable *trösta;* **the paramedics comforted the injured until the ambulance arrived**

commensal [kə'mens(ə)l] *subst. & adj.* (plant *or* animal) which lives on another plant *or* animal, but does not harm it in any way and both may benefit from the association *som lever i kommensalism;* **Candida is a normal commensal in the mouths of 50% of healthy adults**
NOTE: if it causes harm it is a **parasite**

comminuted fracture [ˌkɒmɪnju:tɪd 'fræktʃə] *subst.* fracture where the bone is broken in several places *komminut fraktur, splitterbrott*

commissure ['kɒmɪsjʊə] *subst.* structure which joins two tissues of similar material, such as a group of nerves which crosses from one part of the central nervous system to another *kommissur, fog, söm;* **grey commissure** *or* **white commissure** parts of grey and white matter in the spinal cord nearest the central canal *commisura ventralis resp. alba, grå resp. vit kommissur; see also* CORPUS CALLOSUM

common ['kɒmən] *adj.* **(a)** ordinary *or* not exceptional *or* which happens very frequently *vanlig, allmän;* **accidents are quite common on this part of the motorway; it's a common mistake to believe that cancer is always fatal; common cold** *or* **coryza** = virus infection which causes inflammation of the mucous membrane in the nose and throat *coryza, förkylning, snuva* **(b) (in) common** = belonging to more than one thing *or* person *gemensam;* **haemophilia and Christmas disease have several symptoms in common; common bile duct** = duct leading to the duodenum, formed of the hepatic and cystic ducts *ductus choledochus communis, gemensamma gallgången;* **common carotid artery** = large artery in the lower part of the neck *arteria carotis communis, gemensamma halsartären;* **common hepatic duct** = duct from the liver formed when the right and left hepatic ducts join *ductus hepaticus communis, gemensamma levergången;* **common iliac arteries** = arteries which branch from the aorta and divide into the internal and external iliac arteries *arteriae iliacae communes, stora höftpulsådrorna;* **common iliac veins** = veins draining the legs, pelvis and abdomen, which unite to form the inferior vena cava *venae iliacae communes, gemensamma höftvenerna;* **common mesentery** = double layer of peritoneum attaching the intestine to the abdominal wall *mesenteriet, tarmkäxet;* **final common pathway** = linked neurons which take all impulses from the central nervous system to a muscle *nedre motorneuron*

commonly ['kɒmənli] *adv.* which happens often *vanligen, i allmänhet;* **a cold winter commonly brings a flu epidemic**

communicable disease [kə'mju:nɪkəb(ə)l] *subst.* disease which can be passed from one person to another *or* from an animal to a person *smittsam sjukdom, överförbar sjukdom; see also* CONTAGIOUS, INFECTIOUS

communicate [kə'mju:nɪkeɪt] *vb.* to pass a message to someone *or* something *meddela, stå i förbindelse, hänga ihop (samman);* **autistic children do not communicate, even with their parents; communicating arteries** = arteries which connect the blood supply from each side of the brain, part of the circle of Willis *arteria communicans anterior resp. posterior*

community [kə'mju:nəti] *subst.* group of people who live and work in a district *samhälle;* **the health services serve the local community; community care is an important part of primary health care; community medicine** = study of medical practice which examines groups of people and the health of the community, including housing, pollution and other environmental factors *ung. socialmedicin;* **community physician** = doctor who specializes in community medicine *ung. socialläkare, socialmedicinare;* **Community Psychiatric Nurse (CPN)** = psychiatric nurse who works in a district, visiting various patients in the area *ung. sjuksköterska inom distriktspsykiatri;* **community services** = nursing services which are available to the community *ung. distriktsköterskevård*

compact bone ['kɒmpækt ˌbəʊn] *subst.* type of bone tissue which forms the hard outer layer of bones ⇨ *illustration* BONE STRUCTURE *kompakt ben*

compatibility [kəmˌpætə'bɪləti] *subst.* (i) ability of two drugs not to interfere with each other when administered together *kompatibilitet, blandbarhet, förenlighet;* (ii) ability of a body to accept organs *or* tissue *or* blood from another person and not to reject them *kompatibilitet*

compatible [kəm'pætəb(ə)l] *adj.* able to work together without being rejected *kompatibel, förenlig;* **the surgeons are trying to find a compatible donor** *or* **a donor with a compatible blood group**

compensate ['kɒmpenseɪt] *vb.* *(of an organ)* to make good the failure of another organ *kompensera, uppväga, ersätta;* **the heart has to beat more strongly to compensate for the narrowing of the arteries**

complain [kəm'pleɪn] *vb.* to say that something is not good *klaga;* **the patients have complained about the food; he is complaining of pains in his legs**

complaint [kəm'pleɪnt] *subst.* **(a)** illness *åkomma, sjukdom, besvär;* **he is suffering from a nervous complaint (b)** saying that something is wrong *klagomål, anmärkning;* **the hospital administrator wouldn't listen to the complaints of the consultants**

complement ['kɒmplɪmənt] *subst.* substance which forms part of blood plasma and is essential to the work of antibodies and antigens *komplement;* **complement fixation test (CFT)** = test to measure the amount of complement in antibodies and antigens *komplementbindningsreaktion, KBR*

complex ['kɒmpleks] **1** *subst.* **(a)** *(in psychiatry)* group of ideas which are based on the experience a person has had in the past, and which influence the way he behaves *komplex;* **Electra complex** = condition where a woman feels sexually attracted to her father and sees her mother as an obstacle *elektrakomplex;* **inferiority complex** = condition where the person feels he is inferior to others *mindervärdeskomplex;* **OEdipus complex** = condition where a man feels sexually attracted to his mother and sees his father as an obstacle *oidipuskomplex;* **superiority complex** = condition where the person feels he is superior to others and pays little attention to them *överlägsenhetskomplex* **(b)** group of items *or* buildings *or* organs *komplex, anläggning;* **he works in the new laboratory complex; primary complex** = first lymph node to be infected by TB *primärkomplex;* **Vitamin B complex** = group of vitamins such as folic acid, riboflavine and thiamine *B-vitamin* **(c)** syndrome *or* group of signs and symptoms due to a particular cause *syndrom, symptomkomplex* **2** *adj.* complicated *komplicerad, invecklad, sammansatt;* **a gastrointestinal fistula can cause many complex problems, including fluid depletion**

complexion [kəm'plekʃ(ə)n] *subst.* general colour of the skin on the face *hy, hudfärg, ansiktsfärg;* **he has a red complexion; she has a fine pink complexion; people with fair complexions burn easily in the sun**

complicated fracture [ˌkɒmplɪkeɪtɪd 'fræktʃə] *subst.* fracture with an associated injury of tissue, as where the bone has punctured an artery *fraktur med (komplicerande) vävnadsskada*

complication [ˌkɒmplɪˈkeɪʃ(ə)n] *subst.* **(a)** condition where two or more diseases exist in a patient, and are not always connected *tillstånd med två el. flera samtidiga sjukdomar* **(b)** situation where a patient develops a second disease which changes the course of treatment for the first *komplikation;* **he was admitted to hospital suffering from pneumonia with complications; she appeared to be improving, but complications set in and she died in a few hours**

> QUOTE sickle cell chest syndrome is a common complication of sickle cell disease, presenting with chest pain, fever and leucocytosis
> **British Medical Journal**

> QUOTE venous air embolism is a potentially fatal complication of percutaneous venous catheterization
> **Southern Medical Journal**

component [kəmˈpəʊnənt] *subst.* substance *or* element which forms part of a complete item *komponent, beståndsdel*

compose [kəmˈpəʊz] *vb.* to make up *(tillsammans) bilda, bestå av;* **the lotion is composed of oil, calamine and camphor**

composition [ˌkɒmpəˈzɪʃ(ə)n] *subst.* way in which a compound is formed *komposition, sammansättning, förening;* **chemical composition** = the chemicals which make up a substance *kemisk sammansättning;* **they analysed the blood samples to find out their chemical composition**

compos mentis [ˈkɒmpɒsˈmentɪs] *Latin phrase meaning* of sound mind *or* sane *vid sina sinnens fulla bruk, tillräknelig;* **the patient was non compos mentis when he attacked the doctor**

compound [ˈkɒmpaʊnd] *subst.* chemical substance made up of two or more components *sammansättning, kemisk förening*

compound fracture [ˌkɒmpaʊnd ˈfræktʃə] *subst.* fracture where the skin surface is damaged *or* where the broken bone penetrates the surface of the skin *komplicerad fraktur, öppen fraktur*

compress [ˈkɒmpres; kəmˈpres] **1** *subst.* wad soaked in hot or cold liquid and applied to the skin to relieve pain *or* to force pus out of an infected wound *(fuktig) kompress, omslag* **2** *vb.* to squeeze *or* to press *pressa ihop (samman), trycka ihop (samman), komprimera;* **compressed air sickness** = CAISSON DISEASE

compression [kəmˈpreʃ(ə)n] *subst.* **(a)** squeezing *or* pressing *kompression, tryck;* **the first aider applied compression to the chest of the casualty; compression syndrome** = pain in muscles after strenuous exercise *träningsvärk* **(b)** serious condition where the brain is compressed by blood accumulating in it or by a fractured skull *inklämning*

compulsive [kəmˈpʌlsɪv] *adj.* (feeling) which cannot be stopped *kompulsiv, tvångsmässig;* **she has a compulsive desire to steal; compulsive eating** = psychological condition where the patient has a continual desire to eat *tvångsmässigt ätande; see also* BULIMIA

computer [kəmˈpjuːtə] *subst.* electronic machine for calculating *dator*

computerized axial tomography (CAT) [kəmˈpjuːtəraɪzd ˌæksiəl tə(ʊ)ˈmɒgrəfi (ˌsiːeɪˈtiː)] *subst.* system of scanning a patient's body, where a narrow X-ray beam, guided by a computer, can photograph a thin section of the body *or* of an organ from several angles and uses the computer to build up an image of the section *datortomografi, DT, CT, skiktröntgen*

concave [ˈkɒnkeɪv] *adj.* which curves towards the inside *konkav;* **a concave lens**

conceive [kənˈsiːv] *vb.* to become pregnant *bli gravid, bli med barn (havande); see* CONCEPTION

concentrate [ˈkɒns(ə)ntreɪt] **1** *subst.* **(a)** strength of a solution *koncentration* **(b)** way of showing amounts of a substance in body tissues and fluids *koncentration* **(c)** strong solution which is to be diluted *koncentrat* **2** *vb.* **(a) to concentrate on** = to examine something in particular *koncentrera (sig)* **(b)** to reduce a solution and increase its strength by evaporation *koncentrera*

conception [kənˈsepʃ(ə)n] *subst.* point at which the development of a baby starts *konception, befruktning*

> COMMENT: conception is usually taken to be the moment when the sperm cell fertilizes the ovum, or a few days later, when the fertilized ovum attaches itself to the wall of the womb

conceptus [kənˈseptəs] *subst.* result of the fertilized ovum which will develop into an embryo and fetus *befruktat ägg, konceptionsprodukt*

concha ['kɒŋkə] *subst.* part of the body shaped like a shell *concha, mussla;* **concha auriculae** = part of the outer ear *concha auriculae, öronmusslan;* **nasal conchae** = little projections of bone which form the sides of the nasal cavity *conchae nasales, näsmusslorna*
NOTE: the plural is **conchae**

concretion [kən'kri:ʃ(ə)n, kəŋ'k-] *subst.* mass of hard material which forms in the body (such as a gallstone *or* deposits on bone in arthritis) *konkretion, konkrement*

concussed [kən'kʌst] *adj.* (person) who has been hit on the head and has lost and then regained consciousness *som har utsatts för hjärnskakning;* **he was walking around in a concussed state**

concussion [kən'kʌʃ(ə)n, kəŋ'k-] *subst.* **(a)** applying force to any part of the body *stöt, skakning* **(b)** disturbance of the brain *or* loss of consciousness for a short period, caused by a blow to the head *concussio (cerebri), commotio cerebri, hjärnskakning*

concussive [kən'kʌsɪv] *adj.* which causes concussion *som orsakar hjärnskakning*

condensed [kən'denst] *adj.* made compact *or* more dense *kondenserad, förtätad*

condition [kən'dɪʃ(ə)n] *subst.* **(a)** state (of health *or* of cleanliness) *kondition, tillstånd, skick;* **the arteries are in very good condition; he is ill, and his condition is getting worse; conditions in the hospital are very bad** **(b)** illness *or* injury *or* disorder *besvär, sjukdom, åkomma;* **he is being treated for a heart condition**

conditioned reflex [kən,dɪʃ(ə)nd 'ri:fleks] *subst.* automatic reaction by a person to a stimulus, a normal reaction to a normal stimulus which comes from past experience *betingad reflex*

condom ['kɒndəm] *subst.* rubber sheath worn on the penis during intercourse as a contraceptive and also as a protection against venereal disease *kondom*

conducting system [kən'dʌktɪŋ ,sɪstəm] *subst.* nerve system in the heart which links an atrium to a ventricle, so that the two beat at the same rate *retledningssystemet*

conduction [kən'dʌkʃ(ə)n] *subst.* passing of heat *or* sound *or* nervous impulses from one part of the body to another *ledning, överföring, överledning;* **conduction fibres** = fibres (as in the bundle of His) which transmit impulses *retledningstråd;* **air conduction** = conduction of sounds from the outside to the inner ear through the auditory meatus *luftledning;* **bone conduction** *or* **osteophony** = conduction of sound waves to the inner ear through the bones of the skull *osteofoni, benledning; see also* RINNE'S TEST

conductive [kən'dʌktɪv] *adj.* referring to conduction *konduktiv, lednings-;* **conductive deafness** = deafness caused by a disorder in the conduction of sound into the inner ear, rather than a disorder of the hearing nerves *konduktiv dövhet, ledningshörselnedsättning*

conduit ['kɒndjuɪt] *subst.* channel *or* passage along which a fluid flows *ledning, rör, kanal;* **ileal conduit** = using a loop of the ileum to which one or both ureters are anastomosed, in order to drain urine from the body *konstgjord urinblåsa, Brickerblåsa*

condyle ['kɒndaɪ(ə)l] *subst.* rounded end of a bone which articulates with another *kondyl, ledhuvud, ledknapp;* **occipital condyle** = round part of the occipital bone which joins it to the atlas *condylus occipitalis, nackbenets ledknapp*

condyloid process ['kɒndɪlɔɪd ,prəuses] *subst.* projecting part at each end of the lower jaw which forms the head of the jaw, joining the jaw to the skull *processus condylaris, underkäkens ledutskott*

condyloma [,kɒndɪ'ləumə] *subst.* growth usually found on the vulva *kondylom*

cone [kəun] *subst.* one of two types of cell in the retina of the eye which is sensitive to light *tapp; see also* ROD

COMMENT: cones are sensitive to bright light and colours and do not function in bad light

confined [kən'faɪnd] *adj.* kept in a place *begränsad, bunden till;* **she was confined to bed with pneumonia; since his accident he has been confined to a wheelchair**

confirm [kən'fɜ:m] *vb.* to agree officially that something is true *konfirmera, bekräfta;* **X-rays confirmed the presence of a tumour; the number of confirmed cases of the disease has doubled**

confuse [kən'fju:z] *vb.* to make someone think wrongly; to make things difficult for someone to understand *förvirra;* **the patient was confused by the physiotherapist's instructions; old people can easily become confused if they are moved from their homes; many severely confused patients do not respond to spoken communication**

confusion [kən'fju:ʒ(ə)n] *subst.* being confused *förvirring;* **he has attacks of mental confusion; the absence of any effective treatment for confusion**

congeal [kən'dʒi:(ə)l] *vb. (of fat or blood)* to become solid *koagulera, stelna*

congelatio ⇨ **burn, frostbite**

congenita [kən'dʒenɪtə] *see* AMYOTONIA

congenital [kən'dʒenɪt(ə)l, kɒn-] *adj.* which exists at or before birth *kongenital, medfödd;* **congenital defect** = defect which exists in a baby from birth *medfödd missbildning (defekt);* **congenital dislocation of the hip** = condition where a baby is born with weak ligaments in the hip, so that the femur does not stay in position in the pelvis *kongenital (medfödd) höftledsluxation;* **congenital heart disease** = heart trouble caused by defects present in the heart at birth *vitum organicum cordis congenitum, VOC congenitum, medfött hjärtfel*

COMMENT: a congenital condition is not always inherited from a parent through the genes, as it may be due to abnormalities which develop in the fetus because of factors such as a disease which the mother has (as in the case of German measles) or a drug which she has taken

congenitally [kən'dʒenɪt(ə)li] *adv.* at *or* before birth *före (vid) födelsen;* **the baby is congenitally incapable of absorbing gluten**

congested [kən'dʒestɪd] *adj.* with blood *or* fluid inside *överfylld med blod (vätska), täppt;* **congested face** = red face, caused by blood rushing to the face *rödbrusigt (blodöverfyllt) ansikte*

congestion [kən'dʒestʃ(ə)n] *subst.* accumulation of blood in an organ *kongestion, blodstockning, blodöverfyllnad;* **nasal congestion** = blocking of the nose by inflammation as a response to a cold *or* other infection *nästäppa*

congestive [kən'dʒestɪv] *adj.* (heart failure) caused by congestion *som orsakas av blodstockning*

conization [ˌkɒnaɪ'zeɪʃ(ə)n] *subst.* surgical removal of a cone-shaped piece of tissue *konisation (jfr cervicectomy)*

conjoined twins [kənˌdʒɔɪnd 'twɪnz] *see* SIAMESE TWINS

conjugata ⇨ **conjugate**

conjugate ['kɒn(d)ʒʊgət] *or* **true conjugate** [ˌtru: 'kɒn(d)ʒʊgət] *or* **conjugate diameter** [ˌkɒn(d)ʒʊgət daɪ'æmɪtə] *subst.* measurements of space in the pelvis, used to calculate if normal childbirth is possible *conjugata, bäckenvidd*

conjunctiva [ˌkɒndʒʌŋk'taɪvə] *subst.* membrane which covers the front of the eyeball and the inside of the eyelids *konjunktiva, bindhinnan, bindehinnan*

conjunctival [ˌkɒndʒʌŋk'taɪv(ə)l] *adj.* referring to the conjunctiva *konjunktival, bindhinne-*

conjunctivitis [kənˌdʒʌŋ(k)tɪ'vaɪtɪs] *subst.* inflammation of the conjunctiva *konjunktivit, bindhinneinflammation; see also* PINK EYE

connect [kə'nekt] *vb.* to join *förbinda, förena, ansluta;* **the lungs are connected to the mouth by the trachea; the pulmonary artery connects the heart to the lungs; the biceps is connected to both the radius and the scapula**

connection [kə'nekʃ(ə)n] *subst.* something which joins *förbindelse, förening, anslutning*

connective tissue [kəˌnektɪv 'tɪʃu:] *subst.* tissue which forms the main part of bones and cartilage, ligaments and tendons, in which a large proportion of fibrous material surrounds the tissue cells *bindväv, stödjevävnad*

Conn's syndrome ['kɒnz ˌsɪndrəʊm] *subst.* condition caused by excessive production of aldosterone *Conns syndrom*

consanguinity [ˌkɒnsæŋ'gwɪnəti] *subst.* blood relationship between people *konsangvinitet, blodsband, släktskap*

conscious ['kɒnʃəs] *adj.* awake and knowing what is happening *medveten, vid medvetande;* **he became conscious in the recovery room two hours after the operation; it was two days after the accident before she became conscious**

consciously ['kɒnʃəsli] *adv.* in a conscious way *medvetet*

consciousness ['kɒnʃəsnəs] *subst.* being mentally awake and knowing what is happening *medvetande, medvetenhet;* **to lose consciousness** = to become unconscious *or* to become unable to respond to stimulation by the senses *förlora medvetandet;* **to regain consciousness** = to become conscious after being unconscious *återfå medvetandet, komma till sans*

consent [kən'sent] *subst.* agreement *samtycke, medgivande;* **the parents gave their consent for their son's heart to be used in the transplant operation; the nurses checked the patient's identity bracelet and that his consent had been given; consent form** = form which a patient signs to show he agrees to have the operation *blankett där patient ger sitt samtycke till behandling*

conserve [kən'sɜːv] *vb.* to keep *or* not to waste *bevara, vidmakthålla, spara på;* **the body needs to conserve heat in cold weather**

consolidation [kənˌsɒlɪ'deɪʃ(ə)n] *subst.* (i) stage in mending a broken bone, where the callus formed at the break changes into bone *konsolidering;* (ii) condition where part of the lung becomes solid (as in pneumonia) *förtätning, infiltrat*

constant ['kɒnst(ə)nt] *adj.* **(a)** continuous *or* not stopping *konstant, ständig, oavbruten;* **patients with Alzheimer's disease need constant supervision (b)** level *or* not varying *fast, oförändrad;* **his blood pressure remained constant during the operation**

constipated ['kɒnstɪpeɪtɪd] *adj.* unable to pass faeces often enough *konstiperad, obstiperad, förstoppad*

constipation [ˌkɒnstɪ'peɪʃ(ə)n] *subst.* difficulty in passing faeces often enough *konstipering, obstipation, förstoppning*

> COMMENT: constipated bowel movements are hard, and may cause pain in the anus. One bowel movement per day is the normal frequency. Constipation may be caused by worry *or* by a diet which does not contain enough roughage *or* by lack of exercise, as well as more serious diseases of the intestine

constituent [kən'stɪtjuənt] *subst.* substance which forms part of something *konstituent, beståndsdel;* **the chemical constituents of nerve cells**

constitution [ˌkɒnstɪ'tjuːʃ(ə)n] *subst.* general health and strength of a person *konstitution, kroppskonstitution, fysik;* **she has a strong constitution** *or* **a healthy constitution; he has a weak constitution and is often ill**

constitutional [ˌkɒnstɪ'tjuːʃ(ə)n(ə)l] *adj.* referring to a person's constitution *som avser el. hör till (kropps)konstitution*

constitutionally [ˌkɒnstɪ'tjuːʃ(ə)n(ə)li] *adv.* in a person's constitution *konstitutionell;* **he is constitutionally incapable of feeling tired**

constrict [kən'strɪkt] *vb.* to squeeze *or* to make a passage narrower *dra ihop (samman), snöra ihop (samman)*

constriction [kən'strɪkʃ(ə)n] *subst.* stenosis *or* becoming narrow *konstriktion, stenos, förträngning, sammandragning*

constrictive [kən'strɪktɪv] *adj.* which constricts *konstriktiv, sammandragande, som ger förträngning;* **constrictive pericarditis** = condition where the pericardium becomes thickened and prevents the heart from functioning normally *pericarditis constrictiva, konstriktiv perikardit, pansarhjärta*

constrictor [kən'strɪktə] *subst.* muscle which squeezes an organ *or* which makes an organ contract *konstriktor, sammandragande muskel*

consult [kən'sʌlt] *vb.* to ask someone for his opinion *konsultera, rådfråga;* **he consulted an eye specialist**

consultancy [kən'sʌlt(ə)nsi] *subst.* post of consultant *ung. tjänst som specialistläkare;* **she was appointed to a consultancy with a London hospital**

consultant [kən'sʌlt(ə)nt] *subst.* (i) doctor who is a senior specialist in a particular branch of medicine and who is consulted by a GP *ung. distrikts- el. allmänläkare;* (ii) senior specialized doctor in a hospital *ung. överläkare;* **she was referred to the consultant orthopaedist**

consultation [ˌkɒns(ə)l'teɪʃ(ə)n] *subst.* (i) discussion between two doctors about a case *konsultation;* (ii) meeting with a doctor who examines the patient, discusses his condition with him, and prescribes treatment *konsultation*

consulting room [kən'sʌltɪŋ ruːm] *subst.* room where a doctor sees his patients *mottagningsrum*

consumption [kən'sʌm(p)ʃ(ə)n] *subst.* **(a)** taking food *or* liquid into the body *konsumtion, förtäring, förbrukning;* **the patient's increased consumption of alcohol (b)** former name for pulmonary tuberculosis *lungsot*

consumptive [kən'sʌm(p)tɪv] *adj.* referring to consumption *konsumtions-;*

(patient) suffering from consumption *lungsiktig*

contact ['kɒntækt] **1** *subst.* **(a)** touching someone *or* something *kontakt, beröring;* **to have (physical) contact with someone** *or* **something** = to actually touch someone *or* something *ha (fysisk) kontakt med någon;* **to be in contact with someone** = to be near someone *or* to touch someone *ha (stå i) kontakt med någon;* **the hospital is anxious to trace anyone who may have come into contact with the patient; direct contact** = actually touching an infected person *or* object *direktkontakt;* **indirect contact** = catching a disease by inhaling germs *or* being in contact with a vector *indirekt kontakt;* **contact dermatitis** = inflammation of the skin, caused by touch (as in the case of some types of plant *or* soap, etc.) *kontaktdermatit, kontakteksem* **(b)** person who has been in contact with a person suffering from an infectious disease *person som varit i kontakt med ngn som lider av smittsam sjukdom;* **now that Lassa fever has been diagnosed, the authorities are anxious to trace all contacts which the patient may have met 2** *vb.* to meet *or* to get in touch with (someone) *komma i (stå i, ta) kontakt med*

contact lens ['kɒntækt lenz] *subst.* tiny plastic *or* glass lens which fits over the eyeball (worn instead of spectacles) *kontaktlins*

contagion [kən'teɪdʒ(ə)n] *subst.* spreading of a disease by touching an infected person *or* objects which an infected person has touched *smitta, smittämne;* **the contagion spread through the whole school**

contagious [kən'teɪdʒəs] *adj.* (disease) which can be transmitted by touching an infected person *or* objects which an infected person has touched *kontagiös, smittsam*

contaminant [kən'tæmɪnənt] *subst.* substance which contaminates *smittämne*

contaminate [kən'tæmɪneɪt] *vb.* to make something impure by touching it *or* by adding something to it *kontaminera, smutsa (smitta) ned, förorena;* **supplies of drinking water were contaminated by refuse from the factories; the whole group of tourists fell ill after eating contaminated food**

contamination [kən,tæmɪ'neɪʃ(ə)n] *subst.* action of contaminating *kontamination, nedsmittning, förorening;* **the contamination resulted from drinking polluted water**

content ['kɒntent] *subst.* proportion of a substance in something *innehåll, halt;* **these foods have a high starch content; dried fruit has a higher sugar content than fresh fruit**

continual [kən'tɪnju(ə)l] *adj.* which goes on all the time without stopping *kontinuerlig, ständig, ihållande;* which happens again and again *(ständigt) återkommande;* **he suffered continual recurrence of the disease**

continually [kən'tɪnju(ə)li] *adv.* all the time *kontinuerligt, ständigt, oupphörligt;* **the intestine is continually infected**

continuation [kən,tɪnju'eɪʃ(ə)n] *subst.* part which continues *fortsättning, förlängning;* **the radial artery is a continuation of the brachial artery**

continue [kən'tɪnju:] *vb.* to go on doing something; to do something which was being done before *fortsätta;* **the fever continued for three days; they continued eating as if nothing had happened; the doctor recommended that the treatment should be continued for a further period**

continuous [kən'tɪnjuəs] *adj.* which continues without breaks or stops *kontinuerlig, ständig, ihållande, fortlöpande*

contraception [,kɒntrə'sepʃ(ə)n] *subst.* prevention of pregnancy by using devices (such as a condom *or* an IUD) or drugs (such as the contraceptive pill) or by other means *födelsekontroll, användande av preventivmedel; see also* BIRTH CONTROL

contraceptive [,kɒntrə'septɪv] **1** *adj.* which prevents conception *kontraceptiv, preventiv-;* **a contraceptive device** *or* **contraceptive drug 2** *subst.* drug *or* condom which prevents pregnancy *preventivmedel*

contract [kən'trækt] *vb.* **(a)** *(of muscle)* to become smaller and tighter *kontraheras, dra sig samman;* **as the muscle contracts the limb moves; the diaphragm acts to contract the chest (b) to contract a disease** = to catch a disease *ådra sig;* **he contracted Lassa fever**

contractile tissue [kən,træktaɪ(ə)l 'tɪʃu:] *subst.* tissue in muscle which makes the muscle contract *kontraktil (sammandragande) vävnad*

contraction [kən'trækʃ(ə)n] *subst.* (i) tightening movement which makes a muscle shorter *or* which makes the pupil of the eye smaller *or* which makes the skin wrinkle *kontraktion, sammandragning, hopdragning;* (ii) movement of the muscles of the uterus, marking the beginning of labour *kontraktion, sammandragning, "värk"*

contracture [kən'træktʃə] *subst.* permanent tightening of a muscle caused by fibrosis *kontraktur;* **Dupuytren's contracture**

= condition where the palmar fascia becomes thicker, causing the fingers to bend forwards *Dupuytrens kontraktur;* **Volkmann's contracture** = tightening and fibrosis of the muscles of the forearm because blood supply has been restricted, leading to deformity of the fingers *Volkmanns kontraktur*

contraindication [ˌkɒntrəˌɪndɪ'keɪʃ(ə)n] *subst.* something which suggests that a patient should not be treated with a certain drug *or* not continue to be treated in the same way as at present, because circumstances make that treatment unsuitable *kontraindikation*

contralateral [ˌkɒntrə'læt(ə)r(ə)l] *adj.* affecting the side of the body opposite the one referred to *kontralateral*

contrast medium ['kɒntrɑːst ˌmiːdiəm] *subst.* radio-opaque dye or sometimes gas, put into an organ *or* part of the body so that it will show clearly in an X-ray photograph *kontrast(medel)*

> QUOTE comparing the MRI scan and the CT scan: in the first no contrast medium is required ; in the second iodine-based contrast media are often required
>
> **Nursing 87**

contrecoup ['kɒntrəkuː] *subst.* injury on one side of the brain, caused by a blow received on the opposite side of the head *contre-coup, motstöt*

control [kən'trəʊl] **1** *subst.* power *or* keeping in order *kontroll, styrning;* **the manager has no control over the consultants working in the hospital; the specialists brought the epidemic under control** = they stopped it from spreading *specialisterna fick epidemin under kontroll;* **the epidemic rapidly got out of control** = it spread quickly *epidemin blev snabbt omöjlig att kontrollera; (in experiments)* **control group** = group of people who are not being treated, but whose test data is used as a comparison *kontrollgrupp* **2** *vb.* to keep in order *kontrollera, styra, övervaka;* **the medical authorities are trying to control the epidemic; certain drugs help to control the convulsions; he controls his asthma with a bronchodilator; controlled drugs** *or* **dangerous drugs** = drugs which are on the official list of drugs which are harmful and are not available to the general public *farliga läkemedel som står upptagna på särskild lista (i Storbritannien);* **controlled respiration** = control of a patient's breathing by an anaesthetist during an operation, when normal breathing has stopped *kontrollerad andning (ventilation)*

contused wound [kənˌtjuːzd 'wuːnd] *subst.* wound caused by a blow where the skin is bruised as well as torn and bleeding *vulnus contusum, kontusion(ssår), krossår*

contusion [kən'tjuːʒ(ə)n] *or* **bruise** [bruːz] *subst.* dark painful area on the skin, where blood has escaped into the tissues but not through the skin, following a blow *blåmärke, utgjutning*

conus ['kəʊnəs] *subst.* structure shaped like a cone *conus, kon*

convalesce [ˌkɒnvə'les] *vb.* to get back to good health gradually after an illness *or* operation *tillfriskna, vara på bättringsvägen*

convalescence [ˌkɒnvə'les(ə)ns] *subst.* period of time when a patient is convalescing *konvalescens, tillfrisknande*

convalescent [ˌkɒnvə'les(ə)nt] *adj. & subst.* referring to convalescence *konvalescent(-);* **convalescent patients** *or* **convalescents** = people who are convalescing *konvalescenter;* **convalescent home** = type of hospital where patients can recover from illness *or* surgery *konvalescenthem*

converge [kən'vɜːdʒ] *vb. (of rays)* to come together at a point *konvergera, stråla (löpa) samman*

convergent strabismus [kənˌvɜːdʒ(ə)nt strə'bɪzməs] *or* **squint** [skwɪnt] *subst.* condition where a person's eyes look towards the nose *strabismus convergens (internus), konvergent strabism (skelning), inåtskelning*

conversion [kən'vɜːʃ(ə)n] *subst.* change *konversion, omvandling, förvandling;* **the conversion of nutrients into tissue**

convert [kən'vɜːt] *vb.* to change something into something else *omvandla, förvandla;* **keratinization is the process of converting cells into horny tissue**

convex ['kɒnveks] *adj.* which curves towards the outside *konvex, utåtbuktande;* **a convex lens**

convoluted ['kɒnvəluːtɪd] *adj.* folded and twisted *med många veck (vindlingar);* **convoluted tubules** = coiled parts of a nephron *tubuli renales contorti (oftast förkortat till tubuli)*

convolution [ˌkɒnvə'luːʃ(ə)n] *subst.* twisted shape *veck, vindling, gyrus, hjärnvindling;* **the convolutions of the surface of the cerebrum**

convulsion [kən'vʌlʃ(ə)n] *subst.* fit *or* rapid involuntary contracting and relaxing of the muscles in several parts of the body *konvulsion, kramp(anfall), muskelryckning*
NOTE: often used in the plural: **"the child had convulsions"**

> COMMENT: convulsions in children may be caused by brain disease, such as meningitis, but can often be found at the beginning of a disease (such as pneumonia) which is marked by a sudden rise in body temperature. In adults, convulsions are usually associated with epilepsy

convulsive [kən'vʌlsɪv] *adj.* referring to convulsions *konvulsiv, kramp-;* **he had a convulsive seizure** *see also* ELECTROCONVULSIVE THERAPY

cool [ku:l] **1** *adj.* not very warm *or* quite cold *sval, kylig;* **the patient should be kept cool; keep this bottle in a cool place**
NOTE: **cool - cooler - coolest** **2** *vb.* to become cool *svalna, kylas ned (av)*

Cooleyanemi ⇨ **thalassaemia**

Cooley's anaemia ['ku:liz ə,ni:miə] = THALASSAEMIA

Coombs' test ['ku:mz ,test] *subst.* test for antibodies in red blood cells, used as a test for erythroblastosis foetalis and other haemolytic syndromes *Coombs test*

coordinate [kəʊ'ɔ:dɪneɪt] *vb.* to make things work together *koordinera, samordna, få att samverka;* **he was unable to coordinate the movements of his arms and legs**

> QUOTE there are four recti muscles and two oblique muscles in each eye, which coordinate the movement of the eyes and enable them to work as a pair
> **Nursing Times**

coordination [kəʊ,ɔ:dɪ'neɪʃ(ə)n] *subst.* ability to work together *koordination, samordning, samverkan;* **the patient showed lack of coordination between eyes and hands**

> QUOTE Alzheimer's disease is a progressive disorder which sees a gradual decline in intellectual functioning and deterioration of physical coordination
> **Nursing Times**

cope with ['kəʊp wɪð] *vb.* to deal with *or* to manage *klara (av);* **a hospital administrator has to cope with a lot of forms; he walks with crutches and has difficulty in coping with the stairs**

copper ['kɒpə] *subst.* metallic trace element *koppar, Cu*
NOTE: the chemical symbol is **Cu**

coprolith ['kɒprəlɪθ] *subst.* hard faeces in the bowel *koprolit, sterkolit, fekalit, fekalsten*

coproporphyrin [,kɒprə'pɔ:f(ə)rɪn] *subst.* porphyrin excreted by the liver *koprofyrin*

copulate ['kɒpjʊleɪt] *vb.* to have sexual intercourse *kopulera, ha samlag*

copulation [,kɒpjʊ'leɪʃ(ə)n] *subst.* coitus *or* sexual intercourse *coitus, kopulation, samlag*

cor [kɔ:] *subst.* the heart *cor, hjärtat;* **cor pulmonale** = pulmonary heart disease where the right ventricle is enlarged *cor pulmonale*

coraco-acromial [,kɒrəkəʊə'krəʊmiəl] *adj.* referring to the coracoid process and the acromion *coraco-acromialis, som avser el. hör till både det korpnäbblika utskottet från skulderbladet och akromion (skulderhöjden)*

coraco-acromialis ⇨ **coraco-acromial**

coracobrachialis [,kɒrəkəʊ,bræki'eɪlɪs] *subst.* muscle on the medial side of the upper arm, below the armpit *musculus coracobrachialis*

coracoid process ['kɒrəkɔɪd ,prəʊses] *subst.* projecting part on the shoulder blade *processus coracoideus, korpnäbbsutskottet*

cord [kɔ:d] *subst.* long flexible structure in the body like a thread *korda, sträng, band;* **spermatic cord** = cord formed of the vas deferens, the blood vessels, nerves and lymphatics of the testis, running from the testis to the abdomen *funiculus spermaticus, sädessträngen (som innehåller sädesledaren);* **spinal cord** = part of the central nervous system, running from the medulla oblongata to the filum terminale, in the vertebral canal of the spine *medulla spinalis, ryggmärgen;* **umbilical cord** = cord containing two arteries and one vein which links the fetus inside the womb to the placenta *chorda (funiculus) umbilicalis, navelsträngen;* **vocal cords** = cords in the larynx by which sounds are made as air is forced between them *chordae (plicae) vocales, stämbanden*

cordectomy [kɔ:'dektəmi] *subst.* surgical removal of a vocal cord *operativt avlägsnande av stämband*

cordotomy [kɔːˈdɒtəmi] = CHORDOTOMY

core [kɔː] *subst.* central part *kärna, det innersta (centrala)*

corectopia [ˌkɔːrekˈtəʊpiə] *subst.* ectopia of the pupil *korektopi*

corium [ˈkɔːriəm] *or* **dermis** [ˈdɜːmɪs] *subst.* layer of living tissue beneath the epidermis *corium, korium, dermis, läderhuden*

corn [kɔːn] *or* **heloma** [heˈləʊmə] *subst.* hard painful lump of skin usually on the foot or hand, where something (such as tight shoe) has rubbed or pressed on the skin *helom, liktorn*

cornea [ˈkɔːniə] *subst.* transparent part of the front of the eyeball *cornea, hornhinnan*
NOTE: the plural is **corneae**

corneal [ˈkɔːniəl] *adj.* referring to a cornea *corneal-, korneal-, hornhinne-;* **corneal tissue from donors is used in grafting to replace a damaged cornea; corneal abrasion** = scratch on the cornea, caused by something sharp getting into the eye *abrasio cornae, skrapsår på hornhinnan;* **corneal bank** = place where eyes of dead donors can be kept ready for use in corneal grafts *ögonbank*

corneal graft [ˈkɔːniəl ˌgrɑːft] *or* **keratoplasty** [ˈkerətəʊˌplæsti] *subst.* corneal tissue from a donor *or* dead body, grafted in place of diseased tissue *cornealtransplantat, kornealtransplantat, hornhinnetransplantat*
NOTE: for terms referring to the cornea, see words beginning with **kerat-**

cornealtransplantat ⇨ **corneal graft**

corneum [ˈkɔːniəm] *see* STRATUM

cornification [ˌkɔːnɪfɪˈkeɪʃ(ə)n] *or* **keratinization** [ˌkerətɪnaɪˈzeɪʃ(ə)n] *subst.* process of converting cells into horny tissue *kornifikation, keratinisering, förhorning*

cornu [ˈkɔːnjuː] *subst.* structure in the body which is shaped like a horn *cornu, horn;* **cornua of the thyroid** = four processes of the thyroid cartilage *cornua thyreoidea, sköldbroskhornen*
NOTE: the plural is **cornua**

corona [kəˈrəʊnə] *subst.* structure in the body which is shaped like a crown *corona, kronliknande anatomisk bildning;* **corona capitis** = the crown of the head *or* the top part of the skull *corona capitis, hjässan*

coronal [ˈkɒr(ə)n(ə)l] *adj.* (i) referring to a corona *som avser el. hör till kronliknande anatomisk bildning;* (ii) referring to the crown of a tooth *som avser el. hör till tandkrona;* **coronal plane** = plane at right angles to the median plane, dividing the body into dorsal and ventral halves *frontalplan, tänkt plan genom kroppen vinkelrätt mot medianplanet;* **coronal suture** = horizontal joint across the top of the skull between the parietal and frontal bones ⇨ *illustration* SKULL *sutura coronalis, hjässömmen, kronsömmen*

coronary [ˈkɒr(ə)n(ə)ri] **1** *subst.* *(non-medical term)* coronary thrombosis *or* blood clot in the coronary arteries which leads to a heart attack *"hjärtinfarkt", "hjärtattack";* **he had a coronary and was rushed to hospital 2** *adj.* referring to any structure shaped like a crown, but especially to the arteries which supply blood to the heart muscles *krans-, koronar-, koronarkärls-;* **coronary arteries** = arteries which supply blood to the heart muscles *arteria coronaria dexter resp. sinistra, hjärtats kransartärer, kranskärlen, koronarkärlen;* **coronary bypass graft** *or* **surgery** = surgical operation to treat angina, by grafting a vein to replace a diseased section of a coronary artery *bypassoperation i hjärtats kranskärl;* **coronary circulation** = blood circulation through the arteries and veins of the heart muscles *koronarkärlscirkulationen;* **coronary heart disease (CHD)** = any disease affecting the coronary arteries, which can lead to strain on the heart *or* a heart attack *coronary heart disease, CHD, koronarkärlssjukdom;* **coronary ligament** = folds of peritoneum connecting the back of the liver to the diaphragm *ligamentum coronarium hepatis, bukhinneveck som förbinder leverns baksida med diafragma;* **coronary obstruction** *or* **coronary occlusion** = thickening of the walls of the coronary arteries *or* blood clot in the coronary arteries, which prevents blood reaching the heart muscles and leads to heart failure *koronarkärlsocklusion;* **coronary sinus** = vein which takes most of the venous blood from the heart muscles to the right atrium *sinus coronarius;* **coronary thrombosis** = blood clot which blocks the coronary arteries, leading to a heart attack *koronarkärlstrombos*

> QUOTE coronary heart disease (CHD) patients spend an average of 11.9 days in hospital. Among primary health care services, 1.5% of all GP consultations are due to CHD
> **Health Services Journal**

> QUOTE apart from death, CHD causes considerable morbidity in the form of heart attack, angina and a number of related diseases
> **Health Education Journal**

coronavirus [kəˈrəʊnəˌvaɪ(ə)rəs] *subst.*

virus which causes the common cold *Coronavirus*

coronet ['kɒr(ə)nə] *subst.* public official (either a doctor or a lawyer) who investigates sudden *or* violent deaths *coroner;* **coroner's court** = court where a coroner is the chairman *domstol med coroner som ordförande;* **coroner's inquest** = inquest carried out by a coroner into a death *förhör om dödsorsak*

> COMMENT: coroners investigate deaths which are violent or not expected, deaths which may be murder *or* manslaughter, deaths of prisoners and deaths involving the police

coronoid process ['kɒrənɔɪd ˌprəʊses] *subst.* (i) projecting piece of bone on the ulna *processus coronoideus, utskott på armbågsbenet;* (ii) projecting piece on each of the lower jaw *processus coronoideus, utskott på underkäken*

corpse [kɔːps] *subst.* body of a dead person *lik*

corpus ['kɔːpəs] *subst.* any mass of tissue *corpus, kropp;* **corpus albicans** = scar tissue which replaces the corpus luteum in the ovary *corpus albicans;* **corpus callosum** = tissue which connects the two cerebral hemispheres ➪ *illustration* BRAIN *corpus callosum, hjärnbalken;* **corpus cavernosum** = part of the erectile tissue in the penis and clitoris ➪ *illustration* UROGENITAL SYSTEM (MALE) *corpus cavernosum;* **corpus haemorrhagicum** = blood clot formed in the ovary where a Graafian follicle has ruptured *corpus haemorrhagicum;* **corpus luteum** = body which forms in the ovary after a Graafian follicle has ruptured (the corpora lutea secrete the hormone progesterone to prepare the uterus for implantation of the fertilized ovum) *corpus luteum, gulkropp;* **corpus spongiosum** = part of the penis round the urethra, forming the glans *corpus spongiosum, svällkropp;* **corpus striatum** = part of a cerebral hemisphere *corpus striatum* NOTE: the plural is **corpora**

corpuscle ['kɔːpʌs(ə)l] *subst.* any small round mass *korpuskel, blodkropp;* **red corpuscle** *or* **erythrocyte** = red blood cell which contains haemoglobin and carries oxygen to the tissues and takes carbon dioxide from them *erytrocyt, röd blodkropp;* **white corpuscle** *or* **leucocyte** = white blood cell *or* colourless cell which contains a nucleus but has no haemoglobin *leukocyt, vit blodkropp;* **Krause corpuscles** = encapsulated nerve endings in mucous membrane of mouth, nose, eyes and genitals *inkapslade nervändslut i slemhinnor;* **Meissner's corpuscle** = sensory nerve ending in the skin which is sensitive to touch *corpuscula tactus, Meissners kropp, känselkropp;* **Pacinian corpuscle** = sensory nerve ending in the skin which is sensitive to touch and vibrations ➪ *illustration* SKIN & SENSORY RECEPTORS *Pacinis (känsel)kropp, Vater-Pacinis (känsel)kropp, tryckreceptor;* **renal corpuscle** *or* **Malpighian corpuscle** *or* **Malpighian body** = part of a nephron in the cortex of a kidney *corpusculum renis, Malpighis kropp, njurkropp;* **Ruffini corpuscles** *or* **Ruffini nerve endings** = branching nerve endings in the skin, which are thought to be sensitive to heat ➪ *illustration* SKIN & SENSORY RECEPTORS *nervändslut i huden (som antas känsliga för värme)*

correct [kə'rekt] *vb.* to put faults right *or* to make something work properly *korrigera, rätta till, justera;* **she wears a brace to correct the growth of her teeth; doctors are trying to correct his speech defect**

correction [kə'rekʃ(ə)n] *subst.* showing the mistake in something *påpekande av fel;* making something correct *korrigering, justering, rättelse*

corrective [kə'rektɪv] *subst.* drug which changes the harmful effect of another drug *botemedel*

Corrigan's pulse ['kɒrɪg(ə)nz ˌpʌls] *subst.* type of pulse, where there is a visible rise in pressure followed by a sudden collapse, of the arterial pulse in the neck, caused by aortic regurgitation *pulsus celer et magnus (altus), Corrigans puls (vid hjärtklaffel)*

corrosive [kə'rəʊsɪv] *adj. & subst.* (substance, such as acid *or* alkali) which destroys tissue *frätande (ämne)*

corrugator muscle ['kɒrəgeɪtə ˌmʌs(ə)l] *subst.* muscle which produces vertical wrinkles on the forehead when frowning *musculus corrugator supercilii, ögonbrynsrynkaren*

corset ['kɔːsɪt] *subst.* piece of stiff clothing, worn on the chest *or* over the trunk to support the body as after a back injury *korsett*

cortex ['kɔːteks] *subst.* outer layer of an organ, as opposed to the soft inner medulla *cortex, bark;* **adrenal cortex** = firm outside layer of the adrenal *or* suprarenal glands, which secretes various hormones, including cortisone *cortex suprarenis, binjurebarken;* **cerebellar cortex** = outer covering of grey matter which covers the cerebellum *cortex cerebelli, lillhjärnsbarken;* **cerebral cortex** = outer covering of grey matter which covers the cerebrum *cortex cerebri, hjärnbarken,*

storhjärnsbarken; **olfactory cortex** *or* **visual cortex** = parts of the cerebral cortex which receive information about smell *or* sight *luktcentrum, syncentrum;* **renal cortex** = outer covering of a kidney, immediately beneath the capsule, containing glomeruli ⇨ *illustration* KIDNEY *cortex renis, njurbarken;* **sensory cortex** = area of the cerebral cortex which receives information from nerves in all parts of the body *sensoriska (hjärn)barken*
NOTE: plural is **cortices**

Corti ['kɔːti] *see* ORGAN

cortical ['kɔːtɪk(ə)l] *adj.* referring to a cortex *kortikal;* **(suprarenal) cortical hormones** = hormones (such as cortisone) secreted by the cortex of the adrenal glands *kortikosteroider, binjurebarkhormoner;* **sub-cortical** = beneath the cortex *subkortikal*

corticospinal [ˌkɔːtɪkəʊ'spaɪn(ə)l] *adj.* referring to both the cerebral cortex and the spinal cord *kortikospinal*

corticosteroid [ˌkɔːtɪkəʊ'stɪərɔɪd] *subst.* any steroid hormone produced by the cortex of the adrenal glands *kortikosteroid, binjurebarkhormon*

corticosterone [ˌkɔːtɪkəʊ'stɪərəʊn] *subst.* hormone secreted by the cortex of the adrenal glands *kortikosteron*

corticotrophin [ˌkɔːtɪkəʊ'trəʊfɪn] *or* **adrenocorticotrophic hormone (ACTH)** [əˌdriːnəʊˌkɔːtɪkəʊ'trɒfɪk ˌhɔːməʊn (ˌeɪsiːtiː'eɪtʃ)] *subst.* hormone produced by the anterior pituitary gland, which causes the cortex of the adrenal glands to release corticosteroids *kortikotropin, adrenokortikotropt hormon, ACTH*

cortisol ['kɔːtɪsɒl] *or* **hydrocortisone** [ˌhaɪdrə(ʊ)'kɔːtɪzəʊn] *subst.* steroid hormone produced by the cortex of the adrenal glands *kortisol, hydrokortison*

COMMENT: cortisol is used by the body to maintain blood pressure, connective tissue and break down carbohydrates. It also reduces the body's immune response to infection. Synthetic cortisone is used in the treatment of arthritis, asthma and skin disorders, but can have powerful side-effects on some patients

cortisone ['kɔːtɪzəʊn] *subst.* hormone secreted in small quantities by the adrenal cortex *kortison*

Corynebacterium [kəʊˌraɪnibæk'tɪəriəm] *subst.* genus of bacteria which includes the bacterium which causes diphtheria *Corynebacterium*

coryza [kə'raɪzə] *subst.* nasal catarrh *or* common cold *or* running nose with inflammation of the nasal passages *coryza, förkylning, snuva*

cosmetic surgery [kɒzˌmetɪk 'sɜːdʒ(ə)ri] *subst.* surgical operation carried out to improve the appearance of the patient *kosmetisk operation*

COMMENT: where plastic surgery may be prescribed by a doctor to correct skin *or* bone defects *or* the effect of burns *or* after a disfiguring operation, cosmetic surgery is carried out on the instructions of the patient to remove wrinkles, enlarge breasts, etc.

cost- ['kɒst, ˌ-] *prefix* referring to the ribs *cost(o)-, kost(o)-, revbens-*

costal ['kɒst(ə)l] *adj.* referring to the ribs *kostal, revbens-;* **costal cartilage** = cartilage which forms the end of each rib, and either joins the rib to the breastbone or to the rib above *revbensbrosk;* **costal pleura** = part of the pleura lining the walls of the chest *pleura costalis (parietalis), lungsäckens yttre blad*

costive ['kɒstɪv] **1** *adj.* constipated *or* suffering from difficulty in passing bowel movements *obstiperad, förstoppad* **2** *subst.* drug which causes constipation *obstiperande (förstoppande) medel*

costocervical trunk [ˌkɒstəʊ'sɜːvɪk(ə)l ˌtrʌŋk] *subst.* large artery in the chest *truncus costocervicalis*

costodiaphragmatic [ˌkɒstəʊˌdaɪəfræg'mætɪk] *adj.* referring to the ribs and the diaphragm *som avser el. hör till både revben och diafragma*

costovertebral joints [ˌkɒstəʊ'vɜːtɪbr(ə)l ˌdʒɔɪnts] *subst.* joints between the ribs and the vertebral column *articulationes costovertibrales*

cot death ['kɒt deθ] *or US* **crib death** ['krib deθ] *subst.* sudden infant death syndrome (SIDS) *or* sudden death of a baby in bed *plötslig spädbarnsdöd*

COMMENT: occurs in very young children, up to the age of about 12 months; the cause is still being investigated

co-trimoxazole [ˌkəʊtraɪ'mɒksəzəʊl] *subst.* drug used to combat bacteria in the urinary tract *slags läkemedel (sulfapreparat) mot urinvägsinfektion*

cottage hospital [ˌkɒtɪdʒ 'hɒspɪt(ə)l] *subst.* small local hospital set in pleasant gardens in the country *slags litet sjukhus i lantlig miljö, sjukstuga*

cotton ['kɒt(ə)n] *subst.* fibres from a tropical plant *bomull;* cloth made from cotton thread *bomull(styg);* **she wore a cotton shirt**

cotton wool [ˌkɒt(ə)n 'wʊl] *or* **absorbent cotton** [əbˌsɔːb(ə)nt 'kɒt(ə)n] *subst.* purified fibres from the cotton plant used as a dressing on wounds, etc. *kompress;* **she dabbed the cut with cotton wool soaked in antiseptic; the nurse put a pad of cotton wool over the sore**
NOTE: no plural

cotyledon [ˌkɒtɪ'liːd(ə)n] *subst.* one of the divisions of a placenta *kotyledon*

cotyloid cavity ['kɒtɪlɔɪd ˌkævəti] *or* **acetabulum** [ˌæsɪ'tæbjʊləm] *subst.* part of the pelvic bone, shaped like a cup, into which the head of the femur fits to form the hip joint *acetabulum, höftledspannan*

couch [kaʊtʃ] *subst.* long bed on which a patient lies when being examined by a doctor in a surgery *brits*

couching ['kaʊtʃɪŋ] *subst.* in treatment of cataract, surgical operation to displace the opaque lens of an eye *slags operativ behandling av starr*

cough [kɒf] **1** *subst.* reflex action, caused by irritation in the throat, when the glottis is opened and air is sent out of the lungs suddenly *hosta;* **he gave a little cough to attract the nurse's attention; she has a bad cough and cannot make the speech; cough medicine** *or* **cough linctus** = liquid taken to soothe the irritation which causes a cough *hostmedicin* **2** *vb.* to send air out of the lungs suddenly because the throat is irritated *hosta;* **the smoke made him cough; he has a cold and keeps on coughing and sneezing; coughing fit** = sudden attack of coughing *hostattack, hostanfall*

cough up [ˌkɒf 'ʌp] *vb.* to cough hard to produce a substance from the trachea *hosta upp;* **he coughed up phlegm; she became worried when the girl started coughing up blood**

council ['kaʊns(ə)l, -sɪl] *subst.* group of people elected to manage something *styrelse;* **town council** = elected committee which manages a town *kommunfullmäktige, stadsfullmäktige;* **General Medical Council** = body which registers all practising doctors (without such registration, a doctor cannot practise) *myndighet som registrerar och övervakar läkare i Storbritannien (motsvarande Socialstyrelsen)*

counselling ['kaʊns(ə)lɪŋ] *subst.* method of treating especially psychiatric disorders, where a specialist advises and talks with a patient about his condition and how to deal with it *rådgivning*

counsellor ['kaʊns(ə)lə] *subst.* person who advises and talks with someone about his problems *rådgivare*

count [kaʊnt] **1** *vb.* **(a)** to say numbers in order *räkna;* **the little girl can count up to ten; hold your breath and count to twenty to try to stop a hiccup (b)** to add up to see how many things there are *räkna;* **count the number of tablets left in the bottle (c)** to include *inberäkna, räkna med;* **there were thirty people in the ward if you count the visitors 2** *subst.* act of adding things to see how many there are *(samman)räkning;* **blood count** = test to count the number and types of different blood cells in a certain tiny sample of blood, to give an indication of the condition of the patient's blood as a whole *blodkroppsräkning, blodstatus*

> QUOTE the normal platelet count during pregnancy is described as 150,000 to 400,000 cu mm
> **Southern Medical Journal**

counteract [ˌkaʊntə'rækt] *vb.* to act against something *or* to reduce the effect of something *motverka, neutralisera, förta (verkningarna av något);* **the lotion should counteract the irritant effect of the spray on the skin**

counteraction [ˌkaʊntər'ækʃ(ə)n] *subst. (in pharmacy)* action of one drug which acts against another drug *motverkan, neutralisering*

counterextension [ˌkaʊntərɪk'stenʃ(ə)n] *subst.* orthopaedic treatment, where the upper part of a limb is kept fixed and traction is applied to the lower part of it *slags traktionsbehandling*

counterirritant [ˌkaʊntər'ɪrɪt(ə)nt] *subst.* substance which alleviates the pain in an internal organ, by irritating an area of skin whose sensory nerves are close to those of the organ in the spinal cord *ämne som ger upphov till ytlig irritation, vilken verkar smärtlindrande*

counterirritation [ˌkaʊntərˌɪrɪ'teɪʃ(ə)n] *subst.* skin irritation, applied artificially to alleviate the pain in another part of the body *slags irritation (för smärtminskning)*

counterstain ['kaʊntəsteɪn] **1** *subst.* stain used to identify tissue samples, such as red dye used to identify Gram-negative bacteria *avfärgning* **2** *vb.* to stain specimens with a counterstain, as bacteria with a red stain after having first stained them with violet dye *avfärga; see also* GRAM

course [kɔːs] *subst.* **(a)** passing of time *förlopp, gång;* **his condition has deteriorated in the course of the last few weeks (b)** series of lessons *kurs, studiegång;* series of drugs to be taken *or* of sessions of treatment *serie, följd, kur;* **I'm taking a course in physiotherapy; she's taking a hospital administration course; course of treatment** = series of applications of a treatment (such as a series of injections *or* physiotherapy) *behandlingskur;* **to put someone on a course of drugs** *or* **injections** = to decide that a patient should take a drug *or* should have a number of injections regularly over a certain period of time *sätta ngn på en viss behandling*

court [kɔːt] *subst.* place where a trial is heard *or* where a legal judgement is reached *domstol;* **court order** = order made by a court telling someone to do *or* not to do something *domstolsbeslut;* **he was sent to a mental institution by court order**

cover ['kʌvə] **1** *subst.* **(a)** thing put over something to keep it clean, etc. *lock, skydd;* **keep a cover on the petri dish; cover test** = test for a squint, where an eye is covered and its movements are checked when the cover is taken off *täckprov, test på skelning* **(b)** doing work for someone who is absent *arbete som utförs av ersättare (vikarie, avlösare);* **out-of-hours cover is provided by the other GPs in the practice 2** *vb.* **(a)** to put something over something to keep it clean, etc. *täcka (över), skydda, hölja;* **you should cover the table with a plastic sheet before you start to mix the mouthwash; the fetus is covered with a membrane (b)** to be available to work in place of someone who is absent *ersätta, vikariera (för);* **the other GPs will cover for him while he is on holiday**

covering ['kʌv(ə)rɪŋ] *subst.* layer which covers *or* protects something *skydd, hölje;* **brain covering** = the meninges *meninges, meningerna, hjärnhinnorna*

Cowper's glands ['kuːpəz ˌglændz] *or* **bulbourethral glands** [ˌbʌlbəʊjʊə'riːər(ə)l ˌglændz] *subst.* two glands at the base of the penis which secrete into the urethra *glandulae bulbourethrales, Cowpers körtlar*

cowpox ['kaʊpɒks] *or* **vaccinia** [væk'sɪniə] *subst.* infectious viral disease of cattle *vaccinia, kokoppor*

> COMMENT: the virus can be transmitted to man, and is used as a constituent of the vaccine for smallpox

coxa ['kɒksə] *subst.* the hip joint *coxa, höften*

coxalgia [kɒk'sældʒə] *subst.* pain in the hip joint *koxalgi, höftsmärtor*

coxa plana ⇨ **Legg-Calvé-Perthes disease**

Coxsackie virus [kɒk'sæki ˌvaɪ(ə)rəs] *subst.* one of a group of enteroviruses which enter the cells of the intestines but can cause diseases such as aseptic meningitis and Bornholm disease *Coxsackievirus*

cox vara ⇨ **varus**

CP ⇨ **athetosis, cerebral palsy, paralysis**

CPR [ˌsiːpiː'ɑː] = CARDIOPULMONARY RESUSCITATION

crab (louse) ['kræb (ˌlaʊs)] *or* **pubic louse** ['pjuːbɪk ˌlaʊs] *subst.* louse **Phthirius pubis** which infests the pubic region and other parts of the body with coarse hair *Phthirius (Pediculus) pubis, flatlus*

crack [kræk] **1** *subst.* thin break *spricka;* **there's a crack in one of the bones in the skull 2** *vb.* to make a thin break in something *spräcka;* to split *spricka, ha sönder;* **she cracked a bone in her leg; cracked lips** = lips where the skin has split because of cold *or* dryness *spruckna läppar, nariga läppar*

cradle ['kreɪd(ə)l] *subst.* **(a)** metal frame put over a patient in bed to keep the weight of the bedclothes off the body *filtstöd* **(b)** carrying an injured child by holding him with one arm under the thigh and the other above the waist *slags grepp för att bära skadat barn;* **cradle cap** = yellow deposit on the scalp of babies, caused by seborrhoea *skorv*

cramp [kræmp] *subst.* painful involuntary spasm in the muscles, where the muscle may stay contracted for some time *kramp;* **he went swimming and got cramp in the cold water; menstrual cramps** = cramp in the muscles around the uterus during menstruation *kramp (smärta) vid menstruation;* **stomach cramp** = sharp spasm of the stomach muscles *kramp i magen;* **swimmer's cramp** = spasms in arteries and muscles caused by cold water, or swimming soon after a meal *kramp vid simning;* **writer's cramp** = spasms and pain in the muscles of the wrist and hand, caused by holding a pen for long periods *skrivkramp*

crani- ['kreɪni, ˌ--] *or* **cranio-** ['kreɪniəʊ, ˌ--] *prefix* referring to the skull *crani(o)-, krani(o)-, skall-*

cranial ['kreɪniəl] *adj.* referring to the skull *kranial(-), skall-;* **cranial bone** = one of the bones in the skull *skallben;* **cranial cavity** = space formed by the cranium, inside which the brain is situated *hjärnskålen;* **cranial nerve** = one of the nerves, twelve on each side, which are connected directly to the brain, governing mainly the structures of the head and neck *nervi craniales, kranialnerverna; see* NERVE

craniometry [ˌkreɪnɪ'ɒmetri] *subst.* measuring skulls to find differences in size and shape *kraniometri*

craniopharyngioma [ˌkreɪniəʊfəˌrɪndʒɪ'əʊmə] *subst.* tumour in the brain originating in hypophyseal duct *kraniofaryngiom*

craniostenosis [ˌkreɪniəʊste'nəʊsɪs] *or* **craniosynostosis** [ˌkreɪniəʊsɪnəʊ'stəʊsɪs] *subst.* early closing of the bones in a baby's skull, so making the skull contract *kraniostenos, kraniosynostos*

craniotabes [ˌkreɪniəʊ'teɪbi:z] *subst.* thinness of the bones in the occipital region of a child's skull, caused by rickets, marasmus or syphilis *kraniotabes*

craniotomy [ˌkreɪni'ɒtəmi] *subst.* any surgical operation on the skull, especially cutting away part of the skull *kraniotomi*

cranium ['kreɪniəm] *or* **skull** [skʌl] *subst.* the group of eight bones which surround the brain *cranium, kraniet, skallen*

> COMMENT: the cranium consists of the occipital bone, two parietal bones, two temporal bones and the frontal, ethmoid and sphenoid bones. See also SUTURE

cranky ['kræŋki] *adj. US (informal)* bad-tempered *or* difficult (child) *lynnig, "jobbig"*

crash [kræʃ] **1** *subst.* accident where cars, planes, etc. are damaged *krock, olycka, störtning;* **he was killed in a car crash; none of the passengers was hurt in the crash; crash helmet** = hard hat worn by motorcyclists, etc. *störthjälm* **2** *vb. (of vehicles)* to hit something and be damaged *krocka, krascha, störta;* **the car crashed into the wall; the plane crashed** = the plane hit the ground and was damaged *planet störtade* **3** *adj.* rapid *intensiv, snabb-;* **she took a crash course in physiotherapy** = a course to learn physiotherapy very quickly *hon tog en snabbkurs i sjukgymnastik*

cream [kri:m] *subst.* medicinal oily substance, used to rub on the skin *kräm, salva;* **cold cream** = mixture of almond oil and borax *slags hudkräm*

create [kri'eɪt] *vb.* to make *skapa, åstadkomma*

creatinase ['kri:əti:neɪz] *subst.* enzyme which helps break down creatine into creatinine *kreatinas*

creatine ['kri:əti:n] *subst.* compound of nitrogen found in the muscles and produced by protein metabolism, and excreted as creatinine *kreatin;* **creatine phosphate** = store of energy-giving phosphate in muscles *kreatinfosfat*

creatinine [kri'ætəni:n] *subst.* substance which is the form in which creatine is excreted *kreatinin*

creatinuria [krɪəˌætɪ'njʊəriə] *subst.* excess creatine in the urine *överskottskreatin i urinen*

creatorrhoea [ˌkrɪətə'ri:ə] *subst.* presence of undigested muscle fibre in the faeces, occurring in some pancreatic diseases *kreatorré*

Credé's method [kreɪ'deɪz ˌmeθəd] *subst.* **(a)** method of extracting a placenta, by massaging the uterus through the abdomen *Credés metod (handgrepp)* **(b)** putting silver nitrate solution into the eyes of a baby born to a mother suffering from gonorrhoea, in order to prevent gonococcal conjunctivitis *Credés profylax, Credéprofylax*

creeping eruption [ˌkri:pɪŋ ɪ'rʌpʃ(ə)n] *subst.* itching skin complaint, caused by larvae of various parasites which creep under the skin *slags utslag orsakat av parasitlarver (i tropikerna)*

crepitation [ˌkrepɪ'teɪʃ(ə)n] *or* **rale** [rɑ:l] *subst.* abnormal soft crackling sound heard in the lungs through a stethoscope *krepitation, rassel*

crepitus ['krepɪtəs] *subst.* (i) harsh crackling sound heard through a stethoscope in a patient with inflammation of the lungs *krepitation;* (ii) scratching sound made by a broken bone *or* rough joint *knastrande (skrapande) ljud vid benbrott*

crest [krest] *subst.* long raised part on a bone *crista, kam;* **crest of ilium** *or* **iliac crest** = curved top edge of the ilium *crista iliaca, höftbenskammen*

cretin ['kretɪn] *subst.* patient suffering from congenital hypothyroidism *kretin*

cretinism ['kretɪnɪz(ə)m] *subst.* condition of being a cretin *kretinism*

COMMENT: the condition is due to a defective thyroid gland and affected children, if not treated, develop more slowly than normal, are mentally retarded and have coarse facial features

crib death ['krɪb deθ] *subst. US* = COT DEATH

cribriform plate ['krɪbrɪfɔːm ˌpleɪt] *subst.* top part of the ethmoid bone which forms the roof of the nasal cavity, and part of the roof of the eye sockets *lamina cribrosa, silbensplattan*

cricoid cartilage ['kraɪkɔɪd ˌkɑːt(ə)lɪdʒ] *subst.* ring-shaped cartilage in the lower part of the larynx ⇨ *illustration* LUNGS *cartilago cricoidea, ringbrosket*

cripple ['krɪp(ə)l] **1** *vb.* to make someone physically handicapped *handikappa, lemlästa;* **she was crippled by arthritis; he was crippled in a car crash 2** *subst.* person who is physically disabled *handikappad, krympling;* **cardiac cripple** = person who has a cardiac disease which makes him unable to work normally *hjärtsjuk person*

crippling ['krɪplɪŋ] *adj.* (disease) which makes someone physically handicapped *handikappande;* **arthritis is a crippling disease**

crisis ['kraɪsɪs] *subst.* **(a)** turning point in a disease, after which the patient may start to become better or very much worse *kris, vändpunkt* **(b)** important point *or* time *krisläge;* **mid-life crisis** = MENOPAUSE
NOTE: plural is **crises**

COMMENT: many diseases progress to a crisis and then the patient rapidly gets better; the opposite situation where the patient gets better very slowly is called lysis

crista ['krɪstə] *subst.* crest *crista, kam;* **crista galli** = projection from the ethmoid bone *crista galli, tuppkammen*

critical ['krɪtɪk(ə)l] *adj.* **(a)** referring to crisis *kris-* **(b)** extremely serious *kritisk, krisartad, mycket allvarlig;* **he was taken to hospital in a critical condition; the hospital spokesman said that three of the accident victims were still on the critical list (c)** which criticizes *kritisk, kritiserande;* **the report was critical of the state of aftercare provision**

critically ['krɪtɪk(ə)li] *adv.* in a way which criticizes *kritiskt, mycket allvarligt;* **critically ill** = very seriously ill, where it is not known if the patient will get better *mycket allvarligt sjuk*

criticize ['krɪtɪsaɪz] *vb.* to say what is wrong with something *kritisera, anmärka på;* **the report criticized the state of the hospital kitchens**

CRNA [ˌsiːɑːen'eɪ] = CERTIFIED REGISTERED NURSE ANAESTHETIST

Crohn's disease ['krəʊnz dɪˌziːz] *or* **regional enteritis** [ˌriːdʒ(ə)n(ə)l ˌentə'raɪtɪs] *or* **regional ileitis** [ˌriːdʒ(ə)n(ə)l ˌɪli'aɪtɪs] *see* ILEITIS

cross [krɒs] *subst.* **(a)** shape made with an upright line with another going across it, used as a sign of the Christian church *kors(tecken); (in anatomy)* any cross-shaped structure *korsliknande anatomisk struktur;* **the Red Cross** = international organization which provides emergency medical help *Röda korset* **(b)** mixture of two different breeds *korsning*

cross eye ['krɒs aɪ] *or* **convergent strabismus** [kənˌvɜːdʒ(ə)nt strə'bɪzməs] *subst.* condition where a person's eyes both look towards the nose *strabismus convergens (internus), konvergent strabism (skelning), inåtskelning*

cross-eyed [ˌkrɒs'aɪd] *adj.* strabismal *or* with eyes looking towards the nose *strabistisk, vindögd*

cross-infection [ˌkrɒsɪn'fekʃ(ə)n] *subst.* infection passed from one patient to another in hospital, either directly or from nurses, visitors or equipment *direkt el. indirekt smitta mellan patienter (t.ex. på sjukhus)*

cross match [ˌkrɒs 'mætʃ] *vb. (in transplant surgery)* matching a donor to a recipient as closely as possible to avoid tissue rejection *korstestning, matchning för att förhindra avstötning; see* BLOOD GROUP

cross-section ['krɒsˌsekʃ(ə)n] *subst.* **(a)** sample cut across a specimen for examination under a microscope *tvärsnitt;* **he examined a cross-section of the lung tissue (b)** small part of something, taken to be representative of the whole *tvärsnitt, representativt urval;* **the team consulted a cross-section of hospital ancillary staff**

crotamiton [ˌkrəʊtəˈmaɪtən] *subst.* drug used to treat scabies *or* pruritus *slags läkemedel mot skabb och hudklåda*

crotch [krɒtʃ] *subst.* point where the legs meet the body, where the genitals are *skrevet, grenen*

croup [kru:p] *subst.* children's disease, acute infection of the upper respiratory passages which blocks the larynx *krupp, äkta strypsjuka, difteri*

COMMENT: the patient's larynx swells, and he breathes with difficulty and has a barking cough. Attacks usually occur at night. They can be fatal if the larynx becomes completely blocked

crown [kraʊn] *subst.* (i) top part of a tooth (above the level of the gums); (i) top part of a tooth (above the level of the gums) ⇨ *illustration* TOOTH *krona, tandkrona;* (ii) artificial top attached to a tooth *konstgjord tandkrona;* (iii) top part of the head *hjässan*

crowning [ˈkraʊnɪŋ] *subst.* (i) putting an artificial crown on a tooth *insättning av tandkrona;* (ii) stage in childbirth, where the top of the baby's head becomes visible *det stadium under förlossningen då barnets huvud blir synligt*

cruciate ligament [ˈkru:ʃiət ˌlɪgəmənt] *subst.* any ligament shaped like a cross, especially the ligaments behind the knee, which prevent the knee from bending forwards *ligamentum cruciatum, korsband*

crural [ˈkrʊər(ə)l] *adj.* referring to the thigh, leg or shin *krural*

crus [krʌs] *subst.* long projecting part *crus, skänkel;* **crus cerebri** = one of the nerve tracts between the cerebrum and the medulla oblongata **crura cerebri** *crura cerebri, del av hjärnskänklarna (hjärnstjälkarna);* **crura cerebri** = CEREBRAL PEDUNCLES; **crus of penis** = part of corpus cavernosum attached to the pubic arch *crus penis;* **crura of the diaphragm** = long muscle fibres joining the diaphragm to the lumbar vertebrae *crus dextrum och sinistrum av pars lumbalis* NOTE: the plural is **crura**

crush [krʌʃ] *vb.* to squash *or* to injure with a heavy weight *krossa, klämma (sönder);* **he was crushed by falling stones**

crush syndrome [ˈkrʌʃ ˌsɪndrəʊm] *subst.* condition where the limb of a patient has been crushed, as in an accident *fettembolism, disseminerad intravaskulär koagulation, DIC*

COMMENT: the condition causes kidney failure and shock

crutch [krʌtʃ] *subst.* **(a)** strong support for a patient with an injured leg, formed of a stick with either a holding bar and elbow clasp or with a T-bar which fits under the armpit *krycka;* **human crutch** = method of helping an injured person to walk, where the patient puts his arm round the shoulders of a first aider *mänskligt stöd vid gång* **(b)** = CROTCH

cry [kraɪ] **1** *subst.* sudden vocal sound *rop, skrik* **2** *vb.* to produce tears because of pain *or* shock *or* fear, etc. *gråta;* **she cried when she heard her mother had been killed; the pain made him cry; the baby started crying when it was time for its feed**

cry- [ˈkraɪ, ˌ-] *prefix* referring to cold *cry(o)-, kry(o)-, köld-, frys-*

cryaesthesia [ˌkraɪi:sˈθi:ziə] *subst.* being sensitive to cold *kryestesi*

cryoprecipitat ⇨ **cryoprecipitate**

cryoprecipitate [ˌkraɪəʊprɪˈsɪpɪtət] *subst.* precipitate (such as that from blood plasma) which separates out on freezing and thawing *cryoprecipitat, kryoprecipitat*

COMMENT: cryoprecipitate contains Factor VIII and is used to treat haemophiliacs

cryoprobe [ˈkraɪəʊprəʊb] *subst.* instrument used in cryosurgery, where the tip is kept very cold to destroy tissue *slags sond för kryokirurgi*

cryosurgery [ˌkraɪəʊˈsɜ:dʒ(ə)ri] *subst.* surgery which uses extremely cold instruments to destroy tissue *kryokirurgi, fryskirurgi*

cryotherapy [ˌkraɪəʊˈθerəpi] *subst.* treatment using extreme cold (as in removing a wart with dry ice) *kryoterapi, köldbehandling*

crypt [krɪpt] *subst.* small cavity in the body *krypta;* **crypts of Lieberkuhn** *or* **Lieberkuhn's glands** = small glands in the membrane of the intestines *glandulae intestinales, Lieberkühns körtlar*

crypto- [ˈkrɪptə(ʊ), ˌ--] *prefix* hidden *crypto-, krypto-*

Cryptococcus [ˌkrɪptə(ʊ)ˈkɒkəs] *subst.* one of several single-celled yeasts, which exist

in the soil and can cause disease *Cryptococcus*
NOTE: plural is **Cryptococci**

cryptomenorrhoea [ˌkrɪptə(ʊ)ˌmenə'riːə] *subst.* retention of menstrual flow probably caused by an obstruction *kryptomenorré, falsk amenorré*

cryptorchidism [krɪp'tɔːkɪdɪz(ə)m] *or* **cryptorchism** [krɪp'tɔːkɪz(ə)m] *subst.* condition in a male, where the testicles do not move down into the scrotum *kryptorkism, retentio testis*

crystal ['krɪst(ə)l] *subst.* chemical formation of hard regular-shaped solids *kristall*

crystalline ['krɪstəlaɪn] *adj.* clear like pure crystal *kristallisk, kristallformad*

crystal violet ['krɪst(ə)l ˌva(ɪ)ələt] *or* **gentian violet** ['dʒenʃ(ə)n ˌva(ɪ)ələt] *subst.* blue antiseptic dye used to paint on skin infections *gentian(a)violett (särskilt bra mot svampinfektion)*

Cs *chemical symbol for* caesium *Cs, cesium*

CSF [ˌsiːes'ef] = CEREBROSPINAL FLUID

CT [ˌsiː'tiː] *or* **CAT** [ˌsiːeɪ'tiː] = COMPUTERIZED (AXIAL) TOMOGRAPHY; **CT scanner** = device which directs a narrow X-ray beam at a thin section of the body from various angles, using a computer to build up a complete picture of the cross-section *datortomograf*

Cu *chemical symbol for* copper *Cu, koppar*

cubital ['kjuːbɪt(ə)l] *adj.* referring to the ulna *kubital, armbågs-;* **cubital fossa** = depression in the front of the elbow joint *fossa cubitalis*

cuboidal [kjuː'bɔɪd(ə)l] *adj.* **cuboidal cell** = cube-shaped epithelial cell *kubisk epitelcell*

cuboid bone ['kjuːbɔɪd ˌbəʊn] *subst.* one of the tarsal bones in the foot ⇨ *illustration* FOOT *os cuboideum, tärningsbenet*

cuff [kʌf] *subst.* (i) inflatable ring put round a patient's arm and inflated when blood pressure is being measured *blodtrycksmanschett;* (ii) inflatable ring put round an endotracheal tube to close the passage *kuff*

cuirass respirator [kwɪ'ræs ˌrespəreɪtə] *subst.* type of artificial respirator, which surrounds only the patient's chest *slags respirator*

culdoscope ['kʌldəʊskəʊp] *subst.* instrument used to inspect the interior of the female pelvis, introduced through the vagina *culdoskop, kuldoskop*

culdoscopy [kʌl'dɒskəpi] *subst.* examination of the interior of a woman's pelvis, using a culdoscope *culdoskopi, kuldoskopi*

culdoskop ⇨ **culdoscope**

culdoskopi ⇨ **culdoscopy**

cultivate ['kʌltɪveɪt] *vb.* to make something grow *odla;* **agar is used as a culture medium to cultivate bacteria in a laboratory**

culture ['kʌltʃə] **1** *subst.* bacteria *or* tissues grown in a laboratory *kultur, odling;* **culture medium** *or* **agar** = liquid *or* gel used to grow bacteria *or* tissue *odlingssubstrat;* **stock culture** = basic culture of bacteria from which other cultures can be taken *stamkultur* **2** *vb.* to grow bacteria in a culture medium *odla; see also* SUBCULTURE

cumulative ['kjuːmjʊlətɪv] *adj.* which grows by adding *kumulativ;* **cumulative action** = effect of a drug which is given more often than it can be excreted, and so accumulates in the tissues *kumulation, anhopning, upplagring*

cuneiform bones ['kjuːnɪfɔːm bəʊns] *or* **cuneiforms** ['kjuːnɪfɔːmz] *subst. pl.* three of the tarsal bones in the foot ⇨ *illustration* FOOT *ossa cuneiformia, kilbenen*

cupola ['kjuːp(ə)lə] *subst.* (i) cap *kupol;* (ii) piece of cartilage in a semicircular canal which is moved by the fluid in the canal and connects with the vestibular nerve *cupula cristae ampullaris*

curable ['kjʊərəb(ə)l] *adj.* which can be cured *som går att bota;* **a curable form of cancer** *see also* INCURABLE

curare [kjʊə'rɑːri] *subst.* drug derived from South American plants, used surgically to paralyse muscles during operations *curare*

COMMENT: curare is the poison used to make poison arrows

curative ['kjʊərətɪv] *adj.* which can cure *kurativ, botande, läkande*

curdle ['kɜːd(ə)l] *vb. (of milk)* to coagulate *ysta sig, koagulera*

cure [kjʊə] **1** *subst.* particular way of making a patient well *or* of stopping an illness *kur, behandling, botemedel;* **scientists are trying to develop a cure for the common cold** **2** *vb.* to make a patient healthy *kurera, bota, läka;* **he was completely cured; can the doctors cure his bad circulation? some forms of cancer can't be cured**

curettage [kjʊə'retɪdʒ] *or* **curettement** [kjʊə'retmənt] *subst.* scraping the inside of a hollow organ to remove a growth *or* tissue for examination (often used in connection with the uterus) *curettage, kyrettage, skrapning; see also* D AND C, DILATATION AND CURETTAGE

curette *or US* **curet** [kjʊə'ret] **1** *subst.* surgical instrument like a long thin spoon, used for scraping the inside of an organ *curette, kyrett* **2** *vb.* to scrape with a curette *skrapa med kyrett*

curette ⇨ **curet**

curie ['kjʊəri] *subst.* unit of measurement of radioactivity *curie*
NOTE: with figures usually written as **Ci: 25 Ci**

curvature ['kɜːvətʃə] *subst.* way in which something bends from a straight line *kurva, krökning;* **curvature of the spine** = abnormal bending of the spine forwards or sideways *onormal krökning på ryggraden, skolios, lordos, kyphos;* **greater** *or* **lesser curvature of the stomach** = longer outside convex line of the stomach *or* shorter inside concave line of the stomach *curvatura ventriculi major resp. minor, stora resp. lilla magsäckskrökningen*

curve [kɜːv] **1** *subst.* line which bends round *kurva* **2** *vb.* to make a round shape *böja (kröka) sig;* to bend something round *böja, kröka*

curved [kɜːvd] *adj.* with a shape which is not straight or flat *böjd, krökt;* **a curved line; a curved scalpel**

cushingoid ['kʊʃɪŋɔɪd] *adj.* showing symptoms of Cushing's syndrome *som visar symtom på Cushings sjukdom*

Cushing's disease ['kʊʃɪŋz dɪ,ziːz] *or* **Cushing's syndrome** ['kʊʃɪŋz ˌsɪndrəʊm] *subst.* condition where the adrenal cortex produces too many corticosteroids *Cushings sjukdom (syndrom)*

COMMENT: the syndrome is caused either by a tumour in the adrenal gland, by excessive stimulation of the adrenals by the basophil cells of the pituitary gland, or by a corticosteroid-secreting tumour. The syndrome causes swelling of the face and trunk, the muscles weaken, the blood pressure rises and the body retains salt and water

cusp [kʌsp] *subst.* **(a)** pointed tip of a tooth *kusp, upphöjning på tandkrona* **(b)** flap of membrane forming a valve in the heart *cuspis, flik på hjärtklaff*

cuspid ['kʌspɪd] *or* **canine tooth** ['keɪnaɪn tuːθ] *subst.* one of the four pointed teeth next to the incisors (two in the top jaw and two in the lower jaw) *dens cuspidatus (caninus), hörntand*

cut [kʌt] **1** *subst.* place where the skin has been penetrated by a sharp instrument *snitt, skärsår, huggsår;* **she had a bad cut on her left leg; the nurse will put a bandage on your cut** **2** *vb.* **(a)** to make an opening using a knife, scissors, etc. *skära (bort), göra (in)snitt;* **the surgeon cut the diseased tissue away with a scalpel; she got tetanus after cutting her finger on the broken glass** **(b)** to reduce the number of something *skära ned, reducera, minska;* **accidents have been cut by 10%**

cutaneous [kju'teɪniəs] *adj.* referring to the skin *kutan, hud-;* **cutaneous leishmaniasis** = form of skin disease caused by the tropical parasite Leishmania *Leishmaniasis cutanea, kutan leishmanios*

cuticle ['kjuːtɪk(ə)l] *subst.* (i) epidermis *or* outer layer of skin *epidermis, överhuden;* (ii) strip of epidermis attached at the base of a nail *cuticula unguis, nagelband*

cutis ['kjuːtɪs] *subst.* skin *cutis, huden;* **cutis anserina** = goose pimples *or* reaction of the skin to being cold or frightened, where the skin forms many little bumps *cutis anserina, gåshud*

CVA [ˌsiːviː'eɪ] = CEREBROVASCULAR ACCIDENT

C-vitamin ⇨ **c, ascorbic acid**

CVP ⇨ **central**

cyanide ['sa(ɪ)ənaɪd] *or* **prussic acid** [ˌprʌsɪk 'æsɪd] *subst.* salt of hydrocyanic acid, a poison which kills very rapidly when drunk or inhaled *cyanid, blåsyra*

cyano- ['sa(ɪ)ənəʊ, ˌ---, saɪ'ænə(ʊ)] *prefix* blue *cyano-, blå-*

cyanocobalamin [ˌsa(ɪ)ənəʊkəʊ'bæləmɪn] = VITAMIN B_{12}

cyanokobalamin ⇨ **Vitamin B**

cyanopati ⇨ **cyanotic**

cyanos ⇨ **blueness**

cyanosed ['sa(ɪ)ənəʊst] *adj.* with blue skin *cyanotisk;* **the patient was cyanosed round the lips**

cyanosis [sa(ɪ)ə'nəʊsɪs] *subst.* blue colour of the peripheral skin and mucous membranes, symptom of lack of oxygen in the blood (as in a blue baby) *cyanos*

cyanotic [sa(ɪ)ə'nɒtɪk] *adj.* suffering from cyanosis *cyanotisk;* **cyanotic congenital heart disease** = cyanosis *cyanopati, medfött cyanotiskt hjärtfel*

cyanotisk ⇨ **cyanosed, cyanotic**

cyanvätesyra ⇨ **hydrocyanic acid**

cyclandelate [sɪ'klændəleɪt] *subst.* drug used to treat cerebrovascular disease *cyklandelat*

cycle ['saɪk(ə)l] *subst.* **(a)** series of events which recur regularly *cykel, kretslopp, period;* **menstrual cycle** = period (usually 28 days) during which the endometrium develops, a woman ovulates, and menstruation takes place *menstruationscykel;* **ovarian cycle** = regular changes in the ovary during reproductive life *ovarialcykel* **(b)** bicycle *or* vehicle with two wheels *cykel;* **exercise cycle** = type of cycle which is fixed to the floor, so that someone can pedal on it for exercise *motionscykel*

cyclical ['sɪklɪk(ə)l] *adj.* referring to cycles *cyklisk, periodisk;* **cyclical vomiting** = repeated attacks of vomiting *upprepade kräkningar*

cyclitis [sɪ'klaɪtɪs] *subst.* inflammation of the ciliary body in the eye *cyklit*

cyclizine ['saɪklɪzi:n] *subst.* antihistamine drug used in the treatment of travel sickness *or* pregnancy sickness *or* inner ear disorders *cyklizin*

cyclo- ['saɪkləʊ, ˌ--] *prefix* meaning cyclical *or* referring to cycles *cykl(o)-, cirkel-*

cyclodialysis [ˌsaɪkləʊdaɪ'ælɪsɪs] *subst.* surgical operation to connect the anterior chamber of the eye and the choroid, as treatment of glaucoma *cyklodialys*

cycloplegia [ˌsaɪkləʊ'pli:dʒə] *subst.* paralysis of the ciliary muscle which makes it impossible for the eye to focus properly *cykloplegi*

cyclothymia [ˌsaɪklə(ʊ)'θaɪmiə] *subst.* mild form of manic depression, where the patient suffers from alternating depression and excitement *cyklothymi*

cyclotomy [saɪ'klɒtəmi] *subst.* surgical operation to make a cut in the ciliary body *cyklotomi*

cyes ⇨ **cyesis**

cyesis [saɪ'i:sɪs] *or* **pregnancy** ['pregnənsi] *subst.* condition where a woman is carrying an unborn child in her womb *cyes, graviditet, havandeskap*

cykel ⇨ **cycle**

cyklandelat ⇨ **cyclandelate**

cyklisk ⇨ **cyclical**

cyklit ⇨ **cyclitis**

cyklizin ⇨ **cyclizine**

cyklodialys ⇨ **cyclodialysis**

cykloplegi ⇨ **cycloplegia**

cyklothymi ⇨ **cyclothymia**

cyklotomi ⇨ **cyclotomy**

cykobemin ⇨ **extrinsic, factor, Vitamin B**

cylinder ['sɪlɪndə] *see* OXYGEN

cylinder ⇨ **cast, granular**

cylinderepitelcell ⇨ **columnar**

cyst [sɪst] *subst.* abnormal growth in the body shaped like a pouch, containing liquid *or* semi-liquid substances *cysta;* **branchial cyst** = cyst on the side of the neck of an embryo *gälgångscysta, gälgångsfistel;* **dental cyst** = cyst near the root of a tooth *dentalcysta, cysta nära tandrot;* **dermoid cyst** = cyst found under the skin, usually in the midline, containing hair, sweat glands and sebaceous glands *dermoidcysta;* **ovarian cyst** = cyst which develops in the ovaries *ovarialcysta, äggstockscysta;* **parasitic cyst** = cyst produced by a parasite, usually in the liver *cysta bildad av parasit(er);* **pilonidal cyst** = cyst at the bottom of the spine near the buttocks *pilonidalcysta, hårsäckscysta;* **sebaceous cyst** *or* **wen** = cyst which forms in a sebaceous gland *steatom, aterom, talg(körtel)cysta*

cyst- ['sɪst, ,-] *prefix* referring to the bladder *cyst(o)-, blås-, urinblåse-*

cyst- ⇨ **cystic, vesico-**

cysta ⇨ **cyst**

cystadenoma [ˌsɪstədɪ'nəʊmə] *subst.* adenoma in which fluid-filled cysts form *cystadenom*

cysta, falsk ⇨ **pseudocyst**

cystalgi ⇨ **cystalgia**

cystalgia [sɪ'stældʒə] *subst.* pain in the urinary bladder *cystalgi, urinblåseneuralgi*

cystectomy [sɪ'stektəmi] *subst.* surgical operation to remove all *or* part of the urinary bladder *cystektomi*

cystektomi ⇨ **cystectomy**

cystic ['sɪstɪk] *adj.* **(a)** referring to cysts *cyst-, cystisk* **(b)** referring to a bladder *cyst(o)-, blås-, urinblåse-;* **cystic artery** = artery leading from the hepatic artery to the gall bladder *arteria cystica, gallblåseartären;* **cystic duct** = duct which takes bile from the gall bladder to the bile duct *ductus cysticus, gallblåsegången;* **cystic vein** = vein which drains the gall bladder *vena cystica*

cystica ['sɪstɪkə] *see* SPINA BIFIDA

cysticercosis [ˌsɪstɪsɜː'kəʊsɪs] *subst.* disease caused by infestation of tapeworm larvae from pork *cysticerkos*

cysticercus [ˌsɪstɪ'sɜːkəs] *or* **bladder worm** ['blædəˌwɜːm] *subst.* larva of a tapeworm found in pork, which is enclosed in a cyst, typical of Taenia *cysticerk, dynt, blåsmask*

cysticerk ⇨ **cysticercus**

cysticerkos ⇨ **cysticercosis**

cystic fibrosis [ˌsɪstɪk faɪ'brəʊsɪs] *or* **fibrocystic disease of the pancreas** [ˌfaɪbrəʊ'sɪstɪk dɪˌziːz əv ðə 'pæŋkriəs] *or* **mucoviscidosis** [ˌmjuːkəʊvɪsɪ'dəʊsɪs] *subst.* hereditary disease in which there is malfunction of the exocrine glands, such as the pancreas, in particular those which secrete mucus *cystisk fibros, cystisk pankreasfibros, mukoviskidos*

COMMENT: the thick mucous secretions cause blockage of ducts and many serious secondary effects in the intestines and lungs. Symptoms include loss of weight, abnormal faeces and bronchitis. If diagnosed early, cystic fibrosis can be controlled with vitamins, physiotherapy and pancreatic enzymes

cystine ['sɪstiːn] *subst.* amino acid found in protein, and causing stones to form in urine *cystin*

cystinosis [ˌsɪstɪ'nəʊsɪs] *subst.* defective absorption of amino acids, which results in excessive amounts of cystine accumulating in the kidneys *cystinos*

cystinuria [ˌsɪstɪ'njʊəriə] *subst.* cystine in the urine *cystinuri*

cystisk fibros ⇨ **cystic fibrosis**

cystit ⇨ **cystitis**

cystitis [sɪ'staɪtɪs] *subst.* inflammation of the urinary bladder, which makes a patient pass water often and giving a burning sensation *cystit, blåskatarr*

cystnjure ⇨ **polycystitis**

cystocele ['sɪstəsiːl] *subst.* hernia of the urinary bladder into the vagina *cystocele, vesikocele, urinblåsebråck*

cystografi ⇨ **cystography**

cystogram ['sɪstəgræm] *subst.* X-ray photograph of the urinary bladder *cystogram*

cystography [sɪ'stɒgrəfi] *subst.* examination of the urinary bladder by X-rays after radio-opaque dye has been introduced *cystografi*

cystolithiasis [ˌsɪstəlɪ'θaɪəsɪs] *subst.* condition where stones are formed in the urinary bladder *cystolithiasis*

cystometer [sɪ'stɒmɪtə] *subst.* apparatus which measures the pressure in the bladder *cystometer*

cystometri ⇨ **cystometry**

cystometry [sɪ'stɒmetrɪ] *subst.* measurement of the pressure in the bladder *cystometri*

cystopexi ⇨ **cystopexy**

cystopexy [sɪ'stɒpeksi] *or* **vesicofixation** [ˌvesɪkəʊfɪk'seɪʃ(ə)n] *subst.* surgical operation to fix the bladder in a different position *cystopexi, vesikofixation*

cystoscope ['sɪstəskəʊp] *subst.* instrument made of a long tube with a light at the end, used to inspect the inside of the bladder *cystoskop*

cystoscopy [sɪ'stɒskəpi] *subst.* examination of the bladder using a cystoscope *cystoskopi*

cystoskop ⇨ **cystoscope**

cystoskopi ⇨ **cystoscopy**

cystostomi ⇨ **cystostomy**

cystostomy [sɪ'stɒtəmi] *or* **vesicostomy** [ˌvesɪ'kɒstəmi] *subst.* surgical operation to make an opening between the bladder and the abdominal wall to allow urine to pass without going through the urethra *cystostomi*

cystotomi ⇨ **cystotomy**

cystotomy [sɪ'stɒtəmɪ] *or* **vesicotomy** [ˌvesɪ'kɒtəmi] *subst.* surgical operation to make a cut in a bladder *cystotomi, vesikotomi*

cyt- ['sɪt, ˌ-] *or* **cyto-** ['saɪtə(ʊ), ˌ--] *prefix* referring to cells *cyt(o)-, cell-*

cytarabin ⇨ **cytarabine**

cytarabine [saɪ'teərəbi:n] *subst.* antiviral drug *cytarabin*

cytochemistry [ˌsaɪtə(ʊ)'kemɪstrɪ] *subst.* study of the chemical activity of living cells *studiet av de levande cellernas kemiska aktivitet*

cytogenetics [ˌsaɪtə(ʊ)dʒə'netɪks] *subst.* branch of genetics, which studies the structure and function of cells, especially the chromosomes *cytogenetik*

cytogenetik ⇨ **cytogenetics**

cytokinesis [ˌsaɪtə(ʊ)kɪ'ni:sɪs] *subst.* changes in the cytoplasm of a cell during division *cytokines(i)*

cytologi ⇨ **cytology**

cytological smear [ˌsaɪtə(ʊ)'lɒdʒɪk(ə)l ˌsmɪə] *subst.* sample of tissue taken for examination under a microscope *cytologiskt smear (utstryk)*

cytology [saɪ'tɒlədʒɪ] *subst.* study of the structure and function of cells *cytologi*

cytolys ⇨ **cytolysis**

cytolysis [saɪ'tɒləsɪs] *subst.* breaking down of cells *cytolys*

cytomegalovirus (CMV) [ˌsaɪtə(ʊ)ˌmegələʊ'vaɪ(ə)rəs (ˌsi:em'vi:)] *subst.* virus (one of the herpesviruses) which can cause serious congenital disorders in a fetus if it infects the pregnant mother *cytomegalovirus, CMV*

cytometer [saɪ'tɒmɪtə] *subst.* instrument attached to a microscope, used for measuring and counting the number of cells in a specimen *instrument för räkning av cellantal*

cytopeni ⇨ **cytopenia**

cytopenia [ˌsaɪtə(ʊ)'pi:niə] *subst.* deficiency of cellular elements in blood *or* tissue *cytopeni*

cytoplasm ['saɪtə(ʊ)plæz(ə)m] *subst.* substance inside the cell membrane, which surrounds the nucleus of a cell *cytoplasma*

cytoplasma ⇨ **cytoplasm**

cytoplasmatisk ⇨ **cytoplasmic**

cytoplasmic [ˌsaɪtə(ʊ)'plæzmɪk] *adj.* referring to the cytoplasm of a cell *cytoplasmatisk*

cytosin ⇨ **cytosine**

cytosine ['saɪtə(ʊ)si:n] *subst.* basic element of DNA *cytosin*

cytosom ⇨ **cytosome**

cytosome ['saɪtə(ʊ)səʊm] *subst.* body of a cell, not including the nucleus *cytosom*

cytostatikum ⇨ **anti-cancer drug**

cytotoxic drug [ˌsaɪtə(ʊ)'tɒksɪk ˌdrʌg] *subst.* drug which reduces the reproduction of cells, and is used to treat cancer *cytotoxiskt läkemedel*

cytotoxin [ˌsaɪtə(ʊ)'tɒksɪn] *subst.* substance which has a toxic effect on cells of certain organs *cytotoxin*

Dd

Vitamin D [ˌvɪtəmɪn ˌdi:] *subst.* vitamin which is soluble in fat, and is found in butter, eggs and fish; it is also produced by the skin when exposed to sunlight *D-vitamin*

> COMMENT: Vitamin D helps in the formation of bones, and lack of it causes rickets in children

dab [dæb] *vb.* to touch lightly *badda;* **he dabbed the cut with a piece of absorbent cotton**

da Costa's syndrome [dɑː'kɒstəz ˌsɪndrəʊm] *or* **disordered action of the heart** [dɪsˌɔːdəd 'ækʃ(ə)n əv ðə ˌhɑːt] *subst.* condition where the patient suffers palpitations, breathlessness and dizziness, caused by effort or worry *hjärtneuros*

dacryo- ['dækriəʊ, ˌ---] *prefix* referring to tears *dakry(o)-, tår-*

dacryoadenitis [ˌdækriəʊˌæde'naɪtɪs] *subst.* inflammation of the lacrimal gland *dakry(o)adenit, tårkörtelinflammation*

dacryocystitis [ˌdækriəʊsɪ'staɪtɪs] *subst.* inflammation of the lacrimal sac when the tear duct, which drains into the nose, becomes blocked *dakryocystit, tårsäcksinflammation*

dacryocystography [ˌdækriəʊsɪ'stɒgrəfi] *subst.* contrast radiography to determine the site of an obstruction in the tear ducts *dakryocystografi*

dacryocystorhinostomy [ˌdækriəʊˌsɪstɔːrai'nɒstəmi] *subst.* surgical operation to bypass a blockage from the tear duct which takes tears into the nose *dakryocystorinostomi*

dacryolith ['dækriəʊˌlɪθ] *subst.* stone in the lacrimal sac *dakryolit, tårvägssten, tårvägskonkrement*

dacryoma [ˌdækri'əʊmə] *subst.* benign swelling in one of the tear ducts *godartad svullnad i tårkanal*

dactyl ['dæktɪl] **1** *subst.* finger or toe *dactylus, finger, tå* **2** *prefix* **dactyl-** = referring to fingers or toes *daktyl(o)-, finger-, tå-*

dactylitis [ˌdæktɪ'laɪtɪs] *subst.* inflammation of the fingers or toes, caused by bone infection or rheumatic disease *daktylit*

dactylology [ˌdæktɪ'lɒlədʒi] *subst.* deaf and dumb language *or* signs made with the fingers, used in place of words when talking to a deaf and dumb person, or when a deaf and dumb person wants to communicate *teckenspråk*

dag ⇨ **day, daytime**

dagblindhet ⇨ **hemeralopia**

dagcenter ⇨ **day**

daglig ⇨ **daily, diurnal, quotidian**

dagligen ⇨ **daily, o.d.**

dagpatient ⇨ **day**

dags- ⇨ **diurnal**

dagseende ⇨ **photopic vision**

dagsjukhus ⇨ **day**

dagtid ⇨ **daytime**

dagvård ⇨ **hospital**

DAH [ˌdiːeɪ'eɪtʃ] = DISORDERED ACTION OF THE HEART

daily ['deɪli] **1** *adj.* which happens every day *daglig;* **you should do daily exercises to keep fit** **2** *adv.* every day *dagligen;* **take the medicine twice daily**

dakryocystit ⇨ **dacryocystitis**

dakryocystografi ⇨ **dacryocystography**

dakryocystorinostomi ⇨ **dacryocystorhinostomy**

dakryolit ⇨ **dacryolith**

daktylit ⇨ **dactylitis**

Daltonism ['dɔːlt(ə)nɪz(ə)m] *or* **protanopia** [ˌprəʊtə'nəʊpiə] *subst.* commonest form of colour blindness, where the patient cannot see red *daltonism, protanopi, rödblindhet; compare* DEUTERANOPIA, TRITANOPIA

damage ['dæmɪdʒ] **1** *subst.* harm done to things *skada;* **the disease caused damage to the brain cells; bone damage** *or* **tissue damage** = damage caused to a bone *or* to tissue *benskada, vävnadsskada* NOTE: no plural **2** *vb.* to harm something *skada, tillfoga skada;* **his hearing** *or* **his sense of balance was damaged in the accident; a surgical operation to remove damaged tissue**

dambinda ⇨ **napkin**

dammlunga ⇨ **pneumoconiosis**

damp [dæmp] *adj.* slightly wet *fuktig;* **you should put a damp compress on the bruise**

D and C [ˌdiːənd'siː] = DILATATION AND CURETTAGE

dandruff ['dændrəf] *or* **scurf** ['skɜːf] *or* **pityriasis capitis** [ˌpɪtɪ'ra(ɪ)əsɪs] *subst.* pieces of dead skin which form on the scalp and fall out when the hair is combed *pityriasis capitis, torr seborré, mjäll*

D and V [ˌdiː ənd 'viː] = DIARRHOEA AND VOMITING

dandyfeber ⇨ **dengue**

danger ['deɪn(d)ʒə] *subst.* possibility of harm *or* death *fara, risk;* **unless the glaucoma is treated quickly, there's a danger that the patient will lose his eyesight** *or* **a danger of the patient losing his eyesight; the doctors say she's out of danger** = she is not likely to die *doktorn säger att hon är utom (all) fara*

dangerous ['deɪn(d)ʒ(ə)rəs] *adj.* which can cause harm or death *farlig, vådlig;* **don't touch the electric wires - they're dangerous; cigarettes are dangerous to health; dangerous drugs** = drugs (such as morphine *or* heroin) which are harmful and are not available to the general public, and also poisons which can only be sold to certain persons *farliga läkemedel och gifter (narkotika m m) som bara är tillgängliga för vissa personer*

danssjuka ⇨ **chorea, St Vitus' dance**

dark [dɑːk] **1** *adj.* **(a)** with very little light *mörk;* **switch the lights on - it's getting too dark to read; in the winter it gets dark early; dark adaptation** = change in the retina and pupil of the eye to adapt to dim light after being in normal light *mörkeradap(ta)tion* **(b)** with black or brown hair *mörkhårig;* **he's dark, but his sister is fair**
NOTE: **dark - darker - darkest** **2** *subst.* lack of light *mörker;* **she is afraid of the dark; cats can see in the dark**

darkening ['dɑːk(ə)nɪŋ] *subst.* becoming darker in colour *mörknande;* **darkening of the tissue takes place after bruising**

darkroom ['dɑːkruːm] *subst.* room with no light, in which photographic film can be developed *mörkrum;* **the X-rays are in the darkroom, so they should be ready soon; he hopes to get a job as a darkroom technician**

darra ⇨ **shake, shiver, tremble, vibrate**

darrning ⇨ **fremitus, shivering, trembling, tremor, vibration**

data ['deɪtə] *subst.* any information (in words *or* figures) about a certain subject, especially information which is available on computer *data, information;* **data bank** *or* **bank of data** = store of information in a computer *databank;* **the hospital keeps a data bank of information about possible kidney donors**

databank ⇨ **data**

date [deɪt] *subst.* number of a day or year, name of a month (when something happened) *datum;* **what's the date today? what is the date of your next appointment; do you remember the date of your last checkup?; up-to-date** = very modern *or* using very recent information *or* equipment *modern, aktuell;* **the new hospital is provided with the most up-to-date equipment; out-of-date** = not modern *omodern, föråldrad;* **the surgeons have to work with out-of-date equipment**

dator ⇨ **computer**

datortomografi ⇨ **computerized axial tomography (CAT), scan**

datum ⇨ **date**

daughter ['dɔːtə] *subst.* girl child of a parent *dotter;* **they have two sons and one daughter; daughter cell** = one of the cells which develop by mitosis from a single cell *dottercell*

day [deɪ] *subst.* (i) period of 24 hours *dygn;* (ii) period from morning until night, when it is light *dag;* **he works all day in the office, and then visits patients in the hospital in the evening; take two tablets three times a day; she's attending a day unit for disabled patients; day hospital** = hospital where patients are treated during the day and go home in the evenings *dagsjukhus, växelvård, dagcenter;* **day nursery** = place where small children can be looked after during the daytime, while their parents are at work *daghem, barndaghem;* **day patient** = patient who is in hospital for treatment for a day (i.e. one who does not stay a night) *dagpatient;* **day recovery ward** = ward where day patients who have had minor operations can recover before going home *uppvakningsavdelning*

day blindness ['deɪˌblaɪndnəs] = HEMERALOPIA

daylight ['deɪlaɪt] *subst.* light during the day *dagsljus*

daytime ['deɪtaɪm] *subst.* period of light between morning and night *dag, dagtid;* **he works at night and sleeps during the daytime**

dazed [deɪzd] *adj.* confused in the mind *förvirrad, omtumlad, vimmelkantig;* **she was found walking about in a dazed condition; he was dazed after the accident**

dB [ˌdiː'biː] = DECIBEL

DDS [ˌdiːdiː'es] *US* = DOCTOR OF DENTAL SURGERY

DDT [ˌdiːdiː'tiː] = DICHLORODIPHENYLTRICHLOROETH NE

de- ['diː, ˌdiː, dɪ, də] *prefix* meaning removal *or* loss *de-*

dead [ded] *adj.* **(a)** not alive *död, livlös;* **my grandparents are both dead; when the injured man arrived at hospital he was found to be dead; the woman was rescued from the crash, but was certified dead on arrival at the hospital (b)** not sensitive *domnad, okänslig;* **the nerve endings are dead; his fingers went dead; dead space =** breath in the last part of the inspiration which does not get further than the bronchial tubes *dead space, döda rummet, skadliga rummet*

deaden ['ded(ə)n] *vb.* to make (pain *or* noise) less strong *lindra, dämpa, försvaga;* **the doctor gave him an injection to deaden the pain**

deadly ['dedli] *adj.* likely to kill *dödlig, döds-;* **cyanide is a deadly poison; deadly nightshade =** BELLADONNA

dead (man's) fingers [ˌded (ˌmænz) 'fɪŋgəz] = RAYNAUD'S DISEASE

deaf [def] **1** *adj.* not able to hear *döv;* **you have to shout when you speak to Mr Jones because he's quite deaf; totally deaf** *or* **completely deaf** *or* **stone deaf =** unable to hear any sound at all *totalt (helt, fullständigt) döv, stendöv;* **partially deaf =** able to hear some sounds but not all *hörselskadad, med nedsatt hörsel;* **deaf and dumb =** not able to hear or to speak *dövstum;* **deaf and dumb language** *or* **sign language** *or* **dactylology =** signs made with the fingers, used instead of words when talking to a trained deaf and dumb person, or when a deaf and dumb person wants to communicate *teckenspråk* **2** *subst.* **the deaf** = people who are deaf *de döva;* **hearing aids can be of great use to the partially deaf**

deafen ['def(ə)n] *vb.* to make (someone) deaf for a time *göra döv;* **he was deafened by the explosion**

deafness ['defnəs] *subst.* loss of hearing *hörselnedsättning;* being unable to hear *dövhet;* **conductive deafness =** deafness caused by defective conduction of sound into the inner ear *konduktiv dövhet, ledningshörselnedsättning;* **partial deafness =** (i) being able to hear some tones, but not all *(partiell) hörselnedsättning;* (ii) general dulling of the whole range of hearing *hörselnedsättning;* **progressive deafness =** condition, common in people as they get older, where a person gradually becomes more and more deaf *tilltagande hörselnedsättning;* **perceptive deafness** *or* **sensorineural deafness =** deafness caused by a disorder in the auditory nerves *or* the cochlea *or* the brain centres which receive impulses from the nerves *perceptiv (sensorineural) dövhet (hörselnedsättning);* **total deafness =** being unable to hear any sound at all *total (fullständig) dövhet*

> COMMENT: deafness has many degrees and many causes: old age, viruses, exposure to continuous loud noise or intermittent loud explosions, and diseases such as German measles

deaminate [ˌdiː'æmɪneɪt] *vb.* to remove an amino group from an amino acid, forming ammonia *deaminera*

deamination [diːˌæmɪ'neɪʃ(ə)n] *subst.* removal of an amino group from an amino acid, forming ammonia *deaminering*

> COMMENT: after deamination, the ammonia which is formed is converted to urea by the liver, while the remaining carbon and hydrogen from the amino acid provide the body with heat and energy

deaminera ⇨ **deaminate**

deaminering ⇨ **deamination**

death [deθ] *subst.* dying; end of life *död, dödsfall;* **his sudden death shocked his friends; he met his death in a car crash; death certificate =** official certificate signed by a doctor stating that a person has died, and giving details of the person and the cause of death *dödsattest, dödsbevis;* **death rate =** number of deaths per year per thousand of population *dödstal, dödlighet, mortalitet;* **the death rate from cancer of the liver has remained stable; brain death =** condition where the nerves in the brain stem have died,

and the patient can be certified as dead, although the heart may not have stopped beating *hjärndöd;* **cot death** *or US* **crib death** = sudden death of a baby in bed, with no identifiable cause *plötslig spädbarnsdöd*
NOTE: for terms referring to death see words beginning with **necro-**

debil ⇨ **feebleminded**

debilitate [dɪ'bɪlɪteɪt] *vb.* to make weak *försvaga, tära (på);* **he was debilitated by a long illness; debilitating disease** = disease which makes the patient weak *tärande sjukdom*

debilitet ⇨ **feeblemindedness**

debility [dɪ'bɪləti] *subst.* general weakness *klenhet, svaghet, kraftlöshet*

debridement [dɪ'bri:dmənt] *subst.* removal of dirt *or* dead tissue from a wound to help healing *debridering*

debridering ⇨ **debridement**

debridering (av sår) ⇨ **dehiscence**

decaffeinated [ˌdi:'kæfɪneɪtɪd] *adj.* (coffee) with the caffeine removed *koffeinfri*

decalcification [di:ˌkælsɪfɪ'keɪʃ(ə)n] *subst.* loss of calcium salts from teeth and bones *dekalcifiering, urkalkning*

decapsulation [di:ˌkæpsju'leɪʃ(ə)n] *subst.* surgical operation to remove a capsule from an organ, especially from a kidney *operativt avlägsnande av kapsel*

decay [dɪ'keɪ] **1** *subst.* process by which tissues become rotten, caused by the action of microbes and oxygen *förruttnelse* **2** *vb. (of tissue)* to rot *ruttna;* **the surgeon removed decayed matter from the wound**

decibel ['desɪbel] *subst.* unit of measurement of the loudness of sound, used to compare different levels of sound *decibel*
NOTE: usually written as **dB** after a figure: **20dB:** say 'twenty decibels'

COMMENT: normal conversation is at about 50dB. Very loud noise with a value of over 120dB (such as aircraft engines) can cause pain

decidua [dɪ'sɪdjuə] *subst.* membrane which lines the uterus after fertilization *decidua, yttersta ägghinnan*

COMMENT: the decidua is divided into several parts: the decidua basalis, where the embryo is attached, the decidua capsularis, which covers the embryo and the decidua vera which is the rest of the decidua not touching the embryo; it is expelled after the birth of the baby

deciduous [dɪ'sɪdjuəs] *adj.* **deciduous teeth** *or* **milk teeth** = a child's first twenty teeth, which are gradually replaced by the permanent teeth *dentes decidui, mjölktänderna*

decompensation [ˌdi:ˌkɒmp(ə)n'seɪʃ(ə)n] *subst.* condition where an organ such as the heart cannot cope with extra stress placed on it (and so is unable to circulate the blood properly) *dekompensation*

decompose [ˌdi:kəm'pəʊz] *vb.* to rot *or* to become putrefied *ruttna, lösas upp, falla sönder*

decomposition [ˌdi:ˌkɒmpə'zɪʃ(ə)n] *subst.* process where dead matter is rotted by the action of bacteria *or* fungi *dekomposition, förruttnelse, upplösning, sönderfall*

decompression [ˌdi:kəm'preʃ(ə)n] *subst.* **(a)** reduction of pressure *tryckminskning;* **cardiac decompression** = removal of a haematoma *or* constriction of the heart *avlägsnande av ngt som orsakar hopklämning av hjärtat;* **cerebral decompression** = removal of part of the skull to relieve pressure on the brain *avlägsnande av del av skallen för att minska trycket på hjärnan* **(b)** controlled reduction of atmospheric pressure which occurs as a diver returns to the surface *tryckminskning för att undvika dykarsjuka;* **decompression sickness** = CAISSON DISEASE

decongestant [ˌdi:k(ə)n'dʒest(ə)nt] *adj. & subst.* (drug) which reduces congestion and swelling, sometimes used to unblock the nasal passages *avsvällande medel*

decortication [ˌdi:ˌkɔ:tɪ'keɪʃ(ə)n] *subst.* surgical removal of the cortex of an organ *dekortikering;* **decortication of a lung** *or* **pleurectomy** = surgical operation to remove part of the pleura which has been thickened or made stiff by chronic empyema *dekortikering*

decrease ['di:kri:s; di:'kri:s] **1** *subst.* lowering in numbers *or* becoming less *minskning, nedgång;* **a decrease in the numbers of new cases being notified** **2** *vb.* to become less *or* to make something less *minska(s);* **his blood pressure has decreased to a more normal level; the pressure in the vessel is gradually decreased**

decubitus [dɪ'kju:bɪtəs] *subst.* position of a patient who has been lying down in bed for a long time *dekubitus, trycksår, liggsår;* **decubitus ulcer** = BEDSORE

decussation [ˌdiːkʌˈseɪʃ(ə)n] *subst.* chiasma *or* crossing of nerve fibres in the central nervous system *decussio, chiasma, korsning*

decussio ⇨ **decussation**

deep [diːp] *adj.* **(a)** which goes a long way down *djup;* **be careful - the water is very deep here; the wound is several millimetres deep; take a deep breath** = to inhale a large amount of air *andas in djupt, ta ett djupt andetag* **(b)** inside the body, further from the skin *djup;* **the intercostal muscle is deep to the external; deep vein** = vein which is inside the body near a bone, as opposed to a superficial vein near the skin *djup ven;* **deep vein thrombosis (DVT)** *or* **phlebothrombosis** = thrombus in the deep veins of a leg or the pelvis *djup ventrombos;* **deep facial vein** = small vein which drains from the pterygoid process behind the cheek into the facial vein *vena facialis posterior*
NOTE: the opposite is **superficial.** Note also that a part is **deep to** another part

deeply [ˈdiːpli] *adv.* (breathing) which takes in a large amount of air *djupt;* **he was breathing deeply**

defaecate [ˈdefəkeɪt] *vb.* to pass faeces from the bowels *defekera, tömma tarmen*

defaecation [ˌdefəˈkeɪʃ(ə)n] *subst.* passing out faeces from the bowels *defekation, tarmtömning, avföring*

defect [ˈdiːfekt] *subst.* (i) wrong formation *or* something which is badly formed *defekt, missbildning;* (ii) lack of something which is necessary *brist;* **birth defect** *or* **congenital defect** = malformation which exists in a person's body from birth *medfödd missbildning (defekt)*

defective [dɪˈfektɪv] **1** *adj.* which works badly *or* which is wrongly formed *defekt, missbildad, bristfällig;* **the surgeons operated to repair a defective heart valve 2** *subst.* person suffering from severe mental subnormality *efterbliven (person), förståndshandikappad*

defekation ⇨ **bowel, defaecation**

defekera ⇨ **defaecate**

defekt ⇨ **defect, defective**

defence [dɪˈfens] *subst.* (i) resistance against an attack of a disease *försvar, skydd;* (ii) behaviour of a person which is aimed at protecting him from harm *försvar;* **muscular defence** = rigidity of muscles associated with inflammation such as peritonitis *défense musculair, muskelförsvar;* **defence mechanism** = subconscious reflex by which a person prevents himself from showing emotion *försvarsmekanism*

défense musculaire ⇨ **muscular**

deferens [ˈdef(ə)r(ə)nz] *see* VAS DEFERENS

deferens ⇨ **deferent**

deferent [ˈdef(ə)r(ə)nt] *adj.* (i) which goes away from the centre *deferens, bortförande, avledande;* (ii) referring to the vas deferens *som avser el. hör till vas deferens*

defervescence [ˌdefɜːˈves(ə)ns] *subst.* period during which a fever is subsiding *period då febern går ned*

defibrillation [diːˌfɪbrɪˈleɪʃ(ə)n] *or* **cardioversion** [ˌkɑːdiəʊˈvɜːʃ(ə)n] *subst.* correcting a fibrillating heartbeat by using electrical shocks *elkonvertering, defibrillering*

defibrillator [diːˈfɪbrɪleɪtə] *subst.* apparatus used to give electric shocks to the heart to make it beat regularly *defibrillator*

defibrillering ⇨ **cardioversion**

defibrination [diːˌfaɪbrɪˈneɪʃ(ə)n] *subst.* removal of fibrin from a blood sample to prevent clotting *defibrinering*

defibrinering ⇨ **defibrination**

deficiency [dɪˈfɪʃ(ə)nsi] *subst.* lack *or* not having enough of something *brist;* **deficiency disease** = disease caused by lack of an essential element in the diet (such as vitamins, essential amino and fatty acids, etc.) *bristsjukdom;* **iron deficiency anaemia** = anaemia caused by lack of iron in red blood cells *sideropeni, serumjärnbrist, järnbristanemi;* **vitamin deficiency** = lack of vitamins *vitaminbrist;* **immunodeficiency** = lack of immunity to a disease *nedsatt immunförsvar, immundefekt*

deficient [dɪˈfɪʃ(ə)nt] *adj.* **deficient in something** = not containing the necessary amount of something *utan tillräckligt med ngt, fattig på ngt, med brist på ngt;* **his diet is deficient in calcium** *or* **he has a calcium-deficient diet**

defloration [ˌdiːflɔːˈreɪʃ(ə)n] *subst.* breaking the hymen of a virgin usually at the first sexual intercourse *deflorering*

deflorering ⇨ **defloration**

deflorescence [ˌdiːflɔːˈres(ə)ns] *subst.* disappearance of a rash *deflorescens*

deflorescens ⇨ **deflorescence**

deformans [diːˈfɔːməns] *see* OSTEITIS

deformation [ˌdiːfɔːˈmeɪʃ(ə)n] *subst.* becoming deformed *deformitet, missbildning;* **the later stages of the disease are marked by bone deformation**

deformed [dɪˈfɔːmd] *adj.* not shaped or formed in a normal way *deformerad, missbildad*

deformerad ⇨ **deformed**

deformitet ⇨ **deformation, deformity**

deformity [dɪˈfɔːməti] *subst.* abnormal shape of part of the body *deformitet, missbildning*

degenerate [dɪˈdʒenəreɪt] *vb.* to change so as not to be able to function *degenerera;* **his brain degenerated so much that he was incapable of looking after himself**

degeneration [dɪˌdʒenəˈreɪʃ(ə)n] *subst.* change in the structure of a cell *or* organ so that it no longer works properly *degeneration;* **adipose degeneration** *or* **fatty degeneration** = accumulation of fat in the cells of an organ (such as the heart *or* liver), making the organ less able to perform *degeneratio adiposa, fettdegeneration;* **calcareous degeneration** = deposits of calcium which form at joints in old age *förkalkning, kalkinlagring;* **fibroid degeneration** = change of normal tissue to fibrous tissue (as in cirrhosis of the liver) *fibrös degeneration, fibros, bindvävsvandling*

degenerationsprodukt ⇨ **detritus**

degenerative [dɪˈdʒen(ə)rətɪv, -nəreɪt-] *adj.* (disease) where a part of the body stops functioning *or* functions abnormally *degenerativ*

degenerera ⇨ **degenerate**

deglutition [ˌdiːgluˈtɪʃ(ə)n] *or* **swallowing** [ˈswɒləʊɪŋ] *subst.* action of passing food *or* liquid (sometimes also air) from the mouth into the oesophagus *deglutition, sväljning*

degree [dɪˈgriː] *subst.* **(a)** *(in science)* part of a series of measurements *grad;* **a circle has 360°; the temperature is only 20° Celsius**
NOTE: the word **degree** is written ° after figures: **40 ° C**: say: 'forty degrees Celsius' **(b)** title given by a university or college to a person who has successfully completed a course of studies *grad, examen;* **he has a medical degree from London University; she was awarded a first-class degree in pharmacy** **(c)** level of how important *or* serious something is *grad, mån, nivå;* **to a minor degree** = in a small way *i liten utsträckning (mån);* **degree of burn** = the amount of damage done to the skin and tissue by heat *or* radiation *grad av brännskada;* **first degree burn** = burn where the skin turns red because the epidermis has been affected *combustio erythematosa, första gradens brännskada;* **second degree burn** = burn where the skin becomes very red and blisters *combustio bullosa, andra gradens brännskada;* **third degree burn** = burn where both the epidermis and dermis are destroyed, and a skin graft will be required to repair the damage *necrosis, tredje gradens brännskada*
NOTE: degrees of burn are no longer used officially: burns are now classified into two categories as 'deep burns' and 'superficial burns'

dehiscence [dɪˈhɪs(ə)ns] *subst.* opening wide *öppnande;* **wound dehiscence** = splitting open of a surgical incision *debridering (av sår)*

dehydrate [diːˈhaɪdreɪt] *vb.* to lose water *dehydrera, torka (ut);* **after two days without food or drink, he became dehydrated**

> COMMENT: water is more essential than food for a human being's survival. If someone drinks during the day less liquid than is passed out of the body in urine and sweat, he begins to dehydrate

dehydration [ˌdiːhaɪˈdreɪʃ(ə)n] *subst.* loss of water *dehydrering, uttorkning*

> QUOTE an estimated 60-70% of diarrhoeal deaths are caused by dehydration
> **Indian Journal of Medical Sciences**

dehydrera ⇨ **dehydrate**

dehydrering ⇨ **dehydration**

déjà vu [ˌdeɪʒɑː ˈvuː] *subst.* illusion that a new situation is a previous one being repeated, usually caused by a disease of the brain *déjà vu*

dekalcifiering ⇨ **decalcification**

dekompensation ⇨ **decompensation**

dekomposition ⇨ **decomposition**

dekortikering ⇨ **pleurectomy, decortication**

dekubitalsår ⇨ **bedsore**

dekubitus ⇨ **decubitus, pressure**

dekubitusmadrass, säng med ⇨ **ripple bed**

del ⇨ **pars, part, section**

dela ⇨ **split**

Delhi boil ['deli ˌbɔɪl] *subst.* cutaneous Leishmaniasis, a tropical skin disease caused by the parasite Leishmania *leishmaniasis cutanea, orientböld*

delhudstransplantat ⇨ **split-skin graft**

delicate ['delɪkət] *adj.* (i) easily broken *or* harmed *skör, spröd, gracil;* (ii) easily falling ill *klen, ömtålig;* **the bones of a baby's skull are very delicate; the eye is covered by a delicate membrane; the surgeons carried out a delicate operation to join the severed nerves; his delicate state of health means that he is not able to work long hours**

delirious [dɪ'lɪriəs] *adj.* suffering from delirium *deliriös*

> COMMENT: a person can become delirious because of shock, fear, drugs or fever

delirium [dɪ'lɪriəm] *subst.* mental state where the patient is confused, excited, restless and has hallucinations *delirium;* **delirium tremens (DTs)** *or* **delirium alcoholicum** = state of mental disturbance, especially including hallucinations about insects, trembling and excitement, usually found in chronic alcoholics who attempt to give up alcohol consumption *delirium tremens*

deliver [dɪ'lɪvə] *vb.* to bring something to someone *lämna (fram, över), leverera;* **to deliver a baby** = to help a mother in childbirth *förlösa ett barn;* **the twins were delivered by the midwife**

delivery [dɪ'lɪv(ə)ri] *subst.* birth of a child *förlossning, nedkomst;* **the delivery went very smoothly; breech delivery** = birth where the baby's buttocks appear first *sätesförlossning;* **face delivery** = birth where the baby's face appears first *ansiktsbjudning;* **forceps delivery** *or* **instrumental delivery** = childbirth where the doctor uses forceps to help the baby out of the mother's womb *tångförlossning;* **vertex delivery** = normal birth, where the baby's head appears first *huvudbjudning, kronbjudning, hjässbjudning;* **delivery bed** = special bed on which a mother lies to give birth *förlossningssäng*

delning ⇨ **cleavage, division, fission**

"delning" ⇨ **administration**

delprotes ⇨ **denture**

deltaga ⇨ **attend**

deltamuskeln ⇨ **deltoid (muscle)**

deltoid (muscle) ['deltɔɪd (ˌmʌs(ə)l)] *subst.* big triangular muscle covering the shoulder joint and attached to the humerus, which lifts the arm sideways *musculus deltoideus, deltamuskeln;* **deltoid tuberosity** = raised part of the humerus to which the deltoid muscle is attached *tuberositas deltoidea*

delusion [dɪ'lu:ʒ(ə)n] *subst.* false belief which a person holds which cannot be changed by reason *vanföreställning;* **he suffered from the delusion that he was wanted by the police**

delvis ⇨ **partial, partially, partly**

demens ⇨ **dementia**

dement ⇨ **dementing**

dementia [dɪ'menʃə] *subst.* loss of mental ability and memory, causing disorientation and personality changes, due to organic disease of the brain *demens;* **presenile dementia** = form of mental degeneration affecting adults *presenil demens;* **senile dementia** = form of mental degeneration affecting old people *senil demens, senilitet;* **dementia paralytica** = general paralysis of the insane, a serious condition marking the final stages of syphilis *dementia paralytica;* **dementia praecox** = formerly the name given to schizophrenia *dementia praecox, schizofreni*

dementing [dɪ'mentɪŋ] *adj.* (patient) suffering from dementia *dement*

demografi ⇨ **demography**

demografisk ⇨ **demographic**

demographic [ˌdemə'græfɪk] *adj.* referring to demography *demografisk;* **demographic forecasts** = forecasts of the numbers of people of different ages and sexes in an area at some time in the future *demografiska prognoser (förutsägelser)*

demography [di'mɒgrəfi] *subst.* study of populations and environments *or* changes affecting populations *demografi*

demonstrate ['demənstreɪt] *vb.* to show how something is done *or* is used *demonstrera,* *visa;* **the surgeon demonstrated how to make the incision** *or* **demonstrated the incision**

demonstrator ['demənstreɪtə] *subst.* person who demonstrates, especially in a laboratory *or* surgical department *ung. amanuens*

demonstrera ⇨ **demonstrate**

demulcent [dɪ'mʌls(ə)nt] *subst.* soothing substance which relieves irritation in the stomach *lenande medel*

demyelination [ˌdiːˌma(ɪ)əlɪ'neɪʃ(ə)n] *or* **demyelinating** [diː'ma(ɪ)əlɪneɪtɪŋ] *subst.* destruction of the myelin sheath round nerve fibres *demyelinisering*

COMMENT: can be caused by injury to the head, or is the main result of multiple sclerosis

demyelinisering ⇨ **demyelination**

denatured alcohol [diː'neɪtʃəd ˌælkəhɒl] *see* ALCOHOL

dendrite ['dendraɪt] *subst.* branched process of a nerve cell, which receives impulses from nerve endings of axons of other neurones at synapses ⇨ *illustration* NEURONE *dendrit*

dendritic [den'drɪtɪk] *adj.* referring to a dendrite *dendritisk;* **dendritic ulcer** = branching ulcer on the cornea, caused by herpesvirus *ceratitis dendritica (herpetica); see also* AXODENDRITE

denervation [ˌdiːnə'veɪʃ(ə)n] *subst.* stopping *or* cutting of the nerve supply to a part of the body *denervation, denervering*

denervering ⇨ **denervation**

dengue ['deŋgi] *or* **breakbone fever** ['breɪkbəʊn ˌfiːvə] *subst.* tropical disease caused by an arbovirus, transmitted by mosquitoes, where the patient suffers a high fever, pains in the joints, headache and rash *denguefeber, sjudagarsfeber, dandyfeber*

denguefeber ⇨ **dengue**

Denis Browne splint [ˌdenɪs 'braʊn ˌsplɪnt] *subst.* metal splint used to correct a club foot *slags metallskena för korrigering av klumpfot*

dens [dens] *subst.* tooth *dens, tand;* something shaped like a tooth *tandliknande struktur*

dense [dens] *adj.* compact *or* tightly pressed together *tät, kompakt;* **dense bone** = type of bone tissue which forms the hard outer layer of a bone *pars compacta, kompakt ben(vävnad)*

dental ['dent(ə)l] *adj.* referring to teeth *or* to a dentist *dental, tand-, tandläkar-;* **dental auxiliary** = person who helps a dentist *ung. tandsköterska;* **dental care** = looking after teeth *tandvård;* **dental caries** *or* **dental decay** = rotting of a tooth *karies(angrepp), tandröta;* **dental cyst** = cyst near the root of a tooth *dentalcysta, cysta nära tandrot;* **dental floss** = soft thread used to clean between the teeth *tandtråd;* **dental hygienist** = qualified assistant who cleans teeth and gums *tandhygienist;* **dental plaque** = hard smooth bacterial deposit on teeth, which is the probable cause of caries *plack, tandbeläggning;* **dental practice** = office and patients of a dentist *tandläkarpraktik, tandläkarmottagning;* **dental pulp** = soft tissue inside a tooth *pulpa, tandpulpa;* **dental surgeon** = dentist *or* qualified doctor who practises surgery on teeth *tandläkare;* **dental surgery** = (i) office and operating room of a dentist *tandläkarpraktik, tandläkarmottagning;* (ii) surgery carried out on teeth *tandkirurgi;* **dental technician** = person who makes dentures *tandtekniker*

dentalcysta ⇨ **dental**

dentifrice ['dentɪfrɪs] *subst.* paste *or* powder used with a toothbrush to clean teeth *dentifricium, tandkräm, tandpulver*

dentine ['dentiːn] *subst.* hard substance which surrounds the pulp of teeth, beneath the enamel ⇨ *illustration* TOOTH *dentin, tandben*

dentist ['dentɪst] *subst.* trained doctor who looks after teeth and gums *tandläkare;* **I must go to the dentist - I've got toothache; she had to wait for an hour at the dentist's; I hate going to see the dentist**

dentistry ['dentɪstri] *subst.* profession of a dentist *or* branch of medicine dealing with teeth and gums *tandläkaryrket, odontologi*

dentition [den'tɪʃ(ə)n] *subst.* number, arrangement and special characteristics of all the teeth in a person's jaws *tanduppsättning;* **adult** *or* **permanent dentition** = the thirty-two teeth which an adult has *permanenta tänderna;* **milk** *or* **deciduous dentition** = the twenty teeth which a child has, and which are gradually replaced by the permanent teeth *mjölktänderna*

denture ['den(t)ʃə] *subst.* set of false teeth, fixed to a plate which fits inside the mouth *tandprotes, tandgarnityr;* **partial denture** = part of a set of false teeth, replacing only a few teeth *delprotes*

COMMENT: children have incisors, canines and molars. These are replaced over a period of years by the permanent teeth, which are eight incisors, four canines, eight premolars and twelve molars (the last four molars being called the wisdom teeth)

deodorant [dɪ'əʊd(ə)r(ə)nt] *adj. & subst.* (substance) which hides *or* prevents unpleasant smells *deodorant*

deodorant ▷ **antiperspirant**

deoxygenate [ˌdiː'ɒksɪdʒəneɪt] *vb.* to remove oxygen *ta bort syre;* **deoxygenated blood** *or* **venous blood** = blood from which most of the oxygen has been removed by the tissues and is darker than arterial oxygenated blood *syrefattigt blod, venöst blod*

deoxyribonuclease [ˌdiːɒksɪˌraɪbəʊ'njuːkliːeɪz] *subst.* enzyme which breaks down DNA *de(s)oxyribonukleas*

deoxyribonucleic acid (DNA) [ˌdiːˌɒksɪˌraɪbəʊnjuːˌkliːɪk 'æsɪd (ˌdiːen'eɪ)] *subst.* one of the nucleic acids, the basic genetic material present in the nucleus of each cell *de(s)oxyribonukleinsyra, DNA; see also* RNA

departement ▷ **department**

department [dɪ'pɑːtmənt] *subst.* **(a)** part of a large organization (such as a hospital) *klinik;* **if you want treatment for that cut, you must go to the outpatients department; she is in charge of the physiotherapy department** **(b)** section of the British government *departement, ministerium;* **Department of Health and Social Security (DHSS)** = civil service department which is in charge of the National Health Service *ung. socialdepartementet*

dependant [dɪ'pend(ə)nt] *subst.* person who is looked after *or* supported by someone else *beroende person;* **he has to support a family of six children and several dependants**

dependence [dɪ'pend(ə)ns] *subst.* being dependent on *or* addicted to (a drug) *beroende, missbruk;* **drug dependence** = being addicted to a drug and unable to exist without taking it regularly *läkemedelsberoende, narkotikaberoende, drogberoende;* **physical drug dependence** = state where a person is addicted to a drug (such as heroin) and suffers physical effects if he stops or reduces the drug *fysiskt narkotikaberoende (läkemedelsberoende, drogberoende);* **psychological drug dependence** = state where a person is addicted to a drug (such as cannabis *or* alcohol) but suffers only mental effects if he stops taking it *psykiskt narkotikaberoende (läkemedelsberoende, drogberoende)*

dependent [dɪ'pend(ə)nt] *adj.* **(a)** (i) relying on (a person) *beroende;* (ii) addicted to (a drug) *beroende;* **he is physically dependent on amphetamines; dependent relative** = person who is looked after by another member of the family *person som är beroende (försörjd) av anhörig* **(b)** (part of the body) which is hanging down *nedhängande*

depend on [dɪ'pend ɒn] *vb.* **(a)** to be sure that something will happen *or* that someone will do something *bero på, vara beroende av;* **we depend on the nursing staff in the running of the hospital** **(b)** to rely on something *lita på;* he depends on drugs to relieve the pain *han måste ha (är beroende av) läkemedel för att bli av med smärtan;* the blood transfusion service depends on a large number of donors *blodverksamheten måste ha (är beroende av) ett stort antal givare*

depersonalization [diːˌpɜːs(ə)n(ə)laɪ'zeɪʃ(ə)n] *subst.* psychiatric state where the patient does not believe he is real *depersonalisation*

depilation [ˌdepɪ'leɪʃ(ə)n] *subst.* removal of hair *depilation, depilering, hårborttagning*

depilatory [dɪ'pɪlət(ə)ri, de'p-] *adj. & subst.* (substance) which removes hair *hårborttagnings(medel)*

depilering ▷ **depilation**

deplete [dɪ'pliːt] *vb.* (i) to exhaust the strength *or* the numbers of something *minska kraftigt, tömma;* (ii) to remove a component from a substance *förbruka, göra slut på;* **venous blood is depleted of oxygen by the tissues and returns to the lungs for oxygenation; our nursing staff has been depleted by illness, and the outpatients' unit has had to be closed**

depletion [dɪ'pliːʃ(ə)n] *subst.* being depleted *or* lacking something *förbrukning, förlust;* **salt depletion** = loss of salt from the body, by sweating or vomiting, which causes cramp *saltförlust, saltbrist*

depolarisation ▷ **depolarization**

depolarisering ▷ **depolarization**

depolarization [diːˌpəʊl(ə)raɪˈzeɪʃ(ə)n] *subst.* electrochemical reaction which takes place when an impulse travels along a nerve *depolarisation, depolarisering*

deposit [dɪˈpɒzɪt] **1** *subst.* substance which is attached to part of the body *avlagring, fällning;* **some foods leave a hard deposit on teeth; a deposit of fat forms on the walls of the arteries 2** *vb.* to attach a substance to part of the body *avsätta, avlagra, fälla ut;* **fat is deposited on the walls of the arteries**

depressant [dɪˈpres(ə)nt] *subst.* drug (such as a tranquillizer) which reduces the activity of part of the body *sedativum, lugnande medel, medel med nedsättande effekt;* **thyroid depressant** = drug which reduces the activity of the thyroid gland *tyreostatikum, antityreoid substans*

depressed [dɪˈprest] *adj.* feeling miserable and worried *deprimerad, nedstämd;* **he was depressed after his exam results; she was depressed for some weeks after the death of her husband**

depression [dɪˈpreʃ(ə)n] *subst.* **(a)** mental state where the patient feels miserable and hopeless *depression, nedstämdhet* **(b)** hollow on the surface of a part of the body *impression, fördjupning*

depressive [dɪˈpresɪv] *adj. & subst.* (substance) which causes mental depression *deprimerande, depressiv(t medel);* (state of) depression *deprimerat (tillstånd);* **he is in a depressive state; manic-depressive** = person suffering from a psychological condition where he moves from mania to depression *manisk-depressiv, maniodepressiv*

depressor [dɪˈpresə] *subst.* (i) muscle which pulls part of the body downwards *depressor;* (ii) nerve which inhibits the activity of an organ such as the heart and lowers the blood pressure *depressor;* **tongue depressor** = instrument, usually a thin piece of wood, used by a doctor to hold the patient's tongue down while his throat is being examined *tungspatel, spatel*

deprimerad ▷ **depressed**

deprimerande ▷ **depressive**

deprivation [ˌdeprɪˈveɪʃ(ə)n] *subst.* (i) needing something; (ii) loss of something which is needed *deprivation, förlust;* **maternal deprivation** = psychological condition caused when a child does not have a proper relationship with a mother *modersdeprivation*

deradenitis [dɪˌrædəˈnaɪtɪs] *subst.* inflammation of the lymph nodes in the neck *deradenit*

deranged [dɪˈreɪn(d)ʒd] *adj.* **mentally deranged** = suffering from a mental illness *sinnesrubbad, mentalsjuk, störd*

derangement [dɪˈreɪn(d)ʒmənt] *subst.* disorder *rubbning, störning;* **internal derangement of the knee (IDK)** = condition where the knee cannot function properly because of a torn meniscus *trasig menisk, meniskruptur*

Derbyshire neck [ˈdɑːbɪʃə ˌnek] *subst.* endemic goitre *or* form of goitre which was once widespread in Derbyshire *slags endemisk struma*

Dercum's disease [ˈdɜːkəmz dɪˌziːz] = ADIPOSIS DOLOROSA

derealisation ▷ **derealization**

derealization [diːˌrɪəlaɪˈzeɪʃ(ə)n] *subst.* psychological state where the patient feels the world around him is not real *derealisation*

derivat ▷ **derivative**

derivative [dɪˈrɪvətɪv] *subst.* substance which is derived from another substance *derivat;* **soap is a derivative of petroleum** *see also* PURIFIED

derive [dɪˈraɪv] *vb.* to start from *or* to come into existence from *härleda (sig), härröra, härstamma;* **compounds which derive from** *or* **are derived from sugar; the sublingual region has a rich supply of blood derived from the carotid artery**

derm- [ˈdɜːm, ˌ-] *prefix* referring to skin *derma(to)-, hud-*

dermal [ˈdɜːm(ə)l] *adj.* referring to the skin *dermal, hud-*

dermatitis [ˌdɜːməˈtaɪtɪs] *subst.* inflammation of the skin *dermatit, hudinflammation;* **contact dermatitis** = dermatitis caused by touching something (such as certain types of plant *or* soap) *kontaktdermatit, kontakteksem;* **eczematous dermatitis** = itchy inflammation *or* irritation of the skin due to an allergic reaction to a substance which a person has touched or absorbed *eksematös dermatit;* **exfoliative dermatitis** = typical form of dermatitis where the skin becomes red and comes off in flakes *dermatitis exfoliativa;* **occupational dermatitis** = dermatitis caused by materials touched at work *dermatitis professionalis, yrkesdermatit;* **dermatitis artefacta** = injuries to the skin caused by the patient himself *dermatitis artefacta;* **dermatitis herpetiformis** = type of dermatitis where large itchy blisters form on the skin *dermatitis herpetiformis*

> QUOTE various types of dermal reaction to nail varnish have been noted. Also contact dermatitis caused by cosmetics such as toothpaste, soap, shaving creams
>
> **Indian Journal of Medical Sciences**

dermatofyt ⇨ **dermatophyte**

dermatofytos ⇨ **dermatophytosis**

dermatoglyphics [ˌdɜːmətəʊˈglɪfɪks] *subst.* study which identifies congenital disease from the patterns of ridges on fingerprints, the palms of the hands and the soles of the feet *slags metod att fastställa medfödda sjukdomar utifrån fingeravtryck och mönster på handflator och fotsulor*

dermatographia [ˌdɜːmətəʊˈgreɪfiə] *subst.* swelling on the skin produced by pressing with a blunt instrument, usually an allergic reaction *derm(at)ografi*

dermatolog ⇨ **dermatologist**

dermatological [ˌdɜːmətəˈlɒdʒɪk(ə)l] *adj.* referring to dermatology *dermatologisk*

dermatologist [ˌdɜːməˈtɒlədʒɪst] *subst.* doctor who specializes in the study and treatment of the skin *dermatolog, hudspecialist*

dermatology [ˌdɜːməˈtɒlədʒi] *subst.* study and treatment of the skin and diseases of the skin *dermatologi*

dermatome [ˈdɜːmətəʊm] *subst.* **(a)** special knife used for cutting thin sections of skin for grafting *dermatom* **(b)** area of skin supplied by one spinal nerve *dermatom*

dermatomycosis [ˌdɜːmətəʊmaɪˈkəʊsɪs] *subst.* skin infections caused by a fungus *dermatomykos*

dermatomykos ⇨ **dermatomycosis**

dermatomyositis [ˌdɜːmətəʊˌmaɪəʊˈsaɪtɪs] *subst.* collagen disease with a wasting inflammation of the skin and muscles *dermatomy(os)it*

dermatophyte [ˈdɜːmətəʊfaɪt] *subst.* fungus which affects the skin *dermatofyt*

dermatophytosis [ˌdɜːmətəʊfaɪˈtəʊsɪs] *subst.* fungus infection of the skin *dermatofytos*

dermatoplastik ⇨ **dermatoplasty**

dermatoplasty [ˈdɜːmətəʊplæsti] *or* **skin graft** [ˈskɪn ˌgrɑːft] *subst.* replacing damaged skin by skin taken from another part of the body *or* from a donor *dermatoplastik, hudplastik*

dermatosis [ˌdɜːməˈtəʊsɪs] *subst.* any skin disease *dermatos, hudsjukdom*

dermatospasm ⇨ **goose flesh**

dermis [ˈdɜːmɪs] *or* **corium** [ˈkɔːriəm] *subst.* thick layer of living skin beneath the epidermis ⇨ *illustration* SKIN & SENSORY RECEPTORS *corium, korium, dermis, läderhuden*

dermoid [ˈdɜːmɔɪd] *adj.* referring to the skin *or* like skin *som avser, hör till el. liknar huden;* **dermoid cyst** = cyst found under the skin, usually in the midline, containing hair, sweat glands and sebaceous glands *dermoidcysta*

dermoidcysta ⇨ **dermoid**

desartikulering ⇨ **disarticulation**

Descemet's membrane [desəˈmeɪz ˌmembreɪn] *subst.* one of the deep layers of the cornea *lamina limitans interna, Descemets membran*

descend [dɪˈsend] *vb.* to go down *gå (komma, fara) ned;* **descending aorta** = second part of the aorta as it goes downwards after the aortic arch *aorta descendens;* **descending colon** = third section of the colon which goes down the left side of the body ⇨ *illustration* DIGESTIVE SYSTEM *colon descendens, nedåtgående delen av tjocktarmen;* **descending tract** = tract of nerves which take impulses away from the head *nervbana som leder impulser i riktning från hjärnan*

describe [dɪˈskraɪb] *vb.* to say or write what something *or* someone is like *beskriva, skildra;* **can you describe the symptoms? she described how her right leg suddenly became inflamed**

description [dɪˈskrɪpʃ(ə)n] *subst.* saying or writing what something *or* someone is like *beskrivning, skildring;* **the patient's description of the symptoms**

desensibilisera ⇨ **desensitize**

desensibilisering ⇨ **desensitization**

desensitization [ˌdiːˌsensətaɪˈzeɪʃ(ə)n] *subst.* (i) removal of sensitivity *desensibilisering;* (ii) treatment of an allergy by giving the patient injections of small quantities of the substance to which he is allergic over a period of time until he becomes immune to it *hyposensibilisering*

desensitize [diːˈsensətaɪz] *vb.* (i) to deaden a nerve *or* to remove sensitivity *göra okänslig (mindre känslig);* (ii) to treat a patient suffering from an allergy by giving graduated injections of the substance to which he is allergic over a period of time until he becomes immune to it *desensibilisera;* **the patient was prescribed a course of desensitizing injections**

desinfektion ⇨ **disinfection**

desinfektionsmedel ⇨ **disinfectant**

desinficera ⇨ **disinfect**

desinficering ⇨ **disinfection**

desintegration ⇨ **disintegration**

desintegreras ⇨ **disintegrate**

desire [dɪˈzaɪə] *subst.* wanting greatly to do something *begär, lust;* **he has a compulsive desire to steal**

deskvamation ⇨ **desquamation, ecdysis**

desorienterad ⇨ **disorientated**

desorientering ⇨ **disorientation**

desquamation [ˌdeskwəˈmeɪʃ(ə)n] *subst.* (i) continual process of losing the outer layer of dead skin *deskvamation, fjällning;* (ii) peeling off of the epithelial part of a structure *deskvamation*

destillera ⇨ **distil**

destillering ⇨ **distillation**

destroy [dɪˈstrɔɪ] *vb.* to ruin *or* kill completely *förstöra, döda, bryta ned;* **the nerve cells were destroyed by the infection**

destruction [dɪˈstrʌkʃ(ə)n] *subst.* ruining *or* killing of something completely *förstörelse, dödande, nedbrytning;* **the destruction of the tissue *or* the cells by infection; the destruction of bacteria by phagocytes**

detach [dɪˈtætʃ] *vb.* to separate one thing from another *avskilja, skilja, lösgöra;* **an operation to detach the cusps of the mitral valve; detached retina *or* retinal detachment** = condition where the retina is partially detached from the choroid *ablatio (amotio, solutio) retinae, näthinneavlossning*

> COMMENT: a detached retina can be caused by a blow to the eye, or simply is a condition occurring in old age; if left untreated the eye will become blind. A detached retina can sometimes be attached to the choroid again using lasers

detect [dɪˈtekt] *vb.* to sense *or* to notice (usually something which is very small or difficult to see) *upptäcka, spåra upp;* **an instrument to detect microscopic changes in cell structure; the nurses detected a slight improvement in the patient's condition**

detection [dɪˈtekʃ(ə)n] *subst.* action of detecting something *upptäckt;* **the detection of sounds by nerves in the ears; the detection of a cyst using an endoscope**

detergent [dɪˈtɜːdʒ(ə)nt] *subst.* cleaning substance which removes grease and bacteria *rengöringsmedel, tvättmedel, diskmedel*

> COMMENT: most detergents are not allergenic but some biological detergents which contain enzymes to remove protein stains, can cause dermatitis

deteriorate [dɪˈtɪərɪəreɪt] *vb.* to become worse *försämras;* **the patient's condition deteriorated rapidly**

deterioration [dɪˌtɪərɪəˈreɪʃ(ə)n] *subst.* becoming worse *försämring;* **the nurses were worried by the deterioration in the patient's mental state**

determine [dɪˈtɜːmɪn] *vb.* to find out something correctly *bestämma, fastställa, avgöra;* **health inspectors are trying to determine the cause of the outbreak of Salmonella poisoning**

detet ⇨ **id**

detoxication [ˌdiːˌtɒksɪˈkeɪʃ(ə)n] *or* **detoxification** [ˌdiːˌtɒksɪfɪˈkeɪʃ(ə)n] *subst.* removal of toxic substances to make a poisonous substance harmless *detoxifiering, avgiftning*

detoxifiering ⇨ **detoxication**

detrition [dɪ'trɪʃ(ə)n] *subst.* wearing away by rubbing or use *avnötning*

detritus [dɪ'traɪtəs] *subst.* rubbish produced when something disintegrates *detritus, degenerationsprodukt, avfallsprodukt*

detrusor muscle [dɪ'tru:zə ˌmʌs(ə)l] *subst.* muscular coat of the urinary bladder *musculus detrusor urinae, detrusormuskeln*

detumescence [ˌdi:tju'mes(ə)ns] *subst.* becoming limp (of penis or clitoris after an orgasm); going down (of a swelling) *detumescens*

deuteranopia [ˌdju:tərə'nəʊpiə] *subst.* form of colour blindness, a defect in vision, where the patient cannot see green *deuteranopi, grönblindhet; compare* DALTONISM, TRITANOPIA

develop [dɪ'veləp] *vb.* **(a)** to grow *or* make grow; to mature *utveckla(s);* **the embryo developed quite normally, in spite of the mother's illness; a swelling developed under the armpit; the sore throat developed into an attack of meningitis (b)** to start to get *få;* **she developed a cold; he developed complications and was rushed to hospital**

> QUOTE rheumatoid arthritis is a chronic inflammatory disease which can affect many systems in the body, but mainly the joints. 70% of sufferers develop the condition in the metacarpophalangeal joints
> **Nursing Times**

development [dɪ'veləpmənt] *subst.* thing which develops *or* is being developed; action of becoming mature *utveckling;* **the development of the embryo takes place in the uterus**

developmental [dɪˌveləp'ment(ə)l] *adj.* referring to the development of an embryo *utvecklings-*

deviance ['di:viəns] *subst.* abnormal sexual behaviour *sexuell avvikelse*

deviation [ˌdi:vɪ'eɪʃ(ə)n] *subst.* variation from normal; abnormal position of a joint *or* of the eye (such as strabismus) *deviation, avvikelse*

device [dɪ'vaɪs] *subst.* instrument *or* piece of equipment *anordning, apparat, medel;* **a device for weighing very small quantities of powder; he used a device for examining the interior of the ear**

Devic's disease [də'vɪks dɪˌzi:z] = NEUROMYELITIS OPTICA

dextro- ['dekstrəʊ, ˌ--] *prefix* referring to the right side of the body *or* to the right hand *dextro-, höger-*

dextrocardia [ˌdekstrəʊ'kɑ:diə] *subst.* congenital condition where the apex of the heart is towards the right of the body instead of the left *dextrokardi; compare* LAEVOCARDIA

dextrokardi ▷ **dextrocardia**

dextros ▷ **dextrose, glucose**

dextrose ['dekstrəʊs] *or* **glucose** ['glu:kəʊs] *subst.* simple sugar found in fruit, also broken down in the body from white sugar or carbohydrate and absorbed into the body or excreted by the kidneys *dextros, glukos, druvsocker*

DHA [ˌdi:eɪtʃ'eɪ] = DISTRICT HEALTH AUTHORITY

dhobie itch ['dəʊbi ɪtʃ] *subst.* contact dermatitis (believed to be caused by an allergy to the marking ink used by laundries) *slags kontaktdermatit (kontakteksem)*

DHSS [ˌdi:eɪtʃes'es] = DEPARTMENT OF HEALTH AND SOCIAL SECURITY

diabetes [ˌda(ɪ)ə'bi:ti:z] *subst.* one of a group of diseases, but most commonly used to refer to diabetes mellitus *diabetes;* **diabetes insipidus =** rare disease caused by a disorder of the pituitary gland, making the patient pass large quantities of urine and want to drink more than normal *diabetes insipidus;* **diabetes mellitus =** disease where the body cannot control sugar absorption because the pancreas does not secrete enough insulin *diabetes (mellitus), sockersjuka;* **bronze diabetes =** haemochromatosis *or* hereditary disease where the body absorbs and stores too much iron, giving a dark colour to the skin *hemosideros, hemokromatos, bronsdiabetes;* **gestational diabetes =** diabetes which develops in a pregnant woman *graviditetsdiabetes*

> COMMENT: symptoms of diabetes mellitus are tiredness, abnormal thirst, frequent passing of water and sweet smelling urine. Blood and urine tests will reveal high levels of sugar. Treatment involves keeping to a strict diet, and in some cases the patient needs regular injections of insulin

diabetes- ▷ **diabetic**

diabeteskoma ▷ **diabetic**

diabeteskost ▷ **diabetic**

diabetesretinopati ➪ **diabetic**

diabetic [ˌda(ɪ)əˈbetɪk] **1** *adj.* **(a)** referring to diabetes mellitus *diabetisk, diabetes-;* **diabetic coma** = state of unconsciousness caused by untreated diabetes *diabeteskoma;* **diabetic diet** = diet which is low in carbohydrates and sugar *diabeteskost;* **diabetic retinopathy** = defect in vision caused by diabetes *retinopathia diabetica, diabetesretinopati* **(b)** (food) which contains few carbohydrates and sugar *sockerfri;* **he bought some diabetic chocolate; she lives on diabetic soups** **2** *subst.* person suffering from diabetes *diabetiker*

diabetiker ➪ **diabetic**

diabetisk ➪ **diabetic**

diaclasia [ˌda(ɪ)əˈkleɪziə] *subst.* fracture made by a surgeon to repair an earlier fracture which has set badly *or* to correct a deformity *fraktur som (av ortoped) åstadkoms för att korrigera felläkning el. missbildning*

diadochokinesis [daɪˌædəkɒkaɪˈniːsɪs] *subst.* normal ability to make muscles move limbs in opposite directions *diadochokines(i), diadokokines(i)*

diafores ➪ **diaphoresis**

diaforetikum ➪ **diaphoretic**

diafragma ➪ **diaphragm, midriff**

diafragmabråck ➪ **diaphragmatic, hiatus**

diafragmaliknande ➪ **diaphragmatic**

diafys ➪ **diaphysis, mass, shaft**

diafysär ➪ **diaphyseal**

diagnos ➪ **diagnosis**

diagnose [ˈda(ɪ)əgnəʊz] *vb.* to identify a patient's condition *or* illness, by examining the patient and noting symptoms *diagnosticera, ställa diagnos;* **the doctor diagnosed appendicitis**

diagnosis [ˌda(ɪ)əgˈnəʊsɪs] *subst.* act of diagnosing a patient's condition *or* illness *diagnos;* **the doctor's diagnosis was cancer, but the patient asked for a second opinion; differential diagnosis** = identification of one particular disease from other similar diseases by comparing the range of symptoms of each *differentialdiagnos;* **antenatal** *or* **prenatal diagnosis** = medical examination of a pregnant woman to see if the fetus is developing normally *prenataldiagnostik, fosterdiagnostik* NOTE: plural is **diagnoses**

diagnostic [ˌda(ɪ)əgˈnɒstɪk] *adj.* referring to diagnosis *diagnostisk;* **diagnostic imaging** = scanning for the purpose of diagnosis, as of a pregnant woman to see if the fetus is healthy *visuell diagnostik, t.ex. röntgen, ultraljud, datortomografi;* **diagnostic process** = method of making a diagnosis *diagnostisk process (metod);* **diagnostic test** = test which helps a doctor diagnose an illness *diagnostiskt test (prov); compare* PROGNOSIS

diagnosticera ➪ **diagnose**

diagnostisk ➪ **diagnostic**

diagonal [daɪˈæg(ə)n(ə)l] *adj.* going across at an angle *diagonal*

diagonally [daɪˈæg(ə)n(ə)li] *adv.* crossing at an angle *diagonalt*

diagonalt ➪ **diagonally**

diagram [ˈda(ɪ)əgræm] *subst.* chart *or* drawing which records information as lines or points *diagram, kurva, figur;* **the book gives a diagram of the circulation of blood; the diagram shows the occurrence of cancer in the southern part of the town**

diagram ➪ **chart, graph**

dialys ➪ **dialysis**

dialysapparat ➪ **dialyser, kidney**

dialyser [ˈda(ɪ)əlaɪzə] *subst.* apparatus which uses a membrane to separate solids from liquids, especially a kidney machine *dialysapparat*

dialysis [daɪˈæləsɪs] *subst.* using a membrane as a filter to separate soluble waste substances from the blood *dialys;* **kidney dialysis** *or* **haemodialysis** = removing waste matter from a patient's blood by passing it through a kidney machine *or* dialyser *hemodialys, HD;* **peritoneal dialysis** = removing waste matter from the blood by introducing fluid into the peritoneum which then acts as the filter membrane *peritonealdialys, PD*

diameter [daɪˈæmɪtə] *subst.* distance across a circle (such as a tube *or* blood vessel) *diameter;* **they measured the diameter of the pelvic girdle**

diapedesis [ˌda(ɪ)əpɪˈdiːsɪs] *subst.* movement of white blood cells through the walls of the capillaries into tissues in inflammation *diapedes*

diaper ['da(ɪ)əpə] *subst. US* cloth used to wrap round a baby's bottom and groin, to keep clothing clean and dry *blöja;* **diaper rash** = sore red skin on a baby's buttocks and groin, caused by long contact with ammonia in a wet diaper *blöjdermatit, blöjeksem*
NOTE: GB English is **nappy**

diaphoresis [ˌda(ɪ)əfə'riːsɪs] *subst.* excessive perspiration *diafores, svettning*

diaphoretic [ˌda(ɪ)əfə'retɪk] *adj.* (drug) which causes sweating *diaforetikum, svettdrivande (medel)*

diaphragm ['da(ɪ)əfræm, -frəm] *subst.* **(a)** thin layer of tissue stretched across an opening, especially the flexible sheet of muscle and fibre which separates the chest from the abdomen, and moves to pull air into the lungs in respiration *diafragma, skiljevägg, mellangärdet;* **pelvic diaphragm** = sheet of muscle between the pelvic cavity and the peritoneum *diaphragma pelvis;* **urogenital diaphragm** = fibrous layer beneath the prostate gland through which the urethra passes *diaphragma urogenitalis* **(b) vaginal diaphragm** = circular contraceptive device for women, which is inserted into the vagina and placed over the neck of the uterus before sexual intercourse *pessar, slidpessar*

COMMENT: the diaphragm is a muscle which in breathing expands and contracts with the walls of the chest. The normal rate of respiration is about 16 times a minute

diaphragmatic [ˌda(ɪ)əfræg'mætɪk] *adj.* referring to a diaphragm *som avser el. hör till skiljevägg;* like a diaphragm *diafragmaliknande, skiljeväggsliknande;* **diaphragmatic hernia** = condition where a membrane and organ in the abdomen pass through an opening in the diaphragm into the chest *hernia diaphragmatica, hiatusbråck, diafragmabråck;* **diaphragmatic pleura** = part of the pleura which covers the diaphragm *pleura diapragmatica;* **diaphragmatic pleurisy** = inflammation of the pleura which covers the diaphragm *inflammation i lungsäcken, vätska i lungsäcken;* **diaphragmatic surface of pleura** = surface of the pleura which is in direct contact with the diaphragm *den lungsäcksyta som har direkt kontakt med mellangärdet*

diaphyseal [ˌda(ɪ)ə'fɪziəl] *adj.* referring to a diaphysis *diafysär*

diaphysis [daɪ'æfəsɪs] *subst.* shaft *or* long central part of a long bone *diafys, skaft;* *compare* EPIPHYSIS, METAPHYSIS ⇨ *illustration* BONE STRUCTURE

diaphysitis [ˌda(ɪ)əfə'zaɪtɪs] *subst.* inflammation of the diaphysis, often associated with rheumatic disease *inflammation i diafys (rörbens skaft)*

diarré ⇨ **diarrhoea**

diarré, vattnig ⇨ **ricewater stools**

diarrhoea [ˌda(ɪ)ə'rɪə] *or US* **diarrhea** [ˌda(ɪ)ə'rɪə] *subst.* condition where a patient frequently passes liquid faeces *diarré;* **he had an attack of diarrhoea after going to the restaurant; she complained of mild diarrhoea**

COMMENT: diarrhoea can have many causes: types of food or allergy to food; contaminated or poisoned food; infectious diseases, such as dysentery; sometimes worry or other emotions

diarrhoeal [ˌda(ɪ)ə'riːəl] *adj.* referring to *or* caused by diarrhoea *diarroisk*

diarroisk ⇨ **diarrhoeal**

diarthrosis [ˌdaɪɑː'θrəʊsɪs] *or* **synovial joint** [sɪ'nəʊviəl ˌdʒɔɪnt] *subst.* joint which moves freely in any direction ⇨ *illustration* JOINTS *diart(h)ros*

diastase ['da(ɪ)əsteɪs] *subst.* enzyme which breaks down starch and converts it into sugar *amylas*

diastasis [daɪə'steɪsɪs] *subst.* (i) condition where a bone separates into parts *diastas;* (ii) dislocation of bones at an immovable joint *diastas*

diastole [daɪ'æstəli] *subst.* phase in the beating of the heart between two contractions, where the heart dilates and fills with blood *diastole, utvidgning(sfas);* **the period of diastole lasts about 0.4 seconds in a normal heart rate**

diastolic pressure [ˌdaɪə'stɒlɪk ˌpreʃə] *subst.* blood pressure taken at the diastole *diastoliskt (blod)tryck; compare* SYSTOLE, SYSTOLIC

COMMENT: diastolic pressure is always lower than systolic

diatermi ⇨ **diathermy, electrocoagulation, electrodessication, electrolysis, galvanocautery, thermocoagulation**

diatermislynga ⇨ **snare**

diatermistift ⇨ **diathermy**

diates ⇨ **diathesis**

diathermy [ˌdaɪə'θɜːmi] *subst.* using high frequency electric current to produce heat in body tissue *diatermi;* **medical diathermy** = using heat produced by electricity for treatment of muscle and joint disorders (such as rheumatism) *medicinsk diatermi;* **surgical diathermy** = using a knife *or* electrode which is heated by a strong electric current until it coagulates tissue *kirurgisk diatermi;* **diathermy knife** *or* **diathermy needle** = instrument used in surgical diathermy *diatermistift*

> COMMENT: the difference between medical and surgical uses of diathermy is in the size of the electrodes used. Two large electrodes will give a warming effect over a large area (medical diathermy); if one of the electrodes is small, the heat will be concentrated enough to coagulate tissue (surgical diathermy)

diathesis [daɪ'æθəsɪs] *subst.* general inherited constitution of a person, with his susceptibility to certain diseases *or* allergies *diates, anlag, läggning*

DIC ⇨ **crush syndrome**

dichlorodiphenyltrichloroethane (DDT) 'eθeɪn (ˌdiːdiː'tiː)] *subst.* pesticide, formerly commonly used, but now believed to be poisonous to other animals *dikloridifenyltriklormetylmetan, DDT*

dichromatic [ˌdaɪkrəʊ'mætɪk] *adj.* seeing only two of the three primary colours *dikromatisk; compare* TRICHROMATIC

Dick test ['dɪk ˌtest] *subst.* test to show if a patient is immune to scarlet fever *slags prov för att undersöka immunitet mot scharlakansfeber*

dicrotic pulse [daɪ'krɒtɪk ˌpʌls] *or* **dicrotic wave** [daɪ'krɒtɪk ˌweɪv] *subst.* pulse which beats twice *dikronisk puls, puls med dubbelslag*

dicrotism ['daɪkrətɪz(ə)m] *subst.* condition where the pulse dilates twice with each heartbeat *dikroti(sm), dubbelslag*

didelphys [daɪ'delfɪs] *subst.* **uterus didelphys** = double uterus *or* condition where the uterus is divided in two by a membrane *uterus didelphys, dubbel livmoder*

die [daɪ] **1** *subst.* cast of the patient's mouth taken by a dentist before making a denture *avtryck* **2** *vb.* to stop living *dö, avlida, omkomma;* **his father died last year; she died in a car crash**
NOTE: **dies - dying - died - has died**

diencefalon ⇨ **diencephalon, thalamencephalon**

diencephalon [ˌdaɪen'sefəlɒn, ˌdaɪen'kefəlɒn] *subst.* central part of the forebrain, formed of the thalamus, hypothalamus, pineal gland and third ventricle *diencefalon, thalamencephalon, mellanhjärnan*

diet ['daɪət] **1** *subst.* (i) amount and type of food eaten *föda, kost;* (ii) measured amount of food eaten, usually to try to lose weight *diet;* **he lives on a diet of bread and beer; the doctor asked her to follow a strict diet; he has been on a diet for some weeks, but still hasn't lost enough weight; diet sheet** = list of suggestions for quantities and types of food given to a patient to follow *dietlista;* **balanced diet** = diet which contains the right quantities of basic nutrients *balanserad kost (diet);* **bland diet** = diet in which the patient eats mainly milk-based foods, boiled vegetables and white meat, as a treatment for peptic ulcers *skonkost;* **diabetic diet** = diet which is low in carbohydrates and sugar *diabeteskost;* **low-calorie diet** = diet which provides less than the normal number of calories *kalorifattig kost;* **salt-free diet** = diet which does not contain salt *saltfattig kost* **2** *vb.* to reduce the quantity of food eaten *or* to change the type of food eaten in order to become thinner *or* healthier *följa (hålla) diet, banta;* **she dieted for two weeks before going on holiday; he is dieting to try to lose weight**

diet- ⇨ **dietary, dietetic**

dietary ['daɪət(ə)ri] **1** *subst.* system of nutrition and energy *mathållning, kosthåll;* **the nutritionist supervised the dietaries for the patients 2** *adj.* referring to a diet *diet-, kost-;* **dietary fibre** *or* **roughage** = fibrous matter in food, which cannot be digested *fibrer, kostfibrer*

> COMMENT: dietary fibre is found in cereals, nuts, fruit and some green vegetables. It is believed to be necessary to help digestion and avoid developing constipation, obesity and appendicitis

dietetic [ˌda(ɪ)ə'tetɪk] *adj.* referring to diet *diet-, kost-;* **dietetic principles** = rules concerning the body's needs in food *or* vitamins *or* trace elements *kostprinciper*

dietetics [ˌda(ɪ)əˈtetɪks] *subst.* study of food, nutrition and health, especially when applied to the food intake *die(te)tik*

dieting [ˈda(ɪ)ətɪŋ] *subst.* attempting to reduce weight by reducing the amount of food eaten *bantning*

dietist ⇨ **dietitian, nutritionist**

dietitian [ˌda(ɪ)əˈtɪʃ(ə)n] *subst.* person who specializes in the study of diet, especially an officer in a hospital who supervises dietaries as part of the medical treatment of patients *dietist*

dietlista ⇨ **diet**

Dietl's crisis [ˈdiːt(ə)lz ˌkraɪsɪs] *subst.* painful blockage of the ureter, causing back pressure on the kidney which fills with urine, and swells *slags stopp i uretär*

diff ⇨ **differential**

difference [ˈdɪfr(ə)ns] *subst.* way in which two things are not the same *skillnad, olikhet;* **can you tell the difference between butter and margarine?**

different [ˈdɪfr(ə)nt] *adj.* not the same *olik;* **living in the country is very different from living in the town; he looks quite different since he had the operation**

differential [ˌdɪf(ə)ˈrenʃ(ə)l] *adj.* referring to a difference *differential-;* **differential diagnosis** = identification of one particular disease from other similar diseases by comparing the range of symptoms of each *differentialdiagnos;* **differential blood count** *or* **differential white cell count** = showing the amounts of different types of (white) blood cell in a blood sample *differentialräkning, diff*

differentialdiagnos ⇨ **diagnosis, differential**

differentialräkning ⇨ **differential**

differentiate [ˌdɪf(ə)ˈrenʃɪeɪt] *vb.* to tell the difference between *differentiera, särskilja;* to be different from *skilja sig, vara olik;* **the tumour is clearly differentiated** = the tumour can be easily identified from the surrounding tissue *tumören är klart differentierad*

differentiation [ˌdɪf(ə)renʃɪˈeɪʃ(ə)n] *subst.* development of specialized cells during the early embryo stage *differentiering*

differentiera ⇨ **differentiate**

differentiering ⇨ **differentiation**

difficult [ˈdɪfɪk(ə)lt] *adj.* hard to do *or* not easy *svår, besvärlig;* **the practical examination was very difficult - half the students failed; the heart-lung transplant is a particularly difficult operation; the doctor had to use forceps because the childbirth was difficult**

difficulty [ˈdɪfɪk(ə)lti] *subst.* problem *or* thing which is not easy *svårighet;* **she has difficulty in breathing** *or* **in getting enough vitamins**

diffundera ⇨ **diffuse**

diffus ⇨ **diffuse**

diffuse [dɪˈfjuːz; dɪˈfjuːs] **1** *vb.* to spread through tissue *diffundera;* **some substances easily diffuse through the walls of capillaries** **2** *adj.* (disease) which is widespread in the body *or* which affects many organs *or* cells *diffus, utbredd*

diffusion [dɪˈfjuːʒ(ə)n] *subst.* (i) mixing a liquid with another liquid or a gas with another gas *diffusion;* (ii) passing of a liquid *or* gas through a membrane *diffusion*

difteri ⇨ **croup, diphtheria**

difteribacillen ⇨ **Klebs-Loeffler bacillus**

difteriliknande ⇨ **diphtheroid**

difteroid ⇨ **diphtheroid**

digerdöden ⇨ **black, bubonic plague**

digest [daɪˈdʒest, dɪˈdʒest] *vb.* to break down food in the alimentary tract and convert it into elements which are absorbed into the body *smälta (mat)*

digestible [daɪˈdʒestəb(ə)l, dɪˈdʒestəb(ə)l] *adj.* which can be digested *som kan smältas (brytas ned);* **glucose is an easily digestible form of sugar**

digestion [daɪˈdʒestʃ(ə)n, dɪˈdʒestʃ(ə)n] *subst.* process by which food is broken down in the alimentary tract into elements which can be absorbed by the body *digestion, matspjälkning*

digestionskanalen ⇨ **alimentary canal, digestive, food**

digestionssystemet ⇨ **digestive**

digestive [daɪˈdʒestɪv, dɪˈdʒestɪv] *adj.* referring to digestion *digestiv,* *matspjälknings-;* **digestive enzymes** = enzymes which encourage digestion *matspjälkningsenzymer;* **digestive system** = all the organs in the body (such as the liver and pancreas) which are associated with the digestion of food *digestionssystemet, matspjälkningsapparaten;* **digestive tract** *or* **alimentary tract** = passage from the mouth to the rectum, down which food passes and is digested *canalis alimentarius, digestionskanalen, magtarmkanalen*

COMMENT: the digestive tract is formed of the mouth, throat, oesophagus stomach and small and large intestines. Food is broken down by digestive juices in the mouth, stomach and small intestine, water is removed in the large intestine, and the remaining matter is passed out of the body as faeces

digit ['dɪdʒɪt] *subst.* **(a)** a finger *or* a toe *digitus, finger, tå* **(b)** a number *siffra*

digital ['dɪdʒɪt(ə)l] *adj.* **(a)** referring to fingers *or* toes *digital, finger-, tå-;* **digital veins** = veins draining the fingers *or* toes *venae digitales* **(b) digital computer** = computer which calculates on the basis of numbers *digital dator*

digitalis [ˌdɪdʒɪ'teɪlɪs, ˌdɪdʒɪ'tælɪs] *subst.* poisonous drug extracted from the foxglove plant, used in small doses to treat heart conditions *digitalis*

digitus ⇨ **digit, finger**

digivning ⇨ **lactation**

dikloridifenyltriklormetylmetan ⇨ **dichlorodiphenyltrichloroethane (DDT)**

dikromatisk ⇨ **dichromatic**

dilatation [ˌdaɪleɪ'teɪʃ(ə)n] *or* **dilation** [daɪ'leɪʃ(ə)n, dɪ'leɪʃ(ə)n] *subst.* (i) expansion of a hollow space *or* a passage in the body *dilatation, utvidgning;* (ii) expansion of the pupil of the eye as a reaction to bad light *or* to drugs *pupilldilatation, pupillvidgning;* **dilatation and curettage (D & C)** = surgical operation to scrape the interior of the uterus to obtain a tissue sample *or* to remove a cyst *abrasio mucosae uteri, abrasio, skrapning*

dilatation ⇨ **dilatation, ectasia**

dilatator ⇨ **dilator, divulsor**

dilate [daɪ'leɪt, dɪ'leɪt] *vb.* to swell *dilatera, utvidgas;* **the veins in the left leg have become dilated; the drug is used to dilate the pupil of the eye**

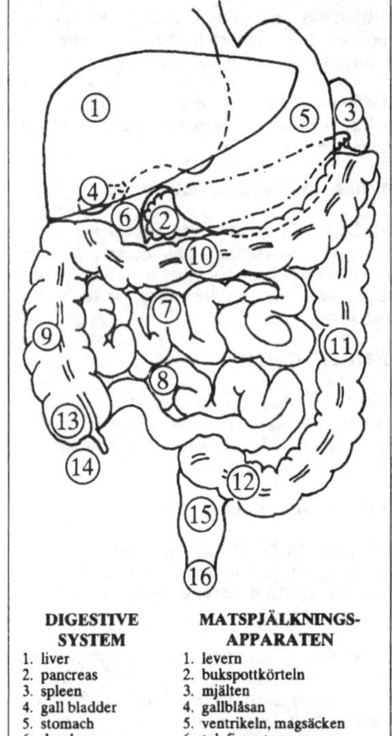

DIGESTIVE SYSTEM	MATSPJÄLKNINGS-APPARATEN
1. liver	1. levern
2. pancreas	2. bukspottkörteln
3. spleen	3. mjälten
4. gall bladder	4. gallblåsan
5. stomach	5. ventrikeln, magsäcken
6. duodenum	6. tolvfingertarmen, tunntarmens första del
7. jejunum	7. tomtarmen, tunntarmens mellersta del
8. ileum	8. ileum, tunntarmens sista del
9. ascending colon	9. uppåtstigande (delen av) tjocktarmen
10. transverse colon	10. tvärgående (delen av) tjocktarmen
11. descending colon	11. nedåtgående (delen av) tjocktarmen
12. sigmoid colon	12. sigmoideum, sigmaformade (delen av) tjocktarmen
13. caecum	13. blindtarmen
14. appendix	14. blindtarmens maskformiga bihang, "blindtarmen"
15. rectum	15. ändtarmen
16. anus	16. analöppningen

dilatera ⇨ **dilate**

dilator [daɪ'leɪtə, dɪ'leɪtə] *subst.* (i) instrument used to widen the entrance to a cavity *dilatator, dilator, stift;* (ii) drug used to make part of the body expand *dilaterande medel;* **dilator pupillae muscle** = muscle in the iris which pulls the iris back and so dilates the pupil *musculus dilatator pupillae*

diluent ['dɪljuənt] *subst.* substance (such as water) which is used to dilute a liquid *utspädningsmedel, förtunningsmedel*

dilute [daɪ'lu:t, dɪ'lu:t] **1** *adj.* with water added *utspädd;* **bathe the wound in a solution of dilute antiseptic 2** *vb.* to add water to a liquid to make it weaker *späda ut;* **the disinfectant must be diluted in four parts of water before it can be used on the skin**

dilution [daɪ'lu:ʃ(ə)n, dɪ'lu:ʃ(ə)n] *subst.* (i) action of diluting *dilution, utspädning, spädning;* (ii) liquid which has been diluted *dilution, lösning*

dimetria [daɪ'mi:triə] *subst.* condition where a woman has a double uterus *uterus didelphys, dubbel livmoder; see also* DIDELPHYS

dimma ⇨ **vapour**

dioptre [daɪ'ɒptə] *or US* **diopter** [daɪ'ɒptə] *subst.* unit of measurement of refraction of a lens *dioptri*

> COMMENT: a one dioptre lens has a focal length of one metre; the greater the dioptre, the shorter the focal length

dioptri ⇨ **dioptre**

dioxide [daɪ'ɒksaɪd] *see* CARBON

diphtheria [dɪf'θɪəriə] *subst.* serious infectious disease of children, caused by the bacillus **Corynebacterium diphtheriae,** with fever and the formation of a fibrous growth like a membrane in the throat which restricts breathing *difteri*

> COMMENT: symptoms of diphtheria begin usually with a sore throat, followed by a slight fever, rapid pulse and swelling of glands in the neck. The "membrane" which forms can close the air passages, and the disease is often fatal, either because the patient is asphyxiated or because the heart becomes fatally weakened. The disease is also highly infectious, and all contacts of the patient must be tested. The Schick test is used to test if a person is immune or susceptible to diphtheria

diphtheroid ['dɪfθərɔɪd] *adj.* (bacterium) like the diphtheria bacterium *difteroid, difteriliknande*

dipl- ['dɪpl, ˌ-] *or* **diplo-** ['dɪpləʊ, ˌ--] *prefix* meaning double *dipl(o)-, dubbel-*

diplacusis [ˌdɪplə'kju:sɪs] *subst.* (i) condition where a patient hears double sounds *diplakusi;* (ii) condition where a patient hears the same sound in a different way in each ear *diplakusi*

diplakusi ⇨ **diplacusis**

diplegi ⇨ **diplegia**

diplegia [daɪ'pli:dʒə] *subst.* paralysis of a similar part on both sides of the body (such as both arms) *diplegi, dubbelsidig förlamning*

diplegic [daɪ'pledʒɪk] *adj.* referring to diplegia *som avser el. hör till diplegi (dubbelsidig förlamning); compare* HEMIPLEGIA

diplococcus [ˌdɪpləʊ'kɒkəs] *subst.* bacterium which occurs in pairs *diplokock*
NOTE: plural is **diplococci**

diploe ['dɪpləʊi:] *subst.* layer of spongy bone tissue filled with red bone marrow, between the inner and outer layers of the skull *diploë*

diploid ['dɪplɔɪd] *adj.* (cell) where each chromosome (except the sex chromosome) occurs twice *diploid; compare* HAPLOID, POLYPLOID

diplokock ⇨ **diplococcus**

diploma [dɪ'pləʊmə] *subst.* certificate showing that a person has successfully finished a course of specialized training *diplom, avgångsbetyg;* **he has a diploma from a College of Nursing; she is taking her diploma exams next week**

diplopia [dɪ'pləʊpiə] *subst.* double vision *or* condition where a patient sees single objects as double *diplopi, dubbelseende; compare* POLYOPIA

dipsomania [ˌdɪpsə(ʊ)'meɪniə] *subst.* uncontrollable desire to drink alcohol *dipsomani*

direct [dɪ'rekt, də'rekt, daɪ'rekt] **1** *adj. & adv.* straight *or* with nothing intervening *direkt;* **his dermatitis is due to direct contact with irritants 2** *vb.* to tell someone what to do *or* how to go somewhere *leda, styra, visa (vägen);* **the police directed the ambulances to the scene of the accident; can you direct me to the outpatients' unit? she spent two years directing the work of the research team**

directly [dɪ'rektlɪ, də'rektli, daɪ'rektli] *adv.* straight *or* with nothing in between *direkt;* **the endocrine or ductless glands secrete hormones directly into the bloodstream; the dressing should not be placed directly on the burn**

director [dɪ'rektə, də'rektə, daɪ'rektə] *subst.* **(a)** person in charge of a department *klinikchef, överläkare;* **he is the director of**

the burns unit **(b)** instrument used to limit the incision made with a surgical knife

direkt ⇨ **direct, directly**

direktkontakt ⇨ **contact**

dirt [dɜːt] *subst.* material which is not clean, like mud, dust, earth, etc. *smuts, orenlighet;* **he allowed dirt to get into the wound which became infected**

dirty [ˈdɜːti] *adj.* not clean *smutsig, oren;* **dirty sheets are taken off the beds every morning; everyone concerned with patient care has to make sure that the wards are not dirty**
NOTE: **dirty - dirtier - dirtiest**

disability [ˌdɪsəˈbɪləti] *subst.* condition where part of the body does not function normally *invaliditet, handikapp;* **deafness is a disability which affects old people; people with severe disabilities can claim grants from the government**

disable [dɪsˈeɪb(ə)l] *vb.* to make someone unable to do some normal activity *invalidisera, handikappa;* **he was disabled by the lung disease; a hospital for disabled soldiers; disabling disease** = disease which makes it impossible for a person to do some normal activity *invalidiserande sjukdom;* **the disabled** = people suffering from a physical *or* mental handicaps which prevent them from doing some normal activity *de handikappade*

disablement [dɪsˈeɪb(ə)lmənt] *subst.* condition where a person has a physical *or* mental handicap *invaliditet, handikapp*

disarticulation [ˌdɪsɑːˌtɪkjʊˈleɪʃ(ə)n] *subst.* amputation of a limb at a joint, which does not involve dividing a bone *desartikulering*

disc [dɪsk] *or US* **disk** [dɪsk] *subst.* flat round structure like a plate *disk, skiva;* **intervertebral disc** round plate of cartilage which separates two vertebrae in the spinal column *discus intervertebralis, intervertebralbrosk, mellankotskiva;* **displaced intervertebral disc** *or* **prolapsed intervertebral disc** *or* **slipped disc** = condition where an intervertebral disc becomes displaced *or* where the soft centre of a disc passes through the hard cartilage outside and presses on a nerve ⇨ *illustration* JOINTS, VERTEBRAL COLUMN *hernia disci intervertebralis, diskbråck, diskprolaps;* **Merkel's discs** = receptor cells in the lower part of the epidermis ⇨ *illustration* SKIN AND SENSORY RECEPTORS *Merkels celler (känselkroppar)*

discharge [dɪsˈtʃɑːdʒ] **1** *subst.* **(a)** (i) secretion of liquid from an opening *flytning, avsöndring, utsöndring;* (ii) release of nervous energy *urladdning;* **vaginal discharge** = flow of liquid from the vagina *vaginalfluor, flytning från slidan* **(b)** sending a patient away from a hospital because the treatment has ended *utskrivning;* **discharge rate** = number of patients with a certain type of disorder who are sent away from hospitals in a certain area (shown as a number per 10,000 of population) *antal utskrivningar i viss sjukdom per 10,000 personer* **2** *vb.* **(a)** to secrete liquid out of an opening *avsöndra, utsöndra, tömma (ut);* **the wound discharged a thin stream of pus (b)** to send a patient away from hospital because the treatment has ended *skriva ut;* **he was discharged from hospital last week; she discharged herself** = she decided to leave hospital and stop taking the treatment provided *hon lät skriva ut sig på eget ansvar*

discoloration [dɪsˌkʌləˈreɪʃ(ə)n] *subst.* change in colour *missfärgning*

discolour [dɪsˈkʌlə] *or US* **discolor** [dɪsˈkʌlər] *vb.* to change the colour of something *missfärga;* **his teeth were discoloured from smoking cigarettes**

> COMMENT: teeth can be discoloured in fluorosis; if the skin on the lips is discoloured it may indicate that the patient has swallowed a poison

discomfort [dɪsˈkʌmfət] *subst.* feeling of not being comfortable *or* not being completely well *obehag;* **she experienced some discomfort after the operation**

discontinue [ˌdɪskənˈtɪnjuː] *vb.* to stop doing something *avbryta, sluta (upphöra) med;* **the doctors decided to discontinue the treatment**

discontinued [ˌdɪskənˈtɪnjuːd] *adj.* no longer done *avbruten, som upphört;* **the use of the drug has been discontinued because of the possibility of side-effects**

discover [dɪsˈkʌvə] *vb.* to find something which was hidden *or* not known before *upptäcka;* **scientists are trying to discover a cure for this disease**

discoverer [dɪˈskʌv(ə)rə] *subst.* person who discovers something *upptäckare;* **who was the discoverer of penicillin?**

discovery [dɪˈskʌv(ə)ri] *subst.* finding something which was not known before *upptäckt;* **the discovery of penicillin completely changed hospital treatment;**

new medical discoveries are reported each week

discrete [dɪ'skriːt] *adj.* separate *or* not joined together *åtskild, enstaka;* **discrete rash** = rash which is formed of many separate spots, which do not join together into one large red patch *utslag med enstaka (ej sammanflytande) fläckar*

disease [dɪ'ziːz] *subst.* illness (of people *or* animals *or* plants, etc.) where the body functions abnormally *sjukdom, fel;* **he caught a disease in the tropics; she is suffering from a very serious disease of the kidneys** *or* **from a serious kidney disease; he is a specialist in occupational diseases** *or* **in diseases which affect workers**

diseased [dɪ'ziːzd] *adj.* (person *or* part of the body) affected by an illness *or* not whole or normal *sjuk, angripen;* **the doctor cut away the diseased tissue**
NOTE: although a particular disease may have few visible characteristic symptoms, the term 'disease' is applied to all physical and mental reactions which make a person ill. Diseases with distinct characteristics have names. For terms referring to disease, see words beginning with **path-** or **patho-**

disfigure [dɪs'fɪgə] *vb.* to change someone's appearance so as to make it less pleasant *vanställa, vanpryda;* **her legs were disfigured by scars**

disinfect [ˌdɪsɪn'fekt] *vb.* to make a place free from germs *or* bacteria *desinficera;* **she disinfected the wound with surgical spirit; all the patient's clothes has to be disinfected**

disinfectant [ˌdɪsɪn'fektənt] *subst.* substance used to kill germs *or* bacteria *desinfektionsmedel*

disinfection [ˌdɪsɪn'fekʃ(ə)n] *subst.* removal of infection caused by germs *or* bacteria *desinfektion, desinficering*
NOTE: the words **disinfect** and **disinfectant** are used for substances which destroy germs on instruments, objects or the skin; substances used to kill germs inside infected people are **antibiotics, drugs, etc.**

disintegrate [dɪs'ɪntɪgreɪt] *vb.* to come to pieces *desintegreras, lösas upp, falla sönder;* **in holocrine glands the cells disintegrate as they secrete**

disintegration [dɪsˌɪntɪ'greɪʃ(ə)n] *subst.* act of disintegrating *desintegration, upplösning, sönderfall*

disk ⇨ **disc**

diskbråck ⇨ **disc**

diskmedel ⇨ **detergent**

diskprolaps ⇨ **disc**

dislike [dɪs'laɪk] **1** *subst.* not liking something *aversion, motvilja, olust;* **he has a strong dislike of cats 2** *vb.* not to like something *tycka illa om, ogilla, ha motvilja mot;* **she dislikes going to the dentist**

dislocate ['dɪslə(ʊ)keɪt] *vb.* to displace a bone from its normal position at a joint *dislokera, luxera, vrida ur led;* **he fell and dislocated his elbow; the shoulder joint dislocates easily** *or* **is easily dislocated**

dislocation [ˌdɪslə(ʊ)'keɪʃ(ə)n] *or* **luxation** [lʌk'seɪʃ(ə)n] *subst.* condition where a bone is displaced from its normal position at a joint *dislokation, luxation, urledvridning;* **pathological dislocation** = dislocation of a diseased joint *patologisk luxation*

dislokation ⇨ **dislocation, displacement, luxation**

dislokera ⇨ **dislocate**

disorder [dɪs'ɔːdə] *subst.* (i) illness *or* sickness *rubbning, störning;* (ii) state where part of the body is not functioning correctly *rubbning, störning;* **the doctor specializes in disorders of the kidneys** *or* **in kidney disorders; the family has a history of mental disorder**

disordered [dɪs'ɔːdəd] *adj.* (i) not functioning correctly *rubbad, störd;* (ii) (organ) affected by a disease *sjuk;* **disordered action of the heart (DAH)** *or* **da Costa's syndrome** = condition where the patient suffers palpitations caused by worry *hjärtneuros*

disorientated [dɪs'ɔːrɪənteɪtɪd] *adj.* (patient) who is confused and does not know where he is *desorienterad, förvirrad*

disorientation [dɪsˌɔːriən'teɪʃ(ə)n] *subst.* condition where the patient is not completely conscious of space *or* time *or* place *desorientering, förvirring, konfusion*

dispensary [dɪ'spens(ə)ri] *subst.* place (part of a chemist's shop *or* department of a hospital) where drugs are prepared *or* mixed and given out according to a doctor's prescription *ung. apotek*

dispensing chemist [dɪ'spensɪŋ ˌkemɪst] *subst.* pharmacist who prepares and provides drugs according to a doctor's prescription *apotekare, farmaceut*

> COMMENT: in the UK, prescriptions can only be dispensed by qualified and registered pharmacists

displace [dɪs'pleɪs] *vb.* to put out of the usual place *förskjuta;* **displaced intervertebral disc** = disc which has moved slightly, so that the soft interior passes through the tougher exterior and causes pressure on a nerve *hernia disci intervertebralis, diskprolaps, diskbråck*

displacement [dɪs'pleɪsmənt] *subst.* movement out of the normal position *dislokation, förskjutning, felläge;* **fracture of the radius together with displacement of the wrist**

disponerad för ⇨ **liable to**

disposable [dɪs'pəʊzəb(ə)l] *adj.* (item) which can be thrown away after use *engångs-;* **disposable syringes; disposable petri dishes**

disposition ⇨ **predisposition**

disproportion [ˌdɪsprə'pɔːʃ(ə)n] *subst.* lack of proper relationships between two things *disproportion, oproportionerligt förhållande;* **cephalopelvic disproportion** = condition where the pelvic opening of the mother is not large enough for the head of the fetus *bäckenträngsel, bäckenförträngning*

dissecans ['dɪsəkæns] *see* OSTEOCHONDRITIS

dissect [dɪ'sekt] *vb.* to cut and separate tissues in a body to examine them *dissekera;* **dissecting aneurysm** = aneurysm which occurs when the inside wall of the aorta is torn, and blood enters the membrane *aneurysma dissecans, dissekerande aneurysm*

dissection [dɪ'sekʃ(ə)n] *subst.* cutting and separating parts of a body *or* an organ as part of a surgical operation *or* as part of an autopsy *or* as part of a course of study *dissektion, dissekering*

> QUOTE renal dissection usually takes from 40 - 60 minutes, while liver and pancreas dissections take from one to three hours. Cardiac dissection takes about 20 minutes and lung dissection takes 60 to 90 minutes
>
> **Nursing Times**

dissekera ⇨ **dissect**

dissekering ⇨ **dissection**

dissektion ⇨ **dissection**

disseminated [dɪ'semɪneɪtɪd] *adj.* occurring in every part of an organ *or* in the whole body *disseminerad, spridd;* **disseminated sclerosis** = MULTIPLE SCLEROSIS; **disseminated lupus erythematosus (DLE)** = inflammatory disease where the skin rash is associated with widespread changes in the central nervous system, the cardiovascular system and many organs *lupus erythematosus el. erythematodes (disseminatus), LED, systemisk lupus erythematosus (erythematodes), SLE*

dissemination [dɪˌsemɪ'neɪʃ(ə)n] *subst.* being widespread throughout the body *dissemination, spridning*

disseminerad ⇨ **disseminated**

disseminerad intravaskulär koagulation ⇨ **crush syndrome**

dissociate [dɪ'səʊsɪeɪt] *vb.* (i) to separate parts *or* functions *dissociera, skilja, sönderdela;* (ii) to separate part of the conscious mind from the rest *dissociera;* **dissociated anaesthesia** = loss of sensitivity to heat *or* pain *or* cold *förlust av vissa sinneskvalitéer*

> COMMENT: patients will dissociate their delusion from the real world around them as a way of escaping from the facts of the real world

dissociation [dɪˌsəʊʃi'eɪʃ(ə)n] *subst.* **(a)** separating of parts *or* functions *dissociation, separation, sönderdelning* **(b)** *(in psychiatry)* condition where part of the consciousness becomes separated from the rest and becomes independent *dissociation, personlighetsklyvning*

dissociera ⇨ **dissociate**

dissolve [dɪ'zɒlv] *vb.* to melt *or* to make something disappear in liquid *upplösa, resorbera;* **the gut used in sutures slowly dissolves in the body fluids**

distal ['dɪst(ə)l] *adj.* further away from the centre of the body *distal, änd-;* **distal phalanges** = the end parts of fingers and toes *distala falangerna, ändfalangerna;* **distal convoluted tubule** = part of the kidney filtering system before the collecting ducts *tubulus renales contorti, distala tubuli*

distally ['dɪst(ə)li] *adv.* placed further from the centre *distalt*

NOTE: the opposite is **proximal.** Note also that you say that a part is distal **to** another part

distalt ⇨ **distally**

distend [dɪs'tend] *vb.* to swell by pressure *spänna(s) ut, tänja(s) ut, utvidga(s);* **distended bladder** = bladder which is full of urine *utspänd blåsa, fylld blåsa*

distension [dɪs'tenʃ(ə)n] *subst.* condition where something is swollen *utvidgning, uttänjning;* **distension of the veins in the abdomen is a sign of blocking of the portal vein; abdominal distension** = swelling of the abdomen (because of gas *or* fluid) *utspänd buk*

distil [dɪ'stɪl] *vb.* to separate the component parts of a liquid by boiling and collecting the condensed vapour *destillera;* **distilled water** *or* **purified water** = water which has been made pure by distillation *destillerat vatten*

distillation [ˌdɪstɪ'leɪʃ(ə)n] *subst.* action of distilling a liquid *destillering*

distinct [dɪ'stɪŋ(k)t] *adj.* separate *or* not to be confused *tydlig, skild, olik;* **the colon is divided into four distinct sections**

distinctive [dɪ'stɪŋ(k)tɪv] *adj.* easily noticed *or* characteristic *typisk, karakteristisk;* **mumps is easily diagnosed by distinctive swellings on the side of the face**

distort [dɪ'stɔːt] *vb.* to twist something into an abnormal shape *stuka, vricka, förvrida;* **his lower limbs were distorted by the disease**

distortion [dɪ'stɔːʃ(ə)n] *subst.* twisting of part of the body out of its normal shape *stukning, vrickning*

distress [dɪ'stres] *subst.* suffering caused by pain *or* worry *oro, plåga;* **attempted suicide is often a sign of the person's mental distress; respiratory distress syndrome** = condition of newborn babies where the lungs do not function properly *idiopatiskt respiratoriskt distress-syndrom, IRDS, syndroma membranorum hyalinorum, hyalina membran*

district ['dɪstrɪkt] *subst.* area *or* part of the country *or* town *distrikt, område;* **district general hospital** = hospital which serves the needs of the population of a district *sjukhus med visst lokalt upptagningsområde (i Storbritannien);* **District Health Authority (DHA)** = administrative unit in the National Health Service which is responsible for all health services provided in a district, including hospitals and clinics *lokal hälsovårdsmyndighet (i Storbritannien);* **district nurse** = nurse who visits patients in their homes in a certain area *distriktssköterska*

distrikt ⇨ **district**

distriktsbarnmorska ⇨ **midwife**

distriktsköterskevård ⇨ **community**

distriktsläkare ⇨ **general practitioner (GP)**

distriktsläkarmottagning ⇨ **health**

distriktssköterska ⇨ **district, home**

disturb [dɪ'stɜːb] *vb.* to worry someone *or* to stop someone working by talking, etc. *störa;* **don't disturb him when he's working; his sleep was disturbed by the other patients in the ward**

disturbance [dɪ'stɜːb(ə)ns] *subst.* being disturbed *störning, rubbning;* **the blow to the head caused disturbance to the brain**

diures ⇨ **diuresis**

diuresis [ˌdaɪjʊ(ə)'riːsɪs] *subst.* increase in the production of urine *diures, urinutsöndring*

diuretic [ˌdaɪjʊ(ə)'retɪk] *adj. & subst.* (substance) which makes the kidneys produce more urine *diuretisk, diuretikum, urindrivande (medel)*

diuretikum ⇨ **diuretic**

diuretisk ⇨ **diuretic**

diurnal [daɪ'ɜːn(ə)l] *adj.* happening in the daytime *or* happening every day *diurnal, daglig, dags-, dygns-*

divergent strabismus [daɪ'vɜːdʒ(ə)nt strəˌbɪzməs] *subst.* condition where a person's eyes both look away from the nose *strabismus divergens (externus), divergent strabism (skelning), utåtskelning*

diverticular disease [ˌdaɪvə'tɪkjʊlə dɪˌziːz] *subst.* disease of the large intestine, where the colon thickens and diverticula form in the walls, causing the patient pain in the lower abdomen *divertikulos, divertikulit*

diverticulitis [ˌdaɪvəˌtɪkju'laɪtɪs] *subst.* inflammation of diverticula formed in the wall of the colon *divertikulit*

diverticulosis [ˌdaɪvəˌtɪkju'ləʊsɪs] *subst.* condition where diverticula form in the intestine but are not inflamed (in the small intestine, this can lead to blind loop syndrome) *divertikulos*

diverticulum [ˌdaɪvə'tɪkjʊləm] *subst.* little sac *or* pouch which develops in the wall of the intestine or other organ *divertikel;* **Meckel's diverticulum** = congenital formation of a diverticulum in the ileum *Meckels divertikel* NOTE: the plural is **diverticula**

divertikel ⇨ **diverticulum**

divertikulit ⇨ **diverticular disease, diverticulitis**

divertikulos ⇨ **diverticular disease, diverticulosis**

divide [dɪ'vaɪd] *vb.* to separate into parts *dela (sig);* **the common carotid divides into two smaller arteries**

division [dɪ'vɪʒ(ə)n] *subst.* cutting into parts *or* splitting into parts *delning;* **cell division** = way in which a cell reproduces itself by mitosis *celldelning*

divulsor [dɪ'vʌlsə] *subst.* surgical instrument used to expand a passage *dilatator, dilator*

dizygoter ⇨ **fraternal twins**

dizygotic twins [ˌdɪzɪ'gɒtɪk ˌtwɪnz] = FRATERNAL TWINS

dizziness ['dɪzinəs] *subst.* feeling that everything is going round because the sense of balance has been affected *yrsel, svindel*

dizzy ['dɪzi] *adj.* having the sense of balance affected *or* feeling that everything is going round *yr;* **after standing in the sun, she became dizzy and had to lie down; he suffers from dizzy spells**

djup ⇨ **deep**

djup(gående) ⇨ **profound**

djupseende ⇨ **stereoscopic vision**

djupt ⇨ **deeply**

djur ⇨ **animal**

djurbett ⇨ **animal**

DLE [ˌdi:el'i:] = DISSEMINATED LUPUS ERYTHEMATOSUS

DMD [ˌdi:em'di:] *US* = DOCTOR OF DENTAL MEDICINE

DNA [ˌdi:en'eɪ] = DEOXYRIBONUCLEIC ACID

DNA-manipulering ⇨ **bioengineering**

DOA [ˌdi:əʊ'eɪ] = DEAD ON ARRIVAL

doctor ['dɒktə] *subst.* **(a)** person who has trained in medicine and is qualified to examine people when they are ill to find out what is wrong with them and to prescribe a course of treatment *doktor, läkare;* **his son is training to be a doctor; if you have a pain in your chest, you ought to see a doctor; he has gone to the doctor's; do you want to make an appointment with the doctor?; family doctor** = general practitioner *or* doctor who looks after the health of people in his area *husläkare, familjeläkare, ung. distriktsläkare* **(b)** title given to a qualified person who is registered with the General Medical Council *legitimerad läkare upptagen i officiellt register i Storbritannien (motsvarande läkarregistret i Sverige);* **I have an appointment with Dr Jones**
NOTE: **doctor** is shortened to **Dr** when written before a name. In the UK surgeons are traditionally not called "Doctor", but are addressed as "Mr", "Mrs", etc. The title "doctor" is also applied to persons who have a high degree from a university in a non-medical subject. So "Dr Jones" may have a degree in music, or in any other subject without a connection with medicine

doft ⇨ **scent**

doktor ⇨ **doctor, medico**

dold ⇨ **occult**

dolichocephalic [ˌdɒlɪkəʊse'fælɪk] *adj.* (person) with a long skull *dolikocefal, långskallig*

dolichocephaly [ˌdɒlɪkəʊ'sefəli] *subst.* condition of a person who has a skull which is longer than normal *dolikocefali, långskallighet*

> COMMENT: in dolichocephaly, the measurement across the skull is less than 75% of the length of the head from front to back

dolikocefal ⇨ **dolichocephalic**

dolikocefali ⇨ **dolichocephaly**

dolor ['dɒlə] *subst.* pain *dolor, smärta, värk, plågor*

dolorimetry [ˌdɒlə'rɪmətri] *subst.* measuring of pain *mätning av smärta*

dolorosa [ˌdɒlə'rəʊsə] *see* ADIPOSIS

domicile ['dɒmɪsaɪ(ə)l] *subst. (in official use)* home *or* place where someone lives *hemort, bostad*

domiciliary [ˌdɒmɪ'sɪliəri] *adj.* at home *or* in the home *bostads-, hem-;* **the doctor made a domiciliary visit** = he visited the patient at home *läkaren gjorde ett hembesök;* **domiciliary midwife** = nurse with special qualification in midwifery, who can assist in childbirth at home *barnmorska som får genomföra hemförlossningar;* **domiciliary services** = nursing services which are available to patients in their homes *hemsjukvård*

dominance ['dɒmɪnəns] *subst.* being more powerful *dominans;* **cerebral dominance** = normal condition where the centres for various functions are located in one cerebral hemisphere *dominans för ena hjärnhalvan;* **ocular dominance** = condition where a person uses one eye more than the other *dominans för ett öga*

dominans ⇨ **dominance**

dominant ['dɒmɪnənt] *adj. & subst.* (genetic trait) which is more powerful than other recessive genes *dominant*

COMMENT: since each physical trait is governed by two genes, if one is recessive and the other dominant, the resulting trait will be that of the dominant gene

dominant ⇨ **dominant, predominant**

dominerande ⇨ **predominant**

domnad ⇨ **dead, numb**

domning ⇨ **numbness**

domstol ⇨ **court**

domstolsbeslut ⇨ **court**

donator ⇨ **donor**

donor ['dəʊnə] *subst.* person who gives his own tissue *or* organs for use in transplants *donator, givare;* **blood donor** = person who gives blood to be used in transfusions *blodgivare;* **kidney donor** = person who gives one of his kidneys as a transplant *njurdonator;* **donor card** = card carried by a person stating that he approves of his organs being used for transplanting after he has died *slags donatorskort*

dopamine ['dəʊpəmi:n] *subst.* substance found in the medulla of the adrenal glands, which also acts as a neurotransmitter, lack of which is associated with Parkinson's disease *dopamin*

dormant ['dɔ:mənt] *adj.* inactive for a time *passiv, inaktiv, latent;* **the virus lies dormant in the body for several years**

dorsal ['dɔ:s(ə)l] *adj.* (i) referring to the back *dorsal;* (ii) referring to the back of the body *dorsal, rygg-;* **dorsal vertebrae** = twelve vertebrae in the back, between the cervical vertebrae and the lumbar vertebrae *vertebrae thoracicae, bröstkotorna* NOTE: the opposite is **ventral**

dorsi- ['dɔ:si, ˌ--] *or* **dorso-** [ˌdɔ:səʊ] *prefix* referring to the back *dorsi-, dorso-, rygg-*

dorsiflexion [ˌdɔ:sɪ'flekʃ(ə)n] *subst.* flexion towards the back of part of the body (such as raising the foot at the ankle, as opposed to plantar flexion) *dorsiflexion*

dorsoventral [ˌdɔ:səʊ'ventr(ə)l] *adj.* (i) referring to the back of the body and the front *dorsoventral;* (ii) extending from the back of the body to the front *dorsoventral*

dorsum ['dɔ:səm] *subst.* back of any part of the body *dorsum, rygg*

dos ⇨ **dosage, dose**

dosage ['dəʊsɪdʒ] *subst.* correct amounts of a drug calculated by a doctor to be necessary for a patient *dos, dosering;* **the doctor decided to increase the dosage of antibiotics; the dosage for children is half that for adults**

dose [dəʊs] **1** *subst.* measured quantity of a drug *or* radiation which is to be administered to a patient at a time *dos, dosering;* **it is dangerous to exceed the prescribed dose 2** *vb.* **to dose with** = to give a patient a drug *medicinera, ge medicin;* **she dosed her son with aspirin and cough medicine before he went to his examination; the patient has been dosing herself with laxatives**

dosering ⇨ **dosage, dose**

dosimeter [dəʊ'sɪmɪtə] *subst.* instrument which measures the amount of X-rays or other radiation received *dosimeter*

dosimetri ⇨ **dosimetry**

dosimetry [dəʊ'sɪmətri] *subst.* measuring the amount of X-rays or radiation received, using a dosimeter *dosimetri*

dotter ⇨ **daughter**

dottercell ⇨ **daughter**

dotterdotter ⇨ **granddaughter**

dotterson ⇨ **grandson**

double ['dʌb(ə)l] *adj.* with two similar parts *dubbel;* **double figures** = numbers from 10 to 99 *tvåsiffriga tal;* **double pneumonia** = pneumonia in both lungs *dubbelsidig lunginflammation;* **double uterus** = DIDELPHYS; **bent double** = bent over completely so that the face is towards the ground *dubbelvikt;* **he was bent double with arthritis**

double-blind [ˌdʌb(ə)l'blaɪnd] *subst.* way of testing a new drug, where neither the people taking the test, nor the people administering it know which patients have had the real drug and which have had the placebo *dubbelblindtest*

double-jointed [ˌdʌb(ə)l'dʒɔɪntɪd] *adj.* able to bend joints to an abnormal degree *som kan böja onormalt mycket i lederna*

double vision [ˌdʌb(ə)l 'vɪʒ(ə)n] = DIPLOPIA

douche [du:ʃ] *subst.* liquid forced into the body to wash out a cavity *sköljning;* device used for washing out a cavity *sköljkanna;* **vaginal douche** = device *or* liquid for washing out the vagina *sköljkanna, slidsköljning*

Douglas bag ['dʌgləs ˌbæg] *subst.* bag used for measuring the volume of air breathed out of the lungs *Douglassäck*

douloureux [du:lu:'ru:] *see* TIC

dov ⇨ **dull**

Down's syndrome ['daʊnz ˌsɪndrəʊm] *or* **trisomy 21** [ˌtraɪsəʊmi twentɪ'wʌn] *subst.* congenital defect, due to existence of three chromosomes at number 21, in which the patient has slanting eyes, a wide face, speech difficulties and is usually mentally retarded *Downs syndrom, tidigare mongolism*
NOTE: sometimes called mongolism because of the shape of the eyes

doze [dəʊz] *vb.* to sleep a little *or* to sleep lightly *dåsa, slumra;* **she dozed off for a while after lunch**

dozy ['dəʊzi] *adj.* sleepy *dåsig, sömnig, slö;* **these antihistamines can make you feel dozy**

DPT [ˌdi:pi:'ti:] = DIPHTHERIA, WHOOPING COUGH, TETANUS; **DPT vaccine** *or* **DPT immunization** = combined vaccine *or* immunization against the three diseases *trippelvaccin(ation)*

dra ⇨ **wheel**

drabba ⇨ **affect**

drabbas (av) ⇨ **suffer**

drachm [dræm] *subst.* measure used in pharmacy (dry weight equals 3.8g, liquid measure equals 3.7ml) *drakmer, c. 3,8 g el. 3,7 ml*

dracontiasis [ˌdrækɒn'taɪəsɪs] *or* **dracunculiasis** [drəˌkʌŋkju'laɪəsɪs] *subst.* tropical disease caused by the guinea worm **Dracunculus medinensis** which enters the body from infected drinking water and forms blisters on the skin, frequently leading to secondary arthritis, fibrosis and cellulitis *dracontiasis*

Dracunculus [drə'kʌŋkjuləs] *or* **guinea worm** ['gɪni wɜ:m] *subst.* parasitic worm which enters the body and rises to the skin to form a blister *Dracunculus medinensis, guineamask, drakmask, medinamask*

dragee [dræ'ʒeɪ] *subst.* sugar-coated drug tablet *or* pill *dragé*

dragerad ⇨ **enteric-coated**

dragering ⇨ **coating**

drag, karakteristiskt ⇨ **trait**

draglakan ⇨ **draw-sheet**

dragning(skraft) ⇨ **attraction**

drain [dreɪn] **1** *subst.* **(a)** pipe for carrying waste water from a house *avlopp(srör), kloak(ledning);* **the report of the health inspectors was critical of the drains (b)** tube to remove liquid from the body *drän, dränagerör, dränageslang* **2** *vb.* to remove liquid from something *dränera, tappa;* **an operation to drain the sinus; they drained the pus from the abscess**

drainage ['dreɪnɪdʒ] *subst.* removal of liquid from the site of an operation *or* pus from an abscess by means of a tube left in the body for a time *dränage, tappning*

drakmask ⇨ **Dracunculus**

drakmer ⇨ **drachm**

drape [dreɪp] *subst.* thin material used to place over a patient about to undergo surgery, leaving the operation site uncovered *operationslakan, operationsklädsel*

draw-sheet ['drɔːʃiːt] *subst.* sheet under a patient in bed, folded so that it can be pulled out as it becomes soiled *draglakan*

dream [driːm] **1** *subst.* images which a person sees when asleep *dröm;* **I had a bad dream about spiders 2** *vb.* to think you see something happening while you are asleep *drömma;* **he dreamt he was attacked by spiders**
NOTE: **dreams - dreaming - dreamed** *or* **dreamt**

dregla ⇨ **dribble**

drepanocyt ⇨ **sickle cell**

drepanocyte ['drepənəʊsaɪt] = SICKLE CELL

drepanocytos ⇨ **sickle cell**

drepanocytosis [ˌdrepənəʊsaɪ'təʊsɪs] = SICKLE-CELL ANAEMIA

dress [dres] *vb.* **(a)** to put on clothes *klä på sig;* **he (got) dressed and then had breakfast; the surgeon was dressed in a green gown; you can get dressed again now (b)** to clean a wound and put a covering over it *lägga om, förbinda;* **nurses dressed the wounds of the accident victims**

dressing ['dresɪŋ] *subst.* covering *or* bandage applied to a wound to protect it *förband, omslag;* **the patient's dressings need to be changed every two hours; gauze dressing** = dressing of thin light material *kompress, gasbinda;* **sterile dressing** = dressing which is sold in a sterile pack, ready for use *sterilt förband;* **adhesive dressing** *see* ADHESIVE

dribble ['drɪb(ə)l] *vb.* to let liquid flow slowly out of an opening, especially saliva out of the mouth *dregla;* **the baby dribbled over her dress**

dribbling ['drib(ə)lɪŋ] *subst.* (i) letting saliva flow out of the mouth *dregel;* (ii) incontinence *or* being unable to keep back the flow of urine *inkontinens*

dricka ⇨ **drink**

drift ⇨ **management; urge**

drill [drɪl] **1** *subst.* tool which rotates very rapidly to make a hole *borr;* surgical instrument used in dentistry to remove caries *tandläkarborr* **2** *vb.* to make a hole with a drill *borra;* **a small hole is drilled in the skull; the dentist drilled one of her molars**

drink [drɪŋk] **1** *subst.* **(a)** liquid which is swallowed *dryck;* **have a drink of water; always have a hot drink before you go to bed; soft drinks** = drinks (like orange juice) with no alcohol in them *läskedryck, juice* **(b)** alcoholic drink *alkoholhaltig dryck* **2** *vb.* **(a)** to swallow liquid *dricka;* **he drinks two cups of coffee for breakfast; you need to drink at least five pints of liquid a day (b)** to drink alcoholic drinks *dricka alkoholhaltiga drycker;* **do you drink a lot?**
NOTE: **drinks - drinking - drank - has drunk**

Drinker respirator ['drɪŋkə ˌrespɪreɪtə] *or* **iron lung** ['aɪən ˌlʌŋ] *subst.* machine which encloses the whole of a patient's body except the head, and in which air pressure is increased and decreased, so forcing the patient to breathe in or out *slags respirator, järnlunga, cuirassrespirator*

drip [drɪp] *subst.* method of introducing liquid slowly and continuously into the body, where a bottle of liquid is held above the patient and the fluid flows slowly down a tube into a needle in a vein *or* into the stomach *dropp, infusion;* **intravenous drip** = drip which goes into a vein *intravenöst dropp;* **saline drip** = drip containing salt solution *saltlösning (elektrolytlösning) för infusion;* **drip feed** = drip containing nutrients *nutritionslösning (för infusion)*

drog ⇨ **drug**

drogberoende ⇨ **addiction, dependence**

drogmissbruk ⇨ **abuse, addiction**

drop [drɒp] **1** *subst.* **(a)** small quantity of liquid *droppe;* **a drop of water fell on the floor; the optician prescribed her some drops for the eyes (b)** reduction *or* fall in quantity of something *fall, sänkning;* **drop in pressure** = sudden reduction in pressure *tryckfall* **2** *vb.* to fall *or* to let something fall *falla, sänkas;* **pressure in the artery dropped suddenly**

drop attack ['drɒp əˌtæk] *subst.* condition where a person suddenly falls down, though he is not unconscious, caused by sudden weakness of the spine *epilepsivariant (med oklar orsak)*

drop foot ['drɒp fʊt] *or* **drop wrist** ['drɒp rɪst] *subst.* conditions, caused by muscular disorder, where the ankle *or* wrist is not strong, and the foot *or* hand hangs limp *droppfot, dropphand, hänghand*

droplet ['drɒplət] *subst.* very small drop of liquid *liten droppe*

drop off [ˌdrɒp 'ɒf] *vb.* to fall asleep *slumra (till), lura till;* **she dropped off in front of the TV**

dropp ⇨ **drip, infusion**

droppe ⇨ **drop, gutta, minim**

droppfinger ⇨ **mallet finger**

droppfot ⇨ **drop foot, foot**

dropphand ⇨ **drop foot, wrist**

dropsy ['drɒpsi] *subst.* swelling of part of the body because of accumulation of fluid in the tissues *hydrops, ödem*

> COMMENT: dropsy is usually caused by kidney failure or heart failure, leading to bad circulation. The legs (especially the ankles) and the arms become very swollen

drown [draʊn] *vb.* to die by inhaling liquid *drunkna;* **he fell into the sea and (was) drowned; six people drowned when the boat sank**

drowning ['draʊnɪŋ] *subst.* act of dying by inhaling liquid *drunkning;* **the autopsy showed that death was due to drowning; dry drowning** = death where the patient's air passage has been constricted because he is under water, though he does not inhale any water *torrdrunkning*

drucken ⇨ **drunk, drunken**

drug [drʌg] *subst.* **(a)** chemical substance (either natural or synthetic) which is used in medicine and affects the way in which organs *or* tissues function *drog, läkemedel;* **the doctors are trying to cure him with a new drug; she was prescribed a course of pain-killing drugs; the drug is being monitored for possible side-effects (b)** habit-forming substance *vanebildande medel, narkotikum;* **he has been taking drugs for several months; the government is trying to stamp out drug pushing; drug abuse** = taking habit-forming drugs *narkotikamissbruk, drogmissbruk, läkemedelsmissbruk;* **a high rate of drug-related deaths** = of deaths associated with the taking of drugs *stort antal dödsfall på grund av narkotikamissbruk; see also* ADDICT, ADDICTION

drugstore ['drʌgstɔː] *subst. US* shop where medicines and drugs can be bought (as well as many other goods) *drugstore, slags apotek*

drum [drʌm] *see* EARDRUM

drunk [drʌŋk] *adj.* intoxicated with too much alcohol *drucken, berusad, full*

drunken ['drʌŋk(ə)n] *adj.* intoxicated *drucken, berusad, full;* **the doctors has to get help to control the drunken patient**
NOTE: drunken is only used in front of a noun, and drunk is usually used after the verb to be: **a drunken patient; that patient is drunk**

drunkna ⇨ **drown**

drunkning ⇨ **drowning**

druvbörd ⇨ **hydatidiform mole**

druvhinnan ⇨ **uveal**

druvsocker ⇨ **dextrose**

dry [draɪ] **1** *adj.* not wet *or* with the smallest amount of moisture *torr;* **the surface of the wound should be kept dry; she uses a cream to soften her dry skin; dry burn** = burn caused by touching a very hot dry surface *brännskada orsakad av beröring med torr, het yta;* **dry gangrene** = condition where the blood supply has been cut off and the tissue becomes black *gangraena sicca, torrt gangrän;* **dry ice** = CARBON DIOXIDE
NOTE: **dry - drier - driest 2** *vb.* to remove moisture from something *torka;* to wipe something until it is dry *torka (av)*

dryck ⇨ **drink**

dryness ['draɪnəs] *subst.* state of being dry *torka, torrhet;* **she complained of dryness in her mouth; dryness in the eyes, accompanied by rheumatoid arthritis**

dry out [ˌdraɪ 'aʊt] *vb.* (i) to dry completely *torka ut;* (ii) /G/ (informal) to treat someone for alcoholism *behandla på "torken" (för alkoholism)*

dråpare ⇨ **killer**

drän ⇨ **drain**

dränage ⇨ **drainage**

dränagebehandling ⇨ **postural**

dränagerör ⇨ **drain**

dränageslang ⇨ **drain**

dränera ⇨ **drain**

dränka ⇨ **flood**

dröm ⇨ **dream**

drömma ⇨ **dream**

DT ⇨ **computerized axial tomography (CAT), scan**

DTs [ˌdiːˈtiːz] = DELIRIUM TREMENS

dubbel ⇨ **double, gemellus**

dubbel- ⇨ **bi-, binary, dipl-**

dubbelartros ⇨ **amphiarthrosis**

dubbelblind ⇨ **double-blind**

dubbelkön ⇨ **intersexuality**

dubbel livmoder ⇨ **uterus**

dubbelseende ⇨ **diplopia, polyopia**

dubbelsidig ⇨ **bilateral**

dubbelslag ⇨ **dicrotism**

dubbelvikt ⇨ **double**

Duchenne muscular dystrophy [duˌʃen ˈmʌskjulə ˌdɪstrəfi] *subst.* hereditary disease of the muscles where some muscles (starting with the legs) swell and become weak *Duchenne-Griesingers sjukdom, muskeldystrofi med pseudohypertrofi*

COMMENT: usually found in young boys. It is carried in the mother's genes

Ducrey's bacillus [duːˈkreɪz bəˌsɪləs] *subst.* type of bacterium causing chancroid *Haemophilus ducreyi, bakterie som orsakar chanker (genitalt sår)*

duct [dʌkt] *subst.* tube which carries liquids, especially one which carries secretions *ductus, gång, rör, kanal;* **bile duct** *or* **cystic duct** *or* **hepatic duct** = tubes which link the gall bladder and liver to the duodenum *gallgång;* **cochlear duct** = spiral channel in the cochlea *ductus cochlearis;* **collecting duct** = part of the kidney filtering system *samlingsrör;* **efferent duct** = duct which carries liquid away from an organ *efferent (avförande) gång, utförsgång;* **ejaculatory ducts** = two ducts formed by the seminal vesicles and vas deferens, which go through the prostate and end in the urethra ⇨ *illustration* UROGENITAL SYSTEM (MALE) *ductus ejaculatorius;* **nasolacrimal duct** *or* **tear duct** = canal which takes tears from the lacrimal sac into the nose *ductus nasolacrimalis, nästårkanalen;* **right lymph duct** = one of the main terminal ducts for carrying lymph, draining the right side of the head and neck *ductus lymphaticus dextra;* **pancreatic duct** = duct leading through the pancreas to the duodenum *ductus pancreaticus;* **semicircular ducts** = ducts in the semicircular canals in the ear ⇨ *illustration* EAR *ductus semicirculares, halvcirkelformiga gångarna;* **thoracic duct** = one of the main terminal ducts carrying lymph, on the left side of the neck *ductus thoracicus, stora bröstgången, stora lymfgången*

ductile [ˈdʌktaɪ(ə)l] *adj.* soft *or* which can bend *böjlig, smidig*

ductless gland [ˈdʌktləs ˌglænd] *or* **endocrine gland** [ˈendə(ʊ)kraɪn ˌglænd] *subst.* gland without a duct which produces hormones which are introduced directly into the bloodstream (such as the pituitary gland, thyroid gland, the adrenals, and the gonads) ⇨ *illustration* GLAND *endokrin (inresekretorisk) körtel, körtel utan utförsgång*

ductule [ˈdʌktjuːl] *subst.* very small duct *mycket fin kanal (gång)*

ductus [ˈdʌktəs] *subst.* duct *ductus, gång, rör, kanal;* **ductus arteriosus** = in a fetus, the blood vessel connecting the left pulmonary artery to the aorta so that blood does not pass through the lungs *ductus arteriosus;* **ductus deferens** *or* **vas deferens** = one of two tubes along which sperm passes from the epididymis to the prostate gland ⇨ *illustration* UROGENITAL SYSTEM (MALE) *(vas) ductus deferens, sädesledaren;* **ductus venosus** = in a fetus, the blood vessel connecting the portal sinus to the inferior vena cava *ductus venosus*

duk ⇨ **tampon, towel**

dull [dʌl] **1** *adj.* (pain) which is not sharp, but continuously painful *dov, malande;* **she complained of a dull throbbing pain in her head; he felt a dull pain in the chest 2** *vb.* to make less sharp *matta, dämpa, försvaga;* **his senses were dulled by the drug**

dumb [dʌm] *adj.* not able to speak *stum*

dumbness [ˈdʌmnəs] *subst.* being unable to speak *stumhet*

dummy [ˈdʌmi] *subst.* rubber teat given to a baby to suck, to prevent it crying *napp, tröstnapp*

NOTE: US English is **pacifier**

dumping syndrome [ˈdʌmpɪŋ ˌsɪndrəʊm] *subst.* rapid passing of the contents of the stomach and duodenum into the jejunum, causing fainting, diarrhoea and sweating in patients who have had a gastrectomy *dumpingsyndrom*

dunka ⇨ **throb**

dunkande ⇨ **throbbing**

dunsa ⇨ **bump**

duoden- ['dju:ə(ʊ)ˌdi:n, ˌ-ˌ-, ˌ-'-] *prefix* referring to the duodenum *duoden(o)-, tolvfingertarms-*

duodenal [ˌdju:ə(ʊ)'di:n(ə)l] *adj.* referring to the duodenum *duodenal, tolvfingertarm-;* **duodenal papillae** = small projecting parts in the duodenum where the bile duct and pancreatic duct open *papillae duodeni;* **duodenal ulcer** = ulcer in the duodenum *ulcus duodeni, sår i tolvfingertarmen*

duodenalfistel ⇨ **duodenostomy**

duodenoscope [ˌdju:əʊ'di:nəʊskəʊp] *subst.* instrument used to examine the inside of the duodenum *duodenoskop*

duodenostomy [ˌdju:əʊdɪ'nɒstəmi] *subst.* permanent opening made between the duodenum and the abdominal wall *duodenostomi, duodenalfistel*

duodenum [ˌdju:ə(ʊ)'di:nəm] *subst.* first part of the small intestine, going from the stomach to the jejunum ⇨ *illustration* DIGESTIVE SYSTEM, STOMACH *duodenum, tolvfingertarmen*

> COMMENT: the duodenum is the shortest part of the small intestine, about 250 mm long. It takes bile from the gall bladder and pancreatic juice from the pancreas and continues the digestive processes started in the mouth and stomach

Dupuytren's contracture [du'pwi:tr(ə)nz kənˌtræktʃə] *subst.* condition where the palmar fascia becomes thicker, causing the fingers (usually the middle and ring fingers) to bend forwards *Dupuytrens kontraktur*

dural [djʊər(ə)l] *adj.* referring to the dura mater *dural*

dura mater [ˌdjʊərə'meɪtə] *subst.* thicker outer meninx covering the brain and spinal cord *dura mater, pakymeninx, hårda hjärnhinnan*

Dutch cap ['dʌtʃ ˌkæp] *subst.* vaginal diaphragm *or* contraceptive device for women, which is placed over the cervix uteri before sexual intercourse *pessar, slidpessar*

duty ['dju:ti] *subst.* requirement for a particular job *or* something which has to be done (especially in a particular job) *or* work which a person has to do *skyldighet, uppgift, tjänst;* **what are the duties of a night sister?; to be on duty** = to be doing official work at a special time *vara i tjänst, vara jourhavande, tjänstgöra, jourtjänstgöra;* **night duty** = work done at night *nattjänstgöring, nattjour;* **Nurse Smith is on night duty this week; duty nurse** = nurse who is on duty *tjänstgörande sjuksköterska;* **a doctor owes a duty of care to his patient** = the doctor has to treat a patient in a proper way, as this is part of the work of being a doctor *en läkare har skyldighet att vårda och behandla patienten på rätt sätt*

dvala ⇨ **lethargy**

D-vitamin ⇨ **Vitamin D**

d.v.t. [ˌdi:vi:'ti:] *or* **DVT** [ˌdi:vi:'ti:] = DEEP VEIN THROMBOSIS

dvärg ⇨ **dwarf**

dvärgväxt ⇨ **dwarfism**

dwarf [dwɔ:f] *subst.* person who is much smaller than normal *dvärg*

dwarfism ['dwɔ:fɪz(ə)m] *subst.* condition where the growth of a person has stopped leaving him much smaller than normal *dvärgväxt*

> COMMENT: may be caused by achondroplasia, where the long bones in the arms and legs do not develop fully but the trunk and head are of normal size. Dwarfism can have other causes, such as rickets *or* deficiency in the pituitary gland

dygn ⇨ **day**

dygns- ⇨ **diurnal**

dykarsjuka ⇨ **caisson disease**

dyna ⇨ **pad**

dynamometer [ˌdaɪnə'mɒmɪtə] *subst.* instrument for measuring the force of muscular contraction *dynamometer*

-dynia [dɪniə] *suffix* meaning pain *-dyni, -smärta*

dynt ⇨ **bladder worm, cysticercus**

dys- [dɪs, 'dɪs, ˌ-] *prefix* meaning difficult *or* defective *dys-*

dysaesthesia [ˌdɪsiːs'θiːziə] *subst.* (i) impairment of a sense, in particular the sense of touch *dysestesi;* (ii) unpleasant feeling of pain experienced when the skin is touched lightly *dysestesi*

dysarthria [dɪs'ɑːθriə] *subst.* difficulty in speaking words clearly, caused by damage to the central nervous system *dysartri*

dysartri ⇨ **dysarthria**

dysbarism ['dɪzbɑːrɪz(ə)m] *subst.* any disorder caused by differences between the atmospheric pressure outside the body and the pressure inside *dysbarism*

dysbasia [dɪs'beɪziə] *subst.* difficulty in walking, especially when caused by a lesion to a nerve *dysbasi, gångsvårighet*

dyschezia [dɪs'kiːziə] *subst.* difficulty in passing faeces *svårighet att tömma tarmen*

dyschondroplasia [ˌdɪskɒndrəʊ'pleɪziə] *subst.* abnormal shortness of long bones *dyskondroplasi*

dyscoria [dɪs'kɔːriə] *subst.* (i) abnormally shaped pupil of the eye *dyskori;* (ii) abnormal reaction of the pupil *dyskori*

dyscrasia [dɪs'kreɪziə] *subst.* old term for any abnormal body condition *dyskrasi*

dysdiadochokinesia [ˌdɪsdaɪˌædəʊkɒkaɪ'niːsiə] *subst.* inability to carry out rapid movements, caused by a disorder *or* lesion of the cerebellum *oförmåga att utföra snabba rörelser pga lillhjärnsskada*

dysenteri ⇨ **dysentery**

dysenteric [ˌdɪs(ə)n'terɪk] *adj.* referring to dysentery *som avser el. hör till dysenteri*

dysentery ['dɪs(ə)ntri] *subst.* infection and inflammation of the colon, causing bleeding and diarrhoea *dysenteri, rödsot*

> COMMENT: dysentery occurs mainly in tropical countries. The symptoms include diarrhoea, discharge of blood and pain in the intestines. There are two main types of dysentery: bacillary dysentery, caused by the bacterium *Shigella* in contaminated food; and amoebic dysentery or amoebiasis, caused by a parasitic amoeba *Entamoeba histolytica* spread through contaminated drinking water

dysestesi ⇨ **dysaesthesia**

dysfagi ⇨ **dysphagia**

dysfasi ⇨ **dysphasia**

dysfoni ⇨ **dysphonia**

dysfunction [dɪs'fʌŋkʃ(ə)n] *subst.* abnormal functioning of an organ *dysfunktion, funktionsrubbning*

dysfunctional uterine bleeding [dɪs'fʌŋkʃ(ə)n(ə)l ˌjuːtəraɪn 'bliːdɪŋ] *subst.* bleeding in the uterus, not caused by a menstrual period *metrorragi, blödning på olaga tid (vilket bör föranleda läkarbesök)*

dysfunktion ⇨ **dysfunction**

dysgenesis [dɪs'dʒenəsɪs] *subst.* abnormal development *dysgenesi*

dysgerminoma [ˌdɪsˌdʒɜːmɪ'nəʊmə] *subst.* malignant tumour of the ovary *or* testicle *dysgerminom*

dysgrafi ⇨ **dysgraphia**

dysgraphia [dɪs'greɪfiə] *subst.* (i) difficulty in writing caused by a brain lesion *dysgrafi;* (ii) writer's cramp *skrivkramp*

dyskinesia [ˌdɪskaɪ'niːziə] *subst.* inability to control voluntary movements *dyskinesi, rörelsesvårigheter*

dyskondroplasi ⇨ **dyschondroplasia**

dyskori ⇨ **dyscoria**

dyskrasi ⇨ **dyscrasia**

dyslali ⇨ **dyslalia**

dyslalia [dɪs'leɪliə] *subst.* disorder of speech, caused by abnormal formation of the tongue *dyslali, talrubbning*

dyslektisk ⇨ **dyslexic**

dyslexi ⇨ **dyslexia**

dyslexia [dɪs'leksiə] *or* **word blindness** ['wɜːd blaɪndnəs] *subst.* disorder of development, where a person is unable to read or write properly and confuses letters *dyslexi, ordblindhet, läs- och skrivsvårigheter*

> COMMENT: caused either by an inherited disability or by a brain lesion; dyslexia does not suggest any lack of normal intelligence

dyslexic [dɪs'leksɪk] **1** *adj.* referring to dyslexia *dyslektisk* **2** *subst.* person suffering from dyslexia *person som lider av läs- och skrivsvårigheter*

dyslogia [dɪs'ləʊdʒə] *subst.* difficulty in putting ideas in words *dyslogi*

dysmenorré ⇨ **dysmenorrhoea**

dysmenorrhoea [ˌdɪsˌmenə'riːə] *subst.* pain experienced at menstruation *dysmenorré, menstruationssmärta;* **primary** *or* **essential dysmenorrhoea** = dysmenorrhoea which occurs at the first menstrual period *essentiell (primär, funktionell) dysmenorré;* **secondary dysmenorrhoea** = dysmenorrhoea which starts at some time after the first menstruation *sekundär (organisk) dysmenorré*

dysostosis [ˌdɪsɒs'təʊsɪs] *subst.* defective formation of bones *dysostosis, defekt benbildning*

dyspareunia [ˌdɪspæ'ruːniə] *subst.* difficult *or* painful sexual intercourse in a woman *dyspareuni*

dyspepsi ⇨ **dyspepsia, indigestion**

dyspepsia [dɪs'pepsiə] *or* **indigestion** [ˌɪndɪ'dʒestʃ(ə)n] *subst.* condition where a person feels pains *or* discomfort in the stomach, caused by indigestion *dyspepsi, indigestion, matspjälkningsbesvär*

dyspeptic [dɪs'peptɪk] *adj.* referring to dyspepsia *som avser el. hör till dyspepsi*

dysphagia [dɪs'feɪdʒiə] *subst.* difficulty in swallowing *dysfagi, sväljningssvårigheter*

dysphasia [dɪs'feɪziə] *subst.* difficulty in speaking and putting words into the correct order *dysfasi*

dysphemia [dɪs'fiːmiə] = STAMMERING

dysphonia [dɪs'fəʊniə] *subst.* difficulty in speaking caused by impairment of the voice *or* vocal cords *or* by laryngitis *dysfoni*

dysplasia [dɪs'pleɪziə] *subst.* abnormal development of tissue *dysplasi*

dyspné ⇨ **dyspnoea**

dyspnoea [dɪsp'niːə] *subst.* difficulty *or* pain in breathing *dyspné, andnöd;* **paroxysmal dyspnoea** = attack of breathlessness at night, caused by heart failure *andnöd pga hjärtsvikt*

dyspraxia [dɪs'præksiə] *subst.* difficulty in carrying out coordinated movements *dyspraxi*

dysrhythmia [dɪs'rɪðmiə] *subst.* abnormal rhythm (either in speaking *or* in electrical impulses in the brain) *rytmrubbning*

dyssynergi ⇨ **asynergia**

dyssynergia [ˌdɪsɪ'nɜːdʒiə] = ASYNERGIA

dystocia [dɪs'təʊsiə] *subst.* difficult childbirth *dystoci, dystoki, svår förlossning;* **fetal dystocia** = difficult childbirth caused by an abnormality *or* malpresentation of the fetus *svår förlossning pga abnormitet hos barnet;* **maternal dystocia** = difficult childbirth caused by an abnormality in the mother *svår förlossning pga abnormitet hos modern*

dystoki ⇨ **dystocia**

dystonia [dɪs'təʊniə] *subst.* disordered muscle tone, causing involuntary contractions which make the limbs deformed *dystoni*

dystrofi ⇨ **dystrophia**

dystrophia [dɪs'trəʊfiə] *or* **dystrophy** ['dɪstrəfi] *subst.* wasting of an organ *or* muscle *or* tissue due to lack of nutrients in that part of the body *dystrofi, förtvining;* **dystrophia adiposogenitalis** = FRÖHLICH'S SYNDROME; **dystrophia myotonica** = hereditary disease with muscle stiffness followed by atrophy of the face and neck muscles *dystrophia myotonica, myotonica atrophica;* **muscular dystrophy** = condition where the tissue of the muscles wastes away *muskeldystrofi*

dysuria [dɪs'jʊəriə] *subst.* difficulty in passing urine *dysuri*

dålig ⇨ **bad, funny, ill, poor, poorly, unwell, upset**

dålig andedräkt ⇨ **bad, halitosis**

dålig kondition, i ⇨ **unfit**

dåsa ⇨ **doze**

dåsig ⇨ **dozy**

däggdjur ⇨ **mammal**

dämpa ⇨ **deaden, dull, suppress**

dö ⇨ **die, expire, pass away**

död ⇨ **dead, death, expiration, necrosed, necrotic**

döda ⇨ **destroy, kill**

dödande ⇨ **destruction**

-dödande ⇨ **-cide**

dödande sjukdom ⇨ **killer**

Döderlein's bacillus ['dedəlaɪnz bə'sɪləs] *subst.* bacterium usually found in the vagina *Döderleins bacill*

dödfödd ⇨ **stillborn**

dödfödsel ⇨ **stillbirth**

dödkött ⇨ **slough**

dödlig ⇨ **deadly, fatal, lethal, terminal**

dödlighet ⇨ **death, mortality (rate)**

dödlighetsstatistik ⇨ **necrology**

dödligt ⇨ **fatally**

döds- ⇨ **deadly, fatal, lethal, necro-**

dödsattest ⇨ **certificate, death**

dödsbevis ⇨ **certificate, death**

dödsfall ⇨ **death, fatality**

dödshjälp ⇨ **euthanasia, mercy killing**

dödsoffer ⇨ **fatality**

dödsolycka ⇨ **fatality**

dödssjuk ⇨ **terminally ill**

dödstal ⇨ **death, mortality (rate)**

döende ⇨ **moribund**

döv ⇨ **deaf**

dövhet ⇨ **deafness**

dövstum ⇨ **deaf**

Ee

vitamin E [ˌvɪtəmɪn 'iː] *subst.* vitamin found in vegetables, vegetable oils, eggs and wholemeal bread *E-vitamin*

ear [ɪə] *subst.* organ which is used for hearing *auris, örat;* **if your ears are blocked, ask a doctor to syringe them; he has gone to see an ear specialist about his deafness; inner ear** = part of the ear inside the head containing the vestibule, the cochlea and the semicircular canals *auris interna, innerörat;* **middle ear** = part of the ear between the eardrum and the inner ear, containing the ossicles *auris media, mellanörat;* **outer ear** *or* **external ear** *or* **pinna** = the ear on the outside of the head together with the passage leading to the eardrum *auris externa, pinna, ytterörat;* **ear canal** = one of several passages in or connected to the ear, especially the external auditory meatus *or* passage from the outer ear to the eardrum *meatus, hörselgången;* **ear ossicle** *or* **auditory ossicle** = one of three small bones (the malleus, the incus and the stapes) in the middle ear *ossiculum auditus, hörselben*
NOTE: for terms referring to the ear see words beginning with **auric-**, **ot-** or **oto-**

> COMMENT: the outer ear is shaped in such a way that it collects sound and channels it to the eardrum. Behind the eardrum, the three ossicles in the middle ear vibrate with sound and transmit the vibrations to the cochlea in the inner ear. From the cochlea, the vibrations are passed by the auditory nerve to the brain

earache ['ɪəreɪk] *or* **otalgia** [əʊ'tældʒiə] *subst.* pain in the ear *otalgi, örsprång, ont i öronen*

eardrum ['ɪədrʌm] *or* **myringa** [mɪ'rɪŋgə] *or* **tympanum** ['tɪmpənəm] *subst.* membrane at the end of the external auditory meatus leading from the outer ear, which vibrates with sound and passes the vibrations on to the ossicles in the middle ear *membrana tympani, myrinx, trumhinnan*
NOTE: for terms referring to the eardrum see words beginning **auric-** or **tympan-**

earwax ['ɪəwæks] *or* **cerumen** [sɪ'ruːmən] *subst.* wax which forms inside the ear *cerumen, öronvax*

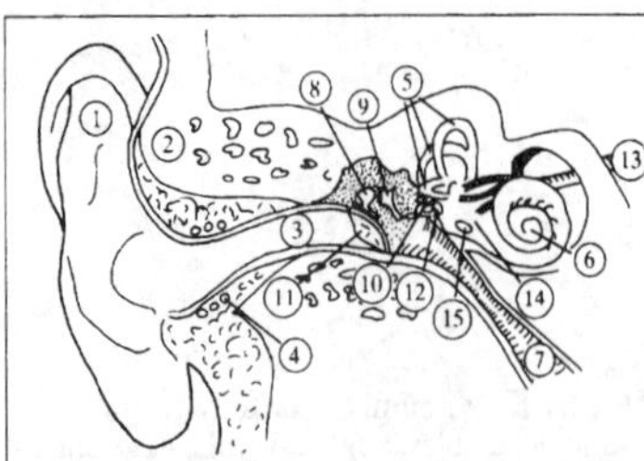

EAR	ÖRAT
1. pinna	1. ytteröra, öronmusslan
2. temporal bone	2. tinningbenet
3. external auditory meatus	3. yttre hörselgången
4. ceruminous glands	4. öronvaxkörtlarna
5. semicircular canals	5. båggångarna
6. cochlea	6. öronsnäckan
7. Eustachian tube	7. örontrumpeten
8. malleus	8. hammaren
9. incus	9. städet
10. stapes	10. stigbygeln
11. tympanic membrane (eardrum)	11. trumhinnan
12. round window	12. runda fönstret
13. auditory nerve	13. 8:e kranialnerven, hörsel- och balansnerven
14. vestibule	14. förgården
15. oval window	15. ovala fönstret

ease [i:z] *vb.* to make (pain *or* worry) less *lindra, lätta (på);* **she had an injection to ease the pain in her leg; the surgeon tried to ease the patient's fears about the results of the scan**

eat [i:t] *vb.* to chew and swallow food *äta;* **I haven't eaten anything since breakfast; the patient must not eat anything for twelve hours before the operation; eating disorders** = illnesses (such as anorexia or bulimia) which are associated with eating *störning i ätbeteendet, besvär förknippade med ätande;* **eating habits** = types of food and quantities of food regularly eaten by a person *kostvanor;* **the dietitian advised her to change her eating habits**
NOTE: **eats - eating - ate - has eaten**

eburnation [ˌi:bəˈneɪʃ(ə)n] *subst.* conversion of cartilage into a hard mass with a shiny surface like bone *slags förbening av brosk*

EB virus [ˌi:ˈbi: ˌvaɪ(ə)rəs] = EPSTEIN-BARR VIRUS

ecbolic [ekˈbɒlɪk] *adj. & subst.* (substance) which produces contraction of the uterus and so induces childbirth *or* abortion *(medel) som orsakar livmodersammandragningar el. abort*

ecchondroma [ˌekənˈdrəʊmə] *subst.* benign tumour on the surface of cartilage *or* bone *ekkondrom, brosksvulst*

ecchymosis [ˌekɪˈməʊsɪs] *or* **bruise** [ˈbru:z] *or* **contusion** [kənˈtju:ʒ(ə)n] *subst.* dark area on the skin, made by blood which has escaped into the tissues after a blow *ekkymom, blåmärke, utgjutning*

eccrine [ˈekrɪn] *or* **merocrine** [ˈmerəʊkraɪn] *adj.* which stays intact during secretion, referring especially to the sweat glands which exist all over the body *ekkrin, merokrin*

eccyesis [ˌeksaɪˈi:sɪs] = ECTOPIC PREGNANCY

ecdysis [ˈekdɪsɪs] *or* **desquamation** [ˌdeskwəˈmeɪʃ(ə)n] *subst.* continuous process of losing the outer layer of dead skin *deskvamation, fjällning*

ECG [ˌi:si:ˈdʒi:] = ELECTROCARDIOGRAM

echinococciasis [ɪˌkaɪnəʊkɒˈkaɪəsɪs] *subst.* disorder caused by a tapeworm **Echinococcus** which forms hydatid cysts in the lungs, liver, kidney or brain *echinococcosis, blåsmasksjuka*

echinococcosis ⇨ **echinococciasis**

Echinococcus granulosus [ˌɪkaɪnəʊˈkɒkəs ˌgrænjuˈləʊsəs] *subst.* type of tapeworm, usually found in animals, but sometimes transmitted to humans, causing hydatid cysts *Echinococcus granulosus*

echo- [ˈekəʊ, ˌ--] *prefix* referring to sound *echo-, eko-*

echocardiogram [ˌekəʊˈkɑ:diə(ʊ)græm] *subst.* recording of heart movements using ultrasound *ekokardiogram*

echocardiography [ˌekəʊˌkɑ:diˈɒgrəfi] *subst.* ultrasonography of the heart *ekokardiografi*

echoencephalography [ˌekəʊenˌkefəˈlɒgrəfi] *subst.* ultrasonography of the brain *ekoencefalografi*

echography [ɪˈkɒgrəfi] *subst.* ultrasonography *or* passing ultrasound waves through the body and recording echoes to show details of internal organs *(ultra)sonografi, ultraljudsundersökning*

echokinesis [ˌekəʊkaɪˈniːsɪs] *subst.* meaningless imitating of another person's actions *ekokinesi*

echolalia [ˌekəʊˈleɪliə] *subst.* repeating words spoken by another person *ekolali, ekofrasi*

echopraxia [ˌekəʊˈpræksiə] *subst.* imitating another person's actions *ekopraxi, ekofrasi*

echovirus [ˌekəʊˈvaɪ(ə)rəs] *subst.* one of a group of viruses which can be isolated from the intestine and which can cause serious illnesses such as aseptic meningitis, gastroenteritis and respiratory infection in small children *ECHO-virus (förkortning av Enteric Cytopathic Human Orphan); compare* REOVIRUS

eclabium [ɪˈkleɪbiəm] *subst.* turning the lips outwards *or* eversion of the lips *eversion (utåtvridning) av läpparna*

eclampsia [ɪˈklæm(p)siə] *subst.* serious condition of pregnant women at the end of pregnancy, where the patient has convulsions and high blood pressure and may go into a coma, caused by toxaemia of pregnancy *eklampsia gravidarum, eklampsi, havandeskapsförgiftning (egentligen pga för högt blodtryck)*

ecmnesia [ekˈniːziə] *subst.* not being able to remember recent events, while remembering clearly events which happened some time ago *minnesförlust för nyligen inträffade händelser pga åldersförändringar, förlust av korttidsminnet*

ecological [ˌiːkəˈlɒdʒɪk(ə)l] *adj.* referring to ecology *ekologisk*

ecologist [ɪˈkɒlədʒɪst] *subst.* scientist who studies ecology *ekolog*

ecology [ɪˈkɒlədʒi] *subst.* study of the environment and the relationship of living organisms to it *ekologi;* **human ecology** = study of man's place in the natural world *humanekologi*

écraseur [ˌeɪkrɑːˈzɜː] *subst.* surgical instrument (usually with a wire loop) used to cut a part *or* a growth off at its base *kirurgiskt instrument (ofta med trådslynga) för att skära av utväxter o.d.*

ecstasy [ˈekstəsi] *subst.* feeling of extreme happiness *extas, hänryckning*

ECT [ˌiːsiːˈtiː] = ELECTROCONVULSIVE THERAPY (electroshock treatment)

ECT ⇨ **electric, electroconvulsive therapy (ECT), electroshock therapy**

ect- [ˈekt, ˌ-] *or* **ecto-** [ˈektəʊ, ˌ--] *prefix* meaning outside *ekt(o)-, yttre*

ectasia [ekˈteɪziə] *subst.* dilatation of a passage *ektasi, dilatation, utvidgning*

ecthyma [ekˈθaɪmə] *subst.* skin disorder *or* serious form of impetigo which penetrates deep under the skin and leaves scars *ekt(h)yma*

ectoderm [ˈektəʊdɜːm] *or* **embryonic ectoderm** [ˌembriˈɒnɪk ˌektəʊdɜːm] *subst.* outer layer of an early embryo *ektoderm, yttre groddbladet*

ectodermal [ˌektəʊˈdɜːm(ə)l] *adj.* referring to the ectoderm *ektodermal*

ectomorph [ˈektəʊmɔːf] *subst.* type of person who tends to be quite thin *ektomorf person*

ectomorphic [ˌektə(ʊ)ˈmɔːfɪk] *adj.* referring to an ectomorph *ektomorf; compare* ENDOMORPH, MESOMORPH

-ectomy [ˈektəmi] *suffix* referring to the removal of a part by surgical operation *-ektomi;* **appendicectomy** = operation to remove the appendix *appendektomi, blindtarmsoperation*

ectoparasite [ˌektəʊˈpærəsaɪt] *subst.* parasite which lives on the skin *ektoparasit, ektosit; compare* ENDOPARASITE

ectopia [ekˈtəʊpiə] *subst.* condition where an organ *or* part of the body is not in its normal position *ektopi, felläge*

ectopic [ekˈtɒpɪk] *adj.* abnormal *or* not in the normal position *ektopisk*

ectopic beat [ekˈtɒpɪk ˌbiːt] *or* **extrasystole** = [ˌekstrəˈsɪstəli] abnormal extra beat of the heart which originates from a point other than the sinoatrial node *ektopiskt slag, extrasystole;* **ectopic pacemaker** = abnormal function of the heart muscle which takes the place of the sinoatrial node *ektopiskt fokus;* **ectopic pregnancy** *or* **extrauterine pregnancy** *or* **eccyesis** = pregnancy where the fetus develops outside the womb, often in one of the Fallopian tubes (tubal pregnancy) *extrauterin (ektopisk) graviditet, utomkvedshavandeskap*
NOTE: the opposite is **entopic**

ectoplasm [ˈektə(ʊ)plæz(ə)m] *subst. (in cells)* outer layer of cytoplasm which is the densest part of the cytoplasm *ektoplasma*

ectro- ['ektrəʊ, ˌ--] *prefix* meaning absence *or* lack of something (usually congenital) *ektro-*

ectrodactyly [ˌektrəʊ'dæktɪli] *subst.* congenital absence of all *or* part of a finger *ektrodaktyli*

ectrogeny [ek'trɒdʒəni] *subst.* congenital absence of a part at birth *medfödd avsaknad av kroppsdel*

ectromelia [ˌektrəʊ'mi:liə] *subst.* congenital absence of one or more limbs *ektromeli*

ectropion [ek'trəʊpiən] *subst.* eversion *or* turning of the edge of an eyelid outwards *ektropi(on), utåtvikning av nedre ögonlocket*

eczema ['eksɪmə] *subst.* non-contagious inflammation of the skin, with itchy rash and blisters *eksem;* **atopic eczema** = type of eczema often caused by hereditary allergy *atopiskt eksem;* **endogenous eczema** = eczema which is caused internally *endogent eksem;* **seborrhoeic eczema** = type of eczema where scales form on the skin, usually on the scalp, and then move down the body *seborroiskt eksem;* **varicose eczema** *or* **hypostatic eczema** = eczema which develops on the legs, caused by bad circulation *hypostatiskt eksem, variköst eksem; see also* PURIFIED

eczematous [ek'semətəs] *adj.* referring to eczema *eksematös;* **eczematous dermatitis** = itchy inflammation *or* irritation of the skin due an allergic reaction to a substance which a person has touched or absorbed *eksematös dermatit*

EDD [ˌi:di:'di:] = EXPECTED DATE OF DELIVERY

edema [ɪ'di:mə] *US* = OEDEMA

edentulous [ɪ'dentjuləs] *adj.* having lost all teeth *tandlös*

edible ['edəb(ə)l] *adj.* which can be eaten *ätbar, ätlig;* **edible fungi** = fungi which can be eaten and are not poisonous *ätliga svampar*

EEG [ˌi:i:'dʒi:] = ELECTROENCEPHALOGRAM

EEG ⇨ **electroencephalogram (EEG), electroencephalography**

EEG-apparat ⇨ **electroencephalograph**

efelider ⇨ **freckles**

effect [ɪ'fekt] **1** *subst.* result of a drug *or* a treatment *or* an action *effekt, verkan;* **the effect of the disease is to make the patient blind; the antiseptic cream has had no effect on the rash; radiotherapy has a positive effect on cancer cells 2** *vb.* to make something happen *åstadkomma, verkställa, utföra;* **the doctors effected a cure**

effective [ɪ'fektɪv] *adj.* which has an effect *effektiv, verksam;* **his way of making the children keep quiet is very effective; embolization is an effective treatment for severe haemoptysis**

effector [ɪ'fektə] *subst.* special nerve ending in muscles *or* glands which is activated to produce contraction *or* secretion *effektor*

effekt ⇨ **action, activity, effect**

effektiv ⇨ **effective, efficient**

effektivt ⇨ **efficiently**

effektor ⇨ **effector**

efferens ['ef(ə)r(ə)ns] *see* VAS EFFERENS

efferent ['ef(ə)r(ə)nt] *adj.* carrying away from part of the body *or* from the centre *efferent, bortförande, utåtledande, avförande;* **efferent duct** = duct which carries a secretion away from a gland *efferent (avförande) gång, utförsgång;* **efferent vessel** = vessel which drains lymph from a gland *vas efferentia, bortförande lymfkärl*
NOTE: the opposite is **afferent**

efficient [ɪ'fɪʃ(ə)nt] *adj.* which works well *or* which functions correctly *effektiv, verksam, ändamålsenlig;* **the new product is an efficient antiseptic; the ward sister is extremely efficient**

efficiently [ɪ'fɪʃ(ə)ntli] *adv.* in an efficient way *effektivt, verksamt, ändamålsenligt;* **she manages all her patients very efficiently**

effleurage [ˌeflu:'rɑ:ʒ] *subst.* form of massage where the skin is stroked in one direction to increase blood flow *effleurage*

effort ['efət] *subst.* using power, either mental or physical *ansträngning;* **he made an effort and lifted his hands above his head; it took a lot of effort to walk even this short distance; if he made an effort he would be able to get out of bed; effort syndrome** *or* **da Costa's syndrome** *or* **disordered action of the heart** = condition where the patient suffers palpitations caused by worry *hjärtneuros*

effusion [ɪ'fju:ʒ(ə)n, e'f-] *subst.* (i) discharge of blood *or* fluid *or* pus into or out of an internal cavity *utgjutning;* (ii) fluid *or* blood *or* pus which is discharged *utgjutning;* **pericardial effusion** = excess of fluid which forms in the pericardial sac *perikardexsudat, utgjutning i hjärtsäcken;* **pleural effusion** = excess of fluid formed in the pleural sac *pleuraexsudat, utgjutning i lungsäcken*

efter- ➪ **after-, post-**

efterbehandling ➪ **aftercare**

efterbild ➪ **after-image**

efterblivenhet ➪ **mental**

efterbörd ➪ **afterbirth**

efterkontroll ➪ **follow-up**

eftersmak ➪ **aftertaste**

efterverkningar ➪ **after-effects**

eftervård ➪ **aftercare**

eftervärkar ➪ **afterpains**

egen- ➪ **auto-, idio-, self-**

egenhet ➪ **idiosyncrasy**

egenskap ➪ **trait**

egentlig ➪ **true**

egenvård ➪ **self-care**

egg [eg] *subst.* **(a)** reproductive cell produced in the female body by the ovary, and which, if fertilized by the male sperm, becomes an embryo *ovum, ägg;* **egg cell** = immature ovum *or* female cell *äggcell* **(b)** **hen's egg** = egg with a hard shell, laid by a chicken, which is used for food *hönsägg;* **he is allergic to eggs**

ego ['i:gəʊ, 'egəʊ] *subst. (in psychology)* part of the mind which is consciously in contact with the outside world and is influenced by experiences of the world *ego, jaget; compare* ID, SUBCONSCIOUS, SUPEREGO

Egyptian ophthalmia [ɪˌdʒɪpʃ(ə)n ɒf'θælmiə] *see* TRACHOMA

egyptiska ögonsjukdomen ➪ **ophthalmia**

EHO [ˌi:eɪtʃ'əʊ] = ENVIRONMENTAL HEALTH OFFICER

EIA [ˌi:aɪ'eɪ] = EXERCISE-INDUCED ASTHMA

eidetic imagery [aɪ'detɪk 'ɪmɪdʒ(ə)ri] *subst.* recalling extremely clear pictures in the mind *eidetiska bilder*

Eisenmenger syndrome ['aɪsenmeŋgəz ˌsɪndrəʊm] *subst.* heart disease caused by a septal defect between the ventricles, with pulmonary hypertension *Eisenmengers komplex*

ejaculate [ɪ'dʒækjuleɪt] *vb.* to send out semen from the penis *ejakulera*

ejaculation [ɪˌdʒækju'leɪʃ(ə)n] *subst.* sending out of semen from the penis *ejakulation, sädesuttömning, sädesavgång;* **premature ejaculation** = situation where the man ejaculates too early during sexual intercourse *ejaculatio praecox, förtidig sädesavgång*

ejaculatio praecox [ɪ'dʒækju'leɪʃiəʊ ˌpri:kɒks] *subst.* situation where the man ejaculates too early during sexual intercourse *ejaculatio praecox, förtidig sädesavgång*

ejaculatory [ɪ'dʒækjʊlət(ə)ri] *adj.* referring to ejaculation *ejakulatorisk;* **ejaculatory ducts** = two ducts, leading from the seminal vesicles and vas deferens, which go through the prostate and end in the urethra ➪ *illustration* UROGENITAL SYSTEM (MALE) *ductus ejaculatorius*

ejakulation ➪ **ejaculation**

ejakulera ➪ **ejaculate**

eject [ɪ'dʒekt] *vb.* to send out something with force *driva (kasta, slunga) ut;* **blood is ejected from the ventricle during systole**

ejection [ɪ'dʒekʃ(ə)n] *subst.* sending out something with force *utdrivning, utstötning*

EKG [ˌi:keɪ'dʒi:] *US* = ELECTROCARDIOGRAM
NOTE: GB English is **ECG**

EKG ➪ **electrocardiogram (ECG), electrocardiography**

EKG-apparat ➪ **electrocardiograph, monitor**

ekkondrom ➪ **ecchondroma**

ekkrin ➪ **eccrine, merocrine**

ekkymom ➪ **bruise, ecchymosis**

eklampsi ➪ **eclampsia**

ekoencefalografi ➪ **echoencephalography**

ekofrasi ➪ **echolalia, echopraxia**

ekokardiografi ➪ **echocardiography**

ekokardiogram ➪ **echocardiogram**

ekokinesi ➪ **echokinesis**

ekolali ➪ **echolalia, palilalia**

ekologi ➪ **ecology**

ekologisk ➪ **ecological**

ekopraxi ➪ **echopraxia**

eksem ➪ **eczema**

eksematös ➪ **eczematous**

ektasi ➪ **ectasia**

ektoderm ➪ **ectoderm**

ektodermal ➪ **ectodermal**

ektomorf ➪ **ectomorphic**

ektoparasit ➪ **ectoparasite**

ektopi ➪ **ectopia**

ektopisk ➪ **ectopic**

ektopiskt fokus ➪ **pacemaker**

ektopiskt hjärtslag ➪ **premature**

ektoplasma ➪ **ectoplasm**

ektosit ➪ **ectoparasite**

ektro- ➪ **ectro-**

ektrodaktyli ➪ **ectrodactyly**

ektromeli ➪ **ectromelia**

ekvilibrium ➪ **equilibrium**

el- ➪ **electric**

elakartad ➪ **malignant, nasty, pernicious, virulent**

elakartad, inte ➪ **non-malignant**

elastic [ɪ'læstɪk] *adj.* which can be stretched and compressed and return to its former shape *elastisk;* **elastic bandage** = type of stretch bandage used to compress varicose tissues *or* to support weak joints *elastiskt förband;* **elastic cartilage** *or* **yellow elastic fibrocartilage** = flexible cartilage such as that in the external ear *elastiskt brosk;* **elastic fibres** *or* **yellow fibres** = basic components of elastic cartilage, also found in the skin and the walls of arteries or the lungs *elastiska fibrer (trådar);* **elastic tissue** = connective tissue, as in the walls of arteries or of the alveoli in the lungs, which contains elastic fibres *elastisk vävnad (bindväv)*

elasticitet ➪ **elasticity**

elasticity [ˌiːlæs'tɪsəti] *subst.* being able to expand and be compressed and to return to the former shape *elasticitet*

elastin [ɪ'læstɪn] *subst.* protein which occurs in elastic fibres *elastin*

elastisk ➪ **elastic**

elation [ɪ'leɪʃ(ə)n] *subst.* being stimulated and excited *upprymdhet*

elbow ['elbəʊ] *subst.* hinged joint where the arm bone (humerus) joins the forearm bones (radius and ulna) *armbågen;* **tennis elbow** *or* *US* **pitcher's elbow** = inflammation of the tendons of the extensor muscles in the hand which are attached to the bone near the elbow *tennisarmbåge*
NOTE: for other terms referring to the elbow, see **cubital**

elchock ➪ **electric, electroconvulsive therapy (ECT), shock**

elderly ['eldəli] *adj. & subst.* old (person) *or* (person) aged over 65 *äldre (person), åldring, pensionär;* **she looks after her two elderly parents; a home for elderly single women; the elderly** = old people *åldringarna, de äldre (gamla), pensionärerna*

eldsmärke ➪ **port wine stain**

elective [ɪ'lektɪv] *adj. elektiv;* (i) (chemical substance) which tends to combine with one particular substance rather than another *(kemiskt ämne) som tenderar att förena sig med vissa ämnen före andra;* (ii) (part of a course in a college *or* university) which a student can choose to take rather than another *valfri, frivillig, tillvals-;* **elective surgery** *or* **elective treatment** = surgery *or* treatment which a patient can choose to have but is not urgently necessary to save his life *elektiv kirurgi resp. behandling*

Electra complex [ɪ'lektrə ˌkɒmpleks] *subst. (in psychology)* condition where a girl feels sexually attracted to her father and sees her mother as an obstacle *elektrakomplex*

electric [ɪ'lektrɪk] *adj.* worked by electricity; used for carrying electricity *elektrisk, el-;* **electric shock** = sudden passage of electricity into the body, causing a nervous spasm or, in severe cases, death *elektrisk stöt;* **electric shock treatment** = treatment of a disorder by giving the patient light electric shocks *ECT, elektrokonvulsiv terapi (behandling), "chockbehandling", "elchock", elbehandling*

electricity [ɪlek'trɪsəti] *subst.* electron energy which can be converted to light *or* heat *or* power *elektricitet;* **the motor is run by electricity; electricity is used to administer shocks to a patient**

electro- [ɪ'lektrə(ʊ), -ˌ--] *prefix* referring to electricity *elektro-*

electrocardiogram (ECG) [ɪˌlektrəʊ'kɑːdiə(ʊ)græm, (ˌiːsiː'dziː)] *subst.* chart which records the electrical impulses in the heart muscle *elektrokardiogram, EKG*

electrocardiograph [ɪˌlektrəʊ'kɑːdiə(ʊ)grɑːf] *subst.* apparatus for measuring and recording the electrical impulses of the muscles of the heart as it beats *elektrokardiograf, EKG-apparat*

electrocardiography [ɪˌlektrəʊˌkɑːdɪ'ɒgrəfi] *subst.* process of recording the electrical impulses of the heart *elektrokardiografi, EKG*

electrocardiophonography [ɪˌlektrəʊˌkɑːdiə(ʊ)fə'nɒgrəfi] *subst.* process of electrically recording the sounds of the heartbeats *fonokardiografi, fonogram*

electrocautery [ɪˌlektrəʊ'kɔːt(ə)ri] = GALVANOCAUTERY

electrochemical [ɪˌlektrəʊ'kemɪk(ə)l] *adj.* referring to electricity and chemicals and their interaction *elektrokemisk*

electrocoagulation [ɪˌlektrəʊkəʊˌægju'leɪʃ(ə)n] *subst.* control of haemorrhage in surgery by coagulation of divided blood vessels by passing a high-frequency electric current through them *elektrokoagulering, elkoagulering, diatermi*

electroconvulsive therapy (ECT) [ɪˌlektrəʊkənˌvʌlsɪv 'θerəpi (ˌiːsiː'tiː)] *or* **electroplexy** [ɪ'lektrəʊˌpleksi] *subst.* treatment of severe depression and some mental disorders by giving the patient small electric shocks in the brain to make him have convulsions *ECT, elektrokonvulsiv terapi (behandling), "chockbehandling", "elchock", elbehandling*

electrode [ɪ'lektrəʊd] *subst.* conductor of an electrical apparatus which touches the body and carries an electric shock *elektrod*

electrodessication [ɪˌlektrəʊˌdesɪ'keɪʃ(ə)n] *or* **fulguration** *subst.* destruction of tissue (such as the removal of a wart) by burning with an electric needle *diatermi*

electroencephalogram (EEG) [ɪˌlektrəʊɪn'sef(ə)ləgræm (ˌiːiː'dʒiː)] *subst.* chart on which are recorded the electrical impulses in the brain *elektroencefalogram, EEG*

electroencephalograph [ɪˌlektrəʊɪn'sef(ə)ləgrɑːf] *subst.* apparatus which records the electrical impulses in the brain *elektroencefalograf, EEG-apparat*

electroencephalography [ɪˌlektrəʊɪnˌsefə'lɒgrəfi] *subst.* process of recording the electrical impulses in the brain *elektroencefalografi, EEG*

electrolysis [ɪlek'trɒləsɪs] *subst.* destruction of tissue (such as removing unwanted hair) by applying an electric current *elektrokoagulering, elkoagulering, diatermi*

electrolyte [ɪ'lektrə(ʊ)laɪt] *subst.* chemical solution of a substance which can conduct electricity *elektrolyt*

electrolytic [ɪˌlektrə(ʊ)'lɪtɪk] *adj.* referring to electrolytes *or* to electrolysis *elektrolytisk*

electromyogram (EMG) [ɪˌlektrə(ʊ)'maɪəʊgræm (ˌiːem'dʒiː)] *subst.* chart showing the electric currents in muscles in action *elektromyogram, EMG*

electromyography [ɪˌlektrəʊmaɪ'ɒgrəfi] *subst.* study of electric currents in active muscles *elektromyografi, EMG*

electron [ɪ'lektrɒn] *subst.* negative particle in an atom *elektron;* **electron microscope (EM)** = microscope which uses a beam of electrons instead of light *elektronmikroskop*

electronic [ɪlek'trɒnɪk] *adj.* referring to electrons *or* working with electrons *elektronisk;* **electronic stethoscope** = stethoscope fitted with an amplifier *elektroniskt stetoskop*

electro-oculography [ɪˌlektrəʊˌɒkjuˈlɒgrəfi] *subst.* recording the electric currents round the eye, induced by eye movements *registrering av de elektriska spänningarna runt ögat vid ögonrörelser*

electrophoresis [ɪˌlektrəʊfəˈriːsɪs] *subst.* analysis of a substance by the movement of charged particles towards an electrode in a solution *elektrofores, elfores*

electroplexy [ɪˈlektrə(ʊ)ˌpleksi] *subst.* *see* ELECTROCONVULSIVE THERAPY

electroretinography [ɪˌlektrəʊˌretɪˈnɒgrəfi] *subst.* process of recording electrical changes in the retina when stimulated by light *elektroretinografi*

electroshock therapy [ɪˈlektrəʊʃɒk ˌθerəpi] *or* **electroshock treatment** [ɪˈlektrəʊʃɒk ˌtriːtment] *or* **electroplexy** [ɪˌlekˈtrɒpleksi] *subst.* electroconvulsive therapy *or* treatment of some mental disorders by giving the patient electric shocks in the brain to make him have convulsions *ECT, elektrokonvulsiv terapi (behandling), "chockbehandling", "elchock", elbehandling*

electrotherapy [ɪˌlektrə(ʊ)ˈθerəpi] *subst.* treatment of a disorder, such as some forms of paralysis, using low-frequency electric current to try to revive the muscles *behandling med elektricitet*

elefantiasis ➪ **elephantiasis**

elektiv ➪ **elective**

elektrakomplex ➪ **Electra complex**

elektricitet ➪ **electricity**

elektrisk ➪ **electric**

elektrod ➪ **electrode**

elektroencefalograf ➪ **electroencephalograph**

elektroencefalografi ➪ **electroencephalography**

elektroencefalogram ➪ **electroencephalogram (EEG)**

elektrofores ➪ **electrophoresis**

elektrokardiograf ➪ **electrocardiograph**

elektrokardiografi ➪ **electrocardiography**

elektrokardiogram ➪ **cardiogram, electrocardiogram (ECG), -gram**

elektrokemisk ➪ **electrochemical**

elektrokoagulering ➪ **electrocoagulation, electrolysis**

elektrolyt ➪ **electrolyte**

elektrolytlösning ➪ **saline**

elektromyografi ➪ **electromyography**

elektromyogram ➪ **electromyogram (EMG)**

elektron ➪ **electron**

elektronisk ➪ **electronic**

elektronmikroskop ➪ **electron**

elektroretinografi ➪ **electroretinography**

element [ˈelɪmənt] *subst.* basic simple chemical substance which cannot be broken down to a simpler substance *grundämne;* **trace element** = substance which is essential to the human body, but only in very small quantities *spårelement, spårämne*

elephantiasis [ˌelɪf(ə)nˈta(ɪ)əsɪs] *subst.* oedematous condition where parts of the body swell and the skin becomes hardened, frequently caused by filariasis (infestation with various species of the parasitic worm **Filaria**) *elefantiasis*

elevation [ˌelɪˈveɪʃ(ə)n] *subst.* raised part *elevation, upphöjning, stegring;* **elevation sling** = sling tied round the neck, used to hold the arm in a high position to prevent bleeding *mitella som håller armen i högläge*

elevator [ˈelɪveɪtə] *subst.* **(a)** muscle which raises part of the body *muskel som lyfter kroppsdel* **(b)** (i) surgical instrument used to lift part of a broken bone *elevatorium;* (ii) instrument used by a dentist to remove a tooth *or* part of a tooth *slags instrument för tandutdragning;* **periosteum elevator** = surgical instrument used to remove the periosteum from a bone *instrument för lyftning av benhinna*

elevatorium ➪ **elevator**

elfores ➪ **electrophoresis**

elicit [ɪ'lɪsɪt] *vb.* to make happen *or* to provoke *framkalla, väcka;* **muscle tenderness was elicited in the lower limbs**

eliminate [ɪ'lɪmɪneɪt] *vb.* to get rid of waste matter from the body *eliminera, avsöndra, utsöndra;* **the excess salts are eliminated through the kidneys**

elimination [ɪˌlɪmɪ'neɪʃ(ə)n] *subst.* removal of waste matter from the body *eliminering, avsöndring, utsöndring*

eliminera ⇨ **eliminate**

eliminering ⇨ **elimination**

elixir [ɪ'lɪksə] *subst.* sweet liquid which hides the unpleasant taste of a drug *elixir*

elkoagulering ⇨ **electrocoagulation, electrolysis**

elkonvertering ⇨ **cardioversion**

elliptocytosis [ɪˌlɪptəʊsaɪ'təʊsɪs] *subst.* condition where abnormal oval-shaped red cells appear in the blood *elliptocytos, ovalocytos*

EM [ˌi:'em] = ELECTRON MICROSCOPE

emaceration ⇨ **emaciation**

emaciated [ɪ'meɪʃieɪtɪd] *adj.* very thin *or* extremely underweight *emac(i)erad, avmagrad, utmärglad;* **anorexic patients become emaciated and may need hospitalization**

emaciation [ɪˌmeɪsɪ'eɪʃ(ə)n] *subst.* being extremely thin; wasting away of body tissue *emaciation, emaceration, avmagring, utmärgling*

emaculation [ɪˌmækju'leɪʃ(ə)n] *subst.* removing spots from the skin *emakulation*

emakulation ⇨ **emaculation**

emalj ⇨ **enamel**

emaljsvulst ⇨ **ameloblastoma**

emasculation [ɪˌmæskju'leɪʃ(ə)n] *subst.* (i) removal of the penis *förlust av penis;* (ii) loss of male characteristics *kastrering*

embalm [ɪm'bɑ:m] *vb.* to preserve a dead body by using special antiseptic chemicals to prevent decay *balsamera*

embolectomy [ˌembə'lektəmi] *subst.* surgical operation to remove a blood clot *embolektomi*

embolektomi ⇨ **embolectomy**

emboli ⇨ **embolism**

embolisering ⇨ **embolization**

embolism ['embəlɪz(ə)m] *subst.* blocking of an artery by a mass of material (usually a blood clot), preventing the flow of blood *emboli;* **air embolism** = interference with the flow of blood in vessels by bubbles of air *luftemboli;* **pulmonary embolism** = blockage of the pulmonary artery *lungemboli*

embolization [ˌembəlaɪ'zeɪʃ(ə)n] *subst.* using emboli inserted down a catheter into a blood vessel to treat internal bleeding *embolisering*

embolus ['embələs] *subst.* mass of material (such as a blood clot *or* air bubble *or* fat globule) which blocks a blood vessel *embolus, blodpropp*
NOTE: plural is **emboli**

> QUOTE once a bleeding site has been located, a catheter is manipulated as near as possible to it, so that embolization can be carried out. Many different materials are used as the embolus
> **British Medical Journal**

embrocation [ˌembrə(ʊ)'keɪʃ(ə)n] *subst.* liniment *or* oily liquid used to rub on the skin, acting as a counterirritant *or* vasodilator *liniment (vätska) för utvärtes frottering*

embryo ['embriəʊ] *subst.* unborn baby during the first eight weeks after conception *embryo* NOTE: after eight weeks, the unborn baby is called a **fetus**

embryologi ⇨ **embryology**

embryological [ˌembriə'lɒdʒɪk(ə)l] *adj.* referring to embryology *embryologisk*

embryologisk ⇨ **embryological**

embryology [ˌembri'ɒlədʒi] *subst.* study of the early stages of the development of the embryo *embryologi*

embryonal ⇨ **embryonic, germinal**

embryonalepitel ⇨ **germinal**

embryonic [ˌembri'ɒnɪk] *adj.* (i) referring to an embryo *embryonal;* (ii) in an early stage of development *outvecklad;* **embryonic membranes** = skins around an embryo providing protection and food supply (the amnion and chorion) *fosterhinnor*

emergency [ɪ'mɜːdʒ(ə)nsi] *subst.* situation where immediate action has to be taken *olycka, olycksfall; US* **emergency medical technician (EMT)** = trained paramedic who gives care to victims at the scene of an accident or in an ambulance *ung. specialutbildad ambulanspersonal;* **emergency ward** = hospital ward which deals with urgent cases (such as accident victims) *akutmottagning, olycksfallsavdelning*

emesis ['eməsɪs] *subst.* vomiting *emes, kräkning, uppkastning*

emetic [ɪ'metɪk] *adj. & subst.* (substance) which causes vomiting *emetisk, emetikum, kräkmedel;* **the doctor administered an emetic**

emetikum ⇨ **emetic**

emetisk ⇨ **emetic**

emfysem ⇨ **emphysema**

EMG [ˌiːem'dʒiː] = ELECTROMYOGRAM

EMG ⇨ **electromyogram (EMG), electromyography**

eminence ['emɪnəns] *subst.* something which protrudes from a surface, such as a lump on a bone *or* swelling on the skin *eminentia, upphöjning; see also* HYPOTHENAR, THENAR

eminentia ⇨ **eminence**

emissary veins ['emɪs(ə)ri ˌveɪnz] *subst.* veins through the skull which connect the venous sinuses with the scalp veins *venae emissariae*

emission [ɪ'mɪʃ(ə)n] *subst.* discharge *or* release of fluid *emission, utsöndring, uttömning;* **nocturnal emission** = production of semen from the penis while a man is asleep *nattlig (sädes)uttöming, pollution*

emmenagogue [ɪ'menəgɒg] *subst.* drug which will help increase menstrual flow *emmenagogum, menstruationspådrivande medel*

emmenagogum ⇨ **emmenagogue**

emmetropia [ˌemɪ'trəʊpiə] *subst.* normal vision *or* correct focusing of light rays by the eye onto the retina *emmetropi, normalseende, normalsyn; compare* AMETROPIA

emolliens ⇨ **emollient**

emollient [ɪ'mɒliənt] *adj. & subst.* (substance) which smooths the skin *emolliens, huduppmjukande (medel)*

emotion [ɪ'məʊʃ(ə)n] *subst.* strong feeling *emotion, känsla*

emotional [ɪ'məʊʃ(ə)n(ə)l] *adj.* showing strong feeling *emotionell, känslomässig;* **emotional disorder** = disorder due to worry *or* stress, etc. *emotionell (känslomässig) störning*

emotionell ⇨ **emotional**

empathy ['empəθi] *subst.* being able to understand the problems and feelings of another person *empati, inlevelse, medkänsla*

empati ⇨ **empathy**

emphysema [ˌemfɪ'siːmə] *subst.* condition where the alveoli of the lungs become enlarged *or* rupture *or* break down, with the result that the surface available for gas exchange is reduced, so reducing the oxygen level in the blood and making it difficult for the patient to breathe *emfysem, lungemfysem*

> COMMENT: emphysema can be caused by smoking or by living in a polluted environment, by old age, asthma or whooping cough

employ [ɪm'plɔɪ] *vb.* **(a)** to use *använda, bruka;* **the dentist usually has to employ force to extract a tooth (b)** to pay a person for regular work *anställa, sysselsätta;* **the local health authority employs a staff of two thousand; she is employed by the dentist as a hygienist; a practice nurse is employed by the practice, not by the health authority**

empty ['em(p)ti] **1** *adj.* with nothing inside *tom;* **the medicine bottle is empty; take this empty bottle and provide a urine sample; the children's ward is never empty** NOTE: opposite is **full 2** *vb.* to take everything out of something *tömma;* **she emptied the water out of the bottle**

empyema [ˌempaɪ'iːmə] *or* **pyothorax** [ˌpaɪəʊ'θɔːræks] *subst.* collection of pus in a cavity, especially in the pleural cavity *empyem, varansamling*

EMT [ˌiːem'tiː] *US* = EMERGENCY MEDICAL TECHNICIAN

emulsion [ɪ'mʌlʃ(ə)n] *subst.* mixture of liquids which do not normally mix (such as oil and water) *emulsion*

EN [ˌiːˈen] = ENROLLED NURSE
NOTE: enrolled nurses are classified according to their area of specialization: **EN(G)** = Enrolled Nurse (General); **EN(M)** = Enrolled Nurse (Mental); **EN(MH)** = Enrolled Nurse (Mental Handicap)

en- ⇨ **mono-, uni-**

enamel [ɪˈnæm(ə)l] *subst.* hard white shiny outer covering of the crown of a tooth ⇨ *illustration* TOOTH *emalj, tandemalj*

enanthema [ˌenənˈθiːmə] *subst.* rash on a mucous membrane, as in the mouth or vagina, produced by the action of toxic substances on small blood vessels *enant(h)em, slemhinneutslag*

enarthrosis [ˌenɑːˈθrəʊsɪs] *subst.* ball and socket joint, such as the hip joint *articulatio sphaeroidea (cotylica), enartros, kulled*

enartros ⇨ **ball and socket joint, enarthrosis**

ENB [ˌiːenˈbiː] = ENGLISH NATIONAL BOARD

encapsulated [ɪnˈkæpsjuleɪtɪd] *adj.* enclosed in a capsule *or* in a sheath of tissue *inkapslad*

encefalin ⇨ **encephalin**

encefalit ⇨ **encephalitis**

encefalocele ⇨ **cephalocele, encephalocele**

encefalografi ⇨ **encephalography, pneumoencephalography, ventriculography**

encefalom ⇨ **encephaloma**

encefalomalaci ⇨ **encephalomalacia**

encefalomyelit ⇨ **encephalomyelitis**

encefalomyelopati ⇨ **encephalomyelopathy**

encefalon ⇨ **brain, encephalon**

encefalopati ⇨ **encephalopathy**

encellig ⇨ **unicellular**

encephal- [ˌenkɪˈfæl, ˌensɪˈfæl] *or* **encephalo-** [enˈkef(ə)lə(ʊ), -ˌ--, enˈsef(ə)lə(ʊ), -ˌ--] *prefix* referring to the brain *encefal(o)-, hjärn-*

encephalin [enˈkefəliːn] *subst.* peptide produced in the brain *encefalin; see also* ENDORPHIN

encephalitis [ˌenkefəˈlaɪtɪs] *subst.* inflammation of the brain *encefalit, hjärninflammation;* **encephalitis lethargica** *or* **lethargic encephalitis** *or* **sleepy sickness** = formerly common type of encephalitis occurring in epidemics *encephalitis epidemica (lethergica), sömnsjuka*

> COMMENT: encephalitis is caused by any of several viruses (viral encephalitis) and is also associated with infectious viral diseases such as measles or mumps

encephalocele [enˈkefələʊsiːl] *subst.* condition where the brain protrudes through a congenital *or* traumatic gap in the skull bones *encefalocele, hjärnbråck*

encephalography [enˌkefəˈlɒgrəfi] *or* **pneumoencephalography** [ˌnjuːməʊenˌkefəˈlɒgrəfi] *subst.* X-ray examination of the ventricles and spaces of the brain after air has been introduced by lumbar puncture *encefalografi, pneumoencefalografi, ventrikulografi, luftskalle*

encephaloid [enˈkefəlɔɪd] **1** *adj.* which looks like brain tissue *hjärnvävnadsliknande* **2** *subst.* large carcinoma of the breast *stort bröstcarcinom*

encephaloma [enˌkefəˈləʊmə] *subst.* tumour of the brain *encefalom, hjärntumör*

encephalomalacia [enˌkefələʊməˈleɪʃiə] *subst.* softening of the brain *encefalomalaci, hjärnuppmjukning*

encephalomyelitis [enˌkefələʊˌmaɪəˈlaɪtɪs] *subst.* group of diseases which cause inflammation of the brain and the spinal cord *encefalomyelit;* **acute disseminated encephalomyelitis** = late reaction to a vaccination *or* disease *akut disseminerad encefalomyelit*

encephalomyelopathy [enˌkefələʊˌmaɪəˈlɒpəθi] *subst.* any condition where the brain and spinal cord are diseased *encefalomyelopati*

encephalon [enˈkefəlɒn] *subst.* the brain *or* the contents of the head *encefalon, cerebrum, hjärnan*

encephalopathy [enˌkefəˈlɒpəθi] *subst.* any disease of the brain *encefalopati,* *hjärnsjukdom; see also* WERNICKE'S ENCEPHALOPATHY

enchondroma [ˌenkən'drəʊmə] *subst.* tumour formed of cartilage growing inside a bone *en(do)kondrom*

enclose [ɪn'kləʊz] *vb.* to surround *or* to keep something inside *omge, innesluta;* **the membrane enclosing the cytoplasm**

encopresis [ˌenkəʊ'pri:sɪs] *subst.* faecal incontinence *or* being unable to control the faeces *enkopres, incontinentia alvi, avföringsinkontinens*

encounter group [ɪn'kaʊntə ˌgru:p] *subst.* form of treatment of psychological disorders, where people meet and talk about their problems in a group *encountergrupp, sensitivitetsträningsgrupp, sensiträningsgrupp*

encourage [ɪn'kʌrɪdʒ] *vb.* to persuade someone that he should do something *uppmuntra, stimulera;* **the surgeon encouraged her to get out of bed and start trying to walk; children should not be encouraged to take medicines by themselves**

encysted [en'sɪstɪd] *adj.* enclosed in a capsule like a cyst *inkapslad*

end [end] **1** *subst.* last part of something *slut;* **end artery** = last section of an artery which does not divide into smaller arteries and does not anastomose with other arteries *ändartär;* **end organ** = nerve ending with encapsulated nerve filaments *ändkropp, nervändkropp;* **end piece** = last part of the tail of a spermatazoon *del av spermiesvans* **2** *vb.* to finish *(av)sluta;* to come to an end *sluta, avslutas, ta slut;* **he ended his talk by showing a series of slides of diseased parts**

end- ['end, ˌ-] *or* **endo-** ['endəʊ, ˌ--] *prefix* meaning inside *end(o)-, inner-*

endanger [ɪn'deɪn(d)ʒə, en-] *vb.* to put at risk *utsätta för fara, äventyra;* **the operation may endanger the life of the patient**

endarterectomy [ˌendɑ:tə'rektəmi] *subst.* surgical removal of the lining of an artery *sotning* NOTE: also called a **rebore**

endarteritis [ˌendɑ:tə'raɪtɪs] *subst.* inflammation of the inner lining of an artery *endarterit;* **endarteritis obliterans** = condition where inflammation in an artery is so severe that it blocks the artery *endarteritis obliterans, Buergers sjukdom*

endemic [en'demɪk] *adj.* (any disease) which is very common in certain places *endemisk;* **this disease is endemic to Mediterranean countries; endemic syphilis** = BEJEL *see also* EPIDEMIC, PANDEMIC

endemiology [enˌdi:mi'ɒlədʒi] *subst.* study of endemic diseases *endemiologi*

endemisk ⇨ **endemic**

end-expiratory [ˌendɪk'spaɪ(ə)t(ə)ri] *see* POSITIVE

ending ['endɪŋ] *subst.* last part of something *slut, avslutning;* **nerve ending** = last part of a nerve, especially of a peripheral nerve ⇨ *illustration* SKIN & SENSORY RECEPTORS *nervändslut*

endo- ['endəʊ, ˌ--] *prefix* meaning inside *end(o)-, inner-*

endocardial [ˌendəʊ'kɑ:diəl] *adj.* referring to the endocardium *endokardiell;* **endocardial pacemaker** = pacemaker attached to the lining of the heart muscle *pacemaker (vanligtvis) fästad vid hjärtats innerhinna*

endocarditis [ˌendəʊkɑ:'daɪtɪs] *subst.* inflammation of the endocardium *or* the membrane lining of the heart *endokardit;* **(subacute) infective endocarditis** = bacterial infection of the heart valves *(subakut) infektiös endokardit*

endocardium [ˌendəʊ'kɑ:diəm] *subst.* membrane which lines the heart ⇨ *illustration* HEART *endokardiet*

endocervicitis [ˌendəʊˌsɜ:vɪ'saɪtɪs] *subst.* inflammation of the membrane in the neck of the uterus *endocervicit*

endocervix [ˌendəʊ'sɜ:vɪks] *subst.* membrane which lines the neck of the uterus *endocervix*

endochondral [ˌendəʊ'kɒndr(ə)l] *adj.* inside a cartilage *endokondral*

endocrine gland ['endəʊkraɪn ˌglænd] *or* **ductless gland** ['dʌktləs ˌglænd] *subst.* gland without a duct which produces hormones which are introduced directly into the bloodstream (such as the pituitary gland, thyroid gland, the adrenals, and the gonads) *endokrin körtel, inresekretorisk körtel;* **endocrine system** = system of related ductless glands *endokrina systemet*

> QUOTE the endocrine system releases hormones in response to a change in concentration of trigger substances in the blood or other body fluids
> **Nursing 87**

endocrinologist [ˌendəʊkrɪˈnɒlədʒɪst] *subst.* doctor who specializes in the study of endocrinology *endokrinolog*

endocrinology [ˌendəʊkrɪˈnɒlədʒi] *subst.* study of the endocrine system, its function and effects *endokrinologi*

endoderm [ˈendəʊdɜːm] *or* **entoderm** [ˈentəʊdɜːm] *subst.* inner of three layers surrounding an embryo *entoderma, inre groddbladet*

> COMMENT: the endoderm gives rise to most of the epithelium of the respiratory system, the alimentary tract, some of the ductless glands, the bladder and part of the urethra

endodermal [ˌendəʊˈdɜːm(ə)l] *or* **entodermal** [ˌentəʊˈdɜːm(ə)l] *adj.* referring to the entoderm *entodermal*

endodontia [ˌendəʊˈdɒnʃiə] *subst.* treatment of chronic toothache by removing the roots of a tooth *avlägsnande av tandrötter som behandling av kronisk tandvärk*

endogenous [enˈdɒdʒ(ə)nəs] *adj.* developing *or* being caused by something inside an organism *endogen;* **endogenous depression** = depression caused by something inside the body *endogen depression;* **endogenous eczema** = eczema which is caused by no obvious external factor *endogent eksem; compare* EXOGENOUS

endokardiell ⇨ **endocardial**

endokardiet ⇨ **endocardium**

endokardit ⇨ **endocarditis**

endokondral ⇨ **endochondral**

endokrinolog ⇨ **endocrinologist**

endokrinologi ⇨ **endocrinology**

endolymph [ˈendəʊlɪmf] *subst.* fluid inside the membranous labyrinth in the inner ear *endolymfa*

endolymphatic duct [ˌendəʊlɪmˈfætɪk ˌdʌkt] *subst.* duct which carries the endolymph inside the membranous labyrinth *del av (gång i) hinnlabyrinten*

endolysin [enˈdɒlɪsɪn] *subst.* substance present in cells, which kills bacteria *endolysin*

endometrial [ˌendəʊˈmiːtriəl] *adj.* referring to the endometrium *som avser el. hör till endometriet (livmoderslemhinnan)*

endometriet ⇨ **endometrium**

endometriosis [ˌendəʊˌmiːtriˈəʊsɪs] *subst.* condition affecting women, where tissue similar to the tissue of the womb is found in other parts of the body *endometrios*

endometritis [ˌendəʊmɪˈtraɪtɪs] *subst.* inflammation of the lining of the uterus *endometrit*

endometrium [ˌendəʊˈmiːtriəm] *subst.* mucous membrane lining the uterus part of which is shed at each menstruation *endometriet, livmoderslemhinnan*

endomorf ⇨ **endomorphic**

endomorph [ˈendəʊmɔːf] *subst.* type of person who tends to be quite fat with large intestines and small muscles *endomorf person*

endomorphic [ˌendəʊˈmɔːfɪk] *adj.* referring to an endomorph *endomorf; see also* ECTOMORPH, MESOMORPH

endomyocarditis [ˌendəʊˌmaɪəʊkɑːˈdaɪtɪs] *subst.* inflammation of the muscle and inner membrane of the heart *endomyokardit*

endomyokardit ⇨ **endomyocarditis**

endomysium [ˌendəʊˈmɪsiəm] *subst.* connective tissue around and between muscle fibres *endomysium*

endoneurium [ˌendəʊˈnjʊəriəm] *subst.* fibrous tissue between the nerve fibres in a nerve trunk *endoneurium*

endoparasite [ˌendəʊˈpærəsaɪt] *subst.* parasite which lives inside its host (as in the intestines) *endoparasit; compare* ECTOPARASITE

endophthalmitis [enˌdɒfθælˈmaɪtɪs] *subst.* inflammation of the interior of the eyeball *endophthalmitis*

endoplasm [ˈendə(ʊ)plæz(ə)m] *subst.* inner layer of the cytoplasm, which is less dense than the rest *endoplasma*

endoplasmic reticulum (ER) [ˌendəʊˈplæzmɪk rɪˈtɪkjʊləm (ˌiːˈɑː)] *subst.* network of vessels forming a membrane in a cytoplasm *reticulum endoplasmaticum, endoplasmatiskt retikel*

endorfin ⇨ **endorphin**

endorphin [en'dɔːfɪn] *subst.* peptide produced by the brain which acts as a natural pain killer *endorfin; see also* ENCEPHALIN

endoscope ['endəskəʊp] *subst.* instrument used to examine the inside of the body, made of a tube which is passed into the body down a passage *endoskop*

endoscopic retrograde cholangiopancreatography (ERCP) [ˌendəʊ'skɒpɪk 'retrə(ʊ)greɪd kəˌlendʒiəʊˌpænkriə'tɒgrəfi (ˌiːɑːsiː'piː)] *subst.* method used to examine the pancreatic duct and bile duct for possible obstructions *endoskopisk retrograd cholangiopankreatografi*

endoscopy [en'dɒskəpi] *subst.* examination of the inside of the body using an endoscope *endoskopi*

endoskeleton [ˌendəʊ'skelɪt(ə)n] *subst.* inner structure of bones and cartilage in an animal *inre skelett el. stödjestruktur; compare* EXOSKELETON

endoskop ⇨ **endoscope, fibrescope**

endospore ['endəʊspɔː] *subst.* spore formed inside a special spore case *spor som bildas i särskild kapsel*

endosteum [en'dɒstiəm] *subst.* membrane lining the bone marrow cavity inside a long bone *endost(eum)*

endotel ⇨ **endothelium**

endothelial [ˌendəʊ'θiːliəl] *adj.* referring to the endothelium *som avser el. hör till endotel*

endothelioma [ˌendəʊˌθiːli'əʊmə] *subst.* malignant tumour originating inside the endothelium *endot(h)eliom*

endothelium [ˌendəʊ'θiːliəm] *subst.* membrane of special cells which lines the heart, the lymph vessels, the blood vessels and various body cavities *endotel; compare* EPITHELIUM

endotoxin [ˌendəʊ'tɒksɪn] *subst.* toxic substance released after the death of a bacterial cell *endotoxin*

endotracheal [ˌendəʊ'treɪkiəl] *adj.* inside the trachea *endotrakeal;* **endotracheal tube** = tube passed down the trachea (through either the nose or mouth) in anaesthesia or to help the patient breathe *endotrakealtub, trakealtub*

endotrakeal ⇨ **endotracheal**

endotrakealtub ⇨ **endotracheal**

end plate ['end ˌpleɪt] *subst.* end of a motor nerve, where it joins muscle fibre *ändplatta, nervändplatta*

enema ['enəmə] *subst.* liquid substance put into the rectum to introduce a drug into the body *or* to wash out the colon before an operation *or* for diagnosis *enema, lavemang;* **enema bag** = bag containing the liquid, attached to a tube into the rectum *påse med lavemangsvätska;* **barium enema** = enema made of barium sulphate, injected into the rectum so as to show up the bowel in X-rays *kolonröntgen*
NOTE: plural is **enemas, enemata**

energetic [ˌenə'dʒetɪk] *adj.* full of energy *or* using energy *energisk, som kräver energi (kraft);* **the patient should not do anything energetic**

energi ⇨ **energy**

energisk ⇨ **energetic**

energivärde ⇨ **energy**

energy ['enədʒi] *subst.* force *or* strength to carry out activities *energi, kraft, ork;* **you need to eat certain types of food to give you energy; energy value** *or* **calorific value** = heat value of food *or* number of Calories which a certain amount of a certain food contains *energivärde;* **the tin of beans has an energy value of 250 calories**

COMMENT: energy is measured in calories, one calorie being the amount of heat needed to raise the temperature of one gram of water by one degree Celsius. The kilocalorie or Calorie is also used as a measurement of the energy content of food, and to show the amount of energy needed by an average person

enervate ['enəveɪt, ɪ'nɜːvɪt] *vb.* to deprive someone of nervous energy *försvaga, göra slö (kraftlös)*

enervation [ˌenə'veɪʃ(ə)n] *subst.* (i) general nervous weakness *allmän nervsvaghet;* (ii) surgical operation to resect a nerve *operativt avlägsnande av (del av) nerv*

engagement [ɪn'geɪdʒmənt] *subst. (in obstetrics)* moment where the presenting part of the fetus (usually the end) enters the pelvis at the beginning of labour *öppningsskedet, utdrivningsskedets inledning*

engelska sjukan ⇨ **rickets**

English National Board (ENB) [ˌɪŋlɪʃ ˈnæʃ(ə)n(ə)l ˌbɔːd (ˌiːenˈbiː)] *subst.* official body responsible for training nurses, for setting nursing examinations and for approving nursing schools *statligt organ som ansvarar för sjuksköterskeutbildningen i Storbritannien*

engorged [ɪnˈgɔːdʒd] *adj.* filled with liquid (usually blood) *överfylld*

engorgement [ɪnˈgɔːdʒmənt] *subst.* congestion *or* excessive filling of a vessel with blood *kongestion, blodöverfyllnad, blodstockning*

engångs- ⇨ **disposable**

engångsblöja ⇨ **nappy**

enhet ⇨ **unit**

enighet ⇨ **agreement**

enkel ⇨ **simple**

enkopres ⇨ **encopresis, incontinence**

enkärnig ⇨ **mononuclear**

enlarge [ɪnˈlɑːdʒ] *vb.* to make larger *or* wider *vidga, förstora;* **operation to enlarge a defective vessel**

enlargement [ɪnˈlɑːdʒmənt] *subst.* (i) widening *vidgning, förstoring;* (ii) point where something becomes wider *utvidgning;* **lumbar enlargement** = point where the spinal cord widens in the lower part of the spine *punkt där ryggmärgens nedre tjockare del börjar*

enligt ⇨ **according to**

enoftalmi ⇨ **enophthalmos**

enophthalmos [ˌenɒfˈθælməs] *subst.* condition where the eyes are very deep in their sockets *enoftalmus, enoftalmi, insjunkna ögon*

enostosis [ˌenəˈstəʊsɪs] *subst.* benign growth inside a bone (usually in the skull *or* in a long bone) *enostos*

enpolig ⇨ **unipolar**

enrolled [ɪnˈrəʊld] *adj.* registered on an official list *registrerad (upptagen) i officiell förteckning;* **(State) Enrolled Nurse (SEN)** = nurse who has passed examinations successfully in one of the special courses of study *ung. legitimerad sjuksköterska*

COMMENT: Enrolled Nurses follow a two year course to qualify in general nursing (ENG), mental nursing (ENM) or nursing mentally handicapped patients (ENMH)

ensamförälder ⇨ **parent**

ensidig ⇨ **mono-, unilateral**

ensiform [ˈensifɔːm] *adj.* shaped like a sword *svärdsliknande;* **ensiform cartilage** *or* **xiphoid process** = bottom part of the breastbone, which in young people is formed of cartilage, but becomes bone by middle age *processus xiphoideus (ensiformis), svärdsutskottet*

enskiktat epitel ⇨ **simple**

enskiktat skivepitel ⇨ **squamous**

enstaka ⇨ **discrete, sporadic**

ENT [ˌiːenˈtiː] = EAR, NOSE AND THROAT **she was sent to see an ENT specialist**

Entamoeba [ˌentəˈmiːbə] *subst.* genus of amoeba which lives in the intestine *Entamoeba, entamöba;* **Entamoeba coli** = harmless intestinal parasite *slags amöba;* **Entamoeba gingivalis** = amoeba living in the gums and tonsils, and causing gingivitis *Entamoeba gingivalis (buccalis);* **Entamoeba histolytica** = intestinal amoeba which causes amoebic dysentery *Entamoeba histolytica (dysenteriae)*

entamöba ⇨ **Entamoeba**

enter- [ˈentə, ˌ--] *or* **entero-** [ˈent(ə)rəʊ, ˌ---] *prefix* referring to the intestine *enter(o)-, tarm-*

enteral [ˈent(ə)r(ə)l] *or* **enteric** [enˈterɪk] *adj.* (i) referring to the intestine, especially the small intestine *enteral, tarm-;* (ii) (drug) which is taken through the intestine *läkemedel som intas genom tarmen*

enteral ⇨ **enteric**

enteralgia [ˌentərˈældʒə] = COLIC

enterectomy [ˌentərˈektəmi] *subst.* surgical removal of part of the intestine *enterektomi, tarmresektion*

enterektomi ⇨ **enterectomy**

enteric [enˈterɪk] *adj.* referring to the intestine *enteral, tarm-;* **enteric fever** = (i) any one of three fevers (typhoid, paratyphoid A and paratyphoid B) *tyfoid el. paratyfoid;* (ii); *US* any febrile disease of the intestines *enterit, tarminflammation*

enteric-coated [en'terɪk,kəʊtɪd] *adj.* (pill) with a coating which prevents it from being digested in the stomach, so that it goes through whole into the intestine and can release the drug there *entero-, dragerad*

enterit ➪ **enteric, enteritis**

enteritis [,entə'raɪtɪs] *subst.* inflammation of the mucous membrane of the intestine *enterit, tarminflammation;* **infective enteritis** = enteritis caused by bacteria *infektiös enterit, bakteriell tarminflammation;* **post-irradiation enteritis** = enteritis caused by X-rays *tarminflammation pga strålning; see also* GASTROENTERITIS

Enterobacter ➪ **Enterobacteria**

Enterobacteria [,entərəʊbæk'tɪəriə] *subst.* important family of bacteria, including Salmonella, Shigella, Escherichia and Klebsiella *Enterobacter*

enterobiasis [,entərəʊ'baɪəsɪs] *or* **oxyuriasis** [,ɒksijuə'raɪəsɪs] *subst.* infection with **Enterobius vermicularis** *or* common children's disease, caused by threadworms in the large intestine which give itching round the anus *springmaskinfektion*

Enterobius [,entə'rəʊbiəs] *subst.* threadworm *or* small thin nematode which infests the large intestine and causes itching round the anus *Enterobius (vermicularis), springmask*

enterocele ['entərəʊsi:l] *subst.* hernia of the intestine *enterocele, tarmbråck*

enterocentesis [,ent(ə)rəʊsen'ti:sɪs] *subst.* surgical puncturing of the intestines where a hollow needle is pushed through the abdominal wall into the intestine to remove gas *or* fluid *enterocentes*

enterococcus [,ent(ə)rəʊ'kɒkəs] *subst.* streptococcus in the intestine *enterokock*

enterocoele [,entərəʊ'si:li] *subst.* the abdominal cavity *cavum abdominis, bukhålan*

enterocolitis [,entərəʊkə'laɪtɪs] *subst.* inflammation of the colon and small intestine *enterokolit*

enterogastrone [,ent(ə)rəʊ'gæstrəʊn] *subst.* hormone released in the duodenum, which controls secretions of the stomach *enterogastron*

enterogen ➪ **enterogenous**

enterogenous [,ent(ə)rəʊ'dʒi:nəs] *adj.* originating in the intestine *enterogen*

enterokock ➪ **enterococcus**

enterokolit ➪ **enterocolitis**

enterolith ['entərəʊlɪθ] *subst.* calculus *or* stone in the intestine *tarmsten*

enteron ['entərɒn] *subst.* the whole intestinal tract *(hela) tarmkanalen*

enteropathy [,entə'rɒpəθi] *subst.* any disorder of the intestine *enteropati, tarmsjukdom;* **gluten enteropathy** = (i) coeliac disease *or* allergic reaction in children to gluten, which prevents the small intestine from absorbing fat *glutenintolerans, celiaki, intestinal infantilism, sprue, malabsorption;* (ii) condition where the villi in the intestine become smaller and so reduce the surface which absorbs nutrients *glutenenteropati*

enteropati ➪ **enteropathy**

enteropeptidase [,ent(ə)rəʊ'peptɪdeɪz] *subst.* enzyme produced by glands in the small intestine *enteropeptidas, peptidas producerat i tunntarmen*

enteroptosis [,entərəʊ'təʊsɪs] *subst.* condition where the intestine is lower than normal in the abdominal cavity *enteroptos, tarmframfall*

enterorrafi ➪ **enterorrhaphy**

enterorrhaphy [,entər'ɔ:rəfi] *subst.* surgical operation to stitch up a perforated intestine *enterorrafi, tarmsutur*

enterospasm ['entərəʊspæz(ə)m] *subst.* irregular painful contractions of the intestine *enterospasm, kramp i tarmen*

enterostomi ➪ **enterostomy**

enterostomy [,ent(ə)'rɒstəmi] *subst.* surgical operation to make an opening between the intestine and the abdominal wall *enterostomi*

enterotomi ➪ **enterotomy**

enterotomy [,entə'rɒtəmi] *subst.* surgical incision of the intestine *enterotomi*

enterotoxin [,entərəʊ'tɒksɪn] *subst.* bacterial exotoxin which particularly affects the intestine *enterotoxin*

enterovirus [ˌentərəʊ'vaɪ(ə)rəs] *subst.* virus which prefers to live in the intestine *enterovirus*

COMMENT: the enteroviruses are an important group of viruses, and include poliomyelitis virus, Coxsackie viruses and the echoviruses

enterozo ⇨ **enterozoon**

enterozoon [ˌenterəʊ'zəʊɒn] *subst.* parasite which infests the intestine *enterozo* NOTE: plural is **enterozoa**

entoderm ['entəʊdɜːm] *or* **endoderm** ['endəʊdɜːm] *subst.* inner of three layers surrounding an embryo *entoderma, inre groddbladet*

COMMENT: the entoderm gives rise to most of the epithelium of the respiratory system, the alimentary tract, some of the ductless glands the bladder and part of the urethra

entoderma ⇨ **entoderm**

entodermal [ˌentəʊ'dɜːm(ə)l] *adj.* referring to the entoderm *entodermal*

entopic [ɪn'tɒpɪk] *adj.* in the normal place *entopisk*
NOTE: the opposite is **ectopic**

entopisk ⇨ **entopic**

entropion [ɪn'trəʊpiən] *subst.* turning of the edge of the eyelid towards the inside *entropion, entropium, inåtvikning av nedre ögonlocket*

entropium ⇨ **entropion**

enucleation [ɪˌnjuːkli'eɪʃ(ə)n] *subst.* (i) surgical removal of all of a tumour *enukleation, utskalning;* (ii) surgical removal of the whole eyeball *enucleatio bulbi*

enukleation ⇨ **enucleation**

enuresis [ˌenjʊə'riːsɪs] *subst.* involuntary passing of urine *enures, ofrivillig urinavgång;* **nocturnal enuresis** *or* **bedwetting** = passing of urine when asleep in bed at night *enuresis nocturna, sängvätning, nattvätning*

enuretic [ˌenju'retɪk] *adj.* referring to enuresis *or* causing enuresis *som avser el. hör till ofrivillig urinavgång*

envenomation [ɪnˌvenə'meɪʃ(ə)n] *subst.* using snake venom as part of a therapeutic treatment *användning av ormgift i sjukdomsbehandling*

environment [ɪn'vaɪ(ə)r(ə)nmənt, en-] *subst.* conditions and influences under which an organism lives *miljö, omgivning, levnadsvillkor*

COMMENT: man's environment can be the country *or* town or house *or* room where he lives; a parasite's environment can be the intestine *or* the scalp and different parasites have different environments

environmental [ɪnˌvaɪ(ə)r(ə)n'ment(ə)l, en-] *adj.* referring to the environment *som avser el. hör till miljö (omgivning, levnadsvillkor), hälsovårds-;* **Environmental Health Officer (EHO)** = official of a local authority who examines the environment and tests for air pollution *or* bad sanitation *or* noise pollution, etc. *ung. hälsovårdsinspektör*

envis ⇨ **persistent, recalcitrant**

enzym ⇨ **enzyme**

enzymatic [ˌenzaɪ'mætɪk] *adj.* referring to enzymes *enzymatisk* NOTE: the names of enzymes mostly end with the suffix **-ase**

enzymatisk ⇨ **enzymatic**

enzyme ['enzaɪm] *subst.* protein substance produced by living cells which catalyzes a biochemical reaction in the body *enzym*

COMMENT: many different enzymes exist in the body, working in the digestive system, in the metabolic processes and helping the synthesis of certain compounds

enäggstvillingar ⇨ **identical, uniovular twins**

eosin ['iːə(ʊ)sɪn] *subst.* red dye used in staining tissue samples *eosin*

eosinofili ⇨ **eosinophilia**

eosinopenia [ˌiːə(ʊ)ˌsɪnə(ʊ)'piːniə] *subst.* reduction in the number of eosinophils in the blood *eosinopeni*

eosinophil [ˌiːə(ʊ)'sɪnəfɪl] *subst.* type of cell which can be stained with eosin *eosinofil leukocyt (vit blodkropp)*

eosinophilia [ˌiːə(ʊ)ˌsɪnə(ʊ)'fɪliə] *subst.* having an excess of eosinophils in the blood *eosinofili*

eparterial [ˌiːpɑː'tɪəriəl] *adj.* situated over *or* on an artery *belägen ovanför el. på en artär (pulsåder)*

ependyma [ɪ'pendɪmə] *subst.* thin membrane which lines the ventricles of the brain and the central canal of the spinal cord *ependym*

ependymal [ɪ'pendɪm(ə)l] *adj.* referring to the ependyma *som avser el. hör till ependym;* **ependymal cell** = one of the cells which form the ependyma *slags epitelcell*

ependymoma [ɪˌpendɪ'məʊmə] *subst.* tumour in the brain originating in the ependyma *ependymom*

epi- ['epɪ, ˌ--] *prefix* meaning on *or* over *epi-, över-*

epiblepharon [ˌepɪ'blefərɒn] *subst.* abnormal fold of skin over the eyelid, which may press the eyelashes against the eyeball *epiblepharon*

epicanthus [ˌepɪ'kænθəs] *or* **epicanthic fold** [ˌepɪˌkænθɪk 'fəʊld] *subst.* large fold of skin in the inner corner of the eye, common in the Far East *epicanthus, epikantus, s.k. mongolveck*

epicardial [ˌepɪ'kɑːdiəl] *adj.* referring to the epicardium *som avser el. hör till hjärtsäckens inre blad;* **epicardial pacemaker** = pacemaker attached to the surface of the ventricle *pacemaker fästad vid hjärtkammarens utsida*

epicardium [ˌepɪ'kɑːdiəm] *subst.* layer of the pericardium which lines the walls of the heart, outside the myocardium ⇨ *illustration* HEART *epikardiet, hjärtsäckens inre blad*

epicondyle [ˌepɪ'kɒndaɪl] *subst.* projecting part of the round end of a bone above the condyle *epikondyl, ledhuvudsutskott;* **lateral and medial epicondyles** = lateral and medial projections on the condyle of the femur and humerus *laterala och mediala epikondylerna*

epicranium [ˌepɪ'kreɪniəm] *subst.* the five layers of the scalp *or* the skin and hair on the head covering the skull *epikraniet, huvudsvålen, skalpen*

epicranius [ˌepɪ'kreɪniəs] *subst.* a scalp muscle *musculus epicranius, skalpmuskeln*

epicritic [ˌepɪ'krɪtɪk] *adj.* referring to the nerves which govern the fine senses of touch and temperature *som avser el. hör till de nerver som reglerar berörings- och temperatursinnet; see also* PROTOPATHIC

epidemic [ˌepɪ'demɪk] *adj. & subst.* (infectious disease) which spreads quickly through a large part of the population *epidemisk;* **the disease rapidly reached epidemic proportions; the health authorities are taking steps to prevent an epidemic of cholera** *or* **a cholera epidemic; epidemic pleurodynia** *or* **Bornholm disease** *see* PLEURODYNIA *see also* ENDEMIC, PANDEMIC

epidemiologi ⇨ **epidemiology**

epidemiology [ˌepɪˌdiːmɪ'ɒlədʒi] *subst.* study of diseases in the community, in particular how they spread and how they can be controlled *epidemiologi*

epidemisjukhus ⇨ **hospital, isolation**

epidemisk ⇨ **epidemic**

epidemisk hjärnhinneinflammation ⇨ **meningococcal**

epidermal [ˌepɪ'dɜːm(ə)l] *adj.* referring to the epidermis *epidermal*

epidermis [ˌepɪ'dɜːmɪs] *subst.* outer layer of skin, including the dead skin on the surface ⇨ *illustration* SKIN & SENSORY RECEPTORS *epidermis, överhuden*

epidermis ⇨ **cuticle**

epidermolysis [ˌepɪdə'mɒlɪsɪs] *subst.* loose condition of the epidermis *epidermolys, överhudsavlossning*

Epidermophyton [ˌepɪdə'mɒfɪtən] *subst.* fungus which grows on the skin and causes athlete's foot among other disorders *Epidermophyton*

epidermophytosis [ˌepɪˌdɜːməʊfaɪ'təʊsɪs] *subst.* fungus infection of the skin, such as athlete's foot *epidermophytosis*

epididymal [ˌepɪ'dɪdəm(ə)l] *adj.* referring to the epididymis *som avser el. hör till bitestikel*

epididymis [ˌepɪ'dɪdəmɪs] *subst.* long twisting thin tube at the back of the testis, which forms part of the efferent duct of the testis, and in which spermatozoa are stored before ejaculation ⇨ *illustration* UROGENITAL SYSTEM (MALE) *epididymis, bitestikel*

epididymitis [ˌepɪˌdɪdɪ'maɪtɪs] *subst.* inflammation of the epididymis *epididymit*

epididymo-orchitis [ˌepɪˌdɪdəməʊɔːˈkaɪtɪs] *subst.* inflammation of the epididymis and the testes *epididymoorkit*

epididymoorkit ⇨ **epididymo-orchitis**

epidural [ˌepɪˈdjʊər(ə)l] *or* **extradural** [ˌekstrəˈdjʊər(ə)l] *adj.* on the outside of the dura mater *epidural;* **epidural block** = analgesia produced by injecting analgesic solution into the space between the vertebral canal and the dura mater *epiduralblockad, epiduralanestesi, epiduralbedövning;* **epidural space** = space between the dura mater (in the spinal cord) and the vertebral canal *epiduralrummet*

epiduralanestesi ⇨ **anaesthetic, caudal, epidural**

epiduralbedövning ⇨ **anaesthetic, caudal, epidural**

epiduralhematom ⇨ **extradural**

epiduralrummet ⇨ **epidural**

epifenomen ⇨ **epiphenomenon**

epifora ⇨ **epiphora**

epifys ⇨ **epiphysis**

epifysbrosk ⇨ **epiphyseal**

epifysen ⇨ **epiphysis, pineal (body)**

epifysplattan ⇨ **epiphyseal**

epifyszonen ⇨ **epiphyseal**

epigastric [ˌepɪˈgæstrɪk] *adj.* referring to the upper abdomen *epigastrisk;* **the patient complained of pains in the epigastric area**

epigastriet ⇨ **epigastrium, gastric**

epigastrisk ⇨ **epigastric**

epigastrium [ˌepɪˈgæstriəm] *subst.* pit of the stomach *or* part of the upper abdomen between the rib cage and the navel *epigastriet, hypogastriet, maggropen*

epigastrocele [ˌepɪˈgæstrəʊsiːl] *subst.* hernia in the upper abdomen *hernia epigastrica*

epiglottis [ˌepɪˈglɒtɪs] *subst.* cartilage at the root of the tongue which moves to block the windpipe when food is swallowed, so that the food does not go down the trachea ⇨ *illustration* THROAT *epiglottis, struplocket*

epiglottit ⇨ **epiglottitis**

epiglottitis [ˌepɪglɒˈtaɪtɪs] *subst.* inflammation and swelling of the epiglottis *epiglottit, struplocksinflammation*

epikantus ⇨ **epicanthus**

epikardiet ⇨ **epicardium, pericardium**

epikondyl ⇨ **epicondyle**

epikraniet ⇨ **epicranium**

epilation [ˌepɪˈleɪʃ(ə)n] *subst.* removing hair by destroying the hair follicles *epilation*

epilepsy [ˈepɪlepsi] *subst.* disorder of the nervous system in which there are convulsions and loss of consciousness due to disordered discharge of cerebral neurones *epilepsi;* **focal epilepsy** = epilepsy arising from a localized area of the brain *epilepsia focalis, fokal (symtomatisk, kortikal) epilepsi;* **Jacksonian epilepsy** = form of epilepsy where the jerking movements start in one part of the body before spreading to others *Jacksonepilepsi;* **idiopathic epilepsy** = epilepsy not caused by lesions of the brain *idiopatisk (genuin, essentiell) epilepsi;* **psychomotor epilepsy** *or* **temporal lobe epilepsy** = epilepsy caused by abnormal discharges from the temporal lobe *epilepsia psychomotorica, epilepsia (regioni) lobi temporalis; see also* TEMPORAL

> COMMENT: the commonest form of epilepsy is major epilepsy or "grand mal", where the patient loses consciousness and falls to the ground with convulsions. A less severe form is minor epilepsy or "petit mal", where attacks last only a few seconds, and the patient appears simply to be hesitating or thinking deeply

epileptic [ˌepɪˈleptɪk] *adj. & subst.* referring to epilepsy *or* (person) suffering from epilepsy *epileptisk, epileptiker;* **epileptic fit** = attack of convulsions (and sometimes unconsciousness) due to epilepsy *epileptiskt anfall*

epileptiform [ˌepɪˈleptɪfɔːm] *adj.* similar to epilepsy *epileptiform*

epileptiker ⇨ **epileptic**

epileptisk ⇨ **epileptic**

epileptogenic [ˌepɪˌleptəʊˈdʒenɪk] *adj.* which causes epilepsy *epileptogen*

epiloia [ˌepɪˈlɔɪə] *subst.* hereditary disease of the brain, where the child is mentally retarded, suffers from epilepsy and has tumours on the kidney and heart *epiloia, sclerosis tuberosis, tuberös skleros*

epiloia ⇨ **tuberose**

epimenorragi ⇨ **epimenorrhagia**

epimenorré ⇨ **epimenorrhoea**

epimenorrhagia [ˌepɪˌmenəˈreɪdʒə] *subst.* very heavy bleeding during menstruation occurring at very short intervals *epimenorragi*

epimenorrhoea [ˌepɪˌmenəˈriːə] *subst.* menstruation at shorter intervals than twenty-eight days *epimenorré*

epimysium [ˌepɪˈmaɪsiəm] *subst.* connective tissue binding striated muscle fibres *epimysium*

epinephrine [ˌepɪˈnefrɪn] *subst. US* adrenaline *or* hormone secreted by the medulla of the adrenal glands which has an effect similar to stimulation of the sympathetic nervous system *adrenalin*

epineurium [ˌepɪˈnjʊəriəm] *subst.* sheath of connective tissue round a nerve *epineurium*

epiphenomenon [ˌepɪfəˈnɒmɪnən] *subst.* strange symptom which may not be caused by a disease *epifenomen, egendomligt symtom som kanske inte orsakas av sjukdom*

epiphora [eˈpɪfərə] *subst.* condition where the eye fills with tears either because the lacrimal duct is blocked or because excessive tears are being secreted *epifora*

epiphyseal [ˌepɪˈfɪziəl] *adj.* referring to an epiphysis *som avser el. hör till epifys;* **epiphyseal cartilage** = type of cartilage in the bones of children and adolescents, which expands and hardens as the bone grows to full size *cartilago epiphysialis, epifysbrosk, tillväxtzon i ben;* **epiphyseal line** = plate of epiphyseal cartilage separating the epiphysis and the diaphysis of a long bone *epifysplattan, epifyszonen, fysen*

epiphysis [eˈpɪfəsɪs] *subst.* centre of bone growth separated from the main part of the bone by cartilage *epifys, epiphysis ossis;* **epiphysis cerebri** = pineal gland ⇨ *illustration* BONE STRUCTURE *corpus pineale, epifysen, övre hjärnbihanget, tallkottkörteln*

epiphysitis [eˌpɪfɪˈsaɪtɪs] *subst.* inflammation of an epiphysis *epifysit; compare* DIAPHYSIS, METAPHYSIS

epiplo- [eˌpɪplə(ʊ)] *prefix* referring to the omentum *epiplo-, bukhinnenäts-*

epiplocele [eˈpɪpləʊsiːl] *subst.* hernia containing part of the omentum *bråck i bukhinnenätet*

epiploic [ˌepɪˈpləʊik] *adj.* referring to the omentum *epiploicus, bukhinnenäts-*

epiploon [eˈpɪpləʊɒn] = OMENTUM

episcleritis [ˌepɪskləˈraɪtɪs] *subst.* inflammation of the outer surface of the sclera in the eyeball *episklerit, sklerit*

episio- [əˈpɪziəʊ, -ˌ--] *adj.* referring to the vulva *episio-, vulva-*

episiorrafi ⇨ **episiorrhaphy**

episiorrhaphy [əˌpɪziˈɔːrəfi] *subst.* stitching of torn labia majora *episiorrafi*

episiotomi ⇨ **episiotomy**

episiotomy [əˌpɪziˈɒtəmi] *subst.* surgical incision of the perineum near the vagina to prevent tearing during childbirth *episiotomi, perinealsnitt*

episklerit ⇨ **episcleritis**

episod ⇨ **episode**

episode [ˈepɪsəʊd] *subst.* separate occurrence of an illness *episod*

episodic [ˌepɪˈsɒdɪk] *adj.* (asthma) which occurs in separate attacks *episodisk, som uppträder i avgränsade perioder*

epispadi ⇨ **epispadias**

epispadias [ˌepɪˈspeɪdiəs] *subst.* congenital defect where the urethra opens on the top of the penis and not at the end *epispadi; compare* HYPOSPADIAS

epispastic [ˌepɪˈspæstɪk] = VESICANT

epistaxis [ˌepɪˈstæksɪs] *subst.* nosebleed *epistaxis, näsblod, näsblödning*

epitel ⇨ **epithelium**

epitel- ⇨ **epithelial**

epitelbildning ⇨ **epithelialization**

epiteliom ⇨ **epithelioma**

epitelisation ⇨ **epithelialization**

epitellager ⇨ **epithelial**

epithalamus [ˌepɪˈθæləməs] *subst.* part of the forebrain containing the pineal body *den del av mellanhjärnan där tallkottkörteln ligger*

epithelial [ˌepɪˈθiːliəl] *adj.* referring to the epithelium *epitel-;* **epithelial layer** = the epithelium *epitellager;* **epithelial tissue** = epithelial cells arranged as a continuous sheet consisting of one or several layers *epitel(vävnad)*

epithelialization [ˌepɪˌθiːliəlaɪˈzeɪʃ(ə)n] *subst.* growth of skin over a wound *epitelisation, epitelbildning*

epithelioma [ˌepɪˌθiːliˈəʊmə] *subst.* tumour arising from epithelial cells *epiteliom*

epithelium [ˌepɪˈθiːliəm] *subst.* layer(s) of cells covering an organ, including the skin and the lining of all hollow cavities except blood vessels, lymphatics and serous cavities *epitel; see also* ENDOTHELIUM, MESOTHELIUM

> COMMENT: epithelium is classified according to the shape of the cells and the number of layers of cells which form it. The types of epithelium according to the number of layers are: simple epithelium (epithelium formed of a single layer of cells) and stratified epithelium (epithelium formed of several layers of cells). The main types of epithelial cells are: columnar epithelium (simple epithelium with long narrow cells, forming the lining of the intestines); ciliated epithelium (simple epithelium where the cells have little hairs, forming the lining of air passages); cuboidal epithelium (with cube-shaped cells, forming the lining of glands and intestines); squamous epithelium or pavement epithelium (with flat cells like scales, which forms the lining of pericardium, peritoneum and pleura)

epituberculosis [ˌepɪtjuːˌbɜːkjuˈləʊsɪs] *subst.* swelling of the lymph node in the thorax, due to tuberculosis *hilustuberkulos, tuberkulos med svullna lymfkörtlar i bröstkorgen*

eponym [ˈepəʊnɪm] *subst.* procedure *or* disease *or* part of the body which is named after a person *eponym*

> COMMENT: an eponym can refer to a disease or condition (Dupuytren's contracture, Guillain-Barré syndrome), a part of the body (circle of Willis), an organism (Leishmania), a surgical procedure (Trendelenburg's operation) or an appliance (Kirschner wire)

eponymous [ɪˈpɒnɪməs] *adj.* named after a person *som är uppkallad efter en viss person*

Epsom salts [ˌepsəm ˈsɔːlts] *subst.* magnesium sulphate *or* white powder which when diluted in water is used as a laxative *magnesiumsulfat*

Epstein-Barr virus [ˌepstaɪnˈbɑː ˌvaɪ(ə)rəs] *or* **EB virus** [ˌiːˈbiː ˌvaɪ(ə)rəs] *subst.* virus which causes glandular fever *Epstein-Barr-virus*

epulid ⇨ **epulis**

epulis [ɪˈpjuːlɪs] *subst.* small fibrous swelling on a gum *epulid, tandköttssvulst*

equal [ˈiːkw(ə)l] **1** *adj.* exactly the same in quantity, size, etc. as something else *lik, likstor;* **the twins are of equal size and weight** **2** *vb.* to be exactly the same as something *vara lik, likna*

equilibrium [ˌiːkwɪˈlɪbriəm] *subst.* state of balance *ekvilibrium, jämvikt, balans*

equina [ɪˈkwaɪnə] *see* CAUDA EQUINA

equinovarus [ɪˌkwaɪnə(ʊ)ˈveərəs] *see* TALIPES

equip [ɪˈkwɪp] *vb.* to provide the necessary apparatus *utrusta, förse med;* **the operating theatre is equipped with the latest scanning devices**

equipment [ɪˈkwɪpmənt] *subst.* apparatus *or* tools which are required to do something *utrustning;* **the centre urgently needs surgical equipment; the surgeons complained about the out-of-date equipment in the hospital**
NOTE: no plural: for one item say **"a piece of equipment"**

ER [ˌiːˈɑː] = ENDOPLASMIC RETICULUM

eradicate [ɪˈrædɪkeɪt] *vb.* to wipe out *or* to remove completely *utrota, lyckas bekämpa, få bukt med;* **international action to eradicate glaucoma**

eradication [ɪˌrædɪˈkeɪʃ(ə)n] *subst.* removing completely *utrotning*

Erb's palsy [ˈɜːbz ˌpɔːlzi] *or* **Erb's paralysis** [ˈɜːbz pəˈræləsɪs] *see* PALSY

ERCP [ˌiːɑːsiːˈpiː] = ENDOSCOPIC RETROGRADE CHOLANGIOPANCREATOGRAPHY

erect [ɪ'rekt] *adj.* stiff and straight *rak, upprätt*

erectile [ɪ'rektaɪ(ə)l] *adj.* which can become erect *erektil;* **erectile tissue** = vascular tissue which can become erect and stiff when engorged with blood (as the corpus cavernosa in the penis) *erektil vävnad, vävnad som kan styvna*

erection [ɪ'rekʃ(ə)n] *subst.* state where a part, such as the penis, becomes swollen because of engorgement with blood *erektion, stånd*

erector spinae [ɪ'rektə ˌspaɪniː] *subst.* large muscle starting at the base of the spine, and dividing as it runs up the spine *musculus erector spinae, ryggsträckarmuskeln*

erektil ⇨ **erectile**

erektion ⇨ **erection**

erepsin [ɪ'repsɪn] *subst.* mixture of enzymes produced by the glands in the intestine, used in the production of amino acids *erepsin, intestinala peptidaser*

erethism ['erəθɪz(ə)m] *subst.* abnormal irritability *eret(h)ism, sjukligt stegrad retbarhet*

erfaren ⇨ **experienced**

erfarenhet ⇨ **experience**

erg [ɜːg] *subst.* unit of measurement of work *or* energy *erg, 10^{-7} joule*

ergograph ['ɜːgəʊgrɑːf] *subst.* apparatus which records the work of one or several muscles *ergograf*

ergometrine [ˌɜːgəʊ'metrin] *subst.* drug derived from ergot, used in obstetrics to reduce bleeding and to produce contractions of the uterus *ergometrin*

ergonomi ⇨ **ergonomics**

ergonomics [ˌɜːgə'nɒmɪks] *subst.* study of man at work *ergonomi*

ergot ['ɜːgət] *subst.* fungus which grows on rye *mjöldryga*

ergotism ['ɜːgətɪz(ə)m] *subst.* poisoning by eating rye which has been contaminated with ergot *ergotism, mjöldrygesjuka*

COMMENT: the symptoms are muscle cramps and dry gangrene in the fingers and toes

erkänna ⇨ **recognize**

erode [ɪ'rəʊd] *vb.* to wear away *or* to break down *erodera, fräta (tära, nöta) på*

erodera ⇨ **erode**

erogen ⇨ **erogenous**

erogenous [ɪ'rɒdʒ(ə)nəs] *subst.* which produces sexual excitement *erogen, erotogen;* **erogenous zone** = part of the body which, if stimulated, produces sexual excitement (such as penis *or* clitoris *or* nipples, etc.) *erogen (erotogen) zon*

erosion [ɪ'rəʊʒ(ə)n] *subst.* wearing away of tissue *or* breaking down of tissue *erosion, ytligt sår;* **cervical erosion** = condition where the epithelium of the mucous membrane lining the cervix uteri extends outside the cervix *eletepi (en normal variant)*

erotogen ⇨ **erogenous**

ersätta ⇨ **compensate, cover, replace**

ersättningsterapi ⇨ **substitution**

eructation [ˌiːrʌk'teɪʃ(ə)n] *subst.* belching *or* allowing air in the stomach to come up through the mouth *eruktation, rap(ning)*

erupt [ɪ'rʌpt] *vb.* to break through the skin *slå ut, bryta ut;* **the permanent incisors erupt before the premolars**

eruption [ɪ'rʌpʃ(ə)n] *subst.* (i) something which breaks through the skin (such as a rash *or* pimple) *eruption, hudutslag;* (ii) appearance of a new tooth in a gum *frambrytande (av tand)*

ery- [ˌerɪ, ɪ'rɪ] *prefix* meaning red *ery-*

erysipelas [ˌerɪ'sɪp(ə)ləs] *subst.* contagious skin disease, where the skin on the face becomes hot and red and painful, caused by **Streptococcus pyogenes** *ros(feber)*

erysipeloid [ˌerɪ'sɪpəlɔɪd] *subst.* bacterial skin infection caused by touching infected fish *or* meat *erysipeloid*

erythema [ˌerɪ'θiːmə] *subst.* redness on the skin, caused by hyperaemia of the blood vessels near the surface *eryt(h)em, hudrodnad;* **erythema ab igne** = pattern of red lines on the skin caused by exposure to heat *erythema ab igne;* **erythema induratum** *or* **Bazin's disease** = tubercular disease where ulcerating nodules appear on the legs of young women *erythema induratum, Bazins sjukdom;* **erythema multiforme** = sudden appearance of inflammatory red patches and sometimes blisters on the skin *erythema multiforme;* **erythema nodosum** = inflammatory disease where red swellings appear on the front of the legs *erythema nodosum, knölros;* **erythema pernio** = CHILBLAIN; **erythema serpens** = bacterial skin infection caused by touching infected fish *or* meat *slags hudinfektion orsakad av kontakt med infekterat kött el. infekterad fisk*

erythematosus [ˌerɪˌθiːməˈtəʊsɪs] *see* DISSEMINATED, LUPUS

erythraemia [ˌerɪˈθriːmiə] *or* **polycythaemia vera** [ˌpɒlɪsaɪˈθiːmiə ˌvɪərə] *subst.* blood disorder where the number of red blood cells increases sharply, together with an increase in the number of white cells, making the blood thicker and slower to flow *polycythaemia (rubra) vera, eryt(h)remi*

erythrasma [ˌerɪˈθræzmə] *subst.* chronic bacterial skin condition in a fold in the skin *or* where two skin surfaces touch (such as between the toes), caused by a Corynebacterium *erythrasma*

erythroblast [ɪˈrɪθrə(ʊ)ˌblæst] *subst.* cell which forms an erythrocyte *or* red blood cell *eryt(h)roblast*

erythroblastosis [ɪˌrɪθrə(ʊ)blæˈstəʊsɪs] *subst.* presence of erythroblasts in the blood, usually found in haemolytic anaemia *eryt(h)roblastos;* **erythroblastosis fetalis** = blood disease affecting newborn babies, caused by a reaction between the rhesus factor of the mother and the fetus *erythroblastosis fetalis (neonatorum)*

> COMMENT: usually this occurs where the mother is rhesus negative and has developed rhesus positive antibodies, which are passed into the blood of a rhesus positive fetus

erythrocyanosis [ɪˌrɪθrə(ʊ)ˌsaɪəˈnəʊsɪs] *subst.* red and purple patches on the skin of the thighs, often accompanied by chilblains and made worse by cold *erythrocyanosis*

erythrocyte [ɪˈrɪθrə(ʊ)saɪt] *subst.* mature non-nucleated red blood cell *or* blood cell which contains haemoglobin and carries oxygen *erytrocyt, röd blodkropp;* **erythrocyte sedimentation rate (ESR)** = diagnostic test to see how fast erythrocytes settle in a sample of blood plasma *sedimentation rate, SR, blodsänkningsreaktion, sänkan*

> QUOTE anemia may be due to insufficient erythrocyte production, in which case the corrected reticulocyte count will be low, or it may be due to hemorrhage or hemolysis, in which cases there should be reticulocyte response
> **Southern Medical Journal**

erythrocytosis [ɪˌrɪθrə(ʊ)saɪˈtəʊsɪs] *subst.* increase in the number of red blood cells in the blood *eryt(h)rocytos*

erythroderma [ɪˌrɪθrə(ʊ)ˈdɜːmə] *subst.* condition where the skin becomes red and flakes off *eryt(h)rodermi, exfoliativ dermatit*

erythroedema [ɪˌrɪθrə(ʊ)ɪˈdiːmə] *or* **pink disease** [ˈpɪŋk dɪˌziːz] *subst.* disease of infants where the child's hands and feet swell and become pink, with a fever and loss of appetite, probably formerly caused by allergic reaction to mercury in lotions *pink disease, erythroedema, akrodyni*

erythroedema ⇨ **acrodynia**

erythrogenesis [ɪˌrɪθrə(ʊ)ˈdʒenəsɪs] *or* **erythropoiesis** [ɪˌrɪθrə(ʊ)pɔɪˈiːsɪs] *subst.* formation of red blood cells in red bone marrow *eryt(h)ropo(i)es*

erythromelalgia [ɪˌrɪθrə(ʊ)melˈældʒə] *subst.* painful swelling of blood vessels in the extremities *eryt(h)romelalgi*

erythromycin [ɪˌrɪθrə(ʊ)ˈmaɪsɪn] *subst.* antibiotic used to combat bacterial infections *eryt(h)romycin*

erythropenia [ɪˌrɪθrə(ʊ)ˈpiːniə] *subst.* condition where a patient has a low number of erythrocytes in his blood *eryt(h)ropeni, anemi, blodbrist*

erythropoiesis [ɪˌrɪθrə(ʊ)pɔɪˈiːsɪs] = ERYTHROGENESIS

erythropoietin [ɪˌrɪθrə(ʊ)ˈpɔɪətɪn] *subst.* hormone which regulates the production of red blood cells *eryt(h)ropo(i)etin*

erythropsia [ˌerɪˈθrɒpsiə] *subst.* condition where the patient sees things as if coloured red *eryt(h)ropsi*

erytrocyt ⇨ **erythrocyte, red**

erytrocytvolymfraktion ⇨ **haematocrit, pack**

Esbach's albuminometer [ˈesbɑːks ælˌbjuːmɪˈnɒmɪtə] *subst.* glass for measuring albumin in urine, using Esbach's method *slags glas för mätning av albumin (äggvita) i urin*

eschar ['eskɑ:] *subst.* dry scab, such as one on a burn *brandskorpa, sårskorpa på brännsår*

escharotic [ˌeskə'rɒtɪk] *subst.* substance which produces an eschar *ämne som ger upphov till brandskorpa*

Escherichia [ˌeʃə'raɪkiə] *subst.* one of the Enterobacteria commonly found in faeces *Escherichia;* **Escherichia coli =** Gram-negative bacillus associated with acute gastroenteritis in infants *Escherichia coli, kolibakterien*

escort [ɪ'skɔ:t] *vb.* to go with someone, especially to go with a patient to make sure he arrives at the right place *eskortera, ledsaga, följa (med);* **escort nurse =** nurse who goes with patients to the operating theatre and back again to the ward *sjuksköterska som följer patient till el. från operation*

Esmarch's bandage ['esmɑ:ks ˌbændɪdʒ] *subst.* rubber band wrapped round a limb as a tourniquet to stop the flow of blood or to drain blood before an operation *Esmarchs binda*

esofagektomi ⇨ **oesophagectomy**

esofagit ⇨ **oesophagitis**

esofagocele ⇨ **oesophagocele**

esofagoskop ⇨ **oesophagoscope**

esofagostomi ⇨ **oesophagostomy**

esofagotomi ⇨ **oesophagotomy**

esofagus ⇨ **oesophagus**

esophagus [i:'sɒfəgəs] *US* = OESOPHAGUS

esotropia [ˌesə(ʊ)'trəʊpiə] *subst.* convergent strabismus *or* type of squint, where the eyes both look towards the nose *esotropi, strabismus convergens (internus), konvergent strabism (skelning), inåtskelning*

espundia [ɪ'spu:ndiə] *see* LEISHMANIASIS

ESR [ˌi:es'ɑ:] = ERYTHROCYTE SEDIMENTATION RATE

essence ['es(ə)ns] *subst.* concentrated oil from a plant, used in cosmetics, and sometimes as analgesics or antiseptics *essens*

essential [ɪ'senʃ(ə)l] *adj.* **(a)** idiopathic *or* (disease) with no obvious cause *essentiell, idiopatisk, utan påtaglig yttre orsak;* **essential hypertension =** high blood pressure without any obvious cause *hypertonia essentialis;* **essential uterine haemorrhage =** heavy uterine bleeding for which there is no obvious cause *kraftiga blödningar från livmodern utan påtaglig yttre orsak* **(b)** extremely important *or* necessary *essentiell, livsnödvändig;* **essential amino acid =** amino acid which is necessary for growth but which cannot be synthesized and has to be obtained from the food supply *essentiell aminosyra;* **essential elements =** chemical elements (such as carbon, oxygen, hydrogen, nitrogen and many others) which are necessary to the body's growth or function *livsnödvändiga grundämnen;* **essential fatty acid (EFA) =** unsaturated fatty acid which is necessary for growth and health *essentiell fettsyra;* **essential oils** *or* **volatile oils =** concentrated oils from a scented plant used in cosmetics or as antiseptics *eteriska oljor, flyktiga oljor*

> COMMENT: the essential amino acids are: isoleucine, leucine, lysine, methionine, phenylalanine, threonine, tryptophan and valine. The essential fatty acids are linoleic acid, linolenic acid and arachidonic acid

essentiell ⇨ **essential, idiopathic**

essentiell tremor ⇨ **tremor**

estradiol ⇨ **oestradiol**

estriol ⇨ **oestriol**

estrogen ['i:strədʒ(ə)n] *US* = OESTROGEN

estrogen ⇨ **oestrogen, oestrogenic hormone**

estron ⇨ **oestrone**

etanol ⇨ **alcohol, ethanol**

eter ⇨ **ether**

eteriska oljor ⇨ **essential**

ethanol ['eθənɒl] *subst.* ethyl alcohol *or* colourless liquid, present in drinking alcohols (whisky *or* gin *or* vodka, etc.) and also used in medicines and as a disinfectant *etylalkohol, etanol*

ether ['i:θə] *subst.* anaesthetic substance, now rarely used *eter, etyleter*

ethical ['eθɪk(ə)l] *adj.* (i) concerning ethics *etisk;* (ii); *US* (drug) available to prescription only *receptbelagd;* **ethical committee =** group of specialists who monitor experiments involving human beings *or* who regulate the way in which members of the medical profession conduct themselves *etisk nämnd*

ethics ['eθɪks] *subst.* code of working which shows how a professional group (such as doctors and nurses) should work, and in particular what type of relationship they should have with their patients *etik*

ethmoidal [eθ'mɔɪd(ə)l] *adj.* referring to the ethmoid bone *or* near to the ethmoid bone *et(h)moidal, silbens-;* **ethmoidal sinuses** = air cells inside the ethmoid bone *sinus ethmoidei, silbenscellerna*

ethmoid bone ['eθmɔɪd ˌbəʊn] *subst.* bone which forms the top of the nasal cavity and part of the orbits *os ethmoidale, silbenet*

ethmoiditis [ˌeθmɔɪ'daɪtɪs] *subst.* inflammation of the ethmoid bone *or* of the ethmoidal sinuses *et(h)moidit*

ethyl alcohol ['eθɪl ˌælkəhɒl] *see* ALCOHOL

ethylene ['eθəli:n] *subst.* gas used as an anaesthetic *etylen*

etik ⇨ **ethics**

etikett ⇨ **label**

etiologi ⇨ **aetiology**

etiology, etiological [ˌi:ti'ɒlədʒi, ˌi:tiə'lɒdʒɪk(ə)l] *US* = AETIOLOGY, AETIOLOGICAL

etisk ⇨ **ethical**

etylalkohol ⇨ **alcohol, ethanol**

etylen ⇨ **ethylene**

etyleter ⇨ **ether**

eu- ['ju:, ˌju:, ju] *prefix* meaning good *eu-*

eubacteria [ˌju:'bæk'tɪəriə] *subst.* true bacteria with rigid cell walls *eubacteria*

eucalyptol [ˌju:kə'lɪptəl] *subst.* substance obtained from eucalyptus oil *eucalyptolum*

COMMENT: eucalyptus oil is used in pharmaceutical products especially to relieve congestion in the respiratory passages

eucalyptolum ⇨ **eucalyptol**

eucalyptus [ˌju:kə'lɪptəs] *subst.* genus of tree growing mainly in Australia, from which a strongly smelling oil is distilled *eucalyptus*

eufori ⇨ **euphoria**

eugenics [ju'dʒenɪks] *subst.* study of how to improve the human race by genetic selection *eugenik, rashygien*

eugenik ⇨ **eugenics**

eunuch ['ju:nək] *subst.* castrated male *eunuck, kastrat*

eunuck ⇨ **eunuch**

eupepsia [ju:'pepsiə] *subst.* good digestion *god matsmältning*

euphoria [ju'fɔ:riə] *subst.* feeling of extreme happiness *eufori*

euplastic [ju'plæstɪk] *subst.* tissue which heals well *bra läkkött*

Eustachian tube [ju'steɪʃ(ə)n ˌtju:b] *or* **syrinx** ['sɪrɪŋ(k)s] *or* **pharyngotympanic tube** [fəˌrɪŋgəʊtɪm'pænɪk ˌtju:b] *subst.* tube which connects the pharynx to the middle ear ⇨ *illustration* EAR *tuba auditiva, otosalpinx, eustachiska röret, örontrumpeten*

COMMENT: the Eustachian tubes balance the air pressure on either side of the eardrum. When a person swallows or yawns, air is forced into the Eustachian tubes and clears them. The tubes can be blocked by an infection (as in a cold) or pressure (as in an aircraft taking off), and if they are blocked, the hearing is impaired

eutanasi ⇨ **euthanasia, mercy killing**

euthanasia [ˌju:θə'neɪziə] *subst.* mercy killing *or* killing of a sick person to put an end to his suffering *eutanasi, dödshjälp*
NOTE: no plural

euthyroidism [ju'θaɪrɔɪdɪz(ə)m] *or* **euthyroid state** [ju'θaɪrɔɪd ˌsteɪt] *adj.* with a normal thyroid gland *euthyroidism*

eutocia [ju'təʊsiə] *subst.* normal childbirth *normal förlossning*

evacuans ⇨ **evacuant**

evacuant [ɪ'vækjuənt] *subst.* medicine which makes a person have a bowel movement *evacuans, avföringsmedel*

evacuate [ɪ'vækjueɪt] *vb.* to discharge faeces from the bowel *or* to have a bowel movement *tömma (tarmen)*

evacuation [ɪˌvækju'eɪʃ(ə)n] *subst.* removing the contents of something, especially discharging faeces from the bowel *evakuering, tömning, utrymning, tarmtömning*

evacuator [ɪ'vækjueɪtə] *subst.* instrument used to empty a cavity such as the bladder *or* bowel *instrument för att evakuera (tömma) kroppshåla*

evakuering ⇨ **evacuation**

evaluate [ɪ'væljueɪt] *vb.* to examine and calculate the quantity *or* level of something *bedöma, uppskatta, utvärdera;* to examine a patient and calculate the treatment required *bedöma;* **the laboratory is still evaluating the results of the tests**

> QUOTE all patients were evaluated and followed up at the hypertension unit
> **British Medical Journal**

evaluation [ɪˌvælju'eɪʃ(ə)n] *subst.* examining and calculating *evaluering, bedömning, utvärdering*

> QUOTE evaluation of fetal age and weight has proved to be of value in the clinical management of pregnancy, particularly in high-risk gestations
> **Southern Medical Journal**

evaluering ⇨ **evaluation**

evaporate [ɪ'væpəreɪt] *vb.* to convert liquid into vapour *evaporera, få att avdunsta, förvandla till gas (ånga)*

evaporation [ɪˌvæpə'reɪʃ(ə)n] *subst.* converting liquid into vapour *evaporation, avdunstning, förgasning, förångning*

evaporator ⇨ **vaporizer**

evaporera ⇨ **evaporate**

eversion [ɪ'vɜːʃ(ə)n] *subst.* turning towards the outside *or* turning inside out *eversion, utåtvridning, vändning ut och in;* **eversion of the cervix** = condition after laceration during childbirth, where the edges of the cervix sometimes turn outwards *cervixeversion*

evertor [ɪ'vɜːtə] *subst.* muscle which makes a limb turn outwards *muskel som vrider kroppsdel utåt*

EVF ⇨ **haematocrit, pack**

evisceration [ɪˌvɪsə'reɪʃ(ə)n] *subst.* (i) surgical removal of the abdominal viscera *evisceration, operativt avlägsnande av organ i bukhålan;* (ii) removal of the contents of an organ *evisceration, utrymning;* **evisceration of the eye** = surgical removal of the contents of an eyeball *evisceratio bulbi*

E-vitamin ⇨ **vitamin E**

evolution [ˌiːvə'luːʃ(ə)n] *subst.* changes in organisms which take place over a long period involving many generations *evolution*

evulsio ⇨ **avulsion**

Ewing's tumour ['juːɪŋz ˌtjuːmə] *or* **Ewing's sarcoma** ['juːɪŋz sɑː'kəʊmə] *subst.* malignant tumour in the marrow of a long bone *Ewingsarkom*

ex- ['eks, ɪks, əks, ɪgz, 'egz] *or* **exo-** ['eksəʊ, ˌ--] *prefix* meaning out of *ex(o)-, ut-*

exacerbate [ɪgz'æsəbeɪt] *vb.* to make a condition more severe *förvärra, försämra;* **the cold damp weather will only exacerbate his chest condition**

exacerbation [ɪgzˌæsə'beɪʃ(ə)n] *subst.* making a condition worse *exacerbation, försämring, förvärrande;* period when a condition becomes worse *exacerbation*

> QUOTE patients were re-examined regularly or when they felt they might be having an exacerbation. Exacerbation rates were calculated from the number of exacerbations during the study
> **Lancet**

exact [ɪg'zækt] *adj.* correct *or* precise *exakt, riktig, precis*

exakt ⇨ **accurate, accurately, exact, precise**

exaltation [ˌegzɔːl'teɪʃ(ə)n] *subst.* sense of being extremely cheerful and excited *exaltation, upphetsning*

examen ⇨ **degree, qualification**

examination [ɪgˌzæmɪ'neɪʃ(ə)n] *subst.* (i) looking at someone *or* something carefully *granskning;* (ii) looking at a patient to find out what is wrong with him *undersökning;* **from the examination of the X-ray photographs, it seems that the tumour has not spread; the surgeon carried out a medical examination before operating**

examine [ɪg'zæmɪn] *vb.* (i) to look at *or* to investigate someone *or* something carefully *examinera, granska;* (ii) to look at and test a patient to find what is wrong with him *undersöka;* **the doctor examined the patient's heart; the tissue samples were examined in the laboratory**

exanthem [ɪg'zænθəm] *subst.* skin rash found with infectious diseases like measles *or* chickenpox *exant(h)em, hudutslag;* **exanthem subitum** = ROSEOLA INFANTUM

exanthematous [ˌeksæn'θemətəs] *adj.* referring to an exanthem *or* like an exanthem *som avser, hör till el. liknar hudutslag*

excavator ['ekskəveɪtə] *subst.* surgical instrument shaped like a spoon *slev*

excavatum ['ekskəveɪtəm] *see* PECTUS

exceed [ɪk'siːd] *vb.* to do more than *or* to be more than *överstiga, överskrida;* **his pulse rate exceeded 100; it is dangerous to exceed the stated dose** = do not take more than the stated dose *det är farligt att överskrida (ta mer än) rekommenderad dos*

exceptional [ɪk'sepʃ(ə)n(ə)l] *adj.* strange *or* not common *exceptionell, ovanlig, sällsynt;* **in exceptional cases, treatment can be carried out in the patient's home**

exceptionell ⇨ **exceptional**

excess [ɪk'ses] *subst.* too much of a substance *överskott;* **the gland was producing an excess of hormones; the body could not cope with an excess of blood sugar; in excess of** = more than *överstigande, mer än;* **short men who weigh in excess of 100 kilos are very overweight**

excessive [ɪk'sesɪv] *adj.* more than normal *överskotts-, onormalt stor (svår, mycket);* **the patient was passing excessive quantities of urine; the doctor noted an excessive amount of bile in the patient's blood**

excessively [ɪk'sesɪvli] *adv.* too much *alltför mycket (högt etc.);* **he has an excessively high blood pressure; if the patient sweats excessively, it may be necessary to cool his body with cold compresses**

exchange [ɪks'tʃeɪn(d)ʒ] **1** *subst.* giving one thing and taking another *utbyte;* **gas exchange** = process where oxygen in air is exchanged in the lungs for waste carbon dioxide from the blood *gasutbyte;* **exchange transfusion** = method of treating leukaemia *or* erythroblastosis in newborn babies, where almost all the abnormal blood is removed from the body and replaced by normal blood *utbytestransfusion* **2** *vb.* to take something away and give something in its place *byta ut;* **in the lungs, carbon dioxide in the blood is exchanged for oxygen from the air**

excidera ⇨ **excise**

excipient [ɪk'sɪpiənt] *subst.* substance added to a drug so that it can be made into a pill *konstituens, hjälpämne*

excise [ɪk'saɪz] *vb.* to cut out *excidera, skära ut (bort)*

excision [ɪk'sɪʒ(ə)n] *subst.* operation by a surgeon to cut and remove part of the body (such as a growth) *excision, utskärning, bortskärning; compare* INCISION

excitans ⇨ **stimulant**

excitation [ˌeksɪ'teɪʃ(ə)n] *subst.* state of being mentally *or* nervously aroused *excitation, upphetsning*

excitation ⇨ **excitation, excitement**

excitatory [ɪk'saɪtət(ə)ri] *adj.* which tends to excite *som retar (stimulerar), upphetsande*

excite [ɪk'saɪt] *vb.* to stimulate *or* to give an impulse to a nerve *or* muscle *reta, stimulera*

excited [ɪk'saɪtɪd] *adj.* (i) very lively and happy *upphetsad, livlig;* (ii) aroused *retad, stimulerad*

excitement [ɪk'saɪtmənt] *subst.* (i) being excited *excitation, retning, upphetsning;* (ii) second stage of anaesthesia *excitationsstadiet*

excoriation [ɪkˌskɔːri'eɪʃ(ə)n] *subst.* raw skin surface *or* mucous membrane after rubbing *or* burning *exkoriation, skavsår, hudavskavning*

excrement ['ekskrəmənt] *subst.* faeces *exkrement(er), f(a)eces, fekalier, avföring*
NOTE: no plural

excrescence [ɪk'skres(ə)ns] *subst.* growth on the skin *exkrescens, utväxt*

excreta [ɪk'skriːtə] *subst pl.* waste material from the body (such as faeces) *exkret, utsöndring*

excrete [ɪk'skriːt] *vb.* to pass waste matter out of the body, especially to discharge faeces *utsöndra, avsöndra, uttömma;* **the urinary system separates waste liquids from the blood and excretes them as urine**

excretion [ɪk'skriːʃ(ə)n] *subst.* passing waste matter (faeces *or* urine *or* sweat) out of the body *utsöndring, avsöndring, uttömning, avföring*

excruciating [ɪk'skru:ʃieɪtɪŋ] *adj.* (pain) which is extremely painful *ytterst plågsam, olidlig;* **he had excruciating pains in his head**

exemplar ⇨ **specimen**

exenteration [eksˌentə'reɪʃ(ə)n] = EVISCERATION

exercise ['eksəsaɪz] **1** *subst.* physical *or* mental activity *or* active use of the muscles as a way of keeping fit *or* to correct a deformity *or* to strengthen a part *motion, träning, övning;* **regular exercise is good for your heart; you should to do five minutes' exercise every morning; he doesn't do** *or* **take enough exercise - that's why he's too fat; exercise cycle** = cycle which is fixed to the floor so that you can pedal on it to get exercise *motionscykel;* **exercise-induced asthma (EIA)** = asthma which is caused by exercise such as running or cycling *astma orsakad av fysisk ansträngning* **2** *vb.* to take exercise *motionera, träna, öva;* **he exercises twice a day to keep fit**

exert [ɪg'zɜ:t] *vb.* to use (force *or* pressure) *använda, utöva, anstränga (sig)*

exertion [ɪg'zɜ:ʃ(ə)n] *subst.* physical activity *ansträngning*

exfoliation [eksˌfəʊli'eɪʃ(ə)n] *subst.* losing layers of tissue (such as sunburnt skin) *exfoliation, flagande, fjällning*

exfoliativ ⇨ **exfoliative**

exfoliative [eks'fəʊlieɪtɪv] *adj.* referring to exfoliation *exfoliativ;* **exfoliative dermatitis** = condition where the skin becomes red and flakes off *dermatitis exfoliativa*

exhalation [ˌekshə'leɪʃ(ə)n] *subst.* (i) expiration *or* breathing out *exhalation, exspiration, utandning;* (ii) air which is breathed out *exhalation, exspiration, utandning*
NOTE: the opposite is = INHALE, INHALATION

exhalation ⇨ **expiration**

exhale [eks'heɪ(ə)l] *vb.* to breathe out *andas ut*

exhaust [ɪg'zɔ:st] *vb.* to tire someone out *överanstränga, utmatta;* to drain energy *uttömma, förbruka;* **he was exhausted by his long walk; the patient was exhausted after the second operation**

exhaustion [ɪg'zɔ:stʃ(ə)n] *subst.* extreme tiredness *or* fatigue *överansträngning, utmattning;* **heat exhaustion** = collapse caused by physical exertion in hot conditions *värmeslag*

exhibitionism [ˌeksɪ'bɪʃ(ə)nɪz(ə)m] *subst.* sexual aberration in which there is a desire to show the genitals to a person of the opposite sex *exhibitionism*

exkoriation ⇨ **excoriation**

exkrement- ⇨ **faecal, scat-, sterco-, stercoraceous**

exkrement, hårt ⇨ **scybalum**

exkrescens ⇨ **excrescence**

exkret ⇨ **excreta**

exo- ['eksəʊ, ˌ--] *prefix* meaning outside *ex(o)-, ut-*

exocrine gland ['eksə(ʊ)kraɪn ˌglænd] *subst.* gland (such as the liver, the sweat glands, the pancreas and the salivary glands) with ducts which channel secretions to particular parts of the body *exokrin körtel;* **exocrine secretions of the pancreas** = enzymes carried from the pancreas to the second part of the duodenum *bukspottskörtelns exokrina sekret*

exoftalmi ⇨ **exophthalmos**

exoftalmus ⇨ **exophthalmos**

exogen ⇨ **exogenous**

exogenous [ek'sɒdʒ(ə)nəs] *adj.* developing *or* caused by something outside the organism *exogen; compare* ENDOGENOUS

exomphalos [ek'sɒmfələs] = UMBILICAL HERNIA

exophthalmic goitre [ˌeksɒf'θælmɪk ˌgɔɪtə] *or* **Graves' disease** ['greɪvz dɪˌzi:z] *see* THYROTOXICOSIS

exophthalmos [ˌeksɒf'θælməs] *subst.* protruding eyeballs *exoftalmus, exoftalmi, glosögdhet*

exoskeleton [ˌeksə(ʊ)'skelɪt(ə)n] *subst.* outer skeleton of some animals such as insects *yttre skelett; compare* ENDOSKELETON

exostosis [ˌeksə(ʊ)'stəʊsɪs] *subst.* benign growth on the surface of a bone *exostos, bensporre, benutväxt*

exotic [ɪg'zɒtɪk] *adj.* (disease) which is not native *or* which comes from a foreign country *främmande, utländsk*

exotoxin [ˌeksəʊ'tɒksɪn] *subst.* poison produced by bacteria, which affects parts of the body away from the place of infection (such as the toxins which cause botulism or tetanus) *exotoxin*

COMMENT: diphtheria is caused by a bacillus; the exotoxin released causes the generalized symptoms of the disease (such as fever and rapid pulse) while the bacillus itself is responsible for the local symptoms in the patient's upper throat

exotropia [ˌeksəʊ'trəʊpiə] *subst.* divergent strabismus *or* form of squint where both eyes look away from the nose *exotropi, strabismus divergens (externus), divergent strabism (skelning), utåtskelning*

expand [ɪk'spænd] *vb.* to spread out *(ut)vidga(s);* **the chest expands as the person breathes in**

expansion [ɪk'spænʃ(ə)n] *subst.* growing larger *or* becoming swollen *utvidgning*

expect [ɪk'spekt] *vb.* to think *or* to hope that something is going to happen *(för)vänta (sig), beräkna;* **she's expecting a baby in June** = she is pregnant and the baby is due to be born in June *hon väntar (skall föda) barn i juni;* **expected date of delivery** = day on which a doctor calculates that the birth will take place *beräknad nedkomst*

expectant mother [ɪkˌspekt(ə)nt 'mʌðə] *subst.* pregnant woman *havande kvinna, blivande mor*

expectorant [ɪk'spektər(ə)nt] *subst.* drug which helps the patient to expectorate *or* to cough up phlegm *expektorans, hostbefrämjande medel, slemlösande medel*

expectorate [ɪk'spektəreɪt] *vb.* to cough up phlegm *or* sputum from the respiratory passages *expektorera, hosta upp*

expectoration [ɪk'spektə'reɪʃ(ə)n] *subst.* coughing up fluid *or* phlegm from the respiratory tract *expektorat, upphostning*

expektorans ▷ **expectorant**

expektorat ▷ **expectoration**

expektorera ▷ **expectorate**

expel [ɪk'spel] *vb.* to send out of the body *stöta (driva) ut;* **air is expelled from the lungs when a person breathes out**

experience [ɪk'spɪəriəns] **1** *subst.* **(a)** having worked in many types of situation, and so knowing how to cope with different problems *erfarenhet, vana;* **he has had six years' experience in tropical medicine; his research is based on his experience as a nurse in a teaching hospital (b)** thing which has happened to someone *upplevelse, händelse;* **he told the complaints board about his experiences as an outpatient 2** *vb.* to live through a situation *uppleva;* **she experienced acute mental disturbance; he is experiencing pains in his right upper leg**

experienced [ɪk'spɪəriənst] *adj.* (person) who has lived through many situations and has learnt how to deal with problems *erfaren, van;* **she is the most experienced member of our nursing staff; we require an experienced nurse to take charge of a geriatric ward**

experiment [ɪk'sperɪmənt] *subst.* scientific test conducted under set conditions *experiment;* **the scientists did some experiments to try the new drug on a small sample of people**

expert ['ekspɜːt] **1** *subst.* person who is trained *or* who has experience in a certain field *expert, specialist;* **he was referred to an expert in tropical diseases; she is an expert in the field of optics; they asked for a second expert opinion 2** *adj.* done well *or* showing experience *sakkunnig, kunnig;* **the clinic offers expert treatment of sexually transmitted diseases**

expiration [ˌekspə'reɪʃ(ə)n] *subst.* (i) breathing out *or* pushing air out of the lungs *exspiration, exhalation, utandning;* (ii) dying *död, sista suck;* **expiration takes place when the chest muscles relax and the lungs become smaller**
NOTE: the opposite is **inspiration**

expire [ɪk'spaɪə, eks-] *vb.* (i) to breathe out *andas ut;* (ii) to die *dö, andas ut sin sista suck*

explain [ɪk'spleɪn] *vb.* to give reasons for something; to make something clear *förklara;* **the doctors cannot explain why he suddenly got better; she tried to explain her symptoms to the doctor**

explanation [ˌekspləˈneɪʃ(ə)n] *subst.* reason for something *förklaring;* **the staff of the hospital could not offer any explanation for the strange behaviour of the consultant**

explant [eks'plɑ:nt] *subst.* tissue taken from a body and grown in a culture in a laboratory *vävnad för odling*

explantation [ˌekspl ɑ:n'teɪʃ(ə)n] *subst.* taking tissue for culture in a laboratory *explantation, odling av vävnad*

exploration [ˌeksplə'reɪʃ(ə)n] *subst.* procedure *or* surgical operation where the aim is to discover the cause of the symptoms *or* the nature and extent of the illness *exploration, undersökning*

explorativ ⇨ **exploratory**

exploratory [ɪk'splɔ:rət(ə)ri] *adj.* referring to an exploration *explorativ;* **exploratory surgery** = surgical operations in which the aim is to discover the cause of the patient's symptoms *or* the nature and extent of the illness *explorativ kirurgi*

explosionsskada ⇨ **blast**

exponering ⇨ **exposure**

expose [ɪk'spəʊz] *vb.* **(a)** to show something which was hidden *visa, avslöja, blotta;* **the operation exposed a generalized cancer; the report exposed a lack of medical care on the part of some of the hospital staff (b)** to place something *or* someone under the influence of something *utsätta (för);* **he was exposed to the disease for two days; she was exposed to a lethal dose of radiation**

exposure [ɪk'spəʊʒə] *subst.* **(a)** being exposed *exponering;* **his exposure to radiation (b)** being damp, cold and with no protection from the weather *utsatthet, strapats, umbärande;* **the survivors of the crash were all suffering from exposure after spending a night in the snow**

expression [ɪk'spreʃ(ə)n] *subst.* **(a)** look on a person's face which shows his emotions *or* what he thinks and feels *uttryck;* **his expression showed that he was annoyed (b)** pushing something out of the body *utpressande, utklämning;* **the expression of the fetus and placenta during childbirth**

exsanguinate [ɪk'sæŋgwɪneɪt] *vb.* to drain blood from the body *tappa blod*

exsanguination [ɪkˌsæŋgwɪ'neɪʃ(ə)n] *subst.* removal of blood from the body *blodtappning*

exspiration ⇨ **exhalation, expiration**

exstirpation ⇨ **extirpation**

exsudat ⇨ **exudate**

exsudation ⇨ **exudation**

exsufflation [ˌeksə'fleɪʃ(ə)n] *subst.* forcing breath out of the body *forcerad utandning*

extend [ɪk'stend] *vb.* to stretch out *sträcka ut;* **the patient is unable to extend his arms fully**

extension [ɪk'stenʃ(ə)n] *subst.* (i) stretching *or* straightening out of a joint *extension, utsträckning;* (ii) stretching of a joint by traction *sträckning*

extensor (muscle) [ɪk'stensə (ˌmʌs(ə)l)] *subst.* muscle which makes a joint become straight *(musculus) extensor, sträckmuskel; compare* FLEXOR

exterior [ɪk'stɪəriə] *subst.* the outside *exterior, exteriör, det yttre;* **the interior of the disc has passed through the tough exterior and is pressing on a nerve**

exteriorization [ɪkˌstɪəriəraɪ'zeɪʃ(ə)n] *subst.* surgical operation to bring an internal organ to the outside surface of the body *extiorisation*

extern ⇨ **external**

externa [ɪk'stɜ:nə] *see* OTITIS

external [ɪk'stɜ:n(ə)l] *adj.* which is outside, especially outside the surface of the body *extern, yttre, utvärtes;* **the lotion is for external use only** = it should only be used on the outside of the body *lösningen är endast för utvärtes bruk;* **external auditory meatus** = passage from the outer ear to the eardrum *meatus acusticus externus, yttre hörselgången;* **external cardiac massage** *or* **external chest** *or* **cardiac compression** = method of making a patient's heart start beating again by rhythmic pressing on the breastbone *yttre hjärtmassage;* **external jugular** = main jugular vein in the neck, leading from the temporal vein *vena jugularis externa, yttre strupvenen;* **external oblique** = outer muscle covering the abdomen *musculus obliquus externus abdominis, bukens yttre snedmuskel*

externally [ɪk'stɜ:n(ə)li] *adv.* on the outside of the body *yttre, utvärtes;* **the ointment should only be used externally** *compare* INTERNAL, INTERNALLY

exteroceptor [ˌekstərəʊ'septə] *subst.* sensory nerve such as those in the eye *or* ear, which is affected by stimuli from outside the body *sensorisk nerv som påverkas av yttre* *stimuli; see also* CHEMORECEPTOR, INTEROCEPTOR, RECEPTOR

extiorisation ⇨ **exteriorization**

extirpation [ˌekstɜːˈpeɪʃ(ə)n] *subst.* total removal of a structure *or* an organ *or* growth by surgery *exstirpation, borttagande*

extra ⇨ **accessory, spare**

extra- [ˈekstrə, ˌ--] *prefix* meaning outside *extra-*

extracapsular [ˌekstrəˈkæpsjʊlə] *adj.* outside a capsule *extrakapsulär;* **extracapsular fracture** = fracture of the upper part of the femur, but which does not involve the capsule round the hip joint *extrakapsulär fraktur*

extracellular [ˌekstrəˈseljʊlə] *adj.* outside cells *extracellulär;* **extracellular fluid** = fluid which surrounds cells *extracellulärvätska*

extracellulärvätska ⇨ **extracellular**

extract [ˈekstrækt; ɪkˈstrækt] **1** *subst.* preparation made by removing water *or* alcohol from a substance, leaving only the essence *extrakt;* **liver extract** = concentrated essence of liver *leverextrakt* **2** *vb.* (i) to take out *ta ut;* (ii) to remove the essence from a liquid *extrahera;* (iii) to pull out a tooth *dra ut;* **adrenaline extracted from the animal's adrenal glands is used in the treatment of asthma**

> QUOTE all the staff are RGNs, partly because they do venesection, partly because they work in plasmapheresis units which extract plasma and return red blood cells to the donor
>
> **Nursing Times**

extraction [ɪkˈstrækʃ(ə)n] *subst.* (i) removal of part of the body, especially a tooth *extraktion, utdragning;* (ii) in obstetrics, delivery, usually a breech presentation, which needs medical assistance *extraktion;* **cataract extraction** = surgical removal of a cataract from the eye *starroperation;* **vacuum extraction** = pulling on the head of the baby with a suction instrument to aid birth *vakuumextraktion*

extradural [ˌekstrəˈdjʊər(ə)l] *or* **epidural** [ˌepɪˈdjʊər(ə)l] *adj.* lying on the outside of the dura mater *extradural, epidural;* **extradural haematoma** = blood clot which forms in the head outside the dura mater, caused by a blow *extraduralhematom, epiduralhematom*

extraduralhematom ⇨ **extradural**

extraembryonal ⇨ **extraembryonic**

extraembryonic [ˌekstrəˌembriˈɒnɪk] *adj.* (part of a fertilized ovum, such as the amnion, allantois and chorion) which is not part of the embryo *extraembryonal*

extrahera ⇨ **extract**

extrakapsulär ⇨ **extracapsular**

extrakt ⇨ **extract**

extraktion ⇨ **extraction**

extrapleural [ˌekstrəˈplʊər(ə)l] *adj.* outside the pleural cavity *utanför lungsäcken, utanför brösthålan*

extrapyramidal [ˌekstrəpɪˈræmɪd(ə)l] *adj.* outside the pyramidal tracts *extrapyramidal;* **extrapyramidal system** *or* **tracts** = motor system which carries motor nerves outside the pyramidal system *extrapyramidala systemet resp. banorna*

extraslag ⇨ **extrasystole**

extrasystole [ˌekstrəˈsɪst(ə)li] *or* **ectopic beat** [ɪkˌtɒpɪk ˈbiːt] *subst.* abnormal extra heartbeat which originates from a point other than the sinoatrial node *extrasystole, extraslag, ektopiskt slag*

extrasystole ⇨ **ectopic beat**

extrauterine pregnancy [ˌekstrəˈjuːtəraɪn ˌpregnənsi] *or* **ectopic pregnancy** [ɪkˈtɒpɪk ˌpregnənsi] *subst.* pregnancy where the embryo develops outside the uterus, often in one of the Fallopian tubes *extrauterin (ektopisk) graviditet, utomkvedshavandeskap*

extravasation [ekˌstrævəˈseɪʃ(ə)n] *subst.* escaping of bodily fluid (such as blood *or* secretions) into tissue *extravasering, utgjutning i vävnaderna (egentligen utanför blodbanan)*

extravasering ⇨ **extravasation**

extraversion [ˌekstrəˈvɜːʃ(ə)n] *subst.* = EXTROVERSION

extreme [ɪksˈtriːm] *adj.* very severe *ytterst stor (svår, sträng), intensiv;* **extreme forms of the disease can cause blindness**

extremiteter ⇨ **extremities, limb**

extremitetsavledning ⇨ **limb**

extremities [ˌɪk'stremətiz] *subst.* parts of the body at the ends of limbs, such as the fingers, toes, nose and ears *extremiteterna*

extrinsic [eks'trɪnsɪk] *adj.* external *or* which originates outside a structure *yttre, som ligger utanför;* **extrinsic allergic alveolitis** = condition where the lungs are allergic to fungus and other allergens *inflammation i lungalveolerna på grund av allergi;* **extrinsic factor** = former term for vitamin B_{12}, which is necessary for the production of red blood cells *extrinsic factor, vitamin B??2??12??, (cyano)kobalamin, cykobemin;* **extrinsic ligament** = ligament between the bones in a joint which is separate from the joint capsule *yttre ligament (ledband);* **extrinsic muscle** = muscle which is some way away from the part of the body (such as the eye) which it operates *muskel som ligger på avstånd från det organ den styr*

extroversion [ˌekstrə'vɜːʃ(ə)n] *subst.* **(a)** *(in psychology)* condition where a person is mainly interested in people and things other than himself *extroversion, utåtriktad läggning* **(b)** congenital turning of an organ inside out *extroversion, medfödd missbildning där organ är ut-och-invänt*

extrovert ['ekstrə(ʊ)vɜːt] *subst.* person who is interested in people and things apart from himself *extrovert, utåtriktad*

extroverted ['ekstrə(ʊ)vɜːtɪd] *adj.* turned inside out *ut-och-invänd; compare* INTROVERSION, INTROVERT

exudate ['eksjudeɪt] *subst.* fluid which is deposited on the surface of tissue as the result of a condition *or* disease *exsudat, utsöndring, uttömning*

exudation [ˌeksju'deɪʃ(ə)n] *subst.* escape of exudate into tissue as a defence mechanism *exsudation, utsöndring, uttömning*

eye [aɪ] *subst.* part of the body with which a person sees *oculus, ögat;* **she has blue eyes; shut your eyes while the doctor gives you an injection; he has got a piece of dust in his eye; she has been having trouble with her eyes** *or* **she has been having eye trouble; he is an outpatient at the local eye hospital; the doctor prescribed some eye drops** *or* **eye ointment; black eye** = darkening and swelling of the tissues round an eye, caused by a blow *blått öga;* **he got two black eyes in the fight; pink eye** *or* **red eye** = epidemic conjunctivitis, common in schools, and caused by the Koch-Weeks bacillus *smittsam konjunktivit;* **eye bath** = small dish into which a solution can be placed for bathing the eye *ögonbad*

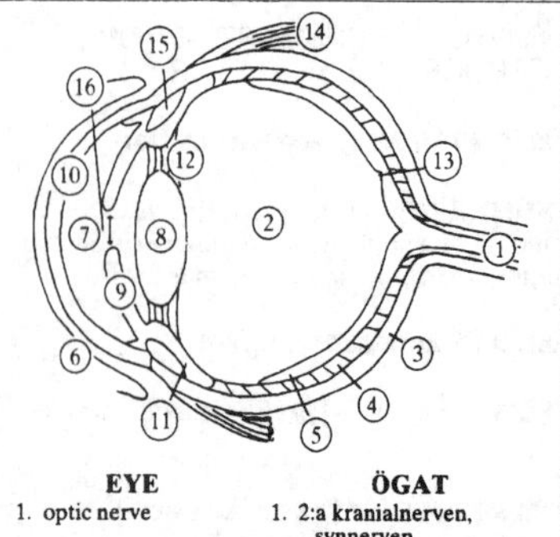

EYE	ÖGAT
1. optic nerve	1. 2:a kranialnerven, synnerven
2. vitreous humour	2. glaskroppen
3. sclera	3. senhinnan
4. choroid	4. åderhinnan
5. retina	5. näthinnan
6. conjunctiva	6. bindehinnan
7. aqueous humour	7. ögonkammarvattnet
8. lens	8. linsen
9. iris	9. regnbågshinnan
10. cornea	10. hornhinnan
11. ciliary body	11. ciliarkroppen, strålkroppen
12. suspensory ligament	12. linsens upphängningstrådar
13. fovea	13. centralgropen
14. muscle	14. övre raka ögonmuskeln
15. ciliary muscle	15. ciliarmuskeln
16. pupil	16. pupillen

eyeball ['aɪbɔːl] *subst.* the receptor part of the eye, a round ball of tissue through which light passes and which is controlled by various muscles *bulbus oculi, ögongloben*

COMMENT: light rays enter the eye through the cornea, pass through the pupil and are refracted through the aqueous humour onto the lens, which then focuses the rays through the vitreous humour onto the retina at the back of the eyeball. Impulses from the retina pass along the optic nerve to the brain

eye bank ['aɪ ˌbæŋk] *subst.* place where parts of eyes given by donors can be kept for use in grafts *ögonbank*

eyebrow ['aɪbraʊ] *subst.* arch of skin with a line of hair above the eye *ögonbrynet;* **he raised his eyebrows** = he looked surprised *han lyfte på ögonbrynet*

eyeglasses ['aɪˌglɑːsɪz] *subst. US* glasses *or* spectacles *glasögon*

eyelash ['aɪlæʃ] *subst.* small hair which grows out from the edge of the eyelid *cilium, ögonfrans, ögonhår*

eyelid ['aɪlɪd] *or* **blepharon** ['blefərɒn] *or* **palpebra** ['pælpɪbrə] *subst.* piece of skin which covers the eye *blepharon,* *ögonlocket* NOTE: for terms referring to the eyelids see words beginning with **blepharo-**

eyesight ['aɪsaɪt] *subst.* being able to see *syn(förmågan), seende;* **he has got very good eyesight; failing eyesight is common in old people**

eyestrain ['aɪstreɪn] *or* **asthenopia** [ˌæsθɪ'nəʊpɪə] *subst.* tiredness in the muscles of the eye, with a headache, caused by reading in bad light, watching television, working on a computer screen, etc. *astenopi, överansträngning av ögonen*

eye tooth ['aɪ ˌtu:θ] *or* **canine tooth** ['keɪnaɪn ˌtu:θ] *subst.* one of the teeth next to the incisors (there are two eye teeth in the upper jaw) *dens cuspidatus (caninus), hörntand* NOTE: plural is **eye teeth** for other terms referring to the eye see words beginning with **oculo-, ophth-** and **opt-**

Ff

F [ef] **1** *abbreviation for* Fahrenheit *F, Fahrenheit* **2** *chemical symbol for* fluorine *F, fluor*

face [feɪs] **1** *subst.* front part of the head, where the eyes, nose and mouth are placed *facies, ansiktet;* **don't forget to wash the patient's face; face delivery** = birth where the baby's face appears first *ansiktsbjudning; (in cosmetic surgery)* **face lift** *or* **face-lifting operation** = surgical operation to remove wrinkles on the face and neck *ansiktslyftning;* **she's gone into hospital for a face lift; face mask** = (i) rubber mask that fits over the patient's nose and mouth and is used to administer an anaesthetic *narkosmask, mask;* (ii) piece of cloth which fits over a doctor's nose and mouth to prevent him breathing out germs when he is performing an operation *munskydd;* **face presentation** = position of a baby in the womb where the face will appear first at birth *ansiktsbjudning* **2** *vb.* to have your face towards *or* to look towards *vända ansiktet mot, stå (vara) vänd mot;* **please face the screen**

COMMENT: the fourteen bones which make up the face are: two maxillae forming the upper jaw; two nasal bones forming the top part of the nose; two lacrimal bones on the inside of the orbit near the nose; two zygomatic or malar bones forming the sides of the cheeks; two palatine bones forming the back part of the top of the mouth; two nasal conchae or turbinate bones which form the sides of the nasal cavity; the mandible or lower jaw; and the vomer in the centre of the nasal septum

facet ['fæsɪt] *subst.* flat surface on a bone *fasett, plan benyta;* **facet syndrome** = condition where a joint in the vertebrae becomes dislocated *(kiropraktorterm för) slags förskjutning av ryggkota*

facial ['feɪʃ(ə)l] *adj.* referring to the face *facial, ansikts-;* **the psychiatrist examined the patient's facial expression; facial bones** = the fourteen bones which form the face *ansiktets ben;* **facial artery** = artery which branches off the external carotid into the face *arteria facialis, ansiktsartären;* **facial nerve** = seventh cranial nerve, which governs the muscles of the face, the taste buds on the front of the tongue, and the salivary and lacrimal glands *nervus facialis, ansiktsnerven, 7:e kranialnerven;* **facial paralysis** *or* **facial palsy** = BELL'S PALSY; **facial vein** = vein which drains down the side of the face into the internal jugular vein *vena facialis communis;* **deep facial vein** = small vein which drains from behind the cheek into the facial vein *vena facialis posterior*

facialispares ▷ **Bell's palsy**

-facient [feɪʃ(ə)nt] *prefix* which makes *-framkallande, som förorsakar;* **abortifacient** = drug or instrument which produces an abortion *abortframkallande*

facies ['feɪʃii:z] *subst.* facial appearance of a patient, used as a guide to diagnosis *utseende (i ansiktet)*

facilitate [fə'sɪləteɪt] *vb.* to help *or* to make something easy *underlätta, förenkla, främja*

facilitation [fəˌsɪlə'teɪʃ(ə)n] *subst.* act where several slight stimuli help a neurone to be activated *facilitation*

facilities [fə'sɪlətiz] *subst pl.* equipment *or* counselling *or* rooms which can be used to do something *anordningar, hjälpmedel, lokaler;* **provision of aftercare facilities**

fack ▷ **field**

fackförbund ▷ **professional**

fact [fækt] *subst.* something which is real and true *faktum;* **it is a fact that the disease is rarely fatal; tell me all the facts of your son's illness so that I can decide what to do; the facts of life** = description of how sexual intercourse is performed and how conception takes place, given to children *hur barn blir till*

factor ['fæktə] *subst.* **(a)** something which has an influence, which makes something else take place *faktor;* **extrinsic factor** = form of vitamin B_{12} *extrinsic factor, vitamin B12, (cyano)kobalamin, cykobemin;* **growth factor** = chemical substance produced in one part of the body which encourages the growth of a type of cell (such as red blood cells) *tillväxtfaktor;* **intrinsic factor** = protein produced in the gastric glands which controls the absorption of extrinsic factor, and the lack of which causes pernicious anaemia *intrinsic factor* **(b)** substance (called Factor I, Factor II, etc.) in the plasma which makes the blood coagulate when a blood vessel is injured *koagulationsfaktor;* **Factor VIII** = substance in plasma which is lacking in haemophiliacs *koagulationsfaktor VIII, antihemofilifaktor A, AHF, AHG;* **Christmas factor** *or* **Factor IX** = substance in plasma, the lack of which causes Christmas disease *koagulationsfaktor IX, antihemofilifaktor B*

faculty ['fæk(ə)lti] *subst.* ability to do something *förmåga;* **mental faculties** = power of the mind to think *or* decide *själsförmögenheter;* **a reduction in blood supply to the brain can have a lasting effect on the mental faculties**

fader ⇨ **father**

fadersbunden ⇨ **fixated**

faecal ['fi:k(ə)l] *adj.* referring to faeces *fekal, sterkoral, exkrement-, avförings-;* **faecal matter** = solid waste matter from the bowels *f(a)eces, fekalier, exkrement(er), avföring*
NOTE: spelt **feces, fecal** especially in the USA. For other terms referring to faeces, see words beginning with **sterco-**

faeces ['fi:si:z] *or* **stools** ['stu:lz] *or* **bowel movements** ['baʊəl ˌmu:vmənt] *subst pl.* solid waste matter passed from the bowels through the anus *f(a)eces, fekalier, exkrement(er), avföring*

fagocyt ⇨ **phagocyte**

fagocyterande ⇨ **phagocytic**

fagocytisk ⇨ **phagocytic**

fagocytos ⇨ **phagocytosis, ingestion**

fagocytär ⇨ **phagocytic**

Fahrenheit ['fær(ə)nhaɪt] *subst.* scale of temperatures where the freezing and boiling points of water are 32° and 212° *Fahrenheit; compare* CELSIUS, CENTIGRADE
NOTE: used in the USA, but less common in the UK. Normally written with an **F** after the degree sign: **32 ° F** (say: 'thirty-two degrees Fahrenheit')

fail [feɪl] *vb.* not to be successful in doing something *or* not to succeed *or* not to do something which you are trying to do *misslyckas;* **the doctor failed to see the symptoms; she has failed her pharmacy exams; he failed his medical and was rejected by the police force**

failure ['feɪljə] *subst.* not a success *svikt, misslyckande;* **the operation to correct the bone defect was a failure; heart failure** = situation where the heart cannot function in a satisfactory way and is unable to circulate blood normally *hjärtsvikt;* **kidney failure** = situation where a kidney does not function properly *njursvikt;* **failure to thrive** = wasting disease of small children who have difficulty in absorbing nutrients *or* who are suffering from malnutrition *failure to thrive*

faint [feɪnt] **1** *vb.* to lose consciousness *or* to stop being conscious for a short time *svimma;* **she fainted when she saw the blood; it was so hot standing in the sun that he fainted 2** *subst.* loss of consciousness for a short period, caused by a temporary reduction in the flow of blood to the brain *svimning;* **he collapsed in a faint 3** *adj.* not very clear *or* difficult to see or hear *svag;* **he could detect a faint improvement in the patient's condition; there's a faint smell of apples in the urine**
NOTE: **faint - fainter - faintest**

fainting ['feɪntɪŋ] *or* **syncope** ['sɪŋkəpi] *subst.* becoming unconscious for a short time *syncope, synkope, svimning;* **fainting fit** *or* **fainting spell** = becoming unconscious for a short time *svimningsanfall;* **she often had fainting fits when she was dieting**

> COMMENT: a fainting spell happens when the supply of blood to the brain is reduced for a short time, and this can be due to many causes, including lack of food, heat exhaustion, standing upright for a long time, and fear

fair [feə] *adj.* light coloured (hair *or* skin) *ljus, ljushårig, blond;* **she's got fair hair; he's dark, but his sister is fair**

Fairbanks' splint ['feəbæŋks ˌsplɪnt] *subst.* special splint used for correcting Erb's palsy *slags skena för korrektion av Erbs förlamning (slags förlossningsskada i armens övre del)*

fair-haired ['feəˌheəd] *adj.* (person) with fair hair *ljus(hårig), blond (person)*

fairly ['feəli] *adv.* quite *ganska, tämligen;* **I'm fairly certain I have met him before; he has been working as a doctor only for a fairly short time**

faktisk ⇨ **actual**

faktor ⇨ **fact, factor**

fakultet ⇨ **school**

falang ⇨ **phalanx**

falangeal ⇨ **phalangeal**

falciform ligament ['fælsɪfɔ:m ˌlɪgəmənt] *subst.* tissue which separates the two lobes of the liver and attaches it to the diaphragm *ligamentum falciforme hepatis*

fall [fɔ:l] **1** *subst.* losing balance and going onto the ground *fall;* **she had a fall and hurt her back; he broke a bone in his hip after a fall 2** *vb.* to drop down onto the ground *falla, ramla (omkull);* **he fell down the stairs; she fell off the wall; don't put the baby's bottle on the cushion - it will fall over** NOTE: **falls - falling - fell - has fallen**

fall ⇨ **case; drop, fall**

falla ⇨ **drop, fall**

fall asleep [ˌfɔ:l ə'sli:p] *vb.* to go to sleep *somna;* **he fell asleep in front of the TV**

falla sönder ⇨ **decompose**

fall ill [ˌfɔ:l 'ɪl] *vb.* to get ill *or* to start to have an illness *bli sjuk, insjukna;* **he fell ill while on holiday and had to be flown home**

fall off [ˌfɔ:l 'ɒf] *vb.* to become less *minska, avta;* **the number of admissions has fallen off this month**

Fallopian tube [fæ'ləʊpiən ˌtju:b] *or* **oviduct** ['əʊvɪdʌkt] *or* **salpinx** ['sælpɪŋks] *or* **uterine tube** ['ju:tərаɪn ˌtju:b] *subst.* one of two tubes which connect the ovaries to the uterus *tuba uterina, salpinx, äggledaren* NOTE: for other terms referring to Fallopian tubes, see words beginning with **salping-** = UROGENITAL SYSTEM (female)

COMMENT: once a month, ova (unfertilized eggs) leave the ovaries and move down the Fallopian tubes to the uterus; at the point where the Fallopian tubes join the uterus an ovum may be fertilized by a sperm cell. Sometimes fertilization and development of the embryo take place in the Fallopian tube itself

falloplastik ⇨ **phalloplasty**

fallos ⇨ **phallus**

Fallot's tetralogy ['fæləts te'trælədʒi] *see* TETRALOGY, WATERSTON'S OPERATION

false [fɔ:ls] *adj.* not true *or* not real *falsk, sken-;* **false pains** = pains which appear to be labour pains but are not *falska värkar;* **false ribs** = ribs which are not attached to the breastbone *de fem understa paren revben;* **false teeth** *or* **dentures** = artificial teeth made of plastic, which fit in the mouth and take the place of teeth which have been extracted *löständer, tandprotes*

falsk ⇨ **false, para-, pseud-**

falx (cerebri) ['fælks (ˌserəbri)] *subst.* fold of the dura mater between the two hemispheres of the cerebrum *falx cerebri, stora hjärnskäran*

familial [fə'mɪliəl] *adj.* referring to a family *familjär, ärftlig;* **familial disorder** = hereditary disorder which affects several members of the same family *familjär sjukdom (rubbning)*

familj ⇨ **family**

familjeläkare ⇨ **family**

familjeplanering ⇨ **planned parenthood, planning**

familjeplaneringsklinik ⇨ **planning**

familjär ⇨ **familial**

family ['fæm(ə)li] *subst.* group of people who are related to each other, especially mother, father and children *familj;* **John is the youngest in our family; they have a very big family - two sons and three daughters; family doctor** = general practitioner, especially one who looks after all the members of a family *husläkare, familjeläkare;* **family planning** = using contraception to control the number of children in a family *familjeplanering;* **family planning clinic** = clinic which gives advice on contraception *familjeplaneringsklinik;* **Family Practitioner Committee** = committee which organizes the management of GPs, dentists, opticians and pharmacists offering their services in an area *i Storbritannien slags organ som administrerar* *privat öppen sjuk- och hälsovård inom visst område*

Fanconi syndrome [fæn'kəʊni ˌsɪndrəʊm] *subst.* kidney disorder where amino acids are present in the urine *Fanconis syndrom*

fantasi ➪ **fantasy, imagery, imagination**

fantasi- ➪ **imaginary**

fantasize ['fæntəsaɪz] *vb.* to imagine that things have happened *fantisera*

fantasy ['fæntəsɪ] *subst.* series of imaginary events which a patient believes really took place *fantasier*

fantisera ➪ **fantasize**

fantomsensation ➪ **phantom**

far ➪ **father**

fara ➪ **danger, risk**

fara, utan ➪ **safely**

farcy ['fɑːsi] *subst.* form of glanders which affects the lymph nodes *slags rots (sjukdom hos häst, som kan överföras till människa)*

farfar ➪ **grandfather**

farföräldrar ➪ **grandparents**

farinaceous [ˌfærɪ'neɪʃəs] *adj.* referring to flour *or* containing starch *mjöl-, stärkelse-;* **farinaceous foods** = foods (such as bread) which are made of flour and have a high starch content *mjölmat, mat med hög halt av stärkelse*

farlig ➪ **dangerous, harmful, noxious, pernicious**

farm [fɑːm] *subst.* land used for growing crops and keeping animals *bondgård, lantbruk;* **he's going to work on the farm during the holidays; you can buy eggs and vegetables at the farm**

farmaceut ➪ **chemist, dispensing chemist, pharmacist**

farmaceutisk ➪ **pharmaceutical**

farmaceutisk specialitet ➪ **proprietary**

farmakolog ➪ **pharmacologist**

farmakologi ➪ **pharmacology**

farmakologisk ➪ **pharmacological**

farmakopé ➪ **formulary, pharmacopoeia**

farmer ['fɑːmə] *subst.* man who looks after or owns a farm *bonde, lantbrukare;* **farmer's lung** = type of asthma caused by an allergy to rotting hay *slags astma*

farmor ➪ **grandmother**

farsightedness [ˌfɑː'saɪtɪdnəs] *or* **longsightedness** [ˌlɒŋ'saɪtɪdnəs] *or* **hypermetropia** [ˌhaɪpəmɪ'trəʊpiə] *or US* **hypertropia** [ˌhaɪpə'trəʊpiə] *subst.* condition where the patient sees clearly objects which are a long way away but cannot see objects which are close *hypermetropi, hyperopi, översynthet, långsynthet*
NOTE: the opposite is **shortsightedness** *or* **myopia**

faryngeal ➪ **pharyngeal**

faryngektomi ➪ **pharyngectomy**

faryngism ➪ **pharyngismus**

faryngit ➪ **pharyngitis**

faryngocele ➪ **pharyngocele**

farynx ➪ **pharynx**

farynx- ➪ **pharyngeal**

farynxtonsillen ➪ **tonsil**

fas ➪ **phase**

fascia ['feɪʃə] *subst.* fibrous tissue covering a muscle or an organ *fascia, bindvävshinna;* **fascia lata** = wide sheet of tissue covering the thigh muscles *fascia lata*
NOTE: plural is **fasciae**

fasciculation [fəˌsɪkju'leɪʃ(ə)n] *subst.* small muscle movements which appear as trembling skin *fascikulation*

fasciculus [fə'sɪkjʊləs] *subst.* bundle of nerve fibres *fascikel, bunt, sträng, nervstråk*
NOTE: plural is **fasciculi**

fascikel ➪ **bundle, fasciculus**

Fasciolopsis [ˌfæsiəʊ'lɒpsɪs] *subst.* type of liver fluke, often found in the Far East, which is transmitted to humans through contaminated waterplants *Fasciolopsis, slags trematod (sugmask)*

fasett ➪ **facet**

FASS ➪ **pharmacopoeia**

fast [fɑːst] **1** *subst.* going without food (either to lose weight *or* for religious reasons) *fasta;* **he went on a fast to lose some weight 2** *vb.* to go without food *fasta, gå (vara) utan mat;* **strict Muslims should fast during the daytime for the month of Ramadan**

fast ➪ **constant, solid, tight, tightly**

fasta ➪ **fast**

fastande ➪ **NPO**

fastigium [fæ'stɪdʒiəm] *subst.* highest temperature during a bout of fever *fastigium, kulmen, höjdpunkt*

fastna ➪ **lodge, stick**

fastsittande ➪ **sessile**

fastställa ➪ **determine, identify**

fastställande ➪ **identification**

fat [fæt] **1** *adj.* big and round in the body *fet, tjock, korpulent;* **you ought to eat less - you're getting too fat; that fat man has a very thin wife; he's the fattest boy in the class**
NOTE: **fat - fatter - fattest 2** *subst.* **(a)** white *or* oily substance in the body, which stores energy and protects the body against cold *fett;* **body fat** *or* **adipose tissue** = tissue where the cells contain fat, which replaces the normal fibrous tissue when too much food is eaten *fettväv(nad), kroppsfett;* **brown fat** = animal fat which can easily be converted to energy, and is believed to offset the effects of ordinary white fat *brunt fett;* **saturated fat** = fat which has the largest amount of hydrogen possible *mättat fett;* **unsaturated fat** = fat which does not have a large amount of hydrogen, and so can be broken down more easily *omättat fett* **(b)** type of food which supplies protein and Vitamins A and D, especially that part of meat which is white *or* solid substances (like lard *or* butter) produced from animals and used for cooking *or* liquid substances like oil *fett, matfett;* **if you don't like the fat on the meat, cut it off; fry the eggs in some fat**

> COMMENT: fat is a necessary part of diet because of the vitamins and energy-giving calories which is contains. Fat in the diet comes from either animal fats or vegetable fats. Animal fats such as butter, fat meat or cream, are saturated fatty acids. It is believed that the intake of unsaturated and polyunsaturated fats (mainly vegetable fats and oils, and fish oil) in the diet, rather than animal fats, helps keep down the level of cholesterol in the blood and so lessens the risk of atherosclerosis. A low-fat diet does not always help to reduce weight

fatal ['feɪt(ə)l] *adj.* which causes *or* results in death *letal, dödlig, döds-;* **he had a fatal accident; cases of bee stings are rarely fatal**

fatality [fə'tæləti] *subst.* case of death *dödsfall, dödsoffer, dödsolycka;* **there were three fatalities during the flooding**

fatally ['feɪt(ə)li] *adv.* in a way which causes death *dödligt, med dödlig utgång;* **his heart was fatally weakened by the lung disease**

father ['fɑːðə] *subst.* man who has a son or daughter *fader, far;* **ask your father if you can borrow his car; she is coming to tea with her father and mother**

fatigue [fə'tiːg] **1** *subst.* very great tiredness *trötthet, utmattning;* **muscle fatigue** *or* **muscular fatigue** = tiredness in the muscles after strenuous exercise *muskeltrötthet* NOTE: no plural **2** *vb.* to tire someone out *trötta ut, utmatta;* **he was fatigued by the hard work**

fat-soluble [ˌfæt'sɒljʊb(ə)l] *adj.* which can dissolve in fat *fettlöslig;* **Vitamin D is fat-soluble**
NOTE: **fat** has no plural when it means the substance; the plural **fats** is used to mean different types of fat for other terms referring to fats see also **lipid** and words beginning with **steato-**

fattig på ngt ➪ **deficient**

fatty ['fæti] *adj.* containing fat *fett-, fetthaltig;* **fatty acid** = acid (such as stearic acid) which is an important substance in the body *fettsyra;* **essential fatty acid** = unsaturated fatty acid which is essential for growth but which cannot be synthesized by the body and has to be obtained from the food supply *essentiell fettsyra;* **fatty degeneration** = accumulation of fat in the cells of an organ (such as the liver *or* heart), making the organ less able to perform *degeneratio adiposa, fettdegeneration*

fauces ['fɔːsiːz] *subst.* opening between the tonsils at the back of the throat, leading to the pharynx *fauces, svalget*

favism ['feɪvɪz(ə)m] *subst.* type of inherited anaemia caused by an allergy to beans *favism, slags ärftlig blodbrist pga intolerans mot bönor*

favus ['feɪvəs] *subst.* highly contagious type of ringworm caused by a fungus which attacks the scalp *favus, skorv*

Fe *chemical symbol for* iron *Fe, järn*

fear [fɪə] *subst.* state where a person is afraid of something happening *rädsla, fruktan;* **he has a morbid fear of flying** *or* **of spiders**

features ['fi:tʃəz] *subst.* appearance of a person's face *(anlets)drag, ansiktsdrag;* **he has heavy features**

feber ⇨ **fever, pyrexia, temperature**

feber- ⇨ **febrile, feverish, pyr-**

feberframkallande ⇨ **pyrogenic**

feberfri ⇨ **afebrile**

feberfrihet ⇨ **apyrexia**

feberkurva ⇨ **chart**

febernedsättande (medel) ⇨ **antipyretic, febrifuge**

febersjukdom ⇨ **febrile, fever**

febertermometer ⇨ **thermometer**

febricula [fe'brɪkjʊlə] *subst.* low fever *febricula, lätt feber*

febrifuge ['febrɪfju:dʒ] *adj. & subst.* (drug such as aspirin) which prevents *or* lowers a fever *antipyretikum, antipyretisk(t medel), febernedsättande (medel)*

febrig ⇨ **feverish**

febril ⇨ **febrile, feverish**

febrile ['fi:braɪ(ə)l] *adj.* referring to a fever *or* caused by a fever *febril, feber-;* **febrile disease** = disease which is accompanied by fever *febersjukdom*

feces ['fi:si:z] *or* **fecal** ['fi:k(ə)l] *US* = FAECES, FAECAL

feeble ['fi:b(ə)l] *adj.* very weak *klen, svag, kraftlös;* **she is old and feeble; some of the patients in the geriatric ward are very feeble**

feebleminded [ˌfi:b(ə)l'maɪndɪd] *adj.* being less than normally intelligent *debil, underbegåvad*

feeblemindedness [ˌfi:b(ə)l'maɪndɪdnəs] *subst.* state of less than normal intelligence *debilitet, underbegåvning*

feed [fi:d] *vb.* to give food (to someone *or* an animal) *mata, ge mat (föda) till, föda, äta;* **he has to be fed with a spoon; the baby has reached the stage when she can feed herself** NOTE: **feeds - feeding - fed - has fed**

feedback ['fi:dbæk] *subst.* linking of the result of an action back to the action itself *feedback, återkoppling;* **negative feedback** = situation where the result represses the process which caused it *negativ feedback;* **positive feedback** = situation where the result stimulates the process again *positiv feedback*

feeding ['fi:dɪŋ] *subst.* action of giving someone something to eat *matning;* **feeding cup** = special cup with a spout, used for feeding patients who cannot feed themselves *pipmugg; see also* BREAST FEEDING, BOTTLE FEEDING, INTRAVENOUS FEEDING

feel [fi:(ə)l] *vb.* **(a)** to touch (usually with your finger) *känna;* **feel how soft the cushion is; when the lights went out we had to feel our way to the door (b)** to give a sensation when touched *kännas;* **the knife felt cold; the floor feels hard (c)** to have a sensation *känna;* **I felt the table move; did you feel the lift go down suddenly? he felt ill after eating the fish; when she saw the report she felt better (d)** to believe *or* to think; to have an opinion *tycka, tro, anse;* **he feels it would be wrong to leave the children alone in the house; the police felt that the accident was the fault of the driver of the car; the doctor feels the patient is well enough to be moved out of intensive care** NOTE: **feels - feeling - felt - felt**

feeling ['fi:(ə)lɪŋ] *subst.* sensation *or* something which you feel *känsla, känsel(förnimmelse);* **I had a feeling that someone was watching me; she had an itchy feeling inside her stomach**

Fehling's solution ['feɪlɪŋz səˌlu:ʃ(ə)n] *subst.* solution used to detect sugar in urine *Fehlings lösning (vätska)*

fekal ⇨ **faecal, stercoraceous**

fekalier ⇨ **excrement, faecal, faeces, stools**

fekalsten ⇨ **coprolith, stercolith**

felaktig ⇨ **incorrect, mis-**

felbehandling ⇨ **malpractice**

felläge ⇨ **displacement, ectopia**

felon ['felən] = WHITLOW

***fel strupe, få ngt i* ⇨ choke**

***felställning* ⇨ malposition**

Felty's syndrome ['felti:z ˌsɪndrəʊm] *subst.* condition where the spleen is enlarged, and the number of white blood cells increases, associated with rheumatoid arthritis *Feltys syndrom*

female ['fi:meɪ(ə)l] *adj. & subst.* (animal *or* plant) of the same sex as a woman or girl *kvinnlig, kvinna;* animal which produces ova and bears young *hona;* **a female cat; a condition found more often in females aged 40 - 60**

***feminisering* ⇨ feminization**

feminization [ˌfemənaɪ'zeɪʃ(ə)n] *subst.* development of female characteristics in a male *feminisering*

***femling* ⇨ quintuplet**

femoral ['fem(ə)r(ə)l] *adj.* referring to the femur *or* to the thigh *femoral(-), lår-, lårbens-;* **femoral artery** = continuation of the external iliac artery, which runs down the front of the thigh and then crosses to the back *arteria femoralis, lårbensartären;* **femoral canal** = inner tube of the sheath surrounding the femoral artery and vein *canalis femoralis, femoralkanalen, kruralkanalen;* **femoral hernia** = hernia of the bowel at the top of the thigh *hernia femoralis (cruralis), femoralbråck;* **femoral nerve** = nerve which governs the muscle at the front of the thigh *nervus femoralis, lårbensnerven;* **femoral triangle** *or* **Scarpa's triangle** = slight hollow at the side of the thigh *trigonum femorale, Scarpas triangel;* **femoral vein** = vein running up the upper leg, a continuation of the popliteal vein *vena femoralis, lårbensvenen*

***femoralbråck* ⇨ femoral**

***femoralkanalen* ⇨ femoral**

femoris ['femərɪs] *subst. see* BICEPS, RECTUS

femur ['fi:mə] *subst.* thighbone *or* bone in the top part of the leg which joins the acetabulum at the hip and the tibia at the knee *femur, lårbenet* NOTE: plural is **femora** = PELVIS

fenestra [fə'nestrə] *subst.* small opening in the ear *fenestra, fönster;* **fenestra ovalis** *or* **fenestra vestibuli** *or* **oval window** = oval opening between the middle ear and the inner ear, closed by a membrane and covered by the stapes *fenestra ovalis, ovala fönstret;* **fenestra rotunda** *or* **fenestra cochleae** *or* **round window** = round opening between the middle ear and the cochlea, and closed by a membrane *fenestra rotunda (cochleae), runda fönstret*

fenestration [ˌfenə'streɪʃ(ə)n] *subst.* surgical operation to relieve deafness by making a small opening in the inner ear *fenestration*

***fenestration* ⇨ Lempert operation**

fennel ['fen(ə)l] *subst.* herb which tastes of aniseed and is used to treat flatulence *fänkål*

***fenobarbital* ⇨ phenobarbitone**

***fenol* ⇨ phenol**

***fenotyp* ⇨ phenotype**

***fenylalanin* ⇨ phenylalanine**

***fenylketonuri* ⇨ phenylketonuria**

***feokromocytom* ⇨ phaeochromocytoma**

fermentation [ˌfɜ:men'teɪʃ(ə)n] *or* **zymosis** [zaɪ'məʊsɪs] *subst.* process where carbohydrates are broken down by enzymes from yeast and produce alcohol *fermentation, jäsning*

***fertil* ⇨ fertile**

fertile ['fɜ:taɪ(ə)l] *adj.* able to bear fruit *or* to produce children *fertil, fruktsam*

***fertilisation* ⇨ fertilization**

***fertilitet* ⇨ fertility**

***fertilitetstal* ⇨ fertility**

fertility [fə'tɪləti] *subst.* being fertile *fertilitet, fruktsamhet;* **fertility rate** = number of births per year, per thousand females aged between 15 and 44 *fertilitetstal, fruktsamhetstal*

fertilization [ˌfɜ:təlaɪ'zeɪʃ(ə)n] *subst.* joining of an ovum and a sperm to form a zygote and so start the development of an embryo *fertilisation, befruktning*

fertilize ['fɜ:təlaɪz] *vb. (of a sperm)* to join with an ovum *befrukta*
NOTE: the opposite is **sterile, sterility, sterilize**

fester ['festə] *vb. (of an infected wound)* to become inflamed and produce pus *bulna, vara sig;* **his legs were covered with festering sores**

festination [ˌfestɪ'neɪʃ(ə)n] *subst.* way of walking where the patient takes short steps, seen in patients suffering from Parkinson's disease *festination*

fet ⇨ **adipose, fat, fleshy, rich**

fetal ['fi:t(ə)l] *see* FETUS

fetal ['fi:t(ə)l] *or* **foetal** ['fi:t(ə)l] *adj.* referring to a fetus *fetal, foster-;* **a sample of fetal blood was examined; fetal position =** position where a person lies curled up on his side, like a fetus in the womb *fosterställning*
NOTE: **fetus** is used to refer to unborn babies from two months after conception until birth. Before then, the baby is an **embryo**

fetichism ['fetɪʃɪz(ə)m] *subst.* psychological disorder where the patient gets sexual satisfaction from touching objects *fetischism*

fetichist ['fetɪʃɪst] *subst.* person suffering from fetichism *fetischist*

fetischism ⇨ **fetichism**

fetischist ⇨ **fetichist**

fetma ⇨ **obesity**

fetoprotein [ˌfi:təʊ'prəʊti:n] *see* ALPHA

fetor ['fi:tə] *or* **foetor** ['fi:tə] *subst.* bad smell *f(o)etor, stank, dålig lukt*

fetoscopy [fɪ'tɒskəpi] *subst.* examination of a fetus inside the womb, taking blood samples to diagnose blood disorders *fetoskopi, slags fosterdiagnostik*

fetoskopi ⇨ **fetoscopy**

fett ⇨ **fat**

fettavsöndrande ⇨ **sebaceous**

fettdegeneration ⇨ **fatty**

fettembolism ⇨ **crush syndrome**

fettfattig kost ⇨ **low**

fetthaltig ⇨ **fatty**

fettkula, liten ⇨ **globule**

fettliknande (ämne) ⇨ **lipoid**

fettlöslig ⇨ **fat-soluble**

fettomsättning ⇨ **lipid**

fettpärla, liten ⇨ **globule**

fettrik ⇨ **adipose**

fettsot ⇨ **lipomatosis**

fettsvulst ⇨ **lipoma**

fettsyra ⇨ **fatty**

fetus ['fi:təs] *or* **foetus** ['fi:təs] *subst.* unborn baby in the womb *fetus, foster*

fever ['fi:və] *or* **pyrexia** [ˌpaɪ(ə)'reksiə] *subst.* (i) rise in the body temperature *pyrexi, feber;* (ii) sickness when the temperature of the body is higher than normal *febersjukdom;* **she is running a slight fever; you must stay in bed until the fever has gone down; intermittent fever =** fever which rises and falls regularly, as in malaria *febris intermittens;* **relapsing fever =** disease caused by a bacterium, where attacks of fever recur from time to time *slags återkommande feber orsakad av bakterie;* **remittent fever =** fever which goes down for a period each day, as in typhoid fever *febris recurrens, återfallsfeber;* **fever sore** *or* **fever blister =** cold sore *or* burning sore, usually on the lips *(mun)sår pga herpes simplex (labialis), förkylningsblåsa*

> COMMENT: normal oral body temperature is about 98.6°F or 37°C and rectal temperature is about 99°F or 37.2°C. A fever often makes the patient feel cold, and is accompanied by pains in the joints. Most fevers are caused by infections; infections which result in fever include cat scratch fever, dengue, malaria, meningitis, psittacosis, Q fever, rheumatic fever, Rocky mountain spotted fever, scarlet fever, septicaemia, typhoid fever, typhus, and yellow fever

feverfew ['fi:vəfju:] *subst.* herb, formerly used to reduce fevers, but now used to relieve migraine *mattram*

feverish ['fi:v(ə)rɪʃ] *adj.* with a fever *febril, febrig, feber-;* **he felt feverish and took an aspirin; she is in bed with a feverish chill**

fiber ⇨ **fibre**

fiberhaltig kost ⇨ **fibre**

fiberliknande ⇨ **fibroid**

fiberoptik ⇨ **fibre optics**

fiberskop ⇨ **fibrescope**

fibr- ['faɪbr, ˌ-] *prefix* referring to fibres *or* fibrous *fibr(o)-, fiber-, tråd-*

fibre ['faɪbə] *or* *US* **fiber** ['faɪbər] *subst.* **(a)** structure in the body shaped like a thread *fiber, tråd;* **collagen fibre** = fibre which is the main component of fasciae, tendons and ligaments and is essential in bones and cartilage *kollagen fiber (tråd);* **elastic fibres** *or* **yellow fibres** = fibres which can expand easily and are found in elastic cartilage, the skin and the walls of arteries and the lungs *elastiska fibrer (trådar);* **nerve fibre** = fibre leading from a nerve cell, carrying nerve impulses *nervfiber, nervtråd;* **optical fibres** = artificial fibres which carry light *or* images *optisk fiber* **(b) dietary fibre** = fibrous matter in food, which cannot be digested *fibrer, kostfibrer;* **high fibre diet** = diet which contains a high percentage of cereals, nuts, fruit and vegetables *fiberhaltig kost* NOTE: no plural for (b)

COMMENT: dietary fibre is found in cereals, nuts, fruit and some green vegetables. There are two types of fibre in food: insoluble fibre (in bread and cereals) which is not digested and soluble fibre (in vegetables and pulses). Foods with the highest proportion of fibre are bread, beans and dried apricots. Fibre is thought to be necessary to help digestion and avoid developing constipation, obesity and appendicitis

fibre optics [ˌfaɪbər 'ɒptɪks] *or* **fibreoptics** [ˌfaɪbər'ɒptɪks] *subst.* examining internal organs using thin fibres which conduct light and images *fiberoptik*

fibrer ⇨ **roughage**

fibrescope ['faɪbəskəʊp] *subst.* device made of bundles of optical fibres which is passed into the body, used for examining internal organs *fiberskop, endoskop*

fibril ['faɪbrɪl] *subst.* very small fibre *fibrill*

fibrill ⇨ **fibril**

fibrillating ['faɪbrɪleɪtɪŋ] *adj.* with fluttering of a muscle *som avser el. hör till flimmer;* **they applied a defibrillator to correct a fibrillating heart beat**

fibrillatio ⇨ **fibrillation**

fibrillation [ˌfaɪbrɪ'leɪʃ(ə)n] *subst.* fluttering of a muscle *fibrillatio, flimmer;* **atrial fibrillation** = rapid uncoordinated fluttering of the atria of the heart, causing an irregular heartbeat *fibrillatio atrii cordis, förmaksflimmer;* **ventricular fibrillation** = serious heart condition where the ventricular muscles flutter and the heart no longer beats to pump blood *fibrillatio ventriculi cordis, ventrikelflimmer, kammarflimmer*

fibrin ['faɪbrɪn] *subst.* protein produced by fibrinogen, which helps make blood coagulate *fibrin;* **fibrin foam** = white material made artificially from fibrinogen, used to prevent bleeding *blodstillande medel framställt av fibrinogen*

COMMENT: removal of fibrin from a blood sample is called defibrination

fibrinogen [faɪ'brɪnədʒ(ə)n] *subst.* substance in blood plasma which produces fibrin when activated by thrombin *fibrinogen*

fibrinolys ⇨ **fibrinolysis**

fibrinolysin [ˌfaɪbrɪ'nɒləsɪn] *or* **plasmin** ['plæzmɪn] *subst.* enzyme which digests fibrin *plasmin, fibrinolysin*

fibrinolysis [ˌfaɪbrɪ'nɒləsɪs] *subst.* removal of blood clots from the system by the action of plasmin on fibrin *fibrinolys*

fibro- ['faɪbrəʊ, ˌ--] *prefix* referring to fibres *fibr(o)-, fiber-*

fibroadenoma [ˌfaɪbrəʊˌædɪ'nəʊmə] *subst.* benign tumour formed of fibrous and glandular tissue *fibroadenom*

fibroblast ['faɪbrəʊblæst] *subst.* long flat cell found in connective tissue, which develops into collagen *fibroblast*

fibrocartilage [ˌfaɪbrəʊ'kɑːtəlɪdʒ] *subst.* cartilage and fibrous tissue combined *fibrocartilago, bindvävsbrosk*

COMMENT: fibrocartilage is found in the discs of the spine. It is elastic like cartilage and pliable like fibre

fibrocartilago ⇨ **fibrocartilage**

fibrochondritis [ˌfaɪbrəʊkɒn'draɪtɪs] *subst.* inflammation of the fibrocartilage *inflammation i bindvävsbrosk*

fibrocyst ['faɪbrəʊsɪst] *subst.* benign tumour of fibrous tissue *godartad bindvävssvulst*

fibrocystic [ˌfaɪbrəʊ'sɪstɪk] *adj.* referring to a fibrocyst *fibrocystisk;* **fibrocystic disease** *or* **cystic fibrosis** = hereditary disease in which there is malfunction of the exocrine glands such as the pancreas, and in particular those which secrete mucus *mukoviskidos, cystisk fibros (pankreasfibros)*

fibrocystisk ⇨ **fibrocystic**

fibrocyte ['faɪbrəʊsaɪt] *subst.* cell which derives from a fibroblast and is found in connective tissue *fibrocyt*

fibroelastosis [ˌfaɪbrəʊˌiːlæ'stəʊsɪs] *subst.* deformed growth of the elastic fibres, especially in the ventricles of the heart *fibroelastos*

fibroid ['faɪbrɔɪd] *adj. & subst.* like fibre *fibroid, fiberliknande, bindvävs-;* **fibroid degeneration** = changing of normal tissue into fibrous tissue (as in cirrhosis of the liver) *fibrös degeneration, bindvävsvandling;* **a fibroid** *or* **fibroid tumour** *or* **fibromyoma** *or* **uterine fibroma** = benign tumour in the muscle fibres of the uterus *fibromyom, uterusfibrom*

fibroma [faɪ'brəʊmə] *subst.* small benign tumour formed in connective tissue *fibrom, bindvävssvulst*

fibromuscular [ˌfaɪbrəʊ'mʌskjʊlə] *adj.* referring to fibrous tissue and muscular tissue *fibromuskulär*

fibromuskulär ⇨ **fibromuscular**

fibromyom ⇨ **fibroid**

fibromyoma [ˌfaɪbrəʊmaɪ'əʊmə] *subst.* benign tumour in the muscle fibres of the uterus *fibromyom*

fibroplasia [ˌfaɪbrəʊ'pleɪziə] *see* RETROLENTAL

fibros ⇨ **degeneration, fibrosis**

fibrosa [faɪ'brəʊsə] *see* OSTEITIS

fibrosarcoma [ˌfaɪbrəʊsɑː'kəʊmə] *subst.* malignant tumour of the connective tissue, common in the legs *fibrosarkom*

fibrosarkom ⇨ **fibrosarcoma**

fibrosis [faɪ'brəʊsɪs] *subst.* replacing damaged tissue by scar tissue *fibros;* **cystic fibrosis** = FIBROCYSTIC DISEASE

fibrosit ⇨ **fibrositis**

fibrositis [ˌfaɪbrə(ʊ)'saɪtɪs] *subst.* painful inflammation of the fibrous tissue which surrounds muscles and joints, especially the muscles of the back *fibrosit, bindvävsinflammation*

fibrous ['faɪbrəs] *adj.* made of fibres *or* like fibre *fibr(o)-, fiber-, tråd-, bindvävs-;* **fibrous capsule** = fibrous tissue surrounding the kidney *njurens bindvävskapsel;* **fibrous joint** = joint where fibrous tissue holds two bones together so that they cannot move (as in the bones of the skull) *syndesmos, bindvävsfog;* **fibrous pericardium** = outer part of the pericardium which surrounds the heart, and is attached to the main blood vessels *hjärtsäckens yttersida;* **fibrous tissue** = tissue made of collagen fibres *fibrös vävnad;* **muscles are attached to bones by bands of strong fibrous tissue called tendons**

> COMMENT: fibrous tissue is the strong white tissue which makes tendons and ligaments; also forms scar tissue

fibula ['fɪbjʊlə] *subst.* long thin bone running between the ankle and the knee, the other thicker bone in the lower leg is the tibia *fibula, vadbenet* NOTE: plural is **fibulae**

fibular ['fɪbjʊlə] *adj.* referring to the fibula *fibulär*

fibulär ⇨ **fibular**

ficka ⇨ **pocket, pouch, recess**

fickklaffarna ⇨ **semilunar**

field [fiːld] *subst.* area of interest *fält, område, fack;* **he specializes in the field of community medicine; don't see that specialist with your breathing problems - his field is obstetrics; field of vision** = area which can be seen without moving the eye *synfält, synkrets*

figur ⇨ **diagram**

fil- ['fɪl, ˌfɪl] *prefix* like a thread *fil-, tråd-*

filament ['fɪləmənt] *subst.* long thin structure like a thread *filament*

filamentous [ˌfɪlə'mentəs] *adj.* like a thread *trådliknande*

Filaria [fɪ'leəriə] *subst.* thin parasitic worm which is found especially in the lymph system, and is passed to humans by mosquitoes *Filaria* NOTE: plural is **Filariae**

> COMMENT: infestation with Filariae in the lymph system causes elephantiasis

filariasis [ˌfɪlə'raɪəsɪs] *subst.* tropical disease caused by parasitic threadworms in the lymph system, transmitted by mosquito bites *filariasis, filarios*

filarios ⇨ **filariasis**

-fili ⇨ **-philia**

filiform ['fɪlɪfɔ:m] *adj.* shaped like a thread *filiform, trådformig;* **filiform papillae =** papillae on the tongue which are shaped like threads, and have no taste buds ⇨ *illustration* TONGUE *papillae filiformes, trådformiga papiller*

filipuncture ['fɪlɪpʌŋtʃə] *subst.* putting a wire into an aneurysm to cause blood clotting *filipunktur*

filipunktur ⇨ **filipuncture**

fill [fɪl] *vb.* **(a)** to make something full *fylla;* **she was filling the bottle with water (b) to fill a tooth** = to put metal into a hole in a tooth after it has been drilled *fylla (plombera) en tand*

filling ['fɪlɪŋ] *subst.* (i) surgical operation carried out by a dentist to fill a hole in a tooth with amalgam *plombering;* (ii) amalgam *or* metallic mixture put into a hole in a tooth by a dentist *fyllning, tandfyllning, plomb;* **I had to have two fillings when I went to the dentist's**

film [fɪlm] *subst.* **(a)** roll of material which is put into a camera for taking photographs *film;* **I must buy a film before I go on holiday; do you want a colour film or a black and white one? (b)** very thin layer of a substance, especially on the surface of a liquid *hinna, tunt skikt (lager);* **a film of oil on the surface of water**

filt ⇨ **blanket**

filter ['fɪltə] **1** *subst.* piece of paper *or* cloth through which a liquid is passed to remove solid substances in it *filter, sil* **2** *vb.* to pass a liquid through a piece of paper *or* cloth to remove solid substances *filtrera, sila;* **impurities are filtered from the blood by the kidneys**

filtrat ⇨ **filtrate**

filtrate ['fɪltreɪt] *subst.* substance which has passed through a filter *filtrat*

filtration [fɪl'treɪʃ(ə)n] *subst.* passing a liquid through a filter *filtrering, silning*

filtrera ⇨ **filter, infiltrate**

filtrering ⇨ **filtration**

filtstöd ⇨ **cradle**

filum ['faɪləm] *subst.* structure which is shaped like a thread *filum, tråd;* **filum terminale** = thin end section of the pia mater in the spinal cord *filum terminale*

fimbria ['fɪmbriə] *subst.* fringe, especially the fringe of hair-like processes at the end of a Fallopian tube near the ovaries *fimbria, frans*
NOTE: plural is **fimbriae**

fimos ⇨ **phimosis**

final ['faɪn(ə)l] *adj.* last *final, slut-, sista;* **this is your final injection; final common pathway** = lower motor neurone *or* linked neurones which take all motor impulses from the spinal cord to a muscle *nedre motorneuron*

fine [faɪn] *adj.* healthy *bra, frisk;* **he was ill last week, but he's feeling fine now**

finger ['fɪŋgə] *subst.* one of the five parts at the end of the hand, but usually not including the thumb *digitus, finger;* **he touched the switch with his finger; finger-nose test** = test of coordination, where the patients is asked to close his eyes, stretch out his arm and then touch his nose with his index finger *finger-näsförsöket*
NOTE: the names of the fingers are **little finger, third finger** *or* **ring finger, middle finger, forefinger** or **index finger (and the thumb)**

> COMMENT: each finger is formed of three finger bones (the phalanges), but the thumb has only two

finger ⇨ **finger, dactyl, digit**

fingeravtryck ⇨ **fingerprint**

fingerled ⇨ **interphalangeal joint**

fingernail ['fɪŋgəneɪ(ə)l] *subst.* hard thin growth covering the end of a finger *fingernagel, nagel;* **she painted her fingernails red**

finger-näsförsöket ⇨ **finger**

fingerprint ['fɪŋgəprɪnt] *subst.* mark left by a finger when you touch something *fingeravtryck;* **the police found fingerprints near the broken window**

fingerstall ['fɪŋgəstɔ:l] *subst.* cover for an infected finger, attached to the hand with strings *fingertuta*

fingertuta ⇨ **fingerstall**

finnar ⇨ **acne**

finnas ⇨ **present**

finne ⇨ **pimple**

finnig ⇨ **pimply, spotty**

fireman's lift ['fa(ɪ)əmənz ˌlɪft] *subst.* way of carrying an injured person by putting him over one's shoulder *slags lyft*

firm [fɜːm] *subst. (informal)* group of doctors and consultants in a hospital (especially one to which a trainee doctor is attached during clinical studies) *slang för grupp av läkare*

first [fɜːst] *adj.* coming before everything else *första;* **first-ever stroke** = stroke which a patient has for the first time in his life *patientens första stroke (slaganfall);* **first intention** = healing of a clean wound where the tissue forms again rapidly and no prominent scar is left *sanatio per primam intentionem, primärläkning*

> QUOTE cerebral infarction (embolic or thrombolic) accounts for about 80% of first-ever strokes
> **British Journal of Hospital Medicine**

first aid [ˌfɜːst 'eɪd] *subst.* help given by an ordinary person to someone who is suddenly ill *or* hurt, given until full-scale medical treatment can be given *första hjälpen;* **she ran to the man who had been knocked down and gave him first aid until the ambulance arrived; first-aid kit** = box with bandages and dressings kept ready to be used in an emergency *förbandslåda;* **first-aid post** *or* **station** = special place where injured people can be taken for immediate attention *plats där första hjälpen ges*

first-aider [ˌfɜːst'eɪdə] *subst.* person who gives first aid to someone who is suddenly ill *or* injured *person som ger första hjälpen*

fish [fɪʃ] *subst.* cold-blooded animal which swims in water, eaten for food *fisk;* **they live on a diet of fish and rice** NOTE: no plural when referring to the food: **you should eat some fish every week**

> COMMENT: fish are high in protein, phosphorus, iodine and vitamins A and D. White fish have very little fat

fisk ⇨ **fish**

fiskfjällssjuka ⇨ **ichthyosis**

fiskleverolja ⇨ **cod liver oil**

fissile ['fɪsaɪ(ə)l] *adj.* which can split *or* can be split *klyvbar*

fission ['fɪʃ(ə)n] *subst.* splitting (as of the cells of bacteria) *fission, klyvning, delning*

fissur ⇨ **fissure**

fissure ['fɪʃə] *subst.* crack or groove in the skin *or* tissue *or* an organ *fissur, spricka, sprickbildning;* **anal fissure** *or* **rectal fissure** *or* **fissure in ano** = crack in the mucous membrane wall of the anal canal *fissura ani, analfissur, rektalfissur;* **horizontal and oblique fissures** = grooves between the lobes of the lungs ⇨ *illustration* LUNGS *fissura horizontalis resp. obliqua;* **lateral fissure** = groove along the side of each cerebral hemisphere *fissura lateralis cerebri, sulcus lateralis;* **longitudinal fissure** = groove separating the two cerebral hemispheres *fissura longitudinalis cerebri*

fist [fɪst] *subst.* hand which is tightly closed *knytnäve, knuten näve (hand);* **the baby held the spoon in its fist; he hit the nurse with his fist**

fistel ⇨ **fistula, sinus**

fistelgång ⇨ **urochesia**

fistula ['fɪstjʊlə] *subst.* passage *or* opening which has been made abnormally between two organs, often near the rectum *or* anus *fistula, fistel;* **anal fistula** *or* **fistula in ano** = fistula which develops between the rectum and the outside of the body after an abscess near the anus *fistula in ano, analfistel;* **biliary fistula** = opening which discharges bile on to the surface of the skin from the gall bladder, bile duct or liver *gallfistel;* **branchial fistula** = cyst on the side of the neck of an embryo *gälgångscysta, gälgångsfistel;* **vesicovaginal fistula** = abnormal opening between the bladder and the vagina *vesikovaginal fistel*

fit [fɪt] **1** *adj.* strong and physically healthy *frisk, kry, pigg, i bästa möjliga form (kondition);* **the manager is not a fit man; you'll have to get fit before the football match; she exercises every day to keep fit; the doctors decided the patient was not fit for surgery; he isn't fit enough to work** = he is still too ill to work *han är inte frisk nog att arbeta*
NOTE: **fit - fitter - fittest** **2** *subst.* sudden attack of a disorder, especially convulsions and epilepsy *anfall, attack;* **she had a fit of coughing; he had an epileptic fit; the baby had a series of fits** **3** *vb.* **(a)** to be the right size *or* shape *passa, vara lagom (stor), sitta (bra);* **he's grown so tall that his trousers don't fit him any more; these shoes don't fit me - they're too tight** **(b)** to attach an appliance correctly *passa i (till, in), anpassa, avpassa;* **the surgeons fitted the artificial hand to the patient's arm** *or* **fitted the patient with an artificial hand** NOTE: you fit someone **with** an appliance

fitness ['fɪtnəs] *subst.* being healthy *kondition, fin form;* **he had to pass a fitness test to join the police force; being in the football team demands a high level of physical fitness**

fix [fɪks] *vb.* **(a)** (i) to fasten *or* to attach *fästa, anbringa;* (ii) to treat a specimen which is permanently attached to a slide *fixera;* **the slide is fixed with an alcohol solution; fixed oils** = liquid fats, especially those used as food *flytande oljor (fett)* **(b)** to arrange *arrangera, ordna;* **the meeting has been fixed for next week**

fixated [fɪk'seɪtɪd] *adj.* (person) with a fixation on a parent *fixerad, (moders)bunden, fadersbunden*

fixation [fɪk'seɪʃ(ə)n] *subst.* (i) psychological disorder where a person does not develop beyond a certain stage *fixering;* (ii) way of preserving a specimen on a slide *fixering, fixation;* **mother-fixation** = condition where a person's development has been stopped at a stage where he remains like a child, dependent on his mother *modersfixering, modersbindning*

fixative ['fɪksətɪv] *subst.* chemical used in the preparation of samples on slides *fixativ, fixermedel, fixeringsmedel*

fixera ⇨ **fix, immobilize, lock, preserve**

fixera sig ⇨ **set**

fixering ⇨ **fixation, immobilization, preservation**

-fixering ⇨ **-pexy**

fixeringsmedel ⇨ **fixative**

fixermedel ⇨ **fixative**

fjäll ⇨ **flake, scale, squama**

fjälla ⇨ **flake, peel, scale off**

fjällig ⇨ **furfuraceous, scaly, squamous**

fjällning ⇨ **desquamation, ecdysis, exfoliation**

fjärrbestrålning ⇨ **teleradiotherapy**

flab [flæb] *subst. informal* soft fat flesh *ung. "bilringar";* **he's doing exercises to try to fight the flab**

flabby ['flæbi] *adj.* with soft flesh *fet och slapp, sladdrig, blekfet;* **she has got flabby from sitting at her desk all day**

flaccid ['flæksɪd] *adj.* soft *or* flabby *sladdrig, slapp*

fladder ⇨ **flutter**

flaga ⇨ **flake, scale, scale off**

flagellate ['flædʒ(ə)lət] *subst.* type of parasitic protozoan which uses whip-like hairs to swim (such as Leishmania) *flagellat, gisseldjur*

flagelltäckt ⇨ **peritrichous**

flagellum [flə'dʒeləm] *subst.* tiny growth on a microorganism, shaped like a whip *flagell, gissel*
NOTE: plural is **flagella**

flagna ⇨ **peel**

flail chest ['fleɪ(ə)l ˌtʃest] *subst.* condition where the chest is not stable, because several ribs have been broken *flail chest*

flake [fleɪk] **1** *subst.* thin piece of tissue *flaga, fjäll;* **dandruff is formed of flakes of dead skin on the scalp 2** *vb.* **to flake off** = to fall off as flakes *flaga, fjälla*

flap [flæp] *subst.* flat piece, especially a piece of skin *or* tissue still attached to the body at one side and used in grafts *flik, spjälkat hudtransplantat*

flare [fleə] *subst.* red colouring of the skin at an infected spot *or* in urticaria *rodnad, hudrodnad, uppblossande*

flaska ⇨ **bottle**

flaskuppfödning ⇨ **bottle**

flat [flæt] *adj. & adv.* level *or* not curved *plan, platt;* **spread the paper out flat on the table; flat foot** *or* **flat feet** *or* **pes planus** = condition where the soles of the feet lie flat on the ground instead of being arched as normal *pes planus, plattfot*

flatlus ⇨ **crab (louse), Pediculus, Phthirius pubis**

flatulence ['flætjʊləns] *subst.* gas *or* air which collects in the stomach *or* intestines causing discomfort *flatulens, gasbildning, väderspänning(ar)*

COMMENT: flatulence is generally caused by indigestion, but can be made worse if the patient swallows air (aerophagy)

flatulens ⇨ **flatulence, flatus, gas, wind**

flatulent ['flætjʊlənt] *adj.* caused by flatulence *flatulent, gasbildande, väderspänd*

flatus ['fleɪtəs] *subst.* air and gas which collects in the intestines and is painful *flatulens, smärtsamma gaser (i magen), väderspänning(ar)*

flatworm ['flætwɜːm] *subst.* any of several types of parasitic worm with a flat body (such as a tapeworm) *plattmask*

flea [fliː] *subst.* tiny insect which sucks blood and is a parasite on animals and humans *loppa*

COMMENT: fleas can transmit disease, most especially bubonic plague which is transmitted by rat fleas

flebektomi ⇨ **phlebectomy**

flebit ⇨ **phlebitis**

flebografi ⇨ **phlebography**

flebogram ⇨ **phlebogram**

flebolit ⇨ **phlebolith**

flebotomi ⇨ **blood, phlebotomy**

flebotrombos ⇨ **phlebothrombosis, venous**

flektera ⇨ **flex**

flerbörd ⇨ **multiple**

flerbördsgraviditet ⇨ **multiple**

fleromättat fett ⇨ **polyunsaturated fat**

flerskiktat epitel ⇨ **stratified**

flesh [fleʃ] *subst.* tissue containing blood, forming the part of the body which is not skin, bone or organs *kött;* **flesh wound** = wound which only affects the fleshy part of the body *köttsår;* **she had a flesh wound in her leg**

fleshy ['fleʃi] *adj.* (i) made of flesh *kött-;* (ii) fat *fet, tjock, korpulent*

flex [fleks] *vb.* to bend *flektera, böja;* **to flex a joint** = to use a muscle to make a joint bend *böja en led*

flexibel ⇨ **flexible**

flexibilitas cerea [ˌfleksɪ'bɪlɪtəs 'sɪəriə] *subst.* condition where if a patient's arms or legs are moved, they remain in that set position for some time *flexibilitas cerea*

flexible ['fleksəb(ə)l] *adj.* which bends easily *flexibel, böjlig, smidig*

flexion ['flekʃ(ə)n] *subst.* bending of a joint *flexion, böjning;* **plantar flexion** = bending of the toes downwards *plantarflexion*

Flexner's bacillus ['fleksnəz bəˌsɪləs] *subst.* bacterium which causes bacillary dysentery *Flexners bacill*

flexor ['fleksə] *subst.* muscle which makes a joint bend *flexor, böjare; compare* EXTENSOR

flexura ⇨ **flexure**

flexure ['flekʃə] *subst.* bend in an organ *flexura, böjning, krök;* fold in the skin *veck;* **hepatic flexure** = bend in the colon, where the ascending and transverse colons join *flexura coli dextra;* **splenic flexure** = bend in the colon where the transverse colon joins the descending colon *flexura coli sinistra (coli lienalis)*

flicka ⇨ **girl**

flik ⇨ **flap**

flik på hjärtklaff ⇨ **cusp**

flimmer ⇨ **fibrillation**

flimmerepitel ⇨ **ciliated epithelium**

flimmerhår ⇨ **cilium**

flimmerskotom ⇨ **amaurosis, fortification figures**

flintskallig ⇨ **bald**

flisa ⇨ **splinter**

float [fləʊt] *vb.* to lie on top of a liquid *or* not to sink *flyta;* **leaves were floating on the lake; floating kidney** = NEPHROPTOSIS; **floating ribs** = the two lowest ribs on each side, which are not attached to the breastbone *costae fluctuans, de två understa paren revben*

floccilegium ⇨ **carphology**

floccitation [ˌflɒksɪˈteɪʃ(ə)n] = CARPHOLOGY

flod ▷ **flood**

flood [flʌd] **1** *subst.* large amount of water over land which is usually dry *högvatten, flod, översvämning;* **after the rainstorm there were floods in the valley 2** *vb.* to cover with a large amount of water *översvämma, dränka;* **the fields were flooded**

flooding [ˈflʌdɪŋ] *or* **menorrhagia** [ˌmenəˈreɪdʒiə] *subst.* very heavy bleeding during menstruation *menorragi, hypermenorré, riklig menstruation*

floppy baby syndrome [ˌflɒpi ˈbeɪbi ˌsɪndrəʊm] = AMYOTONIA CONGENITA

flora [ˈflɔːrə] *subst.* bacteria which exist in a certain part of the body *flora, bakterieflora*

floss [flɒs] **1** *subst.* **dental floss** = soft thread which can be pulled between the teeth to help keep them clean *tandtråd* **2** *vb.* to clean the teeth with floss *använda tandtråd*

flow [fləʊ] **1** *subst.* amount of liquid which is moving *flöde, ström;* **they used a tourniquet to try to stop the flow of blood 2** *vb. (of liquid)* to go past *rinna, strömma, flyta;* **the water flowed down the pipe; blood was flowing from the wound**

flowmeter [ˈfləʊmiːtə] *subst.* meter attached to a pipe (as in anaesthetic equipment) to measure the flow of a liquid *or* gas *flödesmätare*

flu [fluː] *or* **influenza** [ˌɪnfluˈenzə] *subst.* common illness like a bad cold, but with a fever *influensa;* **he's in bed with flu; she caught flu and had to stay at home; there is a lot of flu about this winter; Asian flu** = type of flu which originated in Asia *asiatisk influensa;* **gastric flu** = general term for any mild stomach disorder *magbesvär;* **twenty-four hour flu** = type of flu which lasts for a short period *kortvarig "influensa" ("förkylning")*
NOTE: sometimes written **'flu** to show it is a short form of **influenza**

fluctuation [ˌflʌktʃuˈeɪʃ(ə)n] *subst.* feeling of movement of liquid inside part of the body *or* inside a cyst when pressed by the fingers *fluktuation*

fluga ▷ **fly**

fluid [ˈfluːɪd] *subst.* liquid substance *fluidum, vätska;* **amniotic fluid** = fluid in the amnion in which an unborn baby floats *liquuor amnii, amnionvätska, amnionvatten, fostervatten;* **cerebrospinal fluid (CSF)** = fluid which surrounds the brain and the spinal cord *cerebrospinalvätska;* **pleural fluid** = fluid which forms between the layers of pleura in pleurisy *pleuravätska*

fluke [fluːk] *subst.* parasitic flatworm which settles inside the liver (liver flukes), in the blood stream (Schistosoma), and other parts of the body *levermask, leverflundra*

fluktuation ▷ **fluctuation**

fluor ▷ **fluorine**

fluorescence [flɔːˈres(ə)ns] *subst.* sending out of light from a substance which is receiving radiation *fluorescens*

fluorescens ▷ **fluorescence**

fluorescent [flɔːˈres(ə)nt] *adj.* (substance) which sends out light *fluorescerande*

fluorescerande ▷ **fluorescent**

fluoridation [ˌflʊəraɪˈdeɪʃ(ə)n] *subst.* adding fluoride to drinking water to prevent tooth decay *fluoridering*

> COMMENT: fluoride will reduce decay in teeth, and is often added to drinking water or to toothpaste. Some people object to fluoridation

fluoride [ˈflʊəraɪd] *subst.* chemical compound of fluorine and sodium *or* potassium *or* tin *fluorid*

fluoridering ▷ **fluoridation**

fluorine [ˈflʊəriːn] *subst.* chemical element found in bones and teeth *fluor, F* NOTE: chemical symbol is **F**

fluoros ▷ **fluorosis**

fluoroscope [ˈflʊərəskəʊp] *subst.* apparatus which projects an X-ray image of a part of the body on to a screen, so that the part of the body can be examined as it moves *fluoroskop, apparat för röntgengenomlysning*

fluoroscopy [flɔːˈrɒskəpi] *subst.* examination of the body using X-rays projected onto a screen *fluoroskopi, radioskopi, röntgengenomlysning, genomlysning*

fluorosis [flɔːˈrəʊsɪs] *subst.* condition caused by excessive fluoride in drinking water *fluoros*

COMMENT: at a low level, fluorosis causes discoloration of the teeth, and as the level of fluoride rises, ligaments can become calcified

fluoroskopi ⇨ **fluoroscopy, radioscopy**

flush [flʌʃ] **1** *subst.* red colour in the skin *rodnad, hudrodnad, uppblossande;* **hot flush =** condition in menopausal women, where the patient becomes hot, and sweats, often accompanied by redness of the skin *flush, vallning, blodvallning* **2** *vb.* to turn red *blossa (upp), rodna*

flushed [flʌʃt] *adj.* with red skin (due to heat *or* emotion *or* overeating) *rodnad, blossande;* **his face was flushed and he was breathing heavily**

flutter ['flʌtə] *or* **fluttering** ['flʌt(ə)rɪŋ] *subst.* rapid movement, especially of the atria of the heart, which is not controlled by impulses from the SA node *fladder, hjärtfladder*

flux [flʌks] *subst.* excessive production of liquid from the body *flux, flytning, starkt flöde*

fly [flaɪ] *subst.* small insect with two wings, often living in houses *fluga;* **flies can walk on the ceiling; flies can carry infection onto food**

flygsjuk ⇨ **airsick**

flygsjuka ⇨ **airsickness**

flykten ⇨ **phlyctenule**

flyktig ⇨ **volatile**

flyta ⇨ **float; flow**

flytande ⇨ **liquid**

flytande paraffin ⇨ **paraffin**

flytning ⇨ **discharge, flux**

flytning från slidan ⇨ **vaginal**

flytning från urinröret ⇨ **urethrorrhoea**

flyttbar ⇨ **portable**

flåsa ⇨ **pant**

fläck ⇨ **macula, macule, mark, spot, stain**

fläcka (ned) ⇨ **soil**

fläcktyfus ⇨ **typhus, rickettsial**

flämta ⇨ **gasp, pant**

flämtning ⇨ **gasp**

flöde ⇨ **flow, flux**

flödesmätare ⇨ **flowmeter**

fobi ⇨ **phobia**

fobisk ⇨ **phobic**

focal ['fəʊk(ə)l] *adj.* referring to a focus *fokal(-);* **focal distance** *or* **focal length =** distance between the lens of the eye and the point behind the lens where light is focused *fokaldistans, brännvidd;* **focal epilepsy =** form of epilepsy arising from a localized area of the brain *epilepsia focalis, fokal (symtomatisk, kortikal) epilepsi;* **focal myopathy =** destruction of muscle tissue caused by the substance injected in an intramuscular injection *lokal muskelnedbrytning pga injektion*

focus ['fəʊkəs] **1** *subst.* **(a)** point where light rays converge through a lens *fokus, brännpunkt* **(b)** centre of an infection *fokus, härd* NOTE: plural is **foci** **2** *vb.* to change the lens of an eye so that you see clearly at different distances *fokusera;* **he has difficulty in focusing on the object**

fodra ⇨ **line**

foetalis [fiː'teɪlɪs] *see* ERYTHROBLASTOSIS

foetor ['fiːtə] = FETOR

foetus, foetal ['fiːtəs, 'fiːt(ə)l] = FETUS, FETAL

fog ⇨ **commissure, symphysis**

fokal ⇨ **focal**

fokaldistans ⇨ **focal**

fokomeli ⇨ **phocomelia**

fokus ⇨ **focus**

fokusera ⇨ **focus**

folacin ['fəʊləsɪn] = FOLIC ACID

fold [fəʊld] **1** *subst.* part of the body which is bent so that it lies on top of another part *veck;* **circular folds =** large transverse folds of mucous membrane in the small intestine *plicae circulares (intestini tenuis);* **vestibular folds**

= folds in the larynx above the vocal fold, which are not used for speech (sometimes called "false vocal cords") *plicae vestibulares, falska stämbanden;* **vocal folds** *or* **vocal cords** *see* CORD **2** *vb.* to bend something so that part of it is on top of the rest *vika (ihop), vecka;* **he folded the letter and put it in an envelope; to fold your arms** = to rest one arm on the other across your chest *med armarna i kors*

folic acid [ˌfəʊlɪk 'æsɪd] *subst.* vitamin in the Vitamin B complex found in milk, liver, yeast and green vegetables like spinach, which is essential for creating new blood cells *folsyra, folinsyra*

COMMENT: lack of folic acid can cause anaemia, and it can be caused by alcoholism

folie à deux [ˌfɒlɪ æ 'dɜː] *subst.* rare condition where a psychological disorder is communicated between two people who live together *folie à deux*

folinsyra ⇨ **folic acid**

follicle ['fɒlɪk(ə)l] *subst.* tiny hole *or* sac in the body *follikel;* **atretic follicle** = scarred remains of an ovarian follicle *folliculus atreticus, atretisk follikel (äggstocksblåsa);* **Graafian follicle** *or* **ovarian follicle** = cell which contains the ovum *folliculus ovarii (oophori), Graafs (graafsk) follikel, äggblåsa;* **hair follicle** = tiny hole in the skin with a gland from which a hair grows *folliculus pili, hårfollikel, hårsäck*

COMMENT: an ovarian follicle goes through several stages in its development. The first stage is called a primordial follicle, which then develops into a primary follicle and becomes a mature follicle by the sixth day of the period. This follicle secretes oestrogen until the ovum has developed to the point when it can break out, leaving the corpus luteum behind

follicle-stimulating hormone (FSH) [ˌfɒlɪk(ə)l'stɪmjuleɪtɪŋ ˌhɔːməʊn (ˌefes'eɪtʃ)] *subst.* hormone produced by the pituitary gland which stimulates ova in the ovaries and sperm in the testes *follikelstimulerande hormon, FSH*

follicular [fɒ'lɪkjʊlə] *adj.* referring to follicles *follikular, follikulär*

folliculitis [fɒˌlɪkju'laɪtɪs] *subst.* inflammation of the hair follicles, especially where hair has been shaved *follikulit, hårfollikelinflammation, hårsäcksinflammation*

follikel ⇨ **follicle**

follikular ⇨ **follicular**

follikulit ⇨ **folliculitis**

follikulär ⇨ **follicular**

follow (up) ['fɒləʊ ('ʌp)] *vb.* to check on a patient who has been examined before *följa upp*

follow-up ['fɒləʊʌp] *subst.* check on a patient who has been examined earlier *uppföljning, efterkontroll*

QUOTE length of follow-ups varied from three to 108 months. Thirteen patients were followed for less than one year, but the remainder were seen regularly for periods from one to nine years
New Zealand Medical Journal

folsyra ⇨ **folic acid**

foment ⇨ **poultice**

fomentation [ˌfəʊmen'teɪʃ(ə)n] = POULTICE

fomites ['fəʊmɪtiːz] *subst pl.* objects (such as bedclothes) touched by a patient with a communicable disease which can therefore pass on the disease to others *fomites, smittade föremål*

fonogram ⇨ **electrocardiophonography**

fonokardiografi ⇨ **electrocardiophonography, phonocardiography**

fonokardiogram ⇨ **phonocardiogram**

fontanelle [ˌfɒntə'nel] *subst.* soft cartilage between the bony sections of a baby's skull *fontanell;* **anterior fontanelle** = cartilage at the top of the head where the frontal bone joins the two parietals *fonticulus anterior, stora fontanellen;* **posterior fontanelle** = cartilage at the back of the head where the parietal bones join the occipital *fonticulus posterior, lilla fontanellen; see also* BREGMA

COMMENT: the fontanelles gradually harden over a period of months and by the age of 18 months the baby's skull is usually solid

food [fuːd] *subst.* things which are eaten *föda, mat, näring, kost;* **this restaurant is famous for its food; do you like Chinese food? this food tastes funny; health food** = food with no additives *or* food consisting of

natural cereals, dried fruit and nuts *hälsokost;* **food allergies** = allergies which are caused by food (the commonest are oranges, eggs, tomatoes, strawberries) *födoämnesallergi;* **food canal** *or* **alimentary canal** = passage from the mouth to the rectum through which food passes and is digested *canalis alimentarius, digestionskanalen, magtarmkanalen;* **food poisoning** = illness caused by eating food which is contaminated with bacteria *matförgiftning;* **the hospital had to deal with six cases of food poisoning; all the people at the party went down with food poisoning**
NOTE: **food** is usually used in the singular, but can sometimes be used in the plural

foot [fʊt] *subst.* end part of the leg on which a person stands *pes, foten;* **he has got big feet; you stepped on my foot; athlete's foot** = infectious skin disorder between the toes, caused by a fungus *tinea pedis, fotsvamp;* **drop foot** *or* **foot drop** = being unable to keep the foot at right angles to the leg *droppfot;* **flat foot** *or* **feet** *see* FLAT; **immersion foot** *or* **trench foot** = condition caused by standing in cold water, where the skin of the foot is dead and the toes turn black *skyttegravsfot, köldskada efter långvarig vattenkontakt;* **Madura foot** *see* MADUROMYCOSIS
NOTE: plural is **feet**

> COMMENT: the foot is formed of 26 bones: 14 phalanges in the toes, five metatarsals in the main part of the foot and seven tarsals in the heel

foramen [fəˈreɪmən] *subst.* natural opening inside the body, such as the opening in a bone through which veins or nerves pass *foramen, hål, öppning;* **foramen magnum** = the hole at the bottom of the skull where the brain is joined to the spinal cord *foramen magnum;* **vertebral** *or* **intervertebral foramina** = series of holes in the vertebrae through which the spinal cord passes *foramina intervertebrales;* **foramen ovale** = opening between the two parts of the heart in a fetus *foramen ovale (cordis)*
NOTE: plural is **foramina**

> COMMENT: the foramen ovale normally closes at birth, but if it stays open the blood from the veins can mix with the blood going to the arteries, causing cyanosis (blue baby disease)

forbid [fəˈbɪd] *vb.* to tell someone not to do something *förbjuda;* **smoking is forbidden in the cinema; the health committee has forbidden any contact with the press; she has been forbidden all starchy food; the doctor forbade him to go back to work**
NOTE: **forbids - forbidding - forbade - has forbidden**

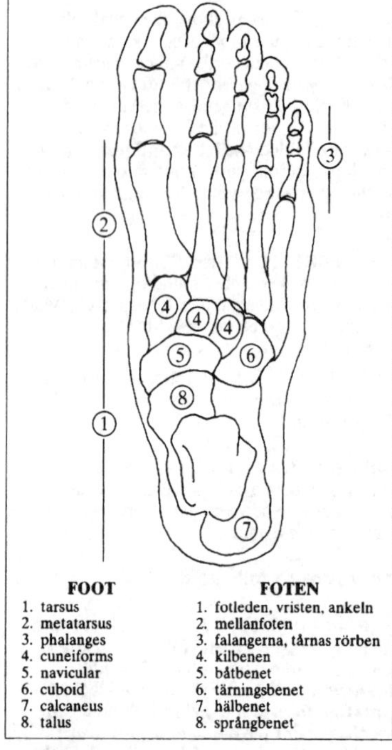

FOOT	FOTEN
1. tarsus	1. fotleden, vristen, ankeln
2. metatarsus	2. mellanfoten
3. phalanges	3. falangerna, tårnas rörben
4. cuneiforms	4. kilbenen
5. navicular	5. båtbenet
6. cuboid	6. tärningsbenet
7. calcaneus	7. hälbenet
8. talus	8. språngbenet

force [fɔːs] **1** *subst.* strength *styrka, kraft;* **the tree was blown down by the force of the wind; he has no force in his right hand 2** *vb.* to make someone do something *tvinga;* **they forced him to lie down on the floor; she was forced to do whatever they wanted**

forceps [ˈfɔːseps] *subst.* surgical instrument like a pair of scissors with spoons at the ends, used for holding and pulling *tång, peang, pincett;* **obstetrical forceps** = type of large forceps used to hold a baby's head during childbirth *förlossningstång*
NOTE: no plural

fore- [ˈfɔː(r), ˌ-] *prefix* in front *fram-, för-*

forearm [ˈfɔːrɑːm] *subst.* lower part of the arm from the elbow to the wrist *underarmen;* **forearm bones** = the ulna and the radius *underarmsbenen*

forebrain [ˈfɔːbreɪn] *subst.* cerebrum *or* front part of the brain in an embryo *prosencephalon, framhjärnan*

forefinger [ˈfɔːˌfɪŋgə] *subst.* first finger on the hand, next to the thumb *index, pekfingret*

foregut ['fɔ:gʌt] *subst.* front part of the gut in an embryo *framtarmen*

forehead ['fɒrɪd, 'fɔ:hed] *subst.* part of the face above the eyes *frons, pannan*

foreign ['fɒr(ə)n] *adj.* not belonging to your own country *utländsk, främmande;* **he speaks several foreign languages; foreign body** = piece of material which is not part of the surrounding tissue, and should not be there, (such as sand in a cut *or* dust in the eye *or* pin which has been swallowed) *corpus alienum, främmande kropp*

foreigner ['fɒr(ə)nə] *subst.* person who comes from another country *utlänning, främling*

forensic medicine [fəˌrensɪk 'med(ə)sɪn] *subst.* medical science concerned with finding solutions to crimes against people (such as autopsies on murdered people *or* taking blood samples from clothes) *forensisk medicin, rättsmedicin*

foreskin ['fɔ:skɪn] *or* **prepuce** ['pri:pju:s] *subst.* skin covering the top of the penis, which can be removed by circumcision *preputiet, förhuden*

forewaters ['fɔ:wɔ:təz] *subst.* fluid which comes out of the vagina at the beginning of childbirth when the amnion bursts *fostervatten*

forget [fə'get] *vb.* not to remember to do something *or* not to remember a piece of information *glömma;* **old people start to forget names; she forgot to take the tablets; he forgot his appointment with the specialist** NOTE: **forgetting - forgot - has forgotten**

forgetful [fə'getf(ə)l] *adj.* (person) who forgets things *glömsk;* **she became very forgetful, and had to be looked after by her sister**

forgetfulness [fə'getf(ə)lnəs] *subst.* condition where someone forgets things *glömska;* **increasing forgetfulness is a sign of old age**

form [fɔ:m] **1** *subst.* **(a)** shape *form, skepnad;* **she has a ring in the form of the letter A (b)** paper with blank spaces which you have to write in *formulär, blankett;* **you have to fill in a form when you are admitted to hospital (c)** state *or* condition *form, kondition;* **our team was in good form and won easily; he's in good form today** = he is very amusing *or* is doing things well *han är i bra form (kondition) idag;* **off form** = not very well *or* slightly ill *i dålig form (kondition), som mår dåligt* **2** *vb.* to make *or* to be the main part of *bilda(s), utgöra;* **calcium is one the elements which forms bones *or* bones are mainly formed of calcium; an ulcer formed in his duodenum; in diphtheria a membrane forms across the larynx**

formaldehyde [fɔ:'mældɪhaɪd] *subst.* strong antiseptic derived from formic acid *formaldehyd*

formalin ['fɔ:m(ə)lɪn] *subst.* solution of formaldehyde in water used to preserve specimens *formalin*

formation [fɔ:'meɪʃ(ə)n] *subst.* action of forming something *bildning;* **drinking milk helps the formation of bones**

formbar ⇨ **plastic**

formel ⇨ **formula**

form, fin ⇨ **fitness**

formication [ˌfɔ:mɪ'keɪʃ(ə)n] *subst.* itching feeling where the skin feels as if it were covered with insects *formikation, myrkrypning(ar)*

formikation ⇨ **formication**

formlös ⇨ **amorphous**

formula ['fɔ:mjulə] *subst.* **(a)** way of indicating a chemical compound using letters and numbers (such as H_2SO_4) *formel* **(b)** instructions how to prepare a drug *recept* **(c)** powdered milk for babies *mjölkersättning* NOTE: plural is **formulae**

formulary ['fɔ:mjuləri] *subst.* book containing formulae for making drugs *farmakopé*

formulär ⇨ **form**

fornix ['fɔ:nɪks] *subst.* arch *fornix, valv;* **fornix cerebri** = section of white matter in the brain between the hippocampus and the hypothalamus ⇨ *illustration* BRAIN *fornix cerebri, hjärnvalvet;* **fornix of the vagina** = space between the cervix of the uterus and the vagina *fornix vaginae, slidvalvet*

forska ⇨ **research**

forskare ⇨ **scientist**

forskning ⇨ **research**

forsla ⇨ **transport**

fortification figures [ˌfɔːtɪfɪˈkeɪʃ(ə)n ˌfɪgəz] *subst.* patterns of coloured light, seen as part of the aura before a migraine attack occurs *fortifikationslinjer, flimmerskotom*

fortifikationslinjer ⇨ **fortification figures**

fortlöpande ⇨ **continuous**

fortplantning ⇨ **propagation, reproduction**

fortplantningsorgan ⇨ **genital, genitalia, reproductive, sex**

fortskridande ⇨ **progression, progressive**

fortsätta ⇨ **continue, keep, persist**

fortsättning ⇨ **continuation**

fosfat ⇨ **phosphate**

fosfatas ⇨ **phosphatase**

fosfatid ⇨ **phospholipid**

fosfaturi ⇨ **phosphaturia**

fosfor ⇨ **phosphorus**

fosforescerande ⇨ **phosphorescent**

fosforescerande urin ⇨ **photuria**

fosfornekros ⇨ **phosphonecrosis**

fosforsyra ⇨ **phosphoric acid**

fossa [ˈfɒsə] *subst.* shallow hollow in a bone *or* the skin *fossa, grop;* **cubital fossa** = depression in the front of the elbow joint *fossa cubitalis;* **glenoid fossa** = socket in the shoulder joint into which the humerus fits *cavitas glenoidalis;* **iliac fossa** = depression on the inner side of the hip bone *fossa iliaca;* **pituitary fossa** = hollow in the upper surface of the sphenoid bone in which the pituitary gland sits *sella turcica, turksadeln;* **temporal fossa** = depression in the side of the head, in the temporal bone above the zygomatic arch *fossa temporalis, tinninggropen*
NOTE: plural is **fossae**

foster ⇨ **fetus**

fosterbjudning ⇨ **presentation**

fosterbjudning, felaktig ⇨ **malpresentation**

fosterdiagnostik ⇨ **diagnosis**

fosterhinna ⇨ **embryonic, chorion, caul**

fosterläge, onormalt ⇨ **malposition**

fostermaceration ⇨ **maceration**

fosterrörelserna, första ⇨ **quickening**

fosterställning ⇨ **fetal**

fostervatten ⇨ **amniotic, forewaters, water**

fostervändning ⇨ **version**

fot- ⇨ **plantar, pod-**

foten ⇨ **foot**

Fothergill's operation [ˈfɒðəgɪlz ˌɒpəˈreɪʃ(ə)n] *subst.* surgical operation to correct prolapse of the womb *slags operation av livmoderframfall*

fotknöl ⇨ **malleolus**

fotleden ⇨ **ankle, tarsus**

fotledsbenen ⇨ **tarsal**

fotledsfraktur ⇨ **ankle**

fotoallergi ⇨ **photodermatosis**

fotodermatit ⇨ **photodermatosis**

fotofobi ⇨ **photophobia**

fotografera ⇨ **photograph**

fotografering ⇨ **photography**

fotokoagulation ⇨ **photocoagulation**

fotoreceptor ⇨ **photoreceptor neurone**

fototerapi ⇨ **phototherapy**

fotryggen ⇨ **instep**

fotryggens bågartär ⇨ **artery**

fotsteg ⇨ **step**

fotsulan ⇨ **sole, planta, plantar**

fotsvamp ⇨ **foot, tinea**

fotvalvet ⇨ **arch**

fotvårdsspecialist ⇨ **chiropodist, podiatrist**

fotvårta ⇨ **plantar**

fourchette [fʊə'ʃet] *subst.* fold of skin at the back of the vulva *rugae vaginalis, slemhinneveck i slidans bakre del*

fovea (centralis) ['fəʊviə (sen,trɑ:lɪs)] *subst.* depression in the retina which is the point where the eye sees most clearly ⇨ *illustration* EYE *fovea centralis, centralgropen*

FPC [,efpi:'si:] = FAMILY PRACTITIONER COMMITTEE

fracture ['fræktʃə] **1** *vb. (of bone)* to break *bryta(s), krossa(s);* **the tibia fractured in two places 2** *subst.* break in a bone *fraktur, brott, benbrott;* **facial fracture** *or* **nasal fracture** *or* **skull fracture; rib fracture** *or* **fracture of a rib; breastbone fracture** *or* **fracture of the breastbone; simple** *or* **closed fracture** = fracture where the skin surface around the damaged bone has not been broken and the broken ends of the bone are close together *sluten fraktur, okomplicerad fraktur;* **Bennett's fracture** *see* BENNETT'S; **Colles' fracture** = fracture of the lower end of the radius with displacement of the wrist backwards, usually when someone has stretched out his hand to try to break a fall *Colles fraktur, distal radiusfraktur;* **comminuted fracture** = fracture where the bone is broken in several places *komminut fraktur, splitterbrott;* **complicated fracture** = fracture with an associated injury of tissue, as where the bone has punctured an artery *fraktur med (komplicerande) vävnadsskada;* **compound fracture** *or* **open fracture** = fracture where the skin surface is damaged *or* where the broken bone penetrates the surface of the skin *öppen fraktur med risk för infektion;* **extracapsular fracture** = fracture of the upper part of the femur, but which does not involve the capsule round the hip joint *extrakapsulär fraktur;* **greenstick fracture** = fracture occurring in children, where a long bone bends but does not break completely *greensticksfraktur, inkomplett (ofullständig) fraktur, infraktion, knickbrott;* **impacted fracture** = fracture where the broken parts of the bones are pushed into each other *inkilad fraktur;* **march fracture** = fracture of one of the metatarsal bones in the foot, caused by too much exercise *marschfraktur, insufficiensfraktur;* **multiple fracture** = condition where a bone is broken in several places *multipel fraktur;* **oblique fracture** = fracture where the bone is broken diagonally *snedfraktur;* **pathological fracture** = fracture of a diseased bone *patologisk fraktur;* **Pott's fracture** = fracture of the end of the fibula together with the end of the malleolus *Potts fraktur;* **stellate fracture** = fracture of the kneecap shaped like a star *fractura stellata, stjärnformad fraktur;* **transverse fracture** = fracture where the bone is broken straight across *tvärfraktur*

fractured ['fræktʃəd] *adj.* broken (bone) *bruten;* **he had a fractured skull; she went to hospital to have her fractured leg reset**

fragil ⇨ **fragile**

fragile ['frædʒaɪ(ə)l] *adj.* easily broken *fragil, skör, bräcklig;* **old people's bones are more fragile than those of adolescents; fragile-X syndrome** = hereditary condition where part of an X chromosome is defective, causing mental defects *fragile-X (syndrom), ärftligt tillstånd med defekt X-kromosom*

fragilitas [frə'dʒɪlɪtəs] *subst.* being fragile *or* brittle *fragilitet, bräcklighet, skörhet;* **fragilitas ossium** *or* **osteogenesis imperfecta** = hereditary condition where the bones are brittle and break easily *fragilitas ossium, osteogenesis imperfecta, benskörhet*

frail [freɪ(ə)l] *adj.* weak *or* easily broken *bräcklig, skör;* **grandfather is getting frail, and we have to look after him all the time; the baby's bones are still very frail**

fraktur ⇨ **break, fracture**

frakturinstrument ⇨ **caliper**

frakturläkning, felaktig ⇨ **malunion**

frakturläkning, utebliven ⇨ **non-union**

framboesi ⇨ **yaws**

framboesia [fræm'bi:ziə] = YAWS

frambrytande ⇨ **eruption**

frame [freɪm] *subst.* main part of a building *or* ship *or* bicycle, etc., which holds it together *stomme, ram, glasögonbåge;* **the bicycle has a very light frame; I've broken the frame of my glasses**

framework ['freɪmwɜ:k] *subst.* main bones which make up the structure of part of the body *stomme, skelett*

framfall ⇨ **procidentia, prolapse, ptosis**

framfallsring ⇨ **pessary**

framgång ⇨ **success**

framgångsrik ⇨ **successful**

framhjärnan ⇨ **forebrain**

framkalla ⇨ **elicit, induce, produce, provoke**

framsida ⇨ **front**

framsteg ⇨ **progress**

framstupa ⇨ **prone, semiprone**

framstupa sidoläge ⇨ **position**

framstående ⇨ **basilic**

framställa ⇨ **synthesize**

framtand ⇨ **incisor (tooth)**

framtarmen ⇨ **foregut**

framträda ⇨ **arise**

framträdande ⇨ **prominent, pronounced**

framåtböjning ⇨ **anteflexion**

framåtvridning ⇨ **anteversion**

frans ⇨ **fimbria**

fransar ⇨ **villus**

fraternal twins [frəˈtɜːn(ə)l ˌtwɪnz] *or* **dizygotic twins** [ˌdɪzɪˌgɒtɪk ˈtwɪnz] *subst.* twins who are not identical (and not always of the same sex) because they come from two different ova fertilized at the same time *dizygoter, tvååggstvillingar; compare* IDENTICAL, MONOZYGOTIC

freckled [ˈfrek(ə)ld] *adj.* with brown spots on the skin *fräknig*

freckles [ˈfrek(ə)lz] *subst pl.* brown spots on the skin, often found in people with fair hair *efelider, fräknar*

freeze [friːz] *vb.* **(a)** to be so cold that water turns to ice *frysa till is;* **it is freezing outside; they say it will freeze tomorrow; I'm freezing** = I'm very cold *jag fryser* **(b)** to make something very cold *or* to become very cold *frysa (ned, till is);* **the surgeon froze the tissue with dry ice**
NOTE: **freezes - freezing - froze - has frozen**

freeze drying [ˌfriːz ˈdraɪɪŋ] *subst.* method of preserving food *or* tissue specimens by freezing rapidly and drying in a vacuum *lyofilisering, frystorkning*

Freiberg's disease [ˈfraɪbɜːgz dɪˌziːz] *subst.* osteochondritis of the head of the second metatarsus *Freibergs-Köhlers sjukdom*

Frei test [ˈfraɪ ˌtest] *subst.* test for the venereal disease lymphogranuloma inguinale *Freis reaktion*

frekvens ⇨ **incidence, rate**

frémissement ⇨ **fremitus, thrill**

fremitus [ˈfremɪtəs] *subst.* trembling *or* vibrating (of part of a patient's body, felt by the doctor's hand or heard through a stethoscope) *fremitus, frémissement, darrning;* **friction fremitus** = scratching felt when the hand is placed on the chest of a patient suffering from pericarditis *frémissement vid hjärtsäcksinflammation;* **vocal fremitus** = vibration of the chest when a person speaks *or* coughs *fremitus vocalis (pectoralis), pektoralfremitus, stämfremitus*

French letter [ˌfren(t)ʃ ˈletə] *subst. informal* = CONDOM

frenektomi ⇨ **phrenicectomy**

frenemfraxis ⇨ **phrenemphraxis**

frenikotomi ⇨ **phrenicotomy**

Frenkel's exercises [ˈfrenk(ə)lz ˌeksəsaɪzɪz] *subst pl.* exercises for patients suffering from locomotor ataxia, to teach coordination of the muscles and limbs *slags övningar för patienter med rubbad samordning av musklerna*

frenulum [ˈfrenjʊləm] *or* **frenum** [ˈfriːnəm] *subst.* fold of mucous membrane (under the tongue *or* by the clitoris) *fren(ul)um, litet slemhinneveck*

fresh [freʃ] *adj.* **(a)** not used *or* not dirty *ren, oanvänd, frisk;* **I'll get some fresh towels; she put some fresh sheets on the bed; fresh air** = open air *frisk luft;* **they came out of the mine into the fresh air (b)** recently made *färsk;* **fresh bread; fresh frozen plasma** = plasma made from freshly donated blood, and kept frozen *färskfrusen plasma* **(c)** not tinned *or* frozen *färsk;* **fresh fish; fresh fruit salad; fresh vegetables are expensive in winter**

fretful [ˈfretf(ə)l] *adj.* (baby) which cries *or* cannot sleep *or* seems unhappy *grinig, retlig*

friars' balsam ['fraɪəz ˌbɔːls(ə)m] *subst.* mixture of various plant oils, including benzoin and balsam, which can be inhaled as a vapour to relieve bronchitis *or* congestion *slags bensoedroppar*

friction ['frɪkʃ(ə)n] *subst.* rubbing together of two surfaces *friktion, gnidning;* **friction fremitus** = scratching felt when the hand is placed on the chest of a patient suffering from pericarditis *frémissement vid hjärtsäcksinflammation;* **friction murmur** = scratching sound around the heart, heard with a stethoscope in patients suffering from pericarditis *gnidningsljud*

Friedländer's bacillus ['friːdlendəz bəˌsɪləs] *subst.* bacterium **Klebsiella pneumoniae** which can cause pneumonia *Friedländers kapselbacill, Klebsiella pneumonia*

Friedman's test ['friːdmənz ˌtest] *subst.* test for pregnancy *Friedmann-Brouhas reaktion (test)*

Friedreich's ataxia ['friːdraɪks ə'tæksiə] *subst.* inherited nervous disease which affects the spinal cord (ataxia is associated with club foot, and makes the patient walk unsteadily and speak with difficulty) *Friedreichs ataxi*

fri från ⇨ **clear**

fri gas i bukhålan ⇨ **pneumoperitoneum**

frighten ['fraɪt(ə)n] *vb.* to make someone afraid *skrämma;* **the noise frightened me; she watched a frightening film about insects which eat people**

frightened ['fraɪt(ə)nd] *adj.* afraid *skrämd, rädd;* **I'm frightened of spiders; don't leave the patient alone - she's frightened of the dark**

frigid ['frɪdʒɪd] *adj.* (woman) who cannot experience orgasm *or* sexual pleasure *frigid*

frigiditet ⇨ **frigidity**

frigidity [frɪ'dʒɪdəti] *subst.* being unable to experience orgasm *or* sexual pleasure *or* who does not feel sexual desire *frigiditet*

frigöra ⇨ **release**

friktion ⇨ **friction**

fringe medicine ['frɪn(d)ʒ ˌmed(ə)sɪn] *subst.* types of medicine which are not part of normal treatment taught in medical schools (such as homeopathy, acupuncture, etc.) *läkekonst som inte hör till skolmedicinen*

frisk ⇨ **fine, fit, fresh, healthy, sound, well**

frisätta ⇨ **release**

frisättning ⇨ **release**

frivillig ⇨ **elective, voluntary, volunteer**

frog [frɒg] *subst.* small animal with no tail, which lives in water or on land and can jump *groda;* **frog plaster** = plaster cast made to keep the legs in a correct position after an operation to correct a dislocated hip *slags gipsförband vid höftledsluxation*

front [frʌnt] *subst.* part of something which faces forwards *framsida;* **the front of the hospital faces south; he spilt soup down the front of his shirt; the Adam's apple is visible in the front of the neck**

frontal ['frʌnt(ə)l] *adj.* referring to the forehead *or* to the front of the head *frontal(-), pann-;* **frontal bone** = bone forming the front of the upper part of the skull behind the forehead ⇨ *illustration* SKULL *os frontale, pannbenet;* **frontal lobe** = front lobe of each cerebral hemisphere *lobus frontalis, frontalloben, pannloben;* **frontal lobotomy** = surgical operation on the brain to treat mental illness by removing part of the frontal lobe *(frontal) lobotomi;* **frontal sinus** = one of two sinuses in the front of the face above the eyes and near the nose *sinus frontalis, pann(bens)hålan* NOTE: the opposite is **occipital**

frontalloben ⇨ **frontal**

frontalplan ⇨ **coronal**

frossbrytning ⇨ **chill, shivering**

frossbrytningar, med ⇨ **algid**

frosseri ⇨ **polyphagia**

frost [frɒst] *subst.* freezing weather when the temperature is below the freezing point of water *frost, köld, kyla;* **there was a frost last night**

frostbite ['frɒstbaɪt] *subst.* injury caused by very severe cold which freezes tissue *congelatio, köldskada, kylskada*

frostbitten ['frɒstˌbɪt(ə)n] *adj.* suffering from frostbite *förfrusen, köldskadad, kylskadad*

COMMENT: in very cold conditions, the outside tissue of the fingers, toes, ears and nose can freeze, becoming white and numb. Thawing of frostbitten tissue can be very painful and must be done very slowly. Severe cases of frostbite may require amputation

frosterytem ▷ **chilblain**

frostskada ▷ **burn, chilblain, cold, pernio**

frottera ▷ **rub**

frozen shoulder [ˌfrəʊz(ə)n 'ʃəʊldə] *subst.* stiffness and pain in the shoulder, caused by inflammation of the membranes of the shoulder joint after injury *or* after the shoulder has been immobile for a time, when deposits may be forming in the tendons *periarthritis humeroscapularis, frozen shoulder*

fructose ['frʌktəʊs] *subst.* fruit sugar found in honey and some fruit, which together with glucose forms sucrose *fruktos, fruktsocker*

fructosuria [ˌfrʌktəʊ'sjʊəriə] *subst.* presence of fructose in the urine *fruktosuri*

fruit [fru:t] *subst.* usually sweet part of a plant which contains the seeds, and is eaten as food *frukt;* **a diet of fresh fruit and vegetables** NOTE: no plural when referring to the food: **you should eat a lot of fruit**

COMMENT: fruit contains fructose and is a good source of vitamin C and some dietary fibre. Dried fruit have a higher sugar content but less vitamin C than fresh fruit

frukost ▷ **breakfast**

fruktan ▷ **fear**

fruktos ▷ **fructose**

fruktosuri ▷ **fructosuria**

fruktsam ▷ **fertile**

fruktsamhet ▷ **fertility**

fruktsamhetstal ▷ **fertility**

fruktsocker ▷ **fructose**

frysa ▷ **freeze**

fryskirurgi ▷ **cryosurgery**

frystorkning ▷ **freeze drying, lyophilization**

frånvarande ▷ **absent**

frånvaro ▷ **absence**

fräknar ▷ **freckles, lentigo**

fräknig ▷ **freckled**

främja ▷ **facilitate**

främmande ▷ **adventitious, exotic, foreign, heterogenous**

främmande kropp ▷ **foreign**

främmande-kroppsinstrument ▷ **spud**

främre ▷ **anterior, pre-**

främre gombågen ▷ **palatoglossal arch**

främst ▷ **primary**

frätande (ämne) ▷ **corrosive**

Fröhlich's syndrome ['freɪlɪks ˌsɪndrəʊm] *or* **dystrophia adiposogenitalis** [dɪ'strəʊfiə ˌædɪˌpəʊzəˌdʒenɪ'tælɪs] *subst.* condition where the patient becomes obese and the genital system does not develop, caused by an adenoma of the pituitary gland *Fröhlichs syndrom*

FSH [ˌefes'eɪtʃ] = FOLLICLE-STIMULATING HORMONE

ftiriasis ▷ **phthiriasis**

ftis ▷ **phthisis**

fugax ['fju:gæks] *see* AMAUROSIS

-fuge [fju:dʒ] *suffix* which drives away *-medel;* **vermifuge** = substance which removes worms *maskfördrivande medel*

fugue [fju:g] *subst.* condition where the patient loses his memory and leaves home *fugue*

fuktig ▷ **damp, moist, wet**

fuktighet ▷ **moisture**

fulguration [ˌfʌlgə'reɪʃ(ə)n] *or* **electrodesiccation** [ɪˌlektrəʊˌdesɪ'keɪʃ(ə)n] *subst.* removal of a growth (such as a wart) by burning with an electric needle *diatermi*

full [fʊl] *adj.* complete *or* with no empty space *full, fylld;* **the hospital cannot take in any more patients - all the wards are full; my appointments book is full for the next two weeks**

full ⇨ **full; drunk, drunken**

fullgångenhet ⇨ **maturity**

full-scale [ˌfʊl'skeɪ(ə)l] *adj.* complete *or* going into all details *omfattande, total;* **the doctors put him through a full-scale medical examination; the local health authority has ordered a full-scale inquiry into the case**

fullständig ⇨ **total**

fullständig abort ⇨ **abortion**

fullständigt ⇨ **absolutely, fully, totally**

full term [ˌfʊl 'tɜːm] *subst.* complete pregnancy of forty weeks *40 veckors graviditet, "tiden ut";* **she has had several pregnancies but none has reached full term**

fully ['fʊli] *adv.* completely *fullt, helt, fullständigt;* **the fetus was not fully developed; is the muscle fully relaxed?**

fulminant ['fʊlmɪnənt] *or* **fulminating** ['fʊlmɪneɪtɪŋ] *adj.* (dangerous disease) which develops very rapidly *fulminant*

> QUOTE the major manifestations of pneumococcal infection in sickle-cell disease are septicaemia, meningitis and pneumonia. The illness is frequently fulminant
>
> **The Lancet**

fulslag ⇨ **whitlow**

fumes [fjuːmz] *subst pl.* gas *or* smoke *rök, gas(er);* **toxic fumes** = poisonous gases or smoke given off by a substance *toxisk (giftig) rök (gas)*

fumigate ['fjuːmɪgeɪt] *vb.* to kill germs *or* insects by using gas *röka ut, desinficera (med gas)*

fumigation [ˌfjuːmɪ'geɪʃ(ə)n] *subst.* killing germs *or* insects by gas *rökning, desinfektion (med gas)*

function ['fʌŋ(k)ʃ(ə)n] **1** *subst.* particular work done by an organ *funktion, uppgift;* **what is the function of the pancreas? the function of an ovary is to form ova 2** *vb.* to work in a particular way *fungera;* **the heart and lungs were functioning normally; his kidneys suddenly stopped functioning**

> QUOTE insulin's primary metabolic function is to transport glucose into muscle and fat cells, so that it can be used for energy
>
> **Nursing '87**

> QUOTE the AIDS virus attacks a person's immune system and damages the ability to fight other disease. Without a functioning immune system to ward off other germs, the patient becomes vulnerable to becoming infected
>
> **Journal of American Medical Association**

functional ['fʌŋ(k)ʃ(ə)n(ə)l] *adj.* (disorder *or* illness) which does not have a physical cause and may have a psychological cause, as opposed to an organic disorder *funktionell;* **functional enuresis** = bedwetting which has a psychological cause *funktionell sängvätning, sängvätning utan organisk orsak*

fundus ['fʌndəs] *subst.* (i) bottom of a hollow organ (such as the uterus) *fundus, botten;* (ii) top section of the stomach (above the body of the stomach) ⇨ *illustration* STOMACH *fundus ventriculi;* **optic fundus** = back part of the inside of the eye, opposite the lens *fundus oculi, ögonbotten*

fungal ['fʌŋg(ə)l] *adj.* referring to fungi *svamp-;* **he had a case of fungal skin infection**

fungera ⇨ **act, function, perform**

fungicid ⇨ **fungicide**

fungicide ['fʌŋgɪsaɪd] *adj. & subst.* (substance) used to kill fungi *fungicid, svampdödande (medel)*

fungiform papillae ['fʌŋgɪfɔːm pə'pɪliː] *subst.* rounded papillae on the tip and sides of the tongue, which have taste buds ⇨ *illustration* TONGUE *papillae fungiformes*

fungoid ['fʌŋgɔɪd] *adj.* like a fungus *fungoid, svampliknande*

fungus ['fʌŋgəs] *subst.* simple plant organism with thread-like cells (such as yeast, mushrooms, mould), and without green chlorophyll *fungus, svamp;* **fungus disease** = disease caused by a fungus *svampsjukdom;* **fungus poisoning** = poisoning by eating a poisonous fungus *svampförgiftning* NOTE: plural is **fungi**. For other terms referring to fungi, see words beginning with **myc-**

> COMMENT: some fungi can become parasites of man, and cause diseases such as thrush. Other fungi, such as yeast, react

with sugar to form alcohol. Some antibiotics (such as penicillin) are derived from fungi

funiculitis [fju,nɪkju'laɪtɪs] *subst.* inflammation of the spermatic cord *funikulit*

funiculus [fju'nɪkjʊləs] *subst.* one of the three parts (lateral *or* anterior *or* posterior funiculus) of the white matter in the spinal cord *funikel, sträng*

funikel ➪ **funiculus**

funikulit ➪ **funiculitis**

funis [fju:nɪs] *subst.* umbilical cord *chorda (funiculus) umbilicus, navelsträngen*

funktion ➪ **function**

funktionell ➪ **functional**

funktionsrubbning ➪ **dysfunction**

funnel chest ['fʌn(ə)l ,tʃest] *or* **pectus excavatum** ['pektəs ,ekskə'veɪtəm] *subst.* congenital deformity, where the chest is depressed in the centre because the lower part of the breastbone is curved backwards *pectus excavatum, trattbröst*

funny ['fʌni] *adj. informal* unwell *konstig, dålig;* **she felt funny after she had eaten the fish; he had a funny turn** = he had a dizzy spell *han kände sig konstig (svimfärdig, yr i huvudet);* **funny bone** = olecranon *or* sharp bone at the end of the ulna at the elbow which gives a shock if it is hit by accident *benutskott vid armbågen som ger upphov till änkestöt vid slag*

fur [fɜ:] *vb. (of the tongue)* to feel as if covered with soft hair *bli (vara) belagd*

COMMENT: the tongue is furred when a patient is feeling unwell, and the papillae on the tongue become covered with a whitish coating

furfuraceous [,fɜ:fjə'reɪʃəs] *adj.* scaly (skin) *fjällig, skorvig, full med mjäll*

Furley stretcher ['fɜ:li ,stretʃə] *see* STRETCHER

furor ['fjʊərɔ:] *subst.* attack of wild violence (especially when mentally deranged) *furor, raseri*

furuncle ['fjʊərʌŋk(ə)l] *or* **boil** [bɔɪl] *subst.* tender raised mass of infected tissue and skin, mainly of a hair follicle, caused by the bacterium Staphylococcus aureus *furunkel, böld*

furunculosis [,fjʊərʌŋkjə'ləʊsɪs] *subst.* condition where several boils appear at the same time *furunkulos*

furunkel ➪ **furuncle**

furunkulos ➪ **furunculosis**

fuse [fju:z] *vb.* to join together to form a single structure *smälta samman, förenas;* **the bones of the joint fused**

fusiform ['fju:zɪfɔ:m] *adj.* (muscles, etc.) shaped like a spindle, with a wider middle section which becomes narrower at each end *fusiform, spolformad*

fusion ['fju:ʒ(ə)n] *subst.* joining, especially a surgical operation to join the bones at a joint permanently so that they cannot move and so relieve pain in the joint *fusion, sammansmältning, förening;* **spinal fusion** = surgical operation to join two vertebrae together to make the spine more rigid *fusionsoperation, slags operation där två ryggkotor förenas*

fusionsoperation ➪ **fusion**

FV-läkare ➪ **house, resident**

fylla ➪ **fill**

fylld ➪ **full**

fylld blåsa ➪ **distend**

fyllning ➪ **filling**

fyrdubbel ➪ **quadruple**

fyrfaldig ➪ **quadruple**

fyrfingrighet ➪ **tetradactyly**

fyrkantig muskel ➪ **quadratus**

fyrling ➪ **quadruplet**

fyrtåighet ➪ **tetradactyly**

fysen ➪ **epiphyseal**

fysikalisk ➪ **physical**

fysikalisk terapi ➪ **physical, physiotherapy**

fysiolog ➪ **physiologist**

fysiologisk ➪ **physiological**

fysioterapi ▷ physical, physiotherapy

fysisk ▷ bodily, physi-, physical

fysiskt ▷ physically

fyt(o)- ▷ phyt-

fytoterapi ▷ herbalism

få ▷ catch, develop, get, obtain, pick up, receive

fåra ▷ groove, sulcus, wrinkle

fällning ▷ deposit, precipitate, precipitation, sediment, sedimentation

färdighet ▷ ability, skill

färdtjänst ▷ mobility

färg ▷ colour

färga ▷ colour, stain

färgblind ▷ colour-blind

färgblindhet ▷ colour blindness

färglös ▷ colourless

färgämne ▷ colouring (matter), pigment, stain

färsk ▷ fresh

fästa ▷ attach, bind, fix

fästa sig ▷ implant

fäste ▷ insertion

fästing ▷ tick

fästställe ▷ insertion

föda ▷ birth; diet, feed, food, nutrition

födande ▷ parturient

föda, närande ▷ nourish

föda upp ▷ bring up

född ▷ born

födelse ▷ birth

födelseattest ▷ birth

födelsedatum ▷ birth

födelsekontroll ▷ birth, contraception

födelsemärke ▷ birthmark, mole

födelsetal ▷ birth

födoämnesallergi ▷ food

följa ▷ monitor

följd ▷ chain, course, succession

följdtillstånd ▷ sequelae

Föllings sjukdom ▷ phenylketonuria

fönstertittarsjuka ▷ claudication

föraning ▷ aura

förband ▷ bandage, dressing, pad

förbandslåda ▷ first aid

förbening ▷ ossification

förbereda ▷ prepare

förbinda ▷ bandage, bind, dress; connect

förbindelse ▷ connection, junction, nexus

förbjuda ▷ ban, forbid

förbrukning ▷ consumption, depletion

förbund ▷ association

förbättras ▷ clear up, improve, progress

förbättring ▷ amelioration, improvement, progress, remission

fördjupning ▷ depression, hollow

förebud ▷ aura

förebygga ▷ prevent

förebyggande ▷ prevention, preventive

förebyggande (medel) ▷ prophylactic

förefalla ▷ appear

föregå ▷ precede

föregående fosterdel ⇨ present

föregångare ⇨ precursor

förekomst ⇨ incidence, occurrence, prevalence

före måltid ⇨ a.c.

förena ⇨ combine, connect, join, knit, link

förenas ⇨ fuse, join

förening ⇨ association; combination, composition, connection, fusion

föreningspunkt ⇨ junction

förenkla ⇨ facilitate

förenlig ⇨ compatible

förenlighet ⇨ compatibility

föreskrift ⇨ prescription, instruction

föreslå ⇨ recommend, suggest

föreställning ⇨ image

företa ⇨ undertake

företagssköterska ⇨ occupational

förete ⇨ present

förfader ⇨ ancestor

förfarande ⇨ procedure

förfluten ⇨ past

förflytta ⇨ refer

förflytta sig ⇨ get around

förfrusen ⇨ frostbitten

förföljelse ⇨ persecution

förgasare ⇨ vaporizer

förgasning ⇨ evaporation

förgiftning ⇨ intoxication, poisoning, toxicosis

förgrening ⇨ arborization, bifurcation, branch

förhandenvarande ⇨ present

förhindra ⇨ inhibit, prevent

förhindrande ⇨ prevention

förhorning ⇨ cornification

förhuden ⇨ foreskin

förhudsförträngning ⇨ phimosis

förhållande ⇨ relationship

förhårdnad ⇨ callosity

förhärskande ⇨ predominant

förhöjd kroppstemperatur ⇨ hyperthermia

förkalkad ⇨ calcified

förkalkning ⇨ calcareous degeneration, calcification

förkasta ⇨ reject

förklara ⇨ certify, explain

förklaring ⇨ explanation, key

förkläde ⇨ apron

förkortning ⇨ retraction

förkrympt ⇨ abortive

förkylning ⇨ cold, coryza, respiratory

förkylningsblåsa ⇨ fever

förlama ⇨ paralyse

förlamad ⇨ palsied, paralytic

förlamning ⇨ palsy, paralysis

förlamning, dubbelsidig ⇨ diplegia, paraplegia

förlamning, ensidig ⇨ monoplegia

förlamning, hysterisk ⇨ pseudoplegia

förlamning, (lättare) ⇨ paresis

förlopp ⇨ course

förlora ⇨ lose, shed

förlossning ⇨ childbirth, delivery, maternity

förlossning, normal ⇨ eutocia

förlossnings- ⇨ obstetric(al)

förlossningsarbete ⇨ labour

förlossningsavdelning ⇨ maternity

förlossningskanalen ⇨ birth

förlossningskonst ⇨ midwifery, obstetrics

förlossningsläkare ⇨ obstetrician

förlossningssjukhus ⇨ maternity

förlossningsskada ⇨ birth

förlossningsstol ⇨ birthing chair

förlossningssäng ⇨ delivery

förlossningstång ⇨ forceps

förlossningsvärkar ⇨ pain

förlust ⇨ depletion, deprivation, loss

förlänga ⇨ prolong

förlängda märgen ⇨ medulla

förmak ⇨ atrium, chamber

förmaksflimmer ⇨ atrial

förmedling ⇨ agency

förmåga ⇨ ability, capacity, faculty

förnimbar ⇨ palpable

förnuft ⇨ reason

förordna ⇨ appoint

förorena ⇨ contaminate, pollute

förorening ⇨ contamination, pollutant, pollution

förorsaka ⇨ induce

förpackning ⇨ pack

förruttnelse ⇨ decay, decomposition, putrefaction

förråd ⇨ supply

förse (med) ⇨ supply

försena ⇨ retard

försening ⇨ retardation

försiktighetsåtgärd ⇨ precaution

förskjuta ⇨ displace

förskjutning ⇨ displacement, shift

förskola ⇨ nursery school

förslag ⇨ suggestion

förslitning ⇨ wear and tear

första ⇨ first, primary

förstadium till cancer ⇨ precancer

första gradens brännskada ⇨ burn

första ordningens neuron ⇨ neurone

förstföderska ⇨ primipara

förstoppad ⇨ constipated, costive

förstoppning ⇨ constipation

förstoring ⇨ enlargement, hyperplasia, hypertrophy

förströelse ⇨ amusement

förstånd ⇨ reason

förståndshandikappad ⇨ defective

förstöra ⇨ destroy

förstörelse ⇨ destruction

försummelse ⇨ malpractice

försvaga ⇨ deaden, debilitate, dull, enervate, impair, weaken

försvarsmekanism ⇨ defence

försvåra ⇨ aggravate

försäkra ⇨ insure, reassure

försäkran ⇨ reassurance

försäkring ⇨ insurance

försämra ⇨ aggravate, exacerbate, impair

försämras ⇨ **deteriorate**

försämring ⇨ **deterioration, exacerbation, impairment**

försök ⇨ **attempt**

försöka ⇨ **attempt**

försörjning ⇨ **supply**

förtidig ⇨ **premature, preterm**

förtidsbörd ⇨ **premature**

förtjockad ⇨ **inspissated**

förtränga ⇨ **stenose**

förträngning ⇨ **coarctation, constriction, isthmus, stenosis, stricture**

förtunnas ⇨ **rarefy**

förtunningsmedel ⇨ **diluent**

förtvina ⇨ **atrophy**

förtvining ⇨ **atrophy, dystrophia, tabes**

förtäring ⇨ **consumption**

förtätad ⇨ **condensed, inspissated**

förtätning ⇨ **consolidation, inspissation**

förutsäga ⇨ **predict**

förutsägelse ⇨ **prediction**

förvaltning ⇨ **administration, service**

förvandla ⇨ **convert**

förvandlas ⇨ **turn**

förvandling ⇨ **conversion**

förvara ⇨ **keep**

förvarning ⇨ **notice, warning**

förvirra ⇨ **confuse**

förvirrad ⇨ **dazed, disorientated**

förvirring ⇨ **confusion, disorientation**

förvrida ⇨ **distort**

förvånande ⇨ **astonishing**

förvåning ⇨ **astonishment**

förvärra ⇨ **aggravate, exacerbate**

förvärvad ⇨ **acquired**

föråldrad ⇨ **date**

förånga(s) ⇨ **vaporize**

förångning ⇨ **evaporation**

förälder ⇨ **parent**

föräldraskap ⇨ **parenthood**

förändring ⇨ **shift**

föräta (sig) ⇨ **overeating**

föröka ⇨ **propagate, breed**

förökning ⇨ **propagation, reproduction**

Gg

g [dʒiː] = GRAM

GABA ['gæbə] = GAMMA AMINOBUTYRIC ACID

gag [gæg] **1** *subst.* instrument placed between a patient's teeth to stop him closing his mouth *munspärr* **2** *vb.* to choke *or* to try to vomit but be unable to do so *få kväljningar, vilja kräkas;* **he gagged on his food; every time the doctor tries to examine her throat, she gags; he started gagging on the endotracheal tube**

gain [geɪn] **1** *subst.* act of adding *or* increasing *ökning, uppgång;* **the baby showed a gain in weight of 25g** *or* **showed a weight gain of 25g 2** *vb.* to add *or* to increase *öka, gå upp, tillta;* **to gain in weight** *or* **to gain weight**

gait [geɪt] *subst.* way of walking *gång, gångart;* **ataxic gait** = way of walking where the patient walks unsteadily due to a disorder of the nervous system *ataktisk gång;* **cerebellar gait** = way of walking where the patient staggers along, caused by a disease of the cerebellum *cerebellär gång;* **spastic gait** = way of walking where the legs are stiff and the feet not lifted off the ground *spastisk gång; see also* FESTINATION

galact- [gə'lækt, -ˌ-] *prefix* referring to milk *galakt(o)-, mjölk-*

galactagogue [gə'læktəˌgɒg] *subst.* substance which stimulates the production of milk *galaktagogum, mjölkdrivande medel*

galactocele [gə'læktə(ʊ)siː(ə)l] *subst.* breast tumour which contains milk *galaktocele, mjölkfylld retentionscysta*

galactorrhoea [gəˌlæktə(ʊ)'rɪə] *subst.* excessive production of milk *galaktorré*

galactosaemia [gəˌlæktə(ʊ)'siːmiə] *subst.* congenital defect where the liver is incapable of converting galactose into glucose, with the result that a baby's development may be affected *galaktosemi*

> COMMENT: the treatment is to remove galactose from the diet

galactose [gə'læktəʊs] *subst.* sugar which forms part of milk, and is converted into glucose by the liver *galaktos*

galaktagogum ⇨ **galactagogue**

galaktocele ⇨ **galactocele**

galaktorré ⇨ **galactorrhoea**

galaktos ⇨ **galactose**

galaktosemi ⇨ **galactosaemia**

galea ['geɪliə] *subst.* (i) any part of the body shaped like a helmet, especially the loose band of tissue in the scalp *galea, hjälmliknande struktur, galeaponeurosen, huvudsvålen;* (ii) type of bandage wrapped round the head *slags förband för huvudet*

galeaponeurosen ⇨ **galea**

galen ⇨ **mad**

gall [gɔːl] *or* **bile** [baɪ(ə)l] *subst.* thick bitter yellowish-brown fluid secreted by the liver and stored in the gall bladder or passed into the stomach, used to digest fatty substances and to neutralize acids *galla*

gall- ⇨ **biliary, bilious, chol-, chole-**

galla ⇨ **gall**

gall bladder ['gɔːl ˌblædə] *subst.* sac situated underneath the liver, in which bile produced by the liver is stored ⇨ *illustration* DIGESTIVE SYSTEM *vesica fellea, gallblåsan*

> COMMENT: bile is stored in the gall bladder until required by the stomach. If fatty food is present in the stomach, bile moves from the gall bladder along the bile duct to the stomach. Since the liver also secretes bile directly into the duodenum, the gall bladder is not an essential organ and can be removed by surgery

gallblåsan ⇨ **gall bladder**

gallblåseartären ⇨ **cystic**

gallblåsegången ⇨ **cystic**

gallblåseinflammation ⇨ **cholecystitis**

gallbrist ⇨ **acholia**

gallfistel ⇨ **biliary**

gallfärgämne ⇨ **bile**

gallgång ⇨ **canal, duct**

gallgångs- ⇨ **choledoch-**

Gallie's operation ['gælɪz ˌɒpə'reɪʃ(ə)n] *subst.* surgical operation where tissues from the patient's thigh are used to hold a hernia in place *slags ljumskbråcksoperation*

gallipot ['gælipɒt] *subst.* little pot for ointment *apoteksburk, liten glaserad lerburk*

gallon ['gælən] *subst.* measurement of liquids which equals eight pints or 4.5 litres *gallon;* **the bucket can hold four gallons; the body contains about two gallons of blood**

gallop rhythm ['gæləp ˌrɪð(ə)m] *subst.* rhythm of heart sounds, three to each cycle, when a patient is experiencing tachycardia *galloperande hjärtrytm, galloprytm*

gallproduktion ⇨ **choleresis**

gallsalter ⇨ **bile**

gallsjuk ⇨ **bilious**

gallstas ⇨ **cholestasis**

gallsten ⇨ **gallstone**

gallstenskolik ⇨ **biliary**

gallstenslidande ⇨ **cholelithiasis**

gallstone ['gɔːlstəʊn] *or* **calculus** ['kælkjʊləs] *subst.* small stone formed from insoluble deposits from bile in the gall bladder *calculus felleus, gallsten*

> COMMENT: gallstones can be harmless, but some cause pain and inflammation and a serious condition can develop if a gallstone blocks the bile duct. Sudden pain going from the right side of the stomach towards the back indicates that a gallstone is passing through the bile duct

gallsyror ⇨ **bile**

gallvägsinflammation ⇨ **cholangitis**

galvanism ['gælvənɪz(ə)m] *subst.* treatment using low voltage electricity *galvanism*

galvanocautery [ˌgælv(ə)nə'kɔːtəri] *or* **electrocautery** [ɪˌlektrə'kɔːtəri] *subst.* removal of diseased tissue using an electrically heated needle *or* loop of wire *diatermi*

gamet ⇨ **gamete, germ**

gamete ['gæmiːt] *subst.* sex cell, either a spermatozoon or an ovum *gamet, könscell*

gametocide [gə'miːtəʊsaɪd] *subst.* drug which kills gametocytes *gametocytdödande medel*

gametocyte [gə'miːtəʊsaɪt] *subst.* cell which is developing into a gamete *gametocyt*

gametogenesis [gəˌmiːtəʊ'dʒenəsɪs] *subst.* process by which a gamete is formed *gametogenes*

gamgee tissue ['gæmdʒiː ˌtɪʃuː] *subst.* surgical dressing, formed of a layer of cotton wool between two pieces of gauze *slags förband*

gamma ['gæmə] *subst.* third letter of the Greek alphabet *gamma*

gamma aminobutyric acid (GABA) [ˌgæmə əˌmiːnəʊbju'tɪrɪk 'æsɪd (gæbə)] *subst.* amino acid found in the brain and many nerve terminals *gamma-amino-smörsyra, Gaba, GABA*

gamma-amino-smörsyra ⇨ **gamma aminobutyric acid (GABA)**

gamma camera ['gæmə ˌkæm(ə)rə] *subst.* camera for taking photographs of parts of the body into which radioactive isotopes have been introduced *gammakamera*

gamma globulins [ˌgæmə'glɒbjʊlɪnz] *subst.* proteins found in plasma, including those which form antibodies as protection against infection *gammaglobuliner*

> COMMENT: gamma globulin injections are sometimes useful as a rapid source of protection against a wide range of diseases

gammakamera ⇨ **gamma camera**

gamma rays ['gæmə reɪz] *subst. pl.* rays which are shorter than X-rays and are given off by radioactive substances *gammastrålar, gammastrålning*

gammastrålning ⇨ **gamma rays**

ganglion ['gæŋgliən] *subst.* **(a)** mass of nerve cell bodies and synapses usually covered in connective tissue, found along the peripheral nerves with the exception of the basal ganglia *ganglion;* **basal ganglia** = masses of grey matter at the base of each cerebral hemisphere which receive impulses from the thalamus and influence the motor impulses from the frontal cortex *basala ganglierna;* **ciliary ganglion** = parasympathetic ganglion in the orbit of the eye, supplying the intrinsic eye muscles *ganglion ciliare;* **coeliac ganglion** = ganglion on each side of the origins of the diaphragm, connected with the coeliac plexus *ganglion coeliacum;* **mesenteric ganglion** = plexus of sympathetic nerve fibres and ganglion cells around the superior mesenteric artery *ganglion mesentericum;* **otic ganglion** = ganglion associated with the mandibular nerve where it leaves the skull *ganglion oticum;* **pterygopalatine ganglion** *or* **sphenopalatine ganglion** = ganglion in the pterygopalatine fossa associated with the maxillary nerve (postganglionic fibres going to the nose, palate, pharynx and lacrimal glands) *ganglion pterygopalatinum (sphenopalatinum);* **spinal ganglion** = cone-shaped mass of cells on the posterior root, the main axons of which form the posterior root of the spinal nerve *ganglion spinale, spinalganglion;* **stellate ganglion** = group of nerve cells in the neck, shaped like a star *ganglion stellatum;* **submandibular ganglion** = ganglion associated with the lingual nerve, relaying impulses to the submandibular and sublingual salivary glands *ganglion submandibulare;* **superior ganglion** = small collection of cells in the jugular foramen *ganglion superius;* **trigeminal ganglion** *or* **Gasserian ganglion** = sensory ganglion containing the cells of origin of the sensory fibres in the fifth cranial nerve *ganglion seminulare, Gassers ganglion;* **vertebral ganglion** = ganglion in front of the origin of the vertebral artery *ganglion vertebrale* **(b)** cyst of a tendon sheath *or* joint capsule (usually at the wrist) which results in a

painless swelling containing fluid *senknut*
NOTE: plural is **ganglia**

ganglionectomy [ˌgæŋgliəˈnektəmi] *subst.* surgical removal of a ganglion *ganglionektomi*

ganglionektomi ⇨ **ganglionectomy**

ganglionic [ˌgæŋgliˈɒnɪk] *adj.* referring to a ganglion *som avser el. hör till ganglion;* **postganglionic neurone** = neurone in a ganglion *or* plexus, the axon of which supplies muscle or glandular tissue directly *postganglionär nervcell*

gangliosidos ⇨ **Tay-Sachs disease**

gangrene [ˈgæŋgriːn] *subst.* condition where tissues die and decay, as a result of bacterial action, because the blood supply has been lost through injury or disease of the artery *gangrän, gangren, kallbrand, brand;* **after he had frostbite, gangrene set in and his toes had to be amputated; dry gangrene** = condition where the blood supply is cut off and the limb becomes black *gangraena sicca, torrt gangrän;* **gas gangrene** = complication of severe wounds in which the bacterium **Clostridium welchii** breeds in the wound and then spreads to healthy tissue which is rapidly decomposed with the formation of gas *gangraena (phlegmone) emphysematosa (gaseosa), gasgangrän, gasflegmone, gasbrand;* **hospital gangrene** = gangrene caused by insanitary hospital conditions *gangraena nosocomialis, hospitalsbrand;* **moist gangrene** = condition where dead tissue decays and swells with fluid because of infection and the tissues have an unpleasant smell *gangraena humida, fuktigt gangrän, kallbrand*

gangrän ⇨ **gangrene, necrosis**

Ganser state [ˈgænsə ˌsteɪt] = PSEUDODEMENTIA

ganska ⇨ **fairly**

gap [gæp] *subst.* space *öppning, lucka, mellanrum;* **there is a gap between his two front teeth; the muscle has passed through a gap in the mucosa**

gap ⇨ **hiatus**

gargle [ˈgɑːg(ə)l] **1** *subst.* mildly antiseptic solution used to clean the mouth *gurgelvatten;* **if diluted with water, the product makes a useful gargle 2** *vb.* to put some antiseptic liquid solution into the back of the mouth and throat and then breathe out air through it *gurgla (sig);* **the doctor recommended gargling twice a day with a saline solution**

gargoylism [ˈgɑːgɔɪlɪz(ə)m] *or* **Hurler's syndrome** [ˈhɜːləz ˌsɪndrəʊm] *subst.* congenital defect of a patient's metabolism which causes polysaccharides and fat cells to accumulate in the body, resulting in mental defects, swollen liver and coarse features *gargoylism, Hurlers syndrom*

garvsyra ⇨ **tannin**

gas [gæs] *subst.* **(a)** (i) state of matter in which particles occupy the whole space in which they occur *gas;* (ii) substance often produced from coal or found underground, and used to cook or heat *gas;* **a gas cooker; we heat our house by gas; gas exchange** = process by which oxygen in air is exchanged in the lungs for waste carbon dioxide carried by the blood *gasutbyte;* **gas gangrene** = complication of severe wounds in which the bacterium **Clostridium welchii** breeds in the wound and then spreads to healthy tissue which is rapidly decomposed with the formation of gas *gangraena (phlegmone) emphysematosa (gaseosa), gasgangrän, gasflegmone, gasbrand;* **gas poisoning** = poisoning by breathing in carbon monoxide or other toxic gas *gasförgiftning* **(b)** gas which accumulates in the stomach or alimentary canal and causes pain *gas;* **gas pains** = flatus *or* excessive formation of gas in the stomach *or* intestine which is painful *flatulens, smärtsamma gaser (i magen), väderspänning(ar)*
NOTE: plural **gases** is only used to mean different types of gas

gasbildande ⇨ **aerogenous, flatulent**

gasbildning ⇨ **flatulence**

gasbildning, medel mot ⇨ **carminative**

gasbinda ⇨ **bandage, dressing, gauze**

gasbrand ⇨ **gangrene, gas**

gaser ⇨ **wind; fumes**

gasflegmone ⇨ **gangrene, gas**

gasförgiftning ⇨ **gas**

gasgangrän ⇨ **gangrene**

gash [gæʃ] **1** *subst.* long cut, as made with a knife *djup skåra, djupt jack (sår);* **she had to have three stitches in the gash in her**

thigh **2** *vb.* to make a long cut *skära (hugga) djupt;* **she gashed her hand on the broken glass**

"gasning" ⇨ **pneumothorax**

gasp [gɑːsp] **1** *subst.* trying to breathe *or* breath taken with difficulty *flämtning, tungt andetag;* **his breath came in short gasps 2** *vb.* to try to breathe taking quick breaths *flämta, dra (kippa) efter andan;* **she was gasping for breath**

Gasserian ganglion [gæˈsɪəriən ˌgæŋgliən] *subst.* trigeminal ganglion *or* sensory ganglion containing the cells of origin of the sensory fibres in the fifth cranial nerve *ganglion seminulare, Gassers ganglion*

gastr- [ˈgæstr, ˌ-] *prefix* referring to the stomach *gastr(o)-, mag-, magsäcks-*

gastralgi ⇨ **gastralgia**

gastralgia [gæˈstrældʒə] *subst.* pain in the stomach *gastralgi, magsmärtor, ont i magen*

gastrectomy [gæˈstrektəmi] *subst.* surgical removal of the stomach *gastrektomi;* **partial gastrectomy** = surgical removal of only the lower part of the stomach *partiell gastrektomi;* **subtotal gastrectomy** = surgical removal of all but the top part of the stomach in contact with the diaphragm *subtotal gastrektomi*

gastrektomi ⇨ **gastrectomy**

gastric [ˈgæstrɪk] *adj.* referring to the stomach *gastrisk, mag-, magsäcks-;* **gastric acid** = hydrochloric acid secreted into the stomach by acid-forming cells *magsyra;* **gastric artery** = artery leading from the coeliac trunk to the stomach *arteria gastrica;* **gastric flu** = general term for any mild stomach disorder *magbesvär;* **gastric juices** = mixture of hydrochloric acid, pepsin, intrinsic factor and mucus secreted by the cells of the lining membrane of the stomach to help the digestion of food *magsaft;* **the walls of the stomach secrete gastric juices; gastric pit** = deep hollow in the mucous membrane forming the walls of the stomach *epigastriet, maggropen;* **gastric ulcer** = ulcer in the stomach *ulcus ventriculus, magsår;* **gastric vein** = vein which follows the gastric artery *vena gastrica*

gastrin [ˈgæstrɪn] *subst.* hormone which is released into the bloodstream from cells in the lower end of the stomach, stimulated by the presence of protein, and which in turn stimulates the flow of acid from the upper part of the stomach *gastrin*

gastrisk ⇨ **gastric**

gastritis [gæˈstraɪtɪs] *subst.* inflammation of the stomach *gastrit, magkatarr*

gastrocele [ˈgæstrəʊsiː(ə)l] *subst.* stomach hernia *or* condition where part of the stomach wall becomes weak and bulges out *gastrocele*

gastrocnemius [ˌgæstrɒkˈniːmiəs] *subst.* large calf muscle *(musculus) gastrocnemius, stora vadmuskeln*

gastrocolic reflex [ˌgæstrəʊˈkɒlɪk ˌriːfleks] *subst.* sudden peristalsis of the colon produced when food is taken into an empty stomach *gastrokoliska reflexen*

gastroduodenal [ˌgæstrəʊˌdjuːəʊˈdiːn(ə)l] *adj.* referring to the stomach and duodenum *gastroduodenal;* **gastroduodenal artery** = artery leading from the gastric artery towards the pancreas *arteria gastroduodenalis*

gastroduodenostomy [ˌgæstrəʊˌdjuːəʊdɪˈnɒstəmi] *subst.* surgical operation to join the duodenum to the stomach so as to bypass a blockage in the pylorus *gastroduodenostomi*

gastroenteritis [ˌgæstrəʊˌentəˈraɪtɪs] *subst.* inflammation of the membrane lining the intestines and the stomach, caused by a viral infection and resulting in diarrhoea and vomiting *gastroenterit, magtarmkatarr*

gastroenterologist [ˌgæstrəʊˌentəˈrɒlədʒɪst] *subst.* doctor who specializes in disorders of the stomach and intestine *gastroenterolog*

gastroenterology [ˌgæstrəʊˌentəˈrɒlədʒi] *subst.* study of the stomach, intestine and other parts of the digestive system and their disorders *gastroenterologi*

gastroenterostomy [ˌgæstrəʊˌentəˈrɒstəmi] *subst.* surgical operation to join the small intestine directly to the stomach so as to bypass a peptic ulcer *gastroenterostomi*

gastroepiploic [ˌgæstrəʊˌepɪˈplɔɪik] *adj.* referring to the stomach and greater omentum *gastroepiploicus;* **gastroepiploic artery** = artery linking the gastroduodenal artery to the splenic artery *arteria gastroepiploica*

gastroileac reflex [ˌgæstrəʊˈɪliæk ˌriːfleks] *subst.* automatic relaxing of the ileocaecal valve when food is present in the stomach *automatisk avslappning av iloecekalklaffen*

gastrointestinal (GI) [ˌgæstrəʊɪn'testɪn(ə)l (ˌdʒiː'aɪ)] *adj.* referring to the stomach and intestine *gastrointestinal;* **he experienced some gastrointestinal (GI) bleeding**

gastrojejunostomy [ˌgæstrəʊˌdʒidʒu'nɒstəmi] *subst.* surgical operation to join the jejunum to the stomach *gastrojejunostomi*

gastrolith ['gæstrəʊlɪθ] *subst.* stone in the stomach *gastrolit*

gastro-oesophageal reflux [ˌgæstrəʊiˌsɒfə'dʒɪəl ˌriːflʌks] *subst.* return of bitter-tasting, partly digested food from the stomach to the oesophagus when the patient has indigestion *refux (återflöde) från magsäcken till matstrupen*

gastropexy ['gæstrəʊˌpeksi] *subst.* attaching the stomach to the wall of the abdomen *gastropexi*

gastroplasty ['gæstrəʊˌplæsti] *subst.* surgery to correct a deformed stomach *plastikoperation av magsäcken*

gastroptosis [ˌgæstrəʊ'təʊsɪs] *subst.* condition where the stomach hangs down *gastroptos*

gastrorrhoea [ˌgæstrə'rɪə] *subst.* excessive flow of gastric juices *alltför starkt magsaftflöde*

gastroscope ['gæstrəskəʊp] *subst.* instrument formed of a tube *or* bundle of glass fibres with a lens attached, by which a doctor can examine the inside of the stomach (it is passed down into the stomach through the mouth) *gastroskop*

gastroscopy [gæ'strɒskəpi] *subst.* examination of the stomach using a gastroscope *gastroskopi*

gastroskopi ⇨ **gastroscopy**

gastrostomi ⇨ **gastrostomy**

gastrostomy [gæ'strɒstəmi] *subst.* surgical operation to create an opening into the stomach from the wall of the abdomen, so that food can be introduced without passing through the mouth and throat *gastrostomi*

gastrotomi ⇨ **gastrotomy**

gastrotomy [gæ'strɒtəmi] *subst.* surgical operation to open up the stomach *gastrotomi*

gasutbyte ⇨ **gas**

gasväv ⇨ **gauze, tulle gras**

gather ['gæðə] *vb.* **(a)** to bring together *or* to collect *samla (ihop), samlas;* **she was gathering material for the study of children suffering from rickets; pus had gathered round the wound; the lecturer gathered up his papers; a group of students gathered round the professor of surgery as he demonstrated the incision (b)** to understand *förstå, sluta sig till;* **did you gather who will be speaking at the ceremony?**

Gaucher's disease ['gəʊʃeɪz dɪˌziːz] *subst.* enzyme disease where fatty substances accumulate in the lymph glands, spleen and liver *Gauchers sjukdom*

> COMMENT: symptoms are anaemia, a swollen spleen and darkening of the skin; the disease can be fatal in children

gauze [gɔːz] *subst.* thin light material used to make dressings *gasväv, gasbinda;* **she put a gauze dressing on the wound; the dressing used was a light paraffin gauze**

gavage [gə'vɑːʒ, 'gævɑːʒ] *subst.* forced feeding of a patient who cannot eat *or* who refuses to eat *sondmatning*

GC [ˌdʒiː'siː] = GONORRHOEA

GDC [ˌdʒiːdiː'siː] = GENERAL DENTAL COUNCIL

ge ⇨ **administer, give, hand, provide**

Gehrig's disease ['geɪrɪgz dɪˌziːz] = AMYOTROPHIC LATERAL SCLEROSIS

Geiger counter ['gaɪgə ˌkaʊntə] *subst.* instrument for detection and measurement of radiation *Geigermätare, Geigerräknare*

gel [dʒel] *subst.* substance that has coagulated to form a jelly-like solid *gel*

gelatin ['dʒelətɪn] *subst.* protein which is soluble in water, made from collagen *gelatin*

> COMMENT: gelatin is used in foodstuffs (such as desserts or meat jellies) and is also used to make capsules in which to put medicine

gelatinliknande ⇨ **gelatinous**

gelatinous [dʒə'lætɪnəs] *adj.* like jelly *gelatinös, gelatinliknande*

gelatinruta ⇨ **lamella**

gelatinös ⇨ **gelatinous**

gemellus [dʒɪˈmeləs] *subst.* twin *or* double *gemellus, dubbel, tvilling;* **gemellus superior** *or* **inferior muscle** = two muscles arising from the ischium *musculus gemellus superior resp. inferior*

gemensam ⇨ **common**

gen ⇨ **gene**

gen- ⇨ **genetic**

-gen ⇨ **-genic**

genast ⇨ **immediately**

gene [dʒiːn] *subst.* unit of DNA on a chromosome which governs the synthesis of one protein, usually an enzyme, and determines a particular characteristic *gen, arvsanlag; see* GENETIC

> COMMENT: genes are either dominant, where the characteristic is always passed on to the child, or recessive, where the characteristic only appears if both parents have contributed the same gene

general [ˈdʒen(ə)r(ə)l] *adj.* not particular; which concerns everything or everybody *allmän;* **general amnesia** = sudden and complete loss of memory *or* state where a person does not even remember who he is *generell (total, allmän) minnesförlust;* **general anaesthesia** = loss of feeling and loss of sensation, after having been given an anaesthetic *narkos, sövning;* **general anaesthetic** = substance given to make a patient lose consciousness so that a major surgical operation can be carried out *narkosmedel;* **General Dental Council (GDC)** = official body which registers and supervises dentists in the UK *myndighet som registrerar och övervakar tandläkare i Storbritannien;* **General Medical Council (GMC)** = official body which registers and supervises doctors in the UK *myndighet som registrerar och övervakar läkare i Storbritannien (motsvarande Socialstyrelsen);* **General Optical Council (GOC)** = official body which registers and supervises opticians in the UK *myndighet som registrerar och övervakar optiker i Storbritannien;* **general paralysis of the insane** (GPI) = widespread damage of the nervous system, marking the final stages of untreated syphilis *dementia paralytica, paralysie générale;* **general practice** = doctor's practice where patients from a district are treated for all types of illness *allmän praktik;* **she qualified as a doctor and went into general practice**

generalized [ˈdʒen(ə)rəlaɪzd] *adj.* occurring throughout the body *allmän, spridd;* **the cancer became generalized** NOTE: the opposite is **localized**

generally [ˈdʒen(ə)rəli] *adv.* normally *i allmänhet, vanligen, för det mesta*

general practitioner (GP) [ˌdʒen(ə)r(ə)l prækˈtɪʃ(ə)nə (ˌdʒiːˈpiː)] *subst.* doctor who treats many patients in a district for all types of illness, though not specializing in any one branch of medicine *allmänpraktiker, allmänpraktiserande läkare, distriktsläkare*
NOTE: plural is **GPs**

> COMMENT: a GP usually has either a MB (bachelor of Medicine) or ChB (Bachelor of surgery) degree. He may also be a MRCS (Member of the Royal College of Surgeons) or LRCP (Licentiate of the Royal College of Physicians). GPs train in hospital as well in general practice, and often have specialist qualifications, such as in obstetrics or child care

generation [ˌdʒenəˈreɪʃ(ə)n] *subst.* all people born at about the same period *generation*

generic [dʒəˈnerɪk] *adj.* (i) referring to a genus *generisk, släkt-;* (ii) (name) given to a drug generally, as opposed to a proprietary name used by the manufacturer *generisk*

generisk ⇨ **generic**

genetic [dʒəˈnetɪk] *adj.* referring to the genes *genetisk, gen-;* **genetic code** = information which determines the synthesis of a cell, is held in the DNA of a cell and is passed on when the cell divides *genetisk kod;* **genetic engineering** = techniques used to change the genetic composition of an organism so that certain characteristics can be created artificially *genteknik*

genetics [dʒəˈnetɪks] *subst.* study of the way the characteristics of an organism are inherited through the genes *genetik*

genetik ⇨ **genetics**

genetisk ⇨ **genetic**

genetiskt urval ⇨ **selection**

-genic [ˈdʒenɪk] *suffix* produced by *or* which produces *-gen;* **photogenic** = produced by light *or* which produces light *fotogen, ljusalstrad, ljusalstrande*

genicular [dʒe'nɪkjʊlə] *adj.* referring to the knee *som avser el. hör till knät*

genital ['dʒenɪt(ə)l] *adj.* referring to reproductive organs *genital(-), köns-, fortplantnings-;* **genital herpes** = venereal infection, caused by a herpesvirus, which forms blisters in the genital region and can have a serious effect on a fetus *herpes genitalis;* **genital organs** *or* **genitals** = external organs for reproduction (penis and testicles in male, vulva in female) *genitalia, genitalorgan, könsorgan, fortplantningsorgan*

genitalia [ˌdʒenɪ'teɪliə] *subst.* genital organs *genitalia, genitalorgan, könsorgan, fortplantningsorgan*

genitalorgan ⇨ **genital, genitalia, reproductive, sex**

genitourinary [ˌdʒenɪtəʊ'jʊərɪnəri] *adj.* referring to both reproductive and urinary systems *urogenital;* **genitourinary system** = organs of reproduction and urination, including the kidneys *urogenitalsystemet*

genklang ⇨ **resonance**

genkomplex ⇨ **genome**

genomborra ⇨ **perforate, stab**

genombrott ⇨ **perforation**

genome ['dʒiːnəʊm] *subst.* (i) basic set of chromosomes in a person *genom, genkomplex;* (ii) set of genes which are inherited from one parent *genuppsättning (som ärvs från ena föräldern)*

genomgripande ⇨ **radical**

genomgå ⇨ **undergo (surgery)**

genomlysning ⇨ **fluoroscopy, radioscopy, transillumination**

genomskinlig ⇨ **transparent**

genomsläpplighet ⇨ **permeability**

genomtränga ⇨ **penetrate**

genomträngande ⇨ **penetration**

genotyp ⇨ **genotype**

genotype ['dʒenətaɪp] *subst.* genetic composition of an organism *genotyp*

genteknik ⇨ **genetic**

gentian violet [ˌdʒenʃ(ə)n 'vaɪələt] *subst.* antiseptic blue dye used to paint on skin infections; dye used to stain specimens *gentian(a)violett*

gentle ['dʒent(ə)l] *adj.* soft *mjuk, varsam;* kind *vänlig, snäll;* **the doctor has gentle hands; you must be gentle when you are holding a little baby; use a gentle antiseptic on the rash** NOTE: **gentle - gentler - gentlest**

genu ['dʒiːnjuː] *subst.* the knee *genu, knät*

genual ['dʒenjʊəl] *adj.* referring to the knee *som avser el. hör till knät*

genupectoral position [ˌdʒenjuː'pekt(ə)r(ə)l pəˌzɪʃ(ə)n] *subst.* position of a patient when kneeling with the chest on the floor *knäbröstläge*

genus ['dʒiːnəs] *subst.* main group of related living organisms *genus, kön;* **a genus is divided into different species**
NOTE: plural is **genera**

genu valgum ['dʒiːnjuː 'vælgəm] *subst.* knock knee *or* state where the knees touch and the ankles are apart when the person is standing straight *genu valgum, kobenthet, X-benthet*

genu varum ['dʒiːnjuː 'veərəm] *subst.* bow leg *or* state where the ankles touch and the knees are apart when the person is standing straight *genu varum, hjulbenthet, O-benthet*

geriatric [ˌdʒeri'ætrɪk] *adj.* referring to old people *geriatrisk, åldrings-;* **geriatric unit** *or* **ward** *or* **hospital** = unit *or* ward *or* hospital which specializes in the treatment of old people *geriatrisk avdelning el. geriatriskt sjukhus*

geriatrician [ˌdʒeriə'trɪʃ(ə)n] *subst.* doctor who specializes in the treatment *or* study of diseases of old people *geriatriker*

geriatrics [ˌdʒeri'ætrɪks] *subst.* study of the diseases and disorders of old people *geriatri(k), gerontologi; compare* PEDIATRICS

geriatriker ⇨ **geriatrician**

geriatrisk ⇨ **geriatric**

germ [dʒɜːm] *subst.* **(a)** microbe (such as a virus *or* bacterium) which causes a disease *bakterie;* **germs are not visible to the naked eye** NOTE: in this sense germ is not a medical term **(b)** part of an organism which develops into a new organism *embryo, grodd;* **germ cell** *or* **gonocyte** = cell which is capable of developing into a spermatozoon or ovum *gamet, könscell;* **germ layers** = two or three layers of cell in animal embryos which form the organs of the body *groddblad*

German measles [ˌdʒɜːmən 'miːz(ə)lz] *or* **rubella** [rʊ'belə] *subst.* common infectious viral disease of children with mild fever, swollen lymph nodes and rash *rubella, röda hund; compare* MEASLES, RUBEOLA

> COMMENT: German measles can cause stillbirth or malformation of an unborn baby if the mother catches the disease while pregnant. It is advisable that girls should catch the disease in childhood, or should be immunized against it

germicide ['dʒɜːmisaɪd] *adj. & subst.* (substance) which can kill germs *bakteriedödande (medel)*

germinal ['dʒɜːmɪn(ə)l] *adj.* (i) referring to a germ *bakterie-;* (ii) referring to an embryo *embryonal, grodd-;* **germinal epithelium** = outer layer of the ovary *embryonalepitel, äggstockens yttersta lager*

gerontologi ⇨ **geriatrics, gerontology**

gerontology [ˌdʒerɒn'tɒlədʒi] *subst.* study of the process of ageing and the diseases of old people *gerontologi, geriatri(k)*

gerontoxon ⇨ **arcus**

Gerstmann's syndrome ['gæːstmænz ˌsɪndrəʊm] *subst.* condition where a patient no longer recognises his body image, cannot tell the difference between left and right, cannot recognise his different fingers and is unable to write *Gerstmanns syndrom*

gestate [dʒe'steɪt] *vb.* to carry a baby in the womb from conception to birth *gå (vara) havande (med)*

gestation [dʒe'steɪʃ(ə)n] *or* **pregnancy** ['pregnənsi] *subst.* period (usually 266 days) from conception to birth, during which the baby develops in the mother's womb *gestation, graviditet, havandeskap, grossess*

> QUOTE evaluation of fetal age and weight has proved to be of value in the clinical management of pregnancy, particularly in high-risk gestations
> **Southern Medical Journal**

gestational diabetes [dʒe'steɪʃ(ə)n(ə)l ˌda(ɪ)ə'biːtiːz] *subst.* form of diabetes mellitus which develops in a pregnant woman *graviditetsdiabetes*

get [get] *vb.* **(a)** to become *bli;* **the muscles get flabby from lack of exercise; she got fat from eating too much; waiting lists for operations are getting longer (b)** (i) to make something happen *få, göra, åstadkomma;* (ii) to pay someone to do something *betala ngn för att göra ngt;* (iii) to persuade someone to do something *övertala ngn att göra ngt;* **he got the hospital to admit the patient as an emergency case; did you get the sister to fill in the form? he got the doctor to repeat the prescription; to have got to** = must *måste;* **you have got to be at the surgery before 9.30; he is leaving early because he has got to drive a long way; has she got to take the tablets every day? (c)** to catch (a disease) *få, ådra sig;* **I think I'm getting a cold; she can't go to work because she's got flu**

get along [ˌget ə'lɒŋ] *vb.* to manage *or* to work *klara sig, reda sig;* **we seem to get along quite well without any electricity**

get around [ˌget ə'raʊnd] *vb.* to move about *röra sig, förflytta sig;* **since she had the accident she gets around on two sticks**

get better [ˌget 'betə] *vb.* to become well again after being ill *bli bättre (frisk), tillfriskna;* **he was seriously ill, but seems to be getting better; her cold has got better; his flu has not got any better, so he will have to stay in bed**

get dressed [ˌget 'drest] *vb.* to put your clothes on *klä på sig;* **he got dressed quickly because he didn't want to be late for work; she was getting dressed when the phone rang; the patient has to be helped to get dressed**

get on [ˌget 'ɒn] *vb.* **(a)** to go into (a bus, etc.) *gå (stiga) på;* **we got on the bus at the post office; she got on her bike and rode away (b)** to become old *bli gammal;* **he's getting on and is quite deaf**

get on with [ˌget 'ɒn wɪð] **(a)** to be friendly with someone *komma bra överens med, trivas med;* **he gets on very well with everyone; I didn't get on with the boss (b)** to continue to do some work *fortsätta med;* **I must get on with the blood tests**

get over [ˌget 'əʊvə] *vb.* to become better after an illness *or* a shock *komma över, övervinna;* **he got over his cold; she never got over her mother's death**

get up [ˌget 'ʌp] *vb.* to stand up *resa sig (upp), ställa sig upp;* to get out of bed *gå upp,* *stiga upp;* **he got up from his chair and walked out of the room; at what time did you get up this morning?**

get well [ˌget ˈwel] *vb.* to become healthy again after being ill *bli bra (frisk), tillfriskna;* **we hope your mother will get well soon; get well card** = card sent to a person who is ill, with good wishes for a rapid recovery *krya-på-dig-kort*

GH [ˌdʒiːˈeɪtʃ] = GROWTH HORMONE

Ghon's focus [ˈgɒnz ˌfəʊkəs] *subst.* spot on the lung produced by the tuberculosis bacillus *slags fläck på lungan pga tbc*

GI [ˌdʒiːˈaɪ] = GASTROINTESTINAL **they diagnosed a GI disease; operation on a GI fistula**

giant [ˈdʒaɪənt] *subst.* very tall person *jätte;* **giant cell** = very large cell such as an osteoclast *or* megakaryocyte *jättecell;* **giant hives** = large flat white blisters caused by an allergic reaction *nässelfeber, nässelutslag, urticaria, stora vita blåsor pga allergi; see also* ARTERITIS, GIGANTISM

Giardia [dʒiːˈɑːdiə] *subst.* microscopic protozoan parasite in the intestine which causes giardiasis *Giardia lamblia (intestinalis)*

giardiasis [ˌdʒiːɑːˈdaɪəsɪs] *or* **lambliasis** [læmˈblaɪəsɪs] *subst.* disorder of the intestine caused by the parasite **Giardia lamblia,** usually with no symptoms, but in heavy infections the absorption of fat may be affected, causing diarrhoea *giardiasis*

gibbosity [gɪˈbɒsəti] *or* **gibbus** [ˈgɪbəs] *subst.* sharp angle in the curvature of the spine caused by the weakening of a vertebra by tuberculosis of the backbone *gibbus, puckel*

giddiness [ˈgɪdinəs] *subst.* condition in which someone feels that everything is turning around, and so cannot stand up *yrsel, svindel;* **he began to suffer attacks of giddiness** *see note at* LABYRINTH

giddy [ˈgɪdi] *adj.* feeling that everything is turning round *yr, vimmelkantig;* **she has had a giddy spell**

gift ⇨ **poison, venom**

gift- ⇨ **tox-, toxico-**

giftgas ⇨ **poisonous**

giftig ⇨ **poisonous, toxic, venomous**

giftstruma ⇨ **goitre, thyrotoxic, thyrotoxicosis, toxic**

gigantism [dʒaɪˈgæntɪz(ə)m] *subst.* condition in which the patient grows very tall, caused by excessive production of growth hormone by the pituitary gland *gigantism, jätteväxt*

gikt ⇨ **gout**

giktknöl ⇨ **tophus, urecchysis**

giljontinsax ⇨ **guillotine, tonsillotome**

Gilliam's operation [ˈgɪliəmz ˌɒpəˈreɪʃ(ə)n] *subst.* surgical operation to correct retroversion of the womb *slags operation för att korrigera bakåtböjning av livmodern*

gingiva [dʒɪnˈdʒaɪvə] *subst.* gum *or* soft tissue covering the part of the jaw which surrounds the teeth ⇨ *illustration* TOOTH *gingiva, tandköttet*

gingivalis [ˌdʒɪndʒɪˈvælɪs] *see* ENTAMOEBA

gingivectomy [ˌdʒɪndʒɪˈvektəmi] *subst.* surgical removal of excess gum tissue *gingivektomi*

gingivektomi ⇨ **gingivectomy**

gingivitis [ˌdʒɪndʒɪˈvaɪtɪs] *subst.* inflammation of the gums as a result of bacterial infection *gingivit, tandköttsinflammation;* **ulcerative** *or* **ulceromembranous gingivitis** = ulceration of the gums which can also affect the membrane of the mouth *Vincents angina, tonsillinflammation*

ginglymus [ˈdʒɪŋglɪməs] *subst.* hinge joint *or* joint (like the knee or elbow) which allows movement in two directions only *ginglymus, gångjärnsled, vinkelled, scharnerled*

ginglymus ⇨ **hinge joint**

gippy tummy [ˈdʒɪpi ˌtʌmi] *subst. informal* diarrhoea which affects people travelling in foreign countries as a result of eating unwashed fruit or drinking water which has not been boiled *slags turistdiarré*

gips ⇨ **plaster, cast**

girdle [ˈgɜːd(ə)l] *subst.* set of bones making a ring or arch *gördel;* **hip girdle** *or* **pelvic girdle** = the sacrum and the two hip bones to which the thigh bones are attached *bäckengördeln, bäckenringen;* **pectoral girdle** *or* **shoulder girdle** = the shoulder bones (scapulae and clavicles) to which the upper arm bones are attached *skuldergördeln*

Girdlestone's operation ['gɜːd(ə)lstəʊnz ˌɒpə'reɪʃ(ə)n] *subst.* surgical operation to relieve osteoarthritis of the hip *Girdlestones operation*

girl [gɜːl] *subst.* female child *flicka;* **she's only got a little girl; they have three children - two boys and a girl**

gisseldjur ➪ **flagellate**

givare ➪ **donor**

give [gɪv] *vb.* **(a)** to pass something to someone *ge;* **he was given a pain-killing injection; the surgeons have given him a new pacemaker (b)** to allow someone time *ge, förunna;* **the doctors have only given her two weeks to live** = the doctors say she will die in two weeks' time *läkarna har bara givit henne två veckor att leva* NOTE: **gives - giving - gave - has given**

give up [ˌgɪv 'ʌp] *vb.* not to do something any more *sluta upp med, avstå från;* **he was advised to give up smoking; she has given up eating chocolate**

glabella [glə'belə] *subst.* rounded area bone in the forehead between the eyebrows *glabella*

gladiolus [ˌglædi'əʊləs] *subst.* middle section of the sternum *gladiolus, mellersta delen av bröstbenet*

gland [glænd] *subst.* **(a)** organ in the body containing cells which secrete substances which act elsewhere (such as a hormone *or* sweat *or* saliva) *glandula, körtel;* **endocrine gland** = gland without a duct which produces hormones which are introduced directly into the bloodstream (such as pituitary gland, thyroid gland, the pancreas, the adrenals, the gonads, the thymus) *endokrin (inresekretorisk) körtel;* **exocrine gland** = gland with a duct down which its secretions pass to a particular part of the body (such as the liver, the sweat glands, the salivary glands) *exokrin körtel;* **adrenal glands** *or* **suprarenal glands** = two endocrine glands at the top of the kidneys which secrete cortisone, adrenaline and other hormones ➪ *illustration* KIDNEY *glandulae suprarenales, binjurarna;* **bulbourethral glands** *or* **Cowper's glands** = two glands at the base of the penis which secrete into the urethra *glandulae bulbourethrales, Cowpers körtlar;* **ceruminous glands** = glands which secrete earwax ➪ *illustration* EAR *glandulae ceruminose, öronvaxkörtlarna;* **lacrimal gland** *or* **tear gland** = gland which secretes tears *glandula lacrimalis, tårkörtel;* **mammary gland** = gland in female mammals which produces milk *glandula mammaria, bröstkörtel, mjölkkörtel;* **meibomian gland** = sebaceous gland on the edge of the eyelid which secretes the liquid which lubricates the eyelid *glandula tarsa, Meiboms körtel;* **parathyroid glands** = four glands in the neck near the thyroid gland, which secrete a hormone which regulates the level of calcium in blood plasma *glandulae parathyreoidae, bisköldkörtlarna;* **parotid gland** = one of the glands which produce saliva, situated in the neck behind the joint of the jaw ➪ *illustration* THROAT *(glandula) parotis, öronspottkörteln;* **pineal gland** *or* **pineal body** = small cone-shaped gland near the midbrain, which produces melatonin and is believed to be associated with Circadian rhythms ➪ *illustration* BRAIN *corpus pineale, epifysen, övre hjärnbihanget, tallkottkörteln;* **pituitary gland** *or* **hypophysis cerebri** = main endocrine gland, about the size of a pea, situated in the sphenoid bone below the hypothalamus, which secretes hormones which stimulate other glands ➪ *illustration* BRAIN *glandula pituitaria (hypophysis), hypophysis cerebri, hypofysen;* **salivary glands** = glands which secrete saliva *glandulae salivarae (salivales, salivares), spottkörtlarna, salivkörtlarna;* **sebaceous gland** = gland which secretes oil at the base of each hair follicle *glandula sebacea, talgkörtel;* **sublingual gland** = salivary gland under the tongue ➪ *illustration* THROAT *glandula sublingualis, undertungsspottkörteln;* **submandibular gland** = salivary gland in the lower jaw ➪ *illustration* THROAT *glandula submandibularis, underkäksspottkörteln;* **sweat gland** = gland which produces sweat, situated beneath the dermis and connected to the skin surface by a sweat duct *glandula sudorifera, svettkörtel;* **thymus gland** = endocrine gland in the front of the top of the thorax, behind the breastbone *t(h)ymus, brässen, halsbrässen;* **thyroid gland** = endocrine gland in the neck, which secretes a hormone which regulates the body's metabolism *glandula thyreoidea, tyreoidea, sköldkörteln;* **greater vestibular glands** *or* **Bartholin's glands** = two glands at the side of the entrance to the vagina, which secrete a lubricating substance *glandulae vestibularis majores, Bartholins körtlar* **(b) lymph** *or* **lymphatic glands** = glands situated in various points of the lymphatic system (especially under the armpits and in the groin) through which lymph passes *nodi lymphatici, lymfkörtlarna*

glanders ['glændəz] *subst.* bacterial disease of horses, which can be caught by humans, with symptoms of high fever and inflammation of the lymph nodes *rots; see also* FARCY

glandula ⇨ **gland**

glandular ['glændjʊlə] *adj.* referring to glands *glandulär*

glandular fever ['glændjʊlə ˌfi:və] *or* **infectious mononucleosis** [ɪnˌfekʃəs ˌmɒnəʊˌnju:kli'əʊsɪs] *subst.* infectious disease where the body has an excessive number of white blood cells *mononucleosis infectiosa, monocytos, mononukleos, körtelfeber*

> COMMENT: the symptoms include sore throat, fever and swelling of the lymph glands in the neck. Glandular fever is probably caused by the Epstein-Barr virus. The test for glandular fever is the Paul-Bunnell reaction

glandulär ⇨ **glandular**

glans [glænz] *or* **glans penis** [ˌglænz 'pi:nɪs] *subst.* bulb at the end of the penis ⇨ *illustration* UROGENITAL SYSTEM (male) *glans (penis), ollonet*

glas ⇨ **glass**

glasbrosk ⇨ **hyaline**

glaskroppen ⇨ **vitreous body**

glass [glɑ:s] *subst.* **(a)** material which you can see through, used to make windows *glas;* **the doors are made of glass; the specimen was kept in a glass jar** NOTE: no plural **some glass, a piece of glass (b)** thing to drink out of, usually made of glass *glas;* **she poured the mixture into a glass (c)** the contents of a glass *glas;* **he drinks a glass of milk every evening; you may drink a small glass of wine with your evening meal** NOTE: plural is **glasses** for (b) and (c)

glasses [glɑ:sɪz] *subst pl.* two pieces of glass or plastic, made into lenses, which are worn in front of the eyes to help the patient see better *glasögon;* **she was wearing dark glasses; he has glasses with gold frames; she needs glasses to read**

glasögon ⇨ **eyeglasses, glasses, spectacles**

glasögonbåge ⇨ **frame**

glatt muskel ⇨ **smooth**

glaucoma [glɔ:'kəʊmə] *subst.* condition of the eyes, caused by abnormally high pressure of fluid inside the eyeball, resulting in disturbances of vision and blindness *glaukom, grön starr*

glaukom ⇨ **glaucoma**

gleet [gli:t] *subst.* thin discharge from the vagina, penis, a wound or an ulcer *tunn avsöndring, tunn utsöndring*

glenohumeral [ˌgli:nəʊ'ju:mər(ə)l] *adj.* referring to both the glenoid cavity and the humerus *glenohumeral;* **glenohumeral joint =** shoulder joint *articulatio humeri, skulderleden, axelleden*

glenoid cavity ['gli:nɔɪd ˌkævəti] *or* **glenoid fossa** ['gli:nɔɪd ˌfɒsə] *subst.* socket in the shoulder blade into which the head of the humerus fits ⇨ *illustration* SHOULDER *cavitas glenoidalis*

glia ['gli:ə] *or* **neuroglia** [nju'rɒgliə] *subst.* connective tissue of the central nervous system, surrounding cell bodies, axons and dendrites *glia, neuroglia, nervlim*

gliaceller ⇨ **glial cells**

glial cells ['gli:əl ˌselz] *subst. pl.* cells in the glia *gliaceller, neurogliaceller*

glida ⇨ **slide**

glio- ['glaɪə(ʊ), ˌ--] *prefix* referring to brain tissue *glio-*

glioblastoma [ˌglaɪəʊblæ'stəʊmə] *or* **spongioblastoma** [ˌspʌndʒiəʊblæ'stəʊmə] *subst.* rapidly developing malignant brain tumour in the glial cells *glioblastom*

glioma [glaɪ'əʊmə] *subst.* any tumour of the glial tissue in the brain *or* spinal cord *gliom*

gliomyoma [ˌglaɪəʊmaɪ'əʊmə] *subst.* tumour of both the nerve and muscle tissue *tumör som utgår från både gliavävnad och muskelvävnad*

globin ['gləʊbɪn] *subst.* protein which combines with other substances to form compounds such as haemoglobin and myoglobin *globin*

globule ['glɒbju:l] *subst.* round drop (of fat) *liten fettpärl, liten fettkula*

globulin ['glɒbjʊlɪn] *subst.* class of protein, present in blood, including antibodies *globulin;* **gamma globulin** *or* **immunoglobulin**

= protein found in plasma, and which forms antibodies as protection against infection *gammaglobulin, immun(o)globulin*

globulinuria [ˌglɒbjulɪ'njʊəriə] *subst.* presence of globulins in the urine *globulinuri, proteinuri, "äggvita"*

globus ['gləʊbəs] *subst.* any ball-shaped part of the body *globus, klot, kula;* **globus hystericus** = lump in the throat, feeling of not being able to swallow caused by worry *or* embarrassment *globus hystericus*

glomangioma [gləˌmændʒi'əʊmə] *subst.* tumour of the skin at the ends of the fingers and toes *glomangiom*

glomerular [gləʊ'merʊlə] *adj.* referring to a glomerulus *glomerulär;* **glomerular capsules** *or* **Bowman's capsules** = expanded ends of a tubule in the kidney which surrounds the glomerular tuft *Bowmans kapslar;* **glomerular tuft** = group of blood vessels in the kidney which filter the blood *glomerulus (kapillärnystan)*

glomerulitis [gləʊˌmerʊ'laɪtɪs] *subst.* inflammation causing lesions of glomeruli in the kidney *glomerulit*

glomerulonefrit ⇨ **Bright's disease, glomerulonephritis**

glomerulonephritis [gləʊˌmerʊləʊnɪ'fraɪtis] *subst.* form of nephritis where the glomeruli in the kidneys are inflamed *glomerulonefrit*

glomerulus [gləʊ'merʊləs] *subst.* group of blood vessels which filter waste matter from the blood in a kidney *glomerulus, njurnystan*
NOTE: plural is **glomeruli**

gloss- ['glɒs, ˌglɒs, glɒs] *prefix* referring to the tongue *gloss(o)-, tung-*

glossa ['glɒsə] *subst.* the tongue *lingua, glossa, tungan*

glossectomy [glɒ'sektəmi] *subst.* surgical removal of the tongue *operativt avlägsnande av tungan*

Glossina [glɒ'saɪnə] *subst.* genus of African flies (such as the tsetse fly), which cause trypanosomiasis *Glossina*

glossitis [glɒ'saɪtɪs] *subst.* inflammation of the surface of the tongue *glossit*

glossodynia [ˌglɒsəʊ'dɪniə] *subst.* pain in the tongue *glossodyni, ont i tungan*

glossopharyngeal nerve [ˌglɒsəʊˌfær(ə)n'dʒiːəl ˌnɜːv] *subst.* ninth cranial nerve which controls the pharynx, the salivary glands and part of the tongue *nervus glossopharyngeus, tung- och svalgnerven, 9:e kranialnerven*

glossoplegia [ˌglɒsəʊ'pliːdʒə] *subst.* paralysis of the tongue *glossoplegi, tungförlamning*

glosögdhet ⇨ **exophthalmos**

glottis ['glɒtɪs] *subst.* opening in the larynx between the vocal cords, which forms the entrance to the main airway from the pharynx *glottis*

glove [glʌv] *subst.* piece of clothing which you wear on your hand *handske;* **the doctor was wearing rubber gloves** *or* **surgical gloves**

gluc- ['gluːk, ˌ-] *prefix* referring to glucose *gluk(o)-, glyk(o)-, glukos-, glykos-*

glucagon ['gluːkəgɒn] *subst.* hormone secreted by the islets of Langerhans in the pancreas, which increases the level of blood sugar by stimulating the breakdown of glycogen *glukagon*

glucocorticoid [ˌgluːkəʊ'kɔːtɪkɔɪd] *subst.* any corticosteroid which breaks down carbohydrates and fats for use by the body, produced by the adrenal cortex *glukokortikoid, glukokortikostereoid*

glucose ['gluːkəʊz] *or* **dextrose** ['dekstrəʊz] *subst.* simple sugar found in some fruit, but also broken down from white sugar or carbohydrate and absorbed into the body or secreted by the kidneys *glukos, dextros, druvsocker;* **blood-glucose level** = amount of glucose present in the blood *blodsockernivå, B-glukosnivå;* **the normal blood-glucose level stays at about 60 to 100 mg of glucose per 100 ml of blood; glucose tolerance test** = test for diabetes mellitus, where the patient eats glucose and his urine and blood are tested at regular intervals *glukosbelastning(sprov)*

COMMENT: combustion of glucose with oxygen to form carbon dioxide and water is the body's main source of energy

glucuronic acid [ˌgluːkju'rɒnɪk 'æsɪd] *subst.* acid formed by glucose and which acts on bilirubin *glukuronsyra*

glue [gluː] **1** *subst.* material which sticks things together *lim;* **glue ear** *or* **secretory otitis media** = condition where fluid forms behind the eardrum and causes deafness *otosalpingit, adhesiv otit, sekretorisk inflammation i mellanörat;* **glue-sniffing** = type of solvent abuse where a person is addicted to inhaling the toxic fumes given off by certain types of glue *sniffning (av lim)* **2** *vb.* to stick things together with glue *limma ihop*

glukagon ⇨ **glucagon**

glukokortikoid ⇨ **glucocorticoid**

glukokortikostereoid ⇨ **glucocorticoid**

glukos ⇨ **glucose**

glukosuri ⇨ **glycosuria**

glukuronsyra ⇨ **glucuronic acid**

glupsk ⇨ **greedy**

glutamic acid [glu:ˌtæmɪk 'æsɪd] *subst.* amino acid in protein *glutaminsyra*

glutaminase [glu:'tæmɪneɪz] *subst.* enzyme in the kidneys, which helps to break down glutamine *glutaminas*

glutamine ['glu:təmi:n] *subst.* amino acid in protein *glutamin*

glutaminsyra ⇨ **glutamic acid**

gluteal ['glu:tiəl] *adj.* referring to the buttocks *gluteal, sätes-;* **superior** *or* **inferior gluteal artery** = arteries supplying the buttocks *arteria glutaea superior resp. inferior;* **superior** *or* **inferior gluteal vein** = veins draining the buttocks *vena glutaea superior resp. inferior;* **gluteal muscles** = muscles in the buttocks *musculus gluteus maximus, medius resp. minimus, sätesmusklerna; see also* GLUTEUS

gluten ['glu:t(ə)n] *subst.* protein found in certain cereals, which makes a sticky paste when water is added *gluten;* **gluten enteropathy** *or* **coeliac disease** = (i) allergic disease (mainly affecting children) in which the lining of the intestine is sensitive to gluten, preventing the small intestine from digesting fat *celiaki, intestinal infantilism, sprue, malabsorption;* (ii) condition in adults where the villi in the intestine become smaller, and so reduce the surface which can absorb nutrients *glutenenteropati*

gluteus ['glu:tiəs] *subst.* one of three muscles in the buttocks, responsible for movements of the hip (the largest is the gluteus maximus, while gluteus medius and minimus are smaller) *musculus gluteus, sätesmuskel*

glyc- *prefix* referring to sugar *gluk(o)-, glyk(o)-, glukos-, glykos-*

glycaemia [glɪ'si:miə] *subst.* normal level of glucose found in the blood *normal blodsockernivå; see also* HYPOGLYCAEMIA, HYPERGLYCAEMIA

glycerin(e) ['glɪs(ə)rɪn] *or* **glycerol** ['glɪsərɒl] *subst.* colourless viscous sweet-tasting liquid present in all fats *glycerin, glycerol*

> COMMENT: synthetic glycerine is used in various medicinal preparations and also as a lubricant in toothpaste, cough medicines, etc. A mixture of glycerine and honey is useful to soothe a sore throat

glycine ['glaɪsi:n] *subst.* amino acid in protein *glycin, glykokoll*

glycocholic acid [ˌglaɪkəʊ'kɒlɪk 'æsɪd] *subst.* one of the bile acids *glykocholsyra, glykokolsyra*

glycogen ['glaɪkədʒ(ə)n] *subst.* type of starch, converted from glucose by the action of insulin, and stored in the liver as a source of energy *glykogen*

glycogenesis [ˌglaɪkəʊ'dʒenəsɪs] *subst.* process by which glucose is converted into glycogen in the liver *glykogenes*

glycogenolysis [ˌglaɪkəʊdʒə'nɒləsɪs] *subst.* process by which glycogen is broken down to form glucose *glykogenolys*

glycosuria [ˌglaɪkəʊ'sjʊəriə] *subst.* high level of sugar in the urine, a symptom of diabetes mellitus *glukosuri*

glykocholsyra ⇨ **glycocholic acid**

glykogen ⇨ **glycogen**

glykogenes ⇨ **glycogenesis**

glykogenolys ⇨ **glycogenolysis**

glykokoll ⇨ **glycine**

glykokolsyra ⇨ **glycocholic acid**

glömma ⇨ **forget**

glömsk ⇨ **forgetful**

glömska ⇨ **forgetfulness**

GMC [ˌdʒiːem'siː] = GENERAL MEDICAL COUNCIL

gnathoplasty ['næθəʊˌplæsti] *subst.* plastic surgery to correct a defect in the jaw *plastikoperation av käken*

gnetter ⇨ **nit**

gnida ⇨ **rub, chafe**

gnidning ⇨ **friction**

gnidningsljud ⇨ **friction**

gnugga ⇨ **rub**

goal [gəʊl] *subst.* that which is expected to be achieved by a certain treatment *mål*

goblet cell ['gɒblət ˌsel] *subst.* tube-shaped cell in the epithelium which secretes mucus *bägarcell*

GOC [ˌdʒiːəʊ'siː] = GENERAL OPTICAL COUNCIL

godartad ⇨ **benign, innocent**

godkänna ⇨ **approve**

go down [ˌgəʊ 'daʊn] *vb.* to become smaller *gå ner, sjunka, minska;* **when the blood sugar level goes down; the swelling has started to go down**

godta ⇨ **approve**

goitre ['gɔɪtə] *or US* **goiter** ['gɔɪtər] *subst.* excessive enlargement of the thyroid gland, seen as a swelling round the neck, caused by a lack of iodine *struma;* **exophthalmic goitre** *or* **Graves' disease** = form of goitre caused by hyperthyroidism, where the heart beats faster, the thyroid gland swells, the eyes protrude and the limbs tremble *tyreotoxikos, giftstruma, Basedows sjukdom, Graves sjukdom*

goitrogen ['gɔɪtrədʒ(ə)n] *subst.* substance which causes goitre *strumaframkallande*

gold [gəʊld] *subst.* soft yellow-coloured precious metal, used as a compound in various drugs, and sometimes as a filling for teeth *guld;* **gold injections** = injections of a solution containing gold, used to relieve rheumatoid arthritis *guldinjektioner* NOTE: the chemical symbol is **Au**

golden ['gəʊld(ə)n] *adj.* coloured like gold *gyllene;* **golden eye ointment** = yellow ointment, made of an oxide of mercury, used to treat inflammation of the eyelids *slags gul salva använd vid ögonlocksinflammation*

Golgi apparatus ['gɒldʒi ˌæpəˌreɪtəs] *subst.* folded membranous structure inside the cell cytoplasm which stores and transports enzymes and hormones *Golgiapparaten, Golgikomplexet*

Golgi cell ['gɒldʒi ˌsel] *subst.* type of nerve cell in the central nervous system, either with long axons (Golgi type 1) or without axons (Golgi type 2) *slags motoriska och sensoriska nervceller*

gom- ⇨ **palato-, uran-**

gombenet ⇨ **palatine**

gombågarna ⇨ **palatine**

gomförlamning ⇨ **palatoplegia**

gomklyvning ⇨ **cleft palate**

gommandel ⇨ **palatine**

gommen ⇨ **palate, roof**

gomphosis [gɒm'fəʊsɪs] *subst.* joint which cannot move, like a tooth in a jaw *gomphosis*

gomspalt ⇨ **cleft palate**

gomspenen ⇨ **uvula**

gomtonsill ⇨ **palatine**

gonad ['gəʊnæd] *subst.* sex gland which produces gametes (the testicles produce spermatozoa in males, and the ovaries produce ova in females) and also sex hormones *gonad, könskörtel*

gonadotrophic hormones [ˌgəʊnədəʊ'trɒfɪk ˌhɔːməʊnz] *subst pl.* hormones (the follicle-stimulating hormone (FSH) and the luteinizing hormone (LH)) produced by the anterior pituitary gland which have an effect on the ovaries in females and on the testes in males *gonadotropa hormoner*

gonadotrophin [ˌgəʊnədəʊ'trəʊfɪn] *subst.* any of a group of hormones produced by the pituitary gland which stimulates the sex glands at puberty *gonadotropin; see also* CHORIONIC

gonadotropin ⇨ **gonadotrophin**

gonagra [gɒ'nægrə] *subst.* form of gout which occurs in the knees *gikt i knät*

goni- ['gəʊni, ˌ--] *prefix* meaning angle *goni(o)-*

goniopuncture [ˌgəʊniəʊ'pʌŋtʃə] *subst.* surgical operation for draining fluid from the eyes of a patient who has glaucoma *slags operation för att minska på trycket vid glaukom*

gonioscope ['gəʊniəskəʊp] *subst.* lens for measuring the angle of the front part of the eye *gonioskop, hornhinnemikroskop*

gonioskop ⇨ **gonioscope**

goniotomy [ˌgəʊni'ɒtəmi] *or* **trabeculotomy** [trəˌbekju'lɒtəmi] *subst.* surgical operation to treat glaucoma by cutting Schlemm's canal *goniotomi*

gonococcal [ˌgɒnə(ʊ)'kɒk(ə)l] *adj.* referring to gonococcus *gonokock-*

gonococcus [ˌgɒnə(ʊ)'kɒkəs] *subst.* type of bacterium, **Neisseria gonorrhoea,** which produces gonorrhoea *gonokock* NOTE: plural is **gonococci**

gonocyte ['gɒnə(ʊ)saɪt] *subst.* germ cell *or* cell which is able to develop into a spermatozoon or an ovum *gonocyt*

gonokock ⇨ **gonococcus**

gonokock- ⇨ **gonococcal**

gonorré ⇨ **gonorrhoea, blennorrhagia, blennorrhoea**

gonorré- ⇨ **gonorrhoeal**

gonorrhoea [ˌgɒnə'rɪə] *subst.* sexually transmitted disease, which produces painful irritation of the mucous membrane and a watery discharge from the vagina or penis *gonorré*

gonorrhoeal [ˌgɒnə'rɪəl] *adj.* referring to gonorrhoea *gonorré-*

gonorroisk uretrit ⇨ **specific**

gonosom ⇨ **sex chromosome**

Goodpasture's syndrome [gʊd'pɑːstʃəz ˌsɪndrəʊm] *subst.* rare lung disease where the patient coughs up blood, is anaemic, and which may result in kidney failure *Goodpastures syndrom*

goose flesh ['guːz fleʃ] *or* **goose pimples** ['guːz ˌpɪmp(ə)lz] *or* **cutis anserina** ['kjuːtɪs ˌænsə'raɪnə] *subst.* reaction of the skin to being cold *or* frightened, where the skin forms many little bumps *cutis anserina, dermatospasm, horripilatio, gåshud, hönshud*

Gordh needle ['gɔːd ˌniːd(ə)l] *subst.* needle with a bag attached, so that several injections can be made one after the other *slags nål med vilken flera injektioner kan ges i följd*

gorget ['gɔːdʒɪt] *subst.* surgical instrument used to remove stones from the bladder *slags slev för att ta ut stenar från gallblåsan med*

gouge [gaʊdʒ] *subst.* surgical instrument like a chisel used to cut bone *gougetång, hålmejsel, skåljärn*

gougetång ⇨ **gouge, rongeur**

goundou ['guːnduː] *subst.* condition caused by yaws, in which growths form on either side of the nose *utväxter på båda sidor av näsan pga framboesi*

gout [gaʊt] *or* **podagra** [pɒ'dægrə] *subst.* disease in which abnormal quantities of uric acid are produced and precipitated as crystals in the cartilage round joints *arthritis urica, podagra, gikt*

> COMMENT: formerly associated with drinking strong wines such as port, but now believed to arise in three ways: excess uric acid in the diet, excess uric acid synthesized by the body and defective secretion of uric acid. It is likely that both overproduction and defective excretion are due to inherited biochemical abnormalities. Excess intake of alcohol can provoke an attack by interfering with the excretion of uric acid

gown [gaʊn] *subst.* long robe worn over other clothes to protect them *rock, skjorta;* **the surgeons were wearing green gowns; the patient lay on his bed in a theatre gown, ready to go to the operating theatre**

GP [ˌdʒiː'piː] *subst.* general practitioner *allmänpraktiker, allmänpraktiserande läkare* NOTE: plural is **GPs**

GPI [ˌdʒiːpiː'aɪ] = GENERAL PARALYSIS OF THE INSANE

gr = GRAIN

Graafian follicle ['græfiən ˌfɒlɪk(ə)l] *see* FOLLICLE

gracil ⇨ **delicate**

gracilis ['greɪsɪlɪs] *subst.* thin muscle running down the inside of the leg from the top of the leg down to the top of the tibia *musculus gracilis, slanka lårmuskeln*

grad ➪ **degree**

graderad ➪ **graduated**

gradtal ➪ **reading**

graduate ['grædʒuət; 'grædʒueɪt] **1** *subst.* person who has completed a university or polytechnic course and has a degree *akademiker, person med akademisk examen;* **she is a graduate from the School of Tropical Medicine 2** *vb.* to finish a course of study at a university or polytechnic and have a degree *avlägga (ta) akademisk examen, bli legitimerad;* **he graduated in Pharmacy last year**

graduated ['grædʒueɪtɪd] *adj.* with marks showing various degrees *or* levels *graderad, mät-;* **a graduated measuring jar**

Graefe's knife ['greɪfi:z ˌnaɪf] *subst.* sharp knife used in operations on cataracts *slags kniv använd vid operation av grå starr*

-graf ➪ **-graph**

-grafi ➪ **-graphy**

graft [grɑ:ft] **1** *subst.* (i) act of transplanting an organ (heart *or* lung *or* kidney) or tissue (bone *or* skin) to replace an organ or tissue which is not functioning or diseased *transplantation;* (ii) organ *or* tissue which is transplanted *graft, transplantat;* **she had to have a skin graft; the corneal graft was successful; the patient was given drugs to prevent the graft being rejected; graft versus host disease** = condition which develops when cells from the grafted tissue react against the patient's own tissue, causing skin disorders *graft-kontra-host-reaktion, antivärdreaktion; see also* AUTOGRAFT, HOMOGRAFT **2** *vb.* to take a healthy organ *or* tissue and transplant it into a patient in place of diseased or defective organ or tissue *transplantera;* **the surgeons grafted a new section of bone at the side of the skull**

grain [greɪn] *subst.* measure of weight equal to .0648 grams *gran*

NOTE: when used with numbers, **grain** is usually written **gr**

gram [græm] measure of weight *gram;* **a thousand grams make one kilogram; I need 5 g of morphine**

NOTE: when used with numbers, **gram** is usually written **g: 50 g** say "fifty grams"

-gram [græm] *suffix* meaning a record in the form of a picture *-gram;* **cardiogram** = X-ray picture of the heart *elektrokardiogram, kardiogram*

gramfärgning ➪ **Gram's stain**

Gram's stain ['græmz ˌsteɪn] *subst.* method of staining bacteria so that they can be identified *Grams färgning, gramfärgning;* **Gram-positive bacterium** = bacterium which retains the first dye and appears blue-black when viewed under the microscope *grampositiv bakterie;* **Gram-negative bacterium** = bacterium which takes up the red counterstain, after the alcohol has washed out the first violet dye *gramnegativ bakterie*

> COMMENT: the tissue sample is first stained with a violet dye, treated with alcohol, and then counterstained with a red dye

gran ➪ **grain**

grandchild ['græntʃaɪ(ə)ld] *subst.* child of a son or daughter *barnbarn* NOTE: plural **grandchildren**

granddaughter ['grænˌdɔ:tə] *subst.* daughter of a son or daughter *sondotter, dotterdotter*

grandes ['grændɪs] *see* MULTIPARA

grandfather ['græn(d)ˌfɑ:ðə] *subst.* father of a mother or father *morfar, farfar*

grand mal [ˌgrɑ: 'mal] *or* **major epilepsy** [ˌmeɪdʒər 'epɪlepsi] *subst.* type of epilepsy, in which the patient becomes unconscious and falls down, while the muscles become stiff and twitch violently *grand mal, epilepsia majora*

grandmother ['grænˌmʌðə] *subst.* mother of a mother of father *farmor, mormor*

grandparents ['græn(d)ˌpeər(ə)nts] *subst pl.* parents of a mother or father *morföräldrar, farföräldrar*

grandson ['grænsʌn] *subst.* son of a son or daughter *sonson, dotterson*

granska ➪ **examine, inspect, study**

granskning ➪ **examination, inspection, study**

granular ['grænjʊlə] *adj.* like grains *granulär, granulös, granulerad, kornig;* **granular cast** = cast composed of cells filled with protein and fatty granules *cylinder, slags* *avgjutning av fett- och proteinkorn;* **granular leucocytes** *or* **granulocytes** = leucocytes with granules (basophils, eosinophils, neutrophils) *granulocyter;* **nongranular leucocytes** = leucocytes without granules (lymphocytes, monocytes) *icke-granulerade leukocyter*

granulation [ˌgrænjuˈleɪʃ(ə)n] *subst.* formation of rough red tissue on the surface of a wound or site of infection, the first stage in the healing process *granulation;* **granulation tissue** *or* **granulations** = soft tissue, consisting mainly of tiny blood vessels and fibres, which forms over a wound *granulationer, granulationsvävnad*

granulationer ⇨ **granulation**

granulationsvävnad ⇨ **granulation, granuloma, proud flesh**

granule [ˈgrænjuːl] *subst.* small particle *or* grain *granulum, litet korn;* **Nissl granules** *or* **Nissl bodies** = coarse granules found in the cytoplasm of the cell bodies of a nerve cell *Nisslpartiklar, Nisslsubstans*

granulerad ⇨ **granular**

granulocyt ⇨ **granular, granulocyte**

granulocyte [ˈgrænjuːləsaɪt] *subst.* type of leucocyte *or* white blood cell which contains granules (such as basophils, eosinophils and neutrophils) *granulocyt*

granulocytopenia [ˌgrænjuːləˌsaɪtəʊˈpiːniə] *subst.* usually fatal disease caused by the lowering of the number of granulocytes in the blood due to a defect in the bone marrow *granulo(cyto)peni*

granuloma [ˌgrænjuˈləʊmə] *subst.* mass of granulation tissue which forms at the site of bacterial infections *granulom, granulationsvävnad;* **granuloma inguinale** = tropical venereal disease affecting the anus and genitals in which the skin becomes covered with ulcers *granuloma inguinale (venereum), ljumskgranulom*
NOTE: plural is **granulomata** or **granulomas**

granulomatosis [ˌgrænjuˌləʊməˈtəʊsɪs] *subst.* chronic inflammation leading to the formation of nodules *granulomatos;* **Wegener's granulomatosis** = disease of the connective tissue in which the nasal passages and lungs are inflamed and ulcerated *granulomatosis Wegener, Wegeners granulomatos*

granulopoiesis [ˌgrænjuːləʊpɔɪˈiːsɪs] *subst.* normal production of granulocytes in the bone marrow *granulopo(i)es, granulocytopo(i)es*

granulum ⇨ **granule**

granulär ⇨ **granular**

granulös ⇨ **granular**

graph [grɑːf, græf] *subst.* diagram which shows the relationship between quantities as a line *grafisk framställning, diagram, kurva;* **temperature graph** = graph showing how a patient's temperature rises and falls *temperaturkurva*

-graph [grɑːf, græf] *suffix* meaning a machine which records as pictures *-graf*

-grapher [grəfə] *suffix* meaning a technician who operates a machine which records *person som sköter registreringsapparat;* **radiographer** = technician who operates an X-ray machine *röntgenassistent*

-graphy [grəfi] *suffix* meaning the technique of study through pictures *-grafi;* **radiography** = X-ray examination of part of the body *radiografi, röntgenografi, röntgenfotografering*

grattage [græˈtɑːʒ] *subst.* scraping the surface of an ulcer which is healing slowly, in order to make it heal more quickly *skrapning av sår som läker långsamt*

grav ⇨ **grave**

grave [greɪv] *subst.* place where a dead person is buried *grav;* **his grave is covered with flowers**

gravel [ˈgræv(ə)l] *subst.* small stones which pass from the kidney to the urinary system, causing pain in the ureter *grus, njurgrus*

Graves' disease [ˈgreɪvz dɪˌziːz] *or* **exophthalmic goitre** [ˌeksɒfˈθælmɪk ˌgɔɪtə] = THYROTOXICOSIS

gravid [ˈgrævɪd] *adj.* pregnant *gravid;* **hyperemesis gravidarum** = vomiting in pregnancy *hyperemesis gravidarum, graviditetskräkningar;* **gravides multiparae** = women who have given birth to at least four live babies *multiparae, mångföderskor*

gravid, bli ⇨ **conceive**

graviditet ⇨ **pregnancy, cyesis, gestation**

graviditetsdiabetes ⇨ **gestational diabetes**

graviditetshormon ⇨ **chorionic**

graviditetskräkningar ⇨ **gravid**

graviditetsperiod ⇨ **term**

graviditetstest ⇨ **pregnancy**

graviditetstid ⇨ **pregnancy**

graviditetstoxikos ⇨ **toxaemia**

Grawitz tumour ['grɑːvɪts ˌtjuːmə] *subst.* malignant tumour in kidney cells *Grawitz tumör*

gray [greɪ] **1** *US* = GREY **2** *subst.* unit of measurement of absorbed radiation *gray, Gy*

graze [greɪz] **1** *subst.* scrape on the skin surface, making some blood flow *skråma, skrubbsår* **2** *vb.* to scrape the skin surface *skrapa (av), skava (av), skrubba*

great [greɪt] *adj.* large *stor;* **great cerebral vein** = median vein draining the choroid plexuses of the lateral and third ventricles *vena cerebri magna;* **great toe** = big toe *or* largest of the five toes, near the inside of the foot *hallux, stortån*
NOTE: **great - greater - greatest**

greater ['greɪtə] *adj.* larger *större;* **greater curvature** = convex line of the stomach *curvatura ventriculi major, stora magsäckskrökningen; see also* OMENTUM, TROCHANTER

greatly ['greɪtli] *adv.* very much *mycket, i hög grad*

greedy ['griːdi] *adj.* always wanting to eat a lot of food *glupsk*
NOTE: **greedy - greedier - greediest**

green [griːn] *adj. & subst.* of a colour like the colour of leaves *grön;* **when he saw the blood he turned green**
NOTE: **green - greener - greenest**

green monkey disease [ˌgriːn 'mʌŋki dɪˌziːz] = MARBURG DISEASE

greenstick fracture ['griːnstɪk ˌfræktʃə] *subst.* type of fracture occurring in children, where a long bone bends, but is not completely broken *greenstícksfraktur, inkomplett (ofullständig) fraktur, infraktion, knickbrott*

greensticksfraktur ⇨ **greenstick fracture**

gren ⇨ **branch, ramus**

grenblock ⇨ **bundle**

grenen ⇨ **crotch**

grey [greɪ] *or US* **gray** [greɪ] *adj. & subst.* of a colour between black and white *grå;* **his hair is quite grey; a grey-haired man; grey commissure** = part of the grey matter nearest to the central canal of the spinal cord, where axons cross over each other *grå kommissur;* **grey matter** = nervous tissue of a dark grey colour, formed of cell bodies and occurring in the central nervous system *substantia grisea, grå substans*

> COMMENT: in the brain, grey matter encloses the white matter, but in the spinal cord, white matter encloses grey matter

griffelliknande ⇨ **styloid**

Griffith's types ['grɪfɪθs ˌtaɪps] *subst.* various types of haemolytic streptococci, classified according to the antigens present in them *olika typer av hemolytiska streptokocker*

grinig ⇨ **fretful**

gripe [graɪp] *subst.* pains in the abdomen *kolik, magknip;* **gripe water** = solution of glucose and alcohol, used to relieve gripe in babies *lösning av druvsocker och alkohol (som förr gavs till spädbarn med kolik)*

grippe [grɪp, griːp] *subst.* influenza *influensa*

gristle ['grɪs(ə)l] *subst.* cartilage *cartilago, brosk*

grocer ['grəʊsə] *subst.* person who sells sugar, butter, tins of food, etc. *specerihandlare*

grocer's itch ['grəʊsəz ˌɪtʃ] *subst.* form of dermatitis on the hands caused by handling flour and sugar *slags hudutslag pga arbete med mjöl och socker*

grodd ⇨ **germ**

groddblad ⇨ **germ**

groddbladet, inre ⇨ **endoderm**

groddbladet, yttre ⇨ **ectoderm**

groddcell ⇨ **blastocyst**

groin [grɔɪn] *subst.* junction at each side of the body where the lower abdomen joins the top of the thighs *inguen, ljumsken;* **he had a dull pain in his groin**
NOTE: for other terms referring to the groin, see **inguinal**

grommet ['grɒmɪt, 'grʌmɪt] *subst.* tube which can be passed from the external auditory meatus into the middle ear *slags rör som kan införas i mellanörat*

groove [gru:v] *subst.* long shallow depression in a surface *sulcus, fåra;* **atrioventricular groove** = groove round the outside of the heart, showing the division between the atria and the ventricles *fåra på hjärtats utsida som visar gränsen mellan förmaken och kamrarna*

grop ⇨ **fossa, lacuna, pit**

gropig ⇨ **pitted**

gross anatomy [ˌgrəʊs ə'nætəmi] *subst.* study of the structure of the body which can be seen without the use of a microscope *makroskopisk anatomi*

grossess ⇨ **gestation, pregnancy**

ground [graʊnd] *subst.* **(a)** soil *or* earth *jord* **(b)** surface of the earth *mark, grund*

ground substance ['graʊnd ˌsʌbstəns] *or* **matrix** ['meɪtrɪks] *subst.* amorphous mass of cells forming the basis of connective tissue *matrix, modervävnad*

group [gru:p] **1** *subst.* **(a)** several people *or* animals *or* things which are all close together *grupp;* **a group of patients were waiting in the surgery; group practice** = practice where several doctors *or* dentists share the same office building and support services *ung. läkargrupp med gemensam praktik;* **group therapy** = type of psychotherapy where a group of people with the same disorder meet together with a therapist to discuss their condition and try to help each other *gruppterapi* **(b)** way of putting similar things together *grupp;* **blood group** = type of blood *blodgrupp;* **age group** = all people of a certain age *åldersgrupp* **2** *vb.* to bring together in a group *gruppera, ordna (föra samman, indela) i grupper;* **the drugs are grouped under the heading "antibiotics"; blood grouping** = classifying patients according to their blood groups *blodgruppering, blodgruppsbestämning*

grov ⇨ **coarse**

grovtarmen ⇨ **colon, large intestine**

grov tremor ⇨ **tremor**

grow [grəʊ] *vb.* **(a)** to become taller *or* bigger *växa;* **your son has grown since I last saw him; he grew three centimetres in one year** **(b)** to become *bli;* **it's growing colder at night now; she grew weak with hunger**
NOTE: **grows - growing - grew - grown**

growing pains ['grəʊɪŋ peɪnz] *subst. pl.* pains associated with adolescence, which can be a form of rheumatic fever *växtvärk*

grown-up ['grəʊnʌp] *subst.* adult *vuxen;* **there are three grown-ups and ten children**

growth [grəʊθ] *subst.* **(a)** increase in size *växt, tillväxt;* **the disease stunts children's growth; the growth in the population since 1960; growth factor** = chemical substance produced in the body which encourages a type of cell (such as a blood cell) to grow *tillväxtfaktor;* **growth hormone (GH)** *or* **somatotrophin** = hormone secreted by the pituitary gland during deep sleep, which stimulates growth of the long bones and protein synthesis *somatotropin, STH, (human) growth hormone, GH, HGH, tillväxthormon* **(b)** lump of tissue which is not natural *or* a cyst *or* a tumour *växt, utväxt, svulst;* **the doctor found she had a cancerous growth on the left breast; he had an operation to remove a small growth from his chin** NOTE: no plural for (a)

grumbling appendix ['grʌmblɪŋ əˌpendɪks] *subst. informal* chronic appendicitis *or* condition where the vermiform appendix is always slightly inflamed *kronisk (recidiverande) appendicit (blindtarmsinflammation)*

grumlig ⇨ **cloudy, opaque**

grumling ⇨ **cloud, opacity**

grundbeståndsdel ⇨ **base, basis**

grundfärg ⇨ **primary**

grundläggande ⇨ **basic**

grundsats ⇨ **principle**

grundval ⇨ **basis**

grundämne ⇨ **element**

grupp ⇨ **group**

gruppterapi ⇨ **group**

grus ⇨ **gravel**

gruvarbetare ⇨ **miner**

grå ⇨ **grey**

gråhårighet ⇨ **canities**

gråta ⇨ **cry**

gräns(värde) ⇨ **limit**

grön ⇨ **green**

grönblindhet ⇨ **deuteranopia**

grötomslag ⇨ **poultice**

GU [ˌdʒiːˈjuː] = GASTRIC ULCER, GENITOURINARY

guanine [ˈgwɑːniːn] *subst.* one of the nitrogen-containing bases in DNA *guanin*

gubernaculum [ˌguːbəˈnækjʊləm] *subst.* fibrous tissue connecting the testes in a fetus (the gonads) to the groin *gubernaculum*

guide [gaɪd] **1** *subst.* person *or* book which shows you how to do something *or* what to do *guide, rådgivare, handbok;* **read this guide to services offered by the local authority; the council has produced a guide for expectant mothers 2** *vb.* to show someone where to go *or* how to do something *ge råd till, visa, (väg)leda*

guide dog [ˈgaɪd dɒg] *subst.* dog which shows a blind person where to go *ledarhund*

Guillain-Barré syndrome [giːˌjænbɑːˈreɪ ˌsɪndrəʊm] *subst.* nervous disorder, in which after a non-specific infection, demyelination of the spinal roots and peripheral nerves takes place, leading to generalized weakness and sometimes respiratory paralysis *Guillain-Barrés syndrom*

guillotine [ˈgɪlətiːn] *subst.* surgical instrument for cutting out tonsils *tonsillotom, giljontinsax*

guineamask ⇨ **Dracunculus**

guinea worm [ˈgɪni wɜːm] = DRACUNCULUS

gul ⇨ **yellow**

gul- ⇨ **xanth-**

gula febern ⇨ **yellow fever**

gula fläcken ⇨ **macula**

guld ⇨ **gold**

gulesäcken ⇨ **vitelline sac**

gulfärgning ⇨ **xanthochromia**

gulkropp ⇨ **luteum**

gullet [ˈgʌlɪt] *or* **oesophagus** [iːˈsɒfəgəs] *subst.* tube down which food and drink passes from the mouth to the stomach *oesophagus, esofagus, matstrupen;* **she had a piece of bread stuck in her gullet**

gulsot ⇨ **acholuric jaundice, icterus**

gum [gʌm] *or* **gingiva** [dʒɪnˈdʒaɪvə] *subst.* part of the mouth, the soft epithelial tissue covering the part of the jaw which surrounds the teeth *gingiva, tandköttet;* **his gums are red and inflamed; a build-up of tartar can lead to gum disease**

gumboil [ˈgʌmbɔɪl] *subst.* abscess on the gum near a tooth *tandböld*
NOTE: for other terms referring to the gums see words beginning with **gingiv-, ul(o)-**

gumma [ˈgʌmə] *subst.* abscess of dead tissue and overgrown scar tissue, which develops in the later stages of syphilis *gumma, syfilom, syfilissvulst*

gummiduk ⇨ **rubber**

gummituta ⇨ **Politzer bag**

gurgelvatten ⇨ **gargle**

gustation [gʌˈsteɪʃ(ə)n] *subst.* act of tasting *smak, avsmakning*

gustatorisk ⇨ **gustatory**

gustatory [ˈgʌstət(ə)ri] *subst.* referring to the sense of taste *gustatorisk, smak-*

gut [gʌt] *subst.* **(a)** *(also informal)* **guts =** digestive tract *or* alimentary canal *or* the intestines, the tubular organ for the digestion and absorption of food *inälvorna, tarmarna, "magen";* **he complained of having a pain in his gut** *or* **he said he had gut pain (b)** type of thread, made from the intestines of sheep, used to sew up internal incisions *catgut, katgut*

Guthrie test [ˈgʌθri ˌtest] *subst.* test used on babies to detect the presence of phenylketonuria *Guthrietest*

gutta [ˈgʌtə] *subst.* drop of liquid (as used in treatment of the eyes) *gutta, droppe*
NOTE: plural is **guttae**

gutter splint [ˈgʌtə splɪnt] *subst.* shaped container in which a broken limb can rest without being completely surrounded *slags stöd för brutet ben el. bruten arm*

Gy ⇨ **gray**

gyllene ⇨ **golden**

gymnastik ⇨ **physical**

gyn- [ˌgaɪn, dʒɪn, dʒaɪn] *prefix* referring to (i) woman *gyn(eko)-, kvinno-;* (ii) the female reproductive system *gyn(eko)-*

gynaecological [ˌgaɪnɪkə'lɒdʒɪk(ə)l] *adj.* referring to the treatment of diseases of women *gynekologisk*

gynaecologist [ˌgaɪnɪ'kɒlədʒɪst] *subst.* doctor who specializes in the treatment of diseases of women *gynekolog*

gynaecology [ˌgaɪnɪ'kɒlədʒi] *subst.* study of female sex organs and the treatment of diseases of women in general *gynekologi*

gynaecomastia [ˌgaɪnɪkə'mæstiə] *subst.* abnormal development of breasts in a male *gynekomasti*
NOTE: words beginning with **gynae-** are spelled **gyne-** in US English

gynekolog ⇨ **gynaecologist**

gynekologi ⇨ **gynaecology**

gynekologisk ⇨ **gynaecological**

gynekologläge ⇨ **lithotomy**

gynekomasti ⇨ **gynaecomastia**

gynna ⇨ **promote**

gyrus ['dʒaɪərəs] *subst.* raised part of the cerebral cortex between the sulci *gyrus, vindel, hjärnvindling;* **postcentral gyrus** sensory area of the cerebral cortex, which receives impulses from receptor cells and senses pain, heat, touch, etc. *gyrus postcentralis, bakre hjärnvindlingen;* **precentral gyrus** motor area of the cerebral cortex *gyrus precentralis, främre hjärnvindlingen*
NOTE: plural is **gyri**

gyrus ⇨ **convolution**

gå ⇨ **walk**

gå ned ⇨ **subside**

gång ⇨ **canal, channel, duct, meatus, passage; gait**

gångjärnsled ⇨ **ginglymus, hinge joint**

gångsvårighet ⇨ **dysbasia**

gåsbröst ⇨ **pigeon chest**

gåshud ⇨ **goose flesh**

gå upp ⇨ **rise**

gälficka ⇨ **pharyngeal**

gälgångscysta ⇨ **branchial cyst**

gälgångsfistel ⇨ **branchial cyst**

gälla ⇨ **apply, involve**

gälspringan ⇨ **branchial pouch**

gäspa ⇨ **yawn**

gäspning ⇨ **yawn**

gördel ⇨ **girdle**

Hh

H *chemical symbol for* hydrogen *H, väte*

HA [ˌeɪtʃ'eɪ] = HEALTH AUTHORITY

habit ['hæbɪt] *subst.* **(a)** action which is an automatic response to a stimulus *automatisk respons* **(b)** regular way of doing something *habitus, vana;* **he got into the habit of swimming every day before breakfast; she's got out of the habit of taking any exercise; from force of habit** = because you do it regularly *av gammal vana;* **I wake up at 6 o'clock from force of habit**

habit-forming ['hæbɪtˌfɔːmɪŋ] *adj.* which makes someone addicted *or* which makes someone get into the habit of taking it *vanebildande;* **habit-forming drugs** = drugs which are addictive *vanebildande läkemedel, narkotika*

habitual [hə'bɪtʃu(ə)l] *adj.* which is done frequently *or* as a matter of habit *habituell;* **habitual abortion** = condition where a woman has abortions with successive pregnancies *abortus habitualis, habituell abort*

habituation [həˌbɪtʃu'eɪʃ(ə)n] *subst.* being psychologically but not physically addicted to *or* dependent on (a drug *or* alcohol, etc.) *psykologiskt beroende, tillvänjning;* **his habituation to nicotine**

habituell ⇨ **habitual**

habituell abort ⇨ **recurrent**

habitus ['hæbɪtəs] *subst.* general physical appearance of the person (including build and posture) *habitus, hållning, yttre kroppsbeskaffenhet*

hack ⇨ **nick, slash**

haem [hi:m] *subst.* molecule containing iron which binds proteins to form haemoproteins such as haemoglobin and myoglobin *hem*

haem- ['hi:m, ˌ-, 'hem, ˌ-] *or* **hem-** ['hi:m, ˌ-, 'hem, ˌ-] *prefix* referring to blood *haem(o)-, hem(o)-, häm(o)-, blod-* NOTE: words beginning with the prefix **haem-** are written **hem-** in US English

haemangioma [hɪˌmændʒɪ'əʊmə] *subst.* benign tumour which forms in blood vessels and appears on the skin as a birthmark *hemangiom;* **cavernous haemangioma** = tumour in connective tissue with wide spaces which contain blood *kavernöst hemangiom*

haemarthrosis [ˌhemɑ:'θrəʊsɪs] *subst.* pain and swelling caused by blood getting into a joint *hemart(h)ros*

haematemesis [ˌhemɑ:'teməsɪs] *subst.* vomiting of blood (usually because of internal bleeding) *hematemes, blodkräkning*

haematin ['hemətɪn] *subst.* substance which forms from haemoglobin when bleeding takes place *hematin*

haematinic [ˌhemə'tɪnɪk] *subst.* drug, such as an iron compound, which increases haemoglobin in blood, used to treat anaemia *slags läkemedel mot blodbrist*

haematocoele ['hi:mətəʊsi:l] *subst.* swelling caused by blood getting into an internal cavity *hematocele, blodbråck*

haematocolpos [ˌhi:mətəʊ'kɒlpəs] *subst.* condition where the vagina is filled with blood at menstruation because the hymen has no opening *hematokolpos*

haematocrit ['hi:mətəʊkrɪt, hɪ'mætəkrɪt] *subst.* (i) volume of red blood cells in a patient's blood, shown as a percentage of the total blood volume *erytrocytvolymfraktion, EVF, hematokrit;* (ii) instrument for measuring haematocrit *hematokritcentrifug*

haematocyst ['hi:mətəʊsɪst] *subst.* cyst which contains blood *hematocystis, blodfylld cysta*

haematogenous [ˌhi:mə'tɒdʒ(ə)nəs] *adj.* (i) which produces blood *blodbildande;* (ii) which is produced by blood *hem(at)ogen*

haematological [ˌhi:mətəʊ'lɒdʒɪk(ə)l] *adj.* referring to haematology *hematologisk*

haematologist [ˌhi:mə'tɒlədʒɪst] *subst.* doctor who specializes in haematology *hematolog*

haematology [ˌhi:mə'tɒlədʒi] *subst.* scientific study of blood, its formation and its diseases *hematologi*

haematoma [ˌhi:mə'təʊmə] *subst.* mass of blood under the skin caused by a blow *or* by the effects of an operation *hematom, blåmärke, utgjutning;* **extradural haematoma** = haematoma in the head, between the dura mater and the skull *extraduralhematom, epiduralhematom;* **intracerebral haematoma** = haematoma inside the cerebrum *intracerebralt hematom;* **perianal haematoma** = haematoma in the anal region *perianalt hematom;* **subdural haematoma** = blood plasma *or* clot between the dura mater and the arachnoid, which displaces the brain, caused by a blow on the head *subduralhematom* NOTE: plural is **haematomata**

haematometra [ˌhi:mə'tɒmɪtrə] *subst.* (i) excessive bleeding in the womb *hematometra;* (ii) swollen womb, caused by haematocolpos *livmodersvullnad pga hematokolpos*

haematomyelia [ˌhi:mətəʊmaɪ'i:liə] *subst.* condition where blood gets into the spinal cord *hematomyeli, spinalblödning*

haematopoiesis [ˌhi:mətəʊpɔɪ'i:sɪs] = HAEMOPOIESIS

haematoporphyrin [ˌhi:mətəʊ'pɔ:fərɪn] *subst.* porphyrin produced from haemoglobin *porfyrin från hemoglobin*

haematosalpinx [ˌhi:mətəʊ'sælpɪŋks] = HAEMOSALPINX

haematozoon [ˌhi:mətəʊ'zəʊɒn] *subst.* parasite living in the blood *hematozo, blodparasit* NOTE: plural is **haematozoa**

haematuria [ˌhi:mə'tjʊəriə] *subst.* abnormal presence of blood in the urine, as a result of injury *or* disease of the kidney or bladder *hematuri*

haemochromatosis [ˌhiːməʊˌkrəʊmə'təʊsɪs] *or* **bronze diabetes** ['brɒnz ˌda(ɪ)ə'biːtiːz] *subst.* hereditary disease in which the body absorbs and stores too much iron, causing cirrhosis of the liver, and giving the skin a dark colour *hemosideros, hemokromatos, bronsdiabetes*

haemoconcentration [ˌhiːməʊˌkɒnsən'treɪʃ(ə)n] *subst.* increase in the percentage of red blood cells because the volume of plasma is reduced *hemokoncentration; opposite of* HAEMODILUTION

haemocytoblast [ˌhiːməʊ'saɪtəʊblæst] *subst.* embryonic blood cell in the bone marrow from which red and white blood cells and platelets develop *hemocytoblast*

haemocytometer [ˌhiːməʊsaɪ'tɒmɪtə] *subst.* glass jar in which a sample of blood is diluted and the blood cells counted *slags glasbehållare som används vid blodkroppsräkning*

haemodialysis [ˌhiːməʊdaɪ'æləsɪs] *subst.* removing waste matter from blood using a dialyser (kidney machine) *hemodialys, HD*

haemodilution [ˌhiːməʊdaɪ'luːʃ(ə)n] *subst.* decrease in the percentage of red blood cells because the volume of plasma has increased *hemodilution; opposite of* HAEMOCONCENTRATION

haemoglobinaemia [ˌhiːməʊˌgləʊbɪ'niːmiə] *subst.* haemoglobin in the plasma *hemoglobinemi*

haemoglobin (Hb) [ˌhiːməʊ'gləʊbɪn, (ˌeɪtʃ'biː)] *subst.* red respiratory pigment (formed of haem and globin) in red blood cells which gives blood its red colour *hemoglobin, Hb; see also* OXYHAEMOGLOBIN

> COMMENT: haemoglobin absorbs oxygen in the lungs and carries it in the blood to the tissues

haemoglobinopathy [ˌhiːməʊˌgləʊbɪ'nɒpəθi] *subst.* inherited disease where production of haemoglobin is abnormal *medfödd sjukdom med onormal hemoglobinproduktion*

haemoglobinuria [ˌhiːməʊˌgləʊbɪ'njʊəriə] *subst.* condition where haemoglobin is found in the urine *hemoglobinuri*

haemogram ['hiːməʊgræm] *subst.* printed result of a blood test *hemogram*

haemolysin [hiː'mɒləsɪn] *subst.* protein which destroys red blood cells *hemolysin*

haemolysis [hiː'mɒləsɪs] *subst.* destruction of red blood cells *hem(at)olys*

haemolytic [ˌhiːməʊ'lɪtɪk] *adj.* (substance, such as snake venom) which destroys red blood cells *hemolytisk;* **haemolytic anaemia** = condition where the destruction of red blood cells is about six times the normal rate, and the supply of new cells from the bone marrow cannot meet the demand *hemolytisk anemi;* **haemolytic disease of the newborn** = condition where the red blood cells of the fetus are destroyed because antibodies in the mother's blood react against the blood of the fetus in the womb *erytroblastos(is) fetalis (neonatorum);* **haemolytic jaundice** = jaundice caused by haemolysis of red blood cells *icterus haemolyticus, hemolytisk ikterus;* **haemolytic uraemic syndrome** = condition in which haemolytic anaemia damages the kidneys *njurskada med hemolys*

haemopericardium [ˌhiːməʊˌperɪ'kɑːdiəm] *subst.* blood in the pericardium *hemoperikardium, hjärttamponad*

haemoperitoneum [ˌhiːməʊˌperitə'niːəm] *subst.* blood in the peritoneal cavity *hemoperitoneum*

haemophilia A [ˌhiːməʊ'fɪliə 'eɪ] *subst.* familial disease, in which inability to synthesize Factor VIII (a clotting factor), means that patient's blood clots very slowly, prolonged bleeding occurs from the slightest wound and internal bleeding can occur without any cause *hemofili A;* **haemophilia B** *or* **Christmas disease** = clotting disorder of the blood, similar to haemophilia A, but in which the blood coagulates badly due to deficiency of Factor IX *hemofili B*

> COMMENT: because haemophilia A is a sex-linked recessive characteristic, it is found only in males, but females are carriers. It can be treated by injections of Factor VIII

haemophiliac [ˌhiːmə(ʊ)'fɪlɪək] *subst.* person who suffers from haemophilia *hemofiliker, blödarsjuk*

haemophilic [ˌhiːməʊ'fɪlɪk] *adj.* referring to haemophilia *hemofilisk*

Haemophilus [hiː'mɒfɪləs] *subst.* genus of bacteria, which need certain factors in the blood to grow *Huemophilus;* **Haemophilus influenzae** = bacterium which lives in healthy throats, but if the patient's resistance is lowered by a bout of flu, then it can cause pneumonia or meningitis *Haemophilus influenzae*

haemophthalmia [ˌhiːmɒfˈθælmiə] *subst.* blood in the eye *hemoftalmus*

haemopneumothorax [ˌhiːməʊˌnjuːməʊˈθɔːræks] = PNEUMOHAEMOTHORAX

haemopoiesis [ˌhiːməʊpɔɪˈiːsɪs] *subst.* continual production of blood cells and blood platelets by the bone marrow *hemopo(i)es, hematopo(i)es, blodbildning*

haemopoietic [ˌhiːməʊpɔɪˈetɪk] *adj.* referring to the formation of blood *hematopoetisk*

haemoptysis [hiːˈmɒptəsɪs] *subst.* condition where the patient coughs blood from the lungs, caused by a serious illness such as anaemia, pneumonia, tuberculosis or cancer *hemoptys, blodupphostning, blodspottning;* **endemic haemoptysis** = PARAGONIMIASIS

haemorrhage [ˈhem(ə)rɪdʒ] **1** *subst.* bleeding where a large quantity of blood is lost, especially bleeding from a burst blood vessel *hemorragi, kraftig blödning;* **she had a haemorrhage and was rushed to hospital; he died of a brain haemorrhage; arterial haemorrhage** = haemorrhage of bright red blood from an artery *artärblödning;* **brain haemorrhage** *or* **cerebral haemorrhage** = bleeding inside the brain from the cerebral artery *hemorrhagia cerebri, hjärnblödning;* **primary haemorrhage** = haemorrhage which occurs immediately after an injury is suffered *primärblödning;* **secondary haemorrhage** = haemorrhage which occurs some time after the injury, due to infection of the wound *sekundärblödning;* **venous haemorrhage** = haemorrhage of dark blood from a vein *venös blödning* **2** *vb.* to bleed heavily *blöda kraftigt;* **the injured man was haemorrhaging from the mouth**

haemorrhagic [ˌheməˈrædʒɪk] *adj.* referring to heavy bleeding *hemorragisk, som avser el. hör till kraftig blödning;* **haemorrhagic disease of the newborn** = disease of babies, which makes them haemorrhage easily, caused by temporary lack of prothrombin *blödning hos spädbarn pga protrombinbrist;* **haemorrhagic stroke** = stroke caused by a burst blood vessel *hjärnblödning*

haemorrhoidectomy [ˌhemərɔɪˈdektəmi] *subst.* surgical removal of haemorrhoids *hemorrojdektomi*

haemorrhoids [ˈhemərɔɪdz] *or* **piles** [paɪlz] *subst pl.* swollen veins in the anorectal passage *hemorrojder;* **external haemorrhoids** = haemorrhoids outside the anus in the skin *yttre hemorrojder;* **internal haemorrhoids** = swollen veins inside the anus *inre hemorrojder;* **first-degree** *or* **second-degree** *or* **third-degree haemorrhoids** = haemorrhoids which remain in the rectum *or* which protrude into the anus but return into the rectum automatically *or* which protrude into the rectum permanently *hemorrojder av olika grader*

haemosalpinx [ˌhiːməʊˈsælpɪŋks] *subst.* blood accumulating in the Fallopian tubes *hem(at)osalpinx*

haemosiderosis [ˌhiːməʊsɪdəˈrəʊsɪs] *subst.* disorder in which iron forms large deposits in the tissue, causing haemorrhaging and destruction of red blood cells *hemosideros*

haemostasis [ˌhiːməʊˈsteɪsɪs] *subst.* stopping bleeding *or* slowing the movement of blood *hemostas, blodstillning, blodstockning*

haemostat [ˈhiːməʊstæt] *subst.* device, such as a clamp, which stops bleeding *klämma e.d. som stoppar blödning*

haemostatic [ˌhiːməʊˈstætɪk] *adj. & subst.* (drug) which stops bleeding *hemostatikum, hemostatisk, blodstillande (medel)*

haemothorax [ˌhiːməʊˈθɔːræks] *subst.* blood in the pleural cavity *hematot(h)orax, hemot(h)orax*

hair [heə] *subst.* **(a)** long thread growing on the body of an animal, from a small pit in the skin called a follicle (hair is mainly made up of a dense form of keratin) *pilus, hår, hårstrå;* **he's beginning to get a few grey hairs; hairs are growing on his chest; hair cell** = cell in the organ of Corti in the ear, which senses sound vibrations in the tectorial membrane *hårcell;* **hair follicle** = tube of epidermal cells containing the root of a hair *folliculus pili, hårfollikel, hårsäck;* **hair papilla** = part of the skin containing capillaries which feed blood to the hair *papilla pili, hårpapill* NOTE: plural **hairs** = SKIN *or* SENSORY RECEPTORS **(b)** mass of hairs growing on the head *håret;* **she's got long black hair; you ought to wash your hair; his hair is too long; he is going to have his hair cut; superfluous** *or* **unwanted hair** = hair which is growing in places where it is not thought to be beautiful (as on the legs) *besvärande hårväxt* NOTE: for other terms referring to hair see words beginning with **pilo-, tricho-** NOTE: no plural

COMMENT: hair is dead tissue and grows out of hair follicles. The follicles are tubes leading into the skin and lined with sebaceous glands which secrete the oil which covers the hair. Hair grows on almost all parts of the body, but is thicker and stronger on the head (the scalp, the eyebrows, inside the nose and ears). After puberty, hair becomes thicker on other parts of the body (the chin, chest and limbs in men, the pubic region and the armpits in both men and women). Hair on the head stops growing in many men in middle age, giving various degrees of baldness. Certain treatments, especially chemotherapy, can cause the hair to fall out. In later middle age, hair loses its natural pigmentation and becomes grey or white

hairy ['heəri] *adj.* covered with hair *hårig;* **he's got hairy arms; hairy cell leukaemia =** form of leukaemia with abnormal white blood cells with thread-like process on them *hårcellsleukemi*

hakan ⇨ **chin**

hakbenet ⇨ **hamate (bone)**

hake ⇨ **hook, retractor**

hakmask ⇨ **Ancylostoma**

haktång ⇨ **volsella**

halitosis [ˌhælɪ'təʊsɪs] *subst.* condition where a person has breath which smells badly *halitos, dålig andedräkt*

COMMENT: halitosis can have several causes: caries in the teeth, infection of the gums, and indigestion are the most usual. The breath can also have an unpleasant smell during menstruation, or in association with certain diseases such as diabetes mellitus and uraemia

hallucinate [hə'lu:sɪneɪt] *vb.* to have hallucinations *hallucinera;* **the patient was hallucinating**

hallucination [həˌlu:sɪ'neɪʃ(ə)n] *subst.* seeing an imaginary scene *or* hearing an imaginary sound as clearly as if it were really there *hallucination;* **he had hallucinations and went into a coma**

hallucinatorisk ⇨ **hallucinatory**

hallucinatory [hə'lu:sɪnət(ə)ri] *adj.* (drug, such as cannabis *or* LSD) which causes hallucinations *hallucinatorisk*

hallucinera ⇨ **hallucinate**

hallucinogen [ˌhælu:'sɪnədʒ(ə)n] *subst.* drug which causes hallucinations (such as cannabis *or* LSD) *hallucinogen*

hallucinogenic [hə'lu:sɪnə'dʒenɪk] *adj.* (substance) which produces hallucinations *hallucinogen;* **a hallucinogenic fungus**

hallux ['hæləks] *subst.* big toe *hallux, stortån;* **hallux valgus =** deformity of the foot, where the big toe turns towards the other toes and a bunion is formed on the protruding joint *hallux valgus*
NOTE: plural is **halluces**

hals ⇨ **cervix, neck**

hals- ⇨ **cervic-, cervical, jugular**

halsbränna ⇨ **heartburn, waterbrash**

halsbrässen ⇨ **thymus (gland)**

halsböld ⇨ **quinsy**

halsen ⇨ **neck, throat**

halsfluss ⇨ **strep throat, tonsillitis**

halsflätan ⇨ **plexus**

halskotorna ⇨ **cervical**

halskrage ⇨ **cervical**

halsnerverna ⇨ **cervical**

halsont ⇨ **sore**

halsplexus ⇨ **plexus**

halsrevben ⇨ **cervical**

halsvenen ⇨ **jugular**

halsvred ⇨ **torticollis**

halt ⇨ **content; lame**

halta ⇨ **limp**

haltande ⇨ **limp, claudication**

halv- ⇨ **hemi-, semi-**

halvblindhet ⇨ **hemianopia**

halvcirkelformig ⇨ **semicircular**

halvfast ⇨ **semi-liquid, semi-solid**

halvmånformig ⇨ **semilunar**

halvsidig ⇨ **hemi-**

halvslummer ⇨ **twilight**

hamamelis [ˌhæməˈmiːlɪs] *see* WITCH HAZEL

hamate (bone) [ˈheɪmeɪt (ˌbəʊn)] *or* **unciform bone** [ˈʌnsɪfɔːm ˌbəʊn] *subst.* one of the eight small carpal bones in the wrist, shaped like a hook ⇨ *illustration* HAND *os hamatum, hakbenet*

hammaren ⇨ **hammer**

hammartå ⇨ **hammer**

hammer [ˈhæmə] *subst.* **(a)** heavy metal tool for knocking nails into wood, etc. *hammare;* **he hit his thumb with the hammer; hammer toe** = toe where the middle joint is permanently bent at right angles *digitus malleus, hammartå* **(b)** malleus *or* one of the three ossicles in the middle ear *malleus, hammaren*

hampa ⇨ **cannabis**

hamstring [ˈhæmstrɪŋ] *subst.* group of tendons behind the knee, which link the thigh muscles to the bones in the lower leg *senor på knäts baksida (till hamstringsmusklerna);* **hamstring muscles** = group of muscles at the back of the thigh, which flex the knee and extend the gluteus maximus *musculus semimembranosus, semitendinosus resp. biceps femoris, hamstringsmusklerna*

hand [hænd] **1** *subst.* terminal part of the arm, beyond the wrist, which is used for holding things *manus, handen;* **he injured his hand with a saw; the commonest hand injuries occur at work 2** *vb.* to pass *räcka, ge;* **can you hand me that book? he handed me the key to the cupboard**

> COMMENT: the hand is formed of twenty-seven bones: fourteen phalanges (in the fingers), five metacarpals in the main part of the hand, and eight carpals in the wrist

handbok ⇨ **guide**

handduk ⇨ **towel, napkin**

handen ⇨ **hand**

handfat ⇨ **basin, bowl**

handflatan ⇨ **palm**

handflate- ⇨ **palmar, volar**

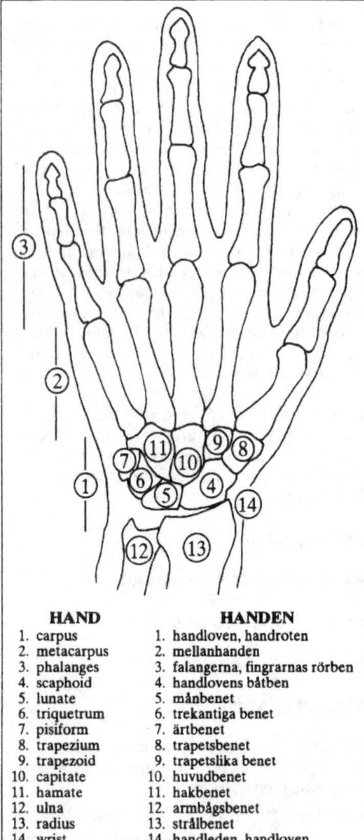

HAND	HANDEN
1. carpus	1. handloven, handroten
2. metacarpus	2. mellanhanden
3. phalanges	3. falangerna, fingrarnas rörben
4. scaphoid	4. handlovens båtben
5. lunate	5. månbenet
6. triquetrum	6. trekantiga benet
7. pisiform	7. ärtbenet
8. trapezium	8. trapetsbenet
9. trapezoid	9. trapetslika benet
10. capitate	10. huvudbenet
11. hamate	11. hakbenet
12. ulna	12. armbågsbenet
13. radius	13. strålbenet
14. wrist	14. handleden, handloven

handflatebågen ⇨ **palmar**

handicap [ˈhændɪkæp] **1** *subst.* physical disability *or* condition which prevents someone from doing some normal activity *handikapp;* **in spite of her handicaps, she tries to live as normal a life as possible; after having both legs amputated, he fought to overcome the handicap 2** *vb.* to prevent someone from doing a normal activity *handikappa;* **he is handicapped by only having one arm**

handicapped [ˈhændɪkæpt] *adj.* (person) who suffers from a handicap *handikappad;* **the handicapped** = people with physical disabilities *de handikappade*

handikapp ⇨ **disability, disablement, handicap, invalidity**

handikappad ⇨ **cripple, disable, handicapped, invalid**

handla ⇨ **act**

handled ⇨ **wrist**

handledare ⇨ **tutor**

handleden ⇨ **joint**

handledning ⇨ **instruction**

handling ⇨ **action**

handlingsoförmåga ⇨ **apraxia**

handlov(e) ⇨ **wrist, carpus**

handlovs- ⇨ **carp-, carpal**

Hand-Schüller Christian disease [ˌhɑntˌʃɪlə ˈkrɪʃ(ə)n dɪˌziːz] *or* **xanthomatosis** [ˌzænθəməˈtəʊsɪs] *subst.* disturbance of cholesterol metabolism in young children which causes defects in membranous bone, mainly in the skull, exophthalmos, diabetes insipidus, and a yellow-brown colour of the skin *(Hand-)Schüller-Christians sjukdom, Hands sjukdom, Christians sjukdom, xanthomatosis generalizata ossium*

handske ⇨ **glove**

hang [hæŋ] *vb.* to attach (something) above the ground (to a nail or hook, etc.) *hänga (upp);* to be attached above the ground (to a nail or hook, etc) *hänga;* **hang your coat on the hook; she hung the photograph over her bed; his hand was almost severed, it was hanging by a band of flesh** NOTE: **hangs - hanging - hung - has hung**

hangnail [ˈhæŋneɪl] *subst.* piece of torn skin at the side of a nail *trasigt nagelband*

hangover [ˈhæŋˌəʊvə] *subst.* condition after having drunk too much alcohol, with dehydration caused by inhibition of the antidiuretic hormone in the kidneys *baksmälla*

> COMMENT: the symptoms of a hangover are pain in the head, inability to stand noise and trembling of the hands

Hansen's bacillus [ˈhænsənz bəˌsɪləs] *or* **Mycobacterium leprae** [ˌmaɪkəʊbækˈtɪəriəm ˈlepriː] *subst.* bacterium which causes leprosy *Mycobacterium leprae, Hansens bacill, leprabacillen*

Hansen's disease [ˈhænsənz dɪˌziːz] = LEPROSY

haploid [ˈhæplɔɪd] *adj.* (cell, such as a gamete) with a single set of unpaired chromosomes *haploid; compare* DIPLOID, POLYPLOID

happen [ˈhæp(ə)n] *vb.* **(a)** to take place *hända, inträffa, ske;* **the accident happened at the corner of the street; how did it happen?; what's happened to his brother?** = what is his brother doing now? *vad har hänt med din bror?* **(b)** to be *or* to do something (by chance) *råka (göra);* **she happened to be standing near the cooker when the fire started; luckily a doctor happened to be passing in the street when the baby fell out of the window; do you happen to have an antidote for snake bites?**

hapten [ˈhæpten] *subst.* substance which causes an allergy, probably by changing a protein so that it becomes antigenic *hapten, inkomplett antigen*

harbour [ˈhɑːbə] *vb.* to hold and protect *härbärgera, innehålla, hysa;* **to harbour a disease** = to hold germs *or* bacteria and allow them to breed and spread disease *ha (och sprida) en sjukdom;* **soiled clothing can harbour dysentery; stagnant water harbours malaria mosquitoes**

hard [hɑːd] **1** *adj.* **(a)** not soft *hård;* **this bed is not too hard - a hard bed is good for someone suffering from back problems; if you have a slipped disc, you will be made to lie on a hard surface for several weeks; hard palate** = front part of the roof of the mouth between the upper teeth *palatum durum, hårda gommen;* **hard water** = tap water which contains a high percentage of calcium *hårt vatten* **(b)** difficult *svår;* **if the exam is too hard, nobody will pass; he's hard of hearing** = he's rather deaf *han hör dåligt (har nedsatt hörsel, är lomhörd)* **(c)** a **hard winter** = a very cold winter *en sträng vinter;* **in a hard winter, old people can suffer from hypothermia**
NOTE: **hard - harder - hardest 2** *adv.* with a lot of effort *hårt, intensivt, kraftigt;* **hit the nail hard with the hammer; if we all work hard, we'll soon overcome the disease**

harden [ˈhɑːd(ə)n] *vb.* to make hard *or* to become hard *hårdna, göra hårdare, indurera*

hardening of the arteries [ˈhɑːd(ə)nɪŋ əv ðɪ ˈɑːt(ə)rɪz] = ARTERIOSCLEROSIS

harelip [ˌheəˈlɪp] *subst.* defect in the upper lip occurring at birth, where the lip is split *lagoch(e)ili, harmynthet, harläpp*

COMMENT: a harelip is often associated with a cleft palate. Both can be successfully corrected by surgery

harkla sig ⇨ **throat**

harm [hɑ:m] **1** *subst.* damage (especially to a person) *skada, ont;* **walking to work every day won't do you any harm; there's no harm in taking the tablets only for one week** = there will be no side effects if you take the tablets for a week *det skadar inte att ta tabletterna en vecka* **2** *vb.* to damage *or* to hurt *skada, göra ont (illa), tillfoga skada;* **walking to work every day won't harm you**

harmful ['hɑ:mf(ə)l] *adj.* which causes damage *skadlig, farlig;* **bright light can be harmful to your eyes; sudden violent exercise can be harmful**

harmless ['hɑ:mləs] *adj.* which causes no damage *oskadlig, ofarlig;* **these herbal remedies are quite harmless**

harmynthet ⇨ **harelip**

harpest ⇨ **tularaemia**

Harrison's sulcus ['hærɪs(ə)nz ˌsʌlkəs] *subst.* hollow on either side of the chest which develops in children who have rickets and breathe in with difficulty *Harrisons fåra*

Harris's operation ['hærɪsɪz ˌɒpəˌreɪʃ(ə)n] *subst.* surgical removal of the prostate gland *slags operativt avlägsnande av prostata*

Hartmann's solution ['hɑ:tmənz səˌlu:ʃ(ə)n] *subst.* chemical solution used in drips to replace body fluids lost in dehydration, particularly as a result of infantile gastroenteritis *vätskeersättning, slags lösning använd mot dehydrering, särskilt hos spädbarn*

Hartnup disease ['hɑ:tnəp dɪˌzi:z] *subst.* condition caused by a hereditary defect in amino acid metabolism, producing thick skin and retarded mental development *Hartnups sjukdom*

harts ⇨ **resin**

hasande gång ⇨ **shuffling walk**

hasch(isch) ⇨ **hashish**

Hashimoto's disease [ˌhæʃɪ'məʊtəz dɪˌzi:z] *subst.* type of goitre in middle-aged women, where the patient is sensitive to secretions from her own thyroid gland, and, in extreme cases, the face swells and the skin turns yellow *struma lymphomatosa, Hashimotos struma*

hashish ['hæʃiʃ] *or* **marijuana** [ˌmærɪ'wɑ:nə] *or* **cannabis** ['kænəbɪs] *subst.* addictive drug made from the leaves or flowers of the Indian hemp plant *hasch(isch)*

hastig ⇨ **rapid**

hastighet ⇨ **rate**

haustrum ['hɔ:strəm] *subst.* sac on the outside of the colon *haustrum coli*
NOTE: plural is **haustra**

havande ⇨ **pregnant, expectant mother**

havandeskap ⇨ **pregnancy, cyesis, gestation**

havandeskapsförgiftning ⇨ **eclampsia, toxaemia**

havandeskapskräkningar ⇨ **morning**

Haversian canal [hə'vɜ:ʃ(ə)n kəˌnæl] *subst.* fine canal which runs through compact bone and contains blood vessels, nerves and lymph ducts *canalis nutricius (ossis), Havers kanal, haver(si)sk kanal*

Haversian system [hə'vɜ:ʃ(ə)n ˌsɪstəm] *subst.* osteon *or* unit of compact bone built around a Haversian canal, made of a series of bony layers which form a cylinder *benstruktur runt en av Havers kanaler*

hay fever ['heɪ ˌfi:və] *or* **allergic rhinitis** [ə'lɜ:dʒɪk raɪ'naɪtɪs] *or* **pollinosis** [ˌpɒlɪ'nəʊsɪs] *subst.* inflammation in the nasal passage and eyes caused by an allergic reaction to flowers and their pollen and scent, also to dust *rhinitis allergica (anaphylactica), pollinos, hösnuva;* **when he has hay fever, he has to stay indoors; the hay fever season starts in May**

Hb [ˌeɪtʃ'bi:] = HAEMOGLOBIN

H band ['eɪtʃ ˌbænd] *subst.* part of pattern in muscle tissue, a light band in the dark A band, seen through a microscope *H-band, H-skiva*

HBV [ˌeɪtʃbi:'vi:] = HEPATITIS B VIRUS

hCG [ˌeɪtʃsi:'dʒi:] = HUMAN CHORIONIC GONADOTROPHIN

HD ⇨ **dialysis**

head [hed] 1 *subst.* **(a)** top part of the body, which contains the eyes, nose, mouth, brain, etc *caput, huvudet;* **can you stand on your head? he hit his head on the low branch; he shook his head** = he moved his head from side to side to mean 'no' *han skakade på huvudet* NOTE: for other terms referring to the head see words beginning with **cephal-** **(b)** first place *topp, första plats;* **he stood at the head of the queue; who's name is at the head of the list?** **(c)** (i) rounded top part of a bone which fits into a socket *ledhuvud, ledkula;* (ii) round main part of a spermatozoon *huvud;* **head of humerus; head of radius; the head of a sperm; head of femur** = rounded projecting end part of the thigh bone which joins the acetabulum at the hip *caput femoris, lårbenshuvudet* **(d)** most important person *chef, ledare;* **he's the head of the anatomy department; she was head of the research unit for some years** 2 *vb.* **(a)** to be the first *or* to lead *leda, stå överst (först, i spetsen för);* **his name heads the list** **(b)** to go towards *gå (ge sig iväg) mot;* **they are heading north; he headed for the administrator's office**

headache ['hedeɪk] *subst.* pain in the head, caused by changes in pressure in the blood vessels feeding the brain which act on the nerves *huvudvärk;* **I must lie down - I've got a headache; she can't come with us because she has got a headache; cluster headache** = headache which occurs behind one eye for a short period *clusterhuvudvärk;* **migraine headache** = very severe throbbing headache which can be accompanied by nausea, vomiting, visual disturbance and vertigo *migrän;* **tension headache** *or* **muscular contraction headache** = headache over all the head, caused by worry *or* stress, and thought to result from chronic contraction of the muscles of the scalp and neck *spänningshuvudvärk*

> COMMENT: headaches can be caused by a blow to the head, by lack of sleep or food, by eye strain, sinus infections and many other causes. Mild headaches can be treated with aspirin and rest. Severe headaches which recur may be caused by serious disorders in the head or nervous system

heal [hi:l] *vb. (of wound)* to mend *or* to become better *läka(s), bota(s);* **after six weeks, his wound had still not healed; a minor cut will heal faster if it is left without a bandage**

healing ['hi:lɪŋ] *subst.* process of getting better *läkning;* **a substance which will accelerate the healing process**

health [helθ] *subst.* being well *or* not being ill; state of being free from physical *or* mental disease *hälsa, hälsotillstånd;* **he's in good health; she had suffered from bad health for some years; the council said that fumes from the factory were a danger to public health; all cigarette packets carry a government health warning; Health and Safety at Work Act** = Act of Parliament which rules how the health of workers should be protected by the companies they work for *ung. arbetarskyddslag (i Storbritannien);* **District Health Authority (DHA** *or* **HA)** = administrative unit in the National Health Service which is responsible for health services, including hospitals and clinics, in a district *lokal hälsovårdsmyndighet (i Storbritannien);* **Regional Health Authority (RHA)** = administrative unit in the National Health Service which is responsible for planning the health service in a region *administrativ enhet inom National Health Service;* **Medical Officer of Health (MOH)** = formerly, a local government official in charge of the health services in an area *tidigare ung. länsläkare el. förste stadsläkare;* **National Health Service (NHS)** = British organization which provides medical services free of charge or at a low cost, to the whole population *allmänna hälso- och sjukvården (i Storbritannien), ung. offentlig sjukvård;* **Environmental Health Officer** *or* **Public Health Inspector** = official of a local authority who examines the environment and tests for air pollution *or* bad sanitation *or* noise levels, etc. *ung. hälsovårdsinspektör;* **health centre** = public building in which a group of doctors practise *or* which contains a children's clinic, etc. *ung. vårdcentral, ung. distriktsläkarmottagning;* **health education** = teaching people (school children and adults) to do things to improve their health, such as taking more exercise, stopping smoking, etc. *hälsoupplysning;* **health insurance** = insurance which pays the cost of treatment for illness, especially when travelling abroad *sjukförsäkring; US* **Health Maintenance Organization (HMO)** = private doctors' practice offering health care to patients who pay a regular subscription *slags privat sjukförsäkring;* **health service** = organization in a district *or* country which is in charge of doctors, hospitals, etc. *hälso- och sjukvården;* **Health Service Commissioner** *or* **Health Service Ombudsman** = official who investigates complains from the public about the National Health Service *slags konsumentombudsman för hälso- och sjukvården (i Storbritannien);* **health visitor** = registered nurse with qualifications in obstetrics, midwifery and preventive medicine, who visits babies and sick patients at home and advises on treatment *slags barnmorska (distriktssköterska) som gör hembesök*

> QUOTE in the UK, the main screen is carried out by health visitors at 6-10 months
> **Lancet**

> QUOTE large numbers of women are dying of cervical cancer in health authorities where the longest backlog of smear tests exists
> **Nursing Times**

> QUOTE the HA told the Health Ombudsman that nursing staff and students now received full training in the use of the nursing process
> **Nursing Times**

> QUOTE occupational health nurses should be part of health care teams in local health centres
> **Nursing Times**

healthy ['helθi] *adj.* (i) well *or* not ill *frisk, vid god hälsa;* (ii) likely to make you well *hälsosam;* **being a farmer is a healthy job; people are healthier than they were fifty years ago; this town is the healthiest place in England; if you eat a healthy diet and take plenty of exercise there is no reason why you should fall ill**
NOTE: **healthy - healthier - healthiest**

hear [hɪə] *vb.* **(a)** to sense sounds with the ears *höra;* **can you hear footsteps? I can't hear what you're saying because of the noise of the aircraft; I heard her shut the front door; he must be getting deaf, because often he doesn't hear the telephone (b)** to get information *höra, få höra (veta);* **have you heard that the Prime Minister has died? where did you hear about the new drug for treating AIDS?**
NOTE: **hears - hearing - heard - has heard**

hearing ['hɪərɪŋ] *subst.* ability to hear *hörseln;* function performed by the ear of sensing sounds and sending sound impulses to the brain *hörseln;* **his hearing is failing; she suffers from bad hearing; hearing aid** = tiny electronic device fitted into or near the ear, to improve the hearing of a deaf person by making sounds louder *hörapparat*
NOTE: for other terms referring to hearing see words beginning with **audi-**

heart [hɑːt] *subst.* main organ in the body, which maintains the circulation of the blood around the body by its pumping action *cor, hjärtat;* **the doctor listened to his heart; she has heart trouble; chambers of the heart** = the two sections (an atrium and a ventricle) of each side of the heart *hjärtats ventriklar (kammare);* **heart block** = slowing of the action of the heart because the impulses from the SA node to the ventricles are delayed or interrupted *hjärtblock;* **heart disease** = any disease of the heart in general *hjärtfel;* **he has a long history of heart disease; heart failure** = failure of the heart to maintain the output of blood to meet the demands of the body *hjärtsvikt;* **heart massage** = treatment to make a heart which has stopped beating start working again *hjärtmassage;* **heart murmur** = abnormal sound made by turbulent flow, usually the result of an abnormality in the structure of the heart *blåsljud;* **heart rate** = number of times the heart beats per minute *hjärtfrekvens;* **heart sounds** = two different sounds made by the heart as it beats *hjärtton;* see LUBB-DUPP; **heart stoppage** = situation where the heart has stopped beating *hjärtstillestånd;* **heart surgery** = surgical operation to remedy a condition of the heart *hjärtkirurgi;* **heart transplant** = surgical operation to transplant a heart into a patient *hjärttransplantation*

> COMMENT: the heart is situated slightly to the left of the central part of the chest, between the lungs. It is divided into two parts by a vertical septum; each half is itself divided into an upper chamber (the atrium) and a lower chamber (the ventricle). The veins bring blood from the body into the right atrium; from there it passes into the right ventricle and is pumped into the pulmonary artery which takes it to the lungs. Oxygenated blood returns from the lungs to the left atrium, passes to the left ventricle and from there is pumped into the aorta for circulation round the arteries. The heart expands and contracts by the force of the heart muscle (the myocardium) under impulses from the sinoatrial node, and a normal heart beats about 70 times a minute; the contracting beat as it pumps blood out (the systole) is followed by a weaker diastole, where the muscles relax to allow blood to flow back into the heart. In a heart attack, part of the myocardium is deprived of blood because of a clot in a coronary artery; this has an effect on the rhythm of the heartbeat and can be fatal. In heart block, impulses from the sinoatrial node fail to reach the ventricles properly; there are either longer impulses (first degree block) or missing impulses (second degree block) or no impulses at all (complete heart block), in which case the ventricles continue to beat slowly and independently of the SA node

heart attack ['hɑːt əˌtæk] *subst.* condition where a coronary artery is blocked by a blood clot (coronary thrombosis), causing myocardial ischaemia and myocardial infarction *hjärtattack, hjärtinfarkt*

heartbeat ['hɑːtbiːt] *subst.* regular noise made by the heart as it pumps blood *hjärtslag*

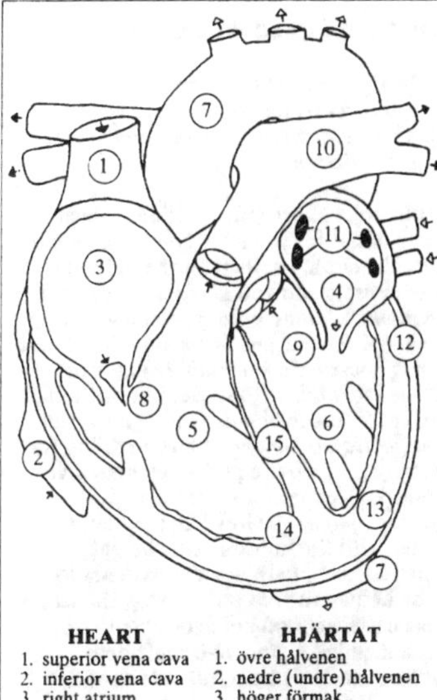

HEART	HJÄRTAT
1. superior vena cava	1. övre hålvenen
2. inferior vena cava	2. nedre (undre) hålvenen
3. right atrium	3. höger förmak
4. left atrium	4. vänster förmak
5. right ventricle	5. höger kammare (ventrikel)
6. left ventricle	6. vänster kammare (ventrikel)
7. aorta	7. aorta, stora kroppspulsådern
8. tricuspid valve	8. trikuspidalklaffen, atrioventrikularklaffen
9. bicuspid valve	9. bikuspidalklaffen, mitralisklaffen
10. pulmonary artery	10. lungartären, pulmonalisartären
11. pulmonary veins	11. lungvenerna, pulmonalisvenerna
12. epicardium	12. epikardiet, hjärtsäckens inre blad
13. myocardium	13. myokardiet, hjärtmuskeln
14. endocardium	14. endokardiet, hjärtats innerhinna
15. septum	15. hjärtskiljeväggen

heartburn ['hɑːtbɜːn] *or* **pyrosis** [paɪ'rəʊsɪs] *subst.* indigestion, causing a burning feeling in the abdomen and oesophagus, and a flow of acid saliva into the mouth *pyros, halsbränna*

heart-lung ['hɑːtlʌŋ] *adj.* referring to both the heart and the lungs *hjärtlung-;* **heart-lung machine** *or* **cardiopulmonary bypass** = machine used to pump blood round the body of a patient and maintain the supply of oxygen to the blood during heart surgery *hjärtlungmaskin;* **heart-lung transplant** = operation to transplant a new heart and lungs into a patient *hjärtlungtransplantation*
NOTE: for other terms referring to the heart, see also words beginning with **card-** or **cardi-**

heat [hiːt] **1** *subst.* being hot *hetta, värme;* **the heat of the sun made the road melt; heat cramp** = cramp produced by loss of salt from the body in very hot conditions *värmekramp;* **heat exhaustion** = collapse due to overexertion in hot conditions *värmeslag;* **heat rash** = MILIARIA; **heat spots** = little red spots which develop on the face in very hot weather *miliaria, värmeutslag;* **heat stroke** = condition where the patient becomes too hot and his body temperature rises abnormally *termoplegi, värmeslag;* **heat treatment** *or* **heat therapy** = using heat (from hot lamps *or* hot water) to treat certain conditions, such as arthritis and bad circulation *termoterapi, värmebehandling* **2** *vb.* to make hot *upphetta, värma (upp);* **the solution should be heated to 25°C**

COMMENT: heat exhaustion involves loss of salt and body fluids; heat stroke is also caused by high outside temperatures, but in this case the body is incapable of producing sweat and the body temperature rises, leading to headaches, stomach cramps and sometimes loss of consciousness

heavily ['hevəli] *adv.* strongly *tungt, mödosamt;* **she was breathing heavily; he was heavily sedated**

heavy ['hevi] *adj.* **(a)** which weighs a lot *tung;* **this box is so heavy I can hardly lift it; people with back trouble should not lift heavy weights; he got a slipped disc from trying to lift a heavy box (b)** strong *stark;* in large quantities *stor, omfattande;* **don't go to bed after you've had a heavy meal; she has a heavy cold and has to stay in bed; the patient was under heavy sedation; heavy smoker** = person who smokes large numbers of cigarettes *storrökare*
NOTE: **heavy - heavier - heaviest**

hebephrenia [ˌhiːbɪ'friːniə] *or* **hebephrenic schizophrenia** [ˌhiːbɪ'frenɪk ˌskɪtsəʊ'friːniə] *subst.* condition where the patient (usually an adolescent) has hallucinations, delusions, and deterioration of personality, talks rapidly and generally acts in a strange manner *schizophrenia hebephrenica, hebefreni*

Heberden's node ['hiːbədənz ˌnəʊd] *subst.* small bony lump which develops on the terminal phalanges of fingers in osteoarthritis *Heberdens knuta*

hebetude ['hebɪtjuːd] *subst.* stupidity *or* dullness of the senses during acute fever *or* being uninterested in one's surroundings and not responding to stimuli *slöhet, avtrubbning*

hectic ['hektɪk] *adj.* feverish or flushed or referring to tuberculosis *hektisk;* **hectic fever** = attack of fever which occurs each day in patients suffering from tuberculosis *febris hectica, hektisk feber*

heel [hiːl] *subst.* **(a)** back part of the foot *hälen;* **heel bone** *or* **calcaneus** = bone forming the heel, beneath the talus *os calcaneum, calcaneus, hälbenet* **(b)** block under the back part of a shoe *häl;* **she wore shoes with very high heels**

Hegar's sign ['heɪgəz ˌsaɪn] *subst.* way of detecting pregnancy, by inserting the fingers into the womb and pressing with the other hand on the pelvic cavity to feel if the neck of the uterus has become soft *Hegars tecken*

height [haɪt] *subst.* **(a)** measurement of how tall *or* how high someone *or* something is *längd;* **he is of above average height; the patient's height is 1.23 m (b)** high place *höjd;* **he has a fear of heights**

hektisk ⇨ **hectic**

hel ⇨ **solid, total**

helavtvättning ⇨ **sponge bath**

helcoplasty ['helkəʊplæsti] *subst.* skin graft to cover an ulcer to aid healing *slags hudtransplantat*

heliotherapy [ˌhiːləʊ'θerəpi] *subst.* treatment of patients by sunlight *or* sunbathing *helioterapi, solbehandling, solbad*

helium ['hiːliəm] *subst.* very light gas used in combination with oxygen, especially to relieve asthma *or* sickness caused by decompression *helium, He*
NOTE: chemical symbol is **He**

helix ['hiːlɪks] *subst.* curved outer edge of the ear *helix, öronmusslan*

helkroppsbestrålning ⇨ **irradiation**

Heller's operation ['heləz ˌɒpə'reɪʃ(ə)n] = CARDIOMYOTOMY

Heller's test ['heləz ˌtest] *subst.* test for protein in the urine *slags undersökning av äggvita i urinen*

helminth ['helmɪnθ] *subst.* general term for a parasitic worm (such as a tapeworm *or* fluke) *helmint, inälvsmask*

helminthiasis [ˌhelmɪn'θaɪəsɪs] *subst.* infestation with parasitic worms *helminthiasis, masksjukdom*

helnykterist ⇨ **abstainer**

heloma [hɪ'ləʊmə] *subst.* corn *or* hard lump of skin, usually on the foot or hand where something has pressed or rubbed against the skin *helom, liktorn*

help [help] **1** *subst.* **(a)** something which makes it easier for you to do something *hjälp, bistånd;* **he cut his nails with the help of a pair of scissors; do you need any help with the patients?; home help** = person who helps an invalid *or* handicapped person in their house by doing housework *hemhjälp* **(b)** making someone safe *hjälpa;* **they went to his help** = they went to rescue him *de gav sig av för att hjälpa (undsätta) honom;* **she was calling for help; they phoned the police for help 2** *vb.* **(a)** to make it easier for someone to do something *hjälpa;* **she has a home help to help her with the housework; she got another nurse to help put the patients to bed; he helped the old lady across the street (b)** (used with **cannot**) not to be able to stop doing something *hjälpa;* **she can't help dribbling; he can't help it if he's deaf 3 help!** = call showing that someone is in difficulties *hjälp!;* **help! help! call a doctor quickly! help, the patient is vomiting blood**

helper ['helpə] *subst.* person who helps *hjälpare, medhjälpare, biträde*

helpful ['helpf(ə)l] *adj.* which helps *hjälpsam*

helpless ['helpləs] *adj.* not able to do anything *hjälplös*

helt ⇨ **absolutely, fully, totally**

hem ⇨ **home; haem**

hem- ['hem, ˌ-] *see* HAEM-

hem- ⇨ **domiciliary**

hemangiom ⇨ **haemangioma, strawberry mark**

hematemes ⇨ **haematemesis**

hematin ⇨ **haematin**

hematocele ⇨ **haematocoele**

hematocystis ⇨ **haematocyst**

hematokolpos ⇨ **haematocolpos**

hematokrit ⇨ **haematocrit, pack**

hematolog ⇨ **haematologist**

hematologi ⇨ **haematology**

hematologisk ⇨ **haematological**

hematom ⇨ **haematoma**

hematometra ⇨ **haematometra**

hematomyeli ⇨ **haematomyelia**

hematopoetisk ⇨ **haemopoietic**

hematozo ⇨ **haematozoon**

hematuri ⇨ **haematuria**

hembesök, göra ⇨ **call**

hemeralopia [ˌhemərəˈləʊpiə] *or* **day blindness** [ˈdeɪ blaɪndnəs] *subst.* being able to see better in bad light than in ordinary daylight (usually a congenital condition) *hemeralopi, dagblindhet*

hemhjälp ⇨ **home**

hemi- [ˈhemi, ˌ--] *prefix* meaning half *hemi-, halv-, halvsidig*

hemialgi ⇨ **hemicrania**

hemianopia [ˌhemiəˈnəʊpiə] *subst.* state of partial blindness, where the patient has only half the normal field of vision in each eye *hemi(an)opsi, halvblindhet*

hemiatrophy [ˌhemiˈætrəfɪ] *subst.* condition where half of the body *or* half of an organ or part is atrophied *hemiatrofi*

hemiballismus [ˌhemibəˈlɪzməs] *subst.* sudden movement of the limbs on one side of the body, caused by a disease of the basal ganglia *hemiballism*

hemicolectomy [ˌhemikəˈlektəmi] *subst.* surgical removal of part of the colon *hemikolektomi*

hemicrania [ˌhemiˈkreɪniə] *subst.* headache *or* migraine in one side of the head *hemikrani, hemialgi, migrän*

hemikolektomi ⇨ **hemicolectomy**

hemikrani ⇨ **hemicrania**

hemimelia [ˌhemiˈmiːliə] *subst.* congenital condition where the patient has excessively short or defective arms and legs *hemimelus*

hemimelus ⇨ **hemimelia**

hemiparesis [ˌhemipəˈriːsɪs] *subst.* slight paralysis of the muscles of one side of the body *hemipares, lättare halvsidig förlamning*

hemiplegia [ˌhemiˈpliːdʒə] *subst.* severe paralysis affecting one side of the body due to damage of the central nervous system *hemiplegi, halvsidig förlamning; compare* DIPLEGIA

hemisfär ⇨ **hemisphere**

hemisphere [ˈhemɪsfɪə] *subst.* half of a sphere *hemisfär;* **cerebral hemisphere** = one half of the cerebrum *hemisphaerum cerebri, storhjärnshemisfär, hjärnhemisfär*

hemligstämpla ⇨ **classify**

hemocytoblast ⇨ **haemocytoblast**

hemodialys ⇨ **dialysis**

hemodilution ⇨ **haemodilution**

hemofili ⇨ **haemophilia A**

hemofiliker ⇨ **haemophiliac**

hemofilisk ⇨ **haemophilic**

hemoftalmus ⇨ **haemophthalmia**

hemoglobin ⇨ **haemoglobin (Hb), respiratory**

hemoglobinemi ⇨ **haemoglobinaemia**

hemoglobinuri ⇨ **haemoglobinuria**

hemogram ⇨ **haemogram**

hemokoncentration ⇨ **haemoconcentration**

hemokromatos ⇨ **haemochromatosis**

hemolysin ⇨ **haemolysin**

hemolytisk ⇨ **haemolytic**

hemoperikardium ⇨ **haemopericardium**

hemoperitoneum ⇨ **haemoperitoneum**

hemopneumothorax ⇨ **pneumohaemothorax**

hemoptys ⇨ **haemoptysis**

hemorragi ▷ **haemorrhage**

hemorragisk ▷ **haemorrhagic**

hemorrojdektomi ▷ **haemorrhoidectomy**

hemorrojder ▷ **haemorrhoids**

hemort ▷ **domicile**

hemosideros ▷ **diabetes, haemochromatosis, haemosiderosis**

hemostas ▷ **haemostasis**

hemostatikum ▷ **haemostatic**

hemostatisk ▷ **haemostatic**

hemp [hemp] *see* INDIAN HEMP

hemsjukvård ▷ **domiciliary**

hemsöka ▷ **infest**

Henle's loop ['henli:z ˌlu:p] *see* LOOP

Henoch's purpura ['henəks ˌpɜ:pjʊrə] *subst.* blood disorder of children, where the skin becomes dark blue and they suffer abdominal pains *purpura allergica (nervosa, rheumatica), Henoch-Schönleins purpura*

hepar ▷ **liver**

heparin ['hep(ə)rɪn] *subst.* anticoagulant substance found in the liver and lungs, and also produced artificially for use in the treatment of thrombosis *heparin*

hepat- [hɪˌpæt] *or* **hepato-** ['hepətə(ʊ), ˌ---] *prefix* referring to the liver *hepat(o)-, lever-*

hepatalgia [ˌhepə'tældʒə] *subst.* pain in the liver *hepatalgi, leversmärtor*

hepatectomy [ˌhepə'tektəmi] *subst.* surgical removal of part of the liver *hepatektomi*

hepatic [hɪ'pætɪk] *adj.* referring to the liver *lever-;* **hepatic artery** = artery which takes the blood to the liver *arteria hepatica (communis);* **hepatic cells** = epithelial cells of the liver acini *leverceller;* **hepatic duct** = duct which links the liver to the bile duct leading to the duodenum *gallgång;* **hepatic flexure** = bend in the colon, where the ascending and transverse colons join *flexura coli dextra;* **hepatic portal system** = group of veins linking to form the portal vein, which brings blood from the pancreas, spleen, gall bladder and the abdominal part of the alimentary canal to the liver *portasystemet;* **hepatic vein** = vein which takes blood from the liver to the inferior vena cava *vena hepatica, leverven*

hepaticostomy [hɪˌpætɪ'kɒstəmi] *subst.* surgical operation to make an opening in the hepatic duct taking bile from the liver *hepatikostomi*

hepatis ['hepətɪs] *see* PORTA

hepatitis [ˌhepə'taɪtɪs] *subst.* inflammation of the liver *hepatit, leverinflammation;* **infectious virus hepatitis** *or* **infective hepatitis** *or* **hepatitis A** = hepatitis transmitted by a carrier through food or drink *hepatit A, hepatitis epidemica (infectiosa), infektiös virushepatit;* **serum hepatitis** *or* **hepatitis B** = hepatitis transmitted by infected blood *or* unsterilized surgical instruments *or* sexual intercourse *hepatit B, serumhepatit, tidigare inokulationshepatit*

> COMMENT: serum hepatitis and infectious hepatitis are caused by different viruses (called A and B), and having had one does not give immunity against an attack of the other. Hepatitis B is more serious than the A form, and can vary in severity from a mild gastrointestinal upset to severe liver failure and death

hepatoblastoma [ˌhepətəʊblæ'stəʊmə] *subst.* malignant tumour in the liver, made up of epithelial-type cells often with areas of immature cartilage and embryonic bone *slags elakartad levertumör*

hepatocele ['hepətəʊsi:(ə)l] *subst.* hernia of the liver through the diaphragm or the abdominal wall *leverbråck*

hepatocellular [ˌhepətəʊ'seljʊlə] *adj.* referring to liver cells *hepatocellulär;* **hepatocellular jaundice** = jaundice caused by injury to *or* disease of the liver cells *icterus hepato-cellularis (parenchymatosus), hepato-cellulär ikterus, parenkymikterus, parenkymatös ikterus*

hepatocirrhosis [ˌhepətəʊsə'rəʊsɪs] = CIRRHOSIS OF THE LIVER

hepatocolic ligament [ˌhepətəʊ'kɒlɪk ˌlɪgəmənt] *subst.* ligament which links the gall bladder and the right flexure of the colon *ligamentum hepatocolicum*

hepatocyte ['hepətəʊsaɪt] *subst.* liver cell which synthesizes and stores substances, and produces bile *slags levercell*

hepatolenticular degeneration [ˌhepətəʊlenˈtɪkjʊlə dɪˈdʒenəˈreɪʃ(ə)n] = WILSON'S DISEASE

hepatoma [ˌhepəˈtəʊmə] *subst.* malignant tumour of the liver formed of mature cells, especially found in patients with cirrhosis *hepatom, slags malign levertumör*

hepatomegaly [ˌhepətəʊˈmegəli] *subst.* condition where the liver becomes very large *hepatomegali, leverförstoring*

hepatotoxic [ˌhepətəʊˈtɒksɪk] *adj.* which destroys the liver cells *hepatotoxisk*

herald patch [ˈher(ə)ld ˌpætʃ] *subst.* small spot of a rash (such as pityriasis rosea) which appears some time before the main rash *primärmedaljong*

herb [hɜːb] *subst.* plant which can be used as a medicine *or* to give a certain taste to food *or* to give a certain scent *herba, ört*

herbal [ˈhɜːb(ə)l] *adj.* referring to herbs *ört-;* **herbal remedies** = remedies made from plants, such as infusions made from dried leaves or flowers in hot water *örtmedicin*

herbalism [ˈhɜːbəlɪz(ə)m] *subst.* science of treatment of illnesses *or* disorders by medicines extracted from plants *fytoterapi, örtmedicin*

herbalist [ˈhɜːbəlɪst] *subst.* person who treats illnesses *or* disorders by medicine extracted from plants *person som behandlar sjukdomar med örtmedicin*

hereditary [həˈredət(ə)ri] *adj.* which is transmitted from parents to children *hereditär, ärftlig*

hereditet ▷ **heredity**

heredity [həˈredəti] *subst.* occurrence of physical *or* mental characteristics in children which are inherited from their parents *hereditet, ärftlighet*

> COMMENT: the characteristics which are most commonly inherited are the pigmentation of skin and hair, eyes (including pigmentation, shortsightedness and other eye defects), blood grouping, and disorders which are caused by defects in blood composition, such as haemophilia

hereditär ▷ **hereditary**

Hering-Breuer reflex [ˌherɪŋˈbrɔɪə ˌriːfleks] *subst.* reflex which regulates breathing *Hering-Breuer-reflex*

hermaphrodite [hɜːˈmæfrədaɪt] *subst.* person with both male and female characteristics *hermafrodit*

hermaphroditism [hɜːˈmæfrədaɪˌtɪz(ə)m] *subst.* condition where a person has both male and female characteristics *hermafroditism*

hernia [ˈhɜːniə] *subst.* condition where an organ bulges through a hole *or* weakness in the wall which surrounds it *hernia, bråck;* **diaphragmatic hernia** = condition where the abdominal contents pass through an opening in the diaphragm into the chest *hernia diaphragmatica, hiatusbråck, diafragmabråck*
NOTE: also called in US English **upside-down stomach** **femoral hernia** = hernia of the bowel at the top of the thigh *hernia femoralis (cruralis), femoralbråck;* **hiatus hernia** = hernia where the stomach bulges through the opening in the diaphragm muscle through which the oesophagus passes *hiatusbråck, diafragmabråck;* **incisional hernia** = hernia which breaks through the abdominal wall at a place where a surgical incision was made during an operation *hernia in cicatrice, ärrbråck;* **inguinal hernia** = hernia where the intestine bulges through the muscles in the groin *hernia inguinalis, ljumskbråck;* **irreducible hernia** = hernia where the organ cannot be returned to its normal position *hernia irreponibilis, irreponibelt bråck;* **reducible hernia** = hernia where the organ can be pushed back into place without an operation *hernia reponibilis, reponibelt bråck;* **strangulated hernia** = condition where part of the intestine is squeezed in a hernia and the supply of blood to it is cut off *hernia incarcerata, inklämt bråck;* **umbilical hernia** *or* **exomphalos** = hernia which bulges at the navel, usually in young children *hernia umbilicalis, omfalocele, navelbråck*

hernial [ˈhɜːniəl] *adj.* referring to a hernia *bråck-;* **hernial sac** = sac formed where a membrane has pushed through a cavity in the body *bråcksäck*

herniated [ˈhɜːnieɪtɪd] *adj.* (organ) which has developed a hernia *med bråck(bildning)*

herniation [ˌhɜːniˈeɪʃ(ə)n] *subst.* development of a hernia *bråckbildning*

hernioplasty [ˈhɜːniəʊˌplæsti] *subst.* surgical operation to reduce a hernia *operativt ingrepp för att minska bråck*

herniorrhaphy [ˌhɜːniˈɔːrəfi] *subst.* radical surgical operation to repair a hernia *radikaloperation av bråck*

herniotomy [ˌhɜːniˈɒtəmi] *subst.* surgical operation to relieve a hernia which results in its reduction *herniotomi, bråckoperation*

heroin [ˈherəʊɪn] *subst.* narcotic drug, a white powder derived from morphine *heroin*

herpangina [ˌhɜːpænˈdʒaɪnə] *subst.* infectious disease of children, where the tonsils and back of the throat become inflamed and ulcerated, caused by a Coxsackie virus *herpangina*

herpes [ˈhɜːpiːz] *subst.* inflammation of the skin or mucous membrane, caused by a virus, where small blisters are formed *herpes;* **herpes simplex (Type I)** *or* **cold sore** = burning sore, usually on the lips *herpes simplex (labialis);* **herpes simplex (Type II)** *or* **genital herpes** = sexually transmitted disease which forms blisters in the genital region *herpes genitalis;* **herpes zoster** *or* **shingles** *or* **zona** = inflammation of a sensory nerve, characterized by pain along the nerve causing a line of blisters to form on the skin, usually found mainly on the abdomen or back, or on the face *herpes zoster, bältros*

> COMMENT: because the same virus causes herpes and chickenpox, anyone who has had chickenpox as a child carries the dormant herpesvirus in his bloodstream and can develop shingles in later life. It is not known what triggers the development of shingles, though it is known that an adult suffering from shingles can infect a child with chickenpox

herpesvirus [ˌhɜːpiːzˈvaɪ(ə)rəs] *subst.* one of a group of viruses which cause herpes (herpesvirus Type I), and genital herpes (herpesvirus Type II) *herpesvirus*

herpetic [hɜːˈpetɪk] *adj.* referring to herpes *herpetisk;* **post herpetic neuralgia** = pains felt after an attack of shingles *smärtor efter bältros*

herpetiformis [həˌpetɪˈfɔːmɪs] *see* DERMATITIS

herpetisk ⇨ **herpetic**

hes ⇨ **hoarse, husky**

heshet ⇨ **hoarseness**

het ⇨ **hot**

hetero- [ˈhet(ə)rəʊ, ˌ--] *prefix* meaning different *heter(o)-, olik-*

heterochromia [het(ə)rəʊˈkrəʊmiə] *subst.* condition where the irises of the eyes are different colours *heterokromi*

heterofori ⇨ **heterophoria**

heterogametic [ˌhet(ə)rəʊgəˈmetɪk] *adj.* (person) who produces gametes with different sex chromosomes (as a human male) *som producerar könsceller med olika könskromosomer; see note at* SEX

heterogen ⇨ **heterogeneous, heterogenous**

heterogeneous [ˌhet(ə)rə(ʊ)ˈdʒiːniəs] *adj.* having different characteristics *or* qualities *heterogen, olikartad*

heterogenous [ˌhetəˈrɒdʒɪnəs] *adj.* coming from a different source *heterogen, främmande*

heterograft [ˈhet(ə)rəʊgrɑːft] *subst.* tissue taken from one species and grafted onto an individual of another species *heterotransplantat, xenograft, xenotransplantat*

heterokromi ⇨ **heterochromia**

heterophoria [ˌhet(ə)rəʊˈfɔːriə] *subst.* condition where if an eye is covered it tends to squint *heterofori*

heteropi ⇨ **heteropsia**

heteropsia [ˌhetəˈrɒpsiə] *subst.* condition where the two eyes see differently *heteropi*

heterosexual [ˌhet(ə)rə(ʊ)ˈsekʃʊ(ə)l] **1** *adj.* referring to the normal relation of the two sexes *heterosexuell* **2** *subst.* person who is sexually attracted to persons of the opposite sex *heterosexuell (person)*

heterosexuality [ˌhet(ə)rə(ʊ)ˌsekʃuˈæləti] *subst.* condition where a person has sexual attraction towards persons of the opposite sex *heterosexualitet; compare* BISEXUAL, HOMOSEXUAL

heterosexuell ⇨ **heterosexual**

heterosis [ˌhetəˈrəʊsɪs] *or* **hybrid vigour** [ˌhaɪbrɪd ˈvɪgə] *subst.* increase in size *or* rate of growth *or* fertility *or* resistance to disease found in offspring of a cross between two species *heterosiseffekt, ökning i styrka, motståndskraft etc. pga korsning mellan olika arter*

heterosiseffekt ⇨ **heterosis**

heterotopia [ˌhet(ə)rəʊ'təʊpiə] *subst.* state where an organ is placed in a different position from normal or is malformed or deformed *or* development of tissue which is not natural to the part in which it is produced *heterotopi*

heterotransplantat ➪ **heterograft, xenograft**

heterotropia [ˌhet(ə)rəʊ'trəʊpiə] *subst.* strabismus *or* condition where the two eyes focus on different points *heterotropi*

hetshunger ➪ **bulimia (nervosa)**

hetta ➪ **heat, calor**

Hg *chemical symbol for* mercury *Hg, kvicksilver*

HGH ➪ **growth**

HIA ➪ **care**

hiatus [haɪ'eɪtəs] *subst.* opening *or* space *hiatus, gap;* **hiatus hernia** *or US* **hiatal hernia** = hernia where the stomach bulges through the opening in the diaphragm muscle through which the oesophagus passes *hernia diaphragmatica, hiatusbråck, diafragmabråck;* **oesophageal hiatus and aortic hiatus** = openings in the diaphragm through which the oesophagus and aorta pass *hiatus oesophagus och hiatus aorticus, matstrupsgapet och aortagapet*

hiatusbråck ➪ **diaphragmatic, hernia**

hiccup ['hɪkʌp] *or* **hiccough** ['hɪkʌp] *or* **singultus** [sɪŋ'gʌltəs] **1** *subst.* spasm in the diaphragm which causes a sudden inhalation of breath followed by sudden closure of the glottis which makes a characteristic sound *singultus, hicka;* **she had an attack of hiccups** *or* **a hiccuping attack; he got the hiccups from laughing too much, and found he couldn't stop them 2** *vb.* to make a hiccup *hicka;* **she patted him on the back when he suddenly started to hiccup; do you know how to stop someone hiccuping? he hiccuped so loudly that everyone in the restaurant looked at him**

> COMMENT: many cures have been suggested for hiccups, but the main treatment is to try to get the patient to think about something else. A drink of water, holding the breath and counting, breathing into a paper bag, are all recommended

hicka ➪ **hiccup**

hidr- [ˌhaɪdr, haɪdr] *prefix* meaning sweat *hidr(o)-, svett-*

hidradenitis [ˌhaɪdrədɪ'naɪtɪs] *subst.* inflammation of the sweat glands *hidradenit, hidro(s)adenit, svettkörtelinflammation*

hidroa ➪ **hydroa**

hidrosis [haɪ'drəʊsɪs] *subst.* (especially excessive) sweating *hidros, svettning*

hidrotic [haɪ'drɒtɪk] **1** *adj.* referring to sweating *som avser el. hör till svett(ning)* **2** *subst.* substance which makes someone sweat *hidrotikum, svettdrivande medel*

Higginson's syringe ['hɪgɪnsənz sɪ'rɪn(d)ʒ] *subst.* syringe with a rubber bulb in the centre that allows flow in one direction only (used mainly to give enemas) *slags spruta som tillåter flöde bara i en riktning*

high [haɪ] *adj.* **(a)** tall *or* reaching far from the ground level *hög;* **the hospital building is 60 m high; the operating theatre has a high ceiling (b)** *(referring to numbers)* big *hög;* **the patient has a very high temperature; there was a high level of glucose in the patient's blood; high blood pressure** *or* **hypertension** = condition where the pressure of blood in the arteries is too high, causing the heart to strain *hypertension, hypertoni, högt blodtryck;* **high energy foods** = foods containing a large number of calories, such as fats or carbohydrates, which give a lot of energy when they are broken down *föda med högt energiinnehåll;* **high temperature short time (HTST) method** = usual method of pasteurizing milk, where the milk is heated to 72°C for 15 seconds and then rapidly cooled *vanlig metod för att pastörisera mjölk*
NOTE:
NOTE: **high - higher - highest**

highly strung ['haɪli ˌstrʌŋ] *adj.* very nervous and tense *mycket nervös (spänd);* **she is highly strung, so don't make comments about her appearance, or she will burst into tears**

Highmore ['haɪmɔː] *subst.* **antrum of Highmore** = MAXILLARY SINUS

high-risk [ˌhaɪ'rɪsk] *adj.* (person) who is very likely to catch a disease *or* develop a cancer *or* suffer an accident *högrisk-;* **high-risk categories of worker; high-risk patient** = patient who has a high risk of catching an infection *högriskpatient*

Hijman van den Berghs reaktion ➪ **van den Bergh test**

hilar ['haɪlə] *adj.* referring to a hilum *hilär, rot-*

hilum ['haɪləm] *subst.* hollow where blood vessels *or* nerve fibres enter an organ such as a kidney *or* lung *hilum, rot* NOTE: the plural is **hila**

hilustuberkulos ➪ **epituberculosis**

hilär ➪ **hilar**

hindbrain ['haɪn(d)breɪn] *subst.* part of brain of an embryo, from which the medulla oblongata, the pons and the cerebellum eventually develop *metencefalon, bakhjärnan*

hinder ➪ **barrier, block, blockage, impediment, obstruction**

hindgut ['haɪndgʌt] *subst.* part of an embryo which develops into the colon and rectum *baktarmen*

hinge joint ['hɪndʒ ˌdʒɔɪnt] *subst.* synovial joint (like the knee) which allows two bones to move in one direction only *ginglymus, gångjärnsled, vinkelled, scharnerled; compare* BALL AND SOCKET JOINT

hinn- ➪ **membranous**

hinna ➪ **coating, film, membrane, tunica**

hinna, tunn ➪ **pellicle**

hinnlabyrinten ➪ **membranous**

hinnsäckar ➪ **otolith**

hip [hɪp] *subst.* ball and socket joint where the thigh bone *or* femur joins the acetabulum of the hip bone *höften;* **hip bath** = small low bath in which a person can sit but not lie down *sittbad(kar);* **hip bone** *or* **innominate bone** = bone made of the ilium, the ischium and the pubis which are fused together, forming part of the pelvic girdle *os ilium, tarmbenet, höftbenet;* **hip fracture** = fracture of the ball at the top of the femur *höftfraktur;* **hip girdle** *or* **pelvic girdle** = the sacrum and the two hip bones *bäckengördeln, bäckenringen;* **hip joint** = joint where the rounded end of the femur joins a socket in the acetabulum ➪ *illustration* PELVIS *articulatio coxae, höftleden;* **hip replacement** = surgical operation to replace the whole ball and socket joint with an artificial one *höftledsplastik*

Hippel-Lindau [ˌhɪp(ə)l'lɪndaʊ] *see* VON HIPPEL-LINDAU

hippocampal formation [ˌhɪpə'kæmp(ə)l fɔː'meɪʃ(ə)n] *subst.* curved pieces of cortex inside each part of the cerebrum *pes hippocampi, ammonshornet*

hippocampus [ˌhɪpə'kæmpəs] *subst.* long rounded elevation projecting into the lateral ventricle in the brain *hippocampus*

Hippocratic oath [ˌhɪpəʊˌkrætɪk 'əʊθ] *subst.* oath sworn by medical students when they become doctors, in which they swear not to do anything to harm their patients and not to tell anyone the details of each patient's case *Hippokrates ed, hippokratiska eden*

hippus ['hɪpəs] *subst.* alternating rapid contraction and dilatation of the pupil of the eye *hippus*

Hirschsprung's disease ['hɪrʃsprʊŋz dɪˌziːz] *subst.* congenital condition where parts of the lower colon lack nerve cells, making peristalsis impossible, so that food accumulates in the upper colon which becomes swollen *megacolon congenitum, megakolon, Hirschsprungs sjukdom*

hirsutism ['hɜːsjuːtɪz(ə)m] *subst.* having excessive hair, especially condition where a woman grows hair on the body in the same way as a man *hirsutism*

hirudin [hɪ'ruːdɪn] *subst.* anticoagulant substance produced by leeches, which is injected into the bloodstream while the leech is feeding *hirudin*

His [hɪs] *subst.* **bundle of His** *or* **atrioventricular bundle** = bundle of modified cardiac muscle which conducts impulses from the atrioventricular node to the septum, and then divides to connect with the ventricles *atrioventrikulära muskelknippet, His bunt (knippe, knut), Hisska bunten (knippet, knutan)*

hiss ➪ **lift**

histaminbelastning ➪ **histamine**

histamine ['hɪstəmiːn] *subst.* substance released from mast cells throughout the body which stimulates tissues in various ways *histamin;* **excess of histamine causes inflammation of the tissues; the presence of substances to which a patient is allergic releases large amounts of histamine into the blood; histamine test** = test to determine the acidity of gastric juice *histaminbelastning, histaminprov*

COMMENT: histamines dilate the blood vessels (giving nettlerash) or constrict the muscles of the bronchi (giving asthmatic attacks)

histaminic [ˌhɪstəˈmɪnɪk] *adj.* referring to histamines *som avser el. hör till histamin;* **histaminic headache** *or* **Horton's disease** = headache affecting the region over the external carotid artery, caused by release of histamines (and associated with rise in temperature and lacrimation) *Hortons syndrom (huvudvärk)*

histaminprov ⇨ **histamine**

histidine [ˈhɪstədiːn] *subst.* amino acid which may be a precursor of histamine *histidin*

histiocyte [ˈhɪstiəʊsaɪt] *subst.* macrophage of the connective tissue, involved in tissue defence *histiocyt*

histiocytoma [ˌhɪstiəʊsaɪˈtəʊmə] *subst.* tumour containing histiocytes *histiocytom*

histiocytosis [ˌhɪstiəʊsaɪˈtəʊsɪs] *subst.* condition where histiocytes are present in the blood *histiocytos;* **histiocytosis X** = any form of histiocytosis (such as Hand-Schüller-Christian disease) where the cause is not known *histiocytosis X*

histo- [ˈhɪstəʊ, ˌ--] *prefix* referring to tissue *histo-, vävnads-*

histochemistry [ˌhɪstəʊˈkemɪstri] *subst.* study of the chemical constituents of cells and tissues and also their function and distribution, using a light or electron microscope to evaluate the stains *histokemi*

histocompatibility [ˌhɪstəʊkəmˌpætəˈbɪləti] *subst.* compatibility between antigens of donors and recipients of transplanted tissues *histokompatibilitet*

histocompatible [ˌhɪstəʊkəmˈpætɪb(ə)l] *adj.* (two organisms) which have tissues which are antigenically compatible *vävnadskompatibla, (vävnader) med så stor immunologisk likhet som möjligt (för att möjliggöra transplantation)*

histogenesis [ˌhɪstəʊˈdʒenəsɪs] *subst.* formation and development of tissue from the embryological germ layer *vävnadsbildning och -utveckling*

histoid [ˈhɪstɔɪd] *adj.* made of *or* developed from a particular tissue *utvecklad ur viss vävnad;* like normal tissue *hist(i)oid*

histokemi ⇨ **histochemistry**

histokompatibilitet ⇨ **histocompatibility**

histologi ⇨ **histology**

histological [ˌhɪstəˈlɒdʒɪk(ə)l] *adj.* referring to histology *histologisk*

histology [hɪˈstɒlədʒɪ] *subst.* study of anatomy of tissue cells and minute cellular structure, done using a microscope after the cells have been stained *histologi*

histolys ⇨ **histolysis**

histolysis [hɪˈstɒləsɪs] *subst.* disintegration of tissue *histolys, vävnadsupplösning*

histolytica [ˌhɪstəˈlɪtɪkə] *see* ENTAMOEBA

histoplasmos ⇨ **histoplasmosis**

histoplasmosis [ˌhɪstəʊplæzˈməʊsɪs] *subst.* lung disease caused by infection with a fungus Histoplasma *histoplasmos*

history [ˈhɪst(ə)ri] *subst.* study of what happened in the past *historia, bakgrund;* **case history** = details of what has happened to a patient under treatment *sjukjournal, sjukdomshistoria;* **medical history** = details of a patient's medical records over a period of time *sjukdomshistoria, sjukhistoria, (medicinsk) anamnes;* **he has a history of serious illness** *or* **a history of Parkinsonism; to take a patient's history** = to ask a patient to tell his case history in his own words on being admitted to hospital *ta upp anamnes på patienten*

> QUOTE these children gave a typical history of exercise-induced asthma
>
> **Lancet**

> QUOTE the need for evaluation of patients with a history of severe heart disease
>
> **Southern Medical Journal**

histotoxic [ˌhɪstəʊˈtɒksɪk] *adj.* (substance) which is poisonous to tissue *toxisk (giftig) för vävnaden*

HIV [ˌeɪtʃaɪˈviː] = HUMAN IMMUNODEFICIENCY VIRUS **tests showed that he was HIV positive; the hospital is carrying out screening tests for HIV infection**

COMMENT: HIV is the virus which causes AIDS

hives [haɪvz] *or* **urticaria** [ˌɜːtɪˈkeəriə] *or* **nettlerash** [ˈnet(ə)lræʃ] *subst.* affection of the skin where white, pink or red patches are formed which itch or sting *urticaria, nässelfeber, nässelutslag;* **giant hives** = ANGIONEUROTIC OEDEMA

hjulbent ➪ **bow-legged**

hjulbenthet ➪ **bow legs**

hjälp ➪ **aid, assistance, help**

hjälp- ➪ **accessory, auxiliary**

hjälpa ➪ **aid, assist, help**

hjälpare ➪ **helper**

hjälplös ➪ **helpless**

hjälpmedel ➪ **aid, appliance, facilities**

hjälpsam ➪ **helpful**

hjälpämne ➪ **excipient**

hjärn- ➪ **cerebr-, cerebral, encephal-**

hjärnan ➪ **brain, cerebrum, encephalon**

hjärnartärerna ➪ **cerebral**

hjärnbalken ➪ **corpus**

hjärnbarken ➪ **cerebral**

hjärnblödning ➪ **cerebrovascular, haemorrhage, haemorrhagic, stroke**

hjärnbryggan ➪ **pons**

hjärnbråck ➪ **cephalocele, encephalocele**

hjärndöd ➪ **brain**

hjärnfeber ➪ **brain fever**

hjärnhemisfär ➪ **cerebral**

hjärnhinnan, hårda ➪ **dura mater**

hjärnhinnan, mjuka ➪ **pia mater**

hjärnhinne- ➪ **mening-, meningeal**

hjärnhinnebråck ➪ **meningocele**

hjärnhinneinflammation ➪ **meningitis**

hjärnhinnorna ➪ **covering, leptomeninges**

hjärninflammation ➪ **encephalitis**

hjärnsjukdom ➪ **encephalopathy**

hjärnskada ➪ **brain damage**

hjärnskadad ➪ **brain-damaged**

hjärnskakning ➪ **concussion**

hjärnskålen ➪ **cranial, neurocranium**

hjärnskänklarna ➪ **cerebral, peduncle**

hjärnstammen ➪ **base, brain stem, stem**

hjärnstjälkarna ➪ **cerebral**

hjärntumör ➪ **brain tumour, encephaloma**

hjärnuppmjukning ➪ **encephalomalacia**

hjärnvalvet ➪ **fornix**

hjärnventrikel ➪ **cerebral, ventricle**

hjärnvindling ➪ **convolution, gyrus**

hjärnvävnadsliknande ➪ **encephaloid**

hjärt- ➪ **cardi-, cardiac, myocardial**

hjärtastma ➪ **asthma**

hjärtat ➪ **heart, cardia, cor**

hjärtattack ➪ **heart attack**

"hjärtattack" ➪ **coronary**

hjärtblock ➪ **heart**

hjärtblåsljud ➪ **cardiac**

hjärtcykeln ➪ **cardiac**

hjärtfel ➪ **heart**

hjärtfladder ➪ **flutter**

hjärtfrekvens ➪ **heart**

hjärtförstoring ➪ **cardiomegaly**

hjärthypertrofi ➪ **cardiomegaly**

hjärtinfarkt ➪ **heart attack, infarction**

"hjärtinfarkt" ⇨ **coronary**

hjärtinfarktavdelning ⇨ **care**

hjärtinflammation ⇨ **carditis**

hjärtintensivavdelning ⇨ **care**

hjärtkateter ⇨ **catheter**

hjärtkatetrisering ⇨ **catheterization**

hjärtkirurg ⇨ **surgeon**

hjärtkirurgi ⇨ **heart**

hjärtkirurgi, öppen ⇨ **open**

hjärtklappning ⇨ **palpitation**

hjärt-kärlsystemet ⇨ **cardiovascular, circulatory**

hjärtlung- ⇨ **heart-lung**

hjärtlungbypass ⇨ **cardiopulmonary bypass**

hjärtlungmaskin ⇨ **cardiopulmonary bypass, heart-lung, lung**

hjärtlungräddning ⇨ **cardiopulmonary resuscitation (CPR)**

hjärtlungtransplantation ⇨ **heart-lung**

hjärtmassage ⇨ **cardiac, heart**

hjärtmuskelinflammation ⇨ **myocarditis**

hjärtmuskeln ⇨ **cardiac, myocardium**

hjärtneuros ⇨ **cardiac, disordered, effort, hyperkinetic syndrome**

hjärtpatient ⇨ **cardiac**

hjärtsjukdom ⇨ **cardiopathy**

hjärtslag ⇨ **heartbeat**

hjärtsmärta ⇨ **cardialgia**

hjärtspecialist ⇨ **cardiologist**

hjärtspetsen ⇨ **apex**

hjärtspetsstöten ⇨ **apex**

hjärtstillestånd ⇨ **cardiac, heart, asystole**

hjärtsvikt ⇨ **cardiac**

hjärtsäcken ⇨ **pericardial, pericardium**

hjärtsäckens inre blad ⇨ **epicardium**

hjärtsäcks- ⇨ **pericard-, pericardial**

hjärtsäcksinflammation ⇨ **pericarditis**

hjärttamponad ⇨ **cardiac, haemopericardium**

hjärtton ⇨ **heart, lubb-dupp**

hjärttrakten ⇨ **precordium**

hjärttransplantation ⇨ **heart**

hjärtventrikel ⇨ **ventricle**

hjärtörat ⇨ **auricle**

hjäss- ⇨ **cephalic**

hjässan ⇨ **bregma, corona, crown, vertex**

hjässbenen ⇨ **parietal**

hjässbens- ⇨ **parietal, biparietal**

hjässbjudning ⇨ **cephalic, vertex**

hjässloben ⇨ **parietal**

hjässömmen ⇨ **coronal**

HLA [ˌeɪtʃel'eɪ] = HUMAN LEUCOCYTE ANTIGEN

> COMMENT: HLA-A is the most important of the antigens responsible for rejection of transplants

HLA system [ˌeɪtʃel'eɪ ˌsɪstəm] *subst.* system of HLA antigens on the surface of cells which need to be histocompatible to allow transplants to take place *HLA-systemet, HL-A-systemet*

HMO [ˌeɪtʃem'əʊ] *US* = HEALTH MAINTENANCE ORGANIZATION

hoarse [hɔːs] *adj.* rough *or* irritated (voice *or* throat) *hes, skrovlig;* **he became hoarse after shouting too much; she spoke in a hoarse whisper**

hoarseness ['hɔːsnəs] *subst.* rough sound of the voice, usually caused by laryngitis *heshet, skrovlighet*

hobnail liver ['hɒbneɪ(ə)l ˌlɪvə] *or* **atrophic cirrhosis** [ə'trɒfɪk sə'rəʊsɪs] *subst.* advanced portal cirrhosis in which the liver has become considerably smaller, where clumps of new cells are formed on the surface of the liver where fibrous tissue has replaced damaged liver cells *atrophia hepatis, atrofisk levercirros, Laënnecs cirros, skrumplever*

Hodgkin's disease ['hɒdʒkɪnz dɪˌziːz] *subst.* malignant disease in which the lymph glands are enlarged and there is an increase in the lymphoid tissues in the liver, spleen and other organs *Hodgkins sjukdom, Sternbergs sjukdom; see also* PEL-EBSTEIN FEVER

COMMENT: the lymph glands swell to a very large size, and the disease can then attack the liver, spleen and bone marrow. It is frequently fatal if not treated early

hoist [hɔɪst] *subst.* device with pulleys and wires for raising a bed *or* a patient *lift, lyftapparat*

hole [həʊl] *subst.* opening *or* space in something *hål;* **hole in the heart** = congenital defect where a hole exists in the wall between the two halves of the heart and allows blood to flow abnormally through the heart and lungs *hål i hjärtat, medfött shuntande vitium*

Holger-Nielsen method [ˌhɒlgə'nɪlsən ˌmeθəd] *subst.* method of giving artificial ventilation by hand, where the patient lies face down and the first aider alternately presses on his back and pulls his arms outwards *slags metod för konstgjord andning*

holistic [hə(ʊ)'lɪstɪk] *adj.* (method of treatment) involving all the patient's mental and family circumstances rather than just dealing with the condition from which he is suffering *holistisk*

holistisk ⇨ **holistic**

hollow ['hɒləʊ] **1** *adj.* (space) which is empty *or* with nothing inside *ihålig;* **the surgeon inserted a hollow tube into the lung; the hollow cavity filled with pus 2** *subst.* place which is lower than the rest of the surface *håla, fördjupning*

holocrine ['hɒlə(ʊ)krɪn] *adj.* (gland) which is secretory only *or* where the secretion is made up of disintegrated cells of the gland itself *holokrin*

holokrin ⇨ **holocrine**

Homans' sign ['həʊmənz ˌsaɪn] *subst.* pain in the calf when the foot is bent back, a sign of deep vein thrombosis *Homans tecken*

home [həʊm] **1** *subst.* **(a)** place where you live *hem;* house which you live in *hem;* **are you going to be at home tomorrow? the doctor told her to stay at home instead of going to work; home help** = person who does housework for an invalid or handicapped person *hemhjälp;* **home nurse** *or* **district nurse** = nurse who visits patients in their homes *distriktssköterska* **(b)** house where people are looked after *hem;* **an old people's home; children's home** = house where children with no parents are looked after *ålderdomshem, barnhem;* **convalescent home** = type of hospital where patients can recover from illness *or* surgery *konvalescenthem;* **nursing home** = house where convalescents or old people can live under medical supervision by a qualified nurse *vårdhem, sjukhem* **2** *adv.* towards the place where you usually live *hem(åt);* **I'm going home; I'll take it home with me; I usually get home at 7 o'clock** = I reach the house where I live *jag brukar komma hem klockan sju;* **she can take the bus home** = she can go to where she lives by bus *hon kan ta bussen hem*

NOTE: used without a preposition: **he went home, she's coming home**

homeo- ['həʊmiə(ʊ), ˌ---] *or* **homoeo-** ['həʊmiə(ʊ), ˌ---] *prefix* meaning like *or* similar *homeo-*

homeopathic [ˌhəʊmiə'pæθɪk] *or* **homoeopathic** [ˌhəʊmiə'pæθɪk] *adj.* **(a)** referring to homeopathy *homeopatisk;* **a homeopathic clinic; she is having a course of homeopathic treatment (b)** (drug) given in very small quantities *homeopatisk*

homeopathist [ˌhəʊmi'ɒpəθɪst] *or* **homoeopathist** [ˌhəʊmi'ɒpəθɪst] *subst.* doctor who practises homeopathy *homeopat*

homeopathy [ˌhəʊmi'ɒpəθi] *or* **homoeopathy** [ˌhəʊmi'ɒpəθi] *subst.* treatment of disorders by giving the patient very small quantities of a substance which, when given to a healthy person, would cause symptoms like those of the disorder being treated *homeopati; compare* ALLOPATHY

homeostasis [ˌhəʊmiəʊ'steɪsɪs] *subst.* process by which the functions and chemistry of a cell *or* internal organ are kept stable, even when external conditions vary greatly *homeostas*

homo- ['həʊmə(ʊ), ˌ--] *prefix* meaning the same *homo-*

homogenize [hə'mɒdʒənaɪz] *vb.* to make something all the same *or* to give something a uniform nature *homogenisera;* **homogenized milk** = milk where the cream has been mixed up into the milk to give the same consistency throughout *homogeniserad mjölk*

homograft ['hɒməgrɑːft] *or* **allograft** ['æləgrɑːft] *subst.* graft of an organ *or* tissue from a donor to a recipient of the same species (as from one person to another) *homograft, allograft, allogent (homologt) transplantat; compare* AUTOGRAFT

homoiothermic [həʊˌmɔɪə'θɜːmɪk] *adj.* (animal) with warm blood *or* warm-blooded (animal) *varmblodig, jämnvarm; compare* POIKILOTHERMIC

> COMMENT: warm-blooded animals are able to maintain a constant body temperature whatever the outside temperature

homolateral ⇨ **ipsilateral**

homologous [hɒ'mɒləgəs] *adj.* (chromosomes) which form a pair *homolog*

homonymous [hə'mɒnɪməs] *adj.* affecting the two eyes in the same way *homonym;* **homonymous hemianopia** = condition where the same half of the field of vision is lost in each eye *homonym hemianopsi*

homoplasty ['həʊməʊˌplæsti] *subst.* surgery to replace lost tissues by grafting similar tissues from another person *hom(e)oplastik*

homosexual [ˌhəʊmə(ʊ)'sekʃu(ə)l] **1** *adj.* referring to homosexuality *homosexuell* **2** *subst.* person who is sexually attracted to people of the same sex, especially a man who experiences sexual attraction for other males *homosexuell (person)*

homosexuality [ˌhəʊmə(ʊ)sekʃu'æləti] *subst.* condition where a person experiences sexual attraction for persons of the same sex *or* has sexual relations with persons of the same sex *homosexualitet*

NOTE: although **homosexual** can apply to both males and females, it is commonly used for males only, and **lesbian** is used for females

compare BISEXUAL, HETEROSEXUAL, LESBIAN

homosexuell ⇨ **homosexual**

hona ⇨ **female**

hook [hʊk] **1** *subst.* surgical instrument with a bent end used for holding structures apart in operations *hake* **2** *vb.* to attach something with a hook *hålla med hake (krok)*

hookworm ['hʊkwɜːm] = ANCYLOSTOMA; **hookworm disease** = ANCYLOSTOMIASIS

hopdragning ⇨ **contraction**

hopklibbning ⇨ **agglutination**

hordeolum [hɔː'dɪələm] *or* **stye** [staɪ] *subst.* infection of the gland at the base of an eyelash *hordeolum, vagel*

horisontell ⇨ **horizontal**

horizontal [ˌhɒrɪ'zɒnt(ə)l] *adj.* which is lying flat *or* at a right angle to the vertical *horisontell, vågrät*

hormonal [hɔː'məʊn(ə)l] *adj.* referring to hormones *hormonell*

hormone ['hɔːməʊn] *subst.* substance which is produced by one part of the body, especially the endocrine glands and is carried to another part of the body by the bloodstream where it has causing particular effects or functions *hormon;* **growth hormone** = hormone which stimulates the growth of long bones *somatotropin, STH, (human) growth hormone, HGH, GH, tillväxthormon;* **sex hormones** = oestrogens and androgens which promote the growth of secondary sexual characteristics *sexualhormoner, könshormoner*

horn [hɔːn] *subst.* **(a)** *(in animals)* hard tissue which protrudes from the head *horn* **(b)** *(in humans)* (i) tissue which grows out of an organ *växt, utväxt, svulst;* (ii) one of the H-shaped limbs of grey matter seen in a cross-section of the spinal cord *horn;* (iii) extension of the pulp chamber of a tooth towards the cusp *en av tandpulpans spetsar*

horn ⇨ **cornu**

horn- ⇨ **horny, kerat-**

Horner's syndrome ['hɔːnəz ˌsɪndrəʊm] *subst.* condition caused by paralysis of the sympathetic nerve in one side of the neck, making the patient's eyelids hang down and the pupils contract *Horners syndrom (triad)*

hornhinnan ⇨ **cornea**

hornhinne- ⇨ **corneal, kerat-**

hornhinnefläck ⇨ **leucoma**

hornhinnegrumling ⇨ **nebula**

hornhinneinflammation ⇨ **keratitis**

hornhinnemikroskop ⇨ **gonioscope**

hornhinnesnitt ⇨ **keratotomy**

hornhinnetransplantation ⇨ **keratoplasty**

hornliknande ⇨ **horny**

hornsvulst ⇨ **keratoma**

horny ['hɔːni] *adj.* like horn *or* hard (skin) *horn-, hornliknande*
NOTE: for terms referring to horny tissue, see words beginning with **kerat-**

hornämne ⇨ **keratin**

horripilatio ⇨ **goose flesh**

horseshoe kidney ['hɔːsʃuː ˌkɪdni] *subst.* congenital defect of the kidney, where sometimes the upper but usually the lower parts of each kidney are joined together *ren arcuatus, hästskonjure*

Horton's disease ['hɔːtənz dɪˌziːz] *or* **Horton's headache** ['hɔːtənz ˌhedeɪk] *subst.* headache repeatedly affecting the region over the external carotid artery, caused by release of histamine in the body *Hortons syndrom (huvudvärk)*

hose [həʊz] *subst.* **(a)** long rubber or plastic tube *slang, tub* **(b)** stocking *strumpa;* **surgical** *or* **elastic hose** = special stocking worn to support and relieve varicose veins *stödstrumpa*

hospice ['hɒspɪs] *subst.* hospital which cares for terminally ill patients *sjukhus för döende patienter*

hospital ['hɒspɪt(ə)l] *subst.* place where sick or injured people are looked after *sjukhus;* **she's so ill she has been sent to hospital; he's been in hospital for several days; the children's hospital is at the end of our street; cottage hospital** = small local hospital set in pleasant gardens in the country *slags litet sjukhus i lantlig miljö, sjukstuga;* **day hospital** = hospital where the patients are treated during the day and go home in the evenings *dagsjukhus, dagvård, växelvård;* **general hospital** = hospital which cares for all types of patient *allmänt sjukhus;* **geriatric hospital** = hospital which specializes in the treatment of old people *geriatriskt sjukhus;* **isolation hospital** = hospital where patients suffering from dangerous infectious diseases can be isolated *epidemisjukhus;* **mental hospital** = hospital for the treatment of mentally ill patients *mentalsjukhus, psykiatriskt sjukhus;* **private hospital** = hospital which takes only paying patients *privatsjukhus;* **teaching hospital** = hospital attached to a medical school where student doctors work and study as part of their training *undervisningssjukhus;* **Hospital Activity Analysis** = regular detailed report on patients in hospitals, including information about treatment, length of stay, death rate. etc. *slags sjukvårdsstatistik;* **hospital bed** = (i) special bed in a hospital *sjukhussäng;* (ii) place in a hospital which can be occupied by a patient *bädd(plats), säng(plats);* **a hospital bed is needed if the patient has to have traction; the reduction in the number of hospital beds over the last few years**

hospitalisera ⇨ **hospitalize**

hospitalization [ˌhɒspɪt(ə)laɪ'zeɪʃ(ə)n] *subst.* sending someone to hospital *hospitalisering, intagning på sjukhus, inläggning på sjukhus;* **the doctor recommended immediate hospitalization**

hospitalize ['hɒspɪt(ə)laɪz] *vb.* to send someone to hospital *hospitalisera, lägga in på sjukhus;* **he is so ill that he has had to be hospitalized**

hospitalsbrand ⇨ **gangrene**

host [həʊst] *subst.* person *or* animal on which a parasite lives *värd, värddjur*

hosta ⇨ **cough, tussis**

hostanfall ⇨ **cough**

hostattack ⇨ **cough**

hosta upp ⇨ **bring up**

hostbefrämjande medel ⇨ **expectorant**

hostdämpande medel ⇨ **antitussive**

hostmedicin ⇨ **antitussive, cough, mixture**

hot [hɒt] *adj.* very warm; of a high temperature *het, varm;* **the water in my bath is too hot; if you're hot, take your coat off; affected skin will feel hot; hot flush** = condition in menopausal women, where the patient becomes hot and sweats, often accompanied by redness of the skin *flush, vallning, blodvallning*
NOTE: **hot - hotter - hottest**

hotande abort ⇨ **abortion**

hour ['a(ʊ)ə] *subst.* period of time lasting sixty minutes *timme;* **there are 24 hours in a day; the hours of work are from 9 to 5; when is your lunch hour?** = when do you stop work for lunch? *när (hur dags) har du lunch?;* **I'll be ready in a quarter of an hour** *or* **in half an hour** = in 15 minutes *or* 30 minutes *jag är färdig om en kvart resp. en halvtimme*

hourglass contraction ['a(ʊ)glɑːs kən'trækʃ(ə)n] *subst.* condition where an organ (such as the stomach) is constricted in the centre *timglasmage etc.*

hourly ['a(ʊ)əli] *adj.* happening every hour *som inträffar varje timme*

house [haʊs] *subst.* building which someone lives in *hus;* **he has a flat in the town and a house in the country; all the houses in our street look the same; his house has six bedrooms; house mite** = small insect living in houses, which can cause an allergic reaction *kvalster;* **house officer** = doctor who works in a hospital (as house surgeon *or* house physician) during the final year of training before registration by the GMC *ung. FV-läkare, läkare under specialistutbildning (specialistträning)*

housemaid's knee [ˌhaʊsmeɪdz 'niː] *or* **prepatellar bursitis** [priːpə'telə ˌbɜː'saɪtɪs] *subst.* condition where the fluid sac in the knee becomes inflamed, caused by kneeling on hard surfaces *bursitis prepatellaris, skurgummeknä*

houseman ['haʊsmən] *subst.* house surgeon *or* house physician *ung. underläkare på sjukhus*
NOTE: the US English is **intern**

HSG ⇨ **Rubin's test**

H-skiva ⇨ **H band**

HTST method [ˌeɪtʃtiːes'tiː ˌmeθəd] = HIGH TEMPERATURE SHORT TIME METHOD

hud- ⇨ **cutaneous, derm-, dermal**

hudavskavning ⇨ **excoriation**

hudblödningar ⇨ **purpura**

hudemfysem ⇨ **surgical**

huden ⇨ **skin**

hudfärg ⇨ **complexion**

hudförhårdnad ⇨ **pad**

hudförtjockning ⇨ **keratosis, pachydermia**

hudgraft ⇨ **skin**

hudinflammation ⇨ **dermatitis**

hudkarcinom ⇨ **rodent ulcer**

hudlös ⇨ **raw**

hudplastik ⇨ **dermatoplasty**

hudrodnad ⇨ **erythema, flare, flush**

hudsjukdom ⇨ **dermatosis**

hudspecialist ⇨ **dermatologist**

hudtorrhet ⇨ **xeroderma**

hudtransplantat ⇨ **skin**

huduppmjukande (medel) ⇨ **emollient**

hudutslag ⇨ **eruption, exanthem, rash**

hugg ⇨ **twinge**

huggsår ⇨ **cut**

Huhner's test ['huːnəz ˌtest] *subst.* test carried out several hours after sexual intercourse to determine the number and motility of spermatozoa *slags undersökning av spermier*

human ['hjuːmən] **1** *adj.* referring to any man, woman or child *human-, människo-;* **a human being** = a person *en människa;* **human chorionic gonadotrophin (hCG)** = hormone produced by the embryo which suppresses the mother's normal menstrual cycle during pregnancy *(humant) choriongonadotropin, HCG, graviditetshormon;* **human immunodeficiency virus (HIV)** = virus which causes AIDS *HIV* **2** *subst.* person *människa, person, individ;* **most animals are afraid of humans**

humanekologi ⇨ **ecology**

humeroulnar joint [ˌhjuːmərəʊ'ʌlnə ˌdʒɔɪnt] *subst.* part of the elbow joint, where the trochlear of the humerus and the trochlear notch of the ulna articulate *articulatio humeroulnaris, humeroulnarleden*

humerus ['hjuːm(ə)rəs] *subst.* top bone in the arm, running from the shoulder to the elbow ⇨ *illustration* SHOULDER *humerus, överarmsbenet*

humour ['hju:mə] *subst.* fluid in the body *vätska;* **aqueous humour** = fluid in the eye between the lens and the cornea *humor aqueus, ögonkammarvatten;* **vitreous humour** = jelly behind the lens in the eye ⇨ *illustration* EYE *humor vitreus, glaskroppen*

humör ⇨ **mind, mood, temper**

hunchback ['hʌn(t)ʃbæk] *subst.* (i) excessive forward curvature of the spine *puckelrygg;* (ii) person suffering from excessive forward curvature of the spine *puckelrygg*

hunger ['hʌŋgə] *subst.* feeling a need to eat *hunger;* **hunger pains** = pains in the abdomen when a person feels hungry (sometimes a sign of a duodenal ulcer) *hungersmärtor;* **air hunger** *see* AIR

hungersmärtor ⇨ **hunger**

hungrig ⇨ **hungry**

hungry ['hʌŋgri] *adj.* wanting to eat *hungrig;* **I'm hungry; are you hungry? you must be hungry after that long walk; the patient will not be hungry after the operation; I'm not very hungry - I had a big breakfast**
NOTE: **hungry - hungrier - hungriest**

Huntington's chorea ['hʌntɪŋtənz kəʊˌrɪə] *see* CHOREA

Hurler's syndrome ['hɜ:ləz ˌsɪndrəʊm] = GARGOYLISM

hurry ['hʌri] **1** *subst.* rush *brådska;* **get out of the way - we're in a hurry!; he's always in a hurry** = he is always rushing about *or* doing things very fast *han har alltid bråttom;* **what's the hurry?** = why are you going so fast? *varför har du så bråttom?* NOTE: no plural **2** *vb.* to go or do something fast *skynda sig;* to make someone go faster *skynda på, påskynda;* **she hurried along the passage; you'll have to hurry if you want to see the doctor, he's just leaving the hospital; don't hurry - we've got plenty of time; don't hurry me, I'm working as fast as I can**

hurt [hɜ:t] **1** *subst. (used by children)* painful spot *ont;* **she has a hurt on her knee** **2** *vb.* (i) to have pain *ha ont;* (ii) to give pain *skada, göra ont, värka;* **he's hurt his hand; where does your foot hurt? his arm is hurting so much he can't write; she fell down and hurt herself; are you hurt? is he badly hurt? my foot hurts; he was slightly hurt in the car crash; two players got hurt in the football game**
NOTE: **hurts - hurting - hurt - has hurt**

hus ⇨ **house**

husky ['hʌski] *adj.* slightly hoarse *hes, skrovlig, beslöjad;* **husky voice**

husläkare ⇨ **family**

Hutchinson-Gilford syndrome ['hʌtʃɪnsən'gɪlfəd ˌsɪndrəʊm] *subst.* progeria *or* premature senility *progeri, Hutchinsons syndrom*

Hutchinson's tooth ['hʌtʃɪnsənz ˌtu:θ] *subst.* narrow upper incisor tooth, with notches along the cutting edge, a symptom of congenital syphilis but also occurring naturally *Hutchinsons tand*

huvud ⇨ **head**

huvud- ⇨ **cephal-, cephalic; key**

huvudbjudning ⇨ **cephalic, vertex**

huvudbronkerna ⇨ **bronchi**

huvuddel ⇨ **body**

huvudkudde ⇨ **pillow**

huvudlus ⇨ **Pediculus**

huvudmätning ⇨ **cephalometry**

huvudsvålen ⇨ **scalp, epicranium, galea**

huvudvärk ⇨ **headache, cephalalgia**

huvudvärkstablett ⇨ **aspirin**

hy ⇨ **complexion**

hyal- ['ha(ɪ)əl, ˌ--] *prefix* like glass *hyal-*

hyalin ['ha(ɪ)əlɪn] *subst.* transparent substance produced from collagen and deposited around blood vessels and scars when certain tissues degenerate *hyalin*

hyaline ['ha(ɪ)əlɪn] *adj.* nearly transparent like glass *hyalin;* **hyaline cartilage** = type of cartilage found in the nose, larynx and joints ⇨ *illustration* JOINTS *hyalint brosk, glasbrosk;* **hyaline membrane disease** *or* **respiratory distress syndrome** = condition of newborn babies, where the lungs do not expand properly *idiopatiskt respiratoriskt distress-syndrom, IRDS, syndrome membranarum hyalinarum, hyalina membran*

hyalitis [ˌha(ɪ)ə'laɪtɪs] *subst.* inflammation of the vitreous humour or the hyaloid membrane in the eye *hyalit*

hyaloid membrane [ˈha(ɪ)əlɔɪd ˌmembreɪn] *subst.* transparent membrane round the vitreous humour in the eye *glashinnan som omger glaskroppen*

hyaluronic acid [ˌha(ɪ)əlʊˌrɒnɪk ˈæsɪd] *subst.* substance which binds connective tissue and is found in the eyes *hyaluronsyra*

hyaluronidase [ˌha(ɪ)əlʊˈrɒnɪdeɪz] *subst.* enzyme which destroys hyaluronic acid *hyaluronidas*

hyaluronsyra ➪ **hyaluronic acid**

hybrid [ˈhaɪbrɪd] *adj. & subst.* cross between two species of plant *or* animal *hybrid, bastard, korsning;* **hybrid vigour** = increase in size *or* rate of growth *or* fertility *or* resistance to disease found in offspring of a cross between two species *heterosiseffekt, ökning i styrka, motståndskraft etc. pga korsning mellan olika arter*

hydatid (cyst) [ˈhaɪdətɪd (ˌsɪst)] *subst.* cyst found in an organ which covers the larvae of the tapeworm Taenia solium *hydatid(cysta)*

hydatid disease [ˈhaɪdətɪd dɪˌziːz] *or* **hydatidosis** [ˌhaɪdətɪˈdəʊsɪs] *subst.* disease caused by hydatid cysts in the lung *or* brain *hydatidsjuka, hydatidos*

hydatidiform mole [ˌhaɪdəˈtɪdɪfɔːm ˌməʊl] *subst.* growth in the uterus, which looks like a hydatid cyst, and is formed of villous sacs swollen with fluid *mola hydatidosa, blåsmola, druvbörd*

hydatidos ➪ **hydatid disease**

hydatidsjuka ➪ **hydatid disease**

hydr- [haɪdr] *prefix* referring to water *hydr(o)-, vatten-*

hydraemia [haɪˈdriːmiə] *subst.* excess of water in the blood *hydremi*

hydragogue [ˈhaɪdrəgɒg] *subst.* laxative *or* substance which produces watery faeces *hydragogum, slags laxermedel*

hydrargyros ➪ **mercurialism, mercury**

hydrarthrosis [ˌhaɪdrɑːˈθrəʊsɪs] *subst.* swelling caused by excess synovial liquid at a joint *hydrartros, vätskeutgjutning i led*

hydro- [ˈhaidrə(u), ˌ--] *prefix* referring to water *hydr(o)-, vatten-*

hydroa [haɪˈdrəʊə] *subst.* eruption of small itchy blisters (as those caused by sunlight) *hidroa*

hydrocefali ➪ **hydrocephalus**

hydrocele [ˈhaɪdrə(ʊ)siː(ə)l] *subst.* collection of watery liquid found in a cavity such as the scrotum *hydrocele, vattenbråck*

hydrocephalus [ˈhaɪdrə(ʊ)ˈkef(ə)ləs] *subst.* excessive quantity of cerebrospinal fluid in the brain *hydrocefali, vattenskalle*

hydrochloric acid [ˌhaɪdrə(ʊ)ˌklɒrɪk ˈæsɪd] *subst.* acid found in the gastric juices which helps the maceration of food *klorvätesyra, saltsyra* NOTE: chemical symbol is **HCl**

hydrocolpos [ˌhaɪdrə(ʊ)ˈkɒlpəs] *subst.* cyst in the vagina containing clear fluid *hydrokolpos, vätskefylld vaginalcysta*

hydrocortisone [ˌhaɪdrə(ʊ)ˈkɔːtɪzəʊn] *subst.* steroid hormone secreted by the adrenal cortex, used to treat rheumatism and inflammatory and allergic conditions *hydrokortison, kortisol*

hydrocyanic acid [ˌhaɪdrə(ʊ)saɪˌænɪk ˈæsɪd] *subst.* acid which forms cyanide *cyanvätesyra, blåsyra*

hydrofobi ➪ **hydrophobia**

hydrogen [ˈhaɪdrədʒ(ə)n] *subst.* chemical element, a gas which combines with oxygen to form water, and with other elements to form acids, and is present in all animal tissue *väte, H* NOTE: chemical symbol is **H**

hydrokolpos ➪ **hydrocolpos**

hydrokortison ➪ **hydrocortisone, cortisol**

hydrometer [haɪˈdrɒmɪtə] *subst.* instrument which measures the density of a liquid *hydrometer*

hydromyelia [ˌhaɪdrəʊmaɪˈiːliə] *subst.* condition where fluid swells the central canal of the spinal cord *hydromyeli*

hydronefros ➪ **hydronephrosis**

hydronephrosis [ˌhaɪdrə(ʊ)nəˈfrəʊsɪs] *subst.* swelling of the pelvis of a kidney caused by accumulation of water due to infection *or* a kidney stone blocking the ureter *hydronefros*

hydropericarditis [ˌhaɪdrə(ʊ)ˌperikɑːˈdaɪtɪs] *or*

hydropericardium [ˌhaɪdrə(ʊ)ˌperiˈkɑːdiəm] *subst.* accumulation of liquid round the heart *hydroperikardit, vatten i hjärtsäcken*

hydrophobia [ˌhaɪdrə(ʊ)ˈfəʊbiə] *or* **rabies** [ˈreɪbiːz] *subst.* frequently fatal virus disease transmitted by infected animals *rabies, hydrofobi, vattuskräck*

> COMMENT: hydrophobia affects the mental balance, and the symptoms include difficulty in breathing or swallowing and a horror of water

hydrops ⇨ **dropsy**

hydrorré ⇨ **hydrorrhoea**

hydrorrhoea [ˌhaɪdrə(ʊ)ˈrɪə] *subst.* discharge of watery fluid *hydrorré*

hydrotherapy [ˌhaɪdrə(ʊ)ˈθerəpi] *subst.* treatment of patients with water, where the patients are put in hot baths *or* are encouraged to swim *hydroterapi, vattenbehandling*

hydrothorax [ˌhaɪdrə(ʊ)ˈθɔːræks] *subst.* collection of liquid in the pleural cavity *hydrot(h)orax, vatten i lungsäcken*

hydroxide [haɪˈdrɒksaɪd] *subst.* chemical compound containing a hydroxyl group *hydroxid;* **aluminium hydroxide** = chemical substance used as an antacid *aluminiumhydroxid*

hygien ⇨ **hygiene, sanitation**

hygiene [ˈhaɪdʒiːn] *subst.* (i) being clean and keeping healthy conditions *hygien, renlighet;* (ii) science of health *hygien, hälsovård, hälsovårdslära;* **nurses have to maintain a strict personal hygiene; dental hygiene** = keeping the teeth clean and healthy *tandhygien*

hygienic [haɪˈdʒiːnɪk] *adj.* (i) clean *hygienisk, ren(lig);* (ii) which produces healthy conditions *hygienisk;* **don't touch the food with dirty hands - it isn't hygienic**

hygienisk ⇨ **hygienic, sanitary**

hygienist [haɪˈdʒiːnɪst] *subst.* person who specializes in hygiene and its application *hygieniker;* **dental hygienist** = person who helps a dentist by cleaning teeth and gums, removing plaque from teeth and giving fluoride treatment *tandhygienist*

hymen [ˈhaɪmen] *subst.* membrane which partially covers the vaginal passage in a virgin *hymen, mödomshinnan*

hymenectomy [ˌhaɪməˈnektəmi] *subst.* surgical removal of the hymen *or* operation to increase the size of the opening of the hymen *or* surgical removal of any membrane *operativt ingrepp i mödomshinnan el. annat membran*

hymenotomy [ˌhaɪməˈnɒtəmi] *subst.* incision of the hymen during surgery *operativt insnitt i mödomshinnan*

hyoglossus [ˌhaɪəʊˈglɒsəs] *subst.* muscle which is attached to the hyoid bone and depresses the tongue *musculus hyoglossus*

hyoid bone [ˈhaɪɔɪd ˌbəʊn] *subst.* small U-shaped bone at the base of the tongue *os hyoideum, tungbenet*

hyoscine [ˈhaɪə(ʊ)siːn] *subst.* drug used as a sedative, in particular for treatment of motion sickness *hyoscin, skopolamin*

hyp- [haɪp, ˌhɪp] *or* **hypo-** [ˈhaɪpə(ʊ), ˌ--] *prefix* meaning less *or* too little *or* too small *hyp(o)-, under-; opposite is* HYPER-

hypaemia [haɪˈpiːmiə] *subst.* insufficient amount of blood in the body *hypemi*

hypalgesia [ˌhaɪpælˈdʒiːziə] *subst.* low sensitivity to pain *hypalgesi*

hypemi ⇨ **hypaemia**

hyper- [ˈhaɪpə, ˌ--] *prefix* meaning higher *or* too much *hyper-, super-, över-; opposite is* HYP- *or* HYPO-

hyperaciditet ⇨ **hyperacidity, hyperchlorhydria**

hyperacidity [ˌhaɪpərəˈsɪdəti] *subst.* increase in acid in the stomach *hyperaciditet*

hyperactive [ˌhaɪpərˈæktɪv] *adj.* being very active *hyperaktiv*

hyperactivity [ˌhaɪpərækˈtɪvəti] *subst.* condition where something (a gland *or* a child) is too active *hyperaktivitet;* **hyperactivity syndrome** = condition where a child is extremely active, restless, breaks things for no reason and will not study *syndrom med hyperaktivitet*

hyperacusis [ˌhaɪpərəˈkjuːsɪs] *or* **hyperacousia** [ˌhaɪpərəˈkjuːziə] *subst.* being very sensitive to sounds *hyperakusi*

hyperaemia [ˌhaɪpərˈiːmiə] *subst.* excess blood in any part of the body *hyperemi*

hyperaesthesia [ˌhaɪpəriːs'θiːziə] *subst.* extremely high sensitivity in the skin *hyperestesi*

hyperaktiv ⇨ **hyperactive**

hyperaktivitet ⇨ **hyperactivity**

hyperakusi ⇨ **hyperacusis**

hyperalgesi ⇨ **hyperalgesia**

hyperalgesia [ˌhaɪpəræl'dʒiːziə] *subst.* increased sensitivity to pain *hyperalgesi*

hyperbaric [ˌhaɪpə'beərɪk] *adj.* (treatment) where a patient is given oxygen at high pressure, used to treat carbon monoxide poisoning *under övertryck, övertrycks-*

hypercalcaemia [ˌhaɪpəkæl'siːmiə] *subst.* excess of calcium in the blood *kalcemi, hyperkalcemi*

hyperchlorhydria [ˌhaɪpəklɔː'haɪdriə] *subst.* excess of hydrochloric acid in the stomach *hyperaciditet, superaciditet*

hyperdactylism [ˌhaɪpə'dæktɪlɪz(ə)m] *or* **polydactylism** [ˌpəʊli'dæktɪlɪz(ə)m] *subst.* having more than the normal number of fingers or toes *polydaktyli, hyperdaktyli*

hyperdaktyli ⇨ **hyperdactylism, polydactylism**

hyperemesis gravidarum [ˌhaɪpər'eməsɪs ˌgrævɪ'deərəm] *subst.* uncontrollable vomiting in pregnancy *hyperemesis gravidarum, graviditetskräkningar*

hyperemi ⇨ **hyperaemia**

hyperestesi ⇨ **hyperaesthesia**

hyperglycaemia [ˌhaɪpəglaɪ'siːmiə] *subst.* excess of glucose in the blood *hyperglykemi*

hyperinsulinism [ˌhaɪpər'ɪnsjʊlɪnɪz(ə)m] *subst.* reaction of a diabetic to an excessive dose of insulin *or* to hypoglycaemia *hyperinsulinism*

hyperkalcemi ⇨ **calcaemia, hypercalcaemia**

hyperkinesia [ˌhaɪpəkɪ'niːziə] *subst.* condition where there is abnormally great strength or movement *hyperkinesi;* **essential hyperkinesia** = condition of children where their movements are excessive and repeated *MBD (minimal brain damage), tillstånd med onormal motorisk aktivitet hos barn*

hyperkinetic syndrome [ˌhaɪpəkɪ'netɪk ˌsɪndrəʊm] *or* **effort syndrome** ['efət ˌsɪndrəʊm] *subst.* condition where the patient experiences fatigue, shortness of breath, pain under the heart and palpitation *hjärtneuros*

hypermenorré ⇨ **flooding, hypermenorrhoea**

hypermenorrhoea [ˌhaɪpəˌmenə'rɪə] *subst.* menstruation in which the flow is excessive *hypermenorré, menorragi*

hypermetrop ⇨ **longsighted**

hypermetropi ⇨ **farsightedness**

hypermetropia [ˌhaɪpəmɪ'trəʊpiə] *or* **longsightedness** [ˌlɒŋ'saɪtɪdnəs] *or US* **hypertropia** [ˌhaɪpə'trəʊpiə] *subst.* condition where the patient sees more clearly objects which are a long way away, but cannot see objects which are close; *compare* MYOPIA *hypermetropi, hyperopi, översynthet*

hypernephroma [ˌhaɪpənə'frəʊmə] = GRAWITZ TUMOUR

hyperopi ⇨ **farsightedness**

hyperostosis [ˌhaɪpərɒ'stəʊsɪs] *subst.* excessive overgrowth on the outside surface of a bone, especially the frontal bone *hyperostos*

hyperpiesis [ˌhaɪpəpaɪ'iːsɪs] *subst.* abnormally high blood pressure *essentiell hypertension, förhöjt blodtryck, Huchards sjukdom*

hyperplasia [ˌhaɪpə'pleɪziə] *subst.* condition in which there is an increase in the number of cells in an organ *hyperplasi, förstoring (genom cellnybildning)*

hyperpyrexia [ˌhaɪpəpaɪ'reksiə] *subst.* high body temperature (above 41.1°C) *hyperpyrexi*

hypersensibilitet ⇨ **hypersensitivity**

hypersensitive [ˌhaɪpə'sensətɪv] *adj.* (person) who reacts more strongly than normal to an antigen *överkänslig*

hypersensitivity [ˌhaɪpəˌsensə'tɪvəti] *subst.* condition where the patient reacts very strongly to something (such as an allergic substance) *hypersensibilitet, överkänslighet, allergi;* **her hypersensitivity to dust;**

anaphylactic shock shows hypersensitivity to an injection

hypertensin ⇨ **angiotensin**

hypertension [ˌhaɪpəˈtenʃ(ə)n] *subst.* high blood pressure *or* condition where the pressure of the blood in the arteries is too high *hypertension, hypertoni, högt blodtryck;* **portal hypertension** = high pressure in the portal vein, caused by cirrhosis of the liver *or* a clot in the vein and causing internal bleeding *portal hypertension;* **pulmonary hypertension** = high blood pressure in the blood vessels supplying the lungs *pulmonell hypertension*

COMMENT: high blood pressure can have many causes: the arteries are too narrow, causing the heart to strain; kidney disease; Cushing's syndrome, etc. High blood pressure is treated with drugs such as beta blockers

hypertensive headache [ˌhaɪpəˌtensɪv ˈhedeɪk] *subst.* headache caused by high blood pressure *huvudvärk pga högt blodtryck*

hypertermi ⇨ **hyperthermia**

hyperthermia [ˌhaɪpəˈθɜːmiə] *subst.* very high body temperature *hypertermi, förhöjd kroppstemperatur*

hyperthyroidism [ˌhaɪpəˈθaɪrɔɪdɪz(ə)m] *subst.* condition where the thyroid gland is too active and swells, as in Graves' disease *hypertyreoidism, hypertyreos*

hypertoni ⇨ **hypertension**

hypertrichosis [ˌhaɪpətraɪˈkəʊsɪs] *subst.* condition where the patient has excessive growth of hair on the body *or* on part of the body *hypertrikos*

hypertrikos ⇨ **hypertrichosis**

hypertrofi ⇨ **hypertrophy**

hypertrophic [ˌhaɪpəˈtrɒfɪk] *adj.* associated with hypertrophy *hypertrofisk;* **hypertrophic rhinitis** = condition where the mucous membranes in the nose become thicker *rinit med slemhinneförtjockning i näsan*

hypertrophy [haɪˈpɜːtrəfi] *subst.* increase in the number or size of cells in a tissue *hypertrofi, förstoring*

hypertropia [ˌhaɪpəˈtrəʊpiə] *subst. US* = HYPERMETROPIA

hypertyreoidism ⇨ **hyperthyroidism**

hypertyreos ⇨ **hyperthyroidism**

hyperventilate [ˌhaɪpəˈventɪleɪt] *vb.* to breathe very fast *hyperventilera;* **we all hyperventilate as an expression of fear or excitement**

hyperventilation [ˌhaɪpəˌventɪˈleɪʃ(ə)n] *subst.* very fast breathing which can be accompanied by dizziness or tetany *hyperventilation*

hypervitaminosis [ˌhaɪpəˌvɪtəmɪˈnəʊsɪs] *subst.* condition caused by taking too many synthetic vitamins, especially Vitamins A and D *hypervitaminos*

hyphaemia [haɪˈfiːmiə] *subst.* (i) insufficient amount of blood in the body *anemi, blodbrist;* (ii) bleeding into the front chamber of the eye *hyphema, hyphemi*

hyphidros ⇨ **hypohidrosis**

hypn- [hɪpn] *prefix* referring to sleep *hypn(o)-, sömn-*

hypnos ⇨ **hypnosis, hypnotism**

hypnosis [hɪpˈnəʊsɪs] *subst.* state like sleep, but caused artificially, where the patient can remember forgotten events in the past *or* will do whatever the hypnotist tells him to do *hypnos*

hypnotherapy [ˌhɪpnə(ʊ)ˈθerəpi] *subst.* treatment by hypnosis, used in treating some addictions *hypnoterapi*

hypnotic [hɪpˈnɒtɪk] *adj.* referring to hypnotism *hypnotisk;* (drug) which causes sleep *hypnotiskt, sömngivande;* (state) which is like sleep but which is caused artificially *hypnotisk*

hypnotikum ⇨ **soporific**

hypnotisera ⇨ **hypnotize**

hypnotisk ⇨ **hypnotic**

hypnotism [ˈhɪpnətɪz(ə)m] *subst.* inducing hypnosis *hypnos*

hypnotist [ˈhɪpnətɪst] *subst.* person who hypnotizes other people *hypnotisör;* **the hypnotist passed his hand in front of her eyes and she went immediately to sleep**

hypnotisör ⇨ **hypnotist**

hypnotize ['hɪpnətaɪz] *vb.* to make someone go into a state where he appears to be asleep, and will do whatever the hypnotist suggests *hypnotisera;* **he hypnotizes his patients, and then persuades them to reveal their hidden problems**

hypo ['haɪpəʊ] *informal* = HYPODERMIC SYRINGE

hypo- ['haɪpə(ʊ), ˌ--] *prefix* meaning less *or* too little *hyp(o)-, under-*

hypoaesthesia [ˌhaɪpəʊiːs'θiːziə] *subst.* condition where the patient has a diminished sense of touch *hyp(o)estesi*

hypocalcaemia [ˌhaɪpəʊkæl'siːmiə] *subst.* abnormally low amount of calcium in the blood, which can cause tetany *hypocalcemi, hypokalcemi*

hypochondria [ˌhaɪpə(ʊ)'kɒndriə] *subst.* condition where a person is too worried about his health and believes he is ill *hypokondri, inbillningssjuka*

hypochondriac [ˌhaɪpə(ʊ)'kɒndrɪæk] **1** *subst.* person who worries about his health too much *hypokondriker* **2** *adj.* **hypochondriac regions** = two parts of the upper abdomen, on either side of the epigastrium below the floating ribs *hypokondriet*

hypochondrium [ˌhaɪpə(ʊ)'kɒndriəm] *subst.* one of the hypochondriac regions in the upper part of the abdomen *hypokondriet*

hypochromic anaemia [ˌhaɪpə(ʊ)ˌkrəʊmɪk ə'niːmiə] *subst.* anaemia where haemoglobin is reduced in proportion to the number of red blood cells, which then appear very pale *hypokrom anemi*

hypodermic [ˌhaɪpə(ʊ)'dɜːmɪk] *adj.* beneath the skin *hypodermatisk, subkutan;* **hypodermic syringe** *or* **a hypodermic** = syringe which injects liquid under the skin *injektionsspruta, spruta;* **hypodermic needle** = needle for injecting liquid under the skin *injektionsnål, nål, kanyl*

hypofysen ⇨ **hypophysis cerebri**

hypofyshormon ⇨ **pituitrin**

hypofysiotropiner ⇨ **hypothalamic**

hypofysloben, främre ⇨ **adenohypophysis**

hypofysstjälken ⇨ **hypophyseal**

hypofysär ⇨ **hypophyseal**

hypogastrium [ˌhaɪpə(ʊ)'gæstriəm] *subst.* part of the abdomen beneath the stomach *hypogastriet*

hypoglossal nerve [ˌhaɪpə(ʊ)'glɒs(ə)l ˌnɜːv] *subst.* twelfth cranial nerve which governs the muscles of the tongue *nervus hypoglossus, 12:e kranialnerven*

hypoglycaemia [ˌhaɪpə(ʊ)glaɪ'siːmiə] *subst.* low concentration of glucose in the blood *hypoglykemi*

hypoglycaemic [ˌhaɪpə(ʊ)glaɪ'siːmɪk] *adj.* suffering from hypoglycaemia *hypoglykemisk;* **hypoglycaemic coma** = state of unconsciousness affecting diabetics after taking an overdose of insulin *hypoglykemiskt koma, hypoglykemisk reaktion, insulinchock*

> COMMENT: hypoglycaemia affects diabetics who feel weak from lack of sugar. A hypoglycaemic attack can be prevented by eating glucose or a lump of sugar when feeling faint

hypohidrosis [ˌhaɪpə(ʊ)haɪ'drəʊsɪs] *or* **hypoidrosis** [ˌhaɪpɔɪ'drəʊsɪs] *subst.* producing too little sweat *hyphidros, nedsatt svettutsöndring*

hypokalaemia [ˌhaɪpə(ʊ)kæ'liːmiə] *subst.* deficiency of potassium in the blood *hypokal(i)emi*

hypokalcemi ⇨ **hypocalcaemia**

hypokondri ⇨ **hypochondria**

hypokondriet ⇨ **hypochondriac, hypochondrium**

hypokondriker ⇨ **hypochondriac**

hypomenorrhoea [ˌhaɪpə(ʊ)ˌmenə'rɪə] *subst.* production of too little blood at menstruation *hypomenorré*

hyponatraemia [ˌhaɪpə(ʊ)næ'triːmiə] *subst.* lack of sodium in the body *hyponatr(i)emi*

hypophyseal [ˌhaɪpə(ʊ)'fɪziəl] *adj.* referring to the hypophysis *or* pituitary gland *hypofysär, hypofys-;* **hypophyseal stalk** = stalk which attaches the pituitary gland to the hypothalamus *hypofysstjälken*

hypophysis cerebri [haɪ'pɒfəsɪs 'serəbri] *or* **pituitary gland** [pɪ'tjuːɪt(ə)ri ˌglænd] *subst.* main endocrine gland in the body *glandula pituitaria (hypophysis), hypophysis cerebri, hypofysen*

COMMENT: the pituitary gland is about the size of a pea, and hangs down from the base of the brain, inside the sphenoid bone on a stalk which attaches it to the hypothalamus. The front lobe of the gland (the adenohypophysis) secretes several hormones (TSH, ACTH) which stimulate the adrenal and thyroid glands, or which stimulate the production of sex hormones, melanin and milk. The rear lobe of the pituitary gland (the neurohypophysis) secretes the antidiuretic hormone ADH and oxytocin. The pituitary gland is the most important gland in the body because the hormones it secretes control the functioning of the other glands

hypoplasia [ˌhaɪpə(ʊ)ˈpleɪziə] *subst.* lack of development *or* defective formation of tissue or an organ *hypoplasi*

hyposensibilisering ➪ **desensitization**

hyposensitive [ˌhaɪpə(ʊ)ˈsensətɪv] *adj.* being less sensitive than normal *mindre känslig än normalt*

hypospadias [ˌhaɪpə(ʊ)ˈspeɪdiəs] *subst.* congenital defect of the wall of the male urethra or the vagina, so that the opening occurs on the under side of the penis or in the vagina *hypospadi; compare* EPISPADIAS

hypostasis [haɪˈpɒstəsɪs] *subst.* condition where fluid accumulates in part of the body because of poor circulation *hypostas*

hypostatic [ˌhaɪpəˈstætɪk] *adj.* referring to hypostasis *hypostatisk;* **hypostatic eczema** = eczema which develops on the legs, caused by bad circulation *hypostatiskt eksem, variköst eksem;* **hypostatic pneumonia =** pneumonia caused by fluid accumulating in the lungs of a bedridden patient with a weak heart *pneumonia hypostatica, hypostatisk lunginflammation*

hypotension [ˌhaɪpə(ʊ)ˈtenʃ(ə)n] *subst.* low blood pressure *hypotension, hypotoni, lågt blodtryck*

hypotermi ➪ **hypothermia**

hypothalamic [ˌhaɪpəʊθəˈlæmɪk] *adj.* referring to the hypothalamus *hypot(h)alamisk;* **hypothalamic hormones** *or* **releasing factors** = substances that cause the pituitary gland to release its hormones *hypofysiotropiner, releasing factors*

hypothalamus [ˌhaɪpə(ʊ)ˈθæləməs] *subst.* part of the brain above the pituitary gland, which controls the production of hormones by the pituitary gland and regulates important bodily functions such as hunger, thirst and sleep ➪ *illustration* BRAIN *hypot(h)alamus*

hypothenar [haɪˈpɒθɪnə] *adj.* referring to the soft fat part of the palm beneath the little finger *som avser el. hör till hypot(h)enar (lillfingervalken);* **hypothenar eminence =** lump on the palm beneath the little finger *hypot(h)enar, lillfingervalken; compare* THENAR

hypothermia [ˌhaɪpə(ʊ)ˈθɜːmiə] *subst.* reduction in body temperature below normal, for official purposes taken to be below 35°C *hypotermi, sänkt kroppstemperatur*

hypothermic [ˌhaɪpə(ʊ)ˈθɜːmɪk] *adj.* suffering from hypothermia *som lider av sänkt kroppstemperatur;* **examination revealed that she was hypothermic, with a rectal temperature of only 29.4°C**

hypothyroidism [ˌhaɪpə(ʊ)ˈθaɪrɔɪdɪz(ə)m] *subst.* underactivity of the thyroid gland *hypotyreoidism, hypotyreos*

hypoton ➪ **hypotonic**

hypotonia [ˌhaɪpə(ʊ)ˈtəʊniə] *subst.* reduced tension in any part of the body *hypotension, hypotoni, lågt blodtryck*

hypotonic [ˌhaɪpə(ʊ)ˈtɒnɪk] *adj.* with reduced tension *med minskat (nedsatt) tryck;* (solution) with lower osmotic pressure than plasma *hypoton*

hypotropia [ˌhaɪpə(ʊ)ˈtrəʊpiə] *subst.* form of squint where one eye looks downwards *slags skelning där ena ögat är riktat nedåt*

hypotyreoidism ➪ **hypothyroidism**

hypotyreos ➪ **hypothyroidism**

hypoventilation [ˌhaɪpə(ʊ)ˌventɪˈleɪʃ(ə)n] *subst.* very slow breathing *hypoventilation*

hypovitaminosis [ˌhaɪpə(ʊ)ˌvɪtəmɪˈnəʊsɪs] *subst.* lack of vitamins *hypovitaminos*

hypoxia [haɪˈpɒksiə] *subst.* inadequate supply of oxygen to tissue or an organ *hypoxi*

hysa ➪ **harbour**

hyster- [hɪstə, ˌhɪstə] *prefix* referring to the womb *hyster(o)-, metr(o)-, uter(o)-, livmoder(s)-*

hysteralgia [ˌhɪstər'ældʒə] *subst.* pain in the womb *metralgi, metrodyni, livmoderssmärta*

hysterectomy [ˌhɪstə'rektəmi] *subst.* surgical removal of the womb, either to treat cancer or because of the presence of fibroids *hysterektomi;* **subtotal hysterectomy =** removal of the womb, but not the cervix *subtotal hysterektomi;* **total hysterectomy =** removal of the whole womb *total hysterektomi*

hysterektomi ➪ **hysterectomy**

hysteria [hɪ'stɪəriə] *subst.* neurotic state, where the patient is unstable, and may scream and wave the arms about, but also is repressed, and may be slow to react to outside stimuli *hysteri*

hysterical [hɪ'sterɪk(ə)l] *adj.* (reaction) of hysteria *hysterisk;* **he burst into hysterical crying; hysterical personality =** mental condition of a person who is unstable, lacks normal feelings and is dependent on others *hysterisk personlighet*

hysterically [hɪ'sterɪk(ə)li] *adv.* in a hysterical way *hysteriskt;* **she was laughing hysterically**

hysterics [hɪ'sterɪks] *subst.* attack of hysteria *hysteriskt anfall;* **she had an attack** *or* **a fit of hysterics** *or* **she went into hysterics**

hystericus [hɪ'sterɪkəs] *see* GLOBUS

hysterisk ➪ **hysterical**

hystero- ['hɪstərə(ʊ), ˌ---] *prefix* referring to the womb *hyster(o)-, metr(o)-, uter(o)-, livmoder(s)-*

hysterocele ['hɪstərə(ʊ)siː(ə)l] *subst.* hernia of the womb *hysterocele, hernia uteri*

hysterocele ➪ **uterocele**

hysterografi ➪ **uterography**

hysteroptosis [ˌhɪstərəʊ'təʊsɪs] *subst.* prolapse of the womb *hysteroptos, metroptos, prolapsus uteri, uterusprolaps, livmoderframfall*

hysterosalpingography [ˌhɪstərə(ʊ)ˌsælpɪŋ'gɒgrəfi] *or* **uterosalpingography** [juːtərəʊˌsælpɪŋ'gɒgrəfi] *subst.* X-ray examination of the womb and Fallopian tubes following injection of radio-opaque material *hysterosalpingografi*

hysteroscope ['hɪstərəskəʊp] *subst.* tube for inspecting the inside of the womb *hysteroskop*

hysterotomy [ˌhɪstə'rɒtəmi] *subst.* surgical incision into the womb (as in Caesarean section *or* for some types of abortion) *hysterotomi*

hågkomst ➪ **recall**

hål ➪ **cavity, foramen, hole, lumen**

håla ➪ **cavity, antrum, hollow, space**

-håla ➪ **-cele, -coele**

hålfoten ➪ **arch**

hålfotsbågen ➪ **arch**

hålhandsbågen ➪ **palmar**

hålkort ➪ **card**

håll ➪ **stitch**

hållning ➪ **habitus, posture**

hållnings- ➪ **postural**

hålmejsel ➪ **gouge**

hålrum ➪ **antrum, sinus**

hålvenen ➪ **vena cava**

hålvenen, övre ➪ **superior**

hår ➪ **hair**

hår- ➪ **pilo-, trich(o)-**

håravfall ➪ **baldness**

hårborttagning ➪ **depilation**

hårbottnen ➪ **scalp**

hårcell ➪ **hair**

hårcellsleukemi ➪ **hairy**

hård ➪ **hard, strict, tight**

hårdna ➪ **harden**

hårfollikel ➪ **follicle**

hårfollikelinflammation ➪ **folliculitis**

hårig ⇨ **hairy**

hårliknande ⇨ **trich(o)-**

hårpapill ⇨ **hair**

hårrörskärl ⇨ **capillary**

hårsjukdom ⇨ **trichosis**

hårstrå ⇨ **hair, pilus**

hårsäck ⇨ **follicle**

hårsäckscysta ⇨ **pilonidal cyst**

hårsäcksinflammation ⇨ **folliculitis**

hårt ⇨ **hard, tightly**

hårtest ⇨ **tuft**

häft- ⇨ **adhesive**

häftförband ⇨ **adhesive, strapping**

häftig ⇨ **acute, lancinating, sharp, violent**

häftplåster ⇨ **adhesive, plaster**

hälbenet ⇨ **heel**

hälen ⇨ **heel**

hälsa ⇨ **health**

hälsokontroll ⇨ **checkup**

hälsokost ⇨ **food, macrobiotic**

hälsosam ⇨ **healthy**

hälsotillstånd ⇨ **health**

hälsoupplysning ⇨ **health**

hälsovådlig ⇨ **insanitary**

hälsovård ⇨ **hygiene**

hälsovårds- ⇨ **sanitary, environmental**

hälsovårdsinspektör ⇨ **health**

hälsovårdslära ⇨ **hygiene**

hälta ⇨ **claudication, lameness, limp**

hämma ⇨ **inhibit, restrict, retard, stunt, suppress**

hämmad ⇨ **abortive**

hämmare ⇨ **inhibitory nerve**

hämning ⇨ **inhibition, retardation, suppression**

hämning, psykomotorisk ⇨ **psychomotor**

häm(o)- ⇨ **haem-**

hämta sig ⇨ **pick up, recuperate**

händelse ⇨ **experience, occurrence**

hänga ⇨ **hang**

hängfinger ⇨ **mallet finger**

hänghand ⇨ **drop foot, wrist**

hänryckning ⇨ **ecstasy**

hänvisa ⇨ **refer**

härbärgera ⇨ **harbour**

härd ⇨ **focus, locus**

härma ⇨ **imitate**

härröra ⇨ **arise, derive, originate**

hästskonjure ⇨ **horseshoe kidney**

höft- ⇨ **ili-, iliac, sciatic**

höftbenet ⇨ **hip, ilium**

höftbens- ⇨ **ili-, iliac**

höftbenskammen ⇨ **iliac**

höftbensmuskeln ⇨ **iliacus**

höften ⇨ **hip, coxa**

höftfraktur ⇨ **hip**

höfthålet ⇨ **obturator**

höfthålsmuskeln ⇨ **obturator**

höftleden ⇨ **hip**

höftledsluxation, kongenital ⇨ **congenital**

höftledspannan ⇨ **acetabulum**

höftledsplastik ⇨ **acetabuloplasty, hip**

höft-ländmuskeln ➪ **iliopsoas**

höftsmärtor ➪ **coxalgia**

hög ➪ **high**

höger ➪ **right, right-hand**

höger- ➪ **dextro-**

högerhänt ➪ **right-handed**

höger-vänstershunt ➪ **shunt**

högrisk- ➪ **high-risk**

högriskpatient ➪ **high-risk**

höja ➪ **raise**

höjd ➪ **height**

höjdpunkt ➪ **fastigium**

höjdsjuka ➪ **mountain sickness**

höjdskräck ➪ **acrophobia**

hölja ➪ **cover**

hölje ➪ **covering, tegmen, theca**

hönsbröst ➪ **pigeon chest**

höra ➪ **hear**

hörapparat ➪ **hearing**

hörbar ➪ **audible**

hörntand ➪ **canine (tooth), cuspid**

hörsel- ➪ **acoustic, audi-, auditory**

hörselbenen ➪ **ear, ossicle**

hörselgången ➪ **ear**

hörselmätare ➪ **audiometer**

hörseln ➪ **hearing**

hörselnedsättning ➪ **deafness**

hörselnerven ➪ **cochlear**

hörselnervsganglion ➪ **spiral**

hörsel- och balansnerven ➪ **vestibulocochlear nerve**

hörselorganet ➪ **organ**

hörselskadad ➪ **deaf**

hörselsten ➪ **otolith**

hösnuva ➪ **hay fever**

Ii

I *chemical symbol for* iodine *I, jod*

iaktta ➪ **observe**

-iasis ['aɪəsɪs] *suffix* meaning disease caused by something *-iasis, -sjukdom;* **amoebiasis** = disease caused by an amoeba *amoebiasis, amöbainfektion*

iatrogenic [aɪˌætrə(ʊ)'dʒenɪk] *adj.* condition which is caused by a doctor's treatment for another disease *or* condition *iatrogen*

> COMMENT: can be caused by a drug (a side-effect), by infection from the doctor, or simply by worry about possible treatment

I band ['aɪˌbænd] *subst.* part of the pattern in muscle tissue, seen through a microscope as a light-coloured band *I-band*

ice [aɪs] *subst.* **(a)** frozen water *is* **(b) dry ice** = solid carbon dioxide *torris, kolsyresnö*

icebag ['aɪsbæg] *or* **ice pack** ['aɪs pæk] *subst.* cold compress made of lumps of ice wrapped in a cloth, put on a bruise *or* swelling to reduce the pain *isblåsa, isomslag*

ice cream [ˌaɪs'kriːm] *subst.* frozen sweet made from cream, water and flavouring *glass;* **after a tonsillectomy, children can be allowed ice cream**

ichor ['aɪkɔː] *subst.* watery liquid which comes from a wound *or* suppurating sore *kor, "elakartat" var*

ichthyosis [ˌɪkθɪ'əʊsɪs] *subst.* hereditary condition where the skin is dry and covered with scales *iktyos, fiskfjällssjuka*

icke-rökare ➪ **non-**

icke-sekretor ➪ **non-secretor**

ICSH [ˌaɪsiːes'eɪtʃ] = INTERSTITIAL CELL STIMULATING HORMONE

icterus ['ɪkt(ə)rəs] = JAUNDICE; **icterus gravis neonatorum** = jaundice associated with erythroblastosis foetalis *icterus, ikterus, gulsot*

ictus ['ɪktəs] *subst.* stroke *or* fit *ictus, iktus, slag, stöt*

ICU [ˌaɪsiː'juː] = INTENSIVE CARE UNIT

id [ɪd] *subst. (in psychology)* basic unconscious drives which exist in hidden forms in a person *detet*

ID-band ⇨ **bracelet, identity, label**

ideal [aɪ'dɪəl] *adj.* very suitable *or* perfect *idealisk, perfekt, önske-;* referring to an idea *tänkt;* **this is an ideal place for a new hospital**

identical [aɪ'dentɪk(ə)l] *adj.* exactly the same *identisk;* **identical twins** *or* **monozygotic twins** = two children born at the same time and from the same ovum, and therefore of the same sex and exactly the same in appearance *monozygoter, enäggstvillingar; compare* FRATERNAL

identifiable [aɪ'dentɪfa(ɪ)əb(ə)l] *adj.* which can be identified *som går att identifiera (fastställa);* **cot deaths have no identifiable cause**

identification [aɪˌdentɪfɪ'keɪʃ(ə)n] *subst.* act of identifying *identifikation, identifiering, fastställande;* **identification with someone** = taking on some characteristics of an older person (such as a parent *or* teacher) *identifiering med ngn*

identifiera ⇨ **identify**

identifiering ⇨ **identification**

identifikation ⇨ **identification**

identify [aɪ'dentɪfaɪ] *vb.* to determine the identity of something *or* someone *identifiera, fastställa;* **the next of kin were asked to identify the body; doctors have identified the cause of the outbreak of dysentery**

identisk ⇨ **identical**

identitet ⇨ **identity**

identitetsband ⇨ **identity**

identity [aɪ'dentəti] *subst.* who a person is *identitet;* **identity bracelet** *or* **label** = label attached to the wrist of a newborn baby *or* patient in hospital, so that he can be identified *identitetsband, ID-band*

idio- ['ɪdiə(ʊ), ˌ--] *prefix* referring to one particular person *idio-, egen-*

idiocy ['ɪdiəsi] *subst.* severe mental subnormality (IQ below 20) *idioti*

idiopathic [ˌɪdiə'pæθɪk] *adj.* (i) referring to idiopathy *idiopatisk;* (ii) (disease) with no obvious cause *idiopatisk, essentiell;* **idiopathic epilepsy** = epilepsy not caused by a brain disorder, beginning during childhood or adolescence *idiopatisk (genuin, essentiell) epilepsi*

idiopathy [ˌɪdi'ɒpəθi] *subst.* condition which develops without any known cause *idiopati*

idiopatisk ⇨ **essential, idiopathic, protopathic**

idiosyncrasy [ˌɪdiə'sɪŋkrəsi] *subst.* (i) way of behaving which is particular to one person *idiosynkrasi, egenhet, karakteristiskt drag;* (ii) one person's strong reaction to treatment *or* to a drug *idiosynkrasi*

idiot ['ɪdiət] *subst.* person suffering from severe mental subnormality *idiot;* **idiot savant** = person with mental subnormality who also possesses a single particular mental ability (such as the ability to play music by ear, to draw remembered objects, to do mental calculations) *idiot savant*

NOTE: the term idiot is no longer used by the medical profession

idioti ⇨ **idiocy**

idioventricular rhythm [ˌɪdiəven'trɪkjʊlə ˌrɪð(ə)m] *subst.* slow natural rhythm in the ventricles of the heart, but not in the atria *idioventrikulär rytm*

IDK [ˌaɪdiː'keɪ] = INTERNAL DERANGEMENT OF THE KNEE

Ig [ˌaɪ'dʒiː] = IMMUNOGLOBULIN

igångsättning av förlossning ⇨ **induction of labour**

IHD [ˌaɪeɪtʃ'diː] = ISCHAEMIC HEART DISEASE

ihålig ⇨ **cavernous, hollow**

ihållande ⇨ **continual, continuous, persistent, recalcitrant**

ihärdig ⇨ **recalcitrant**

IK ⇨ **intelligence**

ikterus ⇨ **icterus, jaundice**

iktus ⇨ **ictus**

iktyos ⇨ **ichthyosis**

ile- ['ɪli, ˌ--] *prefix* referring to the ileum *ile(o)-, ileum-*

ileal ['ɪliəl] *adj.* referring to the ileum *ile(o)-, ileum-;* **ileal bladder** *or* **ileal conduit** = artificial tube formed when the ureters are linked to part of the ileum, and that part is linked to an opening in the abdominal wall *ileumblåsa, Brickerblåsa, kutan uretero-ileostomi*

ileectomy [ˌɪli'ektəmi] *subst.* surgical removal of all *or* part of the ileum *operativt avlägsnande av (del av) ileum*

ileitis [ˌɪli'aɪtɪs] *subst.* inflammation of the ileum *ileit;* **regional ileitis** *or* **regional enteritis** *or* **Crohn's disease** = inflammation of part of the intestine (usually the ileum) resulting in pain, diarrhoea and loss of weight *ileitis terminalis, regional enterit, morbus Crohn, Crohns sjukdom*

> COMMENT: no certain cause has been found for Crohn's disease, where only one section of the intestine becomes inflamed and can be blocked

ileocaecal [ˌɪliəʊ'siːk(ə)l] *adj.* referring to the ileum and the caecum *ileocekal;* **ileocaecal orifice** = point where the small intestine joins the large intestine *ileocaecalporten, punkt där tunntarmen övergår i tjocktarmen*

ileocolic [ˌɪliəʊ'kɒlɪk] *adj.* referring to both the ileum and the colon *ileocekal;* **ileocolic artery** = branch of the superior mesenteric artery *arteria ileocolica*

ileocolitis [ˌɪliəʊkə'laɪtɪs] *subst.* inflammation of both the ileum and the colon *inflammation i både ileum och kolon*

ileocolostomy [ˌɪliəʊkə'lɒstəmi] *subst.* surgical operation to make a link directly between the ileum and the colon *ileokolostomi*

ileoproctostomy [ˌɪliəʊprɒk'tɒstəmi] *subst.* surgical operation to create a link between the ileum and the rectum *ileorektostomi*

ileorectal [ˌɪliəʊ'rekt(ə)l] *adj.* referring to both the ileum and the rectum *ileorektal*

ileorektostomi ⇨ **ileoproctostomy**

ileosigmoidostomy [ˌɪliəʊˌsɪgmɔɪ'dɒstəmi] *subst.* surgical operation to create a link between the ileum and the sigmoid colon *ileosigmoidostomi*

ileostomy [ˌɪli'ɒstəmi] *subst.* surgical operation to make an opening between the ileum and the abdominal wall to act as an artificial opening for excretion of faeces *ileostomi;* **ileostomy bag** = bag attached to the opening after an ileostomy to collect faeces *ileostomipåse*

ileum ['ɪliəm] *subst.* lower part of the small intestine, between the jejunum and the caecum ⇨ *illustration* DIGESTIVE SYSTEM *ileum; compare* ILIUM

> COMMENT: the ileum is the longest section of the small intestine, being about 2.5 metres long

ileumblåsa ⇨ **ileal**

ileus ['ɪliəs] *subst.* obstruction in the intestine, but usually distension caused by loss of muscular action in the bowel (paralytic *or* adynamic ileus) *ileus*

ileus, paralytisk ⇨ **paralytic**

ili- ['ɪli, ˌ--] *prefix* referring to the ilium *ili(o)-, höft-, höftbens-*

iliac ['ɪliæk] *adj.* referring to the ilium *höft-, höftbens-;* **common iliac arteries** = two arteries which branch from the aorta in the abdomen and in turn divide into the internal iliac artery (leading to the pelvis) and the external iliac artery (leading to the leg) *arteriae iliacae communes, stora höftpulsådrorna;* **common iliac veins** = two veins draining the legs, pelvis and abdomen, which join to form the inferior vena cava *venae iliacae communes, gemensamma höftvenerna;* **iliac crest** = curved top edge of the ilium ⇨ *illustration* PELVIS *crista iliaca, höftbenskammen;* **iliac fossa** = depression on the inner side of the hip bone *fossa iliaca;* **iliac regions** = two regions of the lower abdomen, on either side of the hypogastrium *fossa(e) iliaca(e), bukområdena på vardera sidan om hypogastriet;* **iliac spine** = projection at the posterior end of the iliac crest *spina iliaca*

iliacus [ˌɪli'ækəs] *subst.* muscle in the groin which flexes the thigh *musculus iliacus, höftbensmuskeln*

iliococcygeal [ˌɪliəʊkɒk'sɪdʒ(ə)l] *adj.* referring to both the ilium and the coccyx *som avser el. hör till både höft- och svansbenet*

iliolumbar [ˌɪliəʊ'lʌmbə] *adj.* referring to the iliac and lumbar regions *iliolumbar*

iliopectineal [ˌɪliəʊpek'tɪniəl] *or* **iliopubic** [ˌɪliəʊ'pjuːbɪk] *adj.* referring to both the ilium and the pubis *som avser el. hör till både höft- och blygdbenet;* **iliopectineal** *or* **iliopubic eminence** = raised area on the inner surface of the innominate bone *spina iliaca anterior superior*

iliopsoas [ˌɪliəʊˈsəʊəs] *subst.* muscle formed from the iliacus and psoas muscles *musculus iliopsoas, höft-ländmuskeln*

iliotibial [ˌɪliəʊˈtɪbiəl] *adj.* referring to both the ilium and the tibia *or* thigh *som avser el. hör till både höft- och skenbenet el. låret;* **iliotibial tract** = thick fascia on the outside of the tibia *or* thigh *tractus iliotibialis*

ilium [ˈɪliəm] *subst.* top part of each of the hip bones, which form the pelvis ⇨ *illustration* PELVIS *os ilium, höftbenet, tarmbenet; compare* ILEUM

ill [ɪl] *adj.* not well *or* sick *sjuk, dålig;* **eating green apples will make you ill; if you feel ill you ought to see a doctor; he's not as ill as he was last week**
NOTE: **ill - worse - worst**

illamående ⇨ **malaise, nausea, nauseous, sick, sickness**

illegal [ɪˈliːg(ə)l] *adj.* not done according to the law *illegal, olaglig;* **she had an illegal abortion**

illegal abort ⇨ **abortion**

ill health [ˌɪl ˈhelθ] *subst.* not being well *dålig hälsa, ohälsa, sjuklighet;* **he has been in ill health for some time; she has a history of ill health; he had to retire early for reasons of ill health**

illness [ˈɪlnəs] *subst.* **(a)** state of being ill *or* of not being well *sjukdom;* **his illness makes him very tired; most of the children stayed away from school because of illness (b)** type of disease *sjukdom;* **he is in hospital with an infectious tropical illness; scarlet fever is no longer considered to be a very serious illness**

illusion [ɪˈluːʒ(ə)n] *subst.* condition where a person has a wrong perception of external objects *illusion, synvilla;* **optical illusion =** something which is seen wrongly, usually when it is moving, so that it appears to be something else *optisk villa, synvilla*

i.m. [ˌaɪˈem] *or* **IM** [ˌaɪˈem] = INTRAMUSCULAR

image [ˈɪmɪdʒ] *subst.* sensation (such as smell *or* sight *or* taste) which is remembered clearly *bild, föreställning, minnesbild*

imagery [ˈɪmɪdʒ(ə)ri] *subst.* producing visual sensations clearly in the mind *fantasi, fantasiföreställningar*

imaginary [ɪˈmædʒɪn(ə)ri] *adj.* which does not exist but which is imagined *inbillad, fantasi-;* **imaginary playmates** = friends who do not exist but who are imagined by a small child to exist *låtsaslekkamrater*

imagination [ɪˌmædʒɪˈneɪʃ(ə)n] *subst.* being able to see things in your mind *fantasi, inbillning(sförmåga);* **in his imagination he saw himself sitting on a beach in the sun**

imagine [ɪˈmædʒɪn] *vb.* to see *or* hear *or* feel something in your mind *föreställa sig;* **imagine yourself sitting on the beach in the sun; I thought I heard someone shout, but I must have imagined it because there is no one there; to imagine things** = to have delusions *inbilla sig (saker);* **she keeps imagining things; sometimes he imagines he is swimming in the sea**

imaging [ˈɪmɪdʒɪŋ] *subst.* technique for creating pictures of sections of the body, using scanners attached to computers *bildanalys, bildbehandling som vid datortomografi, skiktröntgen;* **magnetic resonance imaging (MRI)** = scanning technique, using magnetic fields and radio waves, for examining soft tissue and cells *magnetisk resonanstomografi, MRT;* **X-ray imaging** = showing X-ray pictures of the inside of part of the body on a screen *röntgengenomlysning*

imbecile [ˈɪmbəsiː(ə)l] *subst.* person who is mentally subnormal *imbecill*

imbecility [ˌɪmbəˈsɪləti] *subst.* mental subnormality (where the IQ is below 50) *imbecillitet*
NOTE: these terms are no longer used by the medical profession

imitate [ˈɪmɪteɪt] *vb.* to do what someone else does *imitera, härma;* **when he walks he imitates his father; she is very good at imitating the English teacher; children learn by imitating adults or older children**

immature [ˌɪməˈtjʊə] *adj.* not mature *immatur, omogen, outvecklad;* **an immature cell** = cell which is still developing *en omogen cell*

immediate [ɪˈmiːdjət] *adj.* which happens now *or* without waiting *omedelbar;* **his condition needs immediate treatment**

immediately [ɪˈmiːdjətli] *adv.* just after *omedelbart, omgående, genast;* **he became ill immediately after he came back from**

holiday; she will phone the doctor immediately (after) her father regains consciousness; if the child's temperature rises, you must call the doctor immediately

immersion foot [ɪ'mɜːʃ(ə)n ˌfʊt] *or* **trench foot** ['tren(t)ʃ ˌfʊt] *subst.* condition, caused by exposure to cold and damp, where the skin of the foot is red and blistered and sometimes becomes affected with gangrene *skyttegravsfot, rodnad hud med blåsor på fötterna pga köld och väta*

immiscible [ɪ'mɪsəb(ə)l] *adj. (of liquids)* which cannot be mixed *inte blandbar*

immobile [ɪ'məʊbaɪ(ə)l, -biːl] *adj.* not moving *or* which cannot move *orörlig*

immobilisera ⇨ **immobilize**

immobilisering ⇨ **immobilization**

immobilization [ɪˌməʊbɪlaɪ'zeɪʃ(ə)n] *subst.* being kept still, without moving *immobilisering, fixering*

immobilize [ɪ'məʊbɪlaɪz] *vb.* to make someone keep still and not move *or* to attach a splint to a joint to prevent the bones moving *immobilisera, fixera*

immovable [ɪ'muːvəb(ə)l] *adj.* (joint) which cannot be moved *orörlig*

immun ⇨ **immune**

immundefekt ⇨ **immune, immunodeficiency**

immune [ɪ'mjuːn] *adj.* protected against an infection *or* allergic disease *immun;* **she seems to be immune to colds; the injection should make you immune to yellow fever; immune deficiency** = lack of immunity to a disease *nedsatt immunförsvar, immundefekt; see also* AIDS; **immune reaction** *or* **immune response** = response of a body where antibodies are produced on introduction of antigens *immunitetsreaktion*

> QUOTE the reason for this susceptibility is a profound abnormality of the immune system in children with sickle-cell disease
>
> **Lancet**

> QUOTE the AIDS virus attacks a person's immune system and damages his or her ability to fight other diseases
>
> **Journal of the American Medical Association**

immunisera ⇨ **immunize**

immunisering ⇨ **immunization**

immunitet ⇨ **immunity**

immunitetsreaktion ⇨ **immune, response**

immunity [ɪ'mjuːnəti] *subst.* ability to resist attacks of a disease because antibodies are produced *immunitet;* **the vaccine gives immunity to tuberculosis; acquired immunity** = immunity which a body acquires (from having caught a disease *or* from immunization), not one which is congenital *förvärvad immunitet;* **active immunity** = immunity which is acquired by catching and surviving an infectious disease *or* by vaccination with a weakened form of the disease which makes the body form antibodies *aktiv immunitet;* **natural immunity** = immunity which a body acquires in the womb or from the mother's milk *naturlig immunitet;* **passive immunity** = immunity which is acquired by the transfer of an immune mechanism from another animal *passiv immunitet*

immunization [ˌɪmjunaɪ'zeɪʃ(ə)n] *subst.* making a person immune to an infection, either by injecting an antiserum (passive immunization) or by giving the body the disease in such a small dose that the body does not develop the disease, but produces antibodies to counteract it *immunisering*

> QUOTE vaccination is the most effective way to prevent children getting the disease. Children up to 6 years old can be vaccinated if they missed earlier immunization
>
> **Health Visitor**

immunize ['ɪmjunaɪz] *vb.* to give someone immunity from an infection *immunisera, vaccinera* NOTE: you immunize someone **against** a disease

immunodeficiency [ˌɪmjunəʊdɪ'fɪʃ(ə)nsi] *subst.* lack of immunity to a disease *nedsatt immunförsvar, immundefekt; see also* HIV

immunoelectrophoresis [ˌɪmjunəʊɪˌletrəʊfə'riːsɪs] *subst.* method of identifying antigens in a laboratory, using electrophoresis *immun(o)elektrofores*

immunoglobulin (Ig) [ˌɪmjunəʊ'glɒbjʊlɪn (ˌel'dʒiː)] *subst.* protein in blood plasma which forms antibodies as protection against infection *immun(o)globulin*

immunologi ⇨ **immunology**

immunological [ˌɪmjunə'lɒdʒɪk(ə)l] *adj.* referring to immunology *immunologisk;* **immunological tolerance** = tolerance of the lymphoid tissues to an antigen *immunologisk tolerans*

immunologisk ⇨ **immunological**

immunology [ˌɪmjuˈnɒlədʒi] *subst.* study of immunity and immunization *immunologi*

immunosuppression [ˌɪmjunəʊsəˈpreʃ(ə)n] *subst.* suppressing the body's natural immune system so that it will not reject a transplanted organ *immunsuppression*

immunosuppressive [ˌɪmjunəʊsəˈpresɪv] *adj. & subst.* (drug) used to counteract the response of the immune system to reject a transplanted organ *immunsuppressiv*

immunotransfusion [ˌɪmjunəʊtrænsˈfjuːʒ(ə)n] *subst.* transfusion of blood, serum or plasma containing immune bodies *transfusion som innehåller antikroppar*

immunsuppression ⇨ **immunosuppression**

immunsuppressiv ⇨ **immunosuppressive**

impacted [ɪmˈpæktɪd] *adj.* tightly pressed *or* firmly lodged against something *inklämd, inkilad, retinerad;* **impacted fracture** = fracture where the broken parts of the bones are driven against each other *inkilad fraktur;* **impacted tooth** = tooth which is held in the jawbone and so cannot grow normally *dens impactus, retinerad (inklämd) tand;* **impacted ureteric calculus** = stone which is lodged in a ureter *inkilad uretärsten*

impaction [ɪmˈpækʃ(ə)n] *subst.* condition where two things are impacted *impaktion, impaktering, inklämning, inkilning;* **dental impaction** = condition where a tooth is impacted in the jaw *retentio dentis, dental impaktering, retinerad (inklämd) tand;* **faecal impaction** = condition where a hardened mass of faeces stays in the rectum *fekal impaktering*

impair [ɪmˈpeə] *vb.* to harm (a sense) so that it does not function properly *försämra, försvaga, nedsätta;* **impaired vision** = eyesight which is not fully clear *nedsatt syn*

impairment [ɪmˈpeəmənt] *subst.* condition where one of the senses is impaired *försämring, försvagning, nedsättning;* **his impairment does not affect his work; the impairment was progressive, but she did not notice that her eyesight was getting worse**

impaktering ⇨ **impaction**

impaktion ⇨ **impaction**

impalpable [ɪmˈpælpəb(ə)l] *adj.* which cannot be felt when touched *impalpabel*

impediment [ɪmˈpedɪmənt] *subst.* obstruction *hinder, fel;* **speech impediment** = condition where a person cannot speak properly because of a deformed mouth *talfel, talrubbning*

imperfecta [ˌɪmpəˈfektə] *see* OSTEOGENESIS

imperforate [ɪmˈpɜːf(ə)rət] *adj.* without an opening *imperforerad, operforerad;* **imperforate anus** = condition where the anus does not have an opening *atresia ani, anus imperforatus, proktatresi;* **imperforate hymen** = membrane in the vagina which has no opening for the menstrual fluid *hymen imperforatus, operforerad mödomshinna*

impetigo [ˌɪmpɪˈtaɪgəʊ] *subst.* irritating and very contagious skin disease caused by staphylococci, which spreads rapidly and is easily passed from one child to another, but can be treated with antibiotics *impetigo, svinkoppor*

implant [ˈɪmplɑːnt; ɪmˈplɑːnt] **1** *subst.* drug *or* tissue inserted under the skin of a patient so that it can be absorbed gradually *implantat* **2** *vb.* to become fixed *fästa sig;* to insert *or* graft in securely *implantera;* **the ovum implants in the wall of the uterus**

implantation [ˌɪmplɑːnˈteɪʃ(ə)n] *or* **nidation** [naɪˈdeɪʃ(ə)n] *subst.* **(a)** inserting of drug *or* tissue into a living body *implantation, implantering;* introduction of one tissue into another surgically *implantation, implantering, transplantation* **(b)** point in the development of an embryo, when the fertilized ovum reaches the uterus and implants in the wall of the uterus *nidation*

impotence [ˈɪmpət(ə)ns] *subst.* inability in a male to have an erection *or* to ejaculate, and so have sexual intercourse *impotens*

impotent [ˈɪmpət(ə)nt] *adj. (of a man)* unable to have sexual intercourse *impotent*

impregnate [ˈɪmpregneɪt] *vb.* **(a)** to make (a female) pregnant *befrukta, göra havande* **(b)** to soak (a cloth) with a liquid *impregnera, dränka in;* **a cloth impregnated with antiseptic**

impregnation [ˌɪmpregˈneɪʃ(ə)n] *subst.* action of impregnating *impregnering, befruktning, indränkning*

impregnera ⇨ **impregnate**

impregnerad ⇨ **waterproof**

impregnering ⇨ **impregnation**

impression [ɪm'preʃ(ə)n] *subst.* **(a)** mould of a patient's jaw made by a dentist before making a denture *avtryck* **(b)** depression on an organ *or* structure into which another organ *or* structure fits *avtryck;* **cardiac impression** = (i) concave area near the centre of the upper surface of the liver under the heart *incisura cardiaca, avtryck av (märke efter) hjärtat på levern;* (ii) depression on the mediastinal part of the lungs where they touch the pericardium *incisura cardiaca, avtryck av (märke efter) hjärtat på lungorna*

impression ⇨ **depression**

improve [ɪm'pru:v] *vb.* to get better *förbättras, bli bättre, repa sig;* to make better *göra bättre, stärka;* **he was very ill, but he is improving now**

improvement [ɪm'pru:vmənt] *subst.* getting better *förbättring;* **the patient's condition has shown a slight improvement; doctors have not detected any improvement in her asthma**

impulse ['ɪmpʌls] *subst.* (i) message transmitted by a nerve *impuls, stöt;* (ii) sudden feeling that you want to act in a certain way *impuls*

impure [ɪm'pjʊə] *adj.* not pure *oren*

impurities [ɪm'pjʊərətɪz] *subst pl.* substances which are not pure *or* clean *orenlighet(er);* **the kidneys filter impurities out of the blood**

inability [ˌɪnə'bɪləti] *subst.* being unable to do something *oförmåga;* **he suffered from a temporary inability to pass water**

inactive [ɪn'æktɪv] *adj.* **(a)** not being active *or* not moving *inaktiv;* **patients must not be allowed to become inactive (b)** which does not work *inaktiv, overksam;* **the serum makes the poison inactive**

inactivity [ˌɪnæk'tɪvəti] *subst.* lack of activity *inaktivitet, overksamhet;* **he has periods of complete inactivity**

inadekvat ⇨ **inadequate**

inadequate [ɪn'ædɪkwət] *adj.* not sufficient *inadekvat, otillräcklig;* **the hospital has inadequate staff to deal with a major accident**

inaktiv ⇨ **dormant, inactive, quiescent**

inaktivitet ⇨ **inactivity**

inandning ⇨ **inhalation, inspiration, sniff**

in articulo mortis [ɪn ɑ:'tɪkjʊləʊ 'mɔ:tɪs] *Latin phrase meaning* "at the onset of death" *in articulo mortis, då döden inträder*

inavel ⇨ **inbreeding**

inbegripa ⇨ **include**

inberäkna ⇨ **count**

inbillad ⇨ **imaginary**

inbillning ⇨ **imagination, phantom**

inbillningssjuka ⇨ **hypochondria**

inblåsning ⇨ **insufflation**

inborn [ˌɪn'bɔ:n] *adj.* which is in the body from birth *medfödd, inneboende, naturlig;* **a body has an inborn tendency to reject transplanted organs**

inbred [ˌɪn'bred] *adj.* suffering from inbreeding *inavlad, som beror på inavel*

inbreeding ['ɪnbri:dɪŋ] *subst.* breeding between a closely related male and female, who have the same parents or grandparents, so making congenital defects spread *inavel*

inbuktning ⇨ **notch**

incapable [ɪn'keɪpəb(ə)l] *adj.* not able to do something *oförmögen;* **she was incapable of feeding herself**

incapacitated [ˌɪnkə'pæsɪteɪtɪd] *adj.* not able to act *oförmögen;* **he was incapacitated for three weeks by his accident**

incarcerated [ɪn'kɑ:səreɪtɪd] *adj.* (hernia) which cannot be corrected by physical manipulation *inkarcererad, inklämd, inkilad*

inception rate [ɪn'sepʃ(ə)n ˌreɪt] *subst.* number of new cases of a disease during a period of time, per thousand of population *incidenstal*

incest ['ɪnsest] *subst.* crime of having sexual intercourse with a close relative (daughter, son, mother, father) *incest*

incestuous [ɪn'sestjuəs] *adj.* referring to incest *incestuös;* **they had an incestuous relationship**

incidence ['ɪnsɪd(ə)ns] *subst.* number of times something happens in a certain population over a period of time *incidens, förekomst, frekvens;* **the incidence of drug-related deaths; men have a higher incidence of stroke than women; incidence rate** = number of new cases of a disease during a given period, per thousand of population *frekvens sjukdomsfall per tusen personer*

incidens ⇨ **incidence**

incidenstal ⇨ **inception rate**

inciderad ⇨ **incised**

incipient [ɪn'sɪpiənt] *adj.* which is just beginning *or* which is in its early stages *begynnande, i första stadiet;* **he has an incipient appendicitis; the tests detected incipient diabetes mellitus**

incised [ɪn'saɪzd] *adj.* which has been cut *inciderad, (upp)skuren;* **incised wound** = wound with clear edges, caused by a sharp knife or razor *vulnus incisum, skärsår*

incision [ɪn'sɪʒ(ə)n] *subst.* cut in a patient's body made by a surgeon using a scalpel *incision, insnitt, snitt;* any cut made with a sharp knife *or* razor *skåra, snitt;* **the first incision is made two millimetres below the second rib** *compare* EXCISION

incisional [ɪn'sɪʒ(ə)n(ə)l] *adj.* referring to an incision *som avser el. hör till incision (snitt);* **incisional hernia** = hernia which breaks through the abdominal wall at a place where a surgical incision was made during an operation *hernia in cicatrice, ärrbråck*

incisor (tooth) [ɪn'saɪzə (tu:θ)] *subst.* one of the front teeth (four each in the upper and lower jaws) which are used to cut off pieces of food ⇨ *illustration* TEETH *dens incisivus, framtand*

incisura ⇨ **notch**

include [ɪn'klu:d] *vb.* to count something *or* someone with others *inkludera, omfatta, inbegripa;* **does the number of cases include the figures for outpatients? the dentist will be on holiday up to and including next Tuesday**

inclusion [ɪn'klu:ʒ(ə)n] *subst.* something enclosed inside something else *inklusion, inneslutning;* **inclusion bodies** = very small particles found in cells infected by virus *inklusionskropp*

incompatibility [ˌɪnkəmˌpætə'bɪləti] *subst.* being incompatible *inkompatibilitet, oförenlighet;* **the incompatibility of the donor's blood with that of the patient**

incompatible [ˌɪnkəm'pætəb(ə)l] *adj.* which does not go together with something else *inkompatibel, oförenlig;* (drugs) which must not be used together because they undergo chemical change and the therapeutic effect is lost *antagonistisk;* (tissue) which is genetically different from other tissue, making it impossible to transplant into that tissue *inkompatibel;* **incompatible blood** = blood from a donor that does not match the blood of the patient receiving the transfusion *inkompatibelt (oförenligt) blod*

incompetence [ɪn'kɒmpət(ə)ns] *subst.* (i) not being able to do a certain act *inkompetens, oförmåga;* (ii); *(of valves)* not closing properly *insufficiens;* **aortic incompetence** = condition where the aortic valve does not close properly, causing regurgitation *aortainsufficiens;* **mitral incompetence** = situation where the mitral valve does not close completely so that blood flows back into the atrium *insufficientia valvulae mitralis, mitralisinsufficiens*

incompetent [ɪn'kɒmpət(ə)nt] *adj.* not able to function *insufficient;* **an incompetent mitral valve**

incomplete [ˌɪnkəm'pli:t] *adj.* which is not complete *inkomplett, ofullständig, partiell;* **incomplete abortion** *see* ABORTION

incontinence [ɪn'kɒntɪnəns] *subst.* inability to control the discharge of urine *inkontinens;* **faecal incontinence** *or* **encopresis** = inability to control the bowel movements *incontinentia alvi, enkopres, avföringsinkontinens;* **stress incontinence** = condition in women where the sufferer is incapable of retaining urine when the intra-abdominal pressure is raised by coughing or laughing *stressinkontinens*

incontinent [ɪn'kɒntɪnənt] *adj.* unable to control the discharge of urine *or* faeces *inkontinent*

incoordination [ˌɪnkəʊˌɔ:dɪ'neɪʃ(ə)n] *subst.* situation where the muscles in various parts of the body do not act together, making it impossible to do certain actions *inkoordination*

incorrect [ˌɪnkə'rekt] *adj.* not correct *inkorrekt, felaktig, oriktig;* **the doctor made**

an incorrect diagnosis; the dosage prescribed was incorrect

increase ['ɪŋkri:s; ɪn'kri:s] **1** *subst.* getting larger *or* higher *ökning;* **an increase in heart rate 2** *vb.* to get larger *or* higher *öka(s);* **his pulse rate increased by 10 per cent**

incubation period [ˌɪŋkju'beɪʃ(ə)n ˌpɪəriəd] *subst.* (i) time during which a virus *or* bacterium develops in the body after contamination *or* infection, before the appearance of the symptoms of the disease *inkubation(stid), latens(tid);* (ii) time during which a bacterial sample grows in a laboratory culture *inkubation*

incubator ['ɪŋkjubeɪtə] *subst.* **(a)** apparatus for growing bacterial cultures *termostat* **(b)** specially controlled container in which a premature baby can be kept in ideal conditions *kuvös*

incurable [ɪn'kjʊərəb(ə)l] *subst. & adj.* (patient) who will never be cured *or* (illness) which cannot be cured *obotlig (person el. sjukdom);* **he is suffering from an incurable disease of the blood; she has been admitted to a hospital for incurables**

incus ['ɪŋkəs] *subst.* one of the three ossicles in the middle ear, shaped like an anvil ➪ *illustration* EAR *incus, städet*

> COMMENT: the incus is the central one of the three bones: the malleus articulates with it, and the incus articulates with the stapes

independent [ˌɪndɪ'pendənt] *adj.* free *or* not controlled by someone else *oberoende, självständig*

independently [ˌɪndɪ'pendəntli] *adv.* not being controlled by anyone *or* anything *oberoende, självständigt;* **the autonomic nervous system functions independently of the conscious will**

index finger ['ɪndeks ˌfɪŋgə] *subst.* first finger next to the thumb *index, pekfingret*

Indian hemp [ˌɪndiən 'hemp] *subst.* tropical plant from which cannabis *or* marijuana *or* hashish can be produced *indisk hampa*

indican ['ɪndikæn] *subst.* potassium salt *indikan, kaliumsalt*

indicate ['ɪndɪkeɪt] *vb.* **(a)** to show *ange, visa;* **the skin reaction indicates a highly allergenic state (b)** to suggest that a certain type of treatment should be given *indicera, motivera;* **a course of antibiotics is indicated; therapeutic intervention was indicated in nine of the patients tested**

indication [ˌɪndɪ'keɪʃ(ə)n] *subst.* sign which suggests that a certain type of treatment should be given *or* that a condition has a particular cause *indikation;* **sulpha drugs have been replaced by antibiotics in many indications** *see also* CONTRAINDICATION

indicator ['ɪndɪkeɪtə] *subst.* substance which shows something, especially a substance secreted in body fluids which shows which blood group a person belongs to *indikator*

indicera ➪ **indicate**

indigestion [ˌɪndɪ'dʒestʃ(ə)n] *or* **dyspepsia** [dɪs'pepsiə] *subst.* disturbance of the normal process of digestion, where the patient experiences pain *or* discomfort in the stomach *indigestion, dyspepsi, matspjälkningsbesvär;* **he is taking tablets to relieve his indigestion** *or* **he is taking indigestion tablets**

indikan ➪ **indican**

indikation ➪ **indication**

indikator ➪ **indicator**

indirect [ˌɪndə'rekt] *adj.* not direct *indirekt;* **indirect contact** = catching a disease by inhaling bacteria *or* by being in contact with a vector, but not in direct contact with an infected person *indirekt kontakt*

indisposed [ˌɪndɪ'spəʊzd] *adj.* slightly ill *indisponerad, opasslig, lätt illamående;* **my mother is indisposed and cannot see any visitors**

indisposition [ˌɪndɪspə'zɪʃ(ə)n] *subst.* slight illness *indisposition, opasslighet, lätt illamående*

individ ➪ **individual, human, person**

individual [ˌɪndɪ'vɪdju(ə)l] *subst. & adj.* one particular person *individ, individuell*

indolent ['ɪnd(ə)lənt] *adj.* (ulcer) which develops slowly and does not heal *indolent, som utvecklas långsamt och inte läker*

indragning ➪ **indrawing, inversion, retraction, withdrawal**

indrawing [ˌɪn'drɔ:ɪŋ] *subst.* pulling towards the inside *indragning*

indrawn [ˌɪn'drɔːn] *adj.* which is pulled inside *indragen*

indrypning ⇨ **instillation**

indränkning ⇨ **impregnation**

induce [ɪn'djuːs] *vb.* to make something happen *framkalla, förorsaka;* **to induce labour** = to make a woman go into labour *sätta igång förlossningsarbete;* **induced abortion** = abortion which is produced by drugs *or* by surgery *abortus provocatus, framkallad abort*

induction of labour [ɪnˌdʌkʃ(ə)n əf 'leɪbə] *subst.* action of starting childbirth artificially *igångsättning av förlossning*

induration [ˌɪndjʊə'reɪʃ(ə)n] *subst.* hardening of tissue *or* of an artery because of pathological change *induration, skleros, cirros*

induratum [ˌɪndjʊə'reɪtəm] *see* ERYTHEMA

indurera ⇨ **harden**

industrial [ɪn'dʌstriəl] *adj.* referring to industries *or* factories *industriell;* **industrial disease** = disease which is caused by the type of work done by a worker (such as by dust produced *or* chemicals used in the factory) *yrkessjukdom, arbetssjukdom*

indwelling catheter [ˌɪn'dwelɪŋ ˌkæθɪtə] *subst.* catheter left in place for a period of time after its introduction *kvarliggande kateter, liggkateter, KAD*

inebriation [ɪˌniːbrɪ'eɪʃ(ə)n] *subst.* state where a person is habitually drunk *berusning*

inertia [ɪ'nɜːʃə] *subst.* complete lack of activity *or* condition of indolence of the body or mind *inertia, tröghet, slapphet*

in extremis [ˌɪnɪks'triːmɪs] *Latin phrase meaning* "at the moment of death" *in extremis, i dödsögonblicket*

infant ['ɪnf(ə)nt] *subst.* small child under two years of age *småbarn, spädbarn;* **infant mortality rate** = number of infants who die per thousand births *spädbarnsdödlighet*

> COMMENT: legally, an infant is a child under eighteen years of age

infantile ['ɪnf(ə)ntaɪ(ə)l] *adj.* (i) referring to small children *infantil, barn-, spädbarns-;* (ii) (disease) which affects children *barn-;* **infantile convulsions** *or* **spasms** = convulsions *or* minor epileptic fits in small children *hypsarytmi (jfr spasmus nutans), slags kramp el. epileptiska anfall hos små barn;* **infantile paralysis** = POLIOMYELITIS

infantilism [ɪn'fæntɪlɪz(ə)m] *subst.* condition where a person keeps some characteristics of an infant when he becomes an adult *infantilism*

infarct ['ɪnfɑːkt] *subst.* area of tissue which is killed when the blood supply is cut off by the blockage of an artery *infarkt*

infarction [ɪn'fɑːkʃ(ə)n] *subst.* killing of tissue by cutting off the blood supply *infarkt;* **cardiac** *or* **myocardial infarction** = death of part of the heart muscle after coronary thrombosis *myokardinfarkt, hjärtinfarkt*

> QUOTE cerebral infarction accounts for about 80% of first-ever strokes
> **British Journal of Hospital Medicine**

> QUOTE apart from death, coronary heart disease causes considerable morbidity in the form of heart attack or myocardial infarction
> **Health Education Journal**

infarkt ⇨ **infarct, infarction**

infect [ɪn'fekt] *vb.* to contaminate with disease-producing microorganisms *or* toxins *infektera;* to transmit infection *smitta (ner);* **the disease infected his liver; the whole arm soon became infected; infected wound** = wound which has become poisoned by bacteria *infekterat sår*

infection [ɪn'fekʃ(ə)n] *subst.* entry of microbes into the body, which then multiply in the body *infektion, smitta;* **as a carrier he was spreading infection to other people in the office; she is susceptible to minor infections**

infectious [ɪn'fekʃəs] *adj.* (disease) which is caused by microbes and can be transmitted to other persons by direct means *infektiös, smittsam;* **this strain of flu is highly infectious; her measles is at the infectious stage; infectious hepatitis** *or* **hepatitis A** = hepatitis transmitted by a carrier through food or drink *hepatit A, hepatitis epidemica (infectiosa), infektiös virushepatit;* **infectious mononucleosis** *or* **glandular fever** = infectious disease where the body has an excessive number of white blood cells *mononucleosis infectiosa, mononukleos, monocytos, körtelfeber*

> COMMENT: the symptoms include sore throat, fever and swelling of the lymph glands in the neck. The disease is caused by the Epstein-Barr virus

infective [ɪn'fektɪv] *adj.* (disease) caused by a microbe, which can be caught from another person but which cannot always be directly transmitted *infektiös, smittsam, bakteriell;* **infective endocarditis** = bacterial infection of the heart valves *infektiös endokardit;* **infective enteritis** = enteritis caused by bacteria *infektiös enterit, bakteriell tarminflammation;* **infective hepatitis** *or* **hepatitis A** = hepatitis transmitted by a carrier through food or drink *hepatit A, hepatitis epidemica (infectiosa), infektiös virushepatit*

infectivity [ˌɪnfek'tɪvəti] *subst.* being infective *smittsamhet;* **the patient's infectivity can last about a week**

infektera ⇨ **infect**

infektion ⇨ **infection**

infektionsficka ⇨ **pocket**

infektionshärd ⇨ **nidus**

infektionssjukdom ⇨ **bug**

infektiös ⇨ **infectious, infective**

inferior [ɪn'fɪəriə] *adj.* lower (part of the body) *inferior, undre, nedre;* **inferior vena cava** = main vein carrying blood from the lower part of the body to the heart *vena cava inferior, nedre (undre) hålvenen*
NOTE: the opposite is **superior**

inferiority [ɪnˌfɪəri'ɒrəti] *subst.* being lower *or* less important *or* less intelligent than others *underlägsenhet, mindervärde;* **inferiority complex** = mental state where the patient feels very inferior to others and compensates for this by behaving violently towards them *mindervärdeskomplex*

infertil ⇨ **infertile, sterile**

infertile [ɪn'fɜːtaɪ(ə)l, -tl] *adj.* not fertile *or* not able to reproduce *infertil, steril, ofruktsam*

infertilitet ⇨ **infertility, sterility**

infertility [ˌɪnfə'tɪləti] *subst.* not being fertile *or* able to reproduce *infertilitet, sterilitet, ofruktsamhet*

infest [ɪn'fest] *vb. (of parasites)* to be present in large numbers *hemsöka, översvämma, angripa (i stort antal);* **the child's hair was infested with lice**

infestation [ˌɪnfes'teɪʃ(ə)n] *subst.* having large numbers of parasites; invasion of the body by parasites *infestation, parasitangrepp;* **the condition is caused by infestation of the hair with lice**

infiltrat ⇨ **consolidation, infiltrate**

infiltrate ['ɪnfɪltreɪt, ɪn'fɪltreɪt] **1** *vb. (of liquid or waste)* to pass from one part of the body to another through a wall *or* membrane and be deposited in the other part *infiltrera, filtrera* **2** *subst.* substance which has infiltrated part of the body *infiltrat*

> QUOTE the chest roentgenogram often discloses interstitial pulmonary infiltrates, but may occasionally be normal
> **Southern Medical Journal**

> QUOTE the lacrimal and salivary glands become infiltrated with lymphocytes and plasma cells. The infiltration reduces lacrimal and salivary secretions which in turn leads to dry eyes and dry mouth
> **American Journal of Nursing**

infiltration [ˌɪnfɪl'treɪʃ(ə)n] *subst.* passing of a liquid through the walls of one part of the body into another part *infiltration;* condition where waste is brought to and deposited round cells *infiltration, inlagring*

infiltrera ⇨ **infiltrate**

infirm [ɪn'fɜːm] *adj.* old and weak *klen, skröplig, svag av ålderdom;* **my grandfather is quite infirm now**

infirmary [ɪn'fɜːm(ə)ri] *subst.* **(a)** room in a school *or* factory where people can go if they are ill *sjukrum, sjukavdelning* **(b)** old name for a hospital *sjukhus*
NOTE: **infirmary** is still used in names of hospitals: **the Glasgow Royal Infirmary**

infirmity [ɪn'fɜːməti] *subst.* (i) being old and weak *ålderdomssvaghet, klenhet, skröplighet;* (ii) illness *krämpa;* **in spite of his infirmities he still reads all the newspapers**

inflame [ɪn'fleɪm] *vb.* to make a tissue react to infection *or* irritation by becoming red and swollen *inflammera;* **the skin has become inflamed around the sore**

inflammation [ˌɪnflə'meɪʃ(ə)n] *subst.* being inflamed *or* having become red and swollen as a reaction to an infection or a blow *inflammation;* **she has an inflammation of the bladder** *or* **a bladder inflammation; the body's reaction to infection took the form of an inflammation of the eyelid**

inflammatory [ɪn'flæmət(ə)ri] *adj.* which makes something become inflamed *som orsakar inflammation;* **inflammatory bowel disease** = CROHN'S DISEASE

inflammera ⇨ **inflame**

inflatable [ɪn'fleɪtəb(ə)l] *adj.* which can be inflated *uppblåsbar*

inflate [ɪn'fleɪt] *vb.* to fill with air *blåsa upp, spänna ut;* **the abdomen is inflated with air before a coelioscopy; in valvuloplasty, a balloon is introduced into the valve and inflated**

influence ['ɪnfluəns] **1** *subst.* being able to have an effect on someone *or* something *inflytande, påverkan* **2** *vb.* to have an effect on someone *or* something *influera, påverka;* **the development of the serum has been influenced by research carried out in the USA**

influensa ▷ **influenza, flu, grippe**

influenza [ˌɪnflu'enzə] *subst.* infectious disease of the upper respiratory tract with fever, malaise and muscular aches, transmitted by a virus, which occurs in epidemics *influensa;* **she is in bed with influenza; half the staff in the office are off work with influenza; the influenza epidemic has killed several people**

COMMENT: influenza virus is spread by droplets of moisture in the air, so the disease can be spread by coughing or sneezing. Influenza can be quite mild, but virulent strains occur from time to time (Spanish influenza, Hong Kong flu) and can weaken the patient so much that he becomes susceptible to pneumonia and other more serious infections

influera ▷ **influence**

inflytande ▷ **influence**

inform [ɪn'fɔːm] *vb.* to tell someone *informera, meddela, underrätta, upplysa;* **have you informed the police that the drugs have been stolen?**

informal [ɪn'fɔːm(ə)l] *adj.* not official *informell;* **informal patient** = patient who has admitted himself to a hospital, without being referred by a doctor *patient som kommer utan remiss (till sjukhus)*

information [ˌɪnfə'meɪʃ(ə)n] *subst.* facts about something *information, upplysning(ar), uppgift(er);* **have you any information about the treatment of sunburn? the police won't give us any information about how the accident happened; you haven't given me enough information about when your symptoms started; that's a very useful piece** *or* **bit of information**

NOTE: no plural **some information; a piece of information**

informera ▷ **inform**

infra- ['ɪnfrə, ˌ--] *prefix* meaning below *infra-*

infraktion ▷ **greenstick fracture**

infraorbital nerve [ˌɪnfrə'ɔːbɪt(ə)l ˌnɜːv] *subst.* continuation of the maxillary nerve below the orbit of the eye *nervus infraorbitalis;* **infraorbital vein** = vessel draining the face through the infraorbital canal to the pterygoid plexus *vena infraorbitale*

infrared rays [ˌɪnfrə'red ˌreɪz] *or* **infrared radiation** [ˌɪnfrə'red ˌreɪdi'eɪʃ(ə)n] *subst.* long invisible rays, below the visible red end of the colour spectrum, used to produce heat in body tissues in the treatment of traumatic and inflammatory conditions *infraröda strålar, infraröd strålning;* **she was advised to take a course of infrared ray treatment**

infundering ▷ **infusion, venoclysis**

infundibulum [ˌɪnfʌn'dɪbjʊləm] *subst.* any part of the body shaped like a funnel, especially the stem which attaches the pituitary gland to the hypothalamus *infundibulum, trattliknande anatomisk bildning*

infusion [ɪn'fjuːʒ(ə)n] *subst.* (i) drink made by pouring boiling water on a dry substance (such as herb tea *or* a powdered drug) *infusion, avkok;* (ii) putting liquid into a body, using a drip *infusion, infundering, dropp; see also* CAVAL

infusion ▷ **drip, venoclysis; tea**

införa ▷ **introduce**

införande ▷ **introduction**

ingestion [ɪn'dʒestʃ(ə)n] *subst.* (i) taking in food *or* drink *or* medicine by the mouth *ingestion, näringsintag;* (ii) process by which a foreign body (such as a bacillus) is surrounded by a cell *fagocytos*

ingjutning, långsam ▷ **venoclysis**

ingredient [ɪn'griːdiənt] *subst.* substance which is used with others to make something (food to eat *or* lotion to put on the skin, etc.) *ingrediens, beståndsdel;* **active ingredient** *see* ACTIVE

ingripande ▷ **intervention**

ingrowing toenail [ˌɪn'grəʊɪŋ ˌtəʊneɪ(ə)l] *subst.* condition where the nail cuts into the tissue at the side of it, and creates inflammation; sepsis and ulceration can also occur *unguis incarnatus, paronyki, inväxt nagel, nageltrång;* **if the nail is slightly ingrown, it can be treated by cutting at the sides**

inguen ⇨ **groin**

inguinal ['ɪŋgwɪn(ə)l] *adj.* referring to the groin *inguinal, ljumsk-;* **inguinal canal** = passage in the lower abdominal wall, carrying the spermatic cord *canalis inguinalis, inguinalkanalen, ljumskkanalen;* **inguinal hernia** = hernia where the intestine bulges through the muscles in the groin, especially through the inguinal canal *hernia inguinalis, ljumskbråck;* **inguinal ligament** *or* **Poupart's ligament** = ligament in the groin, running from the spine to the pubis *ligamentum inguinale, Pouparts ligament, ljumskbandet;* **inguinal region** = groin *or* part of the body where the lower abdomen joins the top of the thigh *regio inguinalis, ljumskregionen*

inguinale [ˌɪŋwɪ'neɪli] *see* GRANULOMA

ingång ⇨ **introitus**

INH ⇨ **isoniazid**

inhalant [ɪn'heɪlənt] *subst.* medicinal substance which is inhaled *inhalationsmedel*

inhalation [ˌɪnhə'leɪʃ(ə)n] *subst.* **(a)** action of breathing in *inhalation, inspiration, inandning;* **smoke inhalation** = breathing in smoke (as in a fire) *inandning av rök* **(b)** action of inhaling a medicinal substance as part of treatment *inhalation;* medicinal substance which is breathed in *inhalationsmedel;* **steam inhalations** = treatment of respiratory disease by making the patient inhale steam with medicinal substances in it *behandling med inandning av ånga, inhalationsbehandling*

inhalation ⇨ **inhalation, inspiration**

inhalationsbehandling ⇨ **inhalation**

inhalationsmedel ⇨ **inhalant, inhalation**

inhalator ⇨ **inhaler**

inhale [ɪn'heɪ(ə)l] *vb.* to breathe in *inhalera, andas in;* **he inhaled some toxic gas fumes and was rushed to hospital; even smoking cigars can be bad for you if you inhale the smoke**

inhaler [ɪn'heɪlə] *subst.* small device for administering medicinal substances into the mouth *or* nose, so that they can be inhaled *inhalator*

NOTE: opposite is **exhale, exhalation**

inhalera ⇨ **inhale**

inherent [ɪn'hɪər(ə)nt] *adj.* thing which is part of the essential character of a person *or* a permanent characteristic of an organism *inneboende, medfödd*

inherit [ɪn'herɪt] *vb.* to receive characteristics from a parent's genes *ärva;* **she inherited her father's red hair; haemophilia is a condition which is inherited through the mother's genes**

inhibera ⇨ **inhibit**

inhibit [ɪn'hɪbɪt] *vb.* to block *or* to prevent an action happening; to stop a functional process *inhibera, hämma, förhindra;* **aspirin inhibits the clotting of blood; to have an inhibiting effect on something** = to block something *or* to stop something happening *ha hämmande inverkan på ngt*

inhibition [ˌɪnhɪ'bɪʃ(ə)n] *subst.* **(a)** action of blocking *or* preventing something happening, especially preventing a muscle *or* organ from functioning properly *inhibition, hämning, blockering* **(b)** *(in psychology)* suppressing a thought which is associated to a sense of guilt *inhibition, hämning;* blocking of a normal spontaneous action by some mental influence *blockering*

inhibitor [ɪn'hɪbɪtə] *subst.* substance which inhibits *inhibitor, blockerande (hämmande) medel*

inhibitory nerve [ɪn'hɪbɪt(ə)ri ˌnɜːv] *subst.* nerve which stops a function taking place *inhibitor, hämmare;* **the vagus nerve is an inhibitory nerve which slows down the action of the heart**

inject [ɪn'dʒekt] *vb.* to put a liquid into a patient's body under pressure, by using a hollow needle inserted into the tissues *injicera, spruta in;* **he was injected with morphine; she injected herself with a drug**

injection [ɪn'dʒekʃ(ə)n] *subst.* **(a)** act of injecting a liquid into the body *injektion;* **intracutaneous injection** = injection of a liquid between the layers of skin (as for a test for an allergy) *intrakutan injektion;* **intramuscular injection** = injection of liquid into a muscle (as for a slow release of a drug) *intramuskulär injektion;* **intravenous injection** = injection of liquid into a vein (as for fast release of a drug) *intravenös injektion;* **hypodermic injection** *or* **subcutaneous**

injection = injection of a liquid beneath the skin (as for pain-killing drugs) *subkutan injektion* **(b)** liquid introduced into the body *injektion;* **he had a penicillin injection**

injektion ➪ **injection, jab, shot**

injektionsnål ➪ **hypodermic**

injektionsspruta ➪ **hypodermic**

injicera ➪ **inject**

injure ['ɪn(d)ʒə] *vb.* to hurt *skada;* **six people were injured in the accident; the injured** = people who have been injured *de skadade;* **all the injured were taken to the nearest hospital**

injury ['ɪn(d)ʒ(ə)ri] *subst.* damage *or* wound caused to a person's body *skada;* **his injuries required hospital treatment; she never recovered from her injuries; he received severe facial injuries in the accident**

ink [ɪŋk] *subst.* coloured liquid which is used for writing *bläck;* **ink blot test** = RORSCHACH TEST

inkapslad ➪ **encapsulated, encysted**

inkarcererad ➪ **incarcerated**

inkilad ➪ **impacted, incarcerated**

inkilning ➪ **impaction**

inkludera ➪ **include**

inklusion ➪ **inclusion**

inklusionskropp ➪ **inclusion**

inklämd ➪ **impacted, incarcerated, strangulated**

inklämning ➪ **compression, impaction, strangulation**

inkompatibilitet ➪ **incompatibility**

inkompetens ➪ **incompetence**

inkomplett ➪ **incomplete**

inkontinens ➪ **dribbling, incontinence**

inkontinent ➪ **incontinent**

inkoordination ➪ **incoordination**

inkorrekt ➪ **incorrect**

inkubation ➪ **incubation period**

inkubationsstadium ➪ **stadium invasioni**

inlagd patient ➪ **inpatient**

inlagring ➪ **infiltration**

inlay ['ɪnleɪ] *subst. (in dentistry)* type of filling for teeth *inlägg*

inlet ['ɪnlet] *subst.* passage *or* opening through which a cavity can be entered *apertura, öppning;* **thoracic inlet** = small opening at the top of the thorax *apertura thoracis superior, övre toraxaperturen (toraxöppningen)*

inlevelse ➪ **empathy**

inlägg ➪ **inlay**

inläggning på sjukhus ➪ **admission, hospitalization**

innate [ˌɪ'neɪt] *adj.* inherited *or* which is present in a body from birth *innatus, medfödd*

inneboende ➪ **inborn, inherent, intrinsic**

innebära ➪ **involve**

innehåll ➪ **content**

inneliggande ➪ **residential**

inner ['ɪnə] *adj.* (part) which is inside *inre, inner-;* **inner ear** = part of the ear inside the head, behind the eardrum, containing the semicircular canals, the vestibule and the cochlea *auris interna, innerörat;* **inner pleura** = membrane attached to the surface of a lung *pleura visceralis (pulmonalis), lungsäckens inre blad* NOTE: the opposite is **outer**

inner- ➪ **end-, endo-, inner**

innermost ['ɪnəməʊst] *adj.* furthest inside *innerst*

innerst ➪ **innermost**

innervation [ˌɪnɜː'veɪʃ(ə)n] *subst.* nerve supply to an organ (both motor nerves and sensory nerves) *innervation, nervförsörjning*

innerörat ➪ **inner, internal**

innesluta ➪ **enclose**

inneslutning ➪ **inclusion**

innocent ['ɪnəs(ə)nt] *adj.* (growth) which is benign *or* not malignant *benign, godartad, oskyldig*

innominate [ɪ'nɒmɪnət] *adj.* with no name *namnlös;* **innominate artery** *or* **brachiocephalic artery** = largest branch of the arch of the aorta, which continues as the right common carotid and right subclavian arteries *arteria brachiocephalica, "namnlösa artären";* **innominate bone** = HIP BONE; **innominate veins** *or* **brachiocephalic veins** = two veins which continue the subclavian and jugular veins to the superior vena cava *vena brachiocephalica dextra resp. sinistra*

inoculate [ɪ'nɒkjuleɪt] *vb.* to introduce vaccine into a person's body in order to make the body create antibodies, so making the person immune to the disease *inokulera, ympa (in), vaccinera;* **the baby was inoculated against diphtheria** NOTE: you inoculate someone **with** or **against** a disease

inoculation [ɪˌnɒkju'leɪʃ(ə)n] *subst.* action of inoculating someone *inokulation, ympning, vaccination;* **has the baby had a diphtheria inoculation?**

inoculum [ɪ'nɒkjʊləm] *subst.* substance (such as a vaccine) used for inoculation *inoculum, medel för ympning (vaccination)*

inokulation ⇨ **inoculation**

inokulationshepatit ⇨ **hepatitis**

inokulera ⇨ **inoculate**

inoperable [ɪn'ɒp(ə)rəb(ə)l] *adj.* (condition) which cannot be operated on *inoperabel;* **the surgeon decided that the cancer was inoperable**

inorganic [ˌɪnɔː'gænɪk] *adj.* (substance) which is not made from animal or vegetable sources *oorganisk*

inotropic [ˌɪnəʊ'trɒpɪk] *adj.* which affects the way muscles contract, especially those of the heart *inotrop*

inpackning ⇨ **pack**

inpatient ['ɪnˌpeɪʃ(ə)nt] *subst.* patient living in a hospital for treatment *or* observation *inlagd patient; compare* OUTPATIENT

inquest ['ɪŋkwest] *subst.* inquiry (by a coroner) into the cause of a death *undersökning av (förhör om) dödsorsak*

> COMMENT: an inquest has to take place where death is violent or not expected, where death could be murder, or where a prisoner dies and when police are involved

inquire [ɪn'kwa(ɪ)ə] *vb.* to ask questions about something *fråga, undersöka;* **he inquired if anything was wrong; she inquired about the success rate of that type of operation; the committee is inquiring into the administration of the District Health Authority**

inquiry [ɪn'kwaɪ(ə)ri] *subst.* official investigation *undersökning, utredning;* **there has been a government inquiry into the outbreak of legionnaires' disease**

inre ⇨ **inner, interior, internal, intrinsic, medial**

inre hörselgången ⇨ **meatus**

inre organen ⇨ **viscera**

inre respiration ⇨ **respiration**

inresekretorisk körtel ⇨ **endocrine gland**

inrättning ⇨ **institution**

insane [ɪn'seɪn] *adj.* mad *or* suffering from a mental disorder *mentalsjuk, sinnessjuk, vansinnig*

insanitary [ɪn'sænət(ə)ri] *adj.* not sanitary *or* unhygienic *hälsovådlig, ohälsosam, ohygienisk;* **cholera spread rapidly because of the insanitary conditions in the town**

insanity [ɪn'sænəti] *subst.* psychotic mental disorder *or* illness *mentalsjukdom, sinnessjukdom, vansinne*

> COMMENT: insanity is the legal term used to describe patients whose mental condition is so unstable that they need to be placed in a hospital to prevent them doing actions which could harm themselves or other people, although some are cared for in the community

insect ['ɪnsekt] *subst.* small animal with six legs and a body in three parts *insekt;* **insects were flying round the lamp; he was stung by an insect; insect bites** = stings caused by insects which puncture the skin to suck blood, and in so doing introduce irritants *insektsbett*

> COMMENT: most insect bites are simply irritating, but some patients can be extremely sensitive to certain types of insect (such as bee stings). Other insect bites can be more serious, as insects can carry the bacteria which produce typhus, sleeping sickness, malaria, filariasis, etc.

insecticide [ɪn'sektɪsaɪd] *subst.* substance which kills insects *insektsmedel, insektsdödande medel*

insekt ⇨ **insect**

insektsbett ⇨ **insect**

insektsmedel ⇨ **insecticide**

insemination [ɪn,semɪ'neɪʃ(ə)n] *subst.* (i) fertilization of an ovum by a sperm *insemination, befruktning;* (ii) introduction of sperm into the vagina *insemination, befruktning;* **artificial insemination =** introduction of semen into a woman's womb by artificial means *artificiell insemination, konstgjord befruktning; see also* AID, AIH

insert [ɪn'sɜ:t] *vb.* to put something into something *sätta (föra, skjuta, sticka) in;* **the catheter is inserted into the passage**

insertion [ɪn'sɜ:ʃ(ə)n] *subst.* (i) point of attachment of a muscle to a bone which *insertion, fäste, fästställe;* (ii) point where an organ is attached to its support *insertion, fäste, fästställe;* (iii) change in the structure of a chromosome, where a segment of the chromosome is introduced into another *slags förändring i kromosomstrukturen*

insides ['ɪnsaɪdz] *subst pl. informal* internal organs, especially the stomach and intestines *inälvor, magen;* **he says he has a pain in his insides; you ought to see the doctor if you think there is something wrong with your insides**

insight ['ɪnsaɪt] *subst.* ability of a patient to realise that he is ill *insikt*

insikt ⇨ **insight**

insipidus [ɪn'sɪpɪdəs] *see* DIABETES

in situ [ɪn'sɪtju:] *adj.* in place *in situ, på platsen*

insjukna ⇨ **fall ill, sicken for**

inskjuten ⇨ **intercalated**

inskränka ⇨ **restrict**

inskränkande ⇨ **restrictive**

inskärning ⇨ **notch**

insnitt ⇨ **incision, section**

insolation ⇨ **sunstroke**

insoluble [ɪn'sɒljʊb(ə)l] *adj.* which cannot be dissolved in liquid *olöslig;* **insoluble fibre** = fibre in bread and cereals, which is not digested, but which swells inside the intestine *olöslig fiber*

insomnia [ɪn'sɒmniə] *subst.* inability to sleep *or* sleeplessness *insomni, sömnlöshet;* **she suffers from insomnia; what does the doctor give you for your insomnia?**

insomniac [ɪn'sɒmniæk] *subst.* person who suffers from insomnia *sömnlös (person)*

inspect [ɪn'spekt] *vb.* to examine *or* to look at something carefully *inspektera, undersöka, granska;* **the doctor inspected the boy's throat; he used a bronchoscope to inspect the inside of the lungs**

inspection [ɪn'spekʃ(ə)n] *subst.* act of examining something *inspektion, undersökning, granskning, besiktning;* **the officials have carried out an inspection of the hospital kitchens**

inspector [ɪn'spektə] *subst.* person who inspects *inspektör;* **Government Health Inspector =** government official who examines offices *or* factories to see if they are clean and healthy *ung. hälsovårdsinspektör*

inspektera ⇨ **inspect**

inspektion ⇨ **inspection**

inspektör ⇨ **inspector**

inspiration [,ɪnspə'reɪʃ(ə)n] *subst.* breathing in *or* taking air into the lungs *inspiration, inhalation, inandning*
NOTE: the opposite is **expiration**

> COMMENT: inspiration takes place when the muscles of the diaphragm contract, allowing the lungs to expand

inspissated [ɪn'spɪseɪtɪd] *adj.* (liquid) which is thickened by removing water from it *förtjockad, förtätad, intorkad*

inspissation [,ɪnspɪ'seɪʃ(ə)n] *subst.* removing water from a solution to make it thicker *inspissation, förtätning, intorkning*

instabil ⇨ **labile, unstable**

instep ['ɪnstep] *subst.* arched top part of the foot *fotryggen*

instick ⇨ **puncture**

instillation [ˌɪnstɪ'leɪʃ(ə)n] *subst.* introducing a liquid into part of the body drop by drop *instillation, indrypning*

instinct ['ɪnstɪŋ(k)t] *subst.* tendency *or* ability which the body has from birth, and does not need to learn *instinkt;* **the body has a natural instinct to protect itself from danger**

instinctive [ɪn'stɪŋ(k)tɪv] *adj.* referring to instinct *instinktiv;* **everyone has an instinctive reaction to move away from fire**

instinkt ➪ **instinct**

instinktiv ➪ **instinctive**

institution [ˌɪnstɪ'tjuːʃ(ə)n] *subst.* hospital *or* clinic, especially a psychiatric hospital *or* children's home *institution, inrättning;* **he has lived all his life in institutions**

institutionalisera ➪ **institutionalize**

institutionalisering ➪ **institutionalization**

institutionalization [ˌɪnstɪ'tjuːʃ(ə)nəlaɪ'zeɪʃ(ə)n] *or* **institutional neurosis** [ˌɪnstɪ'tjuːʃ(ə)n(ə)l nju(ə)ˌrəʊsɪs] *subst.* condition where a patient has become so adapted to life in an institution that it is impossible for him to live outside it *institutionalisering*

institutionalize [ˌɪnstɪ'tjuːʃ(ə)nəlaɪz] *vb.* to put a person into an institution *institutionalisera, lägga in (placera) på institution*

instjälpning ➪ **intussusception, invagination**

instruction [ɪn'strʌkʃ(ə)n] *subst.* teaching how to do something *undervisning, handledning;* **the students are given instruction in dealing with emergency cases; instructions** = words which explain how something is used *or* how to do something *instruktioner, föreskrifter;* **the instructions are written on the medicine bottle; we can't use this machine because we have lost the book of instructions; she gave the taxi driver instructions how to get to the hospital**

instrument ['ɪnstrəmənt] *subst.* piece of equipment *instrument;* tool *verktyg, redskap;* **the doctor had a box of surgical instruments**

instrument ➪ **apparatus, instrument**

instrument- ➪ **instrumental**

instrumental [ˌɪnstrə'ment(ə)l] *adj.* **(a)** using an instrument *instrumentell, instrument-;* **instrumental delivery** = childbirth where the doctor uses forceps to help the baby out of the mother's womb *tångförlossning* **(b) instrumental in** = helping to do something *behjälplig med, som bidrar (medverkar) till;* **she was instrumental in developing the new technique**

instrumentell ➪ **instrumental**

insufficiency [ˌɪnsə'fɪʃ(ə)nsi] *subst.* (i) not being enough to perform normal functions *insufficiens, otillräcklighet;* (ii) incompetence of an organ *insufficiens;* **the patient is suffering from a renal insufficiency**

insufficiens ➪ **incompetence, insufficiency**

insufficiensfraktur ➪ **march fracture**

insufficient ➪ **incompetent**

insufflation [ˌɪnsə'fleɪʃ(ə)n] *subst.* blowing something, such as air *or* a powder, into a cavity in the body *insufflation, inblåsning*

insula ['ɪnsjʊlə] *subst.* part of the cerebral cortex which is covered by the folds of the sulcus *insula, lobus apertus, gyri breves insulae*

insulin ['ɪnsjʊlɪn] *subst.* hormone produced by the islets of Langerhans in the pancreas *insulin*

> COMMENT: insulin controls the way in which the body converts sugar into energy and regulates the level of sugar in the blood; a lack of insulin caused by diabetes mellitus makes the level of glucose in the blood rise. Insulin injections are regularly used to treat diabetes mellitus, but care has to be taken not to exceed the dose as this will cause hyperinsulinism

insulinase ['ɪnsjʊlɪneɪz] *subst.* enzyme which breaks down insulin *insulinas*

insulinchock ➪ **hypoglycaemic**

insulinoma [ˌɪnsjʊlɪ'nəʊmə] *or* **insuloma** [ɪnsjʊ'ləʊmə] *subst.* tumour in the islets of Langerhans *insul(in)om*

insurance [ɪn'ʃʊər(ə)ns] *subst.* agreement with a company that they will pay you money if something is lost or damaged *försäkring;*

accident insurance = insurance which pays out money when an accident happens *olycksfallsförsäkring;* **life insurance** = insurance which pays out money when someone dies *livförsäkring;* **medical insurance** = insurance which pays for private medical treatment *sjukförsäkring;* **National Insurance** = weekly payment from a person's wages (with a supplement from the employer) which pays for state assistance, medical treatment, etc. *socialförsäkring (i Storbritannien)*

insure [ɪn'ʃʊə] *vb.* to agree with a company that they will pay you money if something is lost or damaged *försäkra;* **is your car insured?**

inta ⇨ **take**

intag ⇨ **intake**

intagna (på sjukhus) ⇨ **population**

intagning på sjukhus ⇨ **admission, hospitalization**

intake ['ɪnteɪk] *subst.* taking in (of a substance) *intag, konsumtion;* a high intake of alcohol **she was advised to reduce her intake of sugar**

inte ⇨ **non-, un-**

integration [ˌɪntɪ'greɪʃ(ə)n] *subst.* process where a whole is made into a single unit by the functional combination of the parts *integrering*

COMMENT: there are two modes of integration: nervous and hormonal

integrering ⇨ **integration**

integument [ɪn'tegjumənt] *subst.* covering layer, such as the skin *integument*

intellektet ⇨ **mind, psyche**

intellektuell ⇨ **mental**

intellektuellt ⇨ **mentally**

intelligence [ɪn'telɪdʒ(ə)ns] *subst.* ability to learn and understand quickly *intelligens;* **intelligence quotient (IQ)** = ratio of the mental age as given by an intelligence test, to the actual age of the person *intelligenskvot, IQ, IK;* **intelligence test** = test to see how intelligent someone is, giving a mental age, as opposed to the chronological age of the person *intelligenstest*

COMMENT: the average IQ is between 90 and 110

intelligens ⇨ **intelligence**

intelligenskvot ⇨ **intelligence**

intelligenstest ⇨ **intelligence**

intelligensålder ⇨ **mental**

intelligent [ɪn'telɪdʒ(ə)nt] *adj.* clever *or* able to learn quickly *intelligent;* **he's the most intelligent boy in the class**

intense [ɪn'tens] *adj.* very strong (pain) *intensiv, kraftig;* **she is suffering from intense post herpetic neuralgia**

intensiv ⇨ **extreme, intense; crash**

intensive care [ɪnˌtensɪv 'keə] *subst.* continual supervision and treatment of a patient in a special section of a hospital *intensivvård;* **the patient was put in intensive care; he came out of intensive care and was moved to the general ward; intensive care unit (ICU)** = special section of a hospital which supervises seriously ill patients who need constant supervision *intensivvårdsavdelning, IVA*

intensivvård ⇨ **intensive care**

intensivvårdsavdelning ⇨ **intensive care**

intention [ɪn'tenʃ(ə)n] *subst.* **(a)** healing process *intention, läkning(sprocess);* **healing by first intention** = healing of a clean wound where the tissue reforms quickly *sanatio per primam intentionem, primärläkning;* **healing by second intention** = healing of an infected wound *or* ulcer, which takes place slowly and may leave a permanent scar *sanatio per secundam intentionem, sekundärläkning* **(b)** aiming to do something *intention, avsikt;* **intention tremor** = trembling of the hands when a person makes a voluntary movement to try to touch something *intentionstremor*

intentionstremor ⇨ **intention**

inter- ['ɪntə-, ˌ--] *prefix* meaning between *inter-, mellan-*

interatrial septum [ˌɪntər'eɪtriəl ˌseptəm] *subst.* membrane between the right and left atria in the heart *septum interatriale*

interbreed [ˌɪntə'bri:d] *vb.* to reproduce with another member of the same species *korsa(s)*

intercalated [ɪn'tɜ:kəleɪtɪd] *adj.* inserted between other tissues *inskjuten;* **intercalated disc** = closely applied cell membranes at the end of adjacent cells in cardiac muscle, seen as transverse lines *mellanskiva, Z-skiva*

intercellular [ˌɪntəˈseljʊlə] *adj.* between the cells in tissue *intercellulär*

intercostal [ˌɪntəˈkɒst(ə)l] *adj.* between the ribs *interkostal;* **intercostal muscles** *or* **the intercostals** = muscles between the ribs *musculi intercostales, interkostalmusklerna*

> COMMENT: the intercostal muscles expand and contract the thorax, so changing the pressure in the thorax and making the person breathe in or out. There are three layers of intercostal muscle: external, internal and innermost or intercostalis intimis

intercourse [ˈɪntəkɔːs] *subst.* **(sexual) intercourse** = action of inserting the man's penis into the woman's vagina, releasing spermatozoa from the penis by ejaculation, which may fertilize an ovum from the woman's ovaries *coitus, samlag*

intercurrent disease [ˌɪntəˌkʌr(ə)nt dɪˈziːz] *or* **infection** [ɪnˈfekʃ(ə)n] *subst.* disease *or* infection which affects someone who is suffering from another disease *interkurrent (tillstötande) sjukdom el. infektion*

interdigital [ˌɪntəˈdɪdʒɪt(ə)l] *adj.* referring to the space between the fingers or toes *interdigital*

interest [ˈɪntrəst] **1** *subst.* **(a)** special attention *intresse;* **the consultant takes a lot of interest in his students; she has no interest in what goes on in the ward around her; why doesn't he take more interest in physiotherapy? (b)** something which attracts you particularly *intresse;* **her main interest is the treatment of cardiac patients; do you have any special interests apart from your work? 2** *vb.* to attract someone's attention *intressera;* **he's specially interested in the work of the physiotherapy department; nothing seems to interest her very much**

interesting [ˈɪntrəstɪŋ] *adj.* which attracts your attention *intressant;* **there's an interesting article on the treatment of drug addiction in the magazine**

interfalangealled ⇨ **interphalangeal joint**

interfas ⇨ **interphase**

interfere [ˌɪntəˈfɪə] *vb.* to get involved *or* to stop or hinder a function *interferera, störa*

interference [ˌɪntəˈfɪər(ə)ns] *subst.* act of interfering *interferens, störning*

interferera ⇨ **interfere**

interferon [ˌɪntəˈfɪərɒn] *subst.* protein produced by cells, usually in response to a virus and which then reduces the spread of viruses *interferon*

interior [ɪnˈtɪərɪə] *adj. & subst.* (part) which is inside *interior, inre;* **the interior of the intestine is lined with millions of villi**

interkostal ⇨ **intercostal**

interkostalmusklerna ⇨ **intercostal**

interlobar [ˌɪntəˈləʊbə] *adj.* between lobes *interlobar, interlobär;* **interlobar arteries** = arteries running towards the cortex on each side of a renal pyramid *arteriae interlobares renis*

interlobular [ˌɪntəˈlɒbjʊlə] *adj.* between lobules *interlobular, interlobulär;* **interlobular arteries** = arteries running to the glomeruli of the kidney *arteriae interlobulares renis*

interlobär ⇨ **interlobar**

intermediate [ˌɪntəˈmiːdiət, -dɪeɪt] *adj.* which is in the middle between two things *mellanliggande*

intermedius [ˌɪntəˈmiːdiəs] *see* VASTUS

intermenstrual [ˌɪntəˈmenstru(ə)l] *adj.* between the menstrual periods *intermenstrual*

intermittent [ˌɪntəˈmɪt(ə)nt] *adj.* occurring at intervals *intermittent;* **intermittent claudication** = condition of the arteries causing severe pain in the legs which makes the patient limp after having walked a short distance (the symptoms increase with more walking, but stop after a short rest, and recur when the patient walks again) *claudicatio intermittens, intermittent hälta, fönstertittarsjuka;* **intermittent fever** = fever which rises and falls, like malaria *febris intermittens*

intern [ˈɪntɜːn] *subst. US* medical school graduate who is working in a hospital while at the same time continuing his studies *ung. allmäntjänstgörande läkare, AT-läkare* NOTE: the GB English is **houseman, house officer**

intern ⇨ **internal**

interna [ɪnˈtɜːnɪst] *see* OTITIS

internal [ɪn'tɜ:n(ə)l] *adj.* inside the body *intern, inre, invärtes;* **internal bleeding** = loss of blood from an injury inside the body *inre blödning;* **internal carotid** = artery in the neck, behind the external carotid, which gives off the ophthalmic artery and ends by dividing into the anterior and middle cerebral arteries *arteria carotis interna;* **internal capsule** = broad band of fibres passing to and from the cerebral cortex *capsula interna;* **internal derangement of the knee (IDK)** = condition where the knee cannot function properly because of a torn meniscus *avsliten menisk;* **internal ear** = the part of the ear inside the head, behind the eardrum, containing the semicircular canals, the vestibule and the cochlea *auris interna, innerörat;* **internal jugular** = largest jugular vein in the neck, leading to the brachiocephalic veins *vena jugularis interna, inre strupvenen; US* **internal medicine** = treatment of diseases of the internal organs by specialists *internmedicin, invärtesmedicin;* **internal organs** = organs situated inside the body *inre organ;* **internal oblique** = middle layer of muscle covering the abdomen, beneath the external oblique *musculus obliquus internus abdominis, bukens inre snedmuskel; compare* EXTERNAL

internally [ɪn'tɜ:n(ə)li] *adv.* inside the body *invärtes;* **he was bleeding internally**

interneurone [ˌɪntə'nju:rəʊn] *subst.* neurone with short processes which is a link between two other neurones in sensory *or* motor pathways *interneuron, mellanneuron*

internist [ɪn'tɜ:nɪst] *subst.* specialist who treats diseases of the internal organs *internist, internmedicinare*

internmedicin ⇨ **internal**

internmedicinare ⇨ **internist**

internmedicinsk ⇨ **medical**

internodal [ˌɪntə'nəʊd(ə)l] *adj.* between two nodes *mellan två noder*

internship [ɪn'tɜ:nʃɪp] *subst. US* position of an intern in a hospital *ung. allmäntjänstgöring, AT*

internuncial neurone [ˌɪntə'nʌnʃ(ə)l ˌnju:rəʊn] *subst.* neurone which links two other nerve cells *neuron som binder samman två andra nervceller*

internus [ɪn'tɜ:nəs] *subst.* medial rectus muscle in the orbit of the eye *musculus rectus medialis, mediala (inre) raka ögonmuskeln*

interoceptor [ˌɪntərəʊ'septə] *subst.* nerve cell which reacts to a change taking place inside the body *nervcell som reagerar för förändringar i kroppens inre; see also* CHEMORECEPTOR, EXTEROCEPTOR, PROPRIOCEPTOR, RECEPTOR, VISCEROCEPTOR

interosseous [ˌɪntər'ɒsiəs] *adj.* between bones *mellan ben*

interpeduncular cistern [ˌɪntəpə'dʌŋkjʊlər ˌsɪst(ə)n] *subst.* subarachnoid space between the two cerebral hemispheres beneath the midbrain and the hypothalamus *cisterna interpeduncularis*

interphalangeal joint [ˌɪntəfə'lændʒiəl ˌdʒɔɪnt] *or* **IP joint** [ˌaɪ'pi: ˌdʒɔɪnt] *subst.* joint between the phalanges *articulatio interphalangea manus (pedis), interfalangealled, fingerled, tåled*

interphase ['ɪntəfeɪz] *subst.* stage of a cell between divisions *interfas*

interpubic joint [ˌɪntə'pju:bɪk ˌdʒɔɪnt] *or* **pubic symphysis** [ˌpju:bɪk 'sɪmfəsɪs] *subst.* piece of cartilage which joins the two sections of the pubic bone *symphysis pubica (ossis pubis), symfysen, blygdbensfogen*

interruptus [ˌɪntə'rʌptəs] *see* COITUS

intersexuality [ˌɪntəˌsekʃu'æləti] *subst.* condition where a baby has both male and female characteristics, as in Klinefelter's syndrome and Turner's syndrome *intersexualitet, dubbelkön*

interstices [ɪn'tɜ:stɪsɪz] *subst pl.* small spaces between parts of the body *interstitier, mellanrum*

interstitial [ˌɪntə'stɪʃ(ə)l] *adj.* (tissue) in the spaces between parts of something, especially the tissue between the active tissue in an organ *interstitial(-), interstitiell;* **interstitial cells** *or* **Leydig cells** = testosterone-producing cells between the tubules in the testes *interstitialceller, Leydig-celler, Leydigs (leydigska) celler;* **interstitial cell stimulating hormone (ICSH)** *or* **luteinizing hormone (LH)** = hormone produced by the pituitary gland which stimulates the formation of corpus luteum in females and testosterone in males *insterstitial cell stimulating hormone, ICSH, luteiniserande hormon, LH*

interstitialceller ⇨ **interstitial**

interstitiell ⇨ **interstitial, stroma**

interstitier ▷ **interstices**

intertrigo [ˌɪntəˈtraɪgəʊ] *subst.* irritation which occurs when two skin surfaces rub against each other (as in the armpit *or* between the buttocks) *intertrigo, utslag i hudveck*

intertubercular plane [ˌɪntətjuˈbɜːkjʊlə ˌpleɪn] *subst.* imaginary horizontal line drawn across the lower abdomen at the level of the projecting parts of the iliac bones *tänkt plan genom utskott på höftbenet*

intervention [ˌɪntəˈvenʃ(ə)n] *subst.* treatment *ingripande, behandling;* **medical intervention** *or* **surgical intervention** = treatment of illness by drugs *or* by surgery *medicinsk resp. kirurgisk behandling;* **nursing intervention** = treatment of illness by nursing care, without surgery *omvårdnad(såtgärd)*

interventricular [ˌɪntəvenˈtrɪkjʊlə] *adj.* between ventricles (in the heart *or* brain) *interventrikulär;* **interventricular septum** = wall in the lower part of the heart, separating the ventricles *septum interventriculare;* **interventricular foramen** = opening in the brain between the lateral ventricle and the third ventricle, through which the cerebrospinal fluid passes *foramen interventriculare*

intervertebral [ˌɪntəˈvɜːtɪbr(ə)l] *adj.* between vertebrae *intervertebral;* **intervertebral disc** = thick piece of cartilage which lies between two vertebrae *discus intervertebralis, intervertebralbrosk, mellankotskiva;* **intervertebral foramina** = hole in each vertebra through which the nerves pass *foramina intervertebrales; see also* VERTEBRAL ▷ *illustration* JOINTS, VERTEBRAL COLUMN

intervertebralbrosk ▷ **intervertebral**

intestinal [ɪnˈtestɪn(ə)l] *adj.* referring to the intestine *intestinal, inälvs-, tarm-;* **intestinal anastomosis** = surgical operation to join one part of the intestine to another (after a section has been removed) *tarmanastomos;* **intestinal flora** = bacteria which are always present in the intestine *tarmflora;* **intestinal glands** *or* **glands of Lieberkuhn** = tubular glands found in the mucous membrane of the small and large intestine *glandulae intestinales, Lieberkühns körtlar;* **intestinal infection** = infection in the intestines *tarminfektion;* **intestinal juice** = colourless fluid secreted by the small intestine which contains enzymes that help digestion *tarmsaft;* **intestinal obstruction** = blocking of the intestine *tarmobstruktion, stopp i tarmarna;* **intestinal wall** = layers of tissue which form the intestine *tarmvägg* NOTE: for other terms referring to the intestine see words beginning with **entero-**

intestinal infantilism ▷ **gluten**

intestine [ɪnˈtestɪn] *subst.* **the intestines** = the bowel *or* gut *or* the tract which passes from the stomach to the anus in which food is digested as it passes through *tarmarna;* **small intestine** = section of the intestine from the stomach to the caecum, consisting of the duodenum, the jejunum and the ileum *tunntarmen;* **large intestine** *or* **colon** = section of the intestine from the caecum to the rectum, consisting of the caecum, the ascending, transverse, descending and sigmoid colons and the rectum *colon, kolon, tjocktarmen, grovtarmen*

> COMMENT: absorption of substances in partly digested food is the main function of the small intestine. This is carried out by the little villi in the walls of the intestine which absorb nutrients into the bloodstream. The large intestine absorbs water from the food after it has passed through the small intestine, and the remaining material passes out of the body through the anus as faeces

intima [ˈɪntɪmə] *subst. & adj.* **(tunica) intima** = inner layer of the wall of an artery *or* vein *tunica intima (interna), intiman*

intolerance [ɪnˈtɒlər(ə)ns] *subst.* (i) being unable to endure something, such as pain *intolerans;* (ii) being unable to take certain drugs because of the body's reaction to them *intolerans, överkänslighet;* **he developed an intolerance to penicillin**

intorkad ▷ **inspissated**

intorkning ▷ **inspissation**

intoxicant [ɪnˈtɒksɪk(ə)nt] *subst.* substance, such as an alcoholic drink, which induces a state of intoxication or poisoning *berusningsmedel*

intoxicate [ɪnˈtɒksɪkeɪt] *vb.* to make a person drunk *or* to make a person incapable of controlling his actions, because of the influence of alcohol on his nervous system *berusa;* **he drank six glasses of whisky and became completely intoxicated**

intoxication [ɪnˌtɒksɪˈkeɪʃ(ə)n] *subst.* condition which results from the absorption and diffusion in the body of a poison, such as alcohol *intoxikation, förgiftning, berusning;* **she was driving a bus in a state of intoxication**

intra- ['ɪntrə, ˌ--] *prefix* meaning inside *intra-*

intra-abdominal [ˌɪntrəæb'dɒmɪn(ə)l] *adj.* inside the abdomen *intraabdominal*

intra-articular [ˌɪntrəɑː'tɪkjʊlə] *adj.* inside a joint *intraartikulär*

intracellular [ˌɪntrə'seljʊlə] *adj.* inside a cell *intracellular, intracellulär*

intracerebral haematoma [ˌɪntrə'serəbr(ə)l ˌhiːmə'təʊmə] *subst.* blood clot inside a cerebral hemisphere *intracerebralt hematom*

intracranial [ˌɪntrə'kreɪniəl] *adj.* inside the skull *intrakranial, intrakraniell*

intractable [ɪn'træktəb(ə)l] *adj.* which cannot be treated *svårbehandlad, omedgörlig;* **an operation to relieve intractable pain**

intracutaneous [ˌɪntrəkju'teɪniəs] *or* **intradermal** [ˌɪntrə'dɜːm(ə)l] *adj.* inside layers of skin tissue *intrakutan*

intradural [ˌɪntrə'djʊər(ə)l] *adj.* inside the dura mater *intradural*

intrakranial ⇨ **intracranial**

intrakraniell ⇨ **intracranial**

intrakutan ⇨ **intracutaneous**

intramedullary [ˌɪntrəme'dʌl(ə)ri] *adj.* inside the bone marrow *or* spinal cord *inuti benmärgen el. ryggmärgen*

intramural [ˌɪntrə'mjʊər(ə)l] *adj.* inside the wall of an organ *intramural*

intramuscular [ˌɪntrə'mʌskjʊlə] *adj.* inside a muscle *intramuskulär, i.m.;* **intramuscular injection** = injection made into a muscle *intramuskulär injektion*

intraocular [ˌɪntrə'ɒkjʊlə] *adj.* inside the eye *intraokulär*

intrathecal [ˌɪntrə'θiːk(ə)l] *adj.* inside a sheath *or* inside the intradural or subarachnoid space *intratekal*

intrauterine [ˌɪntrə'juːtəraɪn] *adj.* inside the uterus *intrauterin;* **intrauterine device (IUD)** = plastic coil placed inside the uterus to prevent conception *intrauterint preventivmedel, spiral*

intravenous (IV) [ˌɪntrə'viːnəs (ˌaɪ'viː)] *adj.* into a vein *intravenös, i.v.;* **intravenous feeding** = giving liquid food to a patient by means of a tube inserted into a vein *intravenös (parenteral) nutrition; see also* DRIP; **intravenous injection** = injection into a vein for fast release of a drug *intravenös injektion;* **intravenous pyelogram (IVP)** = series of X-ray photographs of the kidneys using pyelography *intravenöst pyelogram, urografi;* **intravenous pyelography** = X-ray examination of the kidneys after an opaque substance is injected intravenously into the body, and is carried by the blood into the kidneys *intravenös pyelografi, urografi*

intravenously [ˌɪntrə'viːnəsli] *adv.* into a vein *intravenöst;* **a fluid given intravenously**

intravenös ⇨ **intravenous (IV)**

intravenöst ⇨ **intravenously**

intra vitam [ˌɪntrə'vaɪtəm] *Latin phrase meaning* "during life" *intra vitam, under livstiden*

intressant ⇨ **interesting**

intresse ⇨ **interest**

intressera ⇨ **interest**

intrinsic [ɪn'trɪnsɪk] *adj.* referring to the essential nature of an organism *or* included inside an organ or part *inre, inneboende;* **intrinsic factor** = protein produced in the gastric glands which reacts with the the extrinsic factor, and which, if lacking, causes pernicious anaemia *intrinsic factor;* **intrinsic ligament** = ligament which forms part of the capsule surrounding a joint *ligament som utgör del av kapsel runt led;* **intrinsic muscle** = muscle lying completely inside the part or segment, especially of a limb which it moves *helt innesluten muskel*

introduce [ˌɪntrə'djuːs] *vb.* **(a)** to put something into something *föra (stoppa, sticka) in;* **he used a syringe to introduce a medicinal substance into the body; the nurse introduced the catheter into the vein** **(b)** to present two people to one another when they have never met before *presentera;* **can I introduce my new assistant?** **(c)** to start a new way of doing something *introducera, införa;* **the hospital has introduced a new screening process for cervical cancer**

introduction [ˌɪntrə'dʌkʃ(ə)n] *subst.* **(a)** putting something inside *införande;* **the introduction of semen into the woman's uterus; the introduction of an endotracheal tube into the patient's mouth** **(b)** starting a new process *introduktion*

introduktion ⇨ **introduction**

introitus [ɪn'trəʊitəs] *subst.* opening into any hollow organ *or* canal *introitus, ingång*

introversion [ˌɪntrə(ʊ)'vɜːʃ(ə)n] *subst.* condition where a person is excessively interested in himself and his own mental state *introversion, inåtvänd läggning*

introvert [ˌɪntrə(ʊ)'vɜːt] *subst.* person who thinks only about himself and his own mental state *introvert; compare* EXTROVERT, EXTROVERSION

inträffa ⇨ **happen, occur**

inträngande ⇨ **penetration**

intubate ['ɪntjubeit] *vb.* to catheterize *or* to insert a tube into any organ *or* part of the body *intubera*

intubation [ˌɪntju'beɪʃ(ə)n] *subst.* catheterization *or* therapeutic insertion of a tube into the larynx through the glottis to allow passage of air *intubation, intubering*

intubera ⇨ **intubate**

intubering ⇨ **intubation**

intumescence [ˌɪntju'mes(ə)ns] *subst.* swelling of an organ *intumescens, svullnad*

intussusception [ˌɪntəsə'sepʃ(ə)n] *subst.* condition where part of the gastrointestinal tract telescopes with the part beneath, causing an obstruction and strangulation of the part which has been telescoped *intussusception, instjälpning*

intussusception ⇨ **intussusception, invagination**

intyg ⇨ **certificate**

intyga ⇨ **certify**

invagination [ɪnˌvædʒə'neɪʃ(ə)n] *subst.* (i) intussusception *intussusception, instjälpning;* (ii) surgical treatment of hernia, in which a sheath of tissue is made to cover the opening *invagination*

invalid ['ɪnvəliːd] *subst. & adj.* (person) who has had an illness and has not fully recovered from it *sjuklig, sjuk;* (person) who is disabled *invalidiserad, handikappad;* **he has been an invalid since he had the accident six years ago; she is looking after her invalid parents; invalid carriage** = small car, specially made for use by an invalid *invalidfordon;* **invalid chair** *or* **wheelchair** = chair with wheels in which an invalid can sit and move about *rullstol;* **she manages to do all her shopping using her invalid chair; some buildings have special entrances for invalid chairs**

invalidfordon ⇨ **invalid**

invalidisera ⇨ **disable**

invalidiserad ⇨ **invalid**

invaliditet ⇨ **disability, disablement, invalidity**

invalidity [ˌɪnvə'lɪdəti] *subst.* being disabled *invaliditet, handikapp;* **invalidity benefit** = money paid by the government to someone who is permanently disabled *ersättning vid invaliditet*

invasion [ɪn'veɪʒ(ə)n] *subst.* entry of bacteria into a body *or* first attack of a disease *invasion*

invecklad ⇨ **complex**

invent [ɪn'vent] *vb.* **(a)** to make something which has never been made before *uppfinna;* **he invented a new type of catheter (b)** to make up, using your imagination *hitta på, tänka ut;* **he invented the whole story; small children often invent imaginary friends**

invention [ɪn'venʃ(ə)n] *subst.* thing which someone has invented *uppfinning;* **we have seen his latest invention, a brain scanner**

inverkan ⇨ **agency**

inversion [ɪn'vɜːʃ(ə)n] *subst.* being turned towards the inside *or* turning of part of the body (such as the foot) towards the inside *inversion, ut-och-invändning, indragning;* **inversion of the uterus** = condition where the top part of the uterus touches the cervix, as if it were inside out (which may happen after childbirth) *inversion uteri*

invertase [ɪn'vɜːteɪz] *subst.* enzyme in the intestine which splits sucrose *invertas, sackaras*

investigate [ɪn'vestɪgeɪt] *vb.* to examine something to try to find out what caused it *undersöka, utreda;* **health inspectors are investigating the outbreak of legionnaires' disease**

investigation [ɪnˌvestɪ'geɪʃ(ə)n] *subst.* examination to find out the cause of something which has happened *undersökning, utredning;* **the Health Authority ordered an investigation into how the drugs were stolen**

investigative surgery [ɪn'vestɪgeɪtɪv ˌsɜ:dʒəri] *subst.* surgery to investigate the cause of a condition *undersökande (experimentell) kirurgi*

invisible [ɪn'vɪzəb(ə)l] *adj.* which cannot be seen *osynlig;* **the microbes are invisible to the naked eye, but can be clearly seen under a microscope**

in vitro [ɪn ˌvi:trəʊ] *Latin phrase meaning* "in a glass" *in vitro;* **in vitro experiment** = experiment which takes place in the laboratory *experiment in vitro;* **in vitro fertilization (IVF)** = fertilization of a woman's ovum by her husband's sperm in the laboratory *in vitro-fertilisation, provrörsbefruktning; see also* TEST-TUBE BABY

in vivo [ɪn 'vi:vəʊ] *Latin phrase meaning* "in living tissue": experiment which takes place on the living body *in vivo;* **in vivo experiment** = experiment on a living body (such as an animal) *experiment in vivo*

involucrum [ˌɪnvə'lu:krəm] *subst.* covering of new bone which forms over diseased bone *involucrum, benhölje*

involuntary [ɪn'vɒlənt(ə)ri] *adj.* independent of the will *or* done without any mental processes being involved *involuntär, ofrivillig;* **patients are advised not to eat or drink, to reduce the risk of involuntary vomiting while on the operating table; involuntary action** = action where a patient does not use his will power *involuntär (ofrivillig) handling;* **involuntary muscle** = muscle supplied by the autonomic nervous system, and therefore not under voluntary control (such as the muscle which activates a vital organ like the heart) *muskel som styrs av autonoma nervsystemet*

involution [ˌɪnvə'lu:ʃ(ə)n] *subst.* **(a)** return of an organ to normal size, such as the return of the uterus to normal size after childbirth *involution, krympning, tillbakabildning* **(b)** period of decline of organs which sets in after middle age *involution, krympning, tillbakabildning*

involutional [ˌɪnvə'lu:ʃ(ə)n(ə)l] *adj.* referring to involution *som avser el. hör till involution;* **involutional melancholia** = depression which occurs in people (mainly women) after middle age, probably caused by a change of endocrine secretions *slags depression vid menopausen*

involve [ɪn'vɒlv] *vb.* to concern *or* to have to do with *medföra, innebära, gälla;* **the operation involves removing part of the duodenum and attaching the stomach directly to the jejunum**

invärtes ⇨ **internal, internally**

invärtesmedicin ⇨ **internal, medicine**

invärtesmedicinsk ⇨ **medical**

inväxt nagel ⇨ **acronyx**

ingående ⇨ **afferent, centripetal**

inåtskelning ⇨ **cross eye, esotropia**

inälvorna ⇨ **abdominal, gut, insides, viscera**

inälvs- ⇨ **intestinal, splanchnic**

inälvsbukhinnan ⇨ **visceral**

inälvsmask ⇨ **helminth**

inälvsnerv ⇨ **splanchnic**

iodine ['a(ɪ)ədi:n] *subst.* chemical element which is essential to the body, especially to the functioning of the thyroid gland *jod, I;* **tincture of iodine** = weak solution of iodine in alcohol, used as an antiseptic *jodsprit*
NOTE: chemical symbol is **I**

> COMMENT: lack of iodine in the diet can cause goitre

IP [ˌaɪ'pi:] = INTERPHALANGEAL JOINT

ipecacuanha [ˌɪpɪkækju'ænə] *or US* **ipecac** ['ɪpɪkæk] *subst.* drug made from the root of an American plant used as treatment for coughs, and also as an emetic *(radix) ipecacuanhae, kräkrot*

ipsilateral [ˌɪpsɪ'læt(ə)r(ə)l] *adj.* on the same side of the body *ipsilateral, homolateral*

IQ [ˌaɪ'kju:] = INTELLIGENCE QUOTIENT

IRDS ⇨ **hyaline**

irid- [ˌɪrɪd] *prefix* referring to the iris *irid(o)-, regnbågshinne-*

iridectomy [ˌɪrɪ'dektəmi] *subst.* surgical removal of part of the iris *iridektomi, korektomi, sfinkterektomi*

iridektomi ⇨ **iridectomy, sphincterectomy**

iridencleisis [ˌɪrɪdenˈklaɪsɪs] *subst.* operation to treat glaucoma, where part of the iris is used as a drainage channel through a hole in the conjunctiva *iridencleisis*

irideremi ⇨ **aniridia**

iridocyclitis [ˌɪrɪdəʊsɪˈklaɪtɪs] *subst.* inflammation of the iris and the tissues which surround it *iridocyklit, iritis serosa, uveit*

iridodialysis [ˌɪrɪdəʊdaɪˈæləsɪs] *subst.* separation of the iris from its insertion *iridodialys, avlossning av regnbågshinnan*

iridoplegia [ˌɪrɪdəʊˈpliːdʒə] *subst.* paralysis of the iris *iridoplegi*

iridotomy [ˌɪrɪˈdɒtəmi] *subst.* surgical incision into the iris *iridotomi*

iris [ˈaɪ(ə)rɪs] *subst.* coloured ring in the eye, with at its centre the pupil ⇨ *illustration* EYE *iris, regnbågshinnan*

COMMENT: the iris acts as a kind of camera shutter, opening and closing to allow more or less light through the pupil into the eye; the iris acts as a kind of camera shutter, opening and closing to allow more or less light through the pupil into the eye

irisinflammation ⇨ **iritis**

irit ⇨ **iritis**

iritis [aɪ(ə)ˈraɪtɪs] *subst.* inflammation of the iris *irit, irisinflammation*

iron [ˈa(ɪ)ən] *subst.* **(a)** chemical element essential to the body, found in liver, eggs, etc. *järn, Fe* NOTE: chemical symbol is **Fe** **(b)** common grey metal *järn*

COMMENT: iron is an essential part of the red pigment in red blood cells. Lack of iron in haemoglobin results in iron-deficiency anaemia. Storage of too much iron in the body results in haemochromatosis

iron lung [ˈa(ɪ)ən ˌlʌŋ] = DRINKER RESPIRATOR

irradiation [ɪˌreɪdiˈeɪʃ(ə)n] *subst.* **(a)** spread from a centre, as nerve impulses *irradiation, recruitment* **(b)** use of rays to treat patients *or* to kill bacteria in food *strålning, strålbehandling, strålterapi, radioterapi;* **total body irradiation** = treating the whole body with radiation *helkroppsbestrålning*

irreducible [ˌɪrɪˈdjuːsəb(ə)l] *adj.* (hernia) where the organ cannot be returned to its original position without an operation *irreponibel*

irregular [ɪˈregjʊlə] *adj.* not regular *or* abnormal *oregelbunden;* **the patient's breathing was irregular; the nurse noted that the patient had developed an irregular pulse; he has irregular bowel movements**

irreponibel ⇨ **irreducible**

irrigation [ˌɪrɪˈgeɪʃ(ə)n] *subst.* washing out of a cavity in the body *irrigation, sköljning, spolning;* **colonic irrigation** = washing out the large intestine *kolonsköljning, kolonspolning*

irritability [ˌɪrɪtəˈbɪləti] *subst.* state of being irritable *irritabilitet, retbarhet*

irritable [ˈɪrɪtəb(ə)l] *adj.* which can be easily excited *irritabel, retlig, retbar;* **irritable colon** *or* **irritable bowel syndrome** = MUCOUS COLITIS

irritant [ˈɪrɪt(ə)nt] *subst.* substance which can irritate *irriterande (retande) ämne, retmedel;* **irritant dermatitis** = contact dermatitis *or* skin inflammation caused by touching *kontaktdermatit*

irritate [ˈɪrɪteɪt] *vb.* to make something painful *or* itchy *or* sore *irritera, reta;* **some types of wool can irritate the skin**

irritation [ˌɪrɪˈteɪʃ(ə)n] *subst.* action of irritating *irritation, retning*

irritera ⇨ **irritate**

is ⇨ **ice**

isblåsa ⇨ **icebag**

isch- [ɪsk] *prefix* meaning reduction *or* too little *isch-*

ischaemia [ɪˈskiːmiə] *subst.* deficient blood supply to part of the body *ischemi, lokal blodbrist*

ischaemic [ɪˈskiːmɪk] *adj.* lacking in blood *ischemisk;* **ischaemic heart disease (IHD)** = disease of the heart caused by a failure in the blood supply (as in coronary thrombosis) *ischemisk hjärtsjukdom;* **transient ischaemic attack (TIA)** = mild stroke caused by a brief stoppage of blood supply *transitorisk ischemisk attack, TIA*

QUOTE changes in life style factors have been related to the decline in total mortality from IHD. In many studies a sedentary life style has been reported as a risk factor for IHD

Journal of the American Medical Association

QUOTE the term stroke does not refer to a single pathological entity. Stroke may be haemorrhagic or ischaemic: the latter is usually caused by thrombosis or embolism
British Journal of Hospital Medicine

ischemi ⇨ **ischaemia**

ischemisk ⇨ **ischaemic**

ischial ['ɪskiəl] *adj.* referring to the ischium *or* hip joint *som avser el. hör till sittbenet el. höftleden;* **ischial tuberosity** = lump of bone forming the ring of the ischium *tuberositas ischii, sittbensknölen*

ischialgi ⇨ **sciatica**

ischias ⇨ **sciatica**

ischiasnerven ⇨ **sciatic**

ischiocavernosus muscle [ˌɪskiəʊˌkævəˈnəʊsəs ˌmʌs(ə)l] *subst.* muscle along one side of the perineum *musculus ischiocavernosus*

ischiorectal [ˌɪskiəʊˈrekt(ə)l] *adj.* referring to both the ischium and the rectum *ischiorektal;* **ischiorectal abscess** = abscess which forms in fat cells between the anus and the ischium *ischiorektal abscess;* **ischiorectal fossa** = space on either side of the lower end of the rectum and anal canal *fossa ischiorectalis*

ischium ['ɪskiəm] *subst.* lower part of the hip bone in the pelvis ⇨ *illustration* PELVIS *ischium, os ischii, sittbenet*

ischuri ⇨ **ischuria, retention**

ischuria [ɪˈskjʊəriə] *subst.* retention *or* suppression of urine *ischuri, urinretention, urinstämma*

Ishihara test [ˌɪʃɪˈhærə ˌtest] *subst.* test for colour blindness where the patient is asked to identify letters or numbers among a mass of coloured dots *Ishiharas tavlor*

islets of Langerhans [ˌaɪləts əv ˈlæŋəhæns] *or* **islet cells** [ˈaɪlət ˌselz] *subst pl.* groups of cells in the pancreas which secrete the hormones glucagon and insulin *Langerhans cellöar, langerhansska cellöarna*

iso- ['aɪsə(u), ˌ--] *prefix* meaning equal *iso-*

isoantibody [ˌaɪsəʊˈæntɪbɒdi] *subst.* antibody which forms in one person as a reaction to antigens from another person *isoantikropp*

isoantikropp ⇨ **isoantibody**

isograft ['aɪsəʊgrɑːft] *or* **syngraft** ['sɪngrɑːft] *subst.* graft of tissue from an identical twin *isogent (isologt) transplantat, syngent transplantat*

isoimmunization [ˌaɪsəʊˌɪmjunaɪˈzeɪʃ(ə)n] *subst.* immunization of a person with antigens derived from another person *isoimmunisering*

isolate ['aɪsəleɪt] *vb.* **(a)** to keep one patient apart from others (because he has a dangerous infectious disease) *isolera* **(b)** to identify a single virus *or* bacteria among many *isolera, renodla;* **scientists have been able to isolate the virus which causes legionnaires' disease; candida is easily isolated from the mouths of healthy adults**

isolation [ˌaɪsəˈleɪʃ(ə)n] *subst.* separation of a patient, especially one with an infectious disease, from other patients *isolering;* **isolation hospital** *or* **isolation ward** = special hospital *or* special ward in a hospital where patients suffering from infectious dangerous diseases can be isolated *epidemisjukhus, isoleringsavdelning*

isolera ⇨ **isolate**

isolering ⇨ **isolation**

isoleringsavdelning ⇨ **isolation**

isoleucine [ˌaɪsəʊˈluːsɪn] *subst.* essential amino acid *isoleucin*

isometric exercises [ˌaɪsəʊˈmetrɪk ˌeksəsaɪzɪz] *subst.* exercises which strengthen the muscles, where the muscles contract but do not shorten *isometriska övningar*

isomslag ⇨ **icebag**

isoniazid [ˌaɪsəʊˈnaɪəzɪd] *subst.* drug used to treat tuberculosis *isoniazid, INH*

isotonic [ˌaɪsə(ʊ)ˈtɒnɪk] *adj.* (solution, such as a saline drip) with the same pressure as blood, which can therefore be passed directly into the body *isoton*

isotope ['aɪsətəʊp] *subst.* form of a chemical element which has the same chemical properties as other forms, but different atomic mass *isotop;* **radioactive isotope** = isotope which sends out radiation, used in radiotherapy *radioisotop, radioaktiv isotop*

isthmus ['ɪsməs] *subst.* (i) short narrow canal *or* cavity *isthmus, förträngning;* (ii) narrow band of tissue joining two larger masses of similar tissue (such as the section in the centre of the thyroid gland, which joins the two lobes) *isthmus, övergång, mellanparti*

itch [ɪtʃ] **1** *subst.* any irritated place on the skin, which makes a person want to scratch *pruritus, klåda;* **the itch** = scabies *or* infection of the skin caused by a mite, producing violent irritation *skabb* **2** *vb.* to irritate, so that relief can be found by scratching *klia*

itching ['ɪtʃɪŋ] *or* **pruritus** [prʊə'raɪtəs] *subst.* irritation of the skin which makes the patient want to scratch *pruritus, klåda*

itchy ['ɪtʃi] *adj.* which makes someone want to scratch *kliande;* **the main symptom of the disease is an itchy red rash**

-itis ['aɪtɪs] *suffix* meaning inflammation *-it, -inflammation;* **otitis** = inflammation of the ear *otit, öroninflammation;* **rhinitis** = inflammation of the nasal passages *rinit, snuva*

IUD [ˌaɪju:'di:] = INTRAUTERINE DEVICE

IV [ˌaɪ'vi:] = INTRAVENOUS

IVF [ˌaɪvi:'ef] = IN VITRO FERTILIZATION

IVP [ˌaɪvi:'pi:] = INTRAVENOUS PYELOGRAM

i.v. ⇨ **intravenous (IV)**

IVA ⇨ **intensive care**

ivrig ⇨ **anxious, keen**

iögonfallande ⇨ **prominent**

Jj

J [dʒeɪ] *abbreviation for* = JOULE

jab [dʒæb] *subst. informal* injection *or* inoculation *injektion;* **he has had a tetanus jab; go to the doctor to get a cholera jab**

jack ⇨ **nick**

jacket ['dʒækɪt] *subst.* short coat *rock;* **the dentist was wearing a white jacket; bed jacket** = short warm jacket which a patient can wear when sitting in bed *bäddjacka*

jacketkrona ⇨ **cap**

Jacksonian epilepsy [dʒæk'səʊniən ˌepɪlepsi] *see* EPILEPSY

Jacquemier's sign ['dʒækəmɪəz ˌsaɪn] *subst.* sign of early pregnancy, when the vaginal mucosa becomes bluish in colour due to an increased amount of blood in the arteries *slags tidigt graviditetstecken*

jaget ⇨ **ego**

jar [dʒɑ:] **1** *subst.* pot (usually glass) for keeping liquids *or* food in *burk;* **specimens of diseased organs can be kept in glass jars 2** *vb.* to give a shock with a blow *skaka (chocka) genom en stöt;* **the patient fell awkwardly and jarred his spine**

jaundice ['dʒɔ:ndɪs] *or* **icterus** ['ɪktərəs] *subst.* condition where there is an excess of bile pigment in the blood, and where the pigment is deposited in the skin and the whites of the eyes which have a yellow colour *ikterus, gulsot;* **haemolytic jaundice** *or* **prehepatic jaundice** = jaundice caused by haemolysis of the red blood cells *icterus haemolyticus, hemolytisk ikterus;* **hepatocellular jaundice** = jaundice caused by injury to *or* disease of the liver cells *icterus hepato-cellularis (parenchymatosus), hepato-cellulär ikterus, parenkymikterus, parenkymatös ikterus;* **infective jaundice** = jaundice caused by a viral disease such as hepatitis *icterus infectiosus, smittsam gulsot;* **obstructive jaundice** *or* **posthepatic jaundice** = jaundice caused by an obstruction of the bile ducts *icterus obstructivus, obstruktionsikterus, stasikterus, mekanisk ikterus; see also* ACHOLURIC

> COMMENT: jaundice can have many causes, usually relating to the liver: the most common are blockage of the bile ducts by gallstones *or* by disease of the liver, infectious diseases such as the two forms of hepatitis and Weil's disease

jaw [dʒɔ:] *subst.* bones in the face which hold the teeth and form the mouth *käken;* **upper jaw and lower jaw** = the two parts of the jaw, the upper (the maxillae) being fixed parts of the skull, and the lower (the mandible) being attached to the skull with a hinge so that it can move up and down *maxilla, överkäken, mandibula, underkäken;* **teeth are fixed in both the upper and lower jaw; he fell down and broke his jaw** *or* **the punch on his mouth broke his lower jaw**

jawbone ['dʒɔ:bəʊn] *subst.* one of the bones (the maxilla and the mandible) which form the jaw *käkbenet* NOTE: **jawbone** usually refers to the lower jaw or mandible

jejun- [ˌdʒiːdʒun, dʒɪˌdʒuːn] *prefix* referring to the jejunum *jejun(o)-, jejunum-*

jejunal [dʒɪ'dʒuːn(ə)l] *adj.* referring to the jejunum *jejunal;* **jejunal ulcer** = ulcer in the jejunum *sår i tunntarmen*

jejunectomy [ˌdʒiːdʒuː'nektəmi] *subst.* surgical removal of all *or* part of the jejunum *jejunektomi*

jejunoileostomy [dʒɪˌdʒuːnəʊˌɪli'ɒstəmi] *subst.* surgical operation to make an artificial link between the jejunum and the ileum *jejunoileostomi*

jejunostomy [ˌdʒiːdʒu'nɒstəmi] *subst.* surgical operation to make an artificial passage to the jejunum through the wall of the abdomen *jejunostomi*

jejunotomy [ˌdʒiːdʒu'nɒtəmi] *subst.* surgical operation to cut into the jejunum *jejunotomi*

jejunum [dʒiː'dʒuːnəm] *subst.* part of small intestine between the duodenum and the ileum ⇨ *illustration* DIGESTIVE SYSTEM *(intestinum) jejunum, tunntarmen*

COMMENT: the jejunum is about 2 metres long

jerk [dʒɜːk] **1** *subst.* sudden movement of part of the body which indicates that the local reflex arc is intact *reflex;* **ankle jerk** = jerk as a reflex action of the foot when the back of the ankle is tapped *akilles(sene)reflex;* **knee jerk** = jerk made as a reflex action by the knee, when the legs are crossed and the patellar tendon is tapped sharply *patellarreflex* **2** *vb.* to make sudden movements *rycka till;* **some forms of epilepsy are accompanied by jerking of the limbs**

jerky ['dʒɜːki] *adj.* with sudden movement *ryckig;* **the patient made jerky movements with his hand**

jet lag ['dʒet læg] *subst.* condition suffered by people who travel long distances in planes, caused by rapid changes in time zones which affect the metabolism of the body *rubbad dygnsrytm pga lång flygning*
NOTE: does not take **the** or **a**: **"she is suffering from jet lag"; "he took several days to get over his jet lag"**

jigger ['dʒɪgə] = SANDFLEA

"jobbig" ⇨ **cranky**

jod ⇨ **iodine**

jod, proteinbunden ⇨ **protein-bound iodine**

jodsprit ⇨ **iodine**

join [dʒɔɪn] *vb.* to put things together *förena, foga ihop;* to come together *förenas, mötas;* **the bones are joined together by a cartilage; the inflammation started at the point where the ileum joins the caecum**

joint [dʒɔɪnt] *subst.* junction of two or more bones, especially one which allows movement of the bones *articulatio, led, ledgång;* **the elbow is a joint in the arm; arthritis is accompanied by stiffness in the joints; hip joint** *or* **wrist joint** = place where the hip is joined to the upper leg *or* where the wrist joins the arm *articulatio coxae, höftleden, articulatio manus, handleden;* **ball and socket joint** = joint (like the shoulder) where the rounded end of a long bone fits into a socket on another bone *articulatio sphaeroidea (cotylica), enartros, kulled;* **primary cartilaginous joint** = temporary joint where the intervening cartilage is converted into adult bone *synkondros, broskfog;* **secondary cartilaginous joint** = joint where the surfaces of the two bones are connected by a piece of cartilage so that they cannot move (such as the pubic symphysis) *symfys;* **fibrous joint** = joint where two bones are fixed together by fibrous tissue, so that they can move only slightly (as in the bones of the skull) *syndesmos, bindvävsfog;* **hinge joint** = joint (like the knee) which allows the two bones to move in one plane only *ginglymus, gångjärnsled, vinkelled, scharnerled;* **locking joints** = joints (such as the knee *or* elbow) which can be locked in an extended position *spiralleder;* **pivot joint** *or* **trochoid joint** = joint where a bone can rotate easily *articulatio trochoidea, rotationsled, vridled;* **synovial joint** = joint where the two bones are separated by a space filled with synovial fluid which nourishes and lubricates the surfaces of the bones *diart(h)ros;* **joint capsule** = fibrous tissue which surrounds and holds a joint together *capsula articularis, ledkapsel;* **joint mice** = loose pieces of bone *or* cartilage in the knee joint, making the joint lock *ledmus; see also* CHARCOT'S JOINT
NOTE: for other terms referring to joints see words beginning with **arthr-, articul-**

joint-breaker fever ['dʒɔɪntbreɪkə ˌfiːvə] = O'NYONG-NYONG FEVER

jointed ['dʒɔɪntɪd] *adj.* linked with joints *ledad*

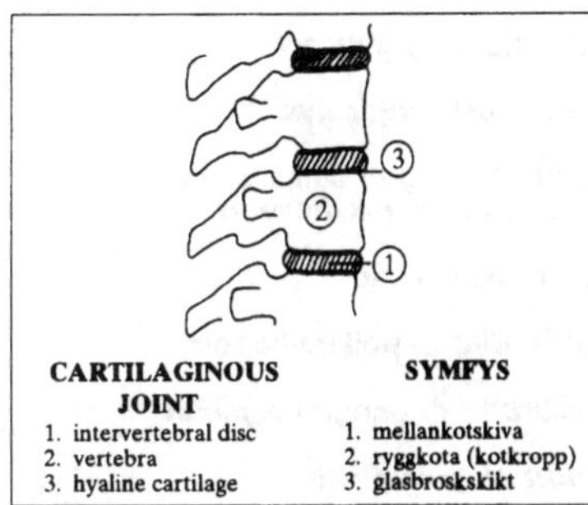

CARTILAGINOUS JOINT	SYMFYS
1. intervertebral disc	1. mellankotskiva
2. vertebra	2. ryggkota (kotkropp)
3. hyaline cartilage	3. glasbroskskikt

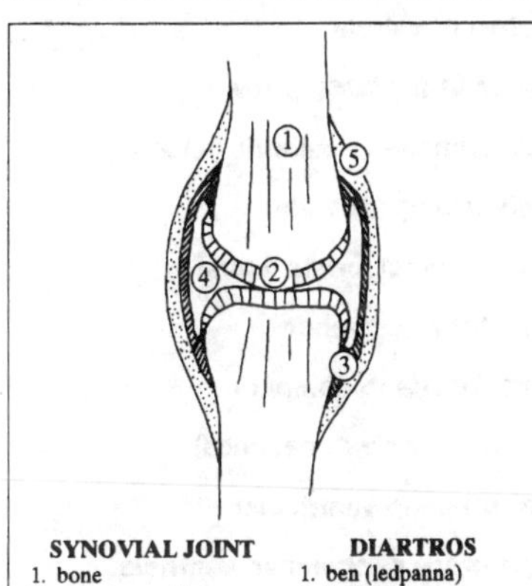

SYNOVIAL JOINT	DIARTROS
1. bone	1. ben (ledpanna)
2. articular cartilage	2. ledbrosk
3. synovial membrane	3. synovialmembran, synovialhinna
4. synovial cavity and fluid	4. ledspalt (ledhåla) och ledvätska
5. joint capsule (ligament)	5. ledkapsel

joule [dʒu:l] *subst.* SI unit for measuring energy and heat *joule, J* NOTE: usually written J with figures: **25J**

> COMMENT: one joule is the amount of energy used to move one kilogram the distance of one metre, using the force of one newton

jourhavande ⇨ **call**

journal ⇨ **record, report**

jourtjänstgöra ⇨ **duty**

jugular ['dʒʌgjʊlə] *adj.* referring to the throat or neck *jugular, hals-;* **jugular nerve** = one of the nerves in the neck *nervus jugularis, halsvenen;* **jugular trunk** = terminal lymph vessel in the neck, draining into the subclavian vein *truncus jugularis;* **jugular vein** *or* **jugular** = one of the veins which pass down either side of the neck *vena jugularis, halsvenen*

> COMMENT: there are three types of jugular vein: the internal jugular is large and leads to the brachiocephalic vein, the external jugular is smaller and leads to the subclavian vein and the anterior jugular is the smallest

juice [dʒu:s] *subst.* fluid secretion of an animal or plant *saft, juice;* **a glass of orange juice** *or* **tomato juice; a tin of grapefruit juice; gastric juice** = acid liquid secreted by the stomach which helps digest food *magsaft;* **intestinal juice** = alkaline liquid secreted by the small intestine which helps digest food *tarmsaft*

junction ['dʒʌŋ(k)ʃ(ə)n] *subst.* joining point *föreningspunkt, förbindelse*

jungfru ⇨ **virgin**

jungfrulighet ⇨ **virginity**

justera ⇨ **correct**

justering ⇨ **correction**

juvenile ['dʒu:vənaɪ(ə)l] *adj.* referring to children *or* adolescents *juvenil, ungdoms-;* **the area has six new cases of juvenile diabetes mellitus**

juxta- [ˌdʒʌkstə] *prefix* meaning beside *or* near *juxta-*

jämn ⇨ **level, smooth**

jämnvarm ⇨ **homoiothermic**

jämvikt ⇨ **equilibrium**

järn ⇨ **iron**

järnbristanemi ⇨ **anaemia, sideropenia**

järnlunga ⇨ **Drinker respirator**

jäsning ⇨ **fermentation**

jäst ⇨ **yeast**

jätte ⇨ **giant**

jättecell ⇨ **giant**

jättecellsarterit ⇨ **arteritis**

jättecellstumör ⇨ **osteoclastoma**

jätteväxt ⇨ **gigantism**

Kk

K [keɪ] 1 *symbol for* potassium *K, kalium* 2 *subst.* **Vitamin K** = vitamin found in green vegetables like spinach and cabbage, and which helps the clotting of blood and is needed to activate prothrombin *K-vitamin*

k *abbreviation for* = one thousand; **kg** = kilogram *kg, kilo(gram);* **kJ** = kilojoule *kJ, kilojoule*

KAD ⇨ **indwelling catheter**

kadaver ⇨ **cadaver**

kadmium ⇨ **cadmium**

kaffesumpsliknande kräkning ⇨ **coffee ground vomit**

Kahn test ['kɑːnz ˌtest] *subst.* test of blood serum to diagnose syphilis *Kahns flockningsreaktion*

kakeki ⇨ **marasmus**

kakexi ⇨ **cachexia**

kala-azar [ˌkæləə'zɑː] *subst.* severe infection, occurring in tropical countries *kala-azar*

> COMMENT: kala-azar is a form of leishmaniasis, caused by the infection of the intestines and internal organs by a parasite *Leishmania* spread by flies. Symptoms are fever, anaemia, general wasting of the body and swelling of the spleen and liver

kalcemi ⇨ **calcaemia, hypercalcaemia**

kalciferol ⇨ **calciferol**

kalcifikation ⇨ **calcification**

kalcitonin ⇨ **calcitonin**

kalcium ⇨ **calcium**

kalium ['keɪliəm] = POTASSIUM

kaliumpermanganat ⇨ **potassium permanganate**

kaliumsalt ⇨ **indican**

kalk ⇨ **calcium; calyx**

kalkinlagring ⇨ **calcareous degeneration, calcification**

kall ⇨ **cold, algid**

kallblodig ⇨ **poikilothermic**

kallbrand ⇨ **gangrene, moist**

kalomel ⇨ **calomel**

kalori ⇨ **calorie**

kalorifattig kost ⇨ **low**

kalorivärde ⇨ **calorific value**

kalvariet ⇨ **calvaria**

kam ⇨ **crest, crista, spine**

kamfer ⇨ **camphor**

kamferolja ⇨ **camphor**

kamliknande ⇨ **pectineal**

kammar- ⇨ **ventricular**

kammare ⇨ **chamber, ventricle**

kammarflimmer ⇨ **ventricular**

kanal ⇨ **canal, channel, conduit, duct, ductus, lumen, passage, tract, vas**

kandidat ⇨ **candidate**

kannformig ⇨ **arytenoid**

kant ⇨ **border, brim, limbus, ridge**

kanto(r)rafi ⇨ **tarsorrhaphy**

kanyl ⇨ **cannula, hypodermic, needle**

kaolin ['keɪəlɪn] *subst.* white powder, the natural form of aluminium silicate *or* china clay *kaolin*

> COMMENT: kaolin is used internally in liquid form to reduce diarrhoea and can also be used externally as a talc or as a poultice

kapacitet ⇨ **capacity**

kapillär ⇨ **capillary**

kapillärblödning ⇨ **capillary**

Kaposi's sarcoma [kə'pəʊzɪz sɑːˌkəʊmə] *subst.* cancer which takes the form of many haemorrhagic nodes affecting the skin, especially on the extremities *Kaposis sarkom*

> COMMENT: formerly a relatively rare disease, found mainly in tropical countries; now more common as it is one of the sequelae of AIDS

kapsel ⇨ **cachet, capsule**

kapsulektomi ⇨ **capsulectomy**

kapsulit ⇨ **capsulitis**

kapsulär ⇨ **capsular**

kapsyl ⇨ **cap**

karakterisera ⇨ **characterize**

karakteristisk ⇨ **characteristic, distinctive, typical**

karaktär ⇨ **character, nature**

karantän ⇨ **quarantine**

karbol(syra) ⇨ **phenol**

karbunkel ⇨ **carbuncle**

karcinogen ⇨ **carcinogenic**

karcinoid ⇨ **carcinoid (tumour)**

karcinom ⇨ **carcinoma**

kardia ⇨ **cardia**

kardialgi ⇨ **cardialgia**

kardiogram ⇨ **cardiogram**

kardiolog ⇨ **cardiologist**

kardiologi ⇨ **cardiology**

kardiomegali ⇨ **cardiomegaly**

kardiomyopati ⇨ **cardiomyopathy**

kardiomyotomi ⇨ **cardiomyotomy**

kardiopati ⇨ **cardiopathy**

kardioskop ⇨ **cardioscope**

kardiospasm ⇨ **cardiospasm, achalasia**

kardiotokografi ⇨ **cardiotocography**

kardiovaskulär ⇨ **cardiovascular**

kardit ⇨ **carditis**

karies ⇨ **caries**

kariesframkallande ⇨ **cariogenic**

kariogen ⇨ **cariogenic**

karminativum ⇨ **carminative**

karoten ⇨ **carotene**

karotin ⇨ **carotene**

karotinemi ⇨ **carotenaemia**

karpalbenen ⇨ **carpal**

karpaltunnelsyndrom ⇨ **carpal**

karpometakarpallederna ⇨ **carpometacarpal joints (CM joints)**

karpopedalspasm ⇨ **carpopedal spasm**

kartilaginär ⇨ **cartilaginous**

kartong ⇨ **pack**

kartotek ⇨ **card index**

kartotekskort ⇨ **card**

karunkel ⇨ **caruncle**

karyotype ['kærɪəʊtaɪp] *subst.* the chromosome complement of a cell, shown as a diagram or as a set of letters and numbers *karyotyp, kromosomuppsättning*

kasein ⇨ **casein**

kasta upp ⇨ **bring up, throw up**

kasta vatten ⇨ **urinate, pass**

kastrat ⇨ **eunuch**

kastrera ⇨ **castrate**

kastrering ⇨ **castration, emasculation**

katabolism ⇨ **catabolism**

katalas ⇨ **catalase**

katalepsi ⇨ **catalepsy**

katalysator ⇨ **catalyst**

katalysera ⇨ **catalyze**

kataplexi ⇨ **cataplexy**

katarakt ⇨ **cataract**

katarr ⇨ **catarrh**

katarral ⇨ **catarrhal**

katarsis ⇨ **catharsis**

katatoni ⇨ **catatonia**

kategori ⇨ **category**

katekolaminer ⇨ **catecholamines**

kateter ⇨ **catheter**

katetrisera ⇨ **catheterize**

katetrisering ⇨ **catheterization**

katgut ⇨ **catgut, gut**

kattfobi ⇨ **ailurophobia**

kaudal ⇨ **caudal**

kaudalblockad ⇨ **caudal**

kausalgi ⇨ **causalgia**

kauter ⇨ **cautery**

kauterisera ⇨ **cauterize**

kauterisering ⇨ **cauterization**

kavern ⇨ **vomica**

kavernös ⇨ **cavernous**

kavitet ⇨ **cavity**

Kayser-Fleischer ring [ˌkaɪzəˈflaɪʃə ˌrɪŋ] *subst.* brown ring on the outer edge of the cornea, which is a diagnostic sign of hepatolenticular degeneration *Kayser-Fleischers ring*

KBR ⇨ **complement**

kcal ⇨ **Cal**

kedjereaktion ⇨ **chain**

keen [kiːn] *adj.* **(a)** eager *or* willing *ivrig, entusiastisk;* **he's keen to go to medical school; she is not at all keen on prescribing placebos (b)** *(of senses)* which can notice differences very well *skarp;* **he has a keen sense of smell; she has keen eyesight** NOTE: **keen - keener - keenest**

keep [kiːp] *vb.* **(a)** to have for a very long time or for ever *behålla, spara, förvara;* **the hospital keeps its medical records for ten years (b)** to continue to do something *fortsätta;* **the pump has to be kept going twenty-four hours a day; keep taking the tablets for ten days (c)** to make someone stay in a state *hålla (kvar);* **the patient must be kept warm and quiet; dangerous medicines should be kept locked in a cupboard** NOTE: **keeps - keeping - kept - has kept**

keep down [ˌkiːp ˈdaʊn] *vb.* to take food and retain it in the stomach *behålla;* **he managed to keep down some soup; she could not even keep a glass of orange juice down**

keep on [ˌkiːp ˈɒn] *vb.* to continue to do something *fortsätta (med);* **the patient kept on calling out in his sleep; you should keep on doing the exercises at home for several weeks**

kefal- ⇨ **cephalic**

kefalhematom ⇨ **cephalhaematoma**

keilit ⇨ **cheilitis**

keil(o)- ⇨ **cheil-**

kejsarsnitt ⇨ **Caesarean section, tomotocia**

kelatkomplexbildare ⇨ **chelating agent**

Keller's operation [ˈkeləz ˌɒpəˌreɪʃ(ə)n] *subst.* operation on the big toe, to remove a bunion *or* correct an ankylosed joint *slags stortåoperation*

keloid [ˈkiːlɔɪd] *subst.* excessive amount of scar tissue at the site of a skin injury *cheloid, keloid, kelom*

kelom ⇨ **keloid**

kemi ⇨ **chemistry**

kemikalie ⇨ **chemical**

kemisk ⇨ **chemical, chem-, chemo-**

kemisk förening ⇨ **compound**

kemist ⇨ **analyst, chemist**

kem(o)- ⇨ **chem-, chemo-**

kemoreceptor ⇨ **chemoreceptor**

kemos ⇨ **chemosis**

kemotaxi ⇨ **chemotaxis**

kemoterapeutikum ⇨ **chemotherapeutic agent**

kemoterapi ⇨ **chemotherapy**

kemotropism ⇨ **chemotaxis**

kerat- ['kerət, ˌ--] *prefix* referring to horn *or* horny tissue *or* the cornea *kerat(o)-, cerat(o)-, horn-, hornhinne-*

keratectasia [ˌkerətek'teɪziə] *subst.* condition where the cornea bulges *keratektasi*

keratectomy [ˌkerət'ektəmi] *subst.* surgical removal of the whole *or* part of the cornea *keratektomi*

keratektasi ⇨ **keratectasia**

keratektomi ⇨ **keratectomy**

keratin ['kerətɪn] *subst.* protein found in horny tissue (such as fingernails *or* hair *or* the outer surface of the skin) *keratin, hornämne*

keratinisering ⇨ **keratinization**

keratinization [ˌkerətɪnaɪ'zeɪʃ(ə)n] *or* **cornification** [ˌkɔːnɪfi'keɪʃ(ə)n] *subst.* appearance of horny characteristics in tissue *keratinisering, kornifikation, förhorning*

keratinize ['kerətɪnaɪz] *vb.* to convert into keratin *or* into horny tissue *omvandla till keratin el. horn;* **the cells are gradually keratinized**

keratit ⇨ **keratitis**

keratitis [ˌkerə'taɪtɪs] *subst.* inflammation of the cornea *keratit, hornhinneinflammation*

keratoacanthoma [ˌkerətəʊˌækən'θəʊmə] *subst.* type of benign skin tumour, which disappears after a few months *keratoakantom*

keratoakantom ⇨ **keratoacanthoma**

keratoconjunctivitis [ˌkerətəʊkənˌdʒʌŋtɪ'vaɪtɪs] *subst.* inflammation of the cornea with conjunctivitis *keratokonjunktivit*

keratoconus [ˌkerətəʊ'kəʊnəs] *subst.* cone-shaped lump on the cornea *keratokonus*

keratoglobus [ˌkerətəʊ'gləʊbəs] *subst.* swelling of the eyeball *keratoglobus, macrocornea*

keratokonjunktivit ⇨ **keratoconjunctivitis**

keratokonus ⇨ **keratoconus**

keratoma [ˌkerə'təʊmə] *subst.* hard thickened growth due to hypertrophy of the horny zone of the skin *keratom, hornsvulst*
NOTE: plural is **keratomata**

keratomalacia [ˌkerətəʊmə'leɪʃə] *subst.* (i) softening of the cornea frequently caused by Vitamin A deficiency *keratomalaci;* (ii) softening of the horny layer of the skin *uppmjukning av hudens hornlager*

keratome ['kerətəʊm] *subst.* surgical knife used for operations on the cornea *keratotom, ceratotom*

keratometer [ˌkerə'tɒmɪtə] *subst.* instrument for measuring the curvature of the cornea *keratometer*

keratometry [ˌkerə'tɒmɪtri] *subst.* process of measuring the curvature of the cornea *keratometri, ceratometri*

keratoplasty ['kerətə(ʊ)ˌplæsti] *or* **corneal graft** ['kɔːniəl ˌgrɑːft] *subst.* grafting corneal tissue from a donor in place of diseased tissue *keratoplastik, hornhinnetransplantation*

keratoscope ['kerətəskəʊp] *or* **Placido's disc** [plə'saɪdəz ˌdɪsk] *subst.* instrument for examining the cornea to see if it has an abnormal curvature *Placidos skiva, keratoskop, ceratoskop, astigmatoskop*

keratosis [ˌkerə'təʊsɪs] *subst.* lesion of the skin *keratos, hudförtjockning*

keratotom ⇨ **keratome**

keratotomy [ˌkerə'tɒtəmi] *subst.* surgical operation to make a cut in the cornea, the first step in many intraocular operations *keratotomi, ceratotomi, hornhinnesnitt*

kerion ['kɪərɪɒn] *subst.* painful soft mass, usually on the scalp, caused by ringworm *kerion celci*

keritinisering ⇨ **cornification**

kernicterus [kə'nɪktərəs] *subst.* yellow pigmentation of the basal ganglia and other nerve cells in the spinal cord and brain, found in children with icterus *kärnikterus*

COMMENT: the symptoms are convulsions, anorexia and drowsiness. The disease can be fatal, and where it is not fatal, spasticity and mental defects appear

Kernig's sign ['kɜ:nɪgz ˌsaɪn] *subst.* symptom of meningitis, when the knee cannot be straightened if the patient is lying down with the thigh brought up against the abdomen *Kernigs symtom (tecken)*

ketoacidosis [ˌki:təʊˌæsɪ'dəʊsɪs] *subst.* accumulation of ketone bodies in tissue in diabetes, causing acidosis *ketoacidos*

ketogenesis [ˌki:təʊ'dʒenəsɪs] *subst.* production of ketone bodies *ketogenes, ketonbildning*

ketogenic diet [ˌki:təʊ'dʒenɪk ˌda(ɪ)ət] *subst.* diet with a high fat content, producing ketosis *ketogen diet (föda)*

ketonaemia [ˌki:təʊ'ni:miə] *subst.* morbid state where ketone bodies exist in the blood *ketonemi*

ketonbildning ⇨ **ketogenesis**

ketone ['ki:təʊn] *subst.* chemical compound containing the group CO attached to two alkyl groups *keton;* **ketone bodies =** ketone compounds formed from fatty acids *ketonkroppar*

ketonemi ⇨ **ketonaemia**

ketonkroppar ⇨ **ketone**

ketonuria [ˌki:təʊ'njʊəriə] *subst.* state where ketone bodies are excreted in the urine *ketonuri*

ketosis [ki:'təʊsɪs] *subst.* state where ketone bodies (such as acetone and acetic acid) accumulate in the tissues, a late complication of juvenile diabetes mellitus *ketos; see also* ACETONE, ACETONURIA

key [ki:] **1** *subst.* **(a)** piece of shaped metal used to open a lock *nyckel;* **she has a set of keys to the laboratory; he signed for the key to the medicine cupboard (b)** part of a piano *or* a typewriter *or* a computer which you push down with your fingers *tangent* **(c)** answer to a problem *or* explanation *lösning, förklaring;* **the key to successful treatment of arthritis is movement 2** *adj.* most important *viktig, huvud-;* **he has the key position in the laboratory; penicillin is the key factor in the treatment of gangrene**

kg = KILOGRAM

kick [kɪk] **1** *subst.* hitting with your foot *spark;* **she could feel the baby give a kick 2** *vb.* to hit something with your foot *sparka;* **she could feel the baby kicking**

kidney ['kɪdni] *subst.* one of two organs situated in the lower part of the back on either side of the spine behind the abdomen, whose function is to maintain normal concentrations of the main constituents of blood, passing the waste matter into the urine *ren, njuren;* **he has a kidney infection; the kidneys have begun to malfunction; she is being treated for kidney trouble; kidney dialysis =** removing waste matter from the blood of a patient by passing it through a kidney machine *hemodialys, HD;* **kidney failure =** situation where a patient's kidneys do not function properly *njursvikt;* **kidney machine =** apparatus through which a patient's blood is passed to be cleaned by dialysis if the patient's kidneys have failed *konstgjord njure, dialysapparat;* **kidney stones =** small hard deposits sometimes formed in the kidney *njurstenar;* **floating kidney =** NEPHROPTOSIS; **horseshoe kidney =** congenital defect of the kidney, where usually the lower parts of each kidney are joined together *ren arcuatus, hästskonjure* NOTE: for other terms referring to the kidney see words beginning with **nephr-, ren-, reno-**

COMMENT: a kidney is formed of an outer cortex and an inner medulla. The nephrons which run from the cortex into the medulla filter the blood and form urine. The urine is passed through the ureters into the bladder. Sudden sharp pain in back of the abdomen, going downwards, is an indication of a kidney stone passing into the ureter

kikhosta ⇨ **whooping cough**

kikhostebakterie ⇨ **Bordetella**

kikning ⇨ **whoop**

kilbenen ⇨ **cuneiform bones**

kilbenet ⇨ **sphenoid bone**

kilbenshålan ⇨ **sphenoid bone**

kill [kɪl] *vb.* to make someone *or* something die *döda;* **she was given the kidney of a person killed in a car crash; heart attacks kill more people every year; antibodies are created to kill bacteria**

killer ['kɪlə] *subst.* person *or* disease which kills *mördare, dråpare, dödande sjukdom;* **virulent typhoid fever can be a killer disease; in the winter, bronchitis is the**

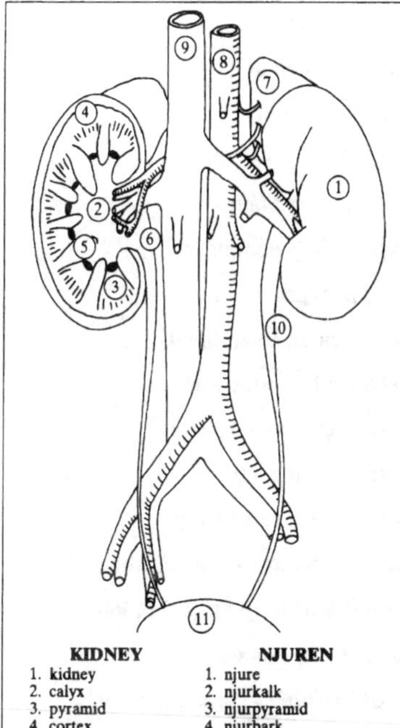

killer of hundreds of old people *see also* PAIN KILLER

Killian's operation ['kɪliənz ˌɒpəˌreɪʃ(ə)n] *subst.* clearing of the frontal sinus by curetting *Killians pannhåleoperation*

COMMENT: in Killian's operation the incision is made in the eyebrow

kilo- ['kɪlə(ʊ)] *prefix* meaning one thousand *kilo-*

kilocalorie ['kɪləʊˌkæl(ə)ri] *subst.* unit of measurement of heat (= 1,000 calories) *kilokalori* NOTE: when used with numbers **kilocalories** is usually written **Cal**

kilogram ['kɪləgræm] *or* **kilo** ['ki:ləʊ] *subst.* measurement of weight (= 1,000 grams) *kilo(gram);* **two kilos of sugar; he weighs 62 kilos (62 kg)** NOTE: when used with numbers **kilos** is usually written **kg**

kilojoule ['kɪlə(ʊ)dʒu:l] *subst.* measurement of energy or heat (= 1,000 joules) *kilojoule* NOTE: with figures usually written **kJ**

kilokalori ⇨ **kilocalorie, Calorie**

Kimmelstiel-Wilson disease [ˌkɪməlsti:l 'wɪls(ə)nz dɪˌzi:z] *or* **syndrome** ['sɪndrəʊm] *subst.* form of nephrosclerosis found in diabetics *Kimmelstiel-Wilsons syndrom, diabetisk glomeruloskleros*

kin [kɪn] *subst.* relatives *or* close members of the family *släkt(ing), anhörig;* **next of kin** = person *or* persons who are most closely related to someone *närmaste anhörig;* **the hospital has notified the next of kin of the death of the accident victim**

kin- [kɪn, kaɪn] *or* **kine-** [ˌkɪni, kaɪ'ni:, -ˌ-] *prefix* meaning movement *kin(e)-*

kinaesthesia [ˌkɪni:s'θi:ziə] *subst.* being aware of the movement and position of parts of the body *kinestesi, muskelsinnet*

COMMENT: kinaesthesia is the result of information from muscles and ligaments which is passed to the brain and which allows the brain to recognize movements *or* touch *or* weight

kinanaesthesia [ˌkɪnæni:s'θi:ziə] *subst.* not being able to sense the movement and position of parts of the body *kinanestesi*

kind- ⇨ **buccal, malar, zygomatic**

kinden ⇨ **cheek**

kindknotan ⇨ **cheekbone, zygoma, zygomatic**

kindmuskeln ⇨ **buccinator**

kindtand, bakre ⇨ **molar**

kindtand, främre ⇨ **premolar**

kinematics [ˌkɪnɪ'mætɪks] *or* **cinematics** [ˌsɪnə'mætɪks] *subst.* science of movement, especially of body movements *kinematik*

kinematik ⇨ **cinematics, kinematics**

kineplasty ['kɪnəplæsti] *or* **cineplasty** ['sɪnəplæsti] *subst.* amputation where the muscles of the stump of the amputated limb are used to operate an artificial limb *kineplastik, kinetiska stumpar*

kinesiology [kaɪˌniːsi'ɒlədʒi] *or* **cinesiology** [saɪˌniːsi'ɒlədʒi] *subst.* study of human movements, referring particularly to their use in treatment *kinetik*

kinetik ⇨ **kinesiology**

kinetochore [kaɪ'niːtəkɔː] = CENTROMERE

kinetos ⇨ **carsickness, seasickness**

kinidin ⇨ **quinidine**

kinin ⇨ **quinine**

kininförgiftning ⇨ **quinine, quininism**

kiropraktik ⇨ **chiropractic**

kiropraktor ⇨ **chiropractor**

Kirschner wire ['kɜːʃnəz ˌwa(ɪ)ə] *subst.* wire attached to a bone and tightened to provide traction to a fracture *Kirschnertråd*

kirurg ⇨ **surgeon**

kirurgavdelning ⇨ **surgical**

kirurgi ⇨ **surgery**

kirurgi, psykiatrisk ⇨ **psychosurgery**

kirurgisk ⇨ **surgical**

kirurgisk diatermi ⇨ **diathermy**

kirurgiskt ⇨ **surgically**

kirurgiskt ingrepp ⇨ **operation**

kissa (på sig) ⇨ **wet**

kiss of life [ˌkɪsəv'laɪf] *subst.* method of artificial respiration where the aider breathes into the patient's lungs (either through the mouth *or* through the nose) *mun-mot-munmetoden;* **he was given the kiss of life**

kit [kɪt] *subst.* equipment put together in a container *utrustning i behållare;* **first-aid kit** = box with bandages and dressings kept ready to be used in an emergency *förbandslåda*

kittlaren ⇨ **clitoris**

kJ = KILOJOULE

kladdig ⇨ **sticky**

klaff ⇨ **valve**

klaff- ⇨ **valvular**

klaffel ⇨ **valvular**

klaff, liten ⇨ **valvula**

klaga ⇨ **complain**

klagomål ⇨ **complaint**

klappa ⇨ **pat**

klar ⇨ **clear, clear, lucid**

klara (av) ⇨ **cope with**

klara sig ⇨ **pull through**

klarna ⇨ **clear up**

klassificera ⇨ **classify**

klassificering ⇨ **classification**

klassifikation ⇨ **classification**

klassisk ⇨ **classic**

klaustrofobi ⇨ **claustrophobia**

klaustrofobiker ⇨ **claustrophobic**

klaustrofobisk ⇨ **claustrophobic**

klavikulär ⇨ **clavicular**

Klebsiella [klebsi'elə] *subst.* form of Gram negative bacteria, one of which, **Klebsiella pneumoniae,** can cause pneumonia *Klebsiella*

Klebs-Loeffler bacillus [ˌklebz'leflə bəˌsɪləs] *subst.* diphtheria bacillus *bacillus diphteriae, difteribacillen*

klen ⇨ **delicate, feeble, infirm, poor, poorly, weak**

klenhet ⇨ **debility, infirmity, weakness**

kleptoman ⇨ **kleptomaniac**

kleptomania [ˌkleptə(ʊ)'meɪniə] *subst.* form of mental disorder where the patient has a compulsive desire to steal things (even things of little value) *kleptomani*

kleptomaniac [ˌkleptə(ʊ)'meɪniæk] *subst.* person who suffers from a compulsive desire to steal *kleptoman*

klia ⇨ **itch**

kliande ➪ **itchy**

klibba ihop (sig) ➪ **agglutinate**

klibbig ➪ **sticky, viscid, viscous**

klient ➪ **client**

klimakterium ➪ **menopause**

Klinefelter's syndrome ['klaɪnfeltəz ˌsɪndrəʊm] *subst.* genetic disorder where a male has an extra female chromosome (making an XXY set), giving sterility and partial female characteristics *Klinefelters syndrom*

klinik ➪ **clinic, department**

klinik- ➪ **clinical**

klinikchef ➪ **director**

kliniker ➪ **clinician**

klinikföreståndare ➪ **matron**

klinisk ➪ **clinical**

klinkorna ➪ **breech, buttocks**

klippbenet ➪ **petrous**

klippbens- ➪ **petrosal, petrous**

klitoris ➪ **clitoris**

kloaken ➪ **cloaca**

kloasma ➪ **chloasma**

klofot ➪ **claw foot**

klohand ➪ **claw hand**

klon ➪ **clone**

kloning ➪ **cloning**

klonisk ➪ **clonic**

klonus ➪ **clonus**

klorering ➪ **chlorination**

klorid ➪ **chloride**

kloroform ➪ **chloroform**

klorofyll ➪ **chlorophyll**

klorokin ➪ **chloroquine**

klorom ➪ **chloroma**

kloros ➪ **chlorosis**

klorpromazin ➪ **chlorpromazine**

klortiazid ➪ **chlorothiazide**

klorvätesyra ➪ **hydrochloric acid**

klotång ➪ **tenaculum**

klumpfot ➪ **club foot**

Klumpke's paralysis ['klu:mpkəz pəˌræləsɪs] *or* **Dejerine-Klumpke's syndrome** [ˌdeʒəˌri:n'klu:mpkəz ˌsɪndrəʊm] *subst.* form of paralysis due to an injury during birth, affecting the forearm and hand *Klumpkes paralys*

kluster ➪ **cluster**

klysma ➪ **proctoclysis**

klyva ➪ **split**

klyvbar ➪ **fissile**

klyvning ➪ **bifurcation, fission**

-klyvning ➪ **-schisis**

klåda ➪ **itch, itching**

klådstillande (medel) ➪ **antipruritic**

klä ➪ **coat**

klä av sig ➪ **strip, undress**

kläder ➪ **clothes**

klädlus ➪ **Pediculus**

klämma ➪ **clamp, clip, pinch, press**

klä på sig ➪ **get dressed**

klösa ➪ **scratch**

knacka (lätt) på ➪ **tap**

knee [ni:] *subst.* joint in the middle of the leg, joining the femur and the tibia *genu, knät;* **water on the knee** = condition where synovial fluid accumulates in the knee joint *vatten i knät (knäna);* **knee jerk** = PATELLAR REFLEX; **knee joint** = joint where the femur and the tibia are joined, covered by the kneecap *articulatio genu, knäleden*

kneecap ['ni:kæp] *or* **patella** [pə'telə] *subst.* small bone in front of the knee joint *patella, knäskålen*

NOTE: for other terms referring to the knee see words beginning with **genu-**

knickbrott ⇨ **greenstick fracture**

knippe ⇨ **bundle**

knit [nɪt] *vb.* **(a)** to make something out of wool, using two long needles *sticka* **(b)** *(of broken bones)* to join together again *förena, få att växa ihop;* **broken bones take longer to knit in old people than in children**
NOTE: **knits - knitting - knit**

knock [nɒk] **1** *subst.* **(a)** sound made by hitting something *knackning* **(b)** hitting of something *slag;* **he was concussed after having had a knock on the head 2** *vb.* to hit something *slå;* **he knocked his head on the floor as he fell**

knock down [ˌnɒk ˈdaʊn] *vb.* to make something fall down by hitting it hard *slå ned;* **he was knocked down by a car**

knock knee [ˈnɒkniː] *or* **genu valgum** [ˈdʒenjuː ˌvælgəm] *subst.* state where the knees touch and the ankles are apart when a person is standing straight *genu valgum, kobenthet, X-benthet*

knock-kneed [ˌnɒkˈniːd] *adj.* (person) whose knees touch when he stands straight with feet slightly apart *kobent, X-bent*

knock out [ˌnɒk ˈaʊt] *vb.* to hit someone so hard that he is no longer conscious *slå ut, slå medvetslös;* **he was knocked out by a blow on the head**

knogarna ⇨ **knuckles**

knopp ⇨ **bud**

knorr(ande) ⇨ **rumbling**

knot [nɒt] **1** *subst.* place where two pieces of string *or* gut are tied together *knut;* **he tied a knot at the end of the piece of string 2** *vb.* to attach with a knot *knyta;* **the nurse knotted the two bandages**
NOTE: **knotting - knotted**

knotig ⇨ **bony**

knottra ⇨ **papule**

knottrig ⇨ **rough**

knuckles [ˈnʌk(ə)lz] *subst pl.* the backs of the joints on a person's hand *knogarna*

knut ⇨ **knot, node**

knutformig ⇨ **tubercular, tuberose, tuberous**

knutig ⇨ **nodular**

knyta ⇨ **knot, tie**

knytnäve ⇨ **fist**

knä- ⇨ **patellar**

knäbröstläge ⇨ **genupectoral position**

knäleden ⇨ **knee**

knäskålen ⇨ **kneecap**

knästräckarmuskeln ⇨ **quadriceps femoris**

knät ⇨ **knee**

knävecket ⇨ **popliteal**

knävecks- ⇨ **popliteal**

knävecksartären ⇨ **popliteal**

knävecksgropen ⇨ **popliteal**

knävecksmuskeln ⇨ **popliteus**

knöl ⇨ **bulb, bump, lump, node, tuber, tubercle**

knölig ⇨ **nodular, tubercular, tuberose, tuberous**

knölros ⇨ **erythema**

koagel ⇨ **clot, coagulum**

koagulation ⇨ **clotting, coagulation**

koagulationsfaktor ⇨ **factor, thromboplastin**

koagulationstid ⇨ **clotting**

koagulera ⇨ **clot, coagulate, congeal, curdle**

koagulering ⇨ **clotting, coagulation**

koan ⇨ **choana**

koanerna ⇨ **nares, nasal**

kobalamin ⇨ **Vitamin B**

kobent ⇨ **knock-kneed**

kobenthet ⇨ **knock knee**

kobolt ➪ **cobalt**

koccidiodomykos ➪ **coccidioidomycosis**

koccy(g)- ➪ **coccy-**

Koch's bacillus ['kəʊks bəˌsɪləs] *subst.* bacillus, **Mycobacterium tuberculosis,** which causes tuberculosis *Kochs bacill, tuberkelbacillen*

Koch-Weeks bacillus [ˌkəʊk'wi:ks bəˌsɪləs] *subst.* bacillus which causes conjunctivitis *Koch-Weeks bacill*

kock ➪ **coccus**

kod ➪ **code**

koda ➪ **code**

kodein ➪ **codeine**

koffein ➪ **caffeine**

koffeinfri ➪ **decaffeinated**

koilonychia [ˌkɔɪləʊ'nɪkiə] *or* **spoon nail** ['spu:n neɪ(ə)l] *subst.* state where the fingernails are brittle and concave, caused by iron-deficiency anaemia *koilonyki, platonyki, skednaglar*

koilonyki ➪ **koilonychia**

koka ➪ **boil**

kokain ➪ **cocaine**

koklear ➪ **cochlear**

koklearnerven ➪ **cochlear**

kokleär ➪ **cochlear**

kokoppor ➪ **cowpox**

koksalt ➪ **salt, sodium**

kol ➪ **carbon, charcoal**

kolangiografi ➪ **cholangiography**

kolangit ➪ **cholangitis**

koldioxid ➪ **carbon dioxide**

kole- ➪ **chole-**

kolecystektomi ➪ **cholecystectomy**

kolecystit ➪ **cholecystitis**

kolecystoduodenostomi ➪ **cholecystoduodenostomy**

kolecystografi ➪ **cholecystography**

kolecystogram ➪ **cholecystogram**

kolecystostomi ➪ **cholecystotomy**

koledoch(o)- ➪ **choledoch-**

koledochostomi ➪ **choledochotomy**

kolektomi ➪ **colectomy**

kolelitotomi ➪ **cholelithotomy**

kolera ➪ **cholera**

kolestas ➪ **cholestasis**

kolesterol ➪ **cholesterol**

kolhydrater ➪ **carbohydrates**

kolibakterien ➪ **Escherichia**

kolik ➪ **colic, gripe**

kolin ➪ **choline**

kolinesteras ➪ **cholinesterase**

kolisk ➪ **colonic**

kolit ➪ **colitis**

kollabera ➪ **collapse**

kollagen ➪ **collagen**

kollagen- ➪ **collagenous**

kollagenos ➪ **collagen**

kollaps ➪ **collapse**

kollapsa ➪ **break down, collapse**

kollateral- ➪ **collateral**

kollateralcirkulation ➪ **circulation (of the blood)**

kollodion ➪ **collodion**

kollodium ➪ **collodion**

kollyrium ➪ **collyrium**

kolobom ➪ **coloboma**

kolon ➪ **colon, large intestine**

kolon- ⇨ colonic

koloni ⇨ colony

kolonröntgen ⇨ barium

kolonsköljning ⇨ colonic

kolonspolning ⇨ colonic

kolostomi ⇨ colostomy

kolostomipåse ⇨ colostomy bag

kolostrum ⇨ colostrum

koloxid ⇨ carbon monoxide

koloxidförgiftning ⇨ carbon monoxide

kolpit ⇨ vaginitis

kolp(o)- ⇨ colp-

kolpopexi ⇨ colpopexy

kolpoptos ⇨ colpoptosis

kolporrafi ⇨ colporrhaphy

kolposkop ⇨ colposcope, vaginoscope

kolposkopi ⇨ colposcopy

kolpotomi ⇨ colpotomy

kolsjuka ⇨ anthracosis

kolsyra ⇨ carbon dioxide

kolsyrad ⇨ carbonated

kolsyresnö ⇨ ice, snow

koluri ⇨ choluria

koma ⇨ coma

komaliknande ⇨ comatose

komatös ⇨ comatose

kombination ⇨ combination

kombinera ⇨ combine

komedon ⇨ blackhead

komma ihåg ⇨ recall, remember

komminut fraktur ⇨ comminuted fracture

kommissur ⇨ commissure

kompakt ⇨ dense

kompatibel ⇨ compatible

kompatibilitet ⇨ compatibility

kompensera ⇨ compensate

kompetens ⇨ qualification

komplement ⇨ complement

komplementbindningsreaktion ⇨ complement

komplex ⇨ complex

komplicerad ⇨ complex

komplicerad fraktur ⇨ open

komplikation ⇨ complication

komponent ⇨ component

komposition ⇨ composition

kompress ⇨ absorbent, compress, cotton wool, dressing, pad

kompression ⇨ compression

komprimera ⇨ compress

kompulsiv ⇨ compulsive

kon ⇨ conus

koncentrat ⇨ concentrate

koncentration ⇨ concentrate

koncentrera ⇨ concentrate

konception ⇨ conception

konceptionsprodukt ⇨ conceptus

kondenserad ⇨ condensed

kondition ⇨ condition, fitness, form

kondom ⇨ condom, protective, rubber, sheath

kondrit ⇨ chondritis

kondr(o)- ⇨ chondr-

kondroblast ⇨ chondroblast

kondrocyt ⇨ chondrocyte

kondrodystrofi ⇨ chondrodysplasia

kondrokalcinos ⇨ chondrocalcinosis

kondrom ⇨ chondroma

kondromalaci ⇨ chondromalacia

kondrosarkom ⇨ chondrosarcoma

konduktiv ⇨ conductive

kondyl ⇨ condyle

kondylom ⇨ condyloma, wart

konfirmera ⇨ confirm

konfusion ⇨ disorientation

kongenital ⇨ congenital

kongestion ⇨ congestion, engorgement

konisation ⇨ cervicectomy

konjunktiva ⇨ conjunctiva

konjunktival ⇨ conjunctival

konjunktivit ⇨ conjunctivitis

konjunktivit, smittsam ⇨ pink

konkav ⇨ concave

konkrement ⇨ calculus, concretion

konkretion ⇨ concretion

konsangvinitet ⇨ consanguinity

konservera ⇨ preserve

konservering ⇨ preservation

konsolidering ⇨ consolidation

konstant ⇨ constant

konstgjord ⇨ artificial, synthetic

konstgjord njure ⇨ kidney

konstgjort ⇨ synthetically

konstiperad ⇨ constipated

konstipering ⇨ constipation

konstituens ⇨ excipient

konstituent ⇨ constituent

konstitution ⇨ constitution

konstitutionell ⇨ constitutionally

konstriktion ⇨ constriction

konstriktiv ⇨ constrictive

konstriktor ⇨ constrictor

konsultation ⇨ consultation

konsultera ⇨ consult

konsumtion ⇨ consumption, intake

konsumtions- ⇨ consumptive

kontagiös ⇨ contagious

kontakt ⇨ contact

kontaktdermatit ⇨ dermatitis, irritant

kontakteksem ⇨ dermatitis

kontaktlins ⇨ contact lens, scleral

kontamination ⇨ contamination

kontaminera ⇨ contaminate

kontinuerlig ⇨ continual, continuous

kontor ⇨ agency

kontraceptiv ⇨ contraceptive

kontraindikation ⇨ contraindication

kontraktion ⇨ contraction

kontraktur ⇨ contracture

kontralateral ⇨ contralateral

kontrast ⇨ meal, solution, contrast medium

kontroll ⇨ control, supervision

kontrollera ⇨ control, manage, monitor, supervise

kontrollgrupp ⇨ control

kontusion(sår) ⇨ contused wound

konvalescens ▷ **convalescence, recuperation**

konvalescent(-) ▷ **convalescent**

konvalescenthem ▷ **convalescent, home**

konvergera ▷ **converge**

konversion ▷ **conversion**

konvex ▷ **convex**

konvulsion ▷ **convulsion**

konvulsiv ▷ **convulsive**

koordination ▷ **coordination**

koordinera ▷ **coordinate**

Koplik's spots ['kɒplɪks spɒts] *subst pl.* small bluish-white spots surrounded by red areola, found in the mouth in the early stages of measles *Kopliks fläckar, kopliska fläckarna*

koppa ▷ **pock**

koppar ▷ **copper**

kopparnäsa ▷ **rhinophyma**

koppning ▷ **scarification**

koppärr ▷ **pockmark**

koprofyrin ▷ **coproporphyrin**

koprolit ▷ **coprolith, stercolith**

kopulation ▷ **coition, coitus, copulation**

kopulera ▷ **copulate**

kor ▷ **ichor**

korda ▷ **chorda, cord**

kordotomi ▷ **chordotomy**

korea ▷ **chorea**

korektomi ▷ **iridectomy, sphincterectomy**

korektopi ▷ **corectopia**

korion ▷ **chorion**

korium ▷ **corium, dermis**

korneal- ▷ **corneal**

kornealgrumling ▷ **nebula**

kornealtransplantat ▷ **corneal graft**

kornifikation ▷ **cornification**

kornig ▷ **granular**

koronar- ▷ **coronary**

koronarkärlen ▷ **coronary**

koronarkärls- ▷ **coronary**

koronarkärlscirkulationen ▷ **coronary**

koronarkärlsocklusion ▷ **coronary**

koronarkärlssjukdom ▷ **coronary**

koronarkärlstrombos ▷ **coronary**

korpnäbbsutskottet ▷ **coracoid process**

korpulent ▷ **fat, fleshy**

korpuskel ▷ **corpuscle**

korrigera ▷ **correct**

korrigering ▷ **correction**

Korsakoff's syndrome ['kɔːsəkɒfs ˌsɪndrəʊm] *subst.* condition where the patient's memory fails and he invents things which have not happened and is confused, caused usually by chronic alcoholism or disorders in which there is a deficiency of vitamin B *Korsakovs (Korsakoffs) syndrom*

korsa(s) ▷ **interbreed**

korsband ▷ **cruciate ligament**

korsbenet ▷ **sacrum**

korsbens- ▷ **sacral, sacro-**

korsbenskotorna ▷ **sacral**

korsbensplexus ▷ **sacral**

korsett ▷ **belt, brace, corset**

korsflätan ▷ **sacral**

korskotorna ▷ **sacral**

korsnerverna ▷ **sacral**

korsning ⇨ **chiasm, cross, decussation, hybrid**

korsryggen ⇨ **lumbar, small of the back**

korstestning ⇨ **cross match**

kortikal ⇨ **cortical**

kortikospinal ⇨ **corticospinal**

kortikosteroid ⇨ **corticosteroid**

kortikosteroider ⇨ **cortical**

kortikosteron ⇨ **corticosterone**

kortikotropin ⇨ **corticotrophin**

kortisol ⇨ **cortisol**

kortison ⇨ **cortisone**

kortregister ⇨ **card index**

kortskallighet ⇨ **brachycephaly**

kortvarig ⇨ **transient**

kost ⇨ **diet, food**

kost- ⇨ **dietary, dietetic**

kostal ⇨ **costal**

kostfibrer ⇨ **dietary**

kosthåll ⇨ **dietary**

kost(o)- ⇨ **cost-**

kostprinciper ⇨ **dietetic**

kostvanor ⇨ **eat**

kot- ⇨ **spondyl-, vertebral**

kota ⇨ **spondyl, vertebra**

kotförskjutning ⇨ **spondylolisthesis**

kotpelaren ⇨ **column**

kotyledon ⇨ **cotyledon**

koxalgi ⇨ **coxalgia**

kraft ⇨ **energy, force, strength, virulence**

kraftig ⇨ **intense, rich, virulent**

kraftigt ⇨ **hard**

kraftlös ⇨ **asthenic, feeble, weak**

kraftlöshet ⇨ **asthenia, debility, weakness**

krage ⇨ **collar**

kramp ⇨ **convulsion, cramp, spasm**

kramp- ⇨ **convulsive, spasmo-**

krampartad ⇨ **spasmodic, spastic**

kramplösande ⇨ **spasmolytic**

krampstillande medel ⇨ **antispasmodic**

kranial(-) ⇨ **cranial**

kranialnerverna ⇨ **cranial**

kranialnervskärna ⇨ **olive**

kraniet ⇨ **cranium**

krani(o)- ⇨ **crani-**

kraniofaryngiom ⇨ **craniopharyngioma**

kraniometri ⇨ **craniometry**

kraniostenos ⇨ **craniostenosis**

kraniosynostos ⇨ **craniostenosis**

kraniotabes ⇨ **craniotabes**

kraniotomi ⇨ **craniotomy**

kranium ⇨ **skull**

krans- ⇨ **coronary**

kranskärlen ⇨ **artery, coronary**

krasslig ⇨ **ailing, unwell**

krauros ⇨ **kraurosis**

kraurosis [krɔːˈrəʊsɪs] *subst.* dryness and shrivelling of a part *krauros, torrhet, skrumpning;* **kraurosis penis** = state where the foreskin becomes dry and shrivelled *kraurosis penis;* **kraurosis vulvae** = condition where the vulva becomes thin and dry due to lack of oestrogen (found usually in elderly women) *kraurosis vulvae*

Krause corpuscles [ˈkraʊzə ˌkɔːpʌs(ə)ls] *subst. pl. see* CORPUSCLE

⇨ *illustration* SKIN AND SENSORY RECEPTORS

krav ⇨ **requirement**

kreatin ⇨ **creatine**

kreatinas ⇨ **creatinase**

kreatinfosfat ⇨ **creatine**

kreatinin ⇨ **creatinine**

kreatorré ⇨ **creatorrhoea**

Krebs cycle ['krebz ˌsaɪk(ə)l] *subst.* = CITRIC ACID CYCLE

krepitation ⇨ **crepitation, crepitus**

kretin ⇨ **cretin**

kretinism ⇨ **cretinism**

kretslopp ⇨ **cycle**

kretsloppet, lilla ⇨ **pulmonary**

kretsloppet, stora ⇨ **systemic**

kris ⇨ **crisis**

kris- ⇨ **critical**

krisartad ⇨ **critical**

krisläge ⇨ **crisis**

kristall ⇨ **crystal**

kristallformad ⇨ **crystalline**

kristallisk ⇨ **crystalline**

kritisera ⇨ **criticize**

kritiserande ⇨ **critical**

kritisk ⇨ **critical**

kritiskt ⇨ **critically**

krock ⇨ **crash**

krom ⇨ **chromium**

kromatid ⇨ **chromatid**

kromatin ⇨ **chromatin**

kromatinfläck ⇨ **chromatin**

kromatografi ⇨ **chromatography**

kromkatgut ⇨ **chromicized catgut**

krom(o)- ⇨ **chrom-**

kromosom ⇨ **chromosome**

kromosomuppsättning ⇨ **karyotype**

krona ⇨ **crown**

kronbjudning ⇨ **cephalic, vertex**

kronisk ⇨ **chronic**

kronisk ledgångsreumatism ⇨ **rheumatoid**

kronsömmen ⇨ **coronal**

kropp ⇨ **body, corpus, soma, system**

kropps- ⇨ **bodily, somat-, systemic**

kroppsbyggnad ⇨ **build**

kroppsdel ⇨ **part**

kroppsfett ⇨ **adipose, body**

kroppskonstitution ⇨ **constitution**

kroppslig ⇨ **bodily, organic, physi-, physical, somatic**

kroppslukt ⇨ **body, odour**

kroppslus ⇨ **Pediculus**

kroppsläge ⇨ **position**

kroppsodör ⇨ **odour**

kroppsställning ⇨ **posture**

kroppsställnings- ⇨ **postural**

kroppstemperatur ⇨ **body, temperature**

kroppsvätskor ⇨ **body**

krossa ⇨ **crush**

krossår ⇨ **contused wound**

Krukenberg tumour ['kruːkənbɜːg ˌtjuːmə] *subst.* malignant tumour in the ovary secondary to a tumour in the stomach *Krukenbergs tumör*

krupp ⇨ **croup**

krupp, falsk ➪ **pseudocroup**

krural ➪ **crural**

kruralkanalen ➪ **canal, femoral**

kry ➪ **fit, well**

krya på sig ➪ **get well, pick up**

krycka ➪ **crutch**

kryestesi ➪ **cryaesthesia**

krympling ➪ **cripple**

krympning ➪ **involution**

kry(o)- ➪ **cry-**

kryokirurgi ➪ **cryosurgery**

kryoprecipitat ➪ **cryoprecipitate**

kryoterapi ➪ **cryotherapy**

krypta ➪ **crypt**

krypto- ➪ **crypto-**

kryptomenorré ➪ **cryptomenorrhoea**

kryptorkism ➪ **cryptorchidism, undescended testis**

kräft- ➪ **carcin-**

kräfta ➪ **cancer**

kräftsvulst ➪ **carcinoma**

kräftsår ➪ **canker**

kräkas ➪ **bring up, puke, throw up, vomit**

kräkmedel ➪ **emetic**

kräkning ➪ **emesis, vomit, vomiting, vomitus**

kräkningsförsök ➪ **retching**

kräkrot ➪ **ipecacuanha**

kräm ➪ **cream, paste**

krämpa ➪ **ailment, infirmity**

kräva ➪ **require**

krävande ➪ **strenuous**

krök ➪ **flexure, loop**

kröka ➪ **bend, curve**

krökning ➪ **curvature**

krökt ➪ **curved**

kubisk epitelcell ➪ **cuboidal**

kubital ➪ **cubital**

kudde ➪ **pillow**

kuff ➪ **cuff**

kula ➪ **globus**

kuldoskop ➪ **culdoscope**

kuldoskopi ➪ **culdoscopy**

kulled ➪ **ball and socket joint, enarthrosis**

kulmen ➪ **fastigium**

kumulation ➪ **cumulative**

kumulativ ➪ **cumulative**

kunnig ➪ **capable, expert**

Kuntscher nail ['kʌntʃə neɪ(ə)l] *or* **Küntscher nail** ['kɪntʃə neɪ(ə)l] *subst.* long steel nail used to pin fractures of long bones through the bone marrow *Küntscherspik*

Kupffer's cells ['kupfəz ˌselz] *subst. pl.* large specialized liver cells which break down haemoglobin into bile *Kupffers celler*

kupol ➪ **cupola**

kur ➪ **course, cure, regimen, remedy, treatment**

kuranstalt ➪ **sanatorium**

kurativ ➪ **curative**

kurator ➪ **medical, almoner**

kurr i magen ➪ **rumbling, borborygmus**

kurs ➪ **course**

kurva ➪ **curvature, curve; chart, diagram, graph**

kusp ➪ **cusp, lobe**

kutan ➪ **cutaneous**

kuvös ⇨ **incubator**

kvadrant ⇨ **quadrant**

kvadrantanopsi ⇨ **quadrantanopia**

kvalificerad ⇨ **skilled**

kvalifikation ⇨ **qualification**

kvalster ⇨ **house**

kvarbliven ⇨ **residual**

kvarhållande ⇨ **retention**

kvarliggande kateter ⇨ **indwelling catheter**

kvartärmalaria ⇨ **quartan fever**

Kveim test ['kvaɪm ˌtest] *subst.* skin test to confirm the presence of sarcoidosis *Kveims reaktion (test)*

kvicksilver ⇨ **mercury**

kvicksilverförgiftning ⇨ **mercurialism, mercury**

kvinna ⇨ **woman, female**

kvinnlig ⇨ **female**

kvinno- ⇨ **gyn-**

kvinnoavdelning ⇨ **woman**

kvinnosjukhus ⇨ **woman**

kvissla ⇨ **pimple**

kvot ⇨ **quotient, ratio**

kväljningar ⇨ **gag, nausea**

kväva ⇨ **asphyxiate, choke, suffocate, strangle**

kväve ⇨ **N, nitrogen**

kväveoxidul ⇨ **laughing gas, nitrous oxide**

kvävning ⇨ **asphyxia, asphyxiation, choking, strangulation, suffocation**

kwashiorkor [kwɒʃi'ɔːkɔː] *subst.* malnutrition of small children, mostly in tropical countries, causing anaemia, wasting of the body and swollen liver *kwashiorkor*

kyfos ⇨ **kyphos, kyphosis**

kyfoskolios ⇨ **kyphoscoliosis**

kyla ⇨ **frost**

kyla ned (av) ⇨ **refrigerate**

kylig ⇨ **cool**

kylknöl ⇨ **pernio**

kylskada ⇨ **chilblain, frostbite**

kylskadad ⇨ **frostbitten**

kylskåp ⇨ **refrigerator**

kylus ⇨ **chyle**

kymotrypsin ⇨ **chymotrypsin**

kymus ⇨ **chyme**

Küntscherspik ⇨ **Kuntscher nail**

kyphos ['kaɪfəs] *subst.* lump on the back in kyphosis *kyfos, puckel*

kyphos ⇨ **curvature**

kyphoscoliosis [ˌkaɪfəʊˌskɒli'əʊsɪs] *subst.* condition where the patient has both forward and lateral curvature of the spine *kyfoskolios*

kyphosis [kaɪ'fəʊsɪs] *or* **hunchback** ['hʌn(t)ʃbæk] *subst.* excessive forward curvature of the spine *kyfos, puckelrygg; see also* LORDOSIS

kyrett ⇨ **curet**

kyrettage ⇨ **curettage**

käkbenet ⇨ **jawbone**

käken ⇨ **jaw**

käkläsa ⇨ **trismus**

källa ⇨ **origin, site, source**

känna ⇨ **feel, sense**

kännbar ⇨ **palpable**

känneteckna ⇨ **characterize**

känsel- ⇨ **sensible, tactile**

känsel(förnimmelse) ⇨ **feeling**

känselkropp ⇨ **Meissner's corpuscle**

känsellös ⇨ **numb**

känsellöshet ⇨ **numbness**

känsel(sinnet) ⇨ **touch**

känsla ⇨ **affection, emotion, feeling**

känslig ⇨ **sensitive, susceptible, vulnerable**

känslighet ⇨ **sensibility, sensitivity, susceptibility**

känslomässig ⇨ **emotional**

kärl ⇨ **vas, vessel**

kärl- ⇨ **angio-, vas-, vascular, vaso-**

kärlbildning ⇨ **vascularization**

kärlinflammation ⇨ **angiitis, vasculitis**

kärlkramp ⇨ **angina (pectoris)**

kärlnystan ⇨ **tuft**

kärlplastik ⇨ **angioplasty**

kärlsammandragande ⇨ **astringent**

kärlsammandragning ⇨ **vasoconstriction**

kärlskada ⇨ **vascular**

kärlspasm ⇨ **angiospasm**

kärlsystemet ⇨ **vascular**

kärlutvidgning ⇨ **angiectasis, vasodilatation**

kärn- ⇨ **nuclear**

kärna ⇨ **core, nucleus**

kärnikterus ⇨ **kernicterus**

kärnkropp ⇨ **nucleolus**

kärnspinnresonans ⇨ **nuclear**

Köhler's disease ['kɜːləz dɪˌziːz] *or* **scaphoiditis** [ˌskæfɔɪ'daɪtɪs] *subst.* degeneration of the navicular bone in children *Köhlers sjukdom, skafoidit*

kölbröst ⇨ **pigeon chest**

köld ⇨ **frost**

köld- ⇨ **cry-**

köldbehandling ⇨ **cryotherapy**

köldfaktor ⇨ **windchill factor**

köldknöl ⇨ **pernio**

köldrysning ⇨ **chill**

köldskada ⇨ **frostbite**

köldskadad ⇨ **frostbitten**

kön ⇨ **genus, sex**

Königs operation ⇨ **Zadik's operation**

könlös ⇨ **asexual, neuter**

köns- ⇨ **genital, reproductive, sexual**

könsbunden ⇨ **sex-linked**

könscell ⇨ **gamete, germ**

könsdrift ⇨ **libido**

könsdriftshöjande (medel) ⇨ **aphrodisiac**

könshormon ⇨ **sex hormone**

könskaraktärer, sekundära ⇨ **secondary**

könsklinik ⇨ **VD**

könskromatin ⇨ **chromatin**

könskromosom ⇨ **sex chromosome**

könskörtel ⇨ **gonad**

könsmognad ⇨ **puberty**

könsorgan ⇨ **genital, genitalia, reproductive, sex**

könssjukdom ⇨ **sexually transmitted disease (STD), social, venereal disease (VD)**

könsumgänge ⇨ **sex, sexual**

körtel ⇨ **gland**

körtelfeber ⇨ **glandular fever**

körtelinflammation ⇨ **adenitis**

körtelliknande ⇨ **adenoid**

körtelsjukdom ⇨ **adenopathy, adenosis**

körtelsvulst ⇨ **adenoma**

kött ⇨ **flesh, meat**

köttsår ⇨ **flesh**

Ll

lab [læb] *subst. informal* = LABORATORY **we'll send the specimens away for a lab test; the lab report is negative; the samples have been returned by the lab**

lab- ['leɪb, ˌ-] *prefix* referring to the lips *or* to labia *labi(o)-, läpp-*

label ['leɪb(ə)l] **1** *subst.* piece of paper *or* card attached to an object *or* person to identify them *etikett, märke;* **identity label** = label attached to the wrist of a newborn baby *or* a patient in hospital, so that he can be identified easily *identitetsband, ID-band* **2** *vb.* to write on a label *or* to attach a label to an object *etikettera, märka;* **the bottle is labelled "poison"**

labia ['leɪbiə] *see* LABIUM

labial ['leɪbiəl] *adj.* referring to the lips *or* to labia *labial, läpp-*

labil ⇨ **labile, unstable**

labile ['leɪbaɪ(ə)l] *adj.* (drug) which is unstable and likely to change if heated or cooled *labil, instabil*

labio- ['leɪbiə(ʊ), ˌ--] *prefix* referring to lips *or* to labia *labi(o)-, läpp-*

labioplasty ['leɪbiə(ʊ)ˌplæsti] *subst.* surgical operation to repair damaged *or* deformed lips *läpplastik*

labium ['leɪbiəm] *subst.* (i) lip *labium, läpp;* (ii) structure which looks like a lip *läppliknande bildning, blygdläpp;* **labia majora** = two large fleshy folds at the outside edge of the vulva *labia majora (pudendi), stora blygdläpparna;* **labia minora** *or* **nymphae** = two small fleshy folds on the inside edge of the vulva ⇨ *illustration* UROGENITAL SYSTEM (female) *labia minora (pudendi), små blygdläpparna*
NOTE: the plural is **labia**

laboratorieföreståndare ⇨ **laboratory**

laboratorieassistent ⇨ **analyst, laboratory**

laboratorium ⇨ **laboratory**

laboratory [lə'bɒrət(ə)ri] *subst.* special room where scientists can do research *or* can test chemical substances *or* can grow tissues in culture, etc. *laboratorium;* **the new drug has passed its laboratory tests; the samples of water from the hospital have been sent to the laboratory for testing; laboratory officer** = qualified person in charge of a laboratory *laboratiorieföreståndare;* **laboratory techniques** = methods *or* skills needed to perform experiments in a laboratory *laboratoriemetoder;* **laboratory technician** = person who does practical work in a laboratory and has particular care of equipment *laboratorieassistent*

labour ['leɪbə] *or US* **labor** ['leɪbər] *subst.*·childbirth, especially the contractions in the womb which take place during childbirth *förlossningsarbete, värkar*

> COMMENT: labour usually starts about nine months (or 266 days) after conception. The cervix expands and the muscles in the uterus contract, causing the amnion to burst. The muscles continue to contract regularly, pushing the baby into, and then through, the vagina

labyrint ⇨ **labyrinth**

labyrinth ['læbərɪnθ] *subst.* interconnecting tubes, especially those in the inside of the ear *labyrint;* **bony labyrinth** *or* **osseous labyrinth** = hard part of the temporal bone surrounding the membranous labyrinth in the inner ear *labyrinthus osseus, benlabyrinten;* **membranous labyrinth** = series of ducts and canals formed of membrane inside the osseous labyrinth *labyrinthus membranaceus, hinnlabyrinten*

> COMMENT: the labyrinth of the inner ear is in three parts: the three semicircular canals, the vestibule and the cochlea. The osseous labyrinth is filled with a fluid (perilymph) and the membranous labyrinth is a series of ducts and canals inside the osseous labyrinth. The membranous labyrinth contains a fluid (endolymph). As the endolymph moves about in the membranous labyrinth it stimulates the vestibular nerve which

communicates the sense of movement of the head to the brain. If a person turns round and round and then stops, the endolymph continues to move and creates the sensation of giddiness

labyrinthitis [ˌlæbərin'θaɪtɪs] *or* **otitis interna** [əʊ'taɪtɪs ɪnˌtɜːnə] *subst.* inflammation of the labyrinth *otitis interna (labyrinthiaca), labyrintit, inre öroninflammation*

labyrintit ➪ **labyrinthitis**

lacerated ['læsəreɪtɪd] *adj.* torn *or* with a rough edge *lacererad, söndersliten, sönderriven;* **lacerated wound** = wound where the skin is torn, as by a rough surface *or* barbed wire *vulnus laceratum, slitsår, rivsår*

laceration [ˌlæsə'reɪʃ(ə)n] *subst.* act of tearing tissue *laceration, sönderrivning, sönderslitning;* wound which has been cut *or* torn with rough edges, and not the result of stabbing *or* pricking *slitsår, rivsår*

lacererad ➪ **lacerated**

lachrymal ['lækrɪm(ə)l] *see* LACRIMAL

lack [læk] **1** *subst.* not having something *brist;* **the children are dying because of lack of food; the hospital had to close two wards because of lack of money 2** *vb.* not to have enough of something *lida brist på, inte ha;* **the children lack winter clothing; their diet lacks essential proteins; he lacks the strength to feed himself** = he isn't strong enough to feed himself *han orkar inte äta själv*

lackmus ➪ **litmus**

lackmuspapper ➪ **litmus**

lacrimal ['lækrɪm(ə)l] *or* **lacrymal** ['lækrɪm(ə)l] *or* **lachrymal** ['lækrɪm(ə)l] *adj.* referring to tears *or* tear ducts *or* tear glands *lakrimal, tår-;* **lacrimal apparatus** *or* **system** = arrangement of glands and ducts which produce and drain tears *tårapparaten;* **lacrimal bones** = two little bones which join with others to form the orbits *ossa lacrimales, tårbenen;* **lacrimal canaliculus** = small canal draining tears into the lacrimal sac *canaliculis lacrimalis, tårröret;* **lacrimal caruncle** = small red point at the inner corner of each eye *caruncula lacrimalis, tårkarunkeln, ögonkarunkeln;* **lacrimal duct** *or* **tear duct** *or* **nasolacrimal duct** = canal which takes tears from the lacrimal sac to the nose *ductus nasolacrimalis, nästårkanalen;* **lacrimal gland** *or* **tear gland** = gland beneath the upper eyelid which secretes tears *glandula lacrimalis, tårkörtel;* **lacrimal puncta** = small openings of the lacrimal canaliculus at the corners of the eyes through which tears drain into the nose *puncta lacrimalia, tårpunkterna;* **lacrimal sac** = sac at the upper end of the nasolacrimal duct, linking it with the lacrimal canaliculus *saccus lacrimalis, tårsäcken*

lacrimation [ˌlækrɪ'meɪʃ(ə)n] *subst.* crying *or* production of tears *tårflöde, tårproduktion*

lacrimator ['lækrɪmeɪtə] *subst.* substance which irritates the eyes and makes tears flow *ämne som irriterar ögonen och orsakar tårflöde*

lact- ['lækt, ˌ-] *prefix* referring to milk *lakt(o)-, mjölk-*

lactase ['lækteɪz] *subst.* enzyme, secreted in the small intestine, which converts milk sugar into glucose and galactose *laktas*

lactate ['lækteɪt] *vb.* to produce milk *avsöndra mjölk*

lactation [læk'teɪʃ(ə)n] *subst.* (i) production of milk *laktation, mjölkavsöndring, amning, digivning;* (ii) period during which a mother is breast feeding a baby *amningsperiod*

COMMENT: lactation is stimulated by the production of the hormone prolactin by the pituitary gland. It starts about three days after childbirth, during which period the breasts secrete colostrum

lacteal ['læktiəl] **1** *adj.* referring to milk *mjölk-* **2** *subst.* lymph vessel in a villus, which helps the digestive process in the small intestine by absorbing fat *lymfkärl i villi (tarmludd)*

lactic acid [ˌlæktɪk 'æsɪd] *subst.* sugar which forms in cells and tissue, also in sour milk, cheese and yoghurt *mjölksyra*

COMMENT: lactic acid is produced as the body uses up sugar during exercise. Excessive amounts of lactic acid in the body can produce muscle cramp

lactiferous [læk'tɪf(ə)rəs] *adj.* which produces *or* secretes *or* carries milk *laktifer, mjölk-, mjölkavsöndrande, mjölkförande;* **lactiferous duct** = duct in the breast which carries milk *ductus lactiferus, mjölkgång;* **lactiferous sinus** = dilatation of the lactiferous duct at the base of the nipple *sinus lactiferus*

Lactobacillus [ˌlæktəʊbə'sɪləs] *subst.* genus of Gram-positive bacteria which can produce lactic acid from glucose and may be found in the digestive tract and the vagina *Lactobacillus*

lactogenic hormone [ˌlæktəʊˈdʒenɪk ˌhɔːməʊn] = PROLACTIN

lactose [ˈlæktəʊs] *or* **milk sugar** [ˈmɪlk ˌʃʊgə] *subst.* sugar found in milk *laktos, mjölksocker;* **lactose intolerance** = condition where a person cannot digest lactose because lactase is absent in the intestine, or because of an allergy to milk, causing diarrhoea *laktosintolerans, laktosmalabsorption*

lactosuria [ˌlæktəʊˈsjʊəriə] *subst.* excretion of lactose in the urine *laktosuri*

lacuna [ləˈkjuːnə] *subst.* small hollow *or* cavity *lakun, hålighet, grop*
NOTE: the plural is **lacunae**

Laennec's cirrhosis [ˌleɪəˈneks səˈrəʊsɪs] *subst.* commonest form of alcoholic cirrhosis of the liver *Laënnecs cirros, atrophia hepatis, atrofisk levercirros, skrumplever*

laevocardia [ˌliːvəʊˈkɑːdiə] *subst.* normal position of the apex of the heart towards the left side of the body *levokardi; compare* DEXTROCARDIA

lag ⇨ **team**

laga ⇨ **mend, repair**

lager ⇨ **coat, layer, stratum**

laglig ⇨ **legal**

lakan ⇨ **sheet**

lakrimal ⇨ **lacrimal**

laktas ⇨ **lactase**

laktasbrist ⇨ **alactasia**

laktation ⇨ **lactation**

laktationshormon ⇨ **prolactin**

laktifer ⇨ **lactiferous**

laktos ⇨ **lactose**

laktosintolerans ⇨ **lactose, sugar**

laktosmalabsorption ⇨ **lactose**

laktosuri ⇨ **lactosuria**

lakun ⇨ **lacuna**

lambda [ˈlæmdə] *subst.* point at the back of the skull where the sagittal suture and lambdoidal suture meet *sutura lambdoidea, punkt där nacksömmen och pilsömmen möts*

lambdasömmen ⇨ **lambdoidal suture**

lambdoid(al) suture [ˈlæmdɔɪd(əl) ˌsuːtʃə] *subst.* horizontal joint across the back of the skull between the parietal and occipital bones ⇨ *illustration* SKULL *sutura lambdoides, lambdasömmen, nacksömmen*

lamblia [ˈlæmbliə] *see* GIARDIA

lambliasis [læmˈblaɪəsɪs] *see* GIARDIASIS

lambå ⇨ **pedicle**

lame [leɪm] *adj.* not able to walk normally because one leg is shorter than the other *or* walking with a limp because of pain *halt;* **he has been lame since his accident**

lamella [ləˈmelə] *subst.* (i) thin sheet of tissue *lamell, blad, tunn skiva;* (ii) thin disc placed under the eyelid to apply a drug to the eye *lamella, gelatinruta*
NOTE: plural is **lamellae**

lameness [ˈleɪmnəs] *subst.* limping *or* walking awkwardly because of pain in a leg *or* because one leg is shorter than the other *hälta*

lamina [ˈlæmɪnə] *subst.* (i) thin membrane *lamina, tunn skiva, tunt lager;* (ii) side part of the posterior arch in a vertebra *lamina arcus vertebrae;* **lamina propria** = connective tissue of mucous membrane containing blood vessels, lymphatics, etc. *lamina propria*
NOTE: the plural is **laminae**

laminectomy [ˌlæmɪˈnektəmi] *or* **rachiotomy** [ˌreɪkiˈɒtəmi] *subst.* surghical operation to cut through the lamina of a vertebra in the spine to get to the spinal cord *laminektomi, raki(o)tomi*

laminektomi ⇨ **laminectomy, rachiotomy**

lamp [læmp] *subst.* electric device which makes light *lampa;* **an electric lamp; an endoscope can have a small lamp at the end of it; the ear specialist shone his lamp into the patient's ear; she lay for thirty minutes under an ultraviolet lamp**

lance [lɑːns] *vb.* to make a cut in a boil *or* abscess to remove the pus *öppna med lancett, sticka hål på*

lancet ['lɑːnsɪt] *subst.* sharp two-edged pointed knife used in surgery *lancett*

lancinate ['lænsɪneɪt] *vb.* to lacerate *or* cut *skära, slita sönder*

lancinating ['lænsɪneɪtɪŋ] *adj.* sharp cutting (pain) *skarp, häftig*

Landry's paralysis ['lændrɪz, pə'ræləsɪs] *see* GUILLAIN-BARRÉ SYNDROME

Langerhans ['læŋgəhænz] *subst.* **islets of Langerhans** = groups of cells in the pancreas which secrete the hormones glucagon, insulin and gastrin *Langerhans cellöar, langerhansska cellöarna*

Lange test ['læŋgi ˌtest] *subst.* method of detecting globulin in the cerebrospinal fluid *metod för att upptäcka globulin i cerebrospinalvätska*

lanolin ['læn(ə)lɪn] *subst.* grease (from sheep's wool) which absorbs water, and is used to rub on dried skin, or in the preparation of cosmetics *lanolin*

lanugo [lə'njuːgəʊ] *subst.* soft hair on the body of a fetus *or* newborn baby *lanugo(hår), ullhår;* soft hair on the body of an adult (except on the palms of the hands, the soles of the feet, and the parts where long hair grows) *mjukt kroppshår*

laparo- ['læpərə(ʊ), ˌ---] *prefix* referring to the lower abdomen *laparo-, buk-*

laparoscope ['læpərəskəʊp] *or* **peritoneoscope** [ˌperi'təʊniəskəʊp] *subst.* surgical instrument which is inserted through a hole in the abdominal wall to allow a surgeon to examine the inside of the abdominal cavity *laparoskop*

laparoscopy [ˌlæpə'rɒskəpi] *or* **peritoneoscopy** [ˌperiˌtəʊni'ɒskəpi] *subst.* using a laparoscope to examine the inside of the abdominal cavity *laparoskopi*

laparoskop ⇨ **laparoscope**

laparoskopi ⇨ **abdominoscopy, coelioscopy, laparoscopy**

laparotomy [ˌlæpə'rɒtəmi] *subst.* surgical operation to cut open the abdominal cavity *laparotomi*

lapis ⇨ **silver nitrate**

lapptest ⇨ **patch test**

large [lɑːdʒ] *adj.* very big *stor;* **he has a large tumour on the right cerebrum**
NOTE: **large - larger - largest**

large intestine [ˌlɑːdʒ ɪn'testɪn] *subst.* section of the digestive system from the caecum to the rectum *colon, kolon, tjocktarmen, grovtarmen*

larva ['lɑːvə] *subst.* stage in the development of an insect *or* tapeworm, after the egg has hatched but before the animal becomes adult *larv*
NOTE: plural is **larvae**

laryng- [lə'rɪndʒ, 'lærɪndʒ, ˌ--] *or* **laryngo-** [lə'rɪŋgəʊ, -ˌ--] *prefix* referring to the larynx *laryng(o)-, strup-, struphuvuds-*

laryngeal [lə'rɪndʒ(ə)l] *adj.* referring to the larynx *laryngeal, struphuvuds-;* **laryngeal inlet** = entrance from the laryngopharynx leading through the vocal cords to the trachea *rima glottidis, ljudspringan, öppningen mellan stämbanden, svalgöppningen i höjd med struphuvudet;* **laryngeal prominence** = Adam's apple *prominentia laryngea, pomum Adami, adamsäpplet;* **laryngeal reflex** = cough *larynxreflex*

laryngectomy [ˌlærɪn'dʒektəmi] *subst.* surgical removal of the larynx, usually as treatment for throat cancer *laryngektomi*

laryngismus (stridulus) [ˌlærɪn'dʒɪzməs (ˌstrɪdjuləs)] *subst.* spasm of the throat muscles with a sharp intake of breath which occurs when the larynx is irritated, as in children suffering from croup *laryngism*

laryngitis [ˌlærɪn'dʒaɪtɪs] *subst.* inflammation of the larynx *laryngit, strupkatarr*

laryngofarynx ⇨ **laryngopharynx**

laryngofissure [ləˌrɪŋgəʊ'fɪʃə] *subst.* surgical operation to make an opening into the larynx through the thyroid cartilage *laryngotomi*

laryngologist [ˌlærɪn'gɒlədʒɪst] *subst.* doctor who specializes in diseases of the larynx, throat and vocal cords *laryngolog*

laryngology [ˌlærɪn'gɒlədʒi] *subst.* study of diseases of the larynx, throat and vocal cords *laryngologi*

laryngopharynx [ˌlærɪŋgəʊ'færɪŋ(k)s] *subst.* part of the pharynx below the hyoid bone *laryngofarynx*

laryngoscope [lə'rɪŋgəskəʊp] *subst.* instrument for examining the inside of the larynx, using a light and mirrors *laryngoskop*

laryngoskop ⇨ **laryngoscope, pharyngoscope**

laryngospasm ['lærɪŋgə(ʊ)spæz(ə)m] *subst.* muscular spasm which suddenly closes the larynx *laryngospasm*

laryngostenosis [ˌlærɪŋgəstə'nəʊsɪs] *subst.* narrowing of the lumen of the larynx *laryngostenos, struphuvudsförträngning*

laryngotomi ⇨ **laryngofissure, laryngotomy**

laryngotomy [ˌlærɪŋ'gɒtəmi] *subst.* surgical operation to make an opening in the larynx through the membrane (especially in an emergency, when the throat is blocked) *laryngotomi*

laryngotracheobronchitis [ləˌrɪŋgəʊˌtreɪkiəʊbrɒŋ'kaɪtɪs] *subst.* inflammation of the larynx, trachea and bronchi, as in croup *inflammation i struphuvudet, luftstrupen och luftrören*

larynx ['lærɪŋ(k)s] *or* **voice box** ['vɔɪs ˌbɒks] *subst.* organ in the throat which produces sounds ⇨ *illustration* THROAT *larynx, struphuvudet*

> COMMENT: the larynx is a hollow passage made of cartilage, containing the vocal cords, situated behind the Adam's apple. It is closed by the epiglottis when swallowing or before coughing

larynxreflex ⇨ **laryngeal**

laser ['leɪzə] *subst.* instrument which produces a highly concentrated beam of light, which can be used to cut or attach tissue, as in operations for detached retina *laser;* **laser probe** = metal probe which is inserted into the body, then heated by a laser beam, used to burn through blocked arteries *lasersond*

lasersond ⇨ **laser**

Lassa fever [ˌlæsə 'fiːvə] *subst.* highly infectious virus disease found in Central and West Africa *Lassa-feber*

> COMMENT: the symptoms are high fever, pains, and ulcers in the mouth. It is often fatal.

Lassar's paste ['læsəz ˌpeɪst] *subst.* ointment made of zinc oxide, used to treat eczema *slags zinksalva mot eksem*

lat ⇨ **lazy**

lata ['lætə] *see* FASCIA

latens(tid) ⇨ **incubation period**

latent ['leɪt(ə)nt] *adj.* (disease) which is present in the body, but does not show any signs *latent;* **the children were tested for latent viral infection**

latent ⇨ **dormant**

lateral ['læt(ə)r(ə)l] *adj.* (i) further away from the midline of the body *lateral, yttre;* (ii) referring to one side of the body *lateral, sido-;* **lateral malleolus** = prominence on the outer surface of the ankle joint *malleolus lateralis, laterala malleolen, yttre fotknölen;* **lateral view** = view of the side of part of the body *sidobild; compare* MEDIAL

lateralis [ˌlætə'reɪlis] *see* VASTUS

lateroversion [ˌlæt(ə)rəʊ'vɜːʃ(ə)n] *subst.* turning (of an organ) to one side *lateroversion*

latissimus dorsi [lə'tɪsɪməs ˌdɔːsi] *subst.* large flat triangular muscle covering the lumbar region and the lower part of the chest *musculus latissimus dorsi, breda ryggmuskeln*

laugh [lɑːf] **1** *subst.* sound made by the throat when a person is amused *skratt;* **he said it with a laugh; she gave a hysterical laugh** **2** *vb.* to make a sound which shows amusement *skratta;* **he started to laugh hysterically**

laughing gas ['lɑːfɪŋ gæs] *subst.* nitrous oxide, gas used in combinations with other gases by dentists as an anaesthetic *kväveoxidul, lustgas*

laundry ['lɔːndri] *subst.* **(a)** place where clothes, etc. are washed *tvättinrättning, tvättstuga;* **the bedclothes will be sent to the hospital laundry to be sterilized** **(b)** clothes, etc. which need to be washed or which have been washed *tvätt(kläder);* **the report criticized the piles of dirty laundry left lying in the wards**

lavage ['lævɪdʒ] *subst.* washing out *or* irrigating an organ, such as the stomach *lavage, sköljning*

lavatory ['lævət(ə)ri] *subst.* toilet *or* place *or* room where one can get rid of water or solid waste from the body *toalett;* **the ladies' lavatory is to the right; there are three lavatories for the ward of ten people**

lavemang ⇨ **enema, proctoclysis**

lavliknande ⇨ **lichenoid**

laxative ['læksətɪv] *subst. & adj.* (medicine) which causes a bowel movement *laxativ, laxermedel, avföringsmedel, laxerande, avförande*

> COMMENT: laxatives are very commonly used without prescription to treat constipation, although they should only be used as a short term solution. Change of diet and regular exercise are better ways of treating most types of constipation

laxerande ⇨ **aperient, cathartic, laxative, purgative**

laxermedel ⇨ **hydragogue, laxative, purgative**

layer ['leɪə] *subst.* flat area of a substance under or over another area *lager, skikt, varv;* **they put three layers of cotton wadding over his eye**

lazy ['leɪzi] *adj.* not wanting to do any work *lat;* **lazy eye** = eye which does not focus properly *nedsatt fokuseringsförmåga*
NOTE: **lazy - lazier - laziest**

lb *see* POUND

LD [ˌel'di:] = LETHAL DOSE

L-dopa [ˌel'dəʊpə] *or* **levodopa** [ˌli:vəʊ'dəʊpə] *subst.* amino acid used in the treatment of Parkinson's disease *L-dopa, levodopa*

l.e. [ˌel'i:] *or* **LE** [ˌel'i:] *abbreviation for* = LUPUS ERYTHEMATOSUS; **LE cells** = white blood cells which show that a patient has lupus erythematosus *LE-celler*

lead [led] *subst.* very heavy soft metallic element, which is poisonous in compounds *bly, Pb;* **lead line** = blue line seen on the gums in cases of lead poisoning *discoloratio gingivae, blysöm* NOTE: chemical symbol is **Pb**

lead-free ['ledfri:] *adj.* with no lead in it *blyfri;* **lead-free paint; lead-free petrol**

lead poisoning ['led ˌpɔɪz(ə)nɪŋ] *or* **plumbism** ['plʌmbɪz(ə)m] *or* **saturnism** ['sætənɪz(ə)m] *subst.* poisoning caused by taking in lead salts *blyförgiftning*

> COMMENT: lead salts are used externally to treat bruises *or* eczema, but if taken internally produce lead poisoning, which can also be caused by paint (children's toys must be painted in lead-free paint) or by lead fumes from car engines (which can be avoided by using lead-free petrol)

leak [li:k] *vb. (of liquids)* to flow out by accident *or* by mistake *läcka;* **blood leaked into the subcutaneous layers**

lecithins ['lesɪθɪnz] *subst. pl.* constituents of all animal and plant cells, involved with the transport and absorption of fats *lecitin*

LED ⇨ **disseminated, systemic**

led ⇨ **articulation, joint**

led- ⇨ **arthr-, articular, synovial**

leda ⇨ **direct, head, manage, transmit**

ledad ⇨ **jointed**

ledarhund ⇨ **guide dog**

ledband ⇨ **ligament**

ledbrosk ⇨ **articular**

led, falsk ⇨ **pseudoarthrosis**

ledgång ⇨ **articulation, joint**

ledgångsinflammation ⇨ **arthritis**

ledgångsinflammation, varig ⇨ **pyarthrosis**

ledgångssjukdom ⇨ **arthropathy**

ledhuvud ⇨ **condyle, head**

ledhuvudsutskott ⇨ **epicondyle**

ledhåla ⇨ **synovial**

ledkapsel ⇨ **capsule**

ledknapp ⇨ **condyle**

ledkula ⇨ **head**

ledmus ⇨ **joint**

ledning ⇨ **conduction, conduit, management**

ledningshörselnedsättning ⇨ **conductive**

ledpanna ⇨ **socket**

ledresektion ⇨ **arthrectomy**

ledsjukdom ⇨ **arthropathy**

ledskål ⇨ **socket**

ledsmärta ⇨ **arthralgia, arthrodynia**

ledstång ⇨ **support**

ledutskott ⇨ **process**

ledvätska ⇨ **synovia**

leech [li:tʃ] *subst.* type of parasitic worm which lives in water and sucks the blood of animals by attaching itself to the skin *blodigel;* **medicinal leech** = leech which is raised specially for use in medicine *blodigel för medicinskt bruk*

> COMMENT: leeches were formerly commonly used in medicine to remove blood from a patient. Today they are used in special cases, where it is necessary to make sure that blood does not build up in part of the body (as in a severed finger which has been sewn back on)

left [left] *adv., adj. & subst.* referring to the side of the body which usually has the weaker hand *vänster;* **he can't write with his left hand; the heart is on the left side of the body**

left-hand [ˌleft'hænd, 'lefthænd] *adj.* on the left side *vänster-;* **look in the left-hand drawer of the desk; the tablets are on the top left-hand shelf in the cupboard**

left-handed [ˌleft'hændɪd] *adj.* using the left hand more often than the right for writing *vänsterhänt;* **she's left-handed; left-handed people need special scissors; about five per cent of the population is left-handed**

left-handedness [ˌleft'hændɪdnəs] *subst.* condition of a person who is left-handed *vänsterhänthet*

leg [leg] *subst.* part of the body with which a person or animal walks and stands *ben;* **she made him stand on one leg and lift the other leg up; he is limping from a leg injury which he received playing football; his left leg is slightly shorter than the right; she complained of pains in her right leg; she fell off the wall and broke her leg**

> COMMENT: the leg is formed of the thigh (with the thighbone or femur), the knee (with the kneecap or patella), and the lower leg (with two bones - the tibia and fibula)

legal ['li:g(ə)l] *adj.* which is allowed by law *laglig, legal;* **legal abortion** = abortion carried out according to the law *abortus legalis, legal abort*

Legg-Calvé-Perthes disease [ˌleg,kælveɪ'pɜ:tɪz dɪˌzi:z] *subst.* degeneration of the upper end of the thighbone in young boys, which prevents the bone growing properly and can result in a permanent limp *Legg-Calvé-Perthes sjukdom, osteochondritis deformans juvenilis, coxa plana*

legionnaires' disease [ˌli:dʒə'neəz dɪˌzi:z] *subst.* bacterial disease similar to pneumonia *legionärssjuka*

> COMMENT: the disease is thought to be transmitted in droplets of moisture in the air, and so the bacterium is found in central air-conditioning systems. It can be fatal to old or sick people, and so is especially dangerous if present in a hospital

legionärssjuka ⇨ **legionnaires' disease**

legitimation ⇨ **licence**

legitimera ⇨ **register**

legitimerad läkare ⇨ **medical**

legitimerad sjuksköterska ⇨ **enrolled**

leiomyoma [ˌlaɪəʊmaɪ'əʊmə] *subst.* tumour of smooth muscle, especially the smooth muscle coating the uterus *leiomyom*

leiomyosarcoma [ˌlaɪəʊˌmaɪəʊsɑ:'kəʊmə] *subst.* sarcoma in which large bundles of smooth muscle are found *leiomyosarkom*

Leishmania [li:ʃ'meɪniə] *subst.* tropical parasite which is passed to humans by the bites of sandflies *Leishmania*

leishmaniasis [ˌli:ʃmə'na(ɪ)əsɪs] *subst.* any of several diseases (such as Delhi boil *or* kala-azar) caused by the parasite **Leishmania,** one form giving disfiguring ulcers, another attacking the liver and bone marrow *leishmanios;* **mucocutaneous leishmaniasis** = disorder affecting the skin and mucous membrane *leishmaniasis mucocutanea, mukokutan leishmanios*

lem ⇨ **limb**

Lembert's suture ['lɑ:mbeəz ˌsu:tʃə] *subst.* suture used to close a wound in the intestine which includes all the coats of the intestine *slags tarmsutur*

lemlästa ⇨ **cripple, maim**

Lempert operation [ˈlempət ˌɒpəˌreɪʃ(ə)n] *subst.* fenestration *or* surgical operation to relieve deafness by making a small opening in the inner ear *fenestration*

lenande medel ⇨ **demulcent**

length [leŋθ] *subst.* measurement of how long something is *längd;* **the small intestine is about 5 metres in length**

lens [lenz] *subst.* **(a)** part of the eye behind the iris and pupil, which focuses light coming from the cornea onto the retina ⇨ *illustration* EYE *lens, linsen* **(b)** piece of shaped glass *or* plastic which forms part of a pair of spectacles *or* microscope *lins;* **contact lens** = tiny glass *or* plastic lens which fits over the eyeball and is worn instead of spectacles *kontaktlins*

COMMENT: the lens in the eye is elastic, and can change its shape under the influence of the ciliary muscle, to allow the eye to focus on objects at different distances

lenticular [lenˈtɪkjʊlə] *adj.* referring to a lens *or* like a lens *lentikulär, lins-, linsformad*

lentigo [lenˈtaɪgəʊ] *subst.* freckle *or* small brown spot on the skin often caused by exposure to sunlight *lentigo, leverfläck, fräken*

lentikulär ⇨ **lenticular**

leper [ˈlepə] *subst.* person suffering from leprosy *spetälsk (person);* **he works in a leper hospital**

lepidosis [ˌlepɪˈdəʊsɪs] *subst.* skin eruption, where pieces of skin fall off in flakes *slags utslag där huden faller av i flagor*

lepra ⇨ **leprosy**

leprabacillen ⇨ **Hansen's bacillus**

leproma [leˈprəʊmə] *subst.* lesion of the skin caused by leprosy *leprom*

leprosy [ˈleprəsi] *or* **Hansen's disease** [ˈhæns(ə)nz dɪˌziːz] *subst.* infectious bacterial disease of skin and peripheral nerve tracts caused by **Mycobacterium leprae,** which destroys the tissues and can cripple the patient if left untreated *lepra, spetälska*

COMMENT: Leprosy attacks the nerves in the skin, and finally the patient loses all feeling in a limb, and parts, such as fingers *or* toes, can drop off

lepto- [ˈleptə(ʊ), ˌ--] *prefix* meaning thin *lepto-*

leptocyte [ˈleptə(ʊ)saɪt] *subst.* thin red blood vessel found in anaemia *smalt blodkärl pga anemi*

leptomeninges [ˌleptə(ʊ)meˈnɪn(d)ʒiːz] *subst.* two inner meninges (pia mater and arachnoid) *leptomeningerna, mjuka hjärnhinnorna*

leptomeningitis [ˌleptə(ʊ)ˌmenɪnˈdʒaɪtɪs] *subst.* inflammation of the leptomeninges *inflammation i leptomingerna (mjuka hjärnhinnorna)*

leptospirosis [ˌleptə(ʊ)spaɪ(ə)ˈrəʊsɪs] *or* **Weil's disease** [ˈvaɪlz dɪˌziːz] *subst.* infectious disease caused by the spirochaete **Leptospira** transmitted to humans from rats, giving jaundice and kidney damage *leptospiros, Weils sjukdom*

leresis [ləˈriːsɪs] *subst.* uncoordinated speech, a sign of dementia *osammanhängande tal*

lesbian [ˈlezbiən] *subst. & adj.* woman who experiences sexual attraction towards other women *lesbisk (kvinna)*

lesbianism [ˈlezbiənɪz(ə)m] *subst.* sexual attraction in one woman for another *lesbianism; compare* HOMOSEXUAL

lesbisk (kvinna) ⇨ **lesbian**

lesion [ˈliːʒ(ə)n] *subst.* wound *or* sore *or* damage to the body *lesion, skada*
NOTE: lesion is used to refer to any damage to the body, from the fracture of a bone to a cut on the skin

lessen [ˈles(ə)n] *vb.* to make less strong *minska, reducera;* **the injection will lessen the pain; modern antibiotics lessen the chance of a patient getting gangrene**

lesser [ˈlesə] *adj.* smaller *mindre;* **lesser trochanter** = projection on the femur which is the insertion of the psoas major muscle *trochanter minor*

letal ⇨ **fatal, lethal**

letalfaktor ⇨ **lethal**

letargi ⇨ **lethargy**

letargisk ⇨ **lethargic**

lethal ['liːθ(ə)l] *adj.* which can kill *letal, dödlig, döds-;* **she took a lethal dose of aspirin; these fumes are lethal if inhaled; lethal gene** = gene which can kill the person who inherits it *letalfaktor*

lethargic [lə'θɑːdʒɪk] *adj.* showing lethargy *letargisk, sömnsjuk;* **lethargic encephalitis** *or* **encephalitis lethargica** = formerly a common type of virus encephalitis occurring in epidemics *encephalitis epidemica (lethargica), sömnsjuka*

lethargy ['leθədʒi] *subst.* mental torpor *or* tired feeling, when the patient has slow movements and is almost inactive *letargi, dvala*

leucine ['luːsiːn] *subst.* essential amino acid *leucin*

leuco- ['luːkə(ʊ), ˌ--] *or* **leuko-** ['luːkə(ʊ), ˌ--] *prefix* meaning white *leuko-, vit*

leucocyte ['luːkə(ʊ)saɪt] *or* **leukocyte** ['luːkə(ʊ)saɪt] *subst.* white blood cell which contains a nucleus but has no haemoglobin *leukocyt, vit blodkropp*

> COMMENT: in normal conditions the blood contains far fewer leucocytes than erythrocytes (red blood cells), but their numbers increase rapidly when infection is present in the body. Leucocytes are either granular (with granules in the cytoplasm) *or* nongranular. The main types of leucocyte are: lymphocytes and monocytes which are nongranular, and neutrophils, eosinophils and basophils which are granular (granulocytes). Granular leucocytes are produced by the bone marrow, and their main function is to remove foreign particles from the blood and fight infection by forming antibodies

leucocytolysis [ˌluːkə(ʊ)saɪ'tɒləsɪs] *subst.* destruction of leucocytes *leuko(cyto)lys*

leucocytosis [ˌluːkə(ʊ)saɪ'təʊsɪs] *subst.* increase in numbers of leucocytes in the blood above the normal upper limit (in order to fight an infection) *leukocytos*

leucoderma [ˌluːkə(ʊ)'dɜːmə] *or* **vitiligo** [ˌvɪti'laɪgəʊ] *subst.* condition where white patches appear on the skin *leukodermi, vitiligo*

leucolysin [ˌluːkəʊ'laɪsɪn] *subst.* protein which destroys white blood cells *slags protein som bryter ned vita blodkroppar*

leucoma [lu'kəʊmə] *subst.* white scar of the cornea *leukom, macula cornea, hornhinnefläck*

leuconychia [ˌluːkə(ʊ)'nɪkiə] *subst.* white marks on the fingernails *leucoma unguium, leukonyki*

leucopenia [ˌluːkə(ʊ)'piːniə] *subst.* reduction in the number of leucocytes in the blood, usually as a result of a disease *leuko(cyto)peni*

leucoplakia [ˌluːkə(ʊ)'plækiə] *subst.* condition where white patches form on mucous membranes (such as on the tongue or inside of the mouth) *leukoplaci, leukoplaki*

leucopoiesis [ˌluːkəʊpɔɪ'iːsɪs] *subst.* production of leucocytes *leukopo(i)es*

leucorrhoea [ˌluːkə'rɪə] *or* **whites** [waɪts] *subst.* excessive discharge of white mucus from the vagina *leukorré, fluor albus, vit flytning*

leucotomy [lu'kɒtəmi] *or* **frontal lobotomy** [ˌfrʌnt(ə)l lə(ʊ)'bɒtəmi] *subst.* surgical operation on the brain to treat mental illness by cutting the nerve fibres at the front of the brain *frontal lobotomi*

leukaemia [lu'kiːmiə] *subst.* any of several malignant diseases where an abnormal number of leucocytes form in the blood *leukemi*

> COMMENT: apart from the increase in the number of leucocytes, the symptoms include swelling of the spleen and the lymph glands. There are several forms of leukaemia: the commonest is acute lymphoblastic leukaemia which occurs in children and can be treated by radiotherapy

leukocyt ⇨ **leucocyte, corpuscle, white**

leukocytos ⇨ **leucocytosis**

leukodermi ⇨ **leucoderma**

leukom ⇨ **leucoma**

leukonyki ⇨ **leuconychia**

leukoplaci ⇨ **leucoplakia**

leukorré ⇨ **leucorrhoea**

leva ⇨ **live**

levande ⇨ **alive, live**

levator [lə'veɪtə] *subst.* **(a)** surgical instrument for lifting pieces of fractured bone *levator, benelevatorium* **(b)** muscle which lifts a limb *or* a part of the body *musculus levator*

level ['lev(ə)l] *adj.* horizontal *or* not rising and falling *jämn;* **her temperature has remained level for the last hour**

lever- ⇨ **hepat-, hepatic**

leverbråck ⇨ **hepatocele**

leverceller ⇨ **hepatic**

levercirros ⇨ **cirrhosis of the liver**

leverflundra ⇨ **fluke, liver**

leverfläck ⇨ **chloasma, lentigo, liver**

leverförstoring ⇨ **hepatomegaly**

leverinflammation ⇨ **hepatitis**

levermask ⇨ **fluke, liver**

levern ⇨ **liver**

leverporten ⇨ **porta**

leversmärtor ⇨ **hepatalgia**

leverven ⇨ **hepatic**

levodopa [ˌliːvə(ʊ)'dəʊpə] *or* **L-dopa** [ˌel'dəʊpə] *subst.* drug used in the treatment of Parkinson's disease *levodopa, L-dopa*

levokardi ⇨ **laevocardia**

levra sig ⇨ **clot**

Leydig cells ['laɪdɪgz ˌselz] *or* **interstitial cells** [ˌɪntə'stɪʃ(ə)l ˌselz] *subst.* testosterone-producing cells between the tubules in the testes *interstitialceller, Leydig-celler, Leydigs (leydigska) celler*

l.g.v. [ˌeldʒiː'viː] = LYMPHOGRANULOMA VENEREUM

LH [ˌel'eɪtʃ] = LUTEINIZING HORMONE

liable to ['la(ɪ)əb(ə)l tʊ] *adj.* likely to catch *or* to suffer from *mottaglig för, disponerad för;* **people in sedentary occupations are liable to digestive disorders**

libido [lɪ'biːdəʊ] *subst.* sexual urge *libido, könsdrift; (in psychology)* force which drives the unconscious mind, used especially referring to the sexual urge *libido*

lice [laɪs] *see* LOUSE

licence ['laɪs(ə)ns] *or US* **license** ['laɪs(ə)ns] *subst.* official document which allows someone to do something (such as allowing a doctor to practise *or* a pharmacist to make and sell drugs; *US* a nurse to practise) *legitimation, tillståndsbevis, legitimation;* **he was practising as a doctor without a licence; she is sitting her registered nurse license examination**

license ['laɪs(ə)ns] *vb.* to give someone a licence to do something *ge ngn tillstånd att göra ngt;* **he is licensed to sell dangerous drugs**

licensure ['laɪsənʃə] *subst. US* act of licensing a nurse to practise nursing *legitimering*

licentiate [laɪ'senʃiət] *subst.* person who has been given a licence to practise as a doctor *ung. legitimerad läkare*

lichen ['laɪk(ə)n, 'lɪtʃ(ə)n] *subst.* type of skin disease with thick skin and small lesions *lichen, revorm;* **lichen planus** = skin disease where itchy purple spots appear on the arms and thighs *lichen planus*

lichenification [laɪˌkenɪfɪ'keɪʃ(ə)n] *subst.* thickening of the skin at the site of a lesion *lichenifiering*

lichenoid ['laɪkənɔɪd] *adj.* like a lichen *lichenoid, lavliknande*

lick [lɪk] *vb.* to make the tongue move over something to taste it *or* to wet it *slicka*

lid [lɪd] *subst.* top which covers a container *lock;* **put the lid back on the jar; a medicine bottle with a child-proof lid**

lida (av) ⇨ **suffer**

lidande ⇨ **suffering**

lidokain ⇨ **lignocaine**

lie [laɪ] **1** *subst.* way in which a fetus is present in the womb *läge;* **transverse lie** = position of the fetus across the body of the mother *tvärläge* **2** *vb.* to be in a flat position *ligga;* **the accident victim was lying on the pavement; make sure the patient lies still and does not move** NOTE: **lies - lying - lay - lain**

Lieberkuhn's glands ['liːbəkuːnz ˌglændz] *or* **crypts of Lieberkuhn** [ˌkrɪpts əv 'liːbəkuːn] *subst.* small glands between the bases of the villi in the small intestine *glandulae intestinales, Lieberkühns körtlar*

lie down [ˌlaɪ 'daʊn] *vb.* to put yourself in a flat position *lägga sig ned;* **she lay down on the floor** *or* **on the bed; the doctor asked him to lie down on the couch; when I was lying down he asked me to lift my legs in the air**

lien ⇨ **spleen**

lienal ⇨ **splenic**

lientery ['laɪəntəri] *or* **lienteric diarrhoea** [ˌlaɪən'terɪk ˌda(ɪ)ə'rɪə] *subst.* form of diarrhoea where the food passes through the intestine rapidly without being digested *slags diarré*

life [laɪf] *subst.* being alive *or* not being dead *liv;* **the surgeons saved the patient's life; his life is in danger because the drugs are not available; the victim showed no sign of life; life expectancy** = number of years a person of a certain age is likely to live *förväntad livslängd;* **life insurance** = insurance against death *livförsäkring;* **life-threatening disease** = disease which may kill the patient *livshotande sjukdom*

lifebelt ['laɪfbelt] *subst.* large ring which helps a person to float in water *livbälte*

life-saving equipment ['laɪfˌseɪvɪŋ ɪˌkwɪpmənt] *subst.* equipment (such as boats *or* stretchers *or* first-aid kit) kept ready in case of an emergency *livräddningsredskap*

lift [lɪft] **1** *subst.* **(a)** machine which takes people from one floor to another in a tall building *hiss* **(b)** way of carrying an injured person *lyft;* **fireman's lift** = way of carrying an unconscious person on the shoulders of one carrier with the carrier's right arm passing between or around the patient's legs and holding the patient's right hand, allowing the carrier's left hand to remain free *slags lyft;* **shoulder lift** = way of carrying a heavy person, where the upper part of his body rests on the shoulders of two carriers *australiensiskt lyft* **2** *vb.* to raise to a higher position *lyfta;* to pick something up *ta (plocka) upp;* **this box is so heavy he can't lift it off the floor; she hurt her back lifting a box down from the shelf**

lift ⇨ **hoist**

ligament ['lɪgəmənt] *subst.* thick band of fibrous tissue which connects the bones at a joint and forms the joint capsule *ligament, ledband; see also* EXTRINSIC, INTRINSIC

ligate ['laɪgeɪt, -'-] *vb.* to tie with a ligature, as to tie a blood vessel to stop bleeding *ligera, underbinda*

ligation [laɪ'geɪʃ(ə)n] *subst.* surgical operation to tie up a blood vessel *ligering, underbindning*

ligature ['lɪgətʃə] *subst.* thread used to tie vessels or a lumen, such as a blood vessel to stop bleeding *ligatur, underbindning*

ligera ⇨ **ligate**

ligering ⇨ **ligation**

ligga ⇨ **lie, site**

"ligga" ⇨ **stay**

liggande ⇨ **recumbent, supine**

ligga på magen ⇨ **pronate**

liggkateter ⇨ **indwelling catheter**

liggsår ⇨ **bedsore, pressure**

light [laɪt] **1** *adj.* **(a)** not heavy *lätt;* **she can carry this box easily - it's quite light; he's not fit, so he can only do light work (b)** bright so that one can see well *ljus;* **at six o'clock in the morning it was just getting light (c)** (hair *or* skin) which is nearer white in colour rather than dark *ljus, blond;* **she has a very light complexion; he has light coloured hair**
NOTE:
NOTE: **light - lighter - lightest 2** *subst.* **(a)** thing which shines and helps one to see *ljus;* **the light of the sun makes plants green; there's not enough light in here to take a photo; light adaptation** = changes in the eye to adapt to an abnormally bright or dim light *or* to adapt to normal light after being in darkness *ljusadap(ta)tion;* **light reflex** = reflex of the pupil of the eye which contracts when exposed to bright light *pupill(ar)reaktion, pupillreflex, ljusreflex;* **light therapy** *or* **light treatment** = treatment of a disorder by exposing the patient to light (sunlight *or* infrared light, etc.) *ljusterapi, ljusbehandling;* **light waves** = waves travelling in all directions from a source of light which stimulate the retina and are visible *ljusvågor* **(b)** object (usually a glass bulb) which gives out light *lampa, belysning, ljus;* **switch on the lights - it's getting dark; the car was travelling with no lights; the endoscope has a small light at the end**

lightening ['laɪt(ə)nɪŋ] *subst.* late stage in pregnancy where the fetus goes down into the pelvic cavity *utdrivningsskiftet*

lighting ['laɪtɪŋ] *subst.* way of giving light *belysning, lyse;* **the lighting in the operating theatre has to be very good**

lightly ['laɪtli] *adv.* without using much pressure *lätt;* **the doctor pressed lightly round the swollen area with the tips of his fingers**

lightning pains ['laɪt(ə)nɪŋ ˌpeɪnz] *subst pl.* sharp pains in the legs in a patient suffering from locomotor ataxia *tabes dorsalis, slags sent symtom vid syfilis*

lignocaine ['lɪgnə(ʊ)keɪn] *or US* **lidocaine** ['laɪdə(ʊ)keɪn] *subst.* drug used as a local anaesthetic *lidokain*

lik ⇨ **cadaver, corpse**

likblek ⇨ **livid**

likna ⇨ **equal, take after**

likstelhet ⇨ **rigor**

likstor ⇨ **equal**

liktorn ⇨ **clavus, corn**

lilla ⇨ **little**

lillfingervalken ⇨ **hypothenar**

lillfingret ⇨ **little**

lillgammal ⇨ **precocious**

lillhjärnan ⇨ **cerebellum**

lillhjärns- ⇨ **cerebellar**

lillhjärnsbarken ⇨ **cortex**

lillhjärnsmasken ⇨ **vermis**

lillhjärnsskänkel ⇨ **peduncle**

lillhjärnsstjälk ⇨ **peduncle**

lillhjärnstältet ⇨ **cerebellum**

lilltån ⇨ **little**

lim ⇨ **glue**

limb [lɪm] *subst.* one of the legs or arms *extremitet, lem;* **lower limbs** = legs *benen;* **upper limbs** = arms *armarna;* **limb lead** = electrode attached to an arm *or* leg when taking an electrocardiogram *extremitetsavledning, armavledning, benavledning*

limbic system ['lɪmbɪk ˌsɪstəm] *subst.* system of nerves in the brain, including the hippocampus, the amygdala and the hypothalamus, which are associated with emotions such as fear and anger *limbiska systemet*

limbiska systemet ⇨ **limbic system**

limbless ['lɪmləs] *adj.* without a limb *utan extremitet(er);* **a limbless ex-soldier**

limbus ['lɪmbəs] *subst.* edge, especially the edge of the cornea where it joins the sclera *limbus, rand, kant*

liminal ['lɪmɪn(ə)l] *adj.* (stimulus) at the lowest level which can be sensed *tröskel-*

limit ['lɪmɪt] **1** *subst.* furthest point *or* place beyond which you cannot go *tröskel, gräns(värde);* **there is a speed limit of 30 miles per hour in towns; there is no age limit for joining the club** = people of all ages can join *det finns ingen åldersgräns för medlemskap i klubben;* **45 is the upper age limit for childbearing** = 45 is the oldest age at which a woman can have a child **2** *vb.* to set a limit to something *begränsa, sätta en gräns;* **you must limit your intake of coffee to two cups a day**

limp [lɪmp] **1** *subst.* way of walking, when one leg is shorter than the other *or* where one leg hurts *haltande, hälta;* **he walks with a limp; the operation has left him with a limp** **2** *vb.* to walk awkwardly, because one leg is shorter than the other *or* because one leg hurts *halta, linka;* **he was still limping three weeks after the accident**

linctus ['lɪŋ(k)təs] *subst.* sweet cough medicine *(söt) hostmedicin*

lindra ⇨ **alleviate, deaden, ease, relieve, soften, soothe**

lindrande ⇨ **palliative, soothing**

lindrig ⇨ **mild, minor, slight**

lindring ⇨ **relief**

line [laɪn] **1** *subst.* ridge *or* mark which connects two points *linje* **2** *vb.* to provide a lining *fodra, beklä;* **the intestine is lined with mucus; the inner ear is lined with fine hairs**

linea ['lɪniə] *subst.* thin line *linea, linje;* **linea alba** = tendon running from the breastbone to the pubic area, to which abdominal muscles are attached *linea alba;* **linea nigra** = dark line on the skin from the navel to the pubis which appears during the later months of pregnancy *linea nigra*

lingual ['lɪŋgw(ə)l] *adj.* referring to the tongue *lingual, tung-;* **lingual artery** = artery which supplies blood to the tongue *arteria lingualis, tungartären;* **lingual tonsil** = lymphoid tissue on the top surface of the back of the tongue ⇨ *illustration* TONGUE *lymfvävnad i tungans bakre övre del;* **lingual vein** = vein which takes blood from the tongue *vena lingualis, tungvenen*

liniment ['lɪnəmənt] *subst.* oily liquid used to rub on the skin, acting as a counterirritant *liniment*

liniment ⇨ **liniment, rub**

lining ['laɪnɪŋ] *subst.* substance *or* tissue on the inside of an organ *invändig beklädnad;* **the thick lining of the aorta**

linje ⇨ **line, linea**

link [lɪŋk] *vb.* to join things together *länka (koppla) ihop, förena;* **the ankle bone links the bones of the lower leg to the calcaneus**

linka ⇨ **limp**

linkage ['lɪŋkɪdʒ] *subst. (of genes)* being close together on a chromosome, and therefore likely to be inherited together *linkage*

linoleic acid [ˌlɪnəʊˌliːɪk 'æsɪd] *subst.* one of the essential fatty acids which cannot be synthesized and has to be taken into the body from food (such as vegetable oil) *linolsyra*

linolenic acid [ˌlɪnəʊˌlenɪk 'æsɪd] *subst.* one of the essential fatty acids *linolensyra, linoljesyra*

linolensyra ⇨ **linolenic acid**

linoljesyra ⇨ **linolenic acid**

linolsyra ⇨ **linoleic acid**

lins ⇨ **lens**

lins- ⇨ **lenticular, phaco-, phako-**

linsformad ⇨ **lenticular**

lint [lɪnt] *subst.* thick flat cotton wadding, used as a surgical dressing *ung. absorptionsförband;* **she put some lint on the wound before bandaging it**
NOTE: no plural

liothyronine [ˌlaɪəʊ'θaɪ(ə)rəʊniːn] *subst.* hormone produced by the thyroid gland, used as a rapid-acting treatment for hypothyroidism *liot(h)yronin, trijodtyronin, T3*

lip [lɪp] *subst.* (i) one of two fleshy muscular parts round the edge of the mouth *läpp;* (ii) flesh round the edge of an opening *vävnad runt öppnings kant;* **her lips were cracked from the cold**
NOTE: for terms referring to lips, see words beginning with **cheil-, lab-, labi-**

lipaemia [lɪ'piːmiə] *subst.* excessive amount of fat (such as cholesterol) in the blood *lipemi*

lipas ⇨ **lipase, steapsin**

lipase ['lɪpeɪz] *subst.* enzyme which breaks down fats in the intestine *lipas*

lipemi ⇨ **lipaemia**

lipid ['lɪpɪd] *subst.* fat *or* fatlike substance which exists in human tissue and forms an important part of the human diet *lipid;* **lipid metabolism** = chemical changes where lipids are broken down into fatty acids *fettomsättning, fettmetabolism*

> COMMENT: lipids are not water soluble. They float in the blood and can attach themselves to the walls of arteries causing atherosclerosis

lipidosis [ˌlɪpɪ'dəʊsɪs] *subst.* disorder of lipid metabolism, where subcutaneous fat is not present in some parts of the body *lipidos*

lipochondrodystrophy [ˌlɪpəʊˌkɒndrəʊ'dɪstrəfi] *subst.* congenital disorder of the lipid metabolism, the bones and main organs, causing mental deficiency and physical deformity *lipokondrodystrofi*

lipodystrophy [ˌlɪpəʊ'dɪstrəfi] *subst.* disorder of lipid metabolism *lipodystrofi*

lipogenesis [ˌlɪpəʊ'dʒenəsɪs] *subst.* production *or* making deposits of fat *lipogenes*

lipoid ['lɪpɔɪd] *subst. & adj.* compound lipid *or* fatty substance (such as cholesterol) which is like a lipid *lipoid, fettliknande (ämne)*

lipoidosis [ˌlɪpɔɪ'dəʊsɪs] *subst.* group of diseases with reticuloendothelial hyperplasia and abnormal deposits of lipoids in the cells *lipoidos*

lipokondrodystrofi ⇨ **lipochondrodystrophy**

lipolysis [lɪ'pɒləsɪs] *subst.* process of breaking down fat by lipase *lipolys*

lipolytic enzyme [ˌlɪpə(ʊ)'lɪtɪk ˌenzaɪm] = LIPASE

lipoma [lɪ'pəʊmə] *subst.* benign tumour formed of fat *lipom, fettsvulst*

lipomatosis [ˌlɪpəʊmə'təʊsɪs] *subst.* excessive deposit of fat in the tissues in tumour-like masses *lipomatos, fettsot*

lipoprotein [ˌlɪpəʊ'prəʊtiːn] *subst.* protein which combines with lipids and carries them in the bloodstream and lymph system *lipoprotein*

liposarcoma [ˌlɪpəʊsɑː'kəʊmə] *subst.* lipoma and sarcoma *liposarkom*

lipotrophic [ˌlɪpəʊ'trɒfɪk] *adj.* (substance) which increases the amount of fat present in the tissues *lipotrofi*

Lippes loop ['lɪpəz ˌluːp] *subst.* type of intrauterine device *Lippes slynga*

lipping ['lɪpɪŋ] *subst.* condition where bone tissue grows over other bones *tillstånd där benvävnad växer över ben*

lipuri ⇨ **chyluria, lipuria**

lipuria [lɪ'pjʊəriə] *subst.* presence of fat *or* oily emulsion in the urine *lipuri, chyluri*

liquid ['lɪkwɪd] *adj. & subst.* matter (like water) which is not solid and is not a gas *flytande, vätska;* **sick patients need a lot of liquids; he was put on a liquid diet; liquid paraffin** = oil used as a laxative *paraffinum liquidum, flytande paraffin, paraffinolja*

liquor ['lɪkə] *subst. (in pharmacy)* solution, usually aqueous, of a pure substance *vattenlösning*

lisp [lɪsp] **1** *subst.* speech defect where the patient has difficulty in pronouncing 's' sounds and replaces them with 'th' *läspning* **2** *vb.* to talk with a lisp *läspa*

list [lɪst] **1** *subst.* number of things written down one after the other *lista;* **there is a list of names in alphabetical order; the names of duty nurses are on the list in the office; he's on the danger list** = he is critically ill *hans tillstånd är kritiskt (livshotande), han är mycket allvarligt sjuk;* **she's off the danger list** = she is no longer critically ill *hennes tillstånd är inte längre kritiskt (livshotande), hon är inte längre allvarligt sjuk* **2** *vb.* to write something in the form of a list *ta med (ta upp, sätta upp, skriva upp) på lista, lista;* **the drugs are listed at the back of the book; the telephone numbers of the emergency services are listed in the yellow pages**

listen ['lɪs(ə)n] *vb.* to pay attention to something heard *lyssna;* **the doctor listened to the patient's chest**

Listeria [lɪ'stɪəriə] *subst.* genus of bacteria found on domestic animals, which can cause uterine infection or meningitis *Listeria*

listless ['lɪstləs] *adj.* weak and tired *apatisk, slö, slapp*

listlessness ['lɪstləsnəs] *subst.* being generally weak and tired *apati, slöhet, slapphet*

liten ⇨ **little, minor, minute, small**

liter ⇨ **litre**

lith- [lɪθ, 'lɪθ, ˌ-] *prefix* meaning stone *lit(h)-, sten-*

lithaemia [lɪ'θiːmiə] *or* **uricacidaemia** [ˌjʊərɪkˌæsə'diːmiə] *subst.* abnormal amount of uric acid in the blood *urikacidemi, förhöjd urinsyrehalt i blodet*

lithiasis [lɪ'θaɪəsɪs] *subst.* forming of stones in an organ *lithiasis, stensjukdom*

litholapaxy [lɪ'θɒləpæksi] *or* **lithotrity** [lɪ'θɒtrɪti] *subst.* evacuation of pieces of a stone in the bladder after crushing it with a lithotrite *lit(h)otripsi, stenkrossning*

lithonephrotomy [ˌlɪθəʊnə'frɒtəmi] *subst.* surgical removal of a stone in the kidney *nefrolitotomi, nefrolitektomi*

lithotomy [lɪ'θɒtəmi] *subst.* surgical removal of a stone from the bladder *lit(h)otomi;* **lithotomy position** = position of a patient for some medical examinations, where the patient lies on his back with his legs flexed and his thighs on his abdomen *litotomiläge, gynekologläge*

lithotrite ['lɪθəʊtraɪt] *subst.* surgical instrument which crushes a stone in the bladder *lit(h)otriptor, lit(h)oklast*

lithotrity [lɪ'θɒtrɪti] = LITHOLAPAXY

lithuresis [ˌlɪθju'riːsɪs] *subst.* passage of small stones from the bladder during urination *passage av små stenar från blåsan vid urinering*

lithuria [lɪ'ɵjʊəriə] *subst.* presence of excessive amounts of uric acid *or* urates in the urine *urin med stora mängder urinsyra el. urat*

litmus ['lɪtməs] *subst.* substance which turns red in acid and blue in alkali *lackmus;* **litmus paper** = small piece of paper impregnated with litmus, used to test for acidity *or* alkalinity *lackmuspapper*

litotomiläge ⇨ **lithotomy**

litre ['li:tə] *subst.* measurement of liquids (equal to 1.76 pints) *liter, l*
NOTE: written l with figures; **2.5 l**

little ['lɪt(ə)l] *adj.* **(a)** small *or* not big *liten, lilla, lill-, små;* **little finger** *or* **little toe** = smallest finger on the hand *or* smallest toe on the foot *lillfingret, digitus minimus, lilltån;* **he has a ring on his little finger; her little toe was crushed by the door (b)** not much *litet, inte mycket;* **she eats very little bread**
NOTE: **little - less - least**

Little's disease ['lɪt(ə)lz dɪˌzi:z] = SPASTIC DIPLEGIA

liv ⇨ **life**

live 1 [laɪv] *adj.* **(a)** living *or* not dead *levande;* **graft using live tissue (b)** carrying electricity *strömförande, spänningsförande;* **he was killed when he touched a live wire 2** [lɪv] *vb.* to be alive *leva;* **he is very ill, and the doctor doesn't think he will live much longer**

livedo [lɪ'vi:dəʊ] *subst.* discoloured spots on the skin *livedo*

liver ['lɪvə] *subst.* large gland in the upper part of the abdomen *hepar, levern;* **she has been suffering from liver trouble; he has been having treatment for a liver infection; liver extract** = food made from animal livers, used as an injection to treat anaemia *leverextrakt;* **liver fluke** = parasitic flatworm which can infest the liver *levermask, leverflundra;* **liver spot** = little brown spot on the skin ⇨ *illustration* DIGESTIVE SYSTEM *leverfläck* NOTE: for other terms referring to the liver, see words beginning with **hepat-**

> COMMENT: the liver is situated in the top part of the abdomen on the right side of the body next to the stomach. It is the largest gland in the body, weighing almost 2 kg. Blood carrying nutrients from the intestines enters the liver by the hepatic portal vein; the nutrients are removed and the blood returned to the heart through the hepatic vein. The liver is the major detoxicating organ in the body; it destroys harmful organisms in the blood, produces clotting agents, secretes bile, stores glycogen and metabolizes proteins, carbohydrates and fats. Diseases affecting the liver include hepatitis and cirrhosis; the symptom of liver disease is often jaundice

livet ⇨ **waist**

livid ['lɪvɪd] *adj.* (skin) with a blue colour because of being bruised *or* because of asphyxiation *livid, blekblå, blå, likblek*

livlös ⇨ **dead**

livmoderframfall ⇨ **hysteroptosis, metroptosis, procidentia**

livmoderhals- ⇨ **cervic-, cervical**

livmoderhalsen ⇨ **cervix**

livmoderhålan ⇨ **uterine**

livmoderinlägg ⇨ **loop**

livmodermunnen ⇨ **vaginal**

livmodern ⇨ **uterus, womb**

livmoder(s)- ⇨ **hyster-, hystero-, metr-, uter-, uterine**

livmoderslemhinnan ⇨ **endometrium**

livmoderväggen ⇨ **myometrium**

livräddningsredskap ⇨ **life-saving equipment**

livsduglig ⇨ **viable**

livsduglighet ⇨ **viability**

livsnödvändig ⇨ **essential, vital**

livsträdet ⇨ **arbor vitae**

ljud ⇨ **sound**

ljud- ⇨ **acoustic**

ljudspringan ⇨ **laryngeal, rima**

ljumsk- ⇨ **inguinal**

ljumskbandet ⇨ **inguinal**

ljumskbråck ⇨ **inguinal**

ljumsken ⇨ **groin**

ljumskgranulom ➪ **granuloma**

ljumskkanalen ➪ **inguinal**

ljumskregionen ➪ **inguinal**

ljus ➪ **light, fair**

ljus- ➪ **phot-**

ljusadapterat seende ➪ **photopic vision**

ljusalstrad ➪ **photogenic**

ljusalstrande ➪ **photogenic**

ljusbehandling ➪ **light**

ljusbrytning ➪ **refraction**

ljushårig ➪ **fair**

ljuskänslig ➪ **photosensitive**

ljuskänslighet ➪ **photophobia, photosensitivity**

ljusreflex ➪ **pupillary**

ljusskygghet ➪ **photophobia**

ljusstråle ➪ **beam**

ljusterapi ➪ **light**

ljusvågor ➪ **light**

lm ➪ **lumen**

Loa loa [ˌləʊə 'ləʊə] *subst.* tropical threadworm which digs under the skin, especially into the eyes, causing loa loa and loiasis *Loa-loa*

loa loa [ˌləʊə 'ləʊə] *subst.* tropical disease of the eyes caused when a threadworm **Loa loa** enters the eye *loiasis*

lobar ['ləʊbə] *adj.* referring to a lobe *lobar, lobär;* **lobar bronchi** *or* **secondary bronchi** = air passages supplying a lobe of a lung *lobbronkerna;* **lobar pneumonia** = infection in one or more lobes of the lung *pneumonia lobaris, lobär lunginflammation*

lobbronkerna ➪ **lobar**

lobe [ləʊb] *subst.* (i) rounded section of an organ, such as the brain *or* lung *or* liver *lob;* (ii) soft fleshy part at the bottom of the ear *orsnibb,* (iii) cusp on the crown of a tooth *kusp, upphöjning på tandkrona;* **frontal lobe** = front lobe of each cerebral hemisphere *lobus frontalis, frontalloben, pannloben;* **occipital lobe** = lobe at the back of each cerebral hemisphere *lobus occipitalis, occipitalloben, nackloben;* **parietal lobe** = lobe at the side and to the top of each cerebral hemisphere *lobus parietalis, parietalloben, hjässloben;* **temporal lobe** = lobe above the ear in each cerebral hemisphere ➪ *illustration* LUNGS *lobus temporalis, temporalloben, tinningloben*

lobectomy [ləʊ'bektəmi] *subst.* surgical removal of one of the lobes of an organ such as the lung *lobektomi*

lobotomy [lə(ʊ)'bɒtəmi] *or* **frontal lobotomy** ['frʌnt(ə)l lə(ʊ)'bɒtəmi] *subst.* surgical operation to treat mental disease by cutting into a lobe of the brain to cut the nerve fibres *(frontal) lobotomi*

lobule ['lɒbju:l] *subst.* small section of a lobe in the lung, formed of acini *lobulus*

lobulus ➪ **lobule**

lobär ➪ **lobar**

local ['ləʊk(ə)l] *adj.* referring to a separate place *lokal;* confined to one part *lokal-;* **local anesthesia** = loss of feeling in a single part of the body *lokalanestesi, lokalbedövning;* **local anaesthetic** *or* **local** = anaesthetic which removes the feeling in a certain part of the body only *lokalanestetikum, lokalbedövningsmedel;* **he had a local for the operation for an ingrowing toenail; the surgeon removed the growth under local anaesthetic**

> QUOTE few parts of the body are inaccessible to modern catheter techniques, which are all performed under local anaesthesia
> **British Medical Journal**

localize ['ləʊkəlaɪz] *vb.* to locate something *or* to find where something is *lokalisera, leta reda på*

> QUOTE these patients may be candidates for embolization of their bleeding point, particularly as angiography will often be necessary to localize that point
> **British Medical Journal**

localized ['ləʊkəlaɪzd] *adj.* (infection) which occurs in one part of the body only *lokal, begränsad* NOTE: the opposite is **generalized**

locate [lə(ʊ)'keɪt, '--] *vb.* (i) to find where something is *lokalisera, leta reda på;* (ii) to be situated in a place *vara belägen (placerad)*

> QUOTE ultrasonography is helpful in determining sites of incompetence and in locating the course of veins in more obese patients
> **British Journal of Hospital Medicine**

> QUOTE the target cells for adult myeloid leukaemia are located in the bone marrow, and there is now evidence that childhood leukaemias also arise in the bone marrow
> **British Medical Journal**

lochia ['ləʊkiə] *subst.* discharge from the vagina after childbirth or abortion *lockier, avslag*

lochial ['ləʊkiəl] *adj.* referring to lochia *lockial, avslags-*

lock [lɒk] *vb.* **(a)** to close a door *or* box, etc. so that it has to be opened with a key *stänga;* **the drugs have to be kept in a locked cupboard (b)** to fix in a position *låsa, fixera;* **locked knee** = displaced piece of cartilage of the knee *or* condition where a piece of the cartilage in the knee slips (the symptom is a sharp pain, and the knee remains permanently bent) *låst knä (ofta efter meniskskada);* **locking of the knee** = condition where the knee joint suddenly becomes rigid *låsningsfenomen*

lock ⇨ **cap, cover, lid**

lockial ⇨ **lochial**

lockier ⇨ **lochia**

lockjaw ['lɒkdʒɔː] = TETANUS

locomotion [ˌləʊkə'məʊʃ(ə)n] *subst.* being able to move *rörelseförmåga*

locomotor ataxia [ˌləʊkəʊˌməʊtər ə'tæksiə] = TABES DORSALIS

loculus ['lɒkjʊləs] *subst.* small space (in an organ) *liten plats, litet ställe*

locum (tenens) ['ləʊkəm ('tenəns)] *subst.* doctor who takes the place of another doctor for a time *vikarie*

locus ['ləʊkəs] *subst.* area *or* point (of infection *or* disease) *locus, plats, ställe, härd;* position on a chromosome where a gene is present *locus*

lodge [lɒdʒ] *vb.* to stay *or* to stick *fastna, bo;* **the piece of bone lodged in her throat; the larvae of the tapeworm lodge in the walls of the intestine**

logoped ⇨ **speech**

loiasis [ləʊ'aɪəsɪs] *subst.* infestation with the threadworm Loa loa, which can infect the eye *loiasis*

loin [lɔɪn] *subst.* lower back part of the body above the buttocks *länd*

lokal ⇨ **local, localized, topical**

lokal- ⇨ **local**

lokalanestesi ⇨ **local**

lokalanestetikum ⇨ **local**

lokalbedövning ⇨ **local**

lokalbedövningsmedel ⇨ **local**

lokalbehandling, läkemedel för ⇨ **topical**

lokalisera ⇨ **localize, locate, site**

lokaliserad ⇨ **situated**

lokal vävnadsdöd ⇨ **necrosis**

longitudinal [ˌlɒn(d)ʒɪ'tjuːdɪn(ə)l] *adj.* lengthwise *or* in the direction of the long axis of the body *longitudinell, längsgående;* **longitudinal arch** = part of the sole of the foot which curves upwards, running along the length of the foot from the heel to the ball of the foot *hålfoten, fotvalvet*

longsighted [ˌlɒŋ'saɪtɪd] *adj.* able to see clearly things which are far away, but not things which are close *hypermetrop, långsynt, översynt*

longsightedness [ˌlɒŋ'saɪtɪdnəs] = HYPERMETROPIA

long-stay [ˌlɒŋ'steɪ] *adj.* staying a long time in hospital *långvårds-;* **patients in long-stay units** *or* **long-stay patients**

longus ['lɒŋgəs] *see* MUSCLE

look after [ˌluk 'ɑːftə] *vb.* to take care of *or* to attend to the needs of (a patient) *ta hand om, vårda;* **the nurses looked after him very well** *or* **he was very well looked after in hospital; she is off work looking after her children who have mumps; some patients need a lot of looking after** = they need continual attention *vissa patienter kräver mycket omvårdnad*

loop [luːp] *subst.* **(a)** curve *or* bend in a line, especially one of the particular curves in a fingerprint *slinga, slynga, krök;* **loop of Henle** = curved tube which forms the main part of a nephron in the kidney *Henles slynga;* **blind loop syndrome** *or* **stagnant loop syndrome** = condition which occurs in cases of diverticulosis or of Crohn's disease, with steatorrhoea, abdominal pain and megaloblastic anaemia *blind loop syndrom* **(b)** curved piece of wire placed in the uterus to prevent contraception *spiral, livmoderinlägg*

loose [luːs] *adj.* not fixed *or* not attached *or* not tight *lös;* **one of my molars has come loose**
NOTE: **loose - looser - loosest**

loosely [ˈluːsli] *adv.* not tightly *löst;* **the bandage was loosely tied round her wrist**

loosen [ˈluːs(ə)n] *vb.* to make loose *lossa (på), lösa (upp);* **loosen the tie round the victim's neck**

loppa ⇨ **flea, Pulex**

lordosis [lɔːˈdəʊsɪs] *subst.* excessive forward curving of the lower part of the spine *lordos, svankrygg; see also* KYPHOSIS

lose [luːz] *vb.* not to have something any longer *förlora;* **he lost the ability to walk; when you have a cold you can easily lose all sense of smell and taste; she has lost weight since last summer** = she has got thinner *hon har gått ned i vikt (magrat) sedan förra sommaren*
NOTE: **loses - losing - lost - has lost**

loss [lɒs] *subst.* not having something any more *förlust, nedsättning;* **loss of appetite** = not having as much appetite as before *aptitförlust, nedsatt aptit;* **loss of sensation** = not being able to feel the limbs any more *förlust av känseln;* **loss of weight** *or* **weight loss** = not weighing as much as before *viktminskning*

lotion [ˈləʊʃ(ə)n] *subst.* medicinal liquid used to rub on the skin *or* to use on the body *lotion, lösning;* **he bathed his eyes in a mild antiseptic lotion; use this lotion on your eczema**

louse [laʊs] *subst.* small insect of the **Pediculus** genus, which sucks blood and lives on the skin as a parasite on animals and humans *lus* NOTE: the plural is **lice**

> COMMENT: there are several forms of louse: the commonest are the body louse, the crab louse and the head louse

low [ləʊ] *adj. & adv.* near the bottom *or* towards the bottom *låg, lågt liggande;* not high *låg;* **he hit his head on the low ceiling; the temperature is too low here for oranges to grow; low blood pressure** *or* **hypotension** condition where the pressure of the blood is abnormally low *hypotension, hypotoni, lågt blodtryck;* **low-calorie diet** = diet with few calories (to help a person to lose weight) *kalorifattig kost;* **lower jaw** = bottom jaw *mandibula, underkäken;* **lower limbs** = legs *benen;* **low-fat diet** = diet with little animal fat (to help skin conditions) *fettfattig kost;* **low-risk patient** = patient not likely to catch a certain disease *lågriskpatient; see also* NEURONE NOTE: opposite is **upper**

lower [ˈləʊə] *vb.* to make something go down *sänka;* to reduce *reducera, minska;* **they covered the patient with wet cloth to try to lower his body temperature**

lozenge [ˈlɒzɪn(d)ʒ] *subst.* sweet medicinal tablet *tablett, pastill;* **she was sucking a cough lozenge**

LPN [ˌelpiːˈen] *US* = LICENSED PRACTICAL NURSE

LRCP [ˌelɑːsiːˈpiː] = LICENTIATE OF THE ROYAL COLLEGE OF PHYSICIANS

LSD [ˌelesˈdiː] *or* **lysergic acid diethylamide** [laɪˌsɜːdʒɪk ˈæsɪd daɪˈeθɪləmaɪd] *subst.* powerful hallucinogenic drug *LSD, lysergsyradietylamid*

lubb-dupp [lʌbˈdʌp] *subst.* two sounds made by the heart, which represent each cardiac cycle when heard through a stethoscope *hjärttonerna*

lubricant [ˈluːbrɪk(ə)nt] *subst.* fluid which lubricates *smörjmedel*

lubricate [ˈluːbrɪkeɪt] *vb.* to make smooth with oil *or* liquid *smörja*

lucid [ˈluːsɪd] *adj.* with a clearly working mind *klar, redig;* **in spite of the pain, he was still lucid**

lucidum [ˈluːsɪdəm] *see* STRATUM

lucka ⇨ **gap**

ludd ⇨ **villus**

luddig ⇨ **villous**

luden ⇨ **villous**

Ludwig's angina [ˈluːdvɪgz ænˌdʒaɪnə] *subst.* cellulitis of the mouth and some parts of the neck which causes the neck to swell and may obstruct the airway *angina Ludovici, Ludwigs angina*

lues ['lu:i:z] *subst.* former name for syphilis *or* the plague *lues, syfilis*

luft ⇨ **air**

luft- ⇨ **pneum-**

luftbråck ⇨ **pneumatocele**

luftemboli ⇨ **air**

luftförorening ⇨ **pollution**

lufthunger ⇨ **air**

luftledning ⇨ **conduction**

luftrör ⇨ **bronchus**

luftrören ⇨ **bronchi, bronchial**

luftrörsastma ⇨ **asthmatic**

luftrörskatarr ⇨ **bronchitis**

luftrörssnitt ⇨ **tracheostomy**

luftsjuk ⇨ **airsick**

luftsjuka ⇨ **airsickness**

luftskalle ⇨ **encephalography, ventriculography**

luftslukande ⇨ **aerophagy**

luftstrupen ⇨ **windpipe**

luftstrups- ⇨ **tracheal**

luftstrupskatarr ⇨ **tracheitis**

lufttryck ⇨ **atmospheric pressure**

luftväg ⇨ **airway, air**

luftvägshinder ⇨ **airway**

lugn ⇨ **calm, rest**

lugnande ⇨ **ataractic, soothing**

lugnande medel ⇨ **depressant, relaxative, sedative, tranquillizer**

lukt ⇨ **odour, scent**

lukt- ⇨ **olfactory**

lukta ⇨ **smell**

luktcentrum ⇨ **cortex**

luktloben ⇨ **olfactory**

luktnerven ⇨ **olfactory**

luktsalt ⇨ **smelling salts**

lukt(sinnet) ⇨ **olfaction, smell**

lumbago [lʌm'beɪgəʊ] *subst.* pain in the lower back *lumbago, ryggskott, ont i ryggen;* **she has been suffering from lumbago for years; he has had an attack of lumbago**

> COMMENT: mainly due to rheumatism, but can be brought on by straining the back muscles or bad posture

lumbal ⇨ **lumbar**

lumbalpunktion ⇨ **spinal**

lumbar ['lʌmbə] *subst.* referring to the lower part of the back *lumbal, länd-;* **lumbar arteries** = four arteries which supply blood to the back muscles and skin *arteriae lumbales;* **lumbar cistern** = subarachnoid space in the spinal cord, where the dura mater ends, filled with cerebrospinal fluid *vätskefyllt rum under spindelvävshinnan vid ryggmärgens bas;* **lumbar enlargement** = wider part of the spinal cord in the lower spine, where the nerves of the lower limbs are attached *punkt där ryggmärgens nedre tjockare del börjar;* **lumbar plexus** = point where several nerves which supply the thighs and abdomen join together, lying in the upper psoas muscle *plexus lumbalis, ländplexus, ländflätan;* **lumbar puncture** *see* PUNCTURE; **lumbar region** = two parts of the abdomen on either side of the umbilical region *korsryggen;* **lumbar vertebrae** = five vertebrae between the thoracic vertebrae and the sacrum *vertebrae lumbales, ländkotorna*

lumbosacral [ˌlʌmbəʊ'seɪkr(ə)l] *adj.* referring to the lumbar vertebrae and the sacrum *lumbosakral;* **lumbosacral joint** = joint at the bottom of the back between the lumbar vertebrae and the sacrum *articulatio lumbosacralis*

lumbricus [lʌm'braɪkəs] *subst.* earthworm *daggmask*

lumen ['lu:mɪn] *subst.* **(a)** SI unit of light emitted per second *lumen, lm* **(b)** (i) inside width of a passage in the body *or* of an instrument (such as an endoscope) *lumen, hål, kanal;* (ii) hole at the end of an instrument (such as an endoscope) *lumen, hål, öppning*

lump [lʌmp] *subst.* mass of hard tissue which rises on the surface *or* under the surface of the skin *bulnad, bula, knöl;* **he has a lump where he hit his head on the low door; she noticed a lump in her right breast and went to see the doctor**

lunate (bone) ['lu:neɪt (ˌbəʊn)] *subst.* one of the eight small carpal bones in the wrist ⇨ *illustration* HAND *os lunatum, månbenet*

lung [lʌŋ] *subst.* one of two organs of respiration in the body into which air is sucked when a person breathes *pulmo, lungan;* **the doctor listened to his chest to see if his lungs were all right; lung cancer** = cancer in the lung *lungcancer;* **lung trouble** = disorder in the lung, such as bronchitis *or* pneumonia, etc. *lungbesvär, lungsjukdom;* **artificial lung** = machine through which the patient's deoxygenated blood is passed to absorb oxygen to take back to the bloodstream *hjärtlungmaskin;* **farmer's lung** = type of asthma caused by an allergy to rotting hay *slags astma;* **shock lung** = serious condition after a blow, where the patient's lungs fail to work *chocklunga* NOTE: for other terms referring to the lungs, see words beginning with **bronch-, pneumo-, pneumon-, pulmo-, pulmon-**

COMMENT: the two lungs are situated in the chest cavity, protected by the rib cage. The heart lies between the lungs. The right lung has three lobes, the left lung only two. Air goes down into the lungs through the trachea and bronchi. It passes to the alveoli where its oxygen is deposited in the blood in exchange for waste carbon dioxide which is exhaled (gas exchange). Lung cancer can be caused by smoking tobacco, and is commonest in people who are heavy smokers

lung- ⇨ **pneum-, pneumon-, pulmo-, pulmonary**

lungan ⇨ **lung**

lungbesvär ⇨ **lung**

lungblåsa ⇨ **air**

lungbråck ⇨ **pneumatocele**

lungcancer ⇨ **lung**

lungemboli ⇨ **pulmonary**

lungemfysem ⇨ **emphysema**

lunginflammation ⇨ **pneumonia**

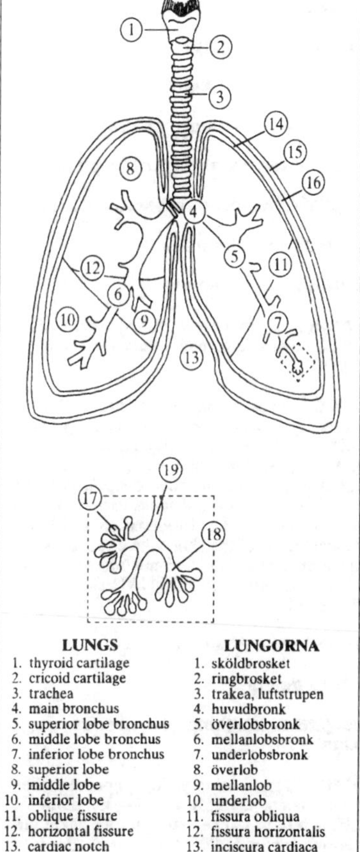

LUNGS	LUNGORNA
1. thyroid cartilage	1. sköldbrosket
2. cricoid cartilage	2. ringbrosket
3. trachea	3. trakea, luftstrupen
4. main bronchus	4. huvudbronk
5. superior lobe bronchus	5. överlobsbronk
6. middle lobe bronchus	6. mellanlobsbronk
7. inferior lobe bronchus	7. underlobsbronk
8. superior lobe	8. överlob
9. middle lobe	9. mellanlob
10. inferior lobe	10. underlob
11. oblique fissure	11. fissura obliqua
12. horizontal fissure	12. fissura horizontalis
13. cardiac notch	13. inciscura cardiaca
14. visceral pleura	14. lungsäckens inre blad
15. parietal pleura	15. lungsäckens yttre blad
16. pleural cavity	16. pleurahålan
17. alveolus	17. alveol, lungblåsa
18. alveolar duct	18. alveolgång
19. bronchiole	19. bronkiol

lungkretsloppet ⇨ **circulation (of the blood), pulmonary**

lungpest ⇨ **pneumonic plague**

lungpulsådrorna ⇨ **pulmonary**

lungsiktig ⇨ **consumptive**

lungsjukdom ⇨ **lung, respiratory**

lungsjukdom, obstruktiv ⇨ **obstructive**

lungsot ➪ **consumption, phthisis**

lungspetsen ➪ **apex**

lungsäcken ➪ **pleura**

lungsäcks- ➪ **pleur-, pleural**

lungsäcksinflammation ➪ **pleurisy**

lungtuberkulos ➪ **tuberculosis (TB)**

lungven ➪ **pulmonary**

lungödem ➪ **pulmonary**

lunula ['lu:njʊlə] *subst.* curved white mark at the base of a fingernail *lunula, måne (på nagel)*

lupus ['lu:pəs] *subst.* type of chronic skin disease *lupus;* **lupus erythematosus acutus (LE)** = one of several collagen diseases *or* a form of lupus, involving the heart and blood vessels *lupus erythematosus el. erythematodes (disseminatus), systemisk lupus erythematosus (erythematodes), SLE;* **lupus vulgaris** = form of tuberculosis of the skin, where red spots appear on the face and become infected *lupus vulgaris; see also* DISSEMINATED, SYSTEMIC

lus ➪ **louse, Pediculus**

lust ➪ **desire**

lustgas ➪ **laughing gas, nitrous oxide**

lutein ['lu:tiɪn] *subst.* yellow pigment in the corpus luteum *lutein;* **luteinizing hormone (LH)** *or* **interstitial cell stimulating hormone** = hormone produced by the pituitary gland, which stimulates the formation of the corpus luteum in females and of testosterone in males *interstitial cell stimulating hormone, ICSH, luteiniserande hormon, LH*

luteum ['lu:tiəm] *subst.* **corpus luteum** = cells which form in the ovary at the place where an ovum has been produced *corpus luteum, gulkropp; see also* MACULA LUTEA

lux [lʌks] *subst.* SI unit of brightness of light shining on a surface *lux, lx*

luxation [lʌk'seɪʃ(ə)n] *subst.* dislocation *or* condition where a bone is displaced from its normal position *luxation, dislokation, urledvridning*

luxera ➪ **dislocate**

lx ➪ **lux**

lyckad ➪ **successful**

lyckas ➪ **succeed**

lyda ➪ **obey**

lyft ➪ **lift**

lyfta ➪ **lift, raise**

lyftapparat ➪ **hoist**

lymf- ➪ **lymphatic**

lymfa ➪ **lymph (fluid), plasma**

lymfadenit ➪ **lymphadenitis**

lymfadenom ➪ **lymphadenoma**

lymfangiografi ➪ **lymphangiography**

lymfangiom ➪ **lymphangioma**

lymfangiosarkom ➪ **lymphangiosarcoma**

lymfangit ➪ **lymphangitis**

lymfaplasi ➪ **Milroy's disease**

lymfatisk ➪ **lymphatic**

lymffollikel ➪ **lymphatic**

lymfgång ➪ **lymphatic**

lymfkapillärer ➪ **lymphatic**

lymfkärl ➪ **lymphatic**

lymfkärlen ➪ **lymphatic, lymph (fluid)**

lymfkärlsinflammation ➪ **lymphangitis**

lymfkärlssvulst ➪ **lymphangioma**

lymfkörtelbesvär ➪ **lymphadenopathy**

lymfkörtelinflammation ➪ **lymphadenitis**

lymfkörtlarna ➪ **lymphatic, lymph (fluid)**

lymfoblast ➪ **lymphoblast**

lymfocyt ➪ **lymphocyte**

lymfocytos ➪ **lymphocytosis**

lymfografi ⇨ **lymphography**

lymfom ⇨ **lymphadenoma, lymphoma**

lymfopeni ⇨ **lymphopenia**

lymforragi ⇨ **lymphorrhagia**

lymforré ⇨ **lymphorrhagia**

lymfosarkom ⇨ **lymphosarcoma**

lymfvätska ⇨ **plasma**

lymfvävnad ⇨ **lymphoid tissue**

lymfödem ⇨ **lymphedema**

lymphadenectomy [lɪm,fædə'nektəmi] *subst.* surgical removal of a lymph node *operativt avlägsnande av lymfkörtel (lymfknuta)*

lymphadenitis [lɪm,fædə'naɪtɪs] *subst.* inflammation of the lymph nodes *lymfadenit, lymfkörtelinflammation*

lymphadenoma [,lɪmfædə'nəʊmə] *subst.* hypertrophy of a lymph node *lymfadenom, lymfom*

lymphadenopathy [lɪm,fædə'nɒpəθi] *subst.* any condition of the lymph nodes *lymfkörtelbesvär*

lymphangiectasis [lɪm,fændʒi'ektəsɪs] *subst.* swelling of the smaller lymph vessels as a result of obstructions in larger vessels *lymf(angi)ektasi*

lymphangiography [lɪm,fændʒi'ɒgrəfi] *subst.* X-ray examination of the lymph vessels following introduction of radio-opaque material *lymfangiografi*

lymphangioma [lɪm,fændʒi'əʊmə] *subst.* tumour formed of lymph tissues *lymfangiom, lymfkärlssvulst*

lymphangioplasty [lɪm,fændʒi'ɒplæsti] *subst.* surgical operation to make artificial lymph channels *operativt ingrepp för att skapa konstgjorda lymfkärl*

lymphangiosarcoma [lɪm,fændʒiəʊsɑː'kəʊmə] *subst.* malignant tumour of the endothelial cells lining the lymph vessels *lymfangiosarkom*

lymphangitis [,lɪmfæn'dʒaɪtɪs] *subst.* inflammation of the lymph vessels *lymfangit, lymfkärlsinflammation*

lymphatic [lɪm'fætɪk] **1** *adj.* referring to lymph *lymfatisk, lymf-;* **lymphatic capillaries** = capillaries which lead from tissue and join lymphatic vessels *lymfkapillärer;* **lymphatic duct** = main channel for carrying lymph *ductus lymphaticus, central lymfbana, lymfgång;* **lymphatic nodes** *or* **lymphatic glands** = glands situated in various points of the lymphatic system, especially under the armpits and in the groin where they produce lymphocytes *nodi lymphatici, lymfkörtlarna;* **lymphatic nodule** = small lymph node found in clusters in tissues *nodulus lymphaticus, lymffollikel;* **lymphatic system** = series of vessels which transport lymph from the tissues through the lymph nodes and into the bloodstream *lymf(kärls)systemet;* **lymphatic vessel** = tube which carries lymph round the body from the tissue to the veins *vas lymphaticum, lymfkärl* **2** *subst.* **the lymphatics** = lymph vessels *vasa lymphtica, lymfkärlen*

lymph (fluid) ['lɪmf (,fluːɪd)] *subst.* colourless liquid containing white blood cells, which circulates in the lymph system from all body tissues, carrying waste matter away from tissues to the veins *lymfa;* **lymph duct** = short trunk entering the junction of the right subclavian and internal jugular veins *ductus lymphaticus dexter, högra lymfgången;* **lymph nodes** *or* **lymph glands** = collections of lymphoid tissue situated in various points of the lymphatic system (especially under the armpits and in the groin) through which lymph passes and in which lymphocytes are produced *nodi lymphatici, lymfkörtlarna;* **lymph vessels** = tubes which carry lymph round the body from the tissues to the veins *vasa lymphatica, lymfkärlen*

> COMMENT: lymph drains from the tissues through capillaries into lymph vessels. It is formed of water, protein and white blood cells (lymphocytes). Waste matter (such as infection) in the lymph is filtered out and destroyed as it passes through the lymph nodes, which then add further lymphocytes to the lymph before it continues in the system. It eventually drains into the innominate veins, and joins the venous bloodstream. Lymph is not pumped round the body like blood but moves by muscle pressure on the lymph vessels. Lymph is an essential part of the body's defence against infection

lymphoblast ['lɪmfəʊblæst] *subst.* abnormal cell which forms in acute lymphatic leukaemia *or* cell formed by the change which takes place in a lymphocyte on contact with an antigen *lymfoblast*

lymphoblastic [ˌlɪmfəʊ'blæstɪk] *adj.* referring to lymphoblasts *or* forming lymphocytes *som avser el. hör till lymfoblast*

lymphocyte ['lɪmfəʊsaɪt] *subst.* type of mature leucocyte *or* white blood cell formed by the lymph nodes, and concerned with the production of antibodies *lymfocyt, slags vit blodkropp;* **T-lymphocyte** = lymphocyte formed in the thymus gland *T-lymfocyt, T-cell*

lymphocytosis [ˌlɪmfəʊsaɪ'təʊsɪs] *subst.* increased number of lymphocytes in the blood *lymfocytos*

lymphoedema [ˌlɪmfəʊɪ'diːmə] *or US* **lymphedema** [ˌlɪmfɪ'diːmə] *subst.* swelling caused by obstruction of the lymph vessels or abnormalities in the development of lymph vessels *lymfödem*

lymphogranuloma inguinale [ˌlɪmfəʊˌgrænju'ləʊmə ˌɪngwineɪli] *or* **lymphogranuloma venereum (l.g.v.)** [ˌlɪmfəʊˌgrænju'ləʊmə ve'nɪəriəm (ˌeldʒiː'viː)] *subst.* venereal disease which causes a swelling of the lymph glands in the groin, occurring in tropical countries *lymphogranuloma inguinale, lymfogranulomatös schanker*

lymphography [lɪm'fɒgrəfi] *subst.* making images of the lymphatic system, after having introduced a radio-opaque substance *lymfografi*

lymphoid tissue ['lɪmfɔɪd ˌtɪʃuː] *subst.* tissue in the lymph nodes, the tonsils and the spleen where masses of lymphocytes are supported by a network of reticular fibres and cells *lymfvävnad*

lymphoma [lɪm'fəʊmə] *subst.* tumour arising from lymphoid tissue *lymfom*

lymphopenia [ˌlɪmfəʊ'piːniə] *or* **lymphocytopenia** [ˌlɪmfəʊˌsaɪtəʊ'piːniə] *subst.* reduction in the number of lymphocytes in the blood *lymfopeni*

lymphopoiesis [ˌlɪmfəʊpɔɪ'iːsɪs] *subst.* production of lymphocytes *or* lymphoid tissue *lymfopo(i)es, utveckling av lymfocyter el. lymfvävnad*

lymphorrhagia [ˌlɪmfə'reɪdʒə] *or* **lymphorrhoea** [ˌlɪmfə'rɪə] *subst.* escape of lymph from ruptured *or* severed lymphatic vessels *lymforragi, lymforré*

lymphosarcoma [ˌlɪmfəʊsɑː'kəʊmə] *subst.* malignant growth arising from lymphocytes and their cells of origin in the lymph nodes *lymfosarkom*

lymphuria [lɪm'fjʊəriə] *subst.* presence of lymph in the urine *lymfa i urinen*

lyofilisering ⇨ **freeze drying, lyophilization**

lyophilization [laɪˌɒfəlaɪ'zeɪʃ(ə)n] *subst.* preserving tissue *or* plasma *or* samples by drying them in a frozen state *lyofilisering, frystorkning*

lys ⇨ **lysis**

lysergic acid diethylamide (LSD) [laɪˌsɜːdʒɪk 'æsɪd daɪ'eθɪləmaɪd (ˌeles'diː)] *subst.* powerful hallucinogenic drug, used in the treatment of severe mental disorders *lysergsyradietylamid, LSD*

lysin ['laɪsɪn] *subst.* protein in the blood which destroys the cell against which it is directed *or* toxin which causes the lysis of cells *lysin; see also* BACTERIOLYSIS, HAEMOLYSIN, LEUCOLYSIN

lysine ['laɪsiːn] *subst.* essential amino acid *lysin*

lysis ['laɪsɪs] *subst.* **(a)** destruction of a cell by a lysin, where the membrane of the cell is destroyed *lysis, upplösning* **(b)** reduction in a fever *or* disease over a period of time *lys, fallande kroppstemperatur vid febersjukdom*

lysol ['laɪsɒl] *subst.* strong disinfectant, made of cresol and soap *lysol*

lysomer ⇨ **body**

lysosome ['laɪsə(ʊ)səʊm] *subst.* particle in a cell which contains enzymes which break down substances (such as bacteria) which enter the cell *lysosom*

lysozyme ['laɪsə(ʊ)zaɪm] *subst.* enzyme found in whites of eggs and in tears, and which destroys certain bacteria *lysozym*

lyssna ⇨ **listen**

låg ⇨ **low, under-**

lågriskpatient ⇨ **low**

långfingret ⇨ **middle finger**

långskallig ⇨ **dolichocephalic**

långskallighet ⇨ **dolichocephaly**

långsynthet ⇨ **farsightedness**

långt framskriden ➪ advanced

långvarig ➪ prolonged

långvårdsavdelning ➪ stay

långvårdspatient ➪ stay

lår- ➪ femoral

lårbenet ➪ thighbone

lårbens- ➪ femoral

lårbensartären ➪ femoral

lårbenshalsen, brott på ➪ collar

lårbenshuvudet ➪ head

lårbensnerven ➪ femoral

lårbensvenen ➪ femoral

låret ➪ thigh

lårmuskeln, fyrkantiga ➪ quadratus

lårmuskeln, slanka ➪ gracilis

låsa ➪ lock

låsningsfenomen ➪ lock

låta ➪ allow; sound

läcka ➪ leak

läderhuden ➪ dermis

läge ➪ lie, position

läge, onormalt ➪ malposition

lägesbeskrivning ➪ topography

lägga om ➪ change

läggdags ➪ bedtime

läka ➪ cure

läkande ➪ curative, remedial

läkar- ➪ medical

läkare ➪ doctor, physician, medico

läkarförbundet, brittiska ➪ British Medical Association (BMA)

läkargrupp ➪ practice

läkarhus ➪ center

läkarintyg ➪ certificate

läkarmottagning ➪ sickbay

läkarsekreterare ➪ medical

läkarundersökning ➪ checkup, medical, physical

läkarvetenskap ➪ medicine, physic

läkarvård ➪ aid

läkekonst ➪ physic

läkemedel ➪ drug, medication, medicinal, medicine, pharmaceutical, preparation, remedy

läkemedels- ➪ pharmaco-

läkemedelsallergi ➪ allergy

läkemedelsberoende ➪ addiction

"läkemedelsdelning" ➪ administration

läkemedelsförordning ➪ Pharmacy Act

läkemedelsläran ➪ Materia Medica

läkemedelsmissbruk ➪ addiction

läkemedelstolerans ➪ tolerance

läkkött, bra ➪ euplastic

läkning ➪ healing, union, intention

länd ➪ loin

länd- ➪ lumbar

ländflätan ➪ lumbar

ländkotorna ➪ lumbar

ländmuskeln, stora ➪ psoas major

ländplexus ➪ lumbar

längd ➪ height, length

längsgående ➪ longitudinal

läpp ➪ lip, labium

läpp- ➪ cheil-, lab-, labial, labio-

läpphypertrofi ➪ macrocheilia

läppinflammation ⇨ **cheilitis**

läpplastik ⇨ **labioplasty**

läppsömmen ⇨ **vermilion border**

lära ⇨ **theory**

lärobok ⇨ **textbook**

läs- och skrivsvårigheter ⇨ **dyslexia**

läspa ⇨ **lisp**

läspning ⇨ **lisp**

lätt ⇨ **light, mild, slight, lightly, mildly**

lätta ⇨ **alleviate, relieve**

lätta (på) ⇨ **ease**

lättnad ⇨ **relief, remission**

"lättsmält" mat ⇨ **predigested food**

lättsmält, vara ⇨ **agree with**

lös ⇨ **loose**

lösas upp ⇨ **decompose**

lösgom ⇨ **plate**

lösgöra ⇨ **detach**

löslig ⇨ **soluble**

lösning ⇨ **dilution, lotion; key, solution**

lösningsmedel ⇨ **solvent**

löständer ⇨ **false**

Mm

maceration [ˌmæsəˈreɪʃ(ə)n] *subst.* softening of a solid by letting it lie in a liquid so that the soluble matter dissolves *maceration, uppmjukning, upplösning;* **neonatal maceration** = softening *or* rotting of fetal tissue after the fetus has died in the womb and has remained in the amniotic fluid *fostermaceration*

Macmillan nurse [məkˈmɪlən ˌnɜːs] *subst.* nurse who specializes in cacer care, employed by the organization Macmillan Cancer Relief *slags sjuksköterska inom onkologisk vård*

macro- [ˈmækrəʊ, ˌ--] *prefix* meaning large *makro-*
NOTE: opposite is **micro-**

macrobiotic [ˌmækrəʊbaɪˈɒtɪk] *subst.* (food) which is healthy *or* which has been produced naturally without artificial additives *or* preservatives *makrobiotisk föda, hälsokost*

> COMMENT: macrobiotic diets are usually vegetarian and are prepared in a special way; they consist of beans, coarse flour, fruit and vegetables. They may not contain enough protein or trace elements, especially to satisfy the needs of children

macrocephaly [ˌmækrəʊˈkef(ə)li] *subst.* having an abnormally large head *makrocefali*

macrocheilia [ˌmækrəʊˈkaɪliə] *subst.* having large lips *makrocheili, läpphypertrofi*

macrocornea ⇨ **keratoglobus**

macrocyte [ˈmækrəʊsaɪt] *subst.* abnormally large red blood cell found in patients suffering from pernicious anaemia *makrocyt*

macrocytosis [ˌmækrəʊsaɪˈtəʊsɪs] *or* **macrocythaemia** [ˌmækrəʊsaɪˈθiːmiə] *subst.* having macrocytes in the blood *makrocytos*

macrodactyly [ˌmækrəʊˈdæktəli] *subst.* hypertrophy of the fingers *or* toes *makrodaktyli*

macrogenitosoma [ˌmækrəʊˌdʒenɪtəˈsəʊmə] *subst.* premature development of the body with the genitals being of an abnormally large size *för tidig kroppslig utveckling med förstorade könsorgan*

macroglobulin [ˌmækrəʊˈglɒbjʊlɪn] *subst.* immunoglobulin *or* globulin protein of high molecular weight, which serves as an antibody *makroglobulin*

macroglossia [ˌmækrəʊˈglɒsiə] *subst.* having an abnormally large tongue *makroglossi*

macrognathia [ˌmækrəʊˈneɪθiə] *subst.* condition in which the jaw is larger than normal *makrognati*

macromastia [ˌmækrəʊˈmæstiə] *subst.* overdevelopment of breasts *makromasti*

macromelia [ˌmækrəʊˈmiːliə] *subst.* having abnormally large limbs *makromeli*

macrophage [ˈmækrəʊfeɪdʒ] *subst.* any of several large cells, which destroy inflammatory tissue, found in connective tissue, wounds, lymph nodes and other parts *makrofag*

macropsia [mæˈkrɒpsiə] *subst.* seeing objects larger than they really are, caused by a defect in the retina *makropsi*

macroscopic [ˌmækrəʊˈskɒpɪk] *adj.* which can be seen with the naked eye *makroskopisk*

macula [ˈmækjʊlə] *subst.* (i) change in the colour of a small part of the body without changing the surface (as in freckles) *makula, fläck;* (ii) area of hair cells inside the utricle and saccule of the ear *macula utriculi och sacculi (jämviktsorgan);* **macula lutea** = yellow spot on the retina, surrounding the fovea, the part of the eye which sees most clearly *macula lutea, gula fläcken*
NOTE: plural is **maculae**

macule [ˈmækjuːl] *subst.* small flat coloured spot on the skin *makula, fläck* NOTE: a spot which is raised above the surface of the skin is a **papule**

maculopapular [ˌmækjuləʊˈpæpjʊlə] *adj.* (rash) made up of macules and papules *makulopapulös*

mad [mæd] *adj.* (person) who is suffering from a mental disorder *vansinnig, galen, tokig*
NOTE: not a medical term

madrass ⇨ **mattress**

madrassutur ⇨ **mattress**

madurafot ⇨ **maduromycosis**

maduromycosis [məˌdjʊərəʊmaɪˈkəʊsɪs] *or* **Madura foot** [məˈdjʊərə fʊt] *or* **maduromycetoma** [məˌdjʊərəʊˌmaɪsəˈtəʊmə] *subst.* tropical fungus infection in the feet, which can destroy tissue and infect bones *madurafot*

mag- ⇨ **gastr-, gastric**

magbesvär ⇨ **gastric, upset**

magen ⇨ **belly, gut, insides, stomach, tummy**

Magendie's foramen [məˈdʒendɪz fəˈreɪmen] *subst.* opening in the fourth ventricle of the brain which allows cerebrospinal fluid to flow *Magendies apertur*

mager ⇨ **skinny, thin**

mager, mycket ⇨ **cadaveric**

maggropen ⇨ **gastric, pit**

magkatarr ⇨ **gastritis**

magknip ⇨ **gripe, stomach, tormina**

magmunnen, nedre ⇨ **pyloric, pylorus**

magna [ˈmægnə] *see* CISTERNA

Magnesia (Milk of) [mægˈniːziə (ˌmɪlk əv)] *subst.* trade name for a mixture of magnesium hydroxide and water, used as a laxative *magnesiumhydroxidsuspension*

magnesium [mægˈniːziəm] *subst.* chemical element found in green vegetables, which is essential especially for the correct functioning of muscles *magnesium, Mg;* **magnesium sulphate** = magnesium salt used as a laxative *magnesiumsulfat;* **magnesium trisilicate** = magnesium compound used to treat peptic ulcers *magnesiumtrisilikat* NOTE: chemical symbol is **Mg**

magnesiumhydroxidsuspension ⇨ **Magnesia (Milk of)**

magnesiumsulfat ⇨ **Epsom salts, magnesium**

magnesiumtrisilikat ⇨ **magnesium**

magnetfält ⇨ **magnetic**

magnetic [mægˈnetɪk] *adj.* having the attraction of a magnet *magnetisk, magnet-;* **magnetic field** = area round a body which is under the influence of its attraction *magnetfält;* **magnetic resonance imaging (MRI)** = scanning technique for examining soft body tissue and cells *magnetisk resonanstomografi, MRT; see also* NUCLEAR MAGNETIC RESONANCE

> QUOTE Magnetic Resonance Imaging scans produce more sensitive images than X-rays, so they are more useful in determining pathophysiology. Although MRI scans are similar to CT scans, they work differently
>
> **Nursing 87**

magnetisk ⇨ **magnetic**

magnum ['mægnəm] *see* FORAMEN

magont ➪ **tummy**

magporten ➪ **pyloric, pylorus**

magports- ➪ **pylor-, pyloric**

magpump ➪ **stomach**

magra ➪ **waste away, weight**

magsaft ➪ **gastric**

magsaftundersökning ➪ **test meal**

magsmärtor ➪ **gastralgia**

magsond ➪ **stomach**

magsyra ➪ **gastric**

magsår ➪ **gastric**

magsår, brustet ➪ **perforate**

magsäcken ➪ **stomach, ventricle**

magsäcks- ➪ **gastr-, gastric**

magsäckskrökningen ➪ **curvature**

magtarmkanalen ➪ **alimentary canal, digestive, food**

magtarmkatarr ➪ **gastroenteritis**

maidenhead ['meɪd(ə)nhed] *subst.* hymen *or* membrane which partially covers the vaginal passage in a virgin *hymen, mödomshinnan*

maim [meɪm] *vb.* to incapacitate someone with a major injury *lemlästa, handikappa;* **the car crash maimed him for life**

maintain [meɪn'teɪn] *vb.* to keep up *upprätthålla, hålla i gång;* **the heart beats regularly to maintain the supply of oxygen to the tissues**

major ['meɪdʒə] *adj.* greater *or* important *or* serious *stor, större, viktig, allvarlig;* **he had to undergo major surgery on his heart; the operation was a major one; labia majora =** two large fleshy folds at the edge of the vulva ➪ *illustration* UROGENITAL SYSTEM (female) *labia majora (pudendi), stora blygdläpparna*
NOTE: the opposite is **minor**

makro- ➪ **macro-**

makrocefali ➪ **macrocephaly**

makrocheili ➪ **macrocheilia**

makrocyt ➪ **macrocyte**

makrocytos ➪ **macrocytosis**

makrodaktyli ➪ **macrodactyly**

makrofag ➪ **macrophage**

makroglobulin ➪ **macroglobulin**

makroglossi ➪ **macroglossia**

makrognati ➪ **macrognathia**

makromasti ➪ **macromastia**

makromeli ➪ **macromelia**

makropsi ➪ **macropsia**

makroskopisk ➪ **macroscopic**

makroskopisk anatomi ➪ **gross anatomy**

makula ➪ **macula, macule**

makulopapulös ➪ **maculopapular**

mal [mɑːl] *subst.* illness *or* disease *sjukdom;* **grand mal =** commonest form of epilepsy, where the patient loses consciousness and falls to the ground with convulsions *grand mal, epilepsia majora;* urinary incontinence is common; **petit mal =** less severe form of epilepsy, where loss of consciousness happens suddenly but lasts a few seconds only and the patient does not fall or urinate *petit mal, epilepsia minora*

mal- [mæl, 'mæl, ˌ-] *prefix* meaning bad *or* abnormal *mal-, onormal*

malabsorption [ˌmæləb'sɔːpʃ(ə)n] *subst.* defective absorption by the intestines of fluids and nutrients in food *malabsorption;* **malabsorption syndrome =** group of symptoms and signs resulting from steatorrhoea and malabsorption of vitamins, protein, carbohydrates and water, including malnutrition, anaemia, oedema, dermatitis *malabsorptionssyndrom*

malabsorption ➪ **coeliac, enteropathy, gluten**

malabsorptionssyndrom ➪ **malabsorption**

malacia [mə'leɪʃə] *subst. & suffix* pathological softening of an organ *or* tissue *malaci, malaki, uppmjukning*

malaise [mə'leɪz] *subst.* feeling of discomfort *illamående, olust(känsla)*

malaki ➪ **malacia**

malande ➪ **dull**

malar ['meɪlə] *adj.* referring to the cheek *kind-;* **malar bone** *or* **zygomatic bone** = cheek bone which forms the prominent part of the cheek and the bottom of the orbit *os zygomaticum, okbenet, kindknotan*

malaria [mə'leəriə] *or* **paludism** ['pælʊdɪz(ə)m] *subst.* tropical disease caused by a parasite **Plasmodium** which enters the body after a bite from a mosquito *malaria*

COMMENT: malaria is a recurrent disease, which produces regular periods of shivering, vomiting, sweating and headaches as the parasites develop in the body; the patient also develops anaemia

malaria- ➪ **malarial, malarious**

malarial [mə'leəriəl] *adj.* referring to malaria *malaria-;* **malarial parasite** = parasite transmitted to human bloodstream by the bite of a mosquito *malariaparasit*

malariamedel ➪ **antimalarial**

malariaparasit ➪ **malarial**

malarious [mə'leəriəs] *adj.* (region) where malaria is endemic *malaria-*

male [meɪl] *subst. & adj.* referring to a man *or* of the same sex as a man *man, manlig, mans-;* **male sex hormone** = testosterone *or* hormone produced by the testes, which causes physical changes to take place in males as they become sexually mature *manligt könshormon (sexualhormon);* **male sex organs** = the testes, epididymis, vasa deferentia, seminal vesicles, ejaculatory ducts and penis *manliga könsorganen (genitalia, genitalorganen, reproduktionsorganen, fortplantningsorganen)*

malformation [ˌmælfɔː'meɪʃ(ə)n] *subst.* abnormal development of a structure *missbildning;* **congenital malformation** = malformation (such as cleft palate) which is present at birth *medfödd missbildning (defekt)*

malformed [ˌmæl'fɔːmd] *adj.* (part of the body) which has been badly formed *missbildad*

malfunction [ˌmæl'fʌŋ(k)ʃ(ə)n] **1** *subst.* abnormal working of an organ *nedsatt funktion;* **his loss of consciousness was due to a malfunction of the kidneys** *or* **to a kidney malfunction 2** *vb.* to work badly *fungera dåligt, "krångla", "strejka";* **during the operation his heart began to malfunction**
NOTE: used more in US English than GB English

malign ➪ **malignant**

malignancy [mə'lɪgnənsi] *subst.* state of being malignant *malignitet;* **the tests confirmed the malignancy of the growth**

QUOTE without a functioning immune system to ward off germs, the patient now becomes vulnerable to becoming infected by bacteria, protozoa, fungi and other viruses and malignancies which may cause life-threatening illness
Journal of the American Medical Association

malignant [mə'lɪgnənt] *adj.* threatening life *or* tending to cause death *or* virulent (tumour) *malign, elakartad;* **malignant tumour** = cancer *or* tumour which is cancerous and can reappear *or* spread into other tissue, even if removed surgically *malign (elakartad) tumör*
NOTE: the opposite is **benign** *or* **non-malignant**

malignitet ➪ **malignancy**

malingering [mə'lɪŋg(ə)rɪŋ] *adj.* pretending to be ill *som simulerar, som låtsas vara sjuk*

malleolus [mə'liːələs] *subst.* one of two bony prominences at each side of the ankle *malleol, fotknöl;* **lateral malleolus** = part of the end of the fibula which protrudes on the outside of the ankle *malleolus lateralis, laterala malleolen, yttre fotknölen;* **medial malleolus** = part of the end of the tibia which protrudes on the inside of the ankle *malleolus medialis, mediala malleolen, inre fotknölen*
NOTE: the plural is **malleoli**

mallet finger ['mælɪt fɪŋgə] *subst.* finger which cannot be straightened because the tendon attaching the top joint has been torn *malletfinger, hängfinger, droppfinger*

malleus ['mælɪəs] *subst.* largest of the three ossicles in the middle ear, shaped like a hammer ➪ *illustration* EAR *malleus, hammaren*

Mallory's stain ['mæləriz ˌsteɪn] *subst.* trichrome stain, used in histology to distinguish collagen, cytoplasm and nuclei *slags histologisk färgmetod*

Mallory-Weiss tears [ˌmæləri'vaɪs ˌteəz] *subst pl.* tearing of the mucous membrane at the junction of the oesophagus and the stomach *symtom vid Mallory-Weiss syndrom*

malnutrition ['mælnju'trɪʃ(ə)n] *subst.* (i) bad nutrition, as a result of starvation *or* wrong diet *or* bad absorption of food *malnutrition, undernäring, näringsrubbning;* (ii) not having enough to eat *svält*

malocclusion [ˌmælə'klu:ʒ(ə)n] *subst.* condition where the teeth in the upper and lower jaws do not meet properly when the patient's mouth is closed *malocklusion, tillslutningsfel; see also* OCCLUSION

Malpighian body [ˌmælˌpɪgiən 'bɒdi] *or* **Malpighian corpuscle** [ˌmælˌpɪgiən 'kɔ:pʌs(ə)l] *or* **renal corpuscle** ['ri:n(ə)l ˌkɔ:pʌs(ə)l] *see* CORPUSCLE

Malpighian glomerulus [ˌmælˌpɪgiən glɒ'merʊləs] *subst.* tuft of capillaries inside the renal corpuscle

Malpighian layer [ˌmælˌpɪgiən 'leiə] *subst.* deepest layer of the epidermis *överhudens innersta lager*

malposition [ˌmælpə'zɪʃ(ə)n] *subst.* wrong position (as of the fetus in the womb *or* of fractured bones) *felställning, onormalt läge, onormalt fosterläge*

malpractice [ˌmæl'præktɪs] *subst.* (i) acting in an unprofessional *or* illegal way *tjänstefel, försummelse;* (ii) wrong treatment of a patient (by a doctor *or* surgeon *or* dentist, etc.) for which the doctor may be tried in court *felbehandling, fall för ansvarsnämnden;* **the surgeon was found guilty of malpractice**

malpresentation [ˌmælˌprez(ə)n'teɪʃ(ə)n] *subst.* abnormal presentation of the fetus in the womb *onormalt fosterläge, felaktig fosterbjudning*

Malta fever ['mɔ:ltə ˌfi:və] = BRUCELLOSIS

maltase ['mɔ:lteɪz] *subst.* enzyme in the small intestine which converts maltose into glucose *maltas*

maltose [mɔ:l'təʊs] *subst.* sugar formed by digesting starch or glycogen *maltos*

malunion [ˌmæl'ju:niən] *subst.* incorrect union of pieces of a broken bone *felaktig frakturläkning*

mamilla [mə'mɪlə] *or* **mammilla** [mə'mɪlə] *or* **nipple** ['nɪp(ə)l] *subst.* protruding part in the centre of the breast, containing the milk ducts through which the milk flows *mammillen, bröstvårtan*

mamillary ['mæmɪl(ə)ri] *or* **mammillary** ['mæmɪl(ə)ri] *adj.* referring to the nipple *mammillar, mammillär, bröst(vårte)-;* **mamillary bodies** = two little projections on the base of the hypothalamus *corpora mammillaria, mammillarkropparna*

mamma ['mæmə] *or* **breast** [brest] *subst.* one of two glands on the chest of a woman which secrete milk *mamma, bröstet, bröstkörteln*

mammal ['mæm(ə)l] *subst.* type of animal (such as the human being) which gives birth to live young, secretes milk to feed them, keeps a constant body temperature and is covered with hair *däggdjur*

mammarplastik ⇨ **mammoplasty**

mammary ['mæm(ə)ri] *adj.* referring to the breast *mammar, mammär, bröst-;* **mammary gland** = gland in females which produces milk *glandula mammaria, bröstkörtel, mjölkkörtel*

mammillarkropparna ⇨ **mamillary**

mammillen ⇨ **mamilla**

mammillär ⇨ **mamillary**

mammografi ⇨ **mammography, xeroradiography**

mammogram ['mæməgræm] *subst.* picture of a breast made using soft-tissue radiography *mammogram*

mammography [mæ'mɒgrəfi] *subst.* examination of the breast, using a special technique *mammografi*

> QUOTE mammography is the most effective technique available today for the detection of occult breast cancer. It has been estimated that mammography can detect a carcinoma two years before it becomes palpable
> **Southern Medical Journal**

mammoplasty ['mæməplæsti] *subst.* plastic surgery to reduce the size of the breasts *mammarplastik*

mammothermography [ˌmæmə(ʊ)θə'mɒgrəfi] *subst.* thermography of a breast *brösttermografi*

mammotropin ⇨ **prolactin**

mammär ⇨ **mammary**

man ⇨ **male**

manage ['mænɪdʒ] *vb.* **(a)** to control *kontrollera;* to be in charge of *sköta, ha hand om, leda;* **she manages the ward very efficiently; we want to appoint someone to manage the group of hospitals; bleeding can usually be managed, but sometimes an operation may be necessary (b)** to be able to do something *kunna, klara (sig);* to succeed in doing something *lyckas (med);* **did you manage to phone the doctor? can she manage at home all by herself? how are we going to manage without the nursing staff?**

management ['mænɪdʒmənt] *subst.* (i) organization *or* running (of a hospital *or* clinic *or* health authority, etc.) *ledning, skötsel, drift;* (ii) organization of a series of different treatments for a patient *behandling*

manager ['mænɪdʒə] *subst.* person in charge of a department in the health service *or* person in charge of a group of hospitals *person med ledningsansvar inom hälso- och sjukvården;* **nurse manager** = nurse who has administrative duties in a hospital *or* the health service *sjuksköterska med administrativa uppgifter, (klinik)föreståndare*

mandel ➪ **tonsil**

mandelkärnan ➪ **amygdala**

mandible ['mændɪb(ə)l] *subst.* lower bone in the jaw ➪ *illustration* SKULL *mandibula, underkäken*

COMMENT: the jaw is formed of two bones, the mandible which is attached to the skull with a hinge joint and can move up and down, and the maxillae which are fixed parts of the skull

mandibula ➪ **mandible**

mandibular [mæn'dɪbjʊlə] *adj.* referring to the lower jaw *mandibular, mandibulär, underkäks-;* **mandibular fossae** = sockets in the skull into which the ends of the lower jaw fit *fossae mandibulares;* **mandibular nerve** = sensory nerve which supplies the teeth in the lower jaw, the temple, the floor of the mouth and the back part of the tongue *nervus mandibularis, tredje trigeminusgrenen*

mane [meɪni] *Latin word meaning* "during the daytime": used on prescriptions *under dagen*
NOTE: the opposite is **nocte**

QUOTE he was diagnosed as having diabetes mellitus at age 14, and was successfully controlled on insulin 15 units mane and 10 units nocte
British Journal of Hospital Medicine

mangan ➪ **manganese**

manganese ['mæŋgəni:z] *subst.* metallic trace element *mangan, Mn*
NOTE: chemical symbol is **Mn**

manhaftighet ➪ **virilism**

mania ['meɪniə] *subst.* state of manic-depressive psychosis where the patient is in a state of excitement, very sure of his own abilities and has increased energy *mani*

-mania ['meɪniə] *suffix* obsession with something *-mani;* **dipsomania** = addiction to alcohol *dipsomani;* **kleptomania** = obsessive stealing of objects *kleptomani*

manic ['mænɪk] *adj.* referring to mania *manisk*

manic-depressive psychosis [,mænɪkdɪ'presɪv saɪ'kəʊsɪs] *subst.* psychological condition where a patient moves between mania and depression and experiences delusion *manisk-depressiv (maniodepressiv) psykos*

manifestation [,mænɪfes'teɪʃ(ə)n] *subst.* sign *or* indication *or* symptom (of a disease) *manifestation, yttring, symtom*

QUOTE the reason for this susceptibility is a profound abnormality of the immune system in children with sickle cell disease. The major manifestations of pneumococcal infection in SCD are septicaemia, meningitis and pneumonia
Lancet

maniodepressiv ➪ **depressive**

manipulate [mə'nɪpjuleɪt] *vb.* to rub *or* to move parts of the body with the hands to treat a joint *or* a slipped disc *or* a hernia *manipulera*

manipulation [mə,nɪpju'leɪʃ(ə)n] *subst.* moving *or* rubbing parts of the body with the hands to treat a disorder of a joint *or* a hernia *manipulation*

manipulera ➪ **manipulate**

manisk ➪ **manic**

manisk-depressiv ➪ **manic-depressive psychosis, depressive**

manlig ➪ **male, virile**

manner ['mænə] *subst.* way of doing something *or* way of behaving *sätt, uppträdande, beteende;* **he was behaving in a strange manner; doctor with a good bedside manner** = doctor who comforts and reassures patients when he examines them in hospital *läkare med ett trevligt (förtroendeingivande) sätt mot patienter*

mannitol ['mænɪtɒl] *subst.* diuretic substance, used to treat oedema *mannitol*

manslemmen ⇨ **penis, phallus**

Mantoux test [mæn'tu: test] *subst.* test for tuberculosis, where the patient is given an intracutaneous injection of tuberculin *Mantoux prov, tuberkulinprov, pure protein derivative, PPD; compare* PATCH TEST

manubrium (sterni) [mə'nu:briəm (ˌstɜ:naɪ)] *subst.* top part of the breastbone *manubrium (sterni), översta delen av bröstbenet*

MAO [ˌemaɪ'əʊ] = MONOAMINE OXIDASE; **MAO inhibitor** = drug used to treat depression by inhibiting the action of MAO, but which also prevents the breakdown of tyramine in the brain and can cause high blood pressure *MAO-hämmare, monoaminooxidashämmare*

marasmus [mə'ræzməs] *or* **failure to thrive** [ˌfeɪljə tʊ 'θraɪv] *subst.* wasting disease which affects small children who have difficulty in absorbing nutrients *or* who are suffering from malnutrition *marasm, kakeki*

marble bone disease ['mɑ:b(ə)l bəʊn dɪˌzi:z] = OSTEOPETROSIS

Marburg virus disease [ˌmɑ:bɜ:g 'vaɪ(ə)rəs dɪˌzi:z] *or* **green monkey disease** [ˌgri:n 'mʌŋki dɪˌzi:z] *subst.* virus disease of green monkeys which is transmitted to humans *Marburgviros*

> COMMENT: because monkeys are used in laboratory experiments, the disease mainly affects laboratory workers. Symptoms include headaches and bleeding from mucous membranes; the disease is often fatal

march fracture ['mɑ:tʃ ˌfræktʃə] *subst.* fracture of one of the metatarsal bones in the foot, caused by excessive exercise to which the body is not accustomed *marschfraktur, insufficiensfraktur*

mardröm ⇨ **nightmare**

Marfan's syndrome [mɑ:'fɑ:nz ˌsɪndrəʊm] *subst.* hereditary condition where the patient has extremely long fingers and toes, with abnormalities of the heart, aorta and eyes *Marfans syndrom*

margarine [ˌmɑ:dʒə'ri:n] *subst.* vegetable fat which looks like butter and is used instead of butter *margarin*

marijuana [ˌmærɪ'wɑ:nə] *or* **cannabis** ['kænəbɪs] *subst.* addictive drug made from the leaves *or* flowers of the Indian hemp plant *cannabis, marijuana, marihuana*

mark [mɑ:k] **1** *subst.* spot *or* small area of a different colour *märke, fläck, prick, ärr;* **there's a red mark where you hit your head; the rash has left marks on the chest and back 2** *vb.* to make a mark *märka;* **the tin is marked 'dangerous'** = it has the word 'dangerous' written on it *burken är märkt "farlig"*

marker ['mɑ:kə] *subst.* (i) label *or* thing which marks a place *markör;* (ii) substance which is part of a chromosome and gives it a genetic mark *genetisk markör*

markerad ⇨ **pronounced**

markör ⇨ **marker**

marmorbensjuka ⇨ **osteopetrosis**

marrow ['mærəʊ] *or* **bone marrow** ['bəʊn ˌmærəʊ] *subst.* soft substance in the centre of a long bone *märg, benmärg;* **bone marrow transplant** = transplant of marrow from a donor to a recipient ⇨ *illustration* BONE STRUCTURE *benmärgstransplantat*

NOTE: for terms referring to bone marrow, see words beginning with **myel-, myelo-**

> COMMENT: two types of bone marrow are to be found: red bone marrow, which forms blood cells and is found in cancellous bone in the vertebrae, the sternum and other flat bones; as a person gets older, fatty yellow bone marrow develops in the central cavity of long bones

marschfraktur ⇨ **march fracture**

masculinization [ˌmæskjʊlɪnaɪ'zeɪʃ(ə)n] *subst.* development of male characteristics (such as body hair and a deep voice) in a woman, caused by hormone deficiency *or* treatment with male hormones *maskulinism*

mask [mɑ:sk] *subst.* (i) metal and rubber frame that fits over the patient's nose and mouth and is used to administer an anaesthetic *mask;* (ii) piece of gauze which fits over the mouth and nose to prevent droplet infection *munskydd;* (iii) cover which fits over the face of a person who has been disfigured in an accident *mask*

mask ⇨ **mask, face; worm**

maskformig ⇨ **vermiform**

maskmedel ⇨ **anthelmintic, vermicide**

masksjukdom ⇨ **helminthiasis**

maskulin ⇨ **virile**

maskulinism ⇨ **masculinization**

masochism ['mæsəkɪz(ə)m] *subst.* abnormal sexual condition where a person takes pleasure in being hurt *or* badly treated *masochism*

masochist ['mæsəkɪst] *subst.* person suffering from masochism *masochist*

masochistic [ˌmæsə'kɪstɪk] *adj.* referring to masochism *masochistisk; compare* SADISM, SADIST, SADISTIC

mass [mæs] *subst.* **(a)** (i) body of matter *massa, resistens;* (ii) mixture for making pills *massa;* (iii) main solid part of bone *diafys* **(b)** large quantity, such as a large number of people *massa, mängd;* **the patient's back was covered with a mass of red spots; mass radiography** = taking X-ray photographs of large numbers of people to check for tuberculosis *skärmbildsundersökning (av stora befolkningsgrupper för att spåra tbc);* **mass screening** = testing large numbers of people for the presence of a disease *massundersökning*

massa ⇨ **mass**

massage ['mæsɑːʒ] **1** *subst.* treatment of muscular conditions which involves rubbing *or* stroking *or* pressing a patient's body with the hands *massage;* **cardiac massage** = rhythmic compression of the heart to maintain circulation when it has stopped beating spontaneously *hjärtmassage* NOTE: no plural, but **a massage** is used to refer to a single treatment: **he had a hot bath and a massage** **2** *vb.* to rub *or* stroke *or* press a patient's body with the hands *massera*

massageapparat ⇨ **vibrator**

massera ⇨ **massage**

masseter (muscle) [mæ'siːtə (ˌmʌs(ə)l)] *subst.* muscle which makes the lower jaw move up or down *masseter, tuggmuskeln*

massive ['mæsɪv] *adj.* very large *mycket stor, omfattande;* **he was given a massive injection of penicillin; she had a massive heart attack**

massundersöka ⇨ **screen**

massundersökning ⇨ **mass**

mast- ['mæst, ˌ-] *prefix* referring to a breast *mast-, bröst-*

mastalgia [mæ'stældʒə] *subst.* pain in the mammary gland *mastalgi, mastodyni*

mastatrofi ⇨ **mastatrophy**

mastatrophy [mæ'stætrəfi] *subst.* atrophy of the mammary gland *mastatrofi*

mast cell ['mæst ˌsel] *subst.* large cell in connective tissue, which carries histamine and reacts to allergens *mastcell*

mastectomy [mæ'stektəmi] *subst.* surgical removal of a breast *mastektomi;* **radical mastectomy** = removal of the breast, and also the associated lymph nodes and muscles *radikal mastektomi*

masticate ['mæstɪkeɪt] *vb.* to chew food *tugga*

mastication [ˌmæstɪ'keɪʃ(ə)n] *subst.* chewing food *mastikation, tuggning*

mastitis [mæs'taɪtɪs] *subst.* inflammation of the breast *mastit, inflammation i bröstkörteln, bröstböld*

mastodyni ⇨ **mastalgia**

mastoid ['mæstɔɪd] *adj.* (i) shaped like a nipple *bröstvårteliknande;* (ii) belonging to the mastoid part of the temporal bone *som avser el. hör till processus mastoideus (vårtutskottet);* **mastoid antrum** *see* ANTRUM; **mastoid (air) cells** = air cells in the mastoid process *hålrummen i processus mastoideus (vårtutskottet);* **mastoid process** *or* **mastoid** = part of the temporal bone which protrudes at the side of the head behind the ear ⇨ *illustration* SKULL *processus mastoideus, vårtutskottet*

mastoidectomy [ˌmæstɔɪ'dektəmi] *subst.* surgical operation to remove part of the mastoid process, as a treatment for mastoiditis *mastoidektomi*

mastoiditis [ˌmæstɔɪ'daɪtɪs] *subst.* inflammation of the mastoid process and air cells *mastoidit*

COMMENT: symptoms are fever, and pain in the ears. The mastoid process can be infected by infection from the middle ear through the mastoid antrum. Mastoiditis can cause deafness and can affect the meninges if not treated

mastoidotomy [ˌmæstɔɪˈdɒtəmi] *subst.* surgical operation to make a cut into the mastoid process to treat infection *mastoidektomi*

masturbate [ˈmæstəbeɪt] *vb.* to excite one's own genitals so as to produce an orgasm *masturbera, onanera*

masturbation [ˌmæstəˈbeɪʃ(ə)n] *subst.* stimulation of one's own genitals to produce an orgasm *masturbation, onani*

masturbera ⇨ **masturbate**

mat ⇨ **food**

mata ⇨ **feed**

match [mætʃ] *vb.* to examine two things to see if they are similar *or* to see if they fit together *matcha, para ihop;* **they are trying to match the donor to the recipient**

> QUOTE bone marrow from donors has to be carefully matched or graft-versus-host disease will ensue
>
> **Hospital Update**

matcha ⇨ **match**

mater [ˈmeɪtə] *see* ARACHNOID, DURA MATER, PIA MATER

materia ⇨ **matter**

material [məˈtɪəriəl] *subst.* **(a)** matter which can be used to make something *material, ämne* **(b)** cloth *tyg;* **the wound should be covered with gauze** *or* **other light material**

Materia Medica [məˈtɪəriə ˈmedɪkə] *Latin words meaning* "medical substance": study of drugs *or* dosages as used in treatment *läkemedelsläran*

maternal [məˈtɜːn(ə)l] *adj.* referring to a mother *moders-, mödra-;* **maternal death** = death of a mother during pregnancy, childbirth or up to twelve months after childbirth *mödradödlighet;* **maternal deprivation** *see* DEPRIVATION; **maternal instincts** = instinctive feelings in a woman to look after and protect her child *modersinstinkt(er)*

maternity [məˈtɜːnəti] *subst.* childbirth *or* becoming a mother *moderskap, förlossning;* **maternity case** = woman who is about to give birth *"förlossningsfall";* **maternity clinic** = clinic where expectant mothers are taught how to look after babies, do exercises and have medical checkups *mödravårdscentral;* **maternity hospital** *or* **maternity ward** *or* **maternity unit** = hospital *or* ward *or* unit which deals only with women giving birth *förlossningssjukhus, förlossningsavdelning, barnbördsavdelning, BB*

matförgiftning ⇨ **food**

mathållning ⇨ **dietary**

matning ⇨ **feeding**

matrix [ˈmeɪtrɪks] *or* **ground substance** [ˈgraʊnd ˌsʌbstəns] *subst.* amorphous mass of cells forming the basis of connective tissue *matrix, modervävnad*

matron [ˈmeɪtr(ə)n] *subst.* woman in charge of a hospital and the nurses in it *ung. sjukhusföreståndare, ung. klinikföreståndare;* **she has been made matron of the maternity hospital; such cases should be reported to the matron**

NOTE: **matron** can be used with names: **Matron Jones**

matsmältning, god ⇨ **eupepsia**

matspjälkning ⇨ **digestion**

matspjälknings- ⇨ **digestive**

matspjälkningsapparaten ⇨ **digestive**

matspjälkningsbesvär ⇨ **dyspepsia**

matspjälkningsenzymer ⇨ **digestive**

matspjälkningskanalen ⇨ **canal**

matstrupen ⇨ **gullet**

matstrups- ⇨ **oesophageal**

matstrupsbråck ⇨ **oesophagocele**

matstrupsgapet ⇨ **oesophageal**

matter [ˈmætə] *subst.* **(a)** substance *materia, substans, ämne;* **grey matter** = nerve tissue which is of a dark grey colour and forms part of the central nervous system *substantia grisea, grå substans;* **white matter** = nerve tissue in the central nervous system which contains more myelin than grey matter *substantia alba, vit substans* **(b) (infected) matter** = pus *var*

mattress ['mætrəs] *subst.* thick soft part of a bed which you lie on *madrass;* **mattress suture** = suture made with a loop on each side of the incision *madrassutur*

maturation [,mætʃu'reɪʃ(ə)n] *subst.* becoming mature *or* fully developed *mognande, mognad*

mature [mə'tʃʊə] *adj.* fully developed *mogen, fullt utvecklad;* **mature follicle** *or* **corpus luteum** = body which forms in the ovary after a Graafian follicle has ruptured *corpus luteum, mogen follikel*

maturing [mə'tʃʊərɪŋ] *adj.* becoming mature *mognande;* **maturing follicle**

maturity [mə'tʃʊərəti] *subst.* **(a)** being fully developed *mognad, fullgångenhet* **(b)** *(in psychology)* being a responsible adult *mognad*

maxilla ⇨ **maxilla (bone)**

maxilla (bone) [mæk'sɪlə (,bəʊn)] *subst.* upper jaw bone ⇨ *illustration* SKULL *maxilla, överkäken* NOTE: the plural is **maxillae.** It is more correct to refer to the upper jaw as the **maxillae** as it is in fact formed of two bones which are fused together

maxillary [mæk'sɪl(ə)ri] *subst.* referring to the maxilla *maxillar, maxillär, överkäks-;* **maxillary air sinus** *or* **maxillary antrum** *or* **antrum of Highmore** = one of two sinuses behind the cheek bones in the upper jaw *antrum Highmori, sinus maxillaris, överkäkshålan*

maxillär ⇨ **maxillary**

maximaldos ⇨ **safe**

MB [,em'bi:] = BACHELOR OF MEDICINE

McBurney's point [mək'bɜ:nɪz ,pɔɪnt] *subst.* point which indicates the normal position of the appendix on the right side of the abdomen, between the hip bone and the navel, which is extremely painful if pressed when the patient has appendicitis *McBurneys punkt, MB*

MCP [,emsi:'pi:] = METACARPOPHALANGEAL

MD [,em'di:] = DOCTOR OF MEDICINE

meal [mi:l] *subst.* eating food at a particular time *mål(tid);* **we have three meals a day - breakfast, lunch and dinner; you should only have a light meal in the evening;** **barium meal** = liquid solution containing barium sulphate which a patient drinks so that an X-ray can be taken of his stomach *kontrast, bariumgröt, bariumsulfat*

measles ['mi:z(ə)lz] *or* **morbilli** [mɔ:'bɪli] *or* **rubeola** [ru'bi:ələ] *subst.* infectious disease of children, where the body is covered with a red rash *morbilli, mässling;* **she's in bed with measles; have you had measles? he's got measles; they caught measles from their friend at school** *see also* GERMAN MEASLES, KOPLIK'S SPOTS

> COMMENT: measles can be a serious disease as it weakens the body's resistance to other diseases, especially bronchitis and ear infections; it can be prevented by immunization. If caught by an adult it can be very serious

measure ['meʒə] **1** *subst.* **(a)** unit of size *or* quantity *or* degree *mått;* **a metre is a measure of length** **(b)** **tape measure** = long tape with centimetres, inches, etc. marked on it *måttband* **2** *vb.* to find out the size of something *mäta;* to be a certain size *vara av viss storlek (längd etc.);* **the room measures 3 metres by 2 metres; a thermometer measures temperature**

measurement ['meʒəmənt] *subst.* size, length, etc. of something which has been measured *mått*

meat [mi:t] *subst.* animal flesh which is eaten *kött*
NOTE: no plural: **some meat, a piece** *or* **a slice of meat; he refuses to eat meat**

meatus [mɪ'eɪtəs] *subst.* opening leading to an internal passage in the body, such as the urethra *or* the nasal cavity *meatus, gång, rör, mynning;* **external auditory meatus** = tube in the skull leading from the outer ear to the eardrum *meatus acusticus externus, yttre hörselgången;* **internal auditory meatus** = channel which takes the auditory nerve through the temporal bone ⇨ *illustration* EAR, SKULL *meatus acusticus internus, inre hörselgången*

mechanism ['mekənɪz(ə)m] *subst.* physical *or* chemical changes by which a function is carried out *or* system in the body which functions in a particular way *mekanism;* **the inner ear is the body's mechanism for balance**

Meckel's diverticulum ['mek(ə)lz ,daɪvə'tɪkjʊləm] *see* DIVERTICULUM

meconium [mɪ'kəʊniəm] *subst.* first dark green faeces produced by a newborn baby *meconium, mekonium, barnbeck*

meddela ⇨ **communicate, inform**

meddelande ⇨ **notice**

medel ⇨ **agent, device, medium, preparation**

medel- ⇨ **medium, mid-**

medellinje ⇨ **midline**

medelålders ⇨ **middle-aged**

medfödd ⇨ **congenital, inborn, inherent, innate**

medföra ⇨ **involve**

medgivande ⇨ **consent**

medhjälpare ⇨ **assistant, auxiliary, helper**

media ['mi:diə] *or* **tunica media** ['tju:nɪkə ˌmi:diə] *subst.* middle layer of the wall of an artery *or* vein *(tunica) media*

medial ['mi:diəl] *adj.* nearer to the central midline of the body *or* to the centre of an organ *medial, inre;* **medial arcuate ligament =** fibrous arch to which the diaphragm is attached *psoasarkaden, slags senbåge;* **medial malleolus =** bone at the end of the tibia which protrudes at the inside of the ankle *malleolus medialis, mediala malleolen, inre fotknölen;* **medial rectus =** muscle arising from the medial part of the common tendinous ring and inserted into the sclera anterior of the eyeball *musculus rectus medialus, inre raka ögonmuskeln; compare* LATERAL

medialis [ˌmi:dɪ'eɪlɪs] *see* VASTUS

median ['mi:diən] *adj.* towards the central midline of the body *or* placed in the middle *median-, mitt-;* **median nerve =** one of the main nerves of the forearm and hand *nervus medianus;* **median plane =** midline at right angles to the coronal plane and dividing the body into right and left parts *medianplan*

medianplan ⇨ **median, sagittal**

mediastinal [ˌmi:diə'staɪn(ə)l] *adj.* referring to the mediastinum *mediastinal;* **the mediastinal surface of pleura or of the lungs**

mediastinitis [ˌmi:diˌæstə'naɪtɪs] *subst.* inflammation of the mediastinum *mediastinit*

mediastinum [ˌmi:diə'staɪnəm] *subst.* section of the chest between the lungs, where the heart, oesophagus, and phrenic and vagus nerves are situated *mediastinum*

medical ['medɪk(ə)l] **1** *adj.* (i) referring to the study of diseases *medicinsk;* (ii) referring to treatment of disease which does not involve surgery *internmedicinsk, invärtesmedicinsk, läkar-;* (iii) (treatment) given by a doctor (as opposed to a surgeon) in a hospital *or* in his surgery *medicinsk;* **a medical student; medical help was provided by the Red Cross; medical assistance =** help provided by a nurse *or* by ambulancemen *or* by a member of the Red Cross, etc. *vård (behandling) som ges av annan än läkare;* **medical certificate =** certificate signed by a doctor, giving a patient permission to be away from work *or* not to do certain types of work *läkarintyg, sjukintyg;* **medical committee =** committee of doctors in a hospital who advise the management on medical matters *slags medicinskt råd;* **medical doctor (MD) =** doctor who practises medicine, but not usually a surgeon *legitimerad läkare, leg. läk.;* **medical examination =** examination of a patient by a doctor *läkarundersökning;* **medical history =** details of a patient's medical records over a period of time *sjukdomshistoria, sjukhistoria, (medicinsk) anamnes;* **Medical Officer of Health (MOH) =** formerly, local government official in charge of the health service in a certain district *tidigare ung. länsläkare el. förste stadsläkare;* **medical practitioner =** person qualified in medicine (a doctor *or* surgeon) *ung. legitimerad läkare;* **Medical Research Council (MRC) =** government body which organizes and pays for medical research *medicinskt forskningsråd i Storbritannien;* **medical secretary =** qualified secretary who specializes in medical documentation, either in a hospital or in a doctor's surgery *läkarsekreterare;* **medical social worker =** person who helps patients with their family problems *or* problems related to their work, which may have an effect on their response to treatment *kurator;* **medical ward =** ward for patients who do not have to undergo surgical operations *medicinavdelning, medicinsk (vård)avdelning* **2** *subst.* official examination of a person by a doctor *läkarundersökning;* **he wanted to join the army, but failed his medical; you will have to have a medical if you take out an insurance policy**

Medic-Alert bracelet [ˌmedɪkə'lɜ:t ˌbreɪslət] *subst.* bracelet worn by a person to show that he suffers from a certain condition (such as diabetes or an allergy) *slags identitetsarmband*

Medicare ['medɪkeə] *subst.* system of public health insurance in the USA *slags sjukförsäkringssystem*

medicated ['medɪkeɪtɪd] *adj.* (talcum powder *or* cough sweet) which contains a medicinal drug *medicinsk;* **medicated**

shampoo = shampoo containing a chemical which is supposed to prevent dandruff *medicinskt schampo*

medication [ˌmedɪ'keɪʃ(ə)n] *subst.* (i) method of treatment by giving drugs to a patient *medicinering;* (ii) medicine *or* drug taken by a patient *medicin, medikament, läkemedel;* **he was given medication by the ambulancemen; what sort of medication has she been taking? 80% of elderly patients admitted to geriatric units are on medication; premedication** = drug given to a patient before an operation *premedicinering*

medicin ⇨ **medication, medicine**

medicinal [mə'dɪs(ə)n(ə)l] *adj.* referring to medicine *or* (substance) with healing properties *medicinal-, medicinsk;* **he has a drink of whisky before he goes to bed for medicinal purposes; medicinal drug** = drug used to treat a disease as opposed to hallucinatory *or* addictive drugs *drog som används av medicinska skäl, läkemedel*

medicinal- ⇨ **medicinal**

medicinally [mə'dɪs(ə)n(ə)li] *adv.* used as a medicine *medicinskt, som medicin (läkemedel);* **the herb can be used medicinally**

medicinare ⇨ **physician**

medicinavdelning ⇨ **medical**

medicine ['meds(ə)n] *subst.* **(a)** drug *or* preparation taken to treat a disease *or* condition *medicin, läkemedel;* **take some cough medicine if your cough is bad; you should take the medicine three times a day; medicine bottle** = special bottle which contains medicine *medicinflaska;* **medicine cabinet** *or* **medicine chest** = cupboard where medicines, bandages, thermometers, etc. can be left locked up, but ready for use in an emergency *medicinskåp* **(b)** (i) study of diseases and how to cure or prevent them *medicin, läkarvetenskap;* (ii) study and treatment of diseases which does not involve surgery *internmedicin, invärtesmedicin;* **he is studying medicine because he wants to be a doctor; clinical medicine** = study and treatment of patients in a hospital ward *or* in the doctor's surgery (as opposed to the operating theatre *or* laboratory) *klinisk medicin*
NOTE: no plural for (b)

medicinera ⇨ **dose**

medicinering ⇨ **medication**

medicinflaska ⇨ **medicine**

medicinflaska, liten ⇨ **phial**

medicinsk ⇨ **medical, medicated, medicinal, medico-**

medicinskåp ⇨ **medicine**

medico ['medɪkəʊ] *subst. informal* doctor *doktor, läkare;* **my medico said I was perfectly fit**

medico- ['medɪkəʊ, ˌ---] *prefix* referring to medicine *or* to doctors *medicinsk*

medicochirurgical [ˌmedɪkəʊˌkaɪ(ə)'rɜːdʒɪk(ə)l] *adj.* referring to both medicine and surgery *som avser el. hör till både medicin och kirurgi*

medikament ⇨ **medication**

medinamask ⇨ **Dracunculus**

medium ['miːdiəm] **1** *adj.* average *or* in the middle *or* at the halfway point *medel-, mitt-* **2** *subst.* substance through which something acts *medium, medel;* **contrast medium** = radio-opaque dye introduced into an organ *or* part of the body so that soft tissue will show clearly on an X-ray photograph *kontrast(medel);* **culture medium** = jelly (such as agar) in which a bacterial culture is grown in a laboratory *odlingssubstrat*

medkänsla ⇨ **empathy**

medroxyprogesterone [medˌrɒksiprə'dʒestərəʊn] *subst.* synthetic female sex hormone used as a contraceptive *medroxiprogesteron*

medulla [me'dʌlə] *subst.* (i) soft inner part of an organ (as opposed to the outer cortex) *märg;* (ii) bone marrow *benmärg;* (iii) any structure similar to bone marrow *benmärgsliknande struktur;* **medulla oblongata** = continuation of the spinal cord going through the foramen magnum into the brain *medulla oblongata, förlängda märgen;* **renal medulla** = inner part of a kidney containing no glomeruli ⇨ *illustration* KIDNEY *medulla renis, njurmärgen;* **adrenal medulla** *or* **suprarenal medulla** = inner part of the adrenal gland which secretes adrenaline and noradrenaline *medulla glandulae suprarenalis, binjuremärgen*

medullarplattan ⇨ **neural**

medullarrännan ⇨ **neural**

medullarröret ⇨ **neural**

medullary [me'dʌl(ə)ri] *adj.* (i) similar to marrow *märgliknande;* (ii) referring to a medulla *medullar, medullär, märg-;* **medullary cavity** = hollow centre of a long bone, containing bone marrow ⇨ *illustration* BONE STRUCTURE *cavum medullare, märghåla;* **medullary cord** = epithelial fibre found near the hilum of the fetal ovary *könssträng (utvecklingsstadium för ovarium och testikel)*

medullated nerve ['medəleɪtɪd ˌnɜːv] *subst.* nerve surrounded by a myelin sheath *myeliniserad nerv*

medulloblastoma [meˌdʌləʊblæ'stəʊmə] *subst.* tumour which develops in the medulla oblongata and the fourth ventricle of the brain in children *medulloblastom*

medullär ⇨ **medullary**

medvetande ⇨ **consciousness, mind**

medvetandet ⇨ **psyche**

medveten ⇨ **conscious**

medvetenhet ⇨ **awareness, consciousness**

medvetet ⇨ **consciously**

medvetslös ⇨ **comatose, unconscious**

medvetslöshet ⇨ **coma, unconsciousness**

medvetslöshet, orsaka ⇨ **overcome**

medvetslös, slå ⇨ **knock out**

mega- ['megə, ˌ--] *or* **megalo-** ['megələʊ, ˌ---] *prefix* meaning large *mega(lo)-* NOTE: the opposite is **micro-**

megacolon [ˌmegə'kəʊlən] *subst.* condition where the lower colon is very much larger than normal, because part of the colon above is constricted, making bowel movements impossible *megacolon congenitum, megakolon, Hirschsprungs sjukdom*

megakaryocyte [ˌmegə'keəriəsaɪt] *subst.* bone marrow cell which produces blood platelets *megakaryocyt*

megakolon ⇨ **megacolon**

megaloblast ['megələʊblæst] *subst.* abnormally large blood cell found in the bone marrow of patients suffering from certain types of anaemia caused by vitamin B_{12} deficiency *megaloblast*

megaloblastanemi ⇨ **megaloblastic**

megaloblastic [ˌmegələʊ'blæstɪk] *adj.* referring to megaloblasts *megaloblastisk, megaloblast-;* **megaloblastic anaemia** = anaemia caused by vitamin B_{12}deficiency *megaloblastanemi*

megaloblastisk ⇨ **megaloblastic**

megalocephaly [ˌmegələʊ'kef(ə)li, ˌmegələʊ'sef(ə)li] *subst.* having an abnormally large head *mega(lo)cefali*

megalocyte ['megələʊsaɪt] *subst.* abnormally large red blood cell, found in pernicious anaemia *megalocyt*

meibomian cyst [maɪ'bəʊmiən ˌsɪst] *or* **chalazion** [kə'leɪziɒn] *subst.* swelling of a sebaceous gland in the eyelid *chalazion, chalazium, kronisk vagel*

meibomian gland [maɪ'bəʊmiən ˌglænd] *or* **tarsal gland** ['tɑːs(ə)l ˌglænd] *subst.* sebaceous gland on the edge of the eyelid which secretes a liquid to lubricate the eyelid *glandula tarsa, Meiboms körtel*

meiosis [maɪ'əʊsɪs] *or US* **miosis** [maɪ'əʊsɪs] *subst.* process of cell division which results in two pairs of haploid cells (cells with only one set of chromosomes) *meios, reduktionsdelning; compare* MITOSIS

Meissner's corpuscle ['maɪsnəz ˌkɔːpʌs(ə)l] *subst.* receptor cell in the skin which is thought to be sensitive to touch ⇨ *illustration* SKIN & SENSORY RECEPTORS *corpuscula tactus, Meissners kropp, känselkropp*

Meissner's plexus ['maɪsnəz ˌpleksəs] *subst.* network of nerve fibres in the wall of the alimentary canal *Meissners plexus*

mekanisk ikterus ⇨ **jaundice**

mekanism ⇨ **mechanism**

mekonium ⇨ **meconium**

melaena [mə'liːnə] *or* **melena** [mə'liːnə] *subst.* black faeces where the colour is caused by bleeding in the intestine *melaena*

melancholia [ˌmelənˈkəʊliə] *subst.* (i) severe depressive illness occurring usually between the ages of 45 and 65 *melankoli;* (ii) clinical syndrome with tendency to delusion, fixed personality, and agitated movements *melankoli;* **involutional melancholia** = depression which occurs in people (mainly women) after middle age, probably caused by a change of endocrine secretions *slags depression vid menopausen*

melanin [ˈmelənɪn] *subst.* dark pigment which gives colour to skin and hair, also found in the choroid of the eye and in certain tumours *melanin*

melanism [ˈmelənɪz(ə)m] *or* **melanosis** [ˌmeləˈnəʊsɪs] *subst.* (i) abnormally depositing of dark pigment *melanism, melanos;* (ii) staining of all body tissue with melanin in a form of carcinoma *grå el. blåsvart missfärgning av huden vid avancerat malignt melanom med dottersvulster*

melanocyt ⇨ **chromatophore, melanocyte**

melanocyte [ˈmelənəʊsaɪt] *subst.* any cell which carries pigment *melanocyt*

melanocyte-stimulating hormone (MSH) [ˌmelənəʊsaɪtˈstɪmjʊleɪtɪŋ ˌhɔːməʊm (ˌem esˈeɪtʃ)] *subst.* hormone produced by the pituitary gland which causes darkening in the colour of the skin *melanocytstimulerande hormon, MSH*

melanoderma [ˌmelənəʊˈdɜːmə] *subst.* (i) abnormally large amount of melanin in the skin *melanodermi;* (ii) discoloration of patches of the skin *fläckvis missfärgning av huden*

melanofor ⇨ **melanophore**

melanoma [ˌmeləˈnəʊmə] *subst.* tumour formed of dark pigmented cells *(malignt) melanom*

melanophore [ˈmelənəʊˌfɔː] *subst.* cell which contains melanin *melanofor*

melanoplakia [ˈmelənəʊˌpleɪkiə] *subst.* areas of pigment in the mucous membrane inside the mouth *melanoplaci, melanoplaki*

melanos ⇨ **melanism**

melanosis [ˌmeləˈnəʊsɪs] *see* MELANISM

melanuria [ˌmeləˈnjʊəriə] *subst.* (i) presence of dark colouring in the urine *mörkfärgning av urinen;* (ii) condition where the urine turns black after being allowed to stand (as in cases of malignant melanoma) *melanuri*

melasma [məˈlæzmə] *subst.* presence of little brown, yellow or black spots on the skin *melasma*

melatonin [ˌmeləˈtəʊnɪn] *subst.* hormone produced by the pineal gland during the hours of darkness, which makes animals sleep during the winter months *melatonin*

> COMMENT: bright light hitting the eye has the effect of stopping the production of melatonin

melena [məˈliːnə] = MELAENA

mellan- ⇨ **inter-, mes-, mid-**

mellanfoten ⇨ **metatarsus**

mellanfots- ⇨ **metatarsal**

mellangärdes- ⇨ **phren-, phrenic**

mellangärdet ⇨ **diaphragm, midriff**

mellanhanden ⇨ **metacarpus**

mellanhandsbenen ⇨ **metacarpal**

mellanhjärnan ⇨ **diencephalon, thalamencephalon**

mellankotskiva ⇨ **intervertebral**

mellanliggande ⇨ **intermediate**

mellanneuron ⇨ **interneurone**

mellannjuren ⇨ **mesonephros**

mellanparti ⇨ **isthmus**

mellanrum ⇨ **gap, interstices, space**

mellanskiva ⇨ **intercalated**

mellanörat ⇨ **middle ear, tympanic, tympanum**

mellitus [ˈmelɪtəs] *see* DIABETES

membran ⇨ **membrane, pellicle**

membrane [ˈmembreɪn] *subst.* thin layer of tissue which lines *or* covers an organ *membran, hinna;* **membrane bone** = bone which develops from tissue and not from cartilage *ben som utvecklas ur annan vävnad än brosk;* **basement membrane** = membrane at the base of an epithelium *basalmembran;* **mucous membrane** = membrane which lines internal passages in the body (such as nose *or* mouth) and secretes mucus *mucosa, mukosa, slemhinna;* **serous membrane** = membrane which lines an internal cavity which does not come into contact with air (such as the peritoneum *or* pericardium) *serosa, serös hinna;* **synovial membrane** = smooth membrane which forms the inner lining of the capsule covering a joint, and secretes the fluid which lubricates the joint *synovialmembran, synovialhinna;* **tectorial membrane** = spiral membrane in the inner ear above the organ of Corti, which contains the hair cells which transmit impulses to the auditory nerve *membrana tectoria (ductus cochlearis), takhinnan;* **tympanic membrane** = eardrum ⇨ *illustration* EAR *membrana tympani, myrinx, trumhinnan*

membranous ['membrənəs] *adj.* referring to membrane *membranös, hinn-;* **membranous labyrinth** = canals round the cochlea *labyrinthus membranaceus, hinnlabyrinten*

memory ['mem(ə)ri] *subst.* ability to remember *minne(sförmåga);* **he has a very good memory for dates; I have no memory for names; he said the whole list from memory; loss of memory** = not being able to remember anything *minnesförlust;* **she was found wandering in the street suffering from loss of memory; he lost his memory after the accident**

men ⇨ **after-effects**

menarche [mə'nɑ:ki] *subst.* start of menstrual periods *menarche, första menstruationen*

mend [mend] *vb.* to repair *laga, reparera;* to make something perfect which has a fault in it *avhjälpa (fel), rätta till;* **the surgeons are trying to mend the defective heart valves**

Mendel's laws ['mend(ə)lz ˌlɔ:z] *subst.* laws of heredity *Mendels (ärftlighets)lagar*

Mendelson's syndrome ['mend(ə)ls(ə)nz ˌsɪndrəʊm] *subst.* sometimes fatal condition where acid fluid from the stomach is brought up into the windpipe and passes into the lungs, occurring mainly in obstetric patients *aspiration*

Ménière's disease [ˌmeni'eəz dɪˌzi:z] *or* **syndrome** ['sɪndrəʊm] *subst.* disease of the middle ear, where the patient becomes dizzy, hears ringing in the ears and may vomit and becomes progressively deaf *Ménières sjukdom (syndrom), otikodini*

> COMMENT: the causes are not certain, but may include infections or allergies, which increase the fluid contents of the labyrinth in the middle ear

mening- [me'nɪn(d)ʒ, -ˌ-] *or* **meningo-** [mə'nɪŋgəʊ, -ˌ--] *prefix* referring to the meninges *mening(o)-, hjärnhinne-, ryggmärgshinne-*

meningeal [me'nɪndʒiəl] *adj.* referring to the meninges *meningeal, hjärnhinne-, ryggmärgshinne-;* **meningeal haemorrhage** = haemorrhage from a meningeal artery *meningeal blödning (apoplexi);* **meningeal sarcoma** = malignant tumour in the meninges *meningealt sarkom*

meningerna ⇨ **covering, meninges**

meninges [me'nɪn(d)ʒi:z] *subst pl.* membranes which surround the brain and spinal cord *meningerna, hjärn- och ryggmärgshinnorna* NOTE: the singular is **meninx**

> COMMENT: the meninges are divided into three layers: the tough outer layer (dura mater) which protects the brain and spinal cord, the middle layer (arachnoid mater) and the delicate inner layer (pia mater) which contains the blood vessels. The cerebrospinal fluid flows in the space (subarachnoid space) between the arachnoid mater and pia mater

meningioma [meˌnɪndʒi'əʊmə] *subst.* benign tumour in the meninges *meningiom*

meningism [me'nɪndʒɪz(ə)m] *subst.* condition where there are signs of meningeal irritation suggesting meningitis, but where there is no pathological change in the cerebrospinal fluid *meningism, pseduomeningit*

meningitis [ˌmenɪn'dʒaɪtɪs] *subst.* inflammation of the meninges, where the patient has violent headaches, fever, and stiff neck muscles, and can become delirious *meningit, hjärnhinneinflammation;* **aseptic meningitis** = relatively mild viral form of meningitis *aseptisk meningit (hjärnhinneinflammation)*

> COMMENT: meningitis is a serious viral or bacterial disease which can cause brain damage and even death. The bacterial form can be treated with antibiotics

meningocele [mə'nɪŋgəʊsi:l] *subst.* condition where the meninges protrude through the vertebral column or skull *meningocele, hjärnhinnebråck, ryggmärgshinnebråck*

meningococcal [məˌnɪŋgəʊ'kɒk(ə)l] *adj.* referring to meningococcus *meningokock-;* **meningococcal meningitis** *or* **spotted fever** = commonest epidemic form of meningitis, caused by a bacterial infection where the meninges become inflamed causing headaches and fever *meningitis cerebrospinalis (epidemica), meningokockmeningit, epidemisk hjärnhinneinflammation*

meningococcus [məˌnɪŋgəʊ'kɒkəs] *subst.* bacterium **Neisseria meningitidis** which causes meningococcal meningitis *Meningococcus* NOTE: plural is **meningococci**

meningoencephalitis [məˌnɪŋgəʊenˌkefə'laɪtɪs] *subst.* inflammation of the meninges and the brain *meningoencefalit*

meningoencephalocele [məˌnɪŋgəʊen'kef(ə)ləʊˌsiː(ə)l] *subst.* condition where part of the meninges and the brain push through a gap in the skull *meningoencefalocele*

meningokockmeningit ⇨ **meningococcal**

meningomyelocele [məˌnɪŋgəʊ'ma(ɪ)ələʊˌsiː(ə)l] *subst.* hernia of part of the meninges and the spinal cord *meningomyelocele*

meningovascular [məˌnɪŋgəʊ'væskjʊlə] *adj.* referring to the meningeal blood vessels *som avser el. hör till hjärn- och ryggmärgshinnornas blodkärl*

meniscectomy [ˌmenɪ'sektəmi] *subst.* surgical removal of a cartilage from the knee *meniskektomi, meniskresektion*

meniscus [mə'nɪskəs] *or* **semilunar cartilage** [ˌsemɪ'luːnə ˌkɑːtəlɪdʒ] *subst.* one of two pads of cartilage (lateral meniscus and medial meniscus) between the femur and tibia in a knee joint *menisk;* **menisci** *cartilagines semilunares, semilunarbrosken, meniskerna*
NOTE: the plural is **menisci**

menisk ⇨ **meniscus**

meniskektomi ⇨ **meniscectomy**

meniskresektion ⇨ **meniscectomy**

meniskruptur ⇨ **derangement**

meno- ['menə(ʊ), ˌ--] *prefix* referring to menstruation *meno-, menstruations-*

menopausal [ˌmenə(ʊ)'pɔːz(ə)l] *adj.* referring to the menopause *som avser el. hör till menopausen*

menopause ['menə(ʊ)pɔːz] *or* **climacteric** [klaɪ'mæktərɪk] *or* **change of life** [ˌtʃeɪn(d)ʃ əv 'laɪf] *subst.* period (usually between 45 and 55 years of age) when a woman stops menstruating and can no longer bear children *menopaus, klimakterium, övergångsålder;* **male menopause** = non-medical term given to a period in a man's life in middle age *manligt klimakterium*

menorragi ⇨ **flooding, hypermenorrhoea, menorrhagia**

menorrhagia [ˌmenə'reɪdʒ(i)ə] *subst.* very heavy bleeding during menstruation *menorragi, hypermenorré*

mens ⇨ **menses, period**

menses ['mensiːz] *subst pl.* blood which flows from the womb during menstruation *mens, menstruation, reglering, månadsblödning*

menstrual ['menstru(ə)l] *adj.* referring to menstruation *menstrual-, menstruations-;* **menstrual cramp** = cramp in the muscles round the uterus during menstruation *kramp (smärta) vid menstruation;* **menstrual cycle** = period (usually 28 days) during which a woman ovulates, then the walls of the uterus swell and bleeding takes place if the ovum has not been fertilized *menstruationscykel;* **menstrual flow** = flow of blood during menstruation *menstruationsflöde*

menstruate ['menstrueɪt] *vb.* to bleed from the uterus during menstruation *menstruera, ha menstruation (mens, reglering, månadsblödning)*

menstruation [ˌmenstru'eɪʃ(ə)n] *subst.* bleeding from the uterus which occurs in a woman each month when the lining of the womb is shed because no fertilized egg is present *mens(truation), reglering, månadsblödning*

menstruationen, första ⇨ **menarche**

menstruations- ⇨ **meno-, menstrual**

menstruationscykel ⇨ **menstrual**

menstruationsflöde ⇨ **menstrual**

menstruationspådrivande medel ⇨ **emmenagogue**

menstruationssmärta ⇨ **dysmenorrhoea**

menstruera ⇨ **menstruate**

menstruum ['menstru:əm] *subst.* liquid used in the extract of active principles from an unrefined drug *lösningsmedel (begrepp från alkemin)*

mental ['ment(ə)l] *adj.* **(a)** referring to the mind *mental, psykisk, psykiatrisk, intellektuell;* **mental age** = age of a person's mental development, measured by intelligence tests *intelligensålder, mental ålder;* **she has a mental age of three; mental block** = temporary inability to remember something *mental blockering (hämning);* **mental deficiency** *or* **defect** *or* **handicap** *or* **retardation** *or* **subnormality** = condition where a person's mind has not developed as fully as the body, so that he is not so mentally advanced as others of the same age *mental (psykisk, intellektuell) utvecklingsstörning, efterblivenhet;* **mental development** = development of the mind *intellektuell utveckling;* **although physically handicapped her mental development is higher than normal for her age; mental hospital** = special hospital for the treatment of mentally ill patients *mentalsjukhus, psykiatriskt sjukhus;* **mental illness** = any disorder which affects the mind *mentalsjukdom, psykisk sjukdom;* **mental patient** = patient suffering from a mental illness *mentalpatient, psykiatrisk patient* **(b)** referring to the chin *som avser el. hör till hakan;* **mental nerve** = nerve which supplies the chin *nervus mentalis*

mental ⇨ **mental, psychological**

mentalis muscle [men'teɪlɪs ˌmʌs(ə)l] *subst.* muscle attached to the front of the lower jaw and the skin of the chin *musculus mentalis*

mentally ['ment(ə)li] *adv.* in the mind *or* referring to the mind *mentalt, psykiskt, intellektuellt;* **by the age of four he was showing signs of being mentally retarded; mentally, she is very advanced for her age**

mentalpatient ⇨ **mental**

mentalsjuk ⇨ **deranged, insane**

mentalsjukdom ⇨ **insanity, mental, psychopathy**

mentalsjukhus ⇨ **mental, psychiatric**

mentalt ⇨ **mentally, psychologically**

menthol ['menθɒl] *subst.* strongly scented compound, produced from peppermint oil, used in cough medicines and in the treatment of neuralgia *mentol*

mentholated ['menθəleɪtɪd] *adj.* impregnated with menthol *mentol-, med mentol*

mentol ⇨ **menthol**

mentol- ⇨ **mentholated**

mentum ['mentəm] *subst.* chin *mentum, hakan*

meproptos ⇨ **procidentia**

meralgia (paraesthetica) [mə'rældʒə (ˌpæres'θetɪkə)] *subst.* pain in the top of the thigh (caused by a pinched nerve) *meralgi*

mercurialism [mə'kjʊəriəlɪz(ə)m] *subst.* mercury poisoning *merkurialism, hydrargyros, kvicksilverförgiftning*

mercurochrome [mə'kjʊərəʊkrəʊm] *subst.* red antiseptic solution *merkurokrom*

mercury ['mɜ:kjʊ(ə)ri] *subst.* poisonous liquid metal, used in thermometers *kvicksilver;* **mercury poisoning** = poisoning by drinking mercury *or* mercury compounds *or* by inhaling mercury vapour *merkurialism, hydrargyros, kvicksilverförgiftning* NOTE: the chemical symbol is **Hg**

mercy killing ['mɜ:si ˌkɪlɪŋ] *subst.* euthanasia *or* killing of a sick person to put an end to suffering *eutanasi, dödshjälp, barmhärtighetsmord*

merit ⇨ **qualification**

Merkel's cells ['mɜ:kelz ˌselz] *or* **discs** [ˌdɪsks] *subst. pl.* epithelial cells in the deeper part of the dermis which form touch receptors *Merkels celler (känselkroppar)*

merkurialism ⇨ **mercurialism, mercury**

merkurokrom ⇨ **mercurochrome**

merocrine ['merəʊkraɪn] *or* **eccrine** ['ekraɪn] *adj.* (gland) which remains intact during secretion, referring especially to the sweat glands *merokrin, ekkrin*

merokrin ⇨ **merocrine**

mes- [mes, 'mes, ˌ-] *or* **meso-** ['mesəʊ, ˌ--] *prefix* meaning middle *mes(o)-, mitt-, mellan-*

mesaortitis [ˌmeseɪɔːˈtaɪtɪs] *subst.* inflammation of the media of the aorta *mesaortit*

mesarteritis [ˌmesɑːtəˈraɪtɪs] *subst.* inflammation of the media of an artery *mesarterit*

mesencephalon [ˌmesenˈkefəlɒn] *or* **midbrain** [ˈmɪdbreɪn] *subst.* small section of the brain stem, above the pons, between the hindbrain and the cerebrum *mesencefalon, mitthjärnan*

mesenterial ⇨ **mesenteric**

mesenteric [ˌmesenˈterɪk] *adj.* referring to the mesentery *mesenterial, tarmkäks-;* **superior** *or* **inferior mesenteric arteries** = arteries which supply the small intestine *or* the transverse colon and rectum *arteria mesenterica superior (inferior);* **mesenteric vein** = vein in the portal system running from the intestine to the portal vein *vena mesenterica superior (inferior)*

mesenterica [ˌmesenˈterɪkə] *see* TABES

mesenteriet ⇨ **mesentery**

mesenteriolum ⇨ **mesoappendix**

mesentery [ˈmesent(ə)ri] *subst.* **common mesentery** = double layer peritoneum which attaches the small intestine and other abdominal organs to the abdominal wall *mesenteriet, tarmkäxet*

mesoappendix [ˌmesəʊəˈpendɪks] *subst.* fold of peritoneum which links the appendix and the ileum *mesoappendix, mesenteriolum, "blindtarmens" tarmkäx*

mesocolon [ˌmesəʊˈkəʊlən] *subst.* fold of peritoneum which supports the colon (in an adult it supports the transverse and sigmoid sections only) *mesokolon, tjocktarmens tarmkäx*

mesoderm [ˈmesəʊdɜːm] *or* **embryonic mesoderm** [ˌembriˈɒnɪk ˌmesəʊdɜːm] *subst.* middle layer of an embryo, which develops into muscles, bones, blood, kidneys, cartilages, urinary ducts, and the cardiovascular and lymphatic systems *mesoderm*

mesodermal [ˌmesəʊˈdɜːm(ə)l] *adj.* referring to the mesoderm *som avser el. hör till mesoderm*

mesokolon ⇨ **mesocolon**

mesometrium [ˌmesəʊˈmiːtriəm] *subst.* muscle layer of the uterus *mesometrium, myometrium, livmoderns muskelvägg*

mesomorf ⇨ **mesomorphic**

mesomorph [ˈmesəʊmɔːf] *subst.* type of person of average height but strong build *mesomorf person*

mesomorphic [ˌmesəʊˈmɔːfɪk] *adj.* like a mesomorph *mesomorf; see also* ECTOMORPH, ENDOMORPH

mesonefros ⇨ **mesonephros**

mesonephros [ˌmesəʊˈnefrɒs] *or* **Wolffian body** [ˈwuːlfiən ˌbɒdi] *subst.* kidney tissue which exists in a human embryo *mesonefros, urnjuren, mellannjuren, wolffska kroppen*

mesosalpinx [ˌmesəʊˈsælpɪŋks] *subst.* upper part of the broad ligament around the Fallopian tubes *mesosalpinx*

mesotel ⇨ **mesothelium**

mesotendon [ˌmesəʊˈtendən] *subst.* synovial membrane connecting the lining of the fibrous sheath to that of a tendon *övergång mellan muskels bindvävshölje och sena*

mesothelium [ˌmesəʊˈθiːliəm] *subst.* layer of cells lining a serous membrane *mesotel; see also* EPITHELIUM, ENDOTHELIUM

mesovarium [ˌmesəʊˈveəriəm] *subst.* fold of peritoneum around the ovaries *mesovarium, bukhinnan runt äggstockarna*

messenger [ˈmes(ə)n(d)ʒə] *subst.* person who brings a message *budbärare;* **messenger RNA** = type of ribonucleic acid which transmits the genetic code from the DNA to the ribosomes which form the proteins coded on the DNA *messenger-RNA, budbärar-RNA*

meta- [ˈmetə, ˌ--] *prefix* which changes *meta-*

metabolic [ˌmetəˈbɒlɪk] *adj.* referring to metabolism *metabol(isk);* **basal metabolic rate (BMR)** = rate at which a person uses energy when at rest (formerly used as a way of testing the thyroid gland) *basalmetabolism, BMB*

metabolisera ⇨ **metabolize**

metabolism [məˈtæbəlɪz(ə)m] *subst.* chemical processes which are continually taking place in the human body and which are essential to life *metabolism, ämnesomsättning;* **basal metabolism** = energy used by a person at rest (i.e. energy needed to keep the body functioning and the temperature normal) *basalmetabolism, basalomsättning, BMB*

> COMMENT: metabolism covers all changes which take place in the body: the building of tissue (anabolism); the breaking down of tissue (catabolism); the conversion of nutrients into tissue; the elimination of waste matter; the action of hormones, etc.

metabolite [mə'tæbəlaɪt] *subst.* substance produced by metabolism *or* substance taken into the body in food and then metabolized *metabolit, ämnesomsättningsprodukt*

metabolize [mə'tæbəlaɪz] *vb.* to change the nature of something by metabolism *metabolisera;* **the liver metabolizes proteins and carbohydrates**

metacarpal [ˌmetə'kɑːp(ə)l] *subst. & adj.* **metacarpal bone** *or* **metacarpal** = one of the five bones in the metacarpus **metacarpal bones** *ossa metacarpalia, metakarpalbenen, mellanhandsbenen*

metacarpophalangeal joint (MCP *or* MP joint) [ˌmetəˌkɑːpəʊfə'læn(d)ʒiəl ˌdʒɔɪnt (ˌemsiː'piː, ˌem'piː ˌdʒɔɪnt)] *subst.* joint between a metacarpal bone and a finger *metakarpofalangealled*

> QUOTE replacement of the MCP joint is usually undertaken to relieve pain, deformity and immobility due to rheumatoid arthritis
> **Nursing Times**

metacarpus [ˌmetə'kɑːpəs] *subst.* the five bones in the hand between the fingers and the wrist ⇨ *illustration* HAND *metacarpus, mellanhanden*

metafas ⇨ **metaphase**

metafys ⇨ **metaphysis**

metakarpalbenen ⇨ **metacarpal**

metakarpofalangealled ⇨ **metacarpophalangeal joint**

metal ['met(ə)l] *subst.* solid material which can carry heat and electricity, some of which are essential for life *metall*

metall ⇨ **metal, metallic**

metallic [me'tælɪk] *adj.* like a metal *or* referring to a metal *metallisk, metall-;* **metallic element** = chemical element which is a metal *metall*

metamorphopsia [ˌmetəmɔː'fɒpsiə] *subst.* condition where the patient sees objects in distorted form, usually due to inflammation of the choroid *metamorfopsi*

metanol ⇨ **methyl alcohol, wood**

metaphase ['metəfeɪz] *subst.* one of the stages in mitosis *or* meiosis *metafas*

metaphysis [me'tæfəsɪs] *subst.* end of the central section of a long bone, where the bone grows and where it joins the epiphysis *metafys*

metaplasia [ˌmetə'pleɪziə] *subst.* change of one tissue to another *metaplasi*

metastasera ⇨ **metastasize**

metastasis [me'tæstəsɪs] *subst.* spreading of a malignant disease from one part of the body to another through the bloodstream *or* the lymph system *metastas, sekundärtumör*
NOTE: the plural is **metastases**

metastasize [me'tæstəsaɪz] *subst.* to spread by metastasis *metastasera*

metastatic [ˌmetə'stætɪk] *adj.* referring to metastasis *metastatisk, metastas-;* **metastatic growths developed in the liver**

metatarsal [ˌmetə'tɑːs(ə)l] *subst. & adj.* one of the five bones in the metatarsus *metatarsal-, mellanfots-;* **metatarsal arch** = arched part of the sole of the foot running across the sole of the foot *tvärgående fotvalvet, hålfoten*

metatarsalgia [ˌmetətɑː'sældʒə] *subst.* pain in the heads of the metatarsal bones *metatarsalgi*

metatarsophalangeal joint [ˌmetəˌtɑːsəʊfə'læn(d)ʒiəl ˌdʒɔɪnt] *subst.* joint between a metatarsal bone and a toe *metatarsofalangealled*

metatarsus [ˌmetə'tɑːsəs] *subst.* the five long bones in the foot between the toes and the tarsus *metatarsus, mellanfoten*

metencefalon ⇨ **hindbrain**

meteorism ['miːtiərɪz(ə)m] *or* **tympanites** [ˌtɪmpə'naɪtiːz] *subst.* condition where gas is present in the stomach or intestines, causing dilatation and pain *meteorism, tympani(sm), väderspänning(ar)*

methaemoglobin [met'hiːməʊˌgləʊbɪn] *subst.* dark brown substance formed from haemoglobin which develops during illness *or* following treatment with certain drugs *methemoglobin*

> COMMENT: methaemoglobin cannot transport oxygen round the body, and so causes cyanosis

methaemoglobinaemia [met,hi:məʊ,gləʊbɪ'ni:miə] *subst.* presence of methaemoglobin in the blood *methemoglobinemi*

methionine [me'θaɪəni:n] *subst.* essential amino acid *metionin*

method ['meθəd] *subst.* way of doing something *metod, sätt, teknik*

methyl alcohol [,meθ(ə)l 'ælkəhɒl] *subst.* wood alcohol (a poisonous alcohol used as fuel) *metylalkohol, metanol, träsprit*

methylated spirits [,meθəleɪtɪd 'spɪrɪts] *subst.* almost pure alcohol, with wood alcohol and colouring added *denaturerad sprit*

methylene blue ['meθəli:n ,blu:] *subst.* blue dye, formerly used as a mild urinary antiseptic, now used to treat drug-induced methaemoglobinaemia *metylenblått*

metionin ⇨ **methionine**

metod ⇨ **method, process, technique**

metr- [metr] *or* **metro-** ['metrə(ʊ), ,--] *prefix* referring to the uterus *metr(o)-, hyster(o)-, uter(o)-, livmoder(s)-*

metralgi ⇨ **hysteralgia, metralgia**

metralgia [me'trældʒə] *subst.* pain in the uterus *metralgi, metrodyni*

metre ['mi:tə] *or US* **meter** ['mi:tər] *subst.* SI unit of length *meter;* **the room is four metres by three**
NOTE: **metre** is usually written **m** with figures: **the colon is 1.3 m long**

metrit ⇨ **metritis, myometritis**

metritis [me'traɪtɪs] *subst.* inflammation of the myometrium *metrit, myometrit, inflammation i livmoderns muskelvägg*

metrocolpocele [,metrə'kɒlpəʊsi:(ə)l] *subst.* condition where the uterus protrudes into the vagina *metrokolpocele*

metrodyni ⇨ **hysteralgia, metralgia**

metrokolpocele ⇨ **metrocolpocele**

metropathia haemorrhagica [,metrə'pæθiə hemə'reɪdʒɪkə] *or* **essential uterine haemorrhage** [ɪ,senʃ(ə)l ,ju:təraɪn 'hem(ə)rɪdʒ] *subst.* abnormal condition of the uterus, where the lining swells and there is heavy menstrual bleeding *kraftiga mensblödningar (orsakade av follikelpersistens)*

metroptos ⇨ **hysteroptosis, metroptosis, uterine**

metroptosis [,metrə'təʊsɪs] *or* **prolapsed womb** [prə'læpst ,wu:m] *or* **prolapse of the uterus** [prəʊ'læps əv ðə ,ju:tərəs] *subst.* condition where the womb has moved downwards out of its normal position *metroptos, hysteroptos, prolapsus uteri, uterusprolaps, livmoderframfall*

metrorragi ⇨ **dysfunctional uterine bleeding, metrorrhagia**

metrorrhagia [,mi:trəʊ'reɪdʒiə] *subst.* abnormal bleeding from the vagina between the menstrual periods *metrorragi*

metrostaxis [,mi:trəʊ'stæksɪs] *subst.* continual light bleeding from the uterus *metrostaxis*

metylalkohol ⇨ **methyl alcohol, wood**

metylenblått ⇨ **methylene blue**

metylkarbonsyra ⇨ **acetic acid**

Mg *chemical symbol for* magnesium *Mg, magnesium*

mg *abbreviation* milligram *mg, milligram*

MI [,em'aɪ] = MITRAL INCOMPETENCE

micelle [m(a)ɪ'sel] *subst.* tiny particle formed by the digestion of fat in the small intestine *micell*

Michel's clips [mɪ'ʃels ,klɪps] *subst. pl.* *see* CLIP

micro- ['maɪkrəʊ, ,--] *prefix* meaning very small *mikro-* NOTE: the opposite is **macro-** *or* **megalo-**

microaneurysm [,maɪkrəʊ'ænjərɪz(ə)m] *subst.* tiny swelling in the wall of a capillary in the retina *mikroaneurysm*

microangiopathy [,maɪkrəʊ,æn(d)ʒɪ'ɒpəθi] *subst.* any disease of the capillaries *mikroangiopati*

microbe ['maɪkrəʊb] *or* **microorganism** [ˌmaɪkrəʊ'ɔːgənɪz(ə)m] *subst.* very small organism which may cause disease and which can only be seen with a microscope *mikrob, mikroorganism*

COMMENT: viruses, bacteria, protozoa and fungi are all forms of microbe

microbial [maɪ'krəʊbiəl] *adj.* referring to microbes *mikrobial, mikrobisk, mikroorganism-;* **microbial disease** = disease caused by a microbe *sjukdom orsakad av mikroorganism;* **microbial ecology** = study of the way in which microbes develop in nature *studiet av mikroorganismernas utveckling i naturen*

microbiological [ˌmaɪkrəʊˌba(ɪ)ə'lɒdʒɪk(ə)l] *adj.* referring to microbiology *mikrobiologisk*

microbiologist [ˌmaɪkrəʊbaɪ'ɒlədʒɪst] *subst.* scientist who specializes in the study of microorganisms *mikrobiolog*

microbiology [ˌmaɪkrəʊbaɪ'ɒlədʒi] *subst.* scientific study of microorganisms *mikrobiologi*

microcephalic [ˌmaɪkrəʊke'fælɪk] *adj.* suffering from microcephaly *mikrocefal(isk)*

microcephaly [ˌmaɪkrəʊ'kef(ə)li] *subst.* condition where a person has an abnormally small head *mikrocefali*

COMMENT: microcephaly in a baby can be caused by the mother having had German measles during pregnancy

microcheilia [ˌmaɪkrəʊ'kaɪliə] *subst.* having abnormally small lips *mikrocheili*

Micrococcus [ˌmaɪkrəʊ'kɒkəs] *subst.* genus of bacterium, some species of which cause arthritis, endocarditis and meningitis *mikrokock*

microcyte ['maɪkrəʊsaɪt] *subst.* abnormally small red blood cell *mikrocyt*

microcytosis [ˌmaɪkrəʊsaɪ'təʊsɪs] *or* **microcythaemia** [ˌmaɪkrəʊsaɪ'θiːmiə] *subst.* presence of excess microcytes in the blood *mikrocytemi*

microdactylia [ˌmaɪkrəʊdæk'tɪliə] *subst.* having abnormally small *or* short fingers or toes *mikrodaktyli*

microdontism [ˌmaɪkrəʊ'dɒntɪz(ə)m] *subst.* having abnormally small teeth *mikrodontism, mikrodentism*

microglia [maɪ'krɒgliə] *subst.* tiny cells in the central nervous system which destroy other cells *mikroglia*

microglossia [ˌmaɪkrəʊ'glɒsiə] *subst.* having an abnormally small tongue *mikroglossi*

micrognathia [maɪkrəʊ'neɪθiə] *subst.* condition where one jaw is abnormally smaller than the other *mikrognati*

micromastia [ˌmaɪkrəʊ'mæstiə] *subst.* having abnormally small breasts *mikromasti*

micromelia [ˌmaɪkrəʊ'miːliə] *subst.* having abnormally small arms *or* legs *mikromeli*

micrometer [maɪ'krɒmɪtə] *subst.* instrument for measuring very small lengths *mikrometer*

micrometre [maɪ'krɒmɪtə] *or* **micron** ['maɪkrɒn] *subst.* measurement of length, one thousandth of a millimetre *mikrometer, mikron*
NOTE: usually written µm with figures: **25** µm

microorganism [ˌmaɪkrəʊ'ɔːgənɪz(ə)m] *or* **microbe** ['maɪkrəʊb] *subst.* very small organism which may cause disease and which can only be seen with a microscope *mikroorganism, mikrob*

micropsia [maɪ'krɒpsiə] *subst.* seeing objects smaller than they really are, caused by a defect in the retina *mikropsi*

microscope ['maɪkrəskəʊp] *subst.* scientific instrument with lenses, which makes very small objects appear larger *mikroskop;* **the tissue was examined under the microscope; under the microscope it was possible to see the cancer cells**

COMMENT: in an ordinary or light microscope, the image is magnified by lenses; an electron microscope uses a beam of electrons instead of light, and so achieves much greater magnification

microscopic [ˌmaɪkrə'skɒpɪk] *subst.* so small that it can only be seen through a microscope *mikroskopisk*

microscopy [maɪ'krɒskəpi] *subst.* science of the use of microscopes *mikroskopi*

Microsporum [maɪ'krɒspərəm] *subst.* type of fungus which causes ringworm of the hair, skin and sometimes nails *mikrosporon, slags trådsvamp*

microsurgery [ˌmaɪkrəʊ'sɜːdʒ(ə)ri] *subst.* surgery on very small parts of the body, using tiny instruments and a microscope *mikrokirurgi*

COMMENT: microsurgery is used in operations on eyes and ears, and also to connect severed nerves and blood vessels

microvillus [ˌmaɪkrəʊˈvɪləs] *subst.* very small process found on the surface of many cells, especially the epithelial cells in the intestine *mikrovillus;* **microvilli** *stavbräm, tarmludd*
NOTE: plural is **microvilli**

micturition [ˌmɪktjuˈrɪʃ(ə)n] *or* **urination** [ˌjʊərɪˈneɪʃ(ə)n] *subst.* passing of urine from the body *ures, miktion, urinering, urinavgång*

mid- [mɪd] *prefix* meaning middle *mitt-, mellan-, medel-*

midbrain [ˈmɪdbreɪn] *or* **mesencephalon** [ˌmesenˈkef(ə)lən] *subst.* small section of the brain stem, above the pons, between the cerebrum and the hindbrain *mesencefalon, mitthjärnan*

midcarpal [mɪdˈkɑːp(ə)l] *adj.* between the two rows of carpal bones *mellan de två raderna av handrotsben*

middle [ˈmɪd(ə)l] *subst.* **(a)** centre *or* central point of something *mitt* **(b)** waist *midjan;* **the water came up to my middle**

middle-aged [ˌmɪd(ə)lˈeɪdʒd] *adj.* not very young and not very old *medelålders;* **a disease which affects middle-aged women**

middle ear [ˌmɪd(ə)l ˈɪə] *subst.* section of the ear between the eardrum and the inner ear *auris media, mellanörat;* **middle ear infection** *or* **otitis media** = infection of the middle ear, usually accompanied by headaches and fever *otitis media, inflammation i mellanörat, örsprång*

COMMENT: the middle ear contains the three ossicles which receive vibrations from the eardrum and transmit them to the cochlea. The middle ear is connected to the throat by the Eustachian tube

middle finger [ˌmɪd(ə)l ˈfɪŋgə] *subst.* the longest of the five fingers *långfingret*

midgut [ˈmɪdgʌt] *subst.* middle part of the gut in an embryo, which develops into the small intestine *mellersta delen av fostrets tarmkanal, vilken utvecklas till tunntarmen*

midjan ⇨ **middle, waist**

mid-life crisis [ˌmɪdlaɪf ˈkraɪsɪs] = MENOPAUSE

midline [ˈmɪdlaɪn] *subst.* imaginary lint drawn down the middle of the body from the head through the navel to the point between the feet *medellinje*

QUOTE patients admitted with acute abdominal pains were referred for study. Abdominal puncture was carried out in the midline immediately above or below the umbilicus

Lancet

midriff [ˈmɪdrɪf] *subst.* the diaphragm *diafragma, mellangärdet*

midstream specimen [ˌmɪdˈstriːm ˌspesəmɪn] *or* **midstream urine** [ˌmɪdˈstriːm ˌjuərɪn] *subst.* urine sample taken in the middle of a flow of urine *mittportion*

midwife [ˈmɪdwaɪf] *subst.* professional person who helps a woman give birth to a child (often at home) *barnmorska;* **community midwife** = midwife who works in a community as part of a primary health care team *distriktsbarnmorska* NOTE: the plural is **midwives**

midwifery [mɪdˈwɪf(ə)ri] *subst.* (i) profession of a midwife *barnmorskeyrket;* (ii) study of practical aspects of obstetrics *obstetrik, förlossningskonst;* **midwifery course** = training course to teach nurses the techniques of being a midwife *barnmorskeutbildning*

COMMENT: to become a Registered Midwife (RM), a Registered General Nurse has to take a further 18 month course, or alternatively can follow a full 3 year course

migraine [ˈmiːgreɪn] *subst.* sharp severe recurrent headache, often associated with vomiting and visual disturbances *migrän;* **he had an attack of migraine and could not come to work; her migraine attacks seem to be worse in the summer**

COMMENT: the cause of migraine is not known. Attacks are often preceded by an "aura", where the patient sees flashing lights *or* the eyesight becomes blurred. The pain is normally intense and situated behind one eye

migrainous [ˈmaɪgreɪnəs] *adj.* (person) who is subject to migraine attacks *som lider av migrän*

migrän ⇨ **headache, hemicrania, migraine**

mikro- ➪ **micro-**

mikroaneurysm ➪ **microaneurysm**

mikroangiopati ➪ **microangiopathy**

mikrob ➪ **microbe**

mikrobiolog ➪ **microbiologist**

mikrobiologi ➪ **microbiology**

mikrobiologisk ➪ **microbiological**

mikrobisk ➪ **microbial**

mikrocefali ➪ **microcephaly**

mikrocheili ➪ **microcheilia**

mikrocyt ➪ **microcyte**

mikrocytemi ➪ **microcytosis**

mikrodaktyli ➪ **microdactylia**

mikrodentism ➪ **microdontism**

mikrodontism ➪ **microdontism**

mikroglia ➪ **microglia**

mikroglossi ➪ **microglossia**

mikrognati ➪ **micrognathia**

mikrokirurgi ➪ **microsurgery**

mikrokock ➪ **Micrococcus**

mikromasti ➪ **micromastia**

mikromeli ➪ **micromelia**

mikrometer ➪ **micrometer; micrometre**

mikron ➪ **micrometre**

mikroorganism ➪ **microbe**

mikroorganism- ➪ **microbial**

mikropsi ➪ **micropsia**

mikroskop ➪ **microscope**

mikroskopi ➪ **microscopy**

mikroskopisk ➪ **microscopic**

mikrosporon ➪ **Microsporum**

mikrovillus ➪ **microvillus**

miktion ➪ **micturition, uresis**

mild [maɪ(ə)ld] *adj.* not severe *or* not cold *or* gentle *mild, lindrig, lätt(are);* **we had a very mild winter; she's had a mild attack of measles; he was off work with a mild throat infection**
NOTE: **mild - milder - mildest**

mild ➪ **bland, mild**

mildly ['maɪ(ə)ldli] *adv.* slightly *or* not strongly *milt, lindrigt, lätt;* **a mildly infectious disease; a mildly antiseptic solution**

mildra ➪ **alleviate, soften, soothe**

miliar ➪ **miliary**

miliaria [ˌmɪli'eəriə] *or* **prickly heat** [ˌprɪkli 'hiːt] *or* **heat rash** ['hiːt rʌʃ] *subst.* itchy red spots which develop on the chest, under the armpits and between the thighs in hot countries, caused by blocked sweat glands *miliaria, värmeutslag*

miliartuberkulos ➪ **miliary, tuberculosis (TB)**

miliary ['mɪliəri] *adj.* small in size, like a seed *miliar, miliär;* **miliary tuberculosis =** tuberculosis which occurs as little nodes in various parts of the body including the meninges of the brain and spinal cord *miliartuberkulos*

milium ['mɪliəm] *subst.* (i) white pinhead-sized tumour on the face in adults *milium;* (ii) retention cyst in infants *retentionscysta hos spädbarn;* (iii) cyst on the skin *liten hudcysta*
NOTE: plural is **milia**

miliär ➪ **miliary**

miljö ➪ **environment, surroundings**

miljöförstöring ➪ **pollution**

milk [mɪlk] *subst.* **(a)** white liquid produced by female mammals to feed their young *mjölk;* **can I have a glass of milk, please? have you enough milk? the patient can only drink warm milk (b)** milk produced by a woman *modersmjölk;* **the milk will start to flow a few days after childbirth** NOTE: no plural **some milk, a bottle of milk** *or* **a glass of milk**

milk leg ['mɪlk leg] *or* **white leg** ['waɪt leg] *or* **phlegmasia alba dolens** [fleg'meɪziə 'ælbə 'dəʊlənz] *subst.* condition which affects women after childbirth, where a leg becomes pale and inflamed *phlegmasia alba dolens*

Milk of Magnesia [ˌmɪlk əv mæg'niːʃə] *subst.* trade name for a mixture of magnesium hydroxide and water, taken as a laxative *magnesiumhydroxidsuspension*

milk sugar ['mɪlk ʃʊgə] = LACTOSE

milk teeth ['mɪlk tiːθ] *or* **deciduous teeth** [dɪ'sɪdjuəs tiːθ] *subst. pl.* a child's first twenty teeth, which are gradually replaced by permanent teeth *dentes decidui, mjölktänderna*
NOTE: for other terms referring to milk see words beginning with **galact-, lact-**

milligram ['mɪligræm] *subst.* measure of weight, one thousandth of a gram *milligram*

millilitre ['mɪliˌliːtə] *subst.* measure of liquid, one thousandth of a litre *milliliter*

millimetre ['mɪliˌmiːtə] *subst.* measure of length, one thousandth of a metre *millimeter*
NOTE: with figures **milligram, millilitre,** and **millimetre** are usually written **mg, ml** and **mm**

Milroy's disease ['mɪlrɔɪz dɪˌziːz] *subst.* hereditary condition where the lymph vessels are blocked and the legs swell *Milroys sjukdom, lymfaplasi*

Minamata disease ['mɪnəmɑːtə dɪˌziːz] *subst.* form of mercury poisoning from eating polluted fish, found first in Japan *slags kvicksilverförgiftning*

mind [maɪnd] *subst.* part of the brain which controls memory *or* consciousness *or* reasoning *medvetande, intellekt, sinne;* **he's got something on his mind** = he's worrying about something *han är bekymrad (går och funderar) över något;* **let's try to take her mind off her exams** = try to stop her worrying about them *låt oss försöka få henne att tänka på något annat än tentorna;* **state of mind** = general feeling *sinnesstämning, humör;* **he's in a very miserable state of mind**
NOTE: for terms referring to mind, see **mental,** and words beginning with **psych-**

***mindervärdeskomplex* ⇨ inferiority**

***mindre* ⇨ lesser**

***mindre (viktig)* ⇨ minor**

miner ['maɪnə] *subst.* person who works in a coal mine *gruvarbetare;* **miner's elbow** = inflammation of the elbow caused by pressure *slags inflammation i armbågen, s.k. studentarmbåge*

mineral ['mɪn(ə)r(ə)l] *subst.* inorganic substance *mineral;* **mineral water** = water taken out of the ground and sold in bottles *mineralvatten*

COMMENT: the most important minerals required by the body are: calcium (found in cheese, milk and green vegetables) which helps the growth of bones and encourages blood clotting; iron (found in bread and liver) which helps produce red blood cells; phosphorus (found in bread and fish) which helps in the growth of bones and the metabolism of fats; iodine (found in fish) is essential to the functioning of the thyroid gland

***mineraloljor* ⇨ oil**

***mineralvatten* ⇨ mineral**

minim ['mɪnɪm] *subst.* liquid measure used in pharmacy (one sixtieth of a drachm) *ung. droppe, 0,0592 ml (Storbritannien), 0,0616 ml (USA)*

***minimal* ⇨ minute**

***minnas* ⇨ recall, remember**

***minne* ⇨ memory, recall**

***minnesbild* ⇨ image**

***minnesförlust* ⇨ amnesia, memory**

minor ['maɪnə] *adj.* not important *liten, obetydlig, mindre (viktig), lindrig;* **minor illness** = illness which is not serious *lindrig sjukdom;* **minor surgery** = surgery which can be undertaken even when there are no hospital facilities *chirurgia minor;* **labia minora** = two small fleshy folds at the edge of the vulva *labia minora (pudendi), små blygdläpparna*
NOTE: the opposite is **major**

QUOTE practice nurses play a major role in the care of patients with chronic disease and they undertake many preventive procedures. They also deal with a substantial amount of minor trauma
Nursing Times

***minska* ⇨ cut, fall off, go down, lessen, lower, reduce, restrict, wear off**

minute [maɪ'njuːt] *adj.* very small *minimal, mycket liten;* **a minute piece of dust got in my eye**

miosis [maɪ'əʊsɪs] *or* **myosis** [maɪ'əʊsɪs] *subst.* **(a)** contraction of the pupil of the eye (as in bright light) *mios,* *pupillförminskning, pupillförträngning, hopdragna pupiller* **(b)** *US* = MEIOSIS

miotic [maɪ'ɒtɪk] *subst.* drug which makes the pupil of the eye become smaller *miotikum, pupillsammandragande medel*

miotikum ⇨ **miotic**

mis- [mɪs] *prefix* meaning wrong *miss-, felaktig*

miscarriage [ˌmɪs'kærɪdʒ] *or* **spontaneous abortion** [spɒn'teɪniəs ə,bɔːʃ(ə)n] *subst.* situation where an unborn baby leaves the womb before the end of the pregnancy, especially during the first seven months of pregnancy *abortus spontaneus, missfall, spontan abort;* **she had two miscarriages before having her first child**

miscarry [ˌmɪs'kærɪ] *vb.* to have a miscarriage *få missfall;* **the accident made her miscarry; she miscarried after catching the infection**

misconduct [mɪs'kɒndʌkt] *subst.* wrong action by a professional person, such as a doctor *tjänstefel, ämbetsbrott;* **professional misconduct** = actions which are considered to be wrong by the body which regulates a profession (such as an action by a doctor which is considered wrong by the Professional Conduct Committee of the General Medical Council) *olämpligt el. olagligt agerande av en yrkesman, tjänstefel*

mismatch [ˌmɪs'mætʃ] *vb.* to match tissues wrongly *felmatcha*

> QUOTE finding donors of correct histocompatible type is difficult but necessary because results using mismatched bone marrow are disappointing
> **Hospital Update**

miss- ⇨ **mis-**

missbildad ⇨ **defective, deformed, malformed**

missbildning ⇨ **defect, deformation, deformity, malformation**

missbildnings- ⇨ **terat-**

missbildningsframkallande ⇨ **teratogen**

missbruk ⇨ **abuse, addiction, dependence, misuse**

missbruka ⇨ **abuse, misuse**

missbrukare ⇨ **addict**

missfall ⇨ **abortion, miscarriage**

missfoster ⇨ **monster**

missfärga ⇨ **discolour**

missfärgning ⇨ **discoloration**

misshandel ⇨ **abuse**

misshandla ⇨ **abuse**

misshandlat barn ⇨ **battered baby**

misslyckande ⇨ **failure**

misslyckas ⇨ **fail**

misstänka ⇨ **suspect**

mist. [mɪst] *or* **mistura** [mɪs'tjʊərə] *see* RE. MIST.

misuse [ˌmɪs'juːs; ˌmɪs'juːz] **1** *subst.* wrong use *missbruk;* **he was arrested for misuse of drugs 2** *vb.* to use (a drug) wrongly *missbruka*

mite [maɪt] *subst.* very small parasite, which causes dermatitis *kvalster;* **harvest mite** *or* **chigger** = tiny parasite which enters the skin near a hair follicle and travels under the skin, causing intense irritation *kvalster av familjen Trombiculidae*

mitella ⇨ **sling, triangular**

mitochondrial [ˌmaɪtə(ʊ)'kɒndriəl] *adj.* referring to mitochondria *som avser el. hör till mitokondrier*

mitochondrion [ˌmaɪtə(ʊ)'kɒndriən] *subst.* tiny rod-shaped part of a cell's cytoplasm responsible for cell respiration **mitochondria** *mitokondrier* NOTE: plural is **mitochondria**

mitokondrier ⇨ **mitochondrion**

mitoshämmare ⇨ **antimitotic**

mitosis [maɪ'təʊsɪs] *subst.* process of cell division, where the mother cell divides into two identical daughter cells *mitos, indirekt celldelning; compare* MEIOSIS

mitral ['maɪtr(ə)l] *adj.* referring to the mitral valve *mitral, mitralis-;* **mitral incompetence (MI)** = situation where the mitral valve does not close completely so that blood goes back into the atrium *insufficientia valvulae mitralis, mitralisinsufficiens;* **mitral stenosis** = condition where the opening in the mitral valve is made smaller because the cusps have stuck together *stenosis valvulae mitralis, mitralisstenos;* **mitral valve** *or* **bicuspid valve** = valve in the heart which allows blood to flow from the left atrium to the left ventricle but not in the opposite direction *valvula mitralis (bicuspidalis), mitralisklaffen, bikuspidalklaffen;* **mitral valvotomy** = surgical operation to detach the cusps of the mitral valve in mitral stenosis *slags operation vid mitralisstenos*

mitralisinsufficiens ⇨ **mitral**

mitralisklaffen ⇨ **mitral**

mitralisstenos ⇨ **mitral**

mitt ⇨ **centre, centrum, middle**

mitt- ⇨ **central, median, medium, mes-, mid-**

mittelschmerz [ˌmɪtel'ʃmeəts] *subst.* pain felt by women in the lower abdomen at ovulation *Mittelschmerz*

mitthjärnan ⇨ **midbrain**

mittportion ⇨ **midstream specimen**

mix [mɪks] *vb.* to put things together *blanda;* **the pharmacist mixed the chemicals in a bottle**

mixture ['mɪkstʃə] *subst.* chemical substances mixed together *mixtur, läkemedelsblandning i flytande form;* **the doctor gave me an unpleasant mixture to drink; take one spoonful of the mixture every three hours; cough mixture** = medicine taken to stop you coughing *hostmedicin*

mjuk ⇨ **soft, gentle**

mjuka upp ⇨ **soften**

mjäll ⇨ **dandruff**

mjält- ⇨ **splen-, splenic**

mjältbrand ⇨ **anthrax, woolsorter's disease**

mjälten ⇨ **spleen**

mjältförstoring ⇨ **splenomegaly**

mjältinflammation ⇨ **splenitis**

mjöldryga ⇨ **ergot**

mjöldrygesjuka ⇨ **ergotism**

mjölk ⇨ **milk**

mjölk- ⇨ **galact-, lact-, lacteal, lactiferous**

mjölkavsöndrande ⇨ **lactiferous**

mjölkavsöndring ⇨ **lactation**

mjölkersättning ⇨ **formula**

mjölkförande ⇨ **lactiferous**

mjölkgång ⇨ **lactiferous**

mjölkkörtel ⇨ **mammary**

mjölksocker ⇨ **lactose**

mjölksyra ⇨ **lactic acid**

mjölktänderna ⇨ **milk teeth, dentition**

mjölmat ⇨ **farinaceous**

ml *abbreviation* = MILLILITRE

MMR [ˌemem'ɑː] = MEASLES, MUMPS AND RUBELLA

Mn *chemical symbol for* manganese *Mn, mangan*

MO [ˌem'əʊ] = MEDICAL OFFICER

Mo *chemical symbol for* molybdenum *Mo, molybden*

mobile ['məʊbaɪ(ə)l] *adj.* able to move about *mobil, rörlig;* **it is important for elderly patients to remain mobile**

mobilisering ⇨ **mobilization**

mobilitet ⇨ **mobility**

mobility [mə(ʊ)'bɪləti] *subst. (of patients)* being able to move about *mobilitet, rörlighet;* **mobility allowance** = government benefit to help disabled people pay for transport *ung. färdtjänst*

mobilization [ˌməʊb(ə)laɪ'zeɪʃ(ə)n] *subst.* making something mobile *mobilisering;* **stapedial mobilization** = operation to relieve deafness by detaching the stapes from the fenestra ovalis *staped(i)olys, stapesmobilisering*

moder ⇨ **mother**

modercell ⇨ **mother, parent**

moderkakan ⇨ **placenta**

modern ⇨ **date**

moders- ⇨ **maternal**

modersbindning ⇨ **mother**

modersdeprivation ⇨ **deprivation**

modersfixering ⇨ **mother**

moderskap ⇨ **maternity**

modersmjölk ⇨ **milk**

modervävnad ⇨ **matrix**

modiolus [mə(ʊ)'di:ələs] *subst.* central stalk in the cochlea *modiolus*

mogen ⇨ **mature**

mognad ⇨ **maturation, maturity**

mognande ⇨ **maturation, maturing**

MOH [ˌeməʊ'eɪtʃ] = MEDICAL OFFICER OF HEALTH

moist [mɔɪst] *adj.* slightly wet *fuktig;* **the compress should be kept moist; moist gangrene** = condition where dead tissue decays and swells with fluid because of infection *gangraena humida, fuktigt gangrän, kallbrand*

moisture ['mɔɪstʃə] *subst.* small quantity of water or other liquid which condenses on a surface *fuktighet;* **moisture can collect in the scar tissue**

mol ⇨ **mole**

molar ['məʊlə] **1** *adj.* referring to mole **(a)** *som avser el. hör till födelsemärke* **(b)** *molar* **2** *subst.* one of the large back teeth, used for grinding food *dens molaris (multicuspidatus), molar, oxeltand, bakre kindtand;* **third molar** *or* **wisdom tooth** = one of the last four molars at the back of the jaw (which sometimes do not appear) ⇨ *illustration* TEETH *dens sapientiae, visdomstand*

COMMENT: in milk teeth there are eight molars, and in permanent teeth there are twelve

molaritet ⇨ **molarity**

molarity [məʊ'lærəti] *subst.* strength of a solution shown as the number of moles of a substance per litre of solution *molaritet*

molass ⇨ **molasses**

molasses [mə'læsɪz] *subst.* dark sweet substance made of sugar before it has been refined *molass*

mole [məʊl] *subst.* **(a)** dark raised spot on the skin *födelsemärke* **(b)** SI unit of amount of a substance *mol*

molecular [mə'lekjʊlə] *adj.* referring to a molecule *molekylar, molekylär(-), molekyl-;* **molecular biology** = study of the molecules of living matter *molekylärbiologi;* **molecular weight** = weight of one molecule of a substance *molekylvikt*

molecule ['mɒlɪkju:l] *subst.* smallest independent mass of a substance *molekyl*

molekyl ⇨ **molecule**

molekyl- ⇨ **molecular**

molekylar ⇨ **molecular**

molekylvikt ⇨ **molecular**

molekylär ⇨ **molecular**

molekylärbiologi ⇨ **molecular**

molluscum [mə'lʌskəm] *subst.* soft round skin tumour *molluscum;* **molluscum contagiosum** = contagious viral skin infection which gives a small soft sore *molluscum contagiosum;* **molluscum fibrosum** = skin tumours of neurofibromatosis *hudtumör vid neurofibromatos (von Recklinghausens sjukdom);* **molluscum sebaceum** = benign skin tumour which disappears after a short time *molluscum sebaceum (pseudocarcinomatosum)*

molybdenum [mɒ'lɪbd(ə)nəm] *subst.* metallic trace element *molybden*
NOTE: the chemical symbol is **Mo**

mongol ['mɒŋg(ə)l] *subst.* former word for a person suffering from Down's syndrome *tidigare benämning på person som lider av Downs syndrom*

mongolism ['mɒŋgəlɪz(ə)m] *subst.* former name for Down's syndrome *tidigare mongolism, Downs syndrom*

mongolveck ⇨ **epicanthus**

Monilia [məʊ'nɪliə] = CANDIDA

moniliasis [ˌmɒni'laɪəsɪs] = CANDIDIASIS

monitor ['mɒnɪtə] **1** *subst.* screen (like a TV screen) on a computer *monitor, bildskärm;* **cardiac monitor** = instrument which checks the functioning of the heart in an intensive care unit *oscilloskop, EKG-apparat* **2** *vb.* to check *or* to examine how a patient is progressing *övervaka, kontrollera, följa*

monitoring ['mɒnɪt(ə)rɪŋ] *subst.* regular examination and recording of a patient's temperature *or* weight *or* blood pressure, etc. *övervakning, patientövervakning*

mono- ['mɒnə(ʊ), ˌ--] *prefix* meaning single *or* one *mono-, en-, ensidig*

monoamine oxidase (MAO) [ˌmɒnəʊ'æmiːn ˌɒksɪdeɪz (ˌemeɪ'əʊ)] *subst.* enzyme which breaks down the catecholamines to their inactive forms *monoaminooxidas, MAO;* **monoamine oxidase inhibitor** *or* **MAO inhibitor** = drug which inhibits monoamine oxidase (used to treat depression, it can also cause high blood pressure) *monoaminooxidashämmare, MAO-hämmare*

monoblast ['mɒnəʊblæst] *subst.* cell which produces a monocyte *monoblast*

monochromat [ˌmɒnə(ʊ)'krəʊmæt] *subst.* colour-blind person *person som lider av total färgblindhet*

monocular [mɒ'nɒkjʊlə] *adj.* referring to one eye *monokular, monokulär;* **monocular vision** = seeing with one eye only, so that the sense of distance is absent *monokulärt seende; compare* BINOCULAR

monocyte ['mɒnə(ʊ)saɪt] *subst.* type of nongranular leucocyte *or* white blood cell with a nucleus shaped like a kidney, which destroys bacterial cells *monocyt*

monocytosis [ˌmɒnəʊsaɪ'təʊsɪs] *or* **mononucleosis** [ˌmɒnəʊˌnjuːkli'əʊsɪs] *or* **glandular fever** ['glændjʊlə ˌfiːvə] *subst.* condition in which there is an abnormally high number of monocytes in the blood *mononucleosis infectiosa, monocytos, mononukleos, körtelfeber*

COMMENT: symptoms include sore throat, swelling of the lymph nodes and fever; it is probably caused by the Epstein-Barr virus

monodactylism [ˌmɒnə(ʊ)'dæktɪlɪz(ə)m] *subst.* congenital condition in which only one finger or toe is present on the hand or foot *monodaktyli*

monokular ⇨ **monocular**

monokulär ⇨ **monocular**

monoliasis ⇨ **perleche**

monomania [ˌmɒnə(ʊ)'meɪnjə] *subst.* deranged state where a person concentrates attention on one idea *monomani*

mononeuritis [ˌmɒnəʊnju'raɪtɪs] *subst.* neuritis which affects one nerve *mononeurit, mononeuropati*

mononeuropati ⇨ **mononeuritis**

mononuclear [ˌmɒnəʊ'njuːkliə] *adj.* (cell, such as a monocyte) which has one nucleus *mononuklear, mononukleär, enkärnig*

mononucleosis [ˌmɒnəʊˌnjuːkli'əʊsɪs] *or* **glandular fever** ['glændjʊlə ˌfiːvə] *see* MONOCYTOSIS

mononuklear ⇨ **mononuclear**

mononukleos ⇨ **monocytosis**

mononukleär ⇨ **mononuclear**

monoplegia ['mɒnəʊˌpliːdʒə] *subst.* paralysis of one part of the body only (i.e. one muscle, one limb) *monoplegi, ensidig förlamning*

monopolar ⇨ **unipolar**

monopolär ⇨ **unipolar**

monorchism ['mɒnɒkɪz(ə)m] *subst.* condition in which only one testis is visible *monorkism*

monosodium glutamate [ˌmɒnə(ʊ)ˌsəʊdiəm 'gluːtəmeɪt] *subst.* a salt, often used to make food taste better *natriumglutamat; see also* CHINESE RESTAURANT SYNDROME

monosomy ['mɒnəʊsəʊmi] *subst.* condition where a person has a chromosome missing from one or more pairs *monosomi*

monosynaptic [ˌmɒnə(ʊ)sɪ'næptɪk] *adj.* nervous pathway with only one synapse *monosynaptisk*

monoxide [mə'nɒksaɪd] *see* CARBON

monozygoter ⇨ **identical, uniovular twins**

monozygotic twins [ˌmɒnə(ʊ)zaɪˌgɒtɪk 'twɪnz] *subst. pl.* = IDENTICAL TWINS

mons pubis [ˌmɒnz 'pju:bɪs] *or* **mons veneris** [ˌmɒnz və'nɪərɪs] *subst.* cushion of fat covering the pubis *mons pubis (Veneris), venusberget*

monster ['mɒnstə] *subst.* deformed fetus which cannot live *missfoster*

Montezuma's revenge [ˌmɒntɪ'zu:məz rɪˌven(d)ʒ] *subst. informal* diarrhoea which affects people travelling in foreign countries, eating unwashed fruit *or* drinking water which has not been boiled *ung. turistsjuka, turistdiarré, faraos hämnd, Djakarta quickstep*

Montgomery's glands [mənt'gʌm(ə)riz ˌglændz] *subst.* sebaceous glands around the nipple which become more marked in pregnancy *glandulae areolares, Montgomerys (bröstvårtgårdens) körtlar*

mood [mu:d] *subst.* a person's mental state (of excitement, depression, euphoria, etc.) *sinnesstämning, humör*

Mooren's ulcer ['məʊrənz ˌʌlsə] *subst.* chronic ulcer of the cornea, found in elderly patients *Moorens ulcus*

mor ⇨ **mother**

morbid ['mɔ:bɪd] *adj.* (i) showing symptoms of being diseased *morbid, sjuk;* (ii) referring to disease *patologisk;* (iii) unhealthy (mental faculty) *morbid, sjuklig, osund;* **the X-ray showed a morbid condition of the kidneys; morbid anatomy** *or* **pathology** = visual study of a diseased body and the changes which the disease has caused to the body *patologi*

> QUOTE adults are considered morbidly obese when they are 45 kg or 100% above their ideal weight
> **Southern Medical Journal**

morbidity [mɔ:'bɪdəti] *subst.* being diseased *or* sick *morbiditet, sjuklighet;* **morbidity rate** = number of cases of a disease per hundred thousand of population *morbiditet, sjukdomsfrekvens*

> QUOTE apart from death, coronary heart disease causes considerable morbidity in the form of heart attack, angina and a number of related diseases
> **Health Education Journal**

morbilli [mɔ:'bɪli] *or* **rubeola** [ru'bi:ələ] = MEASLES

morbilliform [mɔ:'bɪlifɔ:m] *adj.* (rash) similar to measles *morbilliform, mässlingliknande*

morbus Crohn ⇨ **ileitis**

mord ⇨ **murder**

morfar ⇨ **grandfather**

morfea ⇨ **morphea**

morfin ⇨ **morphine**

morfologi ⇨ **morphology**

morföräldrar ⇨ **grandparents**

moribund ['mɒrɪbʌnd] *subst. & adj.* dying (person) *moribund (person), döende (person)*

mormor ⇨ **grandmother**

morning ['mɔ:nɪŋ] *subst.* first part of the day before 12 o'clock noon *morgon och förmiddag;* **morning sickness** = illness (including nausea and vomiting) experienced by women in the early stages of pregnancy when they get up in the morning *illamående under graviditeten, havandeskapskräkningar; (informal)* **morning-after feeling** = HANGOVER; **morning-after pill** = contraceptive pill which is effective if taken after sexual intercourse *oralt preventivmedel som tas efter samlaget*

Moro reflex ['mɔ:rəʊ ˌri:fleks] *subst.* reflex of a newborn baby when it hears a loud noise (the baby is laid on a table and raises its arms if the table is struck) *Moros reflex, omklamringsreflex*

morphea [mɔ:'fiə] *or* **morphoea** [mɔ:'fiə] *subst.* form of scleroderma *or* disease where the skin is replaced by thick connective tissue *morphaea, morfea*

morphine ['mɔ:fi:n] *subst.* alkaloid made from opium, used to relieve pain *morfin;* **the doctor gave him a morphine injection**

morphology [mɔ:'fɒlədʒi] *subst.* study of the structure and shape of living organisms *morfologi*

mortalitet ⇨ **death, mortality (rate)**

mortalitetsstatistik ⇨ **necrology**

mortality (rate) [mɔ:'tæləti (reɪt)] *subst.* number of deaths per year, shown per hundred thousand of population *mortalitet, dödlighet, dödstal*

mortis ['mɔ:tɪs] *see* RIGOR

morula ['mɒrʊlə] *subst.* early stage in the development of an embryo, where the cleavage of the ovum creates a mass of cells *morula, mullbärskula*

mosquito [məsˈkiːtəʊ] *subst.* insect which sucks human blood and passes viruses or parasites into the bloodstream *moskit, mygga*

> COMMENT: in northern countries, an itchy spot is produced; in tropical countries, dengue, filariasis, malaria and yellow fever are transmitted in this way

mot- ⇨ **anti-**

motgift ⇨ **antidote**

mother [ˈmʌðə] *subst.* female parent *moder, mor;* **mother cell** = original cell which splits into daughter cells by mitosis *modercell;* **mother-fixation** = condition where a patient's development has been stopped at a stage where the adult remains like a child, dependent on the mother *modersfixering, modersbindning*

motile [ˈməʊtaɪ(ə)l] *adj.* (cell *or* microbe) which can move spontaneously *rörlig;* **sperm cells are extremely motile**

motility [məʊˈtɪləti] *subst. (of cells or microbes)* being able to move about *motilitet, rörlighet*

motion [ˈməʊʃ(ə)n] *subst.* **(a)** faeces *or* matter which is evacuated in a bowel movement *tarmtömning, avföring* **(b)** movement *rörelse;* **motion sickness** *or* **travel sickness** = illness and nausea felt when travelling *kinetos, rörelsesjuka, åksjuka, ressjuka*

> COMMENT: the movement of liquid inside the labyrinth of the middle ear causes motion sickness, which is particularly noticeable in vehicles which are closed, such as planes, coaches, hovercraft

motion ⇨ **exercise**

motionera ⇨ **exercise**

motionless [ˈməʊʃ(ə)nləs] *subst.* not moving *orörlig;* **catatonic patients can sit motionless for hours**

motionscykel ⇨ **exercise**

motor [ˈməʊtə] *adj.* referring to movement *or* which produces movement *motorisk, motor-;* **motor area** *or* **motor cortex** *or* **pyramidal area** = part of the cortex in the brain which controls voluntary muscle movement by sending impulses to the motor nerves *motoriskt centrum, motoriska (hjärn)barken;* **motor end plate** = end of a motor nerve where it joins muscle fibre *motorisk ändplatta;* **motor nerve** = nerve which carries impulses from the brain to muscles and causes voluntary movement *motorisk nerv, efferent (utåtledande) nerv;* **motor neurone** = neurone which forms part of a motor nerve pathway leading from the brain to a muscle *motorneuron, motorisk nervcell;* **motor neurone disease** = disease of the nerve cells which control the movement of the muscles *sjukdom som angriper de motoriska nervcellerna;* **motor pathway** = series of motor neurones leading from the motor cortex to a muscle *motorisk bana*

> COMMENT: motor neurone disease has three forms: progressive muscular atrophy (PMA), which affects movements of the hands, lateral sclerosis, which is a form of spasticity, and bulbar palsy, which affects the mouth and throat

motorisk ⇨ **motor**

motorisk ändplatta ⇨ **motor, neuromuscular**

motorneuron ⇨ **motor**

motstånd ⇨ **resistance**

motståndskraft ⇨ **resistance**

motståndskraftig ⇨ **resistant**

motställning ⇨ **opposition**

motstöt ⇨ **contrecoup**

motsättning ⇨ **opposition**

motta ⇨ **receive**

mottagare ⇨ **recipient**

mottaglig ⇨ **capable, liable, sensitive, susceptible**

mottaglighet ⇨ **predisposition, responsiveness, sensitivity, susceptibility**

mottagning ⇨ **practice, surgery**

mottagningsrum ⇨ **consulting room**

mottagningssköterska ⇨ **practice**

motverka ⇨ **counteract, neutralize**

motverkan ⇨ **counteraction**

motvilja ⇨ **aversion to, dislike**

mountain fever [ˈmaʊntɪn fiːvə] = BRUCELLOSIS

mountain sickness ['maʊntɪn sɪknəs] *or* **altitude sickness** ['æltɪtju:d sɪknəs] *subst.* condition where a person suffers from oxygen deficiency from being at a high altitude (as on a mountain) where the level of oxygen in the air is low *morbus montanus, bergsjuka, höjdsjuka*

mouth [maʊθ] *subst.* opening at the head of the alimentary canal, through which food and drink are taken in, and through which a person speaks and can breathe *munnen;* **she was sleeping with her mouth open; roof of the mouth** = the palate *or* the top part of the inside of the mouth, which is divided into a hard front part and soft back part *palatum durum, hårda gommen;* **mouth-to-mouth breathing** *or* **mouth-to-mouth ventilation** = method of making a patient start to breathe again, by blowing air through his mouth into his lungs *mun-mot-munmetoden*

mouthful ['maʊθfʊl] *subst.* amount which you can hold in your mouth *munfull, tugga;* **he had a mouthful of soup**

mouthwash ['maʊθwɒʃ] *subst.* antiseptic solution used to treat infection in the mouth *munvatten*
NOTE: for terms referring to the mouth see **oral**, and words beginning with **stomat-**

movement ['mu:vmənt] *subst.* **(a)** act of moving *rörelse;* **active movement** = movement made by a patient using his own will *aktiv rörelse* **(b) bowel movement** = evacuation of faeces from the bowels *tarmtömning, avföring;* **the patient had a bowel movement this morning**

moxybustion [ˌmɒksɪ'bʌstʃ(ə)n] *subst.* treatment used in the Far East, where dried herbs are placed on the skin and set on fire *behandling med moxer (rullar av torkade örter)*

MP [ˌem'pi:] = METACARPOPHALANGEAL (JOINT)

MPS [ˌempi:'es] = MEMBER OF THE PHARMACEUTICAL SOCIETY

MRC [ˌema:'si:] = MEDICAL RESEARCH COUNCIL

MRCGP [ˌema:si:dʒi:'pi:] = MEMBER OF THE ROYAL COLLEGE OF GENERAL PRACTITIONERS

MRCP [ˌema:si:'pi:] = MEMBER OF THE ROYAL COLLEGE OF PHYSICIANS

MRCS [ˌema:si:'es] = MEMBER OF THE ROYAL COLLEGE OF SURGEONS

MRI [ˌema:r'aɪ] = MAGNETIC RESONANCE IMAGING

> QUOTE during a MRI scan, the patient lies within a strong magnetic field as selected sections of his body are stimulated with radio frequency waves. Resulting energy changes are measured and used by the MRI computer to generate images
> **Nursing 87**

MRT ⇨ **imaging, magnetic**

MS [ˌem'es] = MULTIPLE SCLEROSIS, MITRAL STENOSIS

MSH [ˌemes'eɪtʃ] = MELANOCYTE-STIMULATING HORMONE

mucin ['mju:sɪn] *subst.* compound of sugars and protein which is the main substance in mucus *mucin*

muco- ['mju:kəʊ, ˌ--] *prefix* referring to mucus *muko-, slem-*

mucocele ['mju:kəʊsi:(ə)l] *subst.* cavity containing an accumulation of mucus *mukocele, slemcysta*

mucocutaneous [ˌmju:kəʊkju'teɪniəs] *adj.* referring to mucous membrane and the skin *mukokutan*

mucoid ['mjukɔɪd] *adj.* similar to mucus *mukoid, slemliknande*

mucolytic [ˌmjukəʊ'lɪtɪk] *subst.* substance which dissolves mucus *mukolytisk, slemlösande*

mucomembranous colitis [ˌmju:kəʊˌmembrənəs kə(ʊ)'laɪtɪs] = MUCOUS COLITIS

mucoprotein [ˌmju:kəʊ'prəʊti:n] *subst.* form of protein found in blood plasma *slags plasmaprotein*

mucopurulent [ˌmju:kəʊ'pjʊərʊlənt] *adj.* consisting of a mixture of mucus and pus *mukopurulent*

mucopus [ˌmju:kəʊ'pʌs] *subst.* mixture of mucus and pus *blandning av slem och var*

mucormycosis [ˌmju:kɔ:maɪ'kəʊsɪs] *subst.* disease of the ear and throat caused by the fungus Mucor *slags svampsjukdom i näsa och svalg*

mucosa [mju'kəʊzə] *subst.* mucous membrane *mucosa, mukosa, slemhinna*

mucosal [mju'kəʊz(ə)l] *adj.* referring to a mucous membrane *som avser el. hör till slemhinna*

mucous ['mju:kəs] *adj.* referring to mucus *or* covered in mucus *mukös, slem-, slemmig, slemfylld, slemavsöndrande;* **mucous cell** = cell which contains mucinogen which secretes mucin *muköscell, slemcell;* **mucous colitis** *or* **irritable bowel syndrome** *or* **irritable colon** *or* **spastic colon** = inflammation of the mucous membrane in the intestine, where the patient suffers pain caused by spasms in the muscles of the walls of the colon *colica mucosa, colon irritabile, spastisk kolit;* **mucous membrane** *or* **mucosa** = wet membrane which lines internal passages in the body (such as the nose, mouth, stomach and throat) and secretes mucus *mucosa, mukosa, slemhinna;* **mucous plug** = plug of mucus which blocks the cervical canal during pregnancy *slempropp i cervixkanalen hos gravid kvinna*

mucoviscidosis [ˌmju:kəʊˌvɪsi'dəʊsɪs] *or* **cystic fibrosis** [ˌsɪstɪk faɪ'brəʊsɪs] *subst.* hereditary disease in which there is malfunction of the exocrine glands, such as the pancreas, in particular those which secrete mucus *mukoviskidos, cystisk fibros (pankreasfibros)*

mucus ['mju:kəs] *subst.* slippery liquid secreted by mucous membranes inside the body, which protects those membranes *mucus, mukus, slem*
NOTE: for other terms referring to mucus see words beginning with **blenno-**

muko- ➪ **muco-**

mukocele ➪ **mucocele**

mukoid ➪ **mucoid**

mukokutan ➪ **mucocutaneous**

mukolytisk ➪ **mucolytic**

mukopurulent ➪ **mucopurulent**

mukosa ➪ **mucosa, mucous**

mukoviskidos ➪ **mucoviscidosis**

mukus ➪ **mucus**

mukös ➪ **mucous**

muköscell ➪ **mucous**

mullbärskula ➪ **morula**

Mullerian duct [mʌˌlɪəriən 'dʌkt] *or* **Müllerian duct** [mʊˌlɪəriən 'dʌkt] = PARAMESONEPHRIC DUCT

multi- ['mʌlti, ˌ--] *prefix* meaning many *multi-, mång-, fler-*

multianalyser ➪ **analyser**

multifocal lens [ˌmʌlti'fəʊk(ə)l ˌlenz] *subst.* lens in spectacles whose focus changes from top to bottom so that the person wearing the spectacles can see objects clearly at different distances *multifokal lins; compare* BIFOCAL

multiforme ['mʌltifɔ:m] *see* ERYTHEMA

multigravida [ˌmʌlti'grævɪdə] *subst.* pregnant woman who has been pregnant two or more times before *multigravida*

multinucleated [ˌmʌlti'nju:klieɪtɪd] *adj.* (cell) with several nuclei, such as a megakaryocyte *multinukleär, mångkärnig*

multinukleär ➪ **multinucleated**

multipara [mʌl'tɪp(ə)rə] *subst.* woman who has given birth to two or more live children (mainly used for a woman in labour for the second time) *multipara, pluripara, mångföderska;* **gravides multiparae** = women who have had a least four live births *kvinna som har fött minst fyra livsdugliga barn*
NOTE: plural is **multiparae**

multiparae ➪ **multipara**

multiple ['mʌltɪp(ə)l] *adj.* which occurs several times *or* in several places *multipel, mång-, fler-;* **multiple birth** = giving birth to more than one child at the same time *flerbörd;* **multiple fracture** = condition where a bone is broken in several places *multipel fraktur;* **multiple myeloma** = malignant tumour in bone marrow, most often affecting flat bones *multipla myelom;* **multiple pregnancy** = pregnancy where the mother is going to produce more than one baby (i.e. twins, triplets, etc.) *flerbördsgraviditet;* **multiple sclerosis (MS)** *or* **disseminated sclerosis** = disease of the central nervous system which gets progressively worse, where patches of fibres lose their myelin, causing numbness in the limbs, progressive weakness and paralysis *sclerosis disseminata, multipel skleros, MS*

multipolar [ˌmʌlti'pəʊlə] *adj.* (neurone) with several processes *multipolar, multipolär, med flera utskott*

multiresistant [ˌmʌltirɪ'zɪst(ə)nt] *adj.* (disease) which is resistant against several types of antibiotic *multiresistent, som är resistent mot flera olika typer av antibiotika*

mumps [mʌmps] *or* **infectious parotitis** [ɪnˌfekʃəs ˌpærə'taɪtɪs] *subst pl.* infectious disease of children, with fever and swellings in the salivary glands, caused by a paramyxovirus *epidemisk parotit, påssjuka;* **he caught mumps from the children next door; she's in bed with mumps; he can't go to school - he's got mumps**

> COMMENT: mumps is a relatively mild disease in children; in adult males it can have serious complications and cause inflammation of the testicles (mumps orchitis)

mun- ⇨ **oral, stomat-**

Munchhausen's syndrome *or* **Münchhausen's syndrome** ['mʌn(t)ʃhaʊz(ə)nz ˌsɪndrəʊm] *subst.* condition where the patients pretends to be ill in order to be admitted to hospital *Münchhausen-syndrom*

munfull ⇨ **mouthful**

munhålan ⇨ **buccal, oral**

muninflammation ⇨ **stomatitis**

munläsa ⇨ **trismus**

mun-mot-munmetoden ⇨ **kiss of life, mouth, ventilation**

munnen ⇨ **mouth, os, stoma**

munskydd ⇨ **face, mask**

munspärr ⇨ **gag**

muntermometer ⇨ **thermometer**

muntorrhet ⇨ **xerostomia**

muntorsk ⇨ **candidiasis, perleche, thrush**

munvatten ⇨ **mouthwash**

munvinkelragad ⇨ **cheilosis, perleche**

murder ['mɜːdə] **1** *subst.* **(a)** killing someone illegally and intentionally *mord;* **he was charged with murder** *or* **he was found guilty of murder; the murder rate has fallen over the last year** NOTE: no plural **(b)** an act of killing someone illegally and intentionally *mord;* **three murders have been committed during the last week; the police are looking for the knife used in the murder 2** *vb.* to kill someone illegally and intentionally *mörda*

murmur ['mɜːmə] *subst.* sound (usually the sound of the heart), heard through a stethoscope *blåsljud;* **friction murmur =** sound of two serous membranes rubbing together, heard with a stethoscope in patients suffering from pericarditis, pleurisy *gnidningsljud*

Murphy's sign ['mɜːfiz ˌsaɪn] *subst.* sign of an inflamed gall bladder, where the patient will experience pain if the abdomen is pressed while he inhales *slags tecken på inflammation i gallblåsan*

muscae volitantes [ˌmʌskaɪ vɒlɪ'tænteɪz] *subst.* spots *or* shapes which can be seen before the eyes *muscae volitantes, mouches volantes*

muscle ['mʌs(ə)l] *subst.* organ in the body, which contracts to make part of the body move *muskel;* **if you do a lot of exercises you develop strong muscles; the muscles in his legs were still weak after he had spent two months in bed; he had muscle cramp after going into the cold water; muscle fatigue =** tiredness in the muscles after strenuous exercise *muskeltrötthet;* **muscle fibre =** component fibre of muscles (there are two types of fibre which form striated and smooth muscles) *muskelfiber, muskeltråd;* **muscle relaxant =** drug which reduces contractions in the muscles *muskelrelaxans, muskelrelaxerande (muskelavslappande) medel;* **muscle spindles =** sensory receptors which lie along striated muscle fibres *muskelspolar;* **muscle tissue =** tissue which forms the muscles and which is able to expand and contract *muskelvävnad;* **cardiac muscle =** muscle in the heart which makes the heart beat *hjärtmuskeln;* **skeletal muscle =** muscle attached to a bone, which makes a limb move *skelettmuskel;* **smooth muscle** *or* **unstriated muscle =** type of muscle found in involuntary muscles *glatt muskel;* **striated muscle** *or* **striped muscle =** type of muscle found in skeletal muscles whose movements are controlled by the central nervous system *tvärstrimmig muskel;* **visceral muscle =** muscle in the walls of the intestines which makes the intestine contract *glatt muskel i tarmvägg* NOTE: for other terms referring to muscles see words beginning with **my-, myo-**

> COMMENT: there are two types of muscle: voluntary (striated) muscles, which are attached to bones and move parts of the body when made to do so by the brain, and involuntary (smooth) muscles which move essential organs such as the intestines and

bladder automatically. The heart muscle also works automatically

muscular ['mʌskjʊlə] *adj.* referring to muscle *muskulär, muskel-;* **muscular branch** = branch of a nerve to a muscle carrying efferent impulses to produce contraction *efferent (utåtledande) del av nerv;* **muscular defence** = rigidity of muscles associated with inflammation such as peritonitis *défense musculaire, muskelförsvar;* **muscular disorders** = disorders (such as cramp *or* strain) which affect the muscles *muskelstörningar, muskelrubbningar;* **muscular dystrophy** = type of muscle disease where some muscles become weak and are replaced with fatty tissue *muskeldystrofi; see also* DUCHENNE; **muscular relaxant** = drug which relaxes the muscles *muskelrelaxerande (muskelavslappande) medel;* **muscular rheumatism** = pains in the back *or* neck, usually caused by fibrositis or inflammation of the muscles *rhematismus musculorum, muskelreumatism;* **muscular system** = the muscles in the body, usually applied only to striated muscles *muskulaturen;* **muscular tissue** = tissue which forms the muscles and which is able to expand and contract *muskelvävnad*

muscularis [ˌmʌskjʊ'leərɪs] *subst.* muscular layer of an internal organ *organs inre muskellager*

musculocutaneous ['mʌskjʊləʊkju'teɪniəs] *subst.* referring to muscle and skin *som avser el. hör till både muskler och hud;* **musculocutaneous nerve (in the upper limb)** = nerve in the brachial plexus which supplies the muscles in the arm *nervus musculocutaneus*

musculoskeletal [ˌmʌskjʊləʊ'skelit(ə)l] *adj.* referring to muscles and bone *som avser el. hör till både muskler och ben*

musculotendinous [ˌmʌskjʊləʊ'tendɪnəs] *adj.* referring to both muscular and tendinous tissue *som avser el. hör till både muskler och senor*

muskel ⇨ **muscle**

muskel- ⇨ **muscular, my-, myo-**

muskelatrofi ⇨ **amyotrophia**

muskelbråck ⇨ **myocele**

muskeldystrofi ⇨ **muscular**

muskelfiber ⇨ **muscle**

muskelförsvar ⇨ **muscular**

muskelinflammation ⇨ **myositis**

muskelkramp ⇨ **clonus, tetanus**

muskellager ⇨ **coat**

muskelrelaxans ⇨ **muscle**

muskelreumatism ⇨ **muscular**

muskelrubbningar ⇨ **muscular**

muskelryckning ⇨ **convulsion**

muskelsinnet ⇨ **kinaesthesia**

muskelsjukdom ⇨ **myopathy**

muskelsmärta ⇨ **myodynia**

muskelspolar ⇨ **muscle**

muskelspänning ⇨ **tone, tonicity, tonus**

muskelstörningar ⇨ **muscular**

muskelsvulst ⇨ **myoma**

muskeltonus ⇨ **myotonus, tone, tonicity**

muskeltråd ⇨ **muscle**

muskeltrötthet ⇨ **muscle**

muskelvärk ⇨ **myalgia**

muskelvävnad ⇨ **muscle, muscular**

muskulaturen ⇨ **muscular**

muskulär ⇨ **muscular**

mussla ⇨ **concha**

mutant ['mju:t(ə)nt] *subst. & adj.* (i) gene in which mutation has occurred *mutant, muterad gen;* (ii) organism carrying a mutant gene *organism som bär muterad gen*

mutate [mju'teɪt] *vb.* to undergo a genetic change *mutera;* **bacteria can mutate suddenly, and become increasingly able to infect**

mutation [mju'teɪʃ(ə)n] *subst.* change in the DNA which changes the physiological effect of the DNA on the cell *mutation*

mutera ⇨ **mutate**

mutism ['mju:tɪz(ə)m] *subst.* dumbness *or* being unable to speak *mutism, stumhet*

my- [maɪ] *or* **myo-** ['maɪə(ʊ), ˌ--] *prefix* referring to muscle *my(o)-, muskel-*

myalgi ⇨ **myalgia, myodynia**

myalgia [maɪ'ældʒə] *subst.* muscle pain *myalgi, muskelvärk*

myasthenia (gravis) [ˌma(ɪ)əs'θi:niə (ˌgrɑ:vɪs)] *subst.* general weakness and dysfunction of the muscles, caused by defective conduction at the motor end plates *myasthenia gravis*

myc- ['maɪk, ˌ-, 'maɪs, ˌ-] *prefix* referring to fungus *myk(o)-, svamp-*

mycelium [maɪ'si:liəm] *subst.* mass of threads which forms the main part of a fungus *mycel*

mycetoma [ˌmaɪsi'təʊmə] *or* **Madura foot** [mə'du:rə fʊt] = MADUROMYCOSIS

Mycobacterium [ˌmaɪkə(ʊ)bæk'tɪəriəm] *subst.* one of a group of bacteria, including those which cause leprosy and tuberculosis *mykobakterie*

mycology [maɪ'kɒlədʒi] *subst.* study of fungi *mykologi*

Mycoplasma [ˌmaɪkə(ʊ)'plæzmə] *subst.* type of microorganism similar to a bacterium, associated with diseases such as pneumonia and urethritis *mykoplasma*

mycosis [maɪ'kəʊsɪs] *subst.* any disease (such as athlete's foot) caused by a fungus *mykos, svampsjukdom;* **mycosis fungoides** = form of skin cancer, with irritating nodules *mucosis fungoides*

mydriasis [maɪ'dra(ɪ)əsɪs] *subst.* enlargement of the pupil of the eye *mydriasis, pupilldilatation, pupillutvidgning*

mydriatic [ˌmɪdri'ætɪk] *subst.* drug which makes the pupil of the eye become larger *mydriatikum, pupillvidgande medel*

mydriatikum ⇨ **mydriatic**

myectomy [maɪ'ektəmi] *subst.* surgical removal of part *or* all of a muscle *myektomi*

myektomi ⇨ **myectomy, myomectomy**

myel- ['ma(ɪ)əl, ˌ--] *or* **myelo-** ['ma(ɪ)ələ(ʊ), ˌ--] *prefix* referring (i) to bone marrow *myel(o)-, märg-, benmärgs-;* (ii) to the spinal cord *ryggmärgs-*

myelin ['ma(ɪ)əlɪn] *subst.* protective white substance which is formed into a covering (myelin sheath) round nerve fibres by Schwann cells ⇨ *illustration* NEURONE *myelin*

myelinated ['ma(ɪ)əlɪneɪtɪd] *adj.* (nerve fibre) covered by a myelin sheath *myeliniserad*

myelination [ˌma(ɪ)əli'neɪʃ(ə)n] *subst.* process by which a myelin sheath forms round nerve fibres *myelinisation*

myelinisation ⇨ **myelination**

myeliniserad ⇨ **myelinated**

myeliniserad nerv ⇨ **medullated nerve**

myelinskida ⇨ **axon**

myelitis [ˌma(ɪ)ə'laɪtɪs] *subst.* (i) inflammation of the spinal cord *myelit, ryggmärgsinflammation;* (ii) inflammation of bone marrow *benmärgsinflammation*

myeloblast ['ma(ɪ)ələˌblæst] *subst.* precursor of a granulocyte *myeloblast*

myelocele ['ma(ɪ)ələˌsi:(ə)l] *subst.* form of spina bifida where part of the spinal cord passes through a gap in the vertebrae *myelocele, ryggmärgsbråck*

myelocyte ['ma(ɪ)ələˌsaɪt] *subst.* cell in bone marrow which develops into a granulocyte *myelocyt*

myelofibrosis [ˌma(ɪ)ələfaɪ'brəʊsɪs] *subst.* fibrosis of bone marrow, associated with anaemia *myelofibros*

myelografi ⇨ **myelography**

myelogram ['ma(ɪ)ələgræm] *subst.* record of the spinal cord taken by myelography *myelogram*

myelography [ma(ɪ)ə'lɒgrəfi] *subst.* X-ray examination of the spinal cord and subarachnoid space after a radio-opaque substance has been injected *myelografi*

myeloid ['ma(ɪ)əlɔɪd] *adj.* referring to bone marrow *or* to the spinal cord *or* produced by bone marrow *myeloid, benmärgs-;* **myeloid leukaemia** = acute form of leukaemia in adults *myeloisk leukemi;* **myeloid tissue** = red bone marrow *röd benmärg*

myeloma [ˌma(ɪ)ə'ləʊmə] *subst.* malignant tumour in bone marrow *or* at the ends of long bones or in the jaw *myelom, benmärgssvulst*

myelomalacia [ˌma(ɪ)ələʊmə'leɪʃə] *subst.* softening of tissue in the spinal cord *myelomalaki, ryggmärgsuppmjukning*

myelomatosis [ˌma(ɪ)ələʊmə'təʊsɪs] *subst.* disease where malignant tumours infiltrate the bone marrow *myelomatos*

myenteron [maɪ'entərɒn] *subst.* layer of muscles in the small intestine, which produces peristalsis *tunntarmens glatta muskellager*

mygga ⇨ **mosquito**

myiasis ['maɪəsɪs] *subst.* infestation by larvae of flies *myiasis*

mykobakterie ⇨ **Mycobacterium**

mykologi ⇨ **mycology**

mykoplasma ⇨ **Mycoplasma**

mykos ⇨ **mycosis**

mylohyoid [ˌmaɪlə'haɪɔɪd] *subst. & adj.* referring to the molar teeth in the lower jaw and the hyoid bone *som avser el. hör till både oxeltänderna och tungbenet;* **mylohyoid line** = line running along the outside of the lower jawbone, dividing the upper part of the bone which forms part of the mouth from the lower part which is part of the neck *linje på insidan av underkäken (slags muskelfäste)*

mynning ⇨ **aditus, meatus, opening, orifice, ostium, outlet, pore**

myntrulle(bildning) ⇨ **rouleau**

myo- ['maɪə(ʊ), ˌ--] *prefix* meaning muscle *myo-, muskel-*

myoblast ['maɪəˌblæst] *subst.* embryonic cell which develops into muscle *myoblast*

myoblastic [ˌmaɪə(ʊ)'blæstɪk] *adj.* referring to myoblast *som avser el. hör till myoblast*

myocardial [ˌmaɪə(ʊ)'kɑːdiəl] *adj.* referring to the myocardium *myokard-, hjärt-;* **myocardial infarction** = death of part of the heart muscle after coronary thrombosis *myokardinfarkt, hjärtinfarkt*

myocarditis [ˌmaɪə(ʊ)kɑː'daɪtɪs] *subst.* inflammation of the heart muscle *myokardit, hjärtmuskelinflammation*

myocardium [ˌmaɪə(ʊ)'kɑːdiəm] *subst.* middle layer of the wall of the heart, formed of heart muscle ⇨ *illustration* HEART *myokardiet, hjärtmuskeln*

myocele ['maɪəˌsiː(ə)l] *subst.* condition where a muscle pushes through a gap in the surrounding membrane *myocele, muskelbråck*

myoclonic [ˌmaɪə(ʊ)'klɒnɪk] *adj.* referring to myoclonus *myoklonisk;* **myoclonic epilepsy** = form of epilepsy where the limbs jerk frequently *myoklonusepilepsi, Lundborg(-Unverricht)s sjukdom*

myoclonus [maɪ'ɒklənəs] *subst.* muscle spasm which makes a limb give an involuntary jerk *myokloni*

myodynia [ˌmaɪə(ʊ)'dɪniə] *subst.* pain in muscles *myodyni, myalgi, muskelsmärta*

myofibril [ˌmaɪə(ʊ)'faɪbrɪl] *subst.* long thread of striated muscle fibre *myofibrill*

myofibrosis [ˌmaɪə(ʊ)faɪ'brəʊsɪs] *subst.* condition where muscle tissue is replaced by fibrous tissue *myofibros*

myogen ⇨ **myogenic, myosin**

myogenic [ˌmaɪə(ʊ)'dʒenɪk] *adj.* (movement) which comes from an involuntary muscle *myogen*

myoglobin [ˌmaɪə(ʊ)'gləʊbɪn] *subst.* muscle haemoglobin, which takes oxygen from blood and passes it to the muscle *myoglobin*

myoglobinuria
] *subst.* presence of myoglobin in the urine *myoglobinuri*

myograf ⇨ **myograph**

myogram ['maɪə(ʊ)græm] *subst.* record showing how a muscle is functioning *myogram*

myograph ['maɪə(ʊ)grɑːf] *subst.* instrument which records the degree and strength of a muscle contraction *myograf*

myokardiet ⇨ **myocardium**

myokardinfarkt ⇨ **myocardial**

myokardit ⇨ **myocarditis**

myokloni ⇨ **myoclonus**

myoklonisk ⇨ **myoclonic**

myoklonusepilepsi ⇨ **myoclonic**

myokymia [ˌmaɪə(ʊ)'kɪmiə] *subst.* twitching of a certain muscle *myokymi*

myology [maɪ'ɒlədʒi] *subst.* study of muscles and their associated structures and diseases *myologi*

myoma [maɪ'əʊmə] *subst.* benign tumour in a smooth muscle *myom, muskelsvulst*

myomectomy [ˌmaɪə(ʊ)'mektəmi] *subst.* (i) surgical removal of a benign growth from a muscle, especially removal of a fibroid from the uterus *myomektomi, operativt avlägsnande av främst livmodermyom;* (ii) myectomy *myektomi*

myometriet ⇨ **myometrium**

myometritis [ˌmaɪə(ʊ)mə'traɪtɪs] *subst.* inflammation of the myometrium *myometrit, metrit, inflammation i livmoderns muskelvägg*

myometrium [ˌmaɪə(ʊ)'miːtriəm] *subst.* muscular tissue in the uterus *myometriet, livmoderväggen*

myoneural junction [ˌmaɪə(ʊ)'njʊər(ə)l ˌdʒʌŋ(k)ʃ(ə)n] = NEUROMUSCULAR JUNCTION

myopathy [maɪ'ɒpəθi] *subst.* disease of a muscle, especially where the muscle wastes away *myopati, muskelsjukdom;* **focal myopathy** = destruction of muscle tissue caused by the substance injected *lokal muskelnedbrytning pga injektion;* **needle myopathy** = destruction of muscle tissue caused by using a large needle in intramuscular injections *lokal muskelnedbrytning pga användning av grov nål vid injektion*

myopia [maɪ'əʊpiə] *or* **shortsightedness** [ˌʃɔːt'saɪtɪdnəs] *or* **nearsightedness** [ˌnɪə'saɪtɪdnəs] *subst.* condition where a patient can see clearly objects which are close, but not ones which are further away *myopi, närsynthet*

myopic [maɪ'ɒpɪk] *or* **shortsighted** [ˌʃɔːt'saɪtɪd] *or* **nearsighted** [ˌnɪə'saɪtɪd] *adj.* able to see close objects clearly, but not objects which are further away *myop, närsynt*
NOTE: the opposite is **longsightedness** *or* **hypermetropia**

myoplasm ['maɪə(ʊ)plæz(ə)m] *or* **sarcoplasm** ['sɑːkə(ʊ)plæz(ə)m] *subst.* cytoplasm of muscle cells *sarkoplasma*

myoplasty ['maɪə(ʊ)ˌplæsti] *subst.* plastic surgery to repair a muscle *plastikkirurgi av muskel*

myosarcoma [ˌmaɪə(ʊ)sɑː'kəʊmə] *subst.* (i) malignant tumour containing unstriated muscle *myoma sarcomatodes;* (ii) combined myoma and sarcoma *kombinerat myom och sarkom*

myosin ['maɪə(ʊ)sɪn] *subst.* protein in the A bands of muscle fibre which makes muscles elastic *myosin, myogen*

myosis, myotic [maɪ'əʊsɪs, maɪ'ɒtɪk] *see* MIOSIS, MIOTIC

myositis [ˌmaɪə(ʊ)'saɪtɪs] *subst.* inflammation and degeneration of a muscle *myosit, muskelinflammation*

myotactic [ˌmaɪə(ʊ)'tæktɪk] *adj.* referring to the sense of touch in a muscle *som avser el. hör till musklernas beröringssinne;* **myotactic reflex** = reflex action in a muscle which contracts after being stretched *myotatisk reflex, sträckreflex*

myotomy [maɪ'ɒtəmi] *subst.* surgical operation to cut a muscle *myotomi*

myotonia [ˌmaɪə(ʊ)'təʊniə] *subst.* difficulty in relaxing a muscle after exercise *myotoni, tonisk muskelkramp*

myotonic [ˌmaɪə(ʊ)'tɒnɪk] *adj.* referring to tone in a muscle *myotonisk;* **myotonic dystrophy** *or* **dystrophia myotonica** = hereditary disease with muscle stiffness leading to atrophy of the muscles of the face and neck *dystrophia myotonica, myotonia atrophica*

myotonus [maɪ'ɒtənəs] *subst.* muscle tone *muskeltonus*

myringa [mɪ'rɪŋgə] *or* **eardrum** ['ɪədrʌm] *subst.* membrane at the end of the external auditory meatus leading from the outer ear, which vibrates with sound and passes the vibrations on to the ossicles in the middle ear *myrinx, trumhinnan*

myringitis [ˌmɪrɪn'dʒaɪtɪs] *subst.* inflammation of the eardrum *myringit, trumhinneinflammation*

myringoplastik ⇨ **myringoplasty, tympanoplasty**

myringoplasty [mɪ'rɪŋgəʊˌplæsti] *subst.* plastic surgery to correct a defect in the eardrum *myringoplastik, tympanoplastik*

myringotome [mɪˈrɪŋɡəʊtəʊm] *subst.* sharp knife used in myringotomy *myringotom*

myringotomi ⇨ **myringotomy, tympanotomy**

myringotomy [ˌmɪrɪŋˈɡɒtəmi] *subst.* surgical operation to make an opening in the eardrum *myringotomi, tympanotomi, (trumhinne)paracentes*

myrinx ⇨ **eardrum, myringa, tympanic, tympanum**

myrkrypning ⇨ **pins and needles, formication**

myxoedema [ˌmɪksəˈdiːmə] *subst.* condition caused when the thyroid gland does not produce enough thyroid hormone *myxödem*

COMMENT: the patient (usually a middle-aged woman) becomes fat, moves slowly and develops coarse skin; the condition can be treated with thyroxine

myxoedematous [ˌmɪksəˈdemətəs] *adj.* referring to myxoedema *myxödematös*

myxoma [mɪkˈsəʊmə] *subst.* benign tumour of mucous tissue, usually found in subcutaneous tissue of the limbs and neck *myxom, slemhinnesvulst*

myxosarcoma [ˌmɪksəʊsɑːˈkəʊmə] *subst.* malignant tumour of mucous tissue *myxosarkom*

myxovirus [ˌmɪksəʊˈvaɪ(ə)rəs] *subst.* any virus which has an affinity for the mucoprotein receptors in red blood cells (one of which causes influenza) *myxovirus*

myxödem ⇨ **myxoedema**

myxödematös ⇨ **myxoedematous**

mål ⇨ **goal, target**

målbrottet, komma i ⇨ **voice**

målcell ⇨ **target**

månadsblödning ⇨ **catamenia, menses, menstruation, period**

månbenet ⇨ **lunate (bone)**

måne (på nagel) ⇨ **lunula**

mång- ⇨ **multi-, multiple**

mångföderska ⇨ **multipara**

mångkärnig ⇨ **multinucleated**

mått ⇨ **measure, measurement**

måttband ⇨ **measure**

måttstock ⇨ **standard**

mäktig ⇨ **rich**

mängd ⇨ **amount, mass, volume**

människa ⇨ **human, person**

människo- ⇨ **human**

människoloppa ⇨ **Pulex**

märg ⇨ **marrow, medulla, pulp**

märg- ⇨ **medullary, myel-**

märghåla ⇨ **medullary**

märgliknande ⇨ **medullary**

märka ⇨ **label, mark; sense**

märkbar ⇨ **noticeable, visible**

märke ⇨ **label, mark**

märla ⇨ **staple**

mässling ⇨ **measles**

mässlingliknande ⇨ **morbilliform**

mäta ⇨ **measure**

mättat fett ⇨ **saturated fat**

mödomshinnan ⇨ **hymen, maidenhead**

mödra- ⇨ **maternal**

mödradödlighet ⇨ **maternal**

mödravårdscentral ⇨ **maternity**

Mönckeberg's arteriosclerosis [ˈmeŋkənbɜːɡz ɑːˌtɪəriəʊskləˌrəʊsɪs] *subst.* condition of old people, where the media of the arteries in the legs harden, causing limping *Mönckebergs mediaskleros*

mörda ⇨ **murder**

mörk ⇨ **dark**

mörker ⇨ **dark**

mörker- ⇨ **scoto-, scotopic**

mörkeradaptation ⇨ **scotopia**

mörkerseende ⇨ **scotopic**

mörkhårig ⇨ **dark**

mörknande ⇨ **darkening**

mörkrum ⇨ **darkroom**

mörkrädsla ⇨ **nyctaphobia**

mössa ⇨ **cap**

Nn

N 1 *chemical symbol for* nitrogen *N, kväve* **2** *abbreviation for* newton *N, newton*

Na *chemical symbol for* sodium *Na, natrium*

nabothian cyst [nəˈbəʊθiən ˌsɪst] *or* **nabothian follicle** [nəˈbəʊθiən ˌfɒlɪk(ə)l] *or* **nabothian gland** [nəˈbəʊθiən ˌglænd] *subst.* cyst which forms in the cervix of the uterus when the ducts in the cervical glands are blocked *ovula Nabothi, Nabothis ägg*

nack- ⇨ **nuchal, occipital**

nackbenet ⇨ **occipital**

nacken ⇨ **nape, nucha**

nackloben ⇨ **occipital**

nackspärr ⇨ **torticollis**

nackstyvhet ⇨ **neck**

nacksömmen ⇨ **lambdoid(al) suture**

nackvenen, djupa ⇨ **cervical**

naevus [ˈniːv əs] *subst.* birthmark *or* mark on the skin which a baby has at birth and which cannot be removed *naevus, födelsemärke; see also* HAEMANGIOMA, PORT WINE STAIN, STRAWBERRY
NOTE: plural is **naevi**

Naga sore [ˈnɑːgə ˌsɔː] *or* **tropical ulcer** [ˈtrɒpɪk(ə)l ˌʌlsə] *subst.* large area of infection which forms round a wound in tropical countries *slags infekterat sår (som uppstår i tropikerna)*

nagel ⇨ **nail**

nagel- ⇨ **onych-, ungual**

nagelavlossning ⇨ **onychomadesis**

nagelband ⇨ **cuticle**

nagelbitning ⇨ **nail**

nagelböld ⇨ **paronychia, whitlow**

nagelinflammation ⇨ **onychia**

nagelkrökning ⇨ **onychogryphosis**

nagelsax ⇨ **nail**

nagelsjukdom ⇨ **onychosis**

nageltrång ⇨ **ingrowing toenail**

nail [neɪl] *or* **unguis** [ˈʌŋgwɪs] *subst.* hard growth, formed of keratin, which forms on the top surface at the end of each finger and toe *unguis, nagel;* **nail biting** = obsessive chewing of the fingernails, usually a sign of stress *nagelbitning;* **nail scissors** = special curved scissors for cutting nails *nagelsax; see also* FINGERNAIL, TOENAIL
NOTE: for terms referring to nail see words beginning with **onych-**

nalkas ⇨ **approach**

"namnlösa artären" ⇨ **innominate**

namnteckning ⇨ **signature**

nape [neɪp] *or* **nucha** [ˈnjuːkə] *subst.* back of the neck *nacken*

napkin [ˈnæpkɪn] *subst.* soft cloth, used for wiping or absorbing *blöja, liten handduk, trasa;* **sanitary napkin** *or* **sanitary towel** = wad of absorbent cotton material attached by a woman over the vulva to absorb the menstrual flow *dambinda;* **napkin rash** = NAPPY RASH

napp ⇨ **dummy, pacifier, teat**

nappflaska ⇨ **bottle**

nappy [ˈnæpi] *subst.* cloth used to wrap round a baby's bottom and groin to keep clothing clean and dry *blöja;* **disposable nappy** = paper nappy which is thrown away when dirty, and not washed and used again *engångsblöja;* **nappy rash** = sore red skin on a baby's buttocks and groin, caused by reaction to long contact with ammonia in a wet nappy *blöjdermatit, blöjeksem*
NOTE: the US English is **diaper**

narco- ['nɑːkə(ʊ), ˌ--] *prefix* meaning sleep *or* stupor *narko-, bedövnings-*

narcoanalysis [ˌnɑːkəʊə'næləsɪs] *subst.* use of narcotics to induce a comatose state in a patient about to undergo psychoanalysis which may be emotionally disturbing *narkoanalys*

narcolepsy ['nɑːkə(ʊ)ˌlepsi] *subst.* condition where the patient has an uncontrollable tendency to fall asleep at any time *narkolepsi*

narcoleptic [ˌnɑːkə(ʊ)'leptɪk] *subst. & adj.* (substance) which causes narcolepsy *som ger upphov till narkolepsi;* (patient) suffering from narcolepsy *som lider av narkolepsi*

narcosis [nɑː'kəʊsɪs] *subst.* state of stupor induced by a drug *narkos;* **basal narcosis** = making a patient completely unconscious by administering a narcotic before a general anaesthetic *narkosinledning, nedsövning*

narcotic [nɑː'kɒtɪk] *subst. & adj.* (pain-relieving drug) which makes a patient sleep *or* become unconscious *narkotisk, sömngivande, bedövnings-;* **narcotics** *narkotika;* **the doctor put her to sleep with a powerful narcotic; the narcotic side-effects of an antihistamine**

> COMMENT: although narcotics are used medicinally as pain killers, they are highly addictive. The main narcotics are barbiturates, cocaine, and opium and drugs derived from opium, such as morphine, codeine and heroin

nares ['neəriːz] *subst pl.* nostrils *or* two passages in the nose through which air is breathed in or out *nares, näsöppningarna;* **anterior nares** *or* **external nares** = the two nostrils *främre näsöppningarna, näsborrarna;* **internal nares** *or* **posterior nares** *or* **choanae** = two openings shaped like funnels leading from the nasal cavity to the pharynx *koanerna, bakre näsöppningarna*
NOTE: singular is **naris**

narig ⇨ **chapped, crack**

narko- ⇨ **narco-**

narkoanalys ⇨ **narcoanalysis**

narkolepsi ⇨ **narcolepsy**

narkoman ⇨ **addict**

narkomani ⇨ **addiction**

narkos ⇨ **anaesthesia, narcosis**

narkos- ⇨ **anaesthetic**

narkosinledning ⇨ **anaesthetic, narcosis**

narkosläkare ⇨ **anaesthesiologist, anaesthetist**

narkosmask ⇨ **face**

narkosmedel ⇨ **anaesthetic**

narkotika ⇨ **habit-forming, narcotic**

narkotikaberoende ⇨ **addiction, dependence**

narkotikamissbruk ⇨ **abuse, addiction, drug**

narkotikamissbrukare ⇨ **addict**

narkotikarus ⇨ **trip**

narkotikum ⇨ **drug**

narkotisk ⇨ **narcotic**

narrow ['nærəʊ] **1** *adj.* not wide *trång, smal;* **the blood vessel is a narrow channel which takes blood to the tissues; the surgeon inserted a narrow tube into the vein**
NOTE: **narrow - narrower - narrowest** **2** *vb.* to become narrow *smalna, avta, dra ihop sig;* **the bronchial tubes are narrowed causing asthma**

nasal ['neɪz(ə)l] *adj.* referring to the nose *nasal, näs-;* **nasal apertures** *or* **choanae** = two openings shaped like funnels leading from the nasal cavity to the pharynx *koanerna, bakre näsöppningarna;* **nasal bones** = two small bones which form the bridge at the top of the nose ⇨ *illustration* SKULL *os nasale, näsbenet;* **nasal cavity** = cavity behind the nose between the cribriform plates above and the hard palate below, divided in two by the nasal septum, and leading to the nasopharynx ⇨ *illustration* THROAT *cavum nasi, näshålan;* **nasal cartilage** = two cartilages in the nose (the upper is attached to the nasal bone and the front of the maxilla, the lower is thinner and curls round each nostril to the septum) *näsbrosken;* **nasal conchae** *or* **turbinate bones** = three ridges of bone (superior, middle and inferior conchae) which project into the nasal cavity from the side walls *conchae nasales, näsmusslorna;* **nasal congestion** = condition where the nose is blocked by mucus *nästäppa;* **nasal septum** = division between the two part of the nasal cavity, formed of the vomer and the nasal cartilage *septum nasi, nässkiljeväggen*

naso- ['neɪzəʊ, ˌ--] *prefix* referring to the nose *nas(o)-, rin(o)-, näs-*

nasofaryngeal ⇨ **nasopharyngeal**

nasofaryngit ⇨ **nasopharyngitis**

nasofarynx ⇨ **nasopharynx**

nasogastric [ˌneɪzəʊ'gæstrɪk] *adj.* referring to the nose and stomach *som avser el. hör till både näsan och magen;* **nasogastric tube** = tube passed through the nose into the stomach *ventrikelsond*

nasolacrimal [ˌneɪzəʊ'lækrɪm(ə)l] *adj.* referring to the nose and the tear glands *nasolakrimal;* **nasolacrimal duct** = duct which drains tears from the lacrimal sac into the nose *ductus nasolacrimalis, tårkanalen*

nasolakrimal ⇨ **nasolacrimal**

nasopharyngeal [ˌneɪzəʊˌfærɪn'dʒi:əl] *adj.* referring to the nasopharynx *nasofaryngeal*

nasopharyngitis [ˌneɪzəʊˌfærɪn'dʒaɪtɪs] *subst.* inflammation of the mucous membrane of the nasal part of the pharynx *nasofaryngit*

nasopharynx ['neɪzəʊˌfærɪŋ(k)s] *subst.* top part of the pharynx which connects with the nose *nasofarynx, näs-svalgrummet*

nasty ['nɑ:sti] *adj.* unpleasant *obehaglig, elakartad;* **this medicine has a nasty taste; drink some orange juice to take away the nasty taste; this new drug has some nasty side-effects**
NOTE: **nasty - nastier - nastiest**

nates ['neɪti:z] *subst pl.* buttocks *nates, klinkorna, sätet*

National Health Service (NHS) [ˌnæʃ(ə)n(ə)l 'helθ ˌsɜ:vɪs (ˌeneɪtʃ'es)] *subst.* government service in the UK which provides medical services free of charge, or at reduced cost, to the whole population *allmänna hälso- och sjukvården (i Storbritannien), ung. offentlig sjukvård;* **a NHS doctor** = a doctor who works in the National Health Service *läkare som arbetar inom NHS;* **NHS glasses** = cheap spectacles provided by the National Health Service *glasögon som tillhandahålls av NHS;* **on the NHS** = free *or* paid for by the NHS *gratis el. betald av NHS;* **he had his operation on the NHS; she went to see a specialist on the NHS**
NOTE: the opposite of **"on the NHS"** is **"privately"**

> QUOTE figures reveal that 5% more employees in the professional and technical category were working in the NHS compared with three years before
> **Nursing Times**

nativitet ⇨ **birth**

natrium ⇨ **sodium**

natriumbalans ⇨ **sodium**

natriumbikarbonat ⇨ **bicarbonate of soda, sodium**

natriumglutamat ⇨ **monosodium glutamate**

natriumklorid ⇨ **sodium, salt**

natt ⇨ **night**

natt- ⇨ **nocturnal**

nattblindhet ⇨ **nyctalopia**

nattjour ⇨ **duty**

nattjänstgöring ⇨ **duty**

nattlig ⇨ **nocturnal**

nattsjuksköterska ⇨ **night**

nattskräck ⇨ **night**

nattsvett ⇨ **night**

natur ⇨ **nature**

natur- ⇨ **natural**

natural ['nætʃr(ə)l] *adj.* **(a)** normal *or* not surprising *naturlig, normal;* **his behaviour was quite natural; it's natural for old people to go deaf; natural childbirth** = childbirth where the mother is not given pain-killing drugs but is encouraged to give birth to the baby with as little medical assistance as possible *naturlig förlossning;* **natural immunity** = immunity from disease a newborn baby has from birth, which is inherited, acquired in the womb or from the mother's milk *naturlig immunitet* **(b)** not made by men *naturlig;* (thing) which comes from nature *natur-;* **natural gas** = gas which is found in the earth and not made in a factory *naturgas;* **natural history** = study of nature *natur(al)historia*

nature ['neɪtʃə] *subst.* **(a)** (i) essential quality of something *natur, karaktär, beskaffenhet;* (ii) kind *or* sort *typ, slag, sort;* (iii) plants and animals *naturen;* **nature study**

= learning about plant and animal life at school *naturkunskap* **(b) human nature** = general characteristics of human beings *mänskliga naturen*

naturgas ⇨ **natural**

naturlig ⇨ **inborn, natural**

naturopathy [ˌneɪtʃəˈrɒpəθi] *subst.* treatment of diseases and disorders which does not use medical or surgical means, but natural forces such as light, heat, massage, eating natural foods and using herbal remedies *alternativmedicin, naturmedicin*

naturvetenskap ⇨ **science**

naturvetenskaplig ⇨ **scientific**

naturvetenskapsman ⇨ **scientist**

nausea [ˈnɔːsiə] *subst.* feeling sick *or* feeling that you want to vomit *nausea, illamående, kväljning(ar);* **she suffered from nausea in the morning; he felt slight nausea in getting onto the boat**

> COMMENT: nausea can be caused by eating habits, such as eating too much rich food or drinking too much alcohol; it can also be caused by sensations such as unpleasant smells *or* motion sickness. Other causes include stomach disorders, such as gastritis, ulcers and liver infections. Nausea is commonly experienced by women in the early stages of pregnancy, and is called "morning sickness"

nauseated [ˈnɔːsieɪtɪd] *or US* **nauseous** [ˈnɔːsiəs] *adj.* feeling sick *or* feeling about to vomit *illamående, äcklad, med kväljningskänslor;* **the casualty may feel nauseated**

navel [ˈneɪv(ə)l] *or* **omphalus** [ˈɒmfələs] *or* **umbilicus** [ʌmˈbɪlɪkəs] *subst.* scar with a depression in the middle of the abdomen where the umbilical cord was detached after birth *umbilicus, omphalus, naveln*
NOTE: for terms referring to the navel see words beginning with **omphal-**

navel- ⇨ **omphal-, umbilical**

navelblåsan ⇨ **allantois**

navelbråck ⇨ **omphalocele, umbilical**

navelinflammation ⇨ **omphalitis**

naveln ⇨ **belly button, navel, omphalus**

navelområdet ⇨ **umbilical**

navelsträngen ⇨ **umbilical cord, funis**

navicular bone [nəˈvɪkjʊlə bəʊn] *subst.* one of the tarsal bones in the foot ⇨ *illustration* FOOT *os naviculare, båtbenet*

nearsighted [ˌnɪəˈsaɪtɪd] = MYOPIC

nearsightedness [ˌnɪəˈsaɪtɪdnəs] = MYOPIA

nebula [ˈnebjʊlə] *subst.* (i) slightly cloudy spot on the cornea *nebula, kornealgrumling, hornhinnegrumling;* (ii) spray of medicinal solution, applied to the nose or throat using a nebulizer *spray*

nebulisator ⇨ **atomizer**

nebulizer [ˈnebjulaɪzə] = ATOMIZER

Necator [neˈkeɪtə] *subst.* genus of hookworm which infests the small intestine *Necator, slags hakmask*

necatoriasis [neˌkeɪtəˈraɪəsɪs] *subst.* infestation of the small intestine by the parasite Necator *ancylostomiasis, angrepp av inälvsparasiten Necator (americanus)*

neck [nek] *subst.* **(a)** part of the body which joins the head to the body *halsen;* **he is suffering from pains in the neck; the front of the neck is swollen with goitre; the jugular veins run down the side of the neck; stiff neck** = condition where moving the neck is painful, usually caused by a strained muscle *or* by sitting in a cold draught *nackstyvhet, stelhet i nacken;* **neck collar** = special strong collar to support the head of a patient with a fractured neck *halskrage* **(b)** narrow part (of a bone *or* organ) *collum, hals;* **neck of tooth** = point where a tooth narrows slightly, between the crown and the root *tandhals;* **neck of the uterus** = CERVIX NOTE: for terms referring to the neck, see **cervical**

> COMMENT: the neck is formed of the seven cervical vertebrae, and is held vertical by strong muscles. Many organs pass through the neck, including the oesophagus, the larynx and the arteries and veins which connect the brain to the bloodstream

necro- [ˈnekrəʊ, ˌ--] *prefix* meaning death *nekro-, döds-*

necrobiosis [ˌnekrəʊbaɪ'əʊsɪs] *subst.* (i) death of cells surrounded by living tissue *nekrobios, vävnadsdöd;* (ii) gradual localized death of a part or tissue *nekrobios, vävnadsdöd*

necrology [ne'krɒlədʒi] *subst.* scientific study of mortality statistics *mortalitetsstatistik, dödlighetsstatistik*

necrophilia [ˌnekrə(ʊ)'fɪliə] *or* **necrophilism** [ne'krɒfɪlɪz(ə)m] *subst.* (i) abnormal pleasure in corpses *nekrofili;* (ii) sexual attraction to dead bodies *nekrofili*

necropsy ['nekrɒpsi] = POST MORTEM

necrosed ['nekrəʊst] *adj.* dead (tissue *or* bone) *nekrotisk, död (om vävnad)*

necrosis [ne'krəʊsɪs] *subst.* death of a part of the body, such as a bone *or* tissue *or* an organ *nekros, gangrän, lokal vävnadsdöd;* **gangrene is a form of necrosis**

necrospermia [ˌnekrəʊ'spɜːmiə] *subst.* condition where dead sperm exist in the semen *nekrospermi*

necrotic [ne'krɒtɪk] *adj.* referring to necrosis *nekrotisk;* dead (tissue) *död (om vävnad)*

necrotomy [ne'krɒtəmi] *subst.* dissection of a dead body *nekrotomi;* **osteoplastic necrotomy** = surgical removal of a piece of necrosed bone tissue *operativt avlägsnande av nekrotisk benvävnad*

nedbrytning ➪ **destruction**

nedbrytningsprodukt ➪ **breakdown**

nedgång ➪ **decrease**

nedhängande ➪ **dependent**

nedkomst ➪ **delivery, parturition**

nedkylning ➪ **refrigeration**

nedlusning ➪ **pediculosis, phthiriasis**

nedre motorneuron ➪ **pathway**

nedsatt aptit ➪ **loss**

nedsatt funktion ➪ **malfunction**

nedsmittning ➪ **contamination**

nedsmutsning ➪ **pollution**

nedstämd ➪ **depressed**

nedstämdhet ➪ **depression**

nedsätta ➪ **impair**

nedsättning ➪ **impairment, loss**

nedsövning ➪ **narcosis**

needle ['niːd(ə)l] *subst.* (i) thin metal instrument with a hole at one end for attaching a thread, and a sharp point at the other end, used for sewing up surgical incisions *nål;* (ii) thin hollow metal instrument with a point at one end, attached to a hypodermic syringe and used for giving injections *nål, kanyl;* **it is important that needles used for injections should be sterilized; AIDS can be transmitted by using non-sterile needles; stop needle** = needle with a ring round it, so that it can only be pushed a certain distance into the body *nål med (justerbar) stoppring för t.ex. benmärgspunktion;* **surgical needle** = needle for sewing up surgical incisions *kirurgisk nål;* **needle myopathy** = destruction of muscle tissue caused by using a large needle for intramuscular injections *lokal muskelnedbrytning pga användning av grov nål vid injektion*

needlestick ['niːd(ə)lstɪk] *subst.* accidental pricking of one's own skin by a needle (as by a nurse picking up a used syringe) *nålstick*

needling ['niːd(ə)lɪŋ] *subst.* puncture of a cataract with a needle *punktering av grå starr*

nefralgi ➪ **nephralgia**

nefrektomi ➪ **nephrectomy**

nefrit ➪ **nephritis**

nefr(o)- ➪ **nephr-**

nefroblastom ➪ **nephroblastoma**

nefrokalcinos ➪ **nephrocalcinosis**

nefrolitektomi ➪ **lithonephrotomy**

nefrolithiasis ➪ **nephrolithiasis**

nefrolitotomi ➪ **lithonephrotomy, nephrolithotomy**

nefrologi ➪ **nephrology**

nefrom ➪ **nephroma**

nefron ➪ **nephron**

nefropexi ⇨ **nephropexy**

nefroptos ⇨ **nephroptosis**

nefropyelit ⇨ **pyelonephritis**

nefros ⇨ **nephrosis**

nefroskleros ⇨ **nephrosclerosis**

nefrostomi ⇨ **nephrostomy**

nefrotomi ⇨ **nephrotomy**

nefrouretererektomi ⇨ **nephroureterectomy**

negative ['negətɪv] *adj. & subst.* showing 'no' *negativ, nekande;* **the answer is in the negative** = the answer is 'no' *svaret är nekande;* **the test was negative** = the test showed that the patient did not have the disease *provet var negativt;* **negative feedback** = situation where the result of a process represses the process which caused it *negativ feedback*

negativism ['negətɪvɪz(ə)m] *subst.* attitude of a patient who opposes what someone says *negativism*

> COMMENT: there are two types of negativism: active, where the patient does the opposite of what a doctor tells him, and passive, where the patient does not do what he has been asked to do

negra ['ni:grə] *see* LINEA

Negri bodies ['neɪgri ˌbɒdɪz] *subst. pl.* particles found in the cerebral cells of patients suffering from rabies *Negrikroppar*

Neil Robertson stretcher [ˌni:(ə)l 'rɒbəts(ə)n ˌstretʃə] *see* STRETCHER

Neisseria [naɪ'sɪəriə] *subst.* genus of bacteria, including gonococcus which causes gonorrhoea, and meningococcus which causes meningitis *Neisseria*

nekande ⇨ **negative**

nekro- ⇨ **necro-**

nekrobios ⇨ **necrobiosis**

nekrofili ⇨ **necrophilia**

nekros ⇨ **necrosis**

nekrospermi ⇨ **necrospermia**

nekrotisk ⇨ **necrosed, necrotic**

nekrotomi ⇨ **necrotomy**

nematod ⇨ **nematode, roundworm**

nematode ['nemətəʊd] *subst.* type of parasitic roundworm, such as hookworms, pinworms and threadworms *nematod, rundmask, trådmask*

neo- ['ni:ə(ʊ), ˌ--] *prefix* meaning new *neo-, ny-*

neocerebellum [ˌni:əʊˌserə'beləm] *subst.* middle part of the cerebellum *lillhjärnans mittparti*

neomycin [ˌni:əʊ'maɪsɪn] *subst.* type of antibiotic used for treatment of skin disease *neomycin*

neonatal [ˌni:əʊ'neɪt(ə)l] *subst.* referring to the first few weeks after birth *neonatal, nyföddhets-;* **neonatal death rate** number of newborn babies who die, shown per thousand babies born *neonatal mortalitet (dödlighet), spädbarnsdödlighet*

> QUOTE one of the most common routes of neonatal poisoning is percutaneous absorption following topical administration
>
> **Southern Medical Journal**

neonatalavdelning ⇨ **special**

neonate ['ni:ə(ʊ)neɪt] *subst.* newborn baby, less than four weeks old *nyfött barn, spädbarn*

neonatorum [ˌni:əʊneɪ'tɔ:rəm] *see* ASPHYXIA

neoplasm ['ni:əʊplæz(ə)m] *subst.* any new and morbid formation of tissue *neoplasma, tumör, cancer*

> QUOTE testicular cancer comprises only 1% of all malignant neoplasms in the male, but it is one of the most frequently occurring types of tumours in late adolescence
>
> **Journal of American College Health**

nephr- ['nefr, ˌ-] *prefix* referring to the kidney *nefr(o)-, ren(o)-, njur-*

nephralgia [nɪ'frældʒə] *subst.* pain in the kidney *nefralgi, njurkolik*

nephrectomy [nɪ'frektɒmi] *subst.* surgical removal of the whole kidney *nefrektomi*

nephritis [ni'fraɪtɪs] *subst.* inflammation of the kidney *nefrit, njurinflammation*

COMMENT: acute nephritis can be caused by a streptococcal infection. Symptoms can include headaches, swollen ankles, and fever

nephroblastoma [ˌnefrəʊblæ'stəʊmə] *or* **Wilm's tumour** ['wɪlmz ˌtju:mə] *subst.* malignant tumour in the kidneys in young children, usually under the age of 10, leading to swelling of the abdomen, which is treated by removal of the affected kidney *nefroblastom, Wilms tumör*

nephrocalcinosis [ˌnefrəʊˌkælsɪ'nəʊsɪs] *subst.* condition where calcium deposits are found in the kidney *nefrokalcinos*

nephrocapsulectomy [ˌnefrəʊˌkæpsju'lektəmi] *subst.* surgical removal of the capsule round a kidney *operativt avlägsnande av njurens kapsel*

nephrolithiasis [ˌnefrəʊlɪ'θaɪəsɪs] *subst.* condition where stones form in the kidney *nefrolithiasis, njursten(slidande)*

nephrolithotomy [ˌnefrəʊlɪ'θɒtəmi] *subst.* surgical removal of a stone in the kidney *nefrolitotomi*

nephrologist [ne'frɒlədʒɪst] *subst.* doctor who specializes in the study of the kidney and its diseases *njurspecialist*

nephrology [ne'frɒlədʒi] *subst.* study of the kidney and its diseases *nefrologi*

nephroma [ne'frəʊmə] *subst.* tumour in the kidney *or* tumour derived from renal substances *nefrom, njurtumör*

nephron ['nefrɒn] *subst.* tiny structure in the kidney, through which fluid is filtered *nefron*

COMMENT: a nephron is formed of a series of tubules, the loop of Henle, Bowman's capsule and a glomerulus. Blood enters the nephron from the renal artery, and waste materials are filtered out by the Bowman's capsule. Some substances return to the bloodstream by reabsorption in the tubules. Urine is collected in the ducts leading from the tubules to the ureters

nephropexy ['nefrəʊpeksi] *subst.* surgical operation to attach a mobile kidney *nefropexi*

nephroptosis [ˌnefrɒp'təʊsɪs] *or* **floating kidney** [ˌfləʊtɪŋ 'kɪdni] *subst.* condition where the kidney is mobile *nefroptos, vandrande njure, ren mobilis, rörlig njure*

nephrosclerosis [ˌnefrəʊsklə'rəʊsɪs] *subst.* kidney disease due to vascular change *nefroskleros, skrumpnjure*

nephrosis [ne'frəʊsɪs] *subst.* degeneration of the tissue of a kidney *nefros*

nephrostomy [ne'frɒstəmi] *subst.* surgical operation to make a permanent opening into the pelvis of the kidney from the surface *nefrostomi*

nephrotic syndrome [ne'frɒtɪk ˌsɪndrəʊm] *subst.* increasing oedema, albuminuria and raised blood pressure *nefrotiskt syndrom*

nephrotomy [ne'frɒtəmi] *subst.* surgical operation to cut into a kidney *nefrotomi*

nephroureterectomy [ˌnefrəʊˌjʊərɪtə'rektəmi] *or* **ureteronephrectomy** [jʊəˌri:tərəʊne'frektəmi] *subst.* surgical removal of all or part of a kidney and the ureter attached to it *nefroureterektomi*

nerv- ⇨ **nervous, neur-, neural**

nervbana ⇨ **arc, pathway, tract**

nervblockad ⇨ **nerve**

nervcell ⇨ **nerve, neurone**

nervcentrum ⇨ **nerve**

nerve [nɜ:v] *subst.* **(a)** bundle of fibres in a body which take impulses from one part of the body to another (each fibre being the axon of a nerve cell) *nerv;* **cranial nerves** = twelve pairs of nerves which are connected directly to the brain, and govern mainly the structures of the head and neck *nervi craniales, kranialnerverna; see also the list at* CRANIAL; **spinal nerves** = thirty-one pairs of nerves which lead from the spinal cord, and govern mainly the trunk and limbs *nervi spinales, spinalnerverna;* **motor nerve** *or* **efferent nerve** = nerve which carries impulses from the brain and spinal cord to muscles and causes movements *motorisk nerv, efferent (utåtledande) nerv;* **peripheral nerves** = parts of motor and sensory nerves which branch from the brain and spinal cord *perifera nerver;* **sensory nerve** *or* **afferent nerve** = nerve which registers a sensation, such as heat *or* taste *or* smell, etc., and carries impulses to the brain and spinal cord *sensorisk nerv, afferent (inåtledande) nerv;* **vasomotor nerve** = nerve whose impulses make the arterioles become narrower *vasomotorisk nerv* **(b)** *(names of nerves)* **abducent nerve** = sixth cranial nerve which controls the muscle which makes the eyeball turn *(nervus) abducens, 6:e kranialnerven;* **accessory nerve** = eleventh cranial nerve which supplies the muscles in the neck and shoulders *nervus accessorius, 11:e kranialnerven;* **acoustic nerve** *or* **auditory nerve** *or* **vestibulocochlear nerve** = eighth cranial nerve which governs hearing and balance *nervus vestibulo-cochlearis, hörsel- och balansnerven, 8:e kranialnerven;* **circumflex nerve** = sensory and motor nerve in the upper arm *sensorisk och motorisk nerv i överarmen;* **cochlear nerve** = division of the auditory nerve *nervus cochlearis, cochlearisnerven, koklearnerven;* **facial nerve** = seventh cranial nerve which governs the muscles of the face, the taste buds on the front of the tongue and the salivary and lacrimal glands *nervus facialis, ansiktsnerven, 7:e kranialnerven;* **femoral nerve** = nerve which governs the muscle at the front of the thigh *nervus femoralis, lårbensnerven;* **glossopharyngeal nerve** = ninth cranial nerve which controls the pharynx, the salivary glands and part of the tongue *nervus glossopharyngeus, tung- och svalgnerven, 9:e kranialnerven;* **oculomotor nerve** = third cranial nerve which controls the eyeballs and eyelids *nervus oculomotorius, ögonrörelsenerven, 3:e kranialnerven;* **olfactory nerve** = first cranial nerve which controls the sense of smell *nervus olfactorius, luktnerven, 1:a kranialnerven;* **optic nerve** = second cranial nerve which takes sensation of sight from the eye to the brain *nervus opticus, synnerven, 2:a kranialnerven;* **phrenic nerve** = nerve which controls the muscles in the diaphragm *nervus phrenicus;* **pneumogastric nerve** *or* **vagus nerve** = tenth cranial nerve which controls swallowing and nerve fibres in the heart and chest *(nervus) vagus, 10:e kranialnerven;* **radial nerve** = main motor nerve of the arm *nervus radialis, radialnerven;* **sacral nerves** = nerves which branch from the spinal cord in the sacrum and govern the legs, the arms and the genital area *nervi sacrales, sakralnerverna, korsnerverna;* **trigeminal nerve** = fifth cranial nerve which controls the sensory nerves in the forehead and face and the muscles in the jaw *nervus trigeminus, 5:e kranialnerven;* **trochlear nerve** = fourth cranial nerve which controls the muscles of the eyeball *nervus trochlearis, 4:e kranialnerven;* **ulnar nerve** = nerve running from the neck to the elbow, which controls the muscles in the forearm and fingers *nervus ulnaris;* **vestibulocochlear nerve** = eighth cranial nerve which governs hearing and balance *nervus vestibulo-cochlearis, hörsel- och balansnerven, 8:e kranialnerven* **(c) nerve block** = stopping the function of a nerve by injecting an anaesthetic *nervblockad;* **nerve cell** *or* **neurone** = cell in the nervous system, consisting of a cell body, axon(s) and dendrites, which transmits nerve impulses *neuron, nervcell;* **nerve centre** = point at which nerves come together *nervcenter;* **nerve ending** = terminal at the end of a nerve fibre, where a nerve cell connects with another nerve or with a muscle *nervändslut;* **nerve fibre** = fibre leading from a nerve cell, carrying the impulses *nervfiber, nervtråd;* **nerve gas** = gas which attacks the nervous system *nervgas;* **nerve impulse** = electrical impulse which is transmitted by nerve cells *nervimpuls;* **nerve root** = first part of a nerve as it leaves or joins the spinal column (the dorsal nerve root is the entry for a sensory nerve, and the ventral nerve root is the exit for a motor nerve) *nervrot;* **nerve tissue** = tissue which forms nerves, and which is able to transmit the nerve impulses *nervvävnad*

> COMMENT: nerves are the fibres along which impulses are carried. Motor nerves *or* efferent nerves take messages between the central nervous system and muscles, making the muscles move. Sensory nerves *or* afferent nerves transmit impulses (such as sight *or* pain) from the sense organs to the brain

nervfiber ⇨ **nerve**

nervförsörjning ⇨ **innervation**

nervgas ⇨ **nerve**

nervimpuls ⇨ **nerve**

nervinflammation ⇨ **neuritis**

nervlim ⇨ **glia**

nervosa [nəˈvəʊsə] *see* ANOREXIA

nervositet ⇨ **nervousness**

nervous [ˈnɜːvəs] *adj.* **(a)** referring to nerves *nerv-;* **nervous breakdown** = non-medical term for a sudden mental illness, where a patient becomes so depressed and worried that he is incapable of doing anything *nervsammanbrott;* **nervous system** = nervous tissues of the body, including the peripheral nerves, spinal cord, ganglia and nerve centres *nervsystemet;* **autonomic nervous system** = nervous system which regulates the automatic functioning of the structures of the body, such as the heart and lungs *autonoma nervsystemet;* **central nervous system** (CNS) = brain and spinal cord which link together all the nerves *centrala nervsystemet, CNS;* **peripheral nervous system** (PNS) = nervous tissue outside the central nervous system *perifera nervsystemet, PNS; see also*

PARASYMPATHETIC, SYMPATHETIC **(b)** very easily worried *nervös, ängslig, orolig;* **she's nervous about her exams; don't be nervous - the operation is a very simple one**

nervousness ['nɜːvəsnəs] *subst.* state of being nervous *nervositet, ängslan, oro*

nervrot ⇨ **nerve, radicle**

nervsammanbrott ⇨ **nervous**

nervsjukdom ⇨ **neuropathy**

nervsmärta ⇨ **neuralgia**

nervstråk ⇨ **bundle, fasciculus**

nervsutur ⇨ **neurorrhaphy**

nervsvulst ⇨ **neuroma**

nervsystemet ⇨ **nervous**

nervtråd ⇨ **nerve**

nervvävnad ⇨ **tissue**

nervy ['nɜːvi] *adj. informal* worried and nervous *nervös, ängslig, orolig*
NOTE: for other terms referring to nerves see words beginning with **neur-**

nervändkropp ⇨ **end**

nervändplatta ⇨ **end plate**

nervändslut ⇨ **arborization, ending, terminal**

nervös ⇨ **nervous, nervy**

nettlerash ['net(ə)lræʃ] *or* **urticaria** [ˌɜːtɪ'keəriə] *subst.* affection of the skin, with white or red weals which sting or itch, caused by an allergic reaction (often to plants) *urticaria, nässelfeber, nässelutslag*

network ['netwɜːk] *subst.* interconnecting system of lines and spaces, like a net *nätverk;* **a network of fine blood vessels**

neur- ['njʊə(r), ˌ-] *or* **neuro-** ['njʊərəʊ, ˌ--] *prefix* referring to a nerve *or* the nervous system *neur(o)-, nerv-*

neural ['njʊər(ə)l] *adj.* referring to a nerve *or* the nervous system *neural-, nerv-;* **neural arch** = curved part of a vertebra, which forms the space through which the spinal cord passes *arcus vertebrae, ryggkotsbåge;* **neural crest** = ridge of cells in an embryo which forms nerve cells of the sensory and autonomic ganglia *neurallisten;* **neural groove** = groove on the back of an embryo, formed as the neural plate closes to form the neural tube *neuralfåran, medullarrännan;* **neural plate** = thickening of an embryonic disc which folds over to form the neural tube *neuralplattan, medullarplattan;* **neural tube** = tube lined with ectodermal cells running the length of an embryo, which develops into the brain and spinal cord *neuralröret, medullarröret;* **neural tube defect** = congenital defect (such as spina bifida) which occurs when the edges of the neural tube do not close up properly *medfödd missbildning av ryggkotornas bågar*

neuralfåran ⇨ **neural**

neuralgi ⇨ **neuralgia**

neuralgia [njʊ(ə)'rældʒə] *subst.* spasm of pain which runs along a nerve *neuralgi, nervsmärta;* **trigeminal neuralgia** = pain in the trigeminal nerve, which sends intense pains shooting across the face *trigeminusneuralgi*

neurallisten ⇨ **neural**

neuralplattan ⇨ **neural**

neuralröret ⇨ **neural**

neurapraxia [ˌnjʊərə'præksiə] *subst.* lesion of a nerve which leads to paralysis for a very short time, giving a tingling feeling and loss of function *neuropraxi*

neurasteni ⇨ **neurasthenia**

neurasteniker ⇨ **neurasthenic**

neurastenisk ⇨ **neurasthenic**

neurasthenia [ˌnjʊərəs'θiːnjə] *subst.* type of neurosis where the patient is mentally and physically irritable and extremely fatigued *neurasteni*

neurasthenic [ˌnjʊərəs'θenɪk] *subst. & adj.* (person) suffering from neurasthenia *neurasteniker, neurastenisk*

neurectasis [nju'rektəsɪs] *subst.* surgical operation to stretch a peripheral nerve *operativt ingrepp för att sträcka ut perifer nerv*

neurectomy [nju'rektəmi] *subst.* surgical removal of all or part of a nerve *neurektomi*

neurektomi ⇨ **neurectomy**

neurilemma [ˌnjʊəri'lemə] *or* **neurolemma** [ˌnjʊərə(ʊ)'lemə] *subst.* outer sheath formed of Schwann cells, which covers the myelin sheath covering a nerve fibre *neurilemma*

neurilemmoma [ˌnjʊərileˈməʊmə] *or* **neurinoma** [ˌnjʊəriˈnəʊmə] *or* **neurofibroma** [ˌnjʊərəʊfaɪˈbrəʊmə] *subst.* benign tumour of a nerve, formed from the neurilemma *neurilemmom, neurinom, neurofibrom*

neurinom ⇨ **neurilemmoma**

neuritis [nju(ə)ˈraɪtɪs] *subst.* inflammation of a nerve, giving a constant pain *neurit, nervinflammation*

neuroanatomy [ˌnjʊərəʊəˈnætəmi] *subst.* scientific study of the structure of the nervous system *neuroanatomi*

neuroblast [ˈnjʊərəʊˌblæst] *subst.* cell in the embryonic spinal cord which forms a nerve cell *neuroblast*

neuroblastoma [ˌnjʊərəʊblæˈstəʊmə] *subst.* malignant tumour formed from the neural crest, found mainly in young children *neuroblastom*

neurocranium [ˌnjʊərəʊˈkreɪniəm] *subst.* part of the skull which encloses and protects the brain *neurocranium, hjärnskålen*

neurodermatitis [ˌnjʊərəʊˌdɜːməˈtaɪtɪs] *subst.* inflammation of the skin caused by psychological factors *neurodermatit*

neurodermatosis [ˌnjʊərəʊˌdɜːməˈtəʊsɪs] *subst.* nervous condition involving the skin *neurodermatos*

neuroendocrine system [ˌnjʊərəʊˈendəkrɪn ˌsɪstəm] *subst.* system where some organs are controlled by both the nervous system and by hormones *system som reglerar organs funktion med hjälp av både nervimpulser och hormoner*

neuroepitel ⇨ **neuroepithelium**

neuroepiteliom ⇨ **neuroepithelioma**

neuroepithelial [ˌnjʊərəʊˌepiˈθiːliəl] *adj.* referring to the neuroepithelium *som avser el. hör till neuroepitel*

neuroepithelioma [ˌnjʊərəʊˌepiˌθiːliˈəʊmə] *subst.* malignant tumour in the retina *neuroepiteliom*

neuroepithelium [ˌnjʊərəʊˌepiˈθiːliəm] *subst.* epithelial cells forming part of the lining of the mucosa of the nose or the labyrinth of the middle ear *neuroepitel*

neurofibril [ˌnjʊərəʊˈfaɪbrɪl] *subst.* fine thread in the cytoplasm of a neurone *neurofibrill*

neurofibrom ⇨ **neurilemmoma, neurofibroma**

neurofibroma [ˌnjʊərəʊfaɪˈbrəʊmə] *subst.* benign tumour of a nerve, formed from the neurilemma *neurofibrom;* **acoustic neurofibroma** = tumour in the sheath of the auditory nerve *tumör som utgår från hörselnervens skida*

neurofibromatos ⇨ **neurofibromatosis (NF)**

neurofibromatosis (NF) [ˌnjʊərəʊˌfaɪbrəʊməˈtəʊsɪs (ˌenˈef)] *or* **molluscum fibrosum** [məˈlʌskəm faɪˈbrəʊsəm] *or* **von Recklinghausen's disease** [vɒn ˈreklɪŋhaʊzənz dɪˌziːz] *subst.* hereditary condition where the patient has neurofibromata on the nerve trunks, limb plexuses or spinal roots, and pale brown spots appear on the skin *neurofibromatos, von Recklinghausens sjukdom*

neurofysiolog ⇨ **neurophysiologist**

neurofysiologi ⇨ **neurophysiology**

neurogenesis [ˌnjʊərəʊˈdʒenəsɪs] *subst.* development and growth of nerves and nervous tissue *nervernas och nervvävnadens tillväxt och utveckling*

neurogenic [ˌnjʊərəʊˈdʒenɪk] *adj.* (i) coming from the nervous system *neurogen;* (ii) referring to neurogenesis *som avser el. hör till nervernas och nervvävnadens tillväxt och utveckling;* **neurogenic bladder** = condition where a patient cannot control his bladder because of nervous disease *neurogen blåsa*

neuroglandular junction [ˌnjʊərəʊˈglændjʊlə ˌdʒʌŋ(k)ʃ(ə)n] *subst.* point where a nerve joins the gland which it controls *punkt där nerv och den körtel den innerverar möts*

neuroglia [njuˈrɒgliə] *subst.* supporting cells of the spinal cord and brain *neuroglia, glia, nervkitt*

neurogliaceller ⇨ **glial cells**

neurohormone [ˈnjʊərəʊˌhɔːməʊn] *subst.* hormone produced in some nerve cells and secreted from the nerve endings *neurohormon*

neurohypophysis [ˌnjʊərəʊhaɪˈpɒfəsɪs] *subst.* lobe at the back of the pituitary gland, which secretes oxytocin and vasopressin *neurohypofysen*

neurokirurg ⇨ **neurosurgeon**

neurokirurgi ⇨ **neurosurgery**

neurolemma [ˌnjʊərəʊˈlemə] *subst.* = NEURILEMMA

neuroleptic [ˌnjʊərəʊˈleptɪk] *or* **tranquillizer** [ˈtræŋkwəlaɪzə] *subst.* drug which calms a patient and stops him worrying *neuroleptikum*

neurological [ˌnjʊərəˈlɒdʒɪk(ə)l] *adj.* referring to neurology *neurologisk*

neurologist [ˌnju(ə)ˈrɒlədʒɪst] *subst.* doctor who specializes in the study of the nervous system and the treatment of its diseases *neurolog*

neurology [ˌnju(ə)ˈrɒlədʒi] *subst.* scientific study of the nervous system and its diseases *neurologi*

neuroma [njuˈrəʊmə] *subst.* benign tumour formed of nerve cells and nerve fibres *neurom, nervsvulst;* **acoustic neuroma** = tumour in the sheath of the auditory nerve *tumör som utgår från hörselnervens skida*

neuromuscular [ˌnjʊərəʊˈmʌskjʊlə] *adj.* referring to nerves and muscles *neuromuskulär;* **neuromuscular junction** *or* **myoneural junction** = point where a motor nerve joins muscle fibre *motorisk ändplatta*

neuromyelitis optica [ˌnjʊərəʊˌmaɪəˌlaɪtɪs ˈɒptɪkə] *or* **Devic's disease** [dəˈvɪks dɪˌziːz] *subst.* condition similar to multiple sclerosis, where the patient has acute myelitis and the optic nerve is also affected *neuromyelitis optica*

neurone [ˈnjʊərəʊn] *or* **neuron** [ˈnjʊərɒn] *or* **nerve cell** [ˈnɜːv sel] *subst.* cell in the nervous system which transmits nerve impulses *neuron, nervcell;* **bipolar neurone** = neurone with two processes (found in the retina) *bipolart (bipolärt) neuron, bipolar (bipolär) nervcell;* **motor neurone** = neurone which is part of a nerve pathway transmitting impulses from the brain to a muscle or gland *motorneuron, motorisk nervcell;* **upper motor neurone** = neurone which takes impulses from the cerebral cortex *övre (centralt) motorneuron, första ordningens neuron;* **lower motor neurone** = linked neurones which carry motor impulses from the spinal cord to the muscles *nedre (perifert) motorneuron, andra ordningens neuron;* **sensory neurone** = sensory neurone which receives its stimulus directly from the receptor, and passes the impulse to the sensory cortex *sensoriskt neuron, sensorisk nervcell*

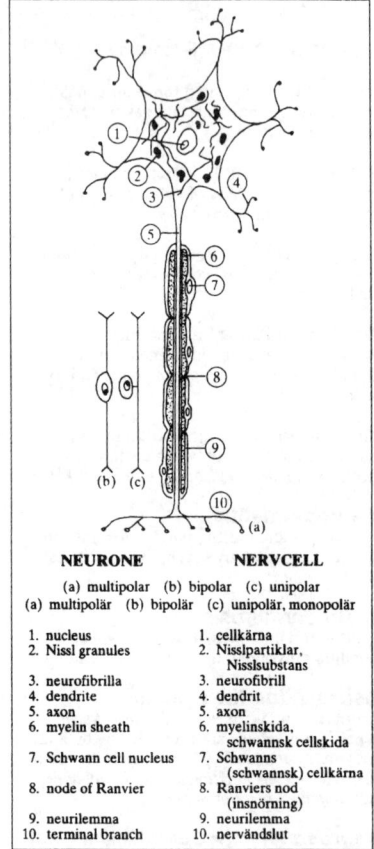

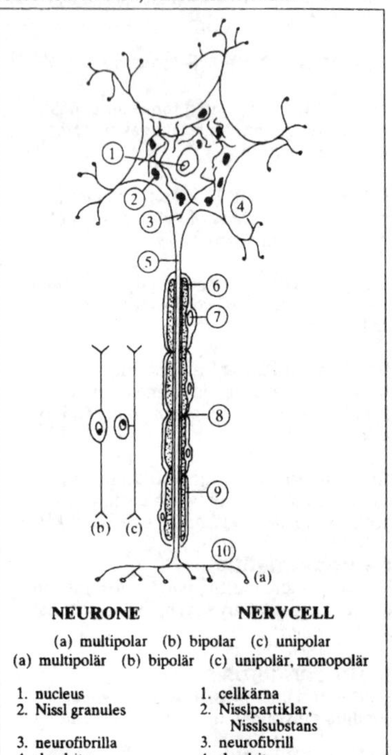

NEURONE **NERVCELL**

(a) multipolar (b) bipolar (c) unipolar
(a) multipolär (b) bipolär (c) unipolär, monopolär

1. nucleus	1. cellkärna
2. Nissl granules	2. Nisslpartiklar, Nisslsubstans
3. neurofibrilla	3. neurofibrill
4. dendrite	4. dendrit
5. axon	5. axon
6. myelin sheath	6. myelinskida, schwannsk cellskida
7. Schwann cell nucleus	7. Schwanns (schwannsk) cellkärna
8. node of Ranvier	8. Ranviers nod (insnörning)
9. neurilemma	9. neurilemma
10. terminal branch	10. nervändslut

neuropathology [ˌnjʊərə(ʊ)pəˈθɒlədʒi] *subst.* study of diseases of the nervous system *neuropatologi*

neuropathy [ˌnjʊəˈrɒpəθi] *subst.* disease involving destruction of the tissues of the nervous system *neuropati, nervsjukdom*

neuropati ⇨ **neuropathy**

neuropatologi ⇨ **neuropathology**

neurophysiologist [ˌnjʊərəʊˌfɪzɪ'ɒlədʒɪst] *subst.* scientist who studies the physiology of the nervous system *neurofysiolog*

neurophysiology [ˌnjʊərəʊfɪzɪ'ɒlədʒi] *subst.* study of the physiology of nerves *neurofysiologi*

neuroplasty ['njʊərəʊˌplæsti] *subst.* surgery to repair damaged nerves *neuroplastik*

neuropsychiatrist [ˌnjʊərəʊsaɪ'ka(ɪ)ətrɪst] *subst.* doctor who specializes in the study and treatment of mental and nervous disorders *specialist på psykiatriska och neurologiska sjukdomar*

neuropsychiatry [ˌnjʊərəʊsaɪ'ka(ɪ)ətri] *subst.* study of mental and nervous disorders *läran om psykiatriska och neurologiska sjukdomar*

neurorrhaphy [nju'rɔːrəfi] *subst.* surgical operation to join by suture a nerve which has been cut *neuro(r)rafi, nervsutur*

neuros ⇨ **neurosis, psychasthenia, psychoneurosis**

neuroscientist [ˌnjʊərəʊ'saɪəntɪst] *subst.* scientist who studies the nervous system *forskare som undersöker nervsystemet*

neurosecretion [ˌnjʊərəʊsɪ'kriːʃ(ə)n] *subst.* (i) substance secreted by a nerve cell *signalsubstans, ämne som utsöndras av nervcell;* (ii) secretion of active substance by nerve cells *neurosekretion*

neurosis [nju(ə)'rəʊsɪs] *subst.* illness of the personality, in which a patient becomes obsessed with something and experiences strong emotions towards it, such as fear of empty spaces, jealousy of a sibling, etc. *neuros, psykoneuros;* **anxiety neurosis** = neurotic condition where the patient is anxious and has morbid fears *ångestneuros* NOTE: plural is **neuroses**

neurosurgeon [ˌnjʊərəʊ'sɜːdʒ(ə)n] *subst.* surgeon who operates on the nervous system, including the brain *neurokirurg*

neurosurgery [ˌnjʊərəʊ'sɜːdʒ(ə)ri] *subst.* surgery on the nervous system, including the brain and spinal cord *neurokirurgi*

neurosyphilis [ˌnjʊərəʊ'sɪf(ə)lɪs] *subst.* syphilis which attacks the nervous system *neurosyfilis*

neurotic [nju(ə)'rɒtɪk] *subst. & adj.* (i) (person) who suffers from neurosis *neurotiker, neurotisk;* (ii) (any person) who is worried or obsessed with something *neurotiker, neurotisk*

neurotically [nju(ə)'rɒtɪk(ə)li] *adv.* in a neurotic way *neurotiskt;* **she is neurotically obsessed with keeping herself clean**

neurotiker ⇨ **neurotic**

neurotisk ⇨ **neurotic**

neurotiskt ⇨ **neurotically**

neurotmesis [ˌnjuːrɒt'miːsɪs] *subst.* cutting a nerve completely *neurotmesis*

neurotomy [njʊ'rɒtəmi] *subst.* surgical operation to cut a nerve *neurotomi*

neurotoxic [ˌnjʊərəʊ'tɒksɪk] *adj.* (substance) which can harm or be poisonous to nerve cells *neurotoxisk*

neurotransmitter [ˌnjʊərəʊtræns'mɪtə] *subst.* chemical substance which transmits nerve impulses from one neurone to another *neurotransmittor, transmittorsubstans, signalsubstans*

neurotripsy ['njʊərəʊˌtrɪpsi] *subst.* surgical bruising *or* crushing of a nerve *neurotripsi*

neurotropic [ˌnjʊərəʊ'trɒpɪk] *adj.* (bacterium) which is attracted to and attacks nerves *neurotrop*

neuter ['njuːtə] *adj.* neither male nor female *neutrum-, könlös*

neutral ['njuːtr(ə)l] *adj.* neither acid nor alkali *neutral;* **a pH factor of 7 is neutral**

neutralisera ⇨ **counteract, neutralize**

neutralize ['njuːtrəlaɪz] *vb.* to counteract the effect of something *neutralisera, motverka; (in bacteriology)* to make a toxin harmless by combining it with the correct amount of antitoxin *neutralisera;* **alkali poisoning can be neutralized by applying acid solution**

neutrofil ⇨ **neutrophil**

neutropenia [ˌnjuːtrə'piːniə] *subst.* condition where there are fewer neutrophils than normal in the blood *neutropeni*

neutrophil ['njuːtrəfɪl] *or* **polymorph** ['pɒlimɔːf] *adj.* type of white blood cell with an irregular nucleus, which can attack and destroy bacteria *neutrofil, polymorfkärnig, polymorfonukleär*

neutrum ⇨ **neuter**

nevus ['niːvəs] *US* = NAEVUS

newborn ['njuːbɔːn] *adj. & subst.* (baby) which has been born recently *nyfödd*

newton ['njuːt(ə)n] *subst.* SI unit of measurement of force *newton* NOTE: written **N** after figures: **the muscle exerted a force of 5N**

> COMMENT: 1 newton is the force required to move 1 kilogram at the speed of 1 metre per second

nexus ['neksəs] *subst.* link *or* point where two organs *or* tissues join *förbindelse, punkt där två organ eller vävnader möts*

NF [ˌen'ef] = NEUROFIBROMATOSIS

NGU ⇨ **non-specific urethritis (NSU)**

NHS [ˌeneɪtʃ'es] = NATIONAL HEALTH SERVICE

niacin ['na(ɪ)əsɪn] *or* **nicotinic acid** [ˌnɪkəˌtɪnɪk 'æsɪd] *subst.* vitamin of the vitamin B complex found in milk, meat, liver, kidney, yeast, beans, peas and bread (lack of niacin can cause mental disorders and pellagra) *niacin, nikotinsyra, vitamin PP*

nick [nɪk] **1** *subst.* little cut *hack, jack;* **he had a nick in his ear lobe which bled 2** *vb.* to make a little cut *skära (sig) litet;* **he nicked his chin while shaving**

nicka ⇨ **nod**

nick(ning) ⇨ **nod**

nickning, ofrivillig ⇨ **nutation**

nickningskramp ⇨ **spasmus nutans**

nicotine ['nɪkətiːn] *subst.* main alkaloid substance found in tobacco *nikotin;* **nicotine poisoning** *or* **nicotinism** = poisoning of the autonomic nervous system with large quantities of nicotine *nikotinism, nikotinförgiftning*

nicotinic acid [ˌnɪkəˌtɪnɪk 'æsɪd] *subst.* = NIACIN

nictation [nɪk'teɪʃ(ə)n] *or* **nictitation** [ˌnɪkti'teɪʃ(ə)n] *subst.* act of winking *nic(ti)tatio, blinkning*

nidation [naɪ'deɪʃ(ə)n] *subst.* **(a)** building of the endometrial layers of the uterus between menstrual periods *livmoderslemhinnans tillväxt mellan menstruationerna* **(b)** implantation *or* point in the development of an embryo, when the fertilized ovum reaches the uterus and implants in the wall of the uterus *nidation, befruktade äggets implantation i livmoderslemhinnan*

nidation ⇨ **implantation**

nidus ['naɪdəs] *subst.* centre of infection *or* site where bacteria can settle and breed *nidus, infektionshärd*

Nielsen ['niː(ə)ls(ə)n] *see* HOLGER

night [naɪt] *subst.* period between sunset and sunrise *or* part of the day when it is dark *natt;* **I don't like going out alone late at night; there are two nurses on duty each night; night blindness** = NYCTALOPIA; **night duty** = being on duty at night *nattjänstgöring;* **night nurse** = nurse who is on duty at night *nattsjuksköterska;* **night sweat** = heavy sweating when asleep at night *nattsvett;* **night terror** = disturbed sleep, which a child does not remember *nattskräck*

nightmare ['naɪtmeə] *subst.* dream which frightens *mardröm;* **the little girl had a nightmare and woke up screaming**

nigra ['naɪgrə] *see* LINEA

nikotin ⇨ **nicotine**

nikotinförgiftning ⇨ **nicotine**

nikotinism ⇨ **nicotine**

nikotinsyra ⇨ **niacin**

ninety-nine (99) [ˌnaɪnti'naɪn] *number* number which a doctor asks someone to say, so that he can inspect the back of the throat *siffror som läkare ber patient säga vid halsundersökning;* **the doctor told him to open his mouth wide and say ninety-nine**

nipple ['nɪp(ə)l] *or* **mammilla** [mə'mɪlə] *subst.* protruding darker part in the centre of the breast, containing the milk ducts through which the milk passes *mammillen, bröstvårtan*

Nissl granules ['nɪs(ə)l ˌgrænjuːlz] *or* **Nissl bodies** ['nɪs(ə)l ˌbɒdiz] *subst. pl.* coarse granules surrounding the nucleus in the cytoplasm of nerve cells ⇨ *illustration* NEURONE *Nisslpartiklar, Nisslsubstans*

nit [nɪt] *subst.* egg or larva of a louse *gnet, gnetter*

nitrogen ['naɪtrədʒ(ə)n] *subst.* chemical element, a gas which is the main component of air and is an essential part of protein *kväve, N*
NOTE: chemical symbol is **N**

> COMMENT: nitrogen is taken into the body by digesting protein-rich foods; excess nitrogen is excreted in urine. When the intake of nitrogen and the excretion rate are equal, the body is in nitrogen balance or protein balance

nitrous oxide ['naɪtrəs ˌɒksaɪd] *or* **laughing gas** ['lɑːfɪŋ gæs] *subst.* gas used in combination with other gases by dentists as an anaesthetic *kväveoxidul, lustgas*

nivå ⇨ **degree**

njur- ⇨ **nephr-, ren-, renal**

njurartärerna ⇨ **renal**

njurbarken ⇨ **renal**

njurbäckenet ⇨ **renal**

njurbäckeninflammation ⇨ **ureteropyelonephritis**

njurbäcken(s)- ⇨ **pyel-**

njurbäckensinflammation ⇨ **pyelitis**

njurclearance ⇨ **clearance**

njurdonator ⇨ **donor**

njuren ⇨ **kidney**

njurgrus ⇨ **gravel**

njurhilus ⇨ **sinus**

njurinflammation ⇨ **nephritis**

njurkalk ⇨ **calyx**

njurkanalerna ⇨ **renal**

njurkapseln ⇨ **capsule**

njurkolik ⇨ **renal, nephralgia**

njurkropp ⇨ **corpuscle**

njurmärgen ⇨ **medulla**

njurnystan ⇨ **glomerulus**

njurspecialist ⇨ **nephrologist**

njursten ⇨ **calculus, kidney**

njursvikt ⇨ **failure**

njurtumör ⇨ **nephroma**

NMR [ˌenem'ɑː] = NUCLEAR MAGNETIC RESONANCE

Nocardia [nəʊ'kɑːdiə] *subst.* genus of bacteria found in soil, some species of which cause nocardiosis and Madura foot *Nocardia, slags strålsvamp*

nocardiosis [nəʊˌkɑːdi'əʊsɪs] *or* **nocardiasis** [ˌnəʊkɑː'daɪəsɪs] *subst.* lung infection which may metastasize to other tissue, caused by Nocardia *nocardios*

nociceptive [ˌnəʊsi'septɪv] *adj.* (nerves) which carry pain to the brain *nociceptiv*

nociceptor [ˌnəʊsi'septə] *subst.* sensory nerve which carries pain to the brain *nociceptor*

nocte ['nɒkti] *Latin word meaning* "at night" (written on prescriptions) *till natten*
NOTE: opposite is **mane**

nocturia [nɒk'tjʊəriə] *subst.* passing abnormally large quantity of urine during the night *nokturi, nykturi*

nocturnal [nɒk'tɜːn(ə)l] *adj.* at night *natt-, nattlig;* **nocturnal enuresis** *or* **bedwetting** = passing urine when asleep in bed at night *enuresis nocturna, sängvätning, nattvätning*

nod [nɒd] **1** *subst.* moving the head forward (as to show agreement) *nick(ning);* **when the nurse asked him if he wanted a drink, he gave a nod 2** *vb.* to move the head forward (as to show agreement) *nicka;* **when she asked if anyone wanted an ice cream, all the children nodded**

nod ⇨ **node**

node [nəʊd] *subst.* (i) small mass of tissue *knut(a), knöl;* (ii) group of nerve cells *nod;* **atrioventricular node** *or* **AV node** = mass of conducting tissue in the right atrium, which continues as the bundle of His, and passes impulses from the atria to the ventricles *atrioventrikularknutan, atrioventrikulärknutan, AV-knutan, AV-noden;* **axillary nodes** = part of the lymphatic system in the arm *axillarknutorna;* **cervical nodes** = lymph nodes in the neck *cervikalknutorna;* **Heberden's nodes** = small bony lumps which develop on the terminal phalanges of fingers in osteoarthritis *Heberdens knutor;* **lymph nodes** = glands of lymphoid tissue situated at various points of the lymphatic system (especially under the armpits and in the groin), through which lymph passes and in which lymphocytes are produced *nodi lymphatici, lymfkörtlarna;* **Osler's nodes** = tender swellings at the ends of fingers and toes in patients suffering from subacute bacterial endocarditis *Oslerknutor;* **node of Ranvier** = one of a series of points along the length of a nerve, where the myelin sheath round the nerve fibre ends and connective tissue touches the axon *Ranviers nod (insnörning)*

nod off [ˌnɒd ˈɒf] *vb. (informal)* to begin to go to sleep *slumra (nicka) till;* **he nodded off in his chair**

nodosa [nə(ʊ)ˈdəʊsə] *see* PERIARTERITIS

nodosum [nə(ʊ)ˈdəʊsəm] *see* ERYTHEMA

nodular [ˈnɒdjʊlə] *adj.* formed of nodules *nodular, nodulär, knutig, knölig*

nodule [ˈnɒdjuːl] *subst.* small node or group of cells *nodulus, liten knuta (knöl);* anterior part of the inferior vermis *nodulus vermis; see also* BOHN

nodulus ⇨ **nodule**

nodulär ⇨ **nodular**

noggrann ⇨ **accurate, precise**

noggrant ⇨ **accurately**

nokturi ⇨ **nocturia**

noma [ˈnəʊmə] *subst.* cancrum oris *or* severe ulcers in the mouth, leading to gangrene *noma, vattenkräfta, fuktig ansiktsbrand*

nomen proprium [ˈnəʊmən ˈprəʊpriəm] *see* N.P.

non- [ˈnɒn, ˌ-] *prefix* meaning not *non-, icke-, inte;* **non-contagious** = not contagious *inte smittsam;* **non-nucleated** = (cell) with no nucleus *som saknar kärna;* **non-smoker** = person who does not smoke *icke-rökare;* **non-venereal disease** = disease which is not a venereal disease *icke-venerisk sjukdom*

non compos mentis [ˌnɒn ˌkɒmpəs ˈmentɪs] *Latin phrase meaning* "not of sound mind": (person) who is mentally incapable of managing his own affairs *otillräknelig*

nongranular leucocytes [ˌnɒnˈgrænjʊlə ˌluːkəʊsaɪts] *subst. pl.* leucocytes (such as lymphocytes *or* monocytes) which have no granules *icke-granulerade leukocyter*

noninvasiv cancer ⇨ **carcinoma**

non-malignant [ˌnɒnməˈlɪgnənt] *adj.* not malignant *inte elakartad;* **a non-malignant growth**

non-medical [ˌnɒnˈmedɪk(ə)l] *adj.* (word) which is not used in specialized medical speech *icke-medicinsk, inte medicinsk, allmänspråklig;* **"nervous breakdown" is a non-medical term for a type of sudden mental illness**

non-secretor [ˌnɒnsɪˈkriːtə] *subst.* person who does not secrete indicators of blood grouping into body fluids *icke-sekretor*

non-specific urethritis (NSU) [ˌnɒnspeˈsɪfɪk ˌjʊərəˈθraɪtɪs (ˌenesˈjuː)] *subst.* sexually transmitted inflammation of the urethra *non gonorrhoisk (icke-gonorroisk, Chlamydia-) uretrit, NGU*

non-sterile [ˌnɒnˈsteraɪ(ə)l] *adj.* (dressing) which is not sterile *or* (instrument) which has not been sterilized *osteril*

non-union [ˌnɒnˈjuːniən] *subst.* condition where the two parts of a fractured bone do not join together and do not heal *utebliven frakturläkning*

noradrenaline [ˌnɔːrəˈdren(ə)lɪn] *or US* **norepinephrine** [ˌnɔːrepiˈnefrɪn] *subst.* hormone secreted by the medulla of the adrenal glands which acts as a vasoconstrictor and is used to maintain blood pressure in shock or haemorrhage or hypotension *noradrenalin*

norm ⇨ **standard**

norma [ˈnɔːmə] *subst.* in anatomy, the skull as seen from a certain angle *skallen sedd ur viss vinkel*

normal [ˈnɔːm(ə)l] *adj.* usual *or* ordinary *or* according to a standard *normal;* **after taking the tablets, his blood pressure went back to normal; her temperature is two degrees above normal; he had an above normal pulse rate; it is normal for a person with myopia to suffer from headaches**

normal ⇨ **natural, standard**

normalkoncentration ⇨ **titre**

normally [ˈnɔːm(ə)li] *adv.* in a normal *or* ordinary way *normalt, vanligen;* **the patients are normally worried before the operation; he was breathing normally**

normalseende ⇨ **emmetropia**

normalstyrka ⇨ **titre**

normalsyn ⇨ **emmetropia, twenty-twenty vision**

normalt ⇨ **normally**

normoblast ['nɔːməʊblæst] *subst.* early form of a red blood cell, normally found only in bone marrow but found in the blood in certain types of leukaemia and anaemia *normoblast*

normocyte ['nɔːməʊsaɪt] *subst.* normal red blood cell *normocyt*

normocytic [ˌnɔːməʊ'saɪtɪk] *adj.* referring to a normocyte *normocytär*

normocytosis [ˌnɔːməʊsaɪ'təʊsɪs] *subst.* having the normal number of red blood cells in the peripheral blood *tillstånd med normalt antal röda blodkroppar i blodet*

normocytär ⇨ **normocytic**

normotension [ˌnɔːməʊ'tenʃ(ə)n] *subst.* normal blood pressure *normotoni, normalt blodtryck*

normotensive [ˌnɔːməʊ'tensɪv] *adj.* (blood pressure) at normal level *normotonisk*

normotoni ⇨ **normotension**

normotonisk ⇨ **normotensive**

nose [nəʊz] *subst.* organ through which a person breathes and smells *nasus, näsan;* **she must have a cold - her nose is running** = liquid mucus is dripping from her nose *hon måste vara förkyld - snuvan rinner;* **he blew his nose** = he blew air through his nose into a handkerchief to get rid of mucus in his nose *han snöt sig;* **to speak through your nose** = to speak as if your nose is blocked, so that you say 'b' instead of 'm' and 'd' instead of 'n' *tala genom näsan*

> COMMENT: the nose is formed of cartilage and small bones making the bridge at the top. It leads into two passages (the nostrils) which in turn lead to the nasal cavity, divided in two by the septum. The nasal passages connect with the sinuses, with the ears through the Eustachian tubes, and with the pharynx. The receptors which detect smell are in the top of the nasal passage.

nosebleed ['nəʊzbliːd] *or* **epistaxis** [ˌepi'stæksɪs] *subst.* bleeding from the nose, usually caused by a blow *or* by sneezing *or* by blowing the nose hard *or* by high blood pressure *epistaxis, näsblod, näsblödning;* **she had a headache, followed by a violent nosebleed**

NOTE: for other terms referring to the nose see **nasal** and words beginning with **naso-, rhin-, rhino-**

noso- ['nɒsə(ʊ), ˌ--] *prefix* referring to diseases *noso-, sjukdoms-*

nosocomial [ˌnɒsəʊ'kəʊmiəl] *adj.* referring to hospitals *nosokomial;* **nosocomial infection** = infection which is passed on to someone in a hospital *nosokomial infektion, sjukhussjuka*

nosokomial ⇨ **nosocomial**

nosologi ⇨ **nosology**

nosology [nɒ'sɒlədʒi] *subst.* classification of diseases *nosologi, sjukdomslära*

nostril ['nɒstr(ə)l] *or* **naris** ['neərɪs] *subst.* one of the two passages in the nose through which air is breathed in or out *naris, näsöppning, näsborre;* **his right nostril is blocked**

notch [nɒtʃ] *subst.* depression on a surface, usually on a bone, but sometimes on an organ *incisura, inbuktning, inskärning;* **cardiac notch** = (i) point in the left lung, where the right inside wall is bent *incisura cardiaca;* (ii) notch at the point where the oesophagus joins the greater curvature of the stomach *vinkeln mellan matstrupen och magsäckens övre del;* **occipital notch** = point on the lower edge of the cerebral hemisphere, where the surface has a notch *inskärning i nacklobens undre kant*

notice ['nəʊtɪs] **1** *subst.* **(a)** piece of writing giving information, usually put in a place where everyone can see it *meddelande;* **he pinned up a notice about the meeting; notices warning the public about the dangers of rabies are posted at every port and airport (b)** warning *varning, förvarning;* **they had to leave with ten minutes' notice; it had to be done at short notice** = with very little warning time *med mycket kort varsel* **(c)** attention *uppmärksamhet;* **take no notice of what he says** = pay no attention to it *or* don't worry about it *bry dig inte om vad han säger;* **she took no notice of what the doctor suggested 2** *vb.* to see *or* to take note of *uppmärksamma, lägga märke till;* **nobody noticed that the patient was sweating; did you notice the development of any new symptoms?**

noticeable ['nəʊtɪsəb(ə)l] *adj.* which can be noticed *märkbar, synlig, synbar;* **the disease has no easily noticeable symptoms**

noticeboard ['nəʊtɪsbɔːd] *subst.* flat piece of wood, etc., on a wall, on which notices can be pinned *anslagstavla*

notifiable disease ['nəʊtɪfa(ɪ)əb(ə)l dɪˌziːz] *subst.* serious infectious disease which in Great Britain has to be reported by a doctor to the Department of Health and Social Security so that steps can be taken to stop it spreading *ung. anmälningspliktig sjukdom*

> COMMENT: the following are notifiable diseases: cholera, diphtheria, dysentery, encephalitis, food poisoning, jaundice, malaria, measles, meningitis, ophthalmia neonatorum, paratyphoid, plague, poliomyelitis, relapsing fever, scarlet fever, smallpox, tuberculosis, typhoid, typhus, whooping cough, yellow fever

notify ['nəʊtɪfaɪ] *vb.* to inform someone officially *anmäla, rapportera;* **the local doctor notified the Health Service of the case of cholera** NOTE: you notify someone of something

nourish ['nʌrɪʃ] *vb.* to give food *or* nutrients to *nära, ge näring åt;* **nourishing food** = food (such as liver *or* brown bread) which supplies nourishment *närande föda*

nourishment ['nʌrɪʃmənt] *subst.* (i) act of supplying nutrients *närande;* (ii) nutrients (such as proteins, fats or vitamins) *näring(sämne)*

noxious ['nɒkʃəs] *adj.* harmful (drug *or* gas) *skadlig, farlig, ohälsosam*

n.p. [ˌen'piː] *abbreviation for the Latin phrase* "nomen proprium": the name of the drug (written on the label of the container) *nomen proprium, preparatnamn*

NPO [ˌenpiː'əʊ] *abbreviation for the Latin phrase* "nil per oram": nothing by the mouth (used to refer to patients being kept without food) *nil per oram, fastande;* **the patient should be kept NPO for five hours before the operation**

NSU [ˌenes'juː] = NON-SPECIFIC URETHRITIS

nucha ['njuːkə] *or* **nape** [neɪp] *subst.* back of the neck *nacken*

nuchal ['njuːk(ə)l] *adj.* referring to the nape *nack-*

nuclear ['njuːklɪə] *adj.* referring to nuclei *nukleär, kärn-;* **nuclear magnetic resonance (NMR)** = scanning technique, using magnetic fields and radio waves, which reveals abnormalities in soft tissue *or* body fluids, etc. *nukleär magnetisk resonans, kärnspinnresonans; see also* MAGNETIC RESONANCE IMAGING

nuclease ['njuːklieɪz] *subst.* enzyme which breaks down the nucleic acids *nukleas*

nucleic acids [njuˌkliːɪk 'æsɪdz] *subst. pl.* organic acids combined with proteins (DNA or RNA) which exist in the nucleus and protoplasm of all cells *nukleinsyror*

nucleolus [nju'kliːələs] *subst.* structure inside a cell nucleus, containing RNA *nukleol, kärnkropp*

nucleoprotein [ˌnjuːkliəʊ'prəʊtiːn] *subst.* compound of protein and nucleic acid, such as chromosomes or ribosomes *nukleoprotein*

nucleus ['njuːkliəs] *subst.* **(a)** central body in a cell, containing DNA and RNA, and controlling the function and characteristics of the cell *nucleus, cellkärna* **(b)** group of nerve cells in the brain or spinal cord *nucleus, kärna;* **basal nuclei** = masses of grey matter at the bottom of each cerebral hemisphere *basala ganglierna;* **nucleus pulposus** = soft central part of an intervertebral disc which disappears in old age ⇨ *illustration* NEURONE *nucleus pulposus*
NOTE: the plural is **nuclei**

nukleas ⇨ **nuclease**

nukleinsyror ⇨ **nucleic acids**

nukleol ⇨ **nucleolus**

nukleoprotein ⇨ **nucleoprotein**

nukleär ⇨ **nuclear**

nullipara [nʌ'lɪp(ə)rə] *subst. & adj.* (woman) who has never had a child *nullipara*

numb [nʌm] *adj.* (limb) which has no feeling *känsellös, domnad;* **her fingers were numb with cold; the tips of his ears went numb** *or* **became numb**

numbness ['nʌmnəs] *subst.* loss of feeling *känsellöshet, domning*

nurse [nɜːs] **1** *subst.* person (usually a woman) who looks after sick people in a hospital *or* helps a doctor in his surgery *sjuksköterska;* **she works as a nurse in the**

local hospital; she's training to be a nurse; charge nurse = nurse who is in charge of a group of patients, a ward or a department in a hospital *ung. avdelningsföreståndare;* **district nurse** *or* **home nurse** = nurse who visits and treats patients in their homes *distriktssköterska;* **escort nurse** = nurse who goes with a patient to the operating theatre and back to the ward *sjuksköterska som följer patient till el. från operation;* **practice nurse** *or* **nurse practitioner** = nurse employed by a clinic *or* doctor's practice who can give advice to patients *sjuksköterska med rådgivande funktion, ung. mottagningssköterska;* **staff nurse** = nurse who is on the permanent staff of a hospital *(fast anställd) sjuksköterska vid sjukhus;* **theatre nurse** = nurse who is specially trained to assist a surgeon during an operation *operationssköterska;* **nurse manager** = nurse who has administrative duties in the health service *or* in a hospital *sjuksköterska med administrativa uppgifter, (klinik)föreståndare* NOTE: although the term nurse applies to both men and women, in popular speech it is used more frequently to refer to women, and **male nurse** is used for men. Nurse can be used as a title before a name: **Nurse Jones 2** *vb.* to look after sick people *vårda, sköta om;* to breast feed a baby *amma;* **when he was ill his mother nursed him until he was better**

> COMMENT: in the UK qualified nurses are either ENs (Enrolled Nurses) or RNs (Registered Nurses). Registered nurses follow a three year course and have to pass the ENB examinations before becoming RGN, RMN or RNMH. RSCNs have a further 6 months or 4 term course before they qualify. Enrolled nurses follow 2 year courses

nursery school ['nɜːs(ə)ri skuːl] *subst.* school for little children *förskola;* **day nursery** = place where small children can be looked after during the daytime, and go home in the evenings *barndaghem, daghem*

nursing ['nɜːsɪŋ] **1** *subst.* work *or* profession of being a nurse *omvårdnad, vård, sjuksköterskeyrket;* **she enjoys nursing; he is taking a nursing course; he has chosen nursing as his career 2** *adj.* **nursing home** = house where convalescents or old people can live, under medical supervision by a qualified nurse *vårdhem, sjukhem;* **nursing mother** = mother who breast feeds her baby *ammande moder;* **nursing officer** = nurse who has administrative duties in the National Health Service *sjuksköterska med vissa administrativa uppgifter inom NHS;* **nursing process** = standard method of treatment carried out by nurses, and its documentation *omvårdnadsprocess;* **nursing practice** = treatment given by nurses *omvårdnad, vård*

> QUOTE all relevant sections of the nurses' care plan and nursing process records had been left blank
> **Nursing Times**

> QUOTE few now dispute the need for clear concise nursing plans to guide nursing practice, provide educational tools and give an accurate legal record
> **Nursing Times**

nutans ['njuːt(ə)ns] *see* SPASMUS

nutation [njuː'teɪʃ(ə)n] *subst.* involuntary nodding of the head *ofrivillig nickning*

nutrient ['njuːtriənt] *subst.* substance (such as protein *or* fat *or* vitamin) in food which is necessary to provide energy or to help the body grow *näring(sämne)*

nutrition [nju'trɪʃ(ə)n] *subst.* (i) study of the supply of nutrients to the body from digesting food *nutrition, näring;* (ii) nourishment *or* food *nutrition, näring(sämne), föda*

nutritional disorder [nju'trɪʃ(ə)n(ə)l dɪsˌɔːdə] *subst.* disorder (such as obesity) related to food and nutrients *nutritionsstörning, näringsrubbning*

nutritionist [nju'trɪʃ(ə)nɪst] *subst.* dietitian *or* person who specializes in the study of nutrition and advises on diets *dietist, näringsexpert*

nutritionslösning (för infusion) ⇨ **drip**

nutritionsstörning ⇨ **nutritional disorder**

ny- ⇨ **neo-**

nyckel ⇨ **key**

nyckelbenet ⇨ **clavicle, collar**

nyckelbens- ⇨ **clavicular**

nyckelbensartären ⇨ **subclavian**

nyckelbensvenen ⇨ **subclavian**

nyctalopia [ˌnɪktə'ləʊpiə] *or* **night blindness** [ˌnaɪt 'blaɪndnəs] *subst.* being unable to see in bad light *nyktalopi, nattblindhet*

nyctaphobia [ˌnɪktə'fəʊbiə] *subst.* fear of the dark *nyktofobi, mörkrädsla*

nyfödd ⇨ **newborn**

nyföddhets- ⇨ **neonatal**

nyfött barn ⇨ **neonate**

nyktalopi ⇨ **nyctalopia**

nykterhet ⇨ **abstinence**

nyktofobi ⇨ **nyctaphobia**

nykturi ⇨ **nocturia**

nymfoman ⇨ **nymphomaniac**

nymfomani ⇨ **nymphomania**

nymphae ['nɪmfiː] *or* **labia minora** [ˌleɪbiə mɪ'mɔːrə] *subst.* two small fleshy folds at the edge of the vulva *labia minora, små blygdläpparna*

nymphomania [ˌnɪmfə'meɪniə] *subst.* obsessive sexual urge in a woman *nymfomani*
NOTE: in a man, called **satyriasis**

nymphomaniac [ˌnɪmfə'meɪniæk] *subst.* woman who has an abnormally obsessive sexual urge *nymfoman*

nypa ⇨ **pinch**

nyp(ning) ⇨ **pinch**

nysa ⇨ **sneeze**

nysmedel ⇨ **sternutatory**

nysning ⇨ **sneeze**

nysningsanfall ⇨ **sneezing fit**

nystagmus [nɪ'stægməs] *subst.* rapid movement of the eyes up and down or from side to side *nystagmus*

> COMMENT: nystagmus can be congenital, but is also a symptom of multiple sclerosis and Ménière's disease

nå (fram till) ⇨ **reach**

nål ⇨ **hypodermic, needle, pin**

nålstick ⇨ **needlestick**

näbbliknande ⇨ **rostral**

närande ⇨ **nourishment**

näring ⇨ **alimentation, food, nourishment, nutrition**

näringsexpert ⇨ **nutritionist**

näringsgula ⇨ **vitellus**

näringsintag ⇨ **alimentation, ingestion**

näringsrubbning ⇨ **malnutrition, nutritional disorder**

näringssubstrat ⇨ **broth**

närmaste anhörig ⇨ **kin**

närsynt ⇨ **myopic**

närsynthet ⇨ **myopia**

närvara ⇨ **attend**

närvarande ⇨ **present**

närvaro ⇨ **presence**

näs- ⇨ **nasal, naso-, rhin-**

näsan ⇨ **nose**

näsbenet ⇨ **nasal**

näsblod ⇨ **nosebleed**

näsborre ⇨ **nostril, nares**

näsbrosken ⇨ **nasal**

näshålan ⇨ **nasal**

näshår ⇨ **vibrissae**

näsmusslorna ⇨ **nasal**

näsryggen ⇨ **bridge**

nässelutslag ⇨ **hives, giant**

nässkiljeväggen ⇨ **nasal**

näs-svalgrummet ⇨ **nasopharynx**

nästårkanalen ⇨ **duct**

nästäppa ⇨ **congestion**

näsöppning ⇨ **nostril, nares**

näthinnan ⇨ **retina**

näthinne- ⇨ **retinal**

näthinneavlossning ⇨ **retinal**

näthinneinflammation ⇨ **retinitis**

nätverk ⇨ **network, plexus**

nötas ⇨ **wear**

Oo

O *symbol for* oxygen *O, syre, syrgas*

o- ⇨ **un-**

oanvänd ⇨ **fresh**

oat cell carcinoma [ˌəʊt sel ˌkɑːsɪˈnəʊmə] *subst.* type of cancer of the bronchi, with distinctive small cells *slags cancer i bronkerna*

oavbruten ⇨ **constant**

obducent ⇨ **pathologist**

obduktion ⇨ **autopsy**

obefintlig ⇨ **absent**

obefruktad ⇨ **unfertilized**

obehag ⇨ **discomfort**

obehaglig ⇨ **nasty**

obehandlad ⇨ **untreated**

obekväm ⇨ **awkward**

oberoende ⇨ **independent, independently**

oberördhet ⇨ **ataraxia**

obese [ə(ʊ)ˈbiːs] **1** *adj.* (person who is) too fat *or* too heavy *adipös, överviktig, tjock* **2** *subst.* **the obese** = overweight people *överviktiga personer*

obesitet ⇨ **obesity**

obesity [ə(ʊ)ˈbiːsəti] *subst.* being overweight *obesitet, adipositet, övervikt, fetma*

COMMENT: obesity is caused by excess fat accumulating under the skin and around organs in the body. It is sometimes due to glandular disorders, but it is usually caused by eating or drinking too much. A tendency to obesity can be hereditary

obetydlig ⇨ **minor**

obey [əˈbeɪ] *vb.* to do what someone *or* a rule says you should do *lyda;* **you ought to obey the doctor's instructions and go to bed; patients must obey the hospital rules**

objektglas ⇨ **slide**

oblandad ⇨ **pure**

obligate [ˈɒblɪgeɪt] *adj.* (organism) which exists and develops in only one way (as viruses which are parasites only inside cells) *obligat, inte fakultativ*

oblique [əˈbliːk] *subst. & adj.* (muscle) which lies at an angle *sned(-), tvärgående;* **oblique fissure** = groove between the lobes of the lungs *fissura obliqua;* **oblique fracture** = fracture where the bone is not broken directly across its axis *snedfraktur;* **oblique muscle** = (i) muscle which controls the eyeball *sned ögonmuskel;* (ii) muscle which controls the abdominal wall *sned bukmuskel;* **external oblique** = outer abdominal muscle *musculus obliquus externus abdominis, bukens yttre snedmuskel;* **internal oblique** = muscle covering the abdomen beneath the external oblique *musculus obliquus internus abdominis, bukens inre snedmuskel*

> QUOTE there are four recti muscles and two oblique muscles in each eye, which coordinate the movement of the eyes and enable them to work as a pair
>
> **Nursing Times**

obliterans [əˈblɪtər(ə)ns] *see* ENDARTERITIS

oblongata [ˌɒblɒŋˈgeɪtə] *see* MEDULLA

obotlig ⇨ **incurable**

observation [ˌɒbzəˈveɪʃ(ə)n] *subst.* examining something over a period of time *observation;* **he was admitted to hospital for observation**

observe [əbˈzɜːv] *vb.* to notice *or* to see something and understand it *observera, iaktta, lägga märke till;* **the nurses observed signs of improvement in the patient's condition; the girl's mother observed symptoms of anorexia and reported them to her doctor**

observera ⇨ **observe**

obsessed [əbˈsest] *adj.* suffering from an obsession *som lider av tvångsföreställningar etc.;* **he is obsessed with the idea that his wife is trying to kill him**

obsession [əbˈseʃ(ə)n] *subst.* mental disorder where the patient has a fixed idea *or* emotion which he cannot get rid of, even if he knows it is wrong or unpleasant *obsession, tvångsföreställning, tvångstanke, tvångshandling;* **she has an obsession about cats**

obsessional [əb'seʃ(ə)n(ə)l] *adj.* referring to an obsession *tvångs-;* **he is suffering from an obsessional disorder**

obsessive [əb'sesɪv] *adj.* showing an obsession *som lider av tvångsföreställningar etc.;* **he has an obsessive desire to steal little objects; obsessive action** = repeated actions (such as washing) which indicate a mental disorder *tvångshandling*

obstetric(al) [əb'stetrɪk(əl)] *adj.* referring to obstetrics *obstetrisk, förlossnings-;* **obstetrical forceps** = type of large forceps used to hold a baby's head during childbirth *förlossningstång;* **obstetric patient** = woman who is being treated by an obstetrician *obstetrisk patient*

obstetrician [ˌɒbstə'trɪʃ(ə)n] *subst.* doctor who specializes in obstetrics *obstetriker, förlossningsläkare*

obstetrics [əb'stetrɪks] *subst.* branch of medicine and surgery dealing with pregnancy, childbirth and the period immediately after childbirth *obstetrik, förlossningskonst*

obstetrik ⇨ **midwifery, obstetrics**

obstetriker ⇨ **obstetrician**

obstetrisk ⇨ **obstetric(al)**

obstipation ⇨ **constipation**

obstiperad ⇨ **constipated, costive**

obstruct [əb'strʌkt] *vb.* to block *obstruera, blockera, stänga, täppa till;* **the artery was obstructed by a blood clot**

obstruction [əb'strʌkʃ(ə)n] *subst.* (i) something which blocks (a passage *or* a blood vessel) *obstruktion, hinder, stopp;* (ii) blocking of a passage *or* blood vessel *obstruktion, tilltäppning, tillsnörning;* **intestinal obstruction** *or* **obstruction of the bowels** = blockage of the intestine *tarmobstruktion, stopp i tarmarna;* **urinary obstruction** = blockage of the urethra, which prevents urine being passed *urinstopp, urinstämma*

obstructive [əb'strʌktɪv] *adj.* caused by an obstruction *obstruktiv;* **obstructive jaundice** = jaundice caused by an obstruction in the bile ducts *icterus obstructivus, obstruktionsikterus, mekanisk ikterus, stasikterus;* **obstructive lung disease** = bronchitis and emphysema *obstruktiv lungsjukdom*

obstruera ⇨ **obstruct**

obstruktion ⇨ **obstruction**

obstruktionsikterus ⇨ **jaundice**

obstruktiv ⇨ **obstructive**

obtain [əb'teɪn] *vb.* to get *få, skaffa sig;* **some amino acids are obtained from food; where did he obtain the drugs?**

obturator ['ɒbtju(ə)reɪtə] *subst.* (i) one of two muscles in the pelvis which govern the movement of the hip and thigh *musculus obturatorius, höfthålsmuskeln;* (ii) device which closes an opening, such as a dental prosthesis which covers a cleft palate *obturator;* (iii) metal bulb which fits into a bronchoscope *or* sigmoidoscope *obturator, propp;* **obturator foramen** = opening in the hip bone near the acetabulum *foramen obturatorium, höfthålet*

obtusion [əb'tjuːʒ(ə)n] *subst.* condition where perception and feelings become dulled *slöhet, tröghet, avtrubbning*

oböjlig ⇨ **stiff**

oböjlighet ⇨ **stiffness**

occipital [ɒk'sɪpɪt(ə)l] *adj.* referring to the back of the head *occipital(-), nack-;* **occipital bone** *or* **occipital** = one of the bones in the skull, the bone at the back of the head *os occipitale, occipitalbenet, nackbenet;* **occipital condyle** = round part of the occipital bone which joins it to the atlas *condylus occipitalis, nackbenets ledknapp;* **occipital lobe** = lobe at the back of each cerebral hemisphere *lobus occipitalis, occipitalloben, nackloben;* **occipital notch** = point on the lower edge of the cerebral hemisphere where the surface has a notch *inskärning i nacklobens undre kant*

occipitalbenet ⇨ **occipital**

occipitalloben ⇨ **occipital**

occipito-anterior [ɒkˌsɪpɪtəʊ æn'tɪəriə] *adj.* (position of a baby at birth) where the baby faces the mother's back *vänd mot moderns ryggsida*

occipito-posterior [ɒkˌsɪpɪtəʊpɒ'stɪəriə] *adj.* (position of a baby at birth) where the baby faces the front *vänd mot moderns buksida*

occiput ['ɒksɪpʌt] *subst.* lower part of the back of the head or skull *occiput, bakhuvudet*

occlusion [ə'klu:ʒ(ə)n] *subst.* **(a)** blockage *or* thing which blocks a passage *or* which closes an opening *ocklusion, blockering, tilltäppning, propp;* **coronary occlusion** = blood clot in the coronary arteries leading to heart failure *koronarkärlsocklusion, blodpropp i hjärtats kranskärl* **(b)** the way in which the teeth in the upper and lower jaws fit together when the jaws are closed *ocklusion, sammanbitning* NOTE: a bad fit between the teeth is a **malocclusion**

occlusive [ə'klu:sɪv] *adj.* referring to occlusion *or* to blocking *som avser el. hör till ocklusion;* **occlusive stroke** = stroke caused by a blood clot *stroke pga blodpropp (i motsats till hjärnblödning);* **occlusive therapy** = treatment of a squint where the good eye is covered up in order to encourage the squinting eye to become straight *slags skelningsbehandling*

occult [ə'kʌlt] *adj.* (i) not easy to see with the naked eye *ockult, som inte syns för blotta ögat;* (ii) (symptom *or* sign) which is hidden *dold, skymd;* **occult blood** = very small quantities of blood in the faeces, which can only be detected by tests *ockult blödning*

occulta [ə'kʌltə] *see* SPINA BIFIDA

occupancy rate ['ɒkjʊp(ə)nsi ˌreɪt] *subst.* number of beds occupied in a hospital, shown as a percentage of all the beds *beläggningsgrad*

occupation [ˌɒkju'peɪʃ(ə)n] *subst.* job *or* work *yrke;* **what is his occupation? people in sedentary occupations are liable to digestive disorders**

occupational [ˌɒkju'peɪʃ(ə)n(ə)l] *adj.* referring to work *yrkes-, arbets-;* **occupational dermatitis** = dermatitis caused by materials with which one comes into contact at work *dermatitis professionalis, yrkesdermatit;* **occupational disease** = disease which is caused by the type of work *or* the conditions in which someone works (such as disease caused by dust *or* chemicals in a factory) *arbetssjukdom, yrkessjukdom;* **occupational health (OH) nurse** = nurse who deals with health problems of people at work *företagssköterska;* **occupational therapist** = qualified therapist who treats people with mental or physical handicaps by using activities such as light work, hobbies, etc. *arbetsterapeut;* **occupational therapy** = light work *or* hobbies used as a means of treatment, especially for handicapped *or* mentally ill patients *arbetsterapi*

occur [ə'kɜ:] *vb.* to happen *or* to take place *inträffa, ske, förekomma;* to be found *påträffas;* **thrombosis occurred in the artery; a form of glaucoma which occurs in infants; one of the most frequently occurring types of tumour**

occurrence [ə'kʌr(ə)ns] *subst.* taking place *or* happening *händelse, förekomst;* **neuralgia is a common occurrence after shingles**

ochronosis [ˌɒkrəʊ'nəʊsɪs] *subst.* condition where cartilage, ligaments and other fibrous tissue become dark as a result of a metabolic disorder, and also the urine turns black on exposure to air *okronos*

ocklusion ⇨ **occlusion**

ockult ⇨ **occult**

ocular ['ɒkjʊlə] *adj.* referring to the eye *okular, okulär, ögon-;* **opticians are trained to detect all kinds of ocular imbalance**

oculi ['ɒkjʊlaɪ] *see* ALBUGINEA, ORBICULARIS

oculist ['ɒkjʊlɪst] *subst.* qualified physician or surgeon who specializes in the treatment of eye disorders *ögonläkare, ögonspecialist*

oculogyric [ˌɒkjuləʊ'dʒɪrɪk] *adj.* which causes eye movements *okulogyr*

oculomotor [ˌɒkjuləʊ'məʊtə] *adj.* referring to movements of the eyeball *okulomotorisk;* **oculomotor nerve** = third cranial nerve which controls the eyeball and upper eyelid *nervus oculomotorius, ögonrörelsenerven, 3:e kranialnerven*

oculonasal [ˌɒkjuləʊ'neɪz(ə)l] *adj.* referring to the eye and the nose *som avser el. hör till både öga och näsa*

o.d. [ˌəʊ'di:] **(a)** *abbreviation for the Latin phrase* "omni die": every day (written on a prescription) *omni die, dagligen* **(b)** *abbreviation for* overdose *överdos*

odiskad ⇨ **unwashed**

odla ⇨ **cultivate, culture**

odling ⇨ **culture**

odlingssubstrat ⇨ **culture**

odont- ['ɒdɒnt, ˌ--] *prefix* meaning teeth *odont-, tand-*

odontalgia [ˌɒdɒn'tældʒə] *subst.* toothache *odontalgi, tandvärk*

odontitis [ˌɒdɒn'taɪtɪs] *subst.* inflammation of the pulpy interior of a tooth *odontit, tandinflammation*

odontoid process [ɒ'dɒntɔɪd ˌprəʊses] *subst.* projecting part of a vertebra, shaped like a tooth *deus axis (utskott på andra halskotan)*

odontologi ➪ **dentistry, odontology**

odontology [ˌɒdɒn'tɒlədʒi] *subst.* study of teeth and associated structures, and their disorders *odontologi*

odontoma [ˌɒdɒn'təʊmə] *or* **odontome** ['ɒdɒntəʊm] *subst.* (i) structure like a tooth which has an abnormal arrangement of its component tissues *slags struktur där ingående vävnader är onormalt ordnade;* (ii) solid or cystic tumour derived from cells concerned with the development of a tooth *odontom, tandsvulst*

odour ['əʊdə] *subst.* smell *odör, lukt;* **body odour** = unpleasant smell produced by a person who has not washed *kroppslukt, kroppsodör*

odynophagia [ˌɒdɪnə(ə)'feɪdʒə] *subst.* condition where pain occurs when food is swallowed *odynofagi, sväljningssmärta*

odör ➪ **odour**

oe- ['iː, ˌiː]
NOTE: words beginning with **oe-** are written **e-** in American English

oedema [ɪ'diːmə] *or US* **edema** [ɪ'diːmə] *subst.* dropsy *or* swelling of part of the body caused by accumulation of fluid in the intercellular tissue spaces *ödem;* **her main problem is oedema of the feet; pulmonary oedema** = collection of fluid in the lungs as in left-sided heart failure *oedema pulmonum, lungödem;* **subcutaneous oedema** = fluid collecting under the skin, usually at the ankles *subkutant ödem*

oedematous [ɪ'demətəs] *adj.* referring to oedema *ödematös*

Oedipus complex ['iːdɪpəs ˌkɒmpleks] *subst. (in psychology)* condition where a boy feels sexually attracted to his mother and sees his father as an obstacle *oidipuskomplex*

oesophageal [iːˌsɒfə'dʒiːəl] *adj.* referring to the oesophagus *esofag(o)-, matstrups-;* **oesophageal hiatus** = opening in the diaphragm through which the oesophagus passes *hiatus oesophageus, matstrupsgapet;* **oesophageal ulcer** = ulcer in the oesophagus *sår i matstrupen*

oesophagectomy [iːˌsɒfə'dʒektəmi] *subst.* surgical removal of part of the oesophagus *esofagektomi*

oesophagitis [iːˌsɒfə'dʒaɪtɪs] *subst.* inflammation of the oesophagus (caused by acid juices from the stomach *or* by infection) *esofagit*

oesophagocele [iː'sɒfəgəʊˌsiː(ə)l] *subst.* condition where the mucous membrane lining the oesophagus protrudes through the wall *esofagocele, matstrupsbråck*

oesophagoscope [iː'sɒfəgəʊskəʊp] *subst.* thin tube with a light at the end, which is passed down the oesophagus to examine it *esofagoskop*

oesophagoscopy [iːˌsɒfə'gɒskəpi] *subst.* examination of the oesophagus with an oesophagoscope *esofagoskopi*

oesophagostomy [iːˌsɒfə'gɒstəmi] *subst.* surgical operation to make an opening in the oesophagus to allow the patient to be fed, usually after an operation on the pharynx *esofagostomi*

oesophagotomy [iːˌsɒfə'gɒtəmi] *subst.* surgical operation to make an opening in the oesophagus to remove something which is blocking it *esofagotomi*

oesophagus [iː'sɒfəgəs] *or US* **esophagus** [ɪ'sɒfəgəs] *subst.* tube down which food passes from the pharynx to the stomach ➪ *illustration* STOMACH, THROAT *oesophagus, esofagus, matstrupen*

oestradiol [ˌiːstrə'daɪɒl] *subst.* type of oestrogen secreted by an ovarian follicle, which stimulates the development of secondary sexual characteristics in females at puberty (a synthetic form is given as treatment for oestrogen deficiency) *estradiol, östradiol*

oestriol ['iːstriɒl] *subst.* placental hormone with oestrogenic properties, found in the urine of pregnant women *estriol, östriol*

oestrogen ['iːstrədʒ(ə)n] *subst.* any substance with the physiological activity of oestradiol *estrogen, östrogen*

COMMENT: synthetic oestrogens form most oral contraceptives, and are also used in the treatment of menstrual and menopausal disorders

oestrogenic hormone [ˌiːstrəˈdʒenɪk ˌhɔːməʊn] *subst.* oestrogen used to treat conditions which develop during menopause *estrogen, östrogen*

oestrone [ˈiːstrəʊn] *subst.* type of oestrogen *estron, östron*

ofarlig ⇨ **harmless, safe**

offentlig sjukvård ⇨ **health**

offer ⇨ **casualty, victim**

-offer ⇨ **sufferer**

official [əˈfɪʃ(ə)l] *adj.* (i) accepted by an authority *officiell, tjänste-;* (ii) (drug) which is permitted by an authority *som godkänts av viss myndighet*

officially [əˈfɪʃ(ə)li] *adv.* (accepted *or* permitted) by an authority *officiellt;* **the drug has been officially listed as a dangerous drug**

officiell ⇨ **official**

officiellt ⇨ **officially**

ofrivillig ⇨ **involuntary**

ofrivillig sädesavgång ⇨ **spermatorrhoea**

ofruktsam ⇨ **infertile, sterile**

ofruktsamhet ⇨ **infertility, sterility**

oft(alm)- ⇨ **ophth-**

oftalmalgi ⇨ **photalgia**

oftalmektomi ⇨ **ophthalmectomy**

oftalmolog ⇨ **ophthalmologist**

oftalmologi ⇨ **ophthalmology**

oftalmoplegi ⇨ **ophthalmoplegia**

oftalmoskop ⇨ **ophthalmoscope**

oftalmoskopi ⇨ **ophthalmoscopy**

oftalmotonometer ⇨ **ophthalmotonometer, tonometer**

oftalmotonometri ⇨ **tonometry**

ofullgången ⇨ **abortive**

ofullständig ⇨ **incomplete, partial**

ofullständig abort ⇨ **abortion**

ofullständigt ⇨ **partially**

ofullständig återbildning ⇨ **subinvolution**

ofödd ⇨ **unborn**

oförenlig ⇨ **incompatible**

oförenlighet ⇨ **incompatibility**

oförmåga ⇨ **inability, incompetence**

oförmögen ⇨ **incapable, incapacitated**

oförändrad ⇨ **constant**

ogenomskinlig ⇨ **opaque**

ogenomskinlighet ⇨ **opacity**

ogilla ⇨ **dislike**

OH [ˌəʊˈeɪtʃ] = OCCUPATIONAL HEALTH **an OH nurse**

ohygienisk ⇨ **insanitary, unhygienic**

ohälsa ⇨ **ill health**

ohälsosam ⇨ **insanitary, noxious, unhealthy**

oidipuskomplex ⇨ **Oedipus complex**

oil [ɔɪl] *subst.* liquid which cannot be mixed with water *oleum, olja;* (there are three types: fixed vegetable *or* animal oils *feta vegetabiliska el. animaliska oljor;* volatile oils *flyktiga oljor;* and mineral oils /ST/ mineraloljor;); **cod liver oil** = oil from the liver of the cod fish, which is rich in calories and in vitamins A and D *torskleverolja, fiskleverolja;* **essential oils** = oils from scented plants used in cosmetics and as antiseptics *eteriska (flyktiga) oljor;* **fixed oil** = oil which is liquid at 20°C *flytande olja (fett)*

oily [ˈɔɪli] *adj.* containing oil *oljig, olje-*

ointment [ˈɔɪntmənt] *subst.* smooth oily medicinal preparation which can be spread on the skin to soothe *or* to protect *salva*

ojämn ⇨ **pitted, rough**

ok- ⇨ **zygomatic**

okbenet ➪ **cheekbone, malar, zygoma**

okbågen ➪ **zygoma, zygomatic**

oklar ➪ **cloudy**

okokt ➪ **unboiled**

okomplicerad ➪ **simple**

okontrollerbar ➪ **uncontrollable**

okoordinerad ➪ **ataxic, uncoordinated**

okronos ➪ **ochronosis**

okular ➪ **ocular**

okulogyr ➪ **oculogyric**

okulomotorisk ➪ **oculomotor**

okulär ➪ **ocular**

okvalificerad ➪ **unqualified**

okänslig ➪ **dead, refractory, resistant**

olaglig ➪ **illegal**

oleaginous [ˌəʊlɪˈædʒɪnəs] *adj.* oily *oljig, olje-*

olecranon (process) [əʊˈlekrənɒn (ˌprəʊsəs)] *subst.* curved process at the end of the ulna *olecranon, armbågsutskottet*
NOTE: usually called **funny bone**

oleic [ˈəʊliːɪk] *adj.* referring to oil *olje-;* **oleic acid** = one of the fatty acids, present in most oils *oljesyra, oleinsyra*

oleinsyra ➪ **oleic**

oleum [ˈəʊliəm] *subst. (term used in pharmacy)* oil *oleum, olja*

olfaction [ɒlˈfækʃ(ə)n] *subst.* (i) sense of smell *lukt(sinnet);* (ii) way in which a person's sensory organs detect smells *luktande*

olfactory [ɒlˈfækt(ə)rɪ] *adj.* referring to the sense of smell *olfaktorisk, lukt-;* **olfactory bulb** = end of the olfactory tract, where the processes of the sensory cells in the nose are linked to the fibres of the olfactory nerve *bulbus olfactorius, luktloben;* **olfactory nerve** = first cranial nerve which controls the sense of smell *nervus olfactorius, luktnerven, 1:a kranialnerven;* **olfactory tract** = nerve tract which takes the olfactory nerve from the nose to the brain *tractus olfactorius*

olfaktorisk ➪ **olfactory**

olidlig ➪ **excruciating**

olig- [ˈɒlɪg, ˌ--] *or* **oligo-** [ˈɒlɪgəʊ, ˌ---] *prefix* meaning few *or* little *olig(o)-*

oligaemia [ˌɒlɪˈgiːmiə] *subst.* condition where the patient has too little blood in his circulatory system *oligemi*

oligemi ➪ **oligaemia**

oligodactylism [ˌɒlɪgəʊˈdæktilɪz(ə)m] *subst.* congenital condition where a baby is born without some fingers or toes *oligodaktyli*

oligodipsia [ˌɒlɪgəʊˈdɪpsiə] *subst.* condition where a patient does not want to drink *oligodipsi*

oligodontia [ˌɒlɪgəʊˈdɒnʃə] *subst.* state in which most of the teeth are lacking *medfött tillstånd med fåtaliga tänder*

oligohydramnios [ˌɒlɪgəʊhaɪˈdræmniəs] *subst.* condition where the amnion surrounding the fetus contains too little amniotic fluid *oligohydramnios*

oligomenorrhoea [ˌɒlɪgəʊˌmenəˈrɪə] *subst.* condition where the patient menstruates infrequently *oligomenorré*

oligospermia [ˌɒlɪgəʊˈspɜːmiə] *subst.* condition where there are too few spermatozoa in the semen *oligospermi*

oliguria [ˌɒlɪˈgjʊəriə] *subst.* condition where the patient does not produce enough urine *oliguri*

olik ➪ **different, distinct**

olik- ➪ **hetero-**

olikartad ➪ **heterogeneous**

olikhet ➪ **difference**

olive [ˈɒlɪv] *subst.* **(a)** fruit of a tree, which gives an edible oil *oliv* **(b)** swelling containing grey matter, on the side of the pyramid of the medulla oblongata *nucleus olivaris, kranialnervskärna*

olja ➪ **oil, oleum**

olje- ➪ **oily, oleaginous, oleic**

oljesyra ⇨ **oleic**

oljig ⇨ **oily, oleaginous**

ollonet ⇨ **glans, balanus, bulb**

olust ⇨ **dislike, malaise**

olycka ⇨ **accident, crash, emergency**

olycksfall ⇨ **accident, casualty, emergency**

olycksfallsavdelning ⇨ **accident, casualty, emergency**

olycksfallsförsäkring ⇨ **insurance**

olycksförebyggande åtgärder ⇨ **prevention**

olyckshändelse ⇨ **accident**

oläkt ⇨ **raw**

olämplig ⇨ **unsuitable**

olöslig ⇨ **insoluble**

o.m. [ˌəʊ'em] *abbreviation for the Latin phrase* "omni mane": every morning (written on a prescription) *omni mane, varje morgon*

-oma ['əʊmə] *suffix* meaning tumour *-om* NOTE: plural is **-omata**

ombesörja ⇨ **provide**

ombesörjande ⇨ **provision**

ombud ⇨ **agent**

Ombudsman ['ɒmbʊdzmən] *see* HEALTH SERVICE COMMISSIONER

omedelbar ⇨ **immediate**

omedelbart ⇨ **immediately**

omedelbar åtgärd, som kräver ⇨ **urgently**

omedgörlig ⇨ **intractable**

omedveten ⇨ **subconscious, subliminal, unconscious**

oment- [əʊ'ment] *prefix* referring to the omentum *oment-, bukhinnenäts-*

omental [əʊ'ment(ə)l] *adj.* referring to the omentum *omental, bukhinnenäts-*

omentectomy [ˌəʊmen'tektəmi] *subst.* surgical removal of part of the omentum *omentektomi*

omentektomi ⇨ **omentectomy**

omentofixation ⇨ **omentopexy**

omentopexy [əʊ'mentəʊˌpeksi] *subst.* surgical operation to attach the omentum to the abdominal wall *omentopexi, omentofixation*

omentum [əʊ'mentəm] *or* **epiploon** [e'pɪpluːn] *subst.* double fold of peritoneum hanging down over the intestines *oment, bukhinnenätet* NOTE: the plural is **omenta.** Note that for the terms referring to the omentum see words beginning with **epiplo-**

> COMMENT: the omentum is in two sections: the greater omentum which covers the intestines, and the lesser omentum which hangs between the liver and the stomach and the liver and the duodenum

omfalit ⇨ **omphalitis**

omfalocele ⇨ **omphalocele, umbilical**

omfatta ⇨ **include**

omfattande ⇨ **full-scale, heavy, massive**

omfång ⇨ **range**

omge ⇨ **enclose, surround**

omgivning ⇨ **environment, surroundings**

omgående ⇨ **immediately**

omklamringsreflex ⇨ **Moro reflex**

omkomma ⇨ **die**

omodern ⇨ **date**

omogen ⇨ **immature**

omphal- ['ɒmfəl, ˌ--] *prefix* referring to the navel *omfal(o)-, navel-*

omphalitis [ˌɒmfə'laɪtɪs] *subst.* inflammation of the navel *omfalit, navelinflammation*

omphalocele ['ɒmfələˌsiː(ə)l] *subst.* hernia where part of the intestine protrudes through the abdominal wall near the navel *hernia umbilicalis, omfalocele, navelbråck*

omphalus ['ɒmfələs] *or* **navel** ['neɪv(ə)l] *or* **umbilicus** [ʌm'bɪlikəs] *subst.* scar with a depression in the middle of the abdomen where the umbilical cord was detached after birth *omphalus, umbilicus, naveln*

område ➪ **area, district, field, region, zona, zone**

omskära ➪ **circumcise**

omskärelse ➪ **circumcision, peritomy**

omslag ➪ **compress, dressing, pad, poultice**

omsorg ➪ **attention, care**

omtumlad ➪ **dazed**

omvandla ➪ **convert**

omvandling ➪ **conversion**

omvårdnad ➪ **care, nursing**

omvårdnadsplan ➪ **care plan**

omvårdnadsprocess ➪ **nursing**

omvårdnad(såtgärd) ➪ **intervention**

omättat fett ➪ **unsaturated fat**

o.n. [ˌəʊ'en] *abbreviation for the Latin phrase* "omni nocte": every night (written on a prescription) *omni nocte, till natten*

onanera ➪ **masturbate**

onani ➪ **masturbation, onanism**

onanism ['əʊnənɪz(ə)m] *subst.* masturbation *onani, masturbation*

Onchocerca [ˌɒŋkəʊ'sɜːkə] *subst.* genus of tropical parasitic threadworm *Onchocerca*

onchocerciasis [ˌɒŋkəʊsɜː'ka(ɪ)əsɪs] *subst.* infestation with **Onchocerca** where the larvae can move into the eye, causing river blindness *onchocerciasis*

onco- ['ɒŋkə(ʊ), ˌ--] *prefix* referring to tumours *onko-, tumör-*

oncogene ['ɒŋkədʒiːn] *subst.* part of the genetic system which causes malignant tumours to develop *onkogen*

> QUOTE all cancers may be reduced to fundamental mechanisms based on cancer risk genes or oncogenes within ourselves. An oncogene is a gene that encodes a protein that contributes to the malignant phenotype of the cell
> **British Medical Journal**

oncogenesis [ˌɒŋkə'dʒenəsɪs] *subst.* origin and development of a tumour *onkogenes*

oncogenic [ˌɒŋkə'dʒenɪk] *adj.* (substance *or* virus) which causes tumours to develop *onkogen, tumörframkallande*

oncology [ɒŋ'kɒlədʒi] *subst.* scientific study of new growths *onkologi*

oncolysis [ɒŋ'kɒləsɪs] *subst.* destruction of a tumour *or* of tumour cells *onkolys*

oncotic [ɒŋ'kɒtɪk] *adj.* referring to a tumour *onkotisk*

onko- ➪ **onco-**

onkogen ➪ **oncogene, oncogenic**

onkogenes ➪ **oncogenesis**

onkologi ➪ **oncology**

onkolys ➪ **oncolysis**

onkotisk ➪ **oncotic**

onormal ➪ **aberrant, abnormal, anomalous, mal-**

onset ['ɒnset] *subst.* beginning *början, angrepp;* **the onset of the illness is marked by sudden high temperature**

> QUOTE a follow-up study of 84 patients with early onset pre-eclampsia (before 37 weeks' gestation) showed a high prevalence of renal disease
> **British Medical Journal**

ont ➪ **harm, hurt**

ont, göra ➪ **ache**

ont, ha ➪ **suffer**

ont i halsen ➪ **sore**

ontogenes ➪ **ontogeny**

ontogeni ➪ **ontogeny**

ontogeny [ɒn'tɒdʒəni] *subst.* origin and development of an individual organism *ontogenes, ontogeni*

onych- [ˌɒnɪk] *prefix* referring to nails *onyk-, nagel-*

onychauxis [ˌɒnɪ'kɔːksɪs] *subst.* overgrowth of the nails of the fingers or toes *alltför kraftig nagelväxt*

onychia [ɒ'nɪkiə] *subst.* abnormality of the nails, caused by inflammation of the matrix *onykit, onyxit, nagelinflammation*

onychogryphosis [ˌɒnɪkəugrɪ'fəusɪs] *subst.* condition where the nails are bent or curved over the ends of the fingers or toes *onykogrypos, nagelkrökning*

onycholysis [ˌɒnɪ'kɒləsɪs] *subst.* condition where a nail becomes separated from its bed, without falling out *onykolys*

onychomadesis [ˌɒnɪkəumə'diːsɪs] *subst.* condition where the nails fall out *nagelavlossning*

onychomycosis [ˌɒnɪkəumaɪ'kəusɪs] *subst.* infection of the nail with a fungus *onykomykos*

onychosis [ˌɒnɪ'kəusɪs] *subst.* any disease of the nails *onyki, nagelsjukdom*

onyk- ⇨ **onych-**

onyki ⇨ **onychosis**

onykit ⇨ **onychia**

onykogrypos ⇨ **onychogryphosis**

onykolys ⇨ **onycholysis**

onykomykos ⇨ **onychomycosis**

o'nyong-nyong fever [əuni'ɒŋniɒŋ ˌfiːvə] *or* **joint-breaker fever** ['dʒɔɪntbreɪkə ˌfiːvə] *subst.* infectious virus disease prevalent in East Africa, spread by mosquitoes *sjukdom orsakad av arbovirus, spridd genom moskiter*

> COMMENT: the symptoms are high fever, inflammation of the lymph nodes and excruciating pains in the joints

onyxit ⇨ **onychia**

oo- ['əuə, ˌ-] *prefix* referring to an ovum *or* to an embryo *oo-, ägg-*

oocyesis [ˌəuəsaɪ'iːsɪs] *subst.* pregnancy which develops in the ovary *X, extrauterin graviditet, ektopisk graviditet (utomkvedshavandeskap) i äggstock*

oocyte ['əuəsaɪt] *subst.* cell which forms from an oogonium and becomes an ovum by meiosis *oocyt*

ooforalgi ⇨ **oophoralgia**

ooforektomi ⇨ **oophorectomy, ovariectomy, ovariotomy**

ooforit ⇨ **oophoritis, ovaritis**

ooforom ⇨ **oophoroma**

ooforon ⇨ **oophoron**

ooforopexi ⇨ **oophoropexy**

ooforosalpingektomi ⇨ **oophorosalpingectomy**

ooforosalpingit ⇨ **salpingo-oophoritis**

ooforotomi ⇨ **ovariotomy**

oogenesis [ˌəuə'dʒenəsɪs] *subst.* formation and development of ova *oogenes, äggbildning*

oogenetic [ˌəuədʒə'netɪk] *adj.* referring to oogenesis *som avser el. hör till äggbildningen*

oogonium [ˌəuə'gəuniəm] *subst.* cell produced at the beginning of the development of an ovum *oogonium, primordialägg, urägg*
NOTE: the plural is **oogonia**

> COMMENT: in oogenesis, an oogonium produces an oocyte which develops through several stages to produce a mature ovum. Polar bodies are also formed which do not develop into ova

oopho- ['əuəfə(u), ˌ--] *or* **oophoro-** [əu'ɒfərə(u), -ˌ---] *prefix* referring to the ovaries *oofor(o)-, ovari(o)-, ovarial-, äggstocks-*

oophoralgia [ˌəuəfə'rældʒə] *subst.* pain in the ovaries *ooforalgi, ovarialsmärta*

oophorectomy [ˌəuəfə'rektəmi] *or* **ovariectomy** [əuˌveəri'ektəmi] *subst.* surgical removal of an ovary *ooforektomi, ovariektomi*

oophoritis [ˌəuəfə'raɪtɪs] *or* **ovaritis** [ˌəuvə'raɪtɪs] *subst.* inflammation in an ovary, which can be caused by mumps *ooforit, ovarit, äggstocksinflammation*

oophoroma [ˌəuəfə'rəumə] *subst.* rare

ovarian tumour, occurring in middle age *ooforom, elakartad äggstockstumör*

oophoron [əʊ'ɒfərɒn] *or* **ovary** ['əʊv(ə)ri] *subst.* one of two organs in a woman which produce ova *or* egg cells and secrete the female hormone oestrogen *ooforon, ovarium, äggstock*

oophoropexy [əʊ'ɒfərəˌpeksi] *subst.* surgical operation to attach an ovary *ooforopexi*

oophorosalpingectomy [əʊˌɒfərəˌsælpɪn'dʒektəmi] *subst.* surgical removal of an ovary and the Fallopian tube attached to it *ooforosalpingektomi, ovariosalpingektomi, salpingooforektomi, salpingovariektomi*

oorganisk ⇨ **inorganic**

oorganiska syror ⇨ **acid**

ooze [u:z] *vb. (of pus or blood)* to flow slowly *sippra, rinna långsamt*

OP [ˌəʊ'pi:] = OUTPATIENT

opacity [ə(ʊ)'pæsəti] *subst.* (i) not allowing light to pass through *opacitet, ogenomskinlighet;* (ii) area in the eye which is not clear *opacitet, grumling*

opak ⇨ **opaque**

opaque [ə(ʊ)'peɪk] *adj.* not transparent *opak, ogenomskinlig, grumlig;* **radio-opaque dye** = liquid which appears on an X-ray, and which is introduced into soft organs (such as the kidney) so that they show up clearly on an X-ray photograph *röntgenkontrast(medel), röntgentätt medel*

oparig ⇨ **azygos**

opasslig ⇨ **ailing, indisposed**

opasslighet ⇨ **indisposition**

opastöriserad ⇨ **unpasteurized**

open ['əʊp(ə)n] *adj.* not closed *öppen;* **open fracture** *or* **compound fracture** = fracture where the skin surface is damaged *or* where the broken bone penetrates the surface of the skin *öppen fraktur, komplicerad fraktur;* **open heart surgery** = surgery to repair part of the heart *or* one of the coronary arteries, performed while the heart has been bypassed and the blood is circulated by a pump *öppen hjärtkirurgi;* **open visiting** = arrangement in a hospital where visitors can enter the wards at any time *obegränsad besökstid*

opening ['əʊp(ə)nɪŋ] *subst.* place where something opens *öppning, mynning*

operable ['ɒp(ə)rəb(ə)l] *adj.* (condition) which can be treated by an operation *operabel;* **the cancer is still operable**

operate ['ɒpəreɪt] *vb.* **to operate on a patient** = to treat a patient's condition by cutting open his body and removing a part which is diseased *or* repairing a part which is not functioning correctly *operera;* **the patient was operated on yesterday; the surgeons decided to operate as the only way of saving the baby's life; operating microscope** = special microscope with two eyepieces and a light, used in very delicate surgery *operationsmikroskop;* **operating theatre** *or US* **operating room (OR)** = special room in a hospital where surgeons carry out operations *operationssal;* **operating table** = special table on which the patient is placed while an operation is being carried out *operationsbord*

operation [ˌɒpə'reɪʃ(ə)n] *subst.* (i) way in which a drug acts *verkan;* (ii) surgical intervention *or* act of cutting open a patient's body to treat a disease *or* disorder *operation, operativt ingrepp, kirurgiskt ingrepp;* **she's had an operation on her foot; the operation to remove the cataract was successful; a team of surgeons performed the operation; heart operations are always difficult** NOTE: a surgeon **performs** an operation **on** a patient

operations- ⇨ **surgical**

operationsbord ⇨ **operate, table**

operationsförberedelser ⇨ **prep, preparation**

operationshandskar ⇨ **surgical**

operationsklädsel ⇨ **drape**

operationskniv ⇨ **scalpel**

operationslakan ⇨ **drape**

operationsmikroskop ⇨ **operate**

operationsrock ⇨ **theatre**

operationssal ⇨ **operate, surgery**

operationsskjorta ⇨ **theatre**

operationssköterska ⇨ **nurse**

operculum [ə(ʊ)'pɜ:kjʊləm] *subst.* (i) part of the cerebral hemisphere which overlaps the insula *operculum;* (ii) plug of mucus which can block the cervical canal during pregnancy *slempropp (i livmoderhalsen under havandeskap)*

operera ⇨ **operate**

operforerad ⇨ **imperforate**

operon ['ɒpəˌrɒn] *subst.* group of genes which controls the production of enzymes *slags gen som styr enzymproduktionen, gen som styr andra gener*

ophth- [ɒfθ, ɒpθ] *prefix* referring to the eye *oft(alm)-, ögon-*

ophthalmectomy [ˌɒfθæl'mektəmi] *subst.* surgical removal of an eye *oftalmektomi*

ophthalmia [ɒf'θælmiə] *subst.* inflammation of the eye *oftalmi(t), ögoninflammation;* **ophthalmia neonatorum** = conjunctivitis of a newborn baby, beginning 21 days after birth, caused by infection in the birth canal *ögoninflammation hos nyfödda (ofta orsakad av Chlamydia el. gonorré);* **Egyptian ophthalmia** *or* **trachoma** = virus disease of the eyes, common in tropical countries *trakom, egyptiska ögonsjukdomen*

ophthalmic [ɒf'θælmɪk] *adj.* referring to the eye *oftalm(isk)-, ögon-;* **ophthalmic practitioner** *or* **optician** = qualified person who specializes in testing eyes and prescribing lenses *ung. legitimerad optiker;* **ophthalmic surgeon** = surgeon who specializes in surgery to treat eye disorders *ögonkirurg;* **ophthalmic nerve** = branch of the trigeminal nerve, supplying the eyeball, the upper eyelid, the brow and one side of the scalp *nervus ophtalmicus, gren av 5:e kranialnerven (trigeminus)*

ophthalmitis [ˌɒfθæl'maɪtɪs] *subst.* inflammation of the eye *oftalmi(t), ögoninflammation*

ophthalmological [ˌɒfθælmə'lɒdʒɪk(ə)l] *adj.* referring to ophthalmology *som avser el. hör till oftalmologi*

ophthalmologist [ˌɒfθæl'mɒlədʒɪst] *subst.* doctor who specializes in the study of the eye and its diseases *oftalmolog, ögonspecialist*

ophthalmology [ˌɒfθæl'mɒlədʒi] *subst.* study of the eye and its diseases *oftalmologi*

ophthalmoplegia [ɒfˌθælmə'pliːdʒə] *subst.* paralysis of the muscles of the eye *oftalmoplegi, ögonmuskelförlamning*

ophthalmoscope [ɒf'θælməskəʊp] *subst.* instrument containing a bright light and small lenses, used by a doctor to examine the inside of an eye *oftalmoskop, ögonspegel*

ophthalmoscopy [ˌɒfθæl'mɒskəpi] *subst.* examination of the inside of an eye using an ophthalmoscope *oftalmoskopi, ögonspegling*

ophthalmotomy [ˌɒfθæl'mɒtəmi] *subst.* surgical operation to make a cut in the eyeball *operativt snitt i ögongloben*

ophthalmotonometer [ɒfˌθælmətə'nɒmɪtə] *or* **tonometer** [tə(ʊ)'nɒmɪtə] *subst.* instrument which measures pressure inside the eye *tonometer, oftalmotonometer*

-opia ['əʊpiə] *suffix* referring to a defect in the eye *-opi, -seende, -syn(thet);* **myopia** = being shortsighted *myopi, närsynthet*

opiate ['əʊpiət] *subst.* sedative which is prepared from opium, such as morphine or codeine *opiat*

opinion [ə'pɪnjən] *subst.* what someone thinks about something *åsikt, uppfattning, utlåtande;* **what's the surgeon's opinion of the case? the doctor asked the consultant for his opinion as to the best method of treatment; she has a very high** *or* **very low opinion of her doctor** = she thinks he is very good *or* very bad *hon har en mycket hög (låg) tanke om läkaren, hon har en mycket hög (låg) uppfattning om läkaren;* **to ask for a second opinion** = to ask another doctor *or* consultant to examine a patient and give his opinion on diagnosis *or* treatment *be att få höra någon annans åsikt*

opium ['əʊpiəm] *subst.* substance made from poppies, used in the preparation of codeine and heroin *opium*

opponens [ə'pəʊnəns] *subst.* muscles in the fingers which tend to draw these fingers opposite to other fingers *musculus opponens digiti, opponent*

opponent ⇨ **opponens**

opportunist(ic) [ˌɒpə'tjuːnɪst (ˌɒpətjuː'nɪstɪk] *adj.* (parasite *or* microbe) which senses that an organism is weak and then attacks it *som avser el. hör till opportunist (slags mikroorganism)*

opposition [ˌɒpə'zɪʃ(ə)n] *subst.* movement of the hand muscles where the tip of the thumb is made to touch the tip of another finger so as to hold something *opposition, motställning, motsättning*

opsonic index [ɒp'sɒnɪk ˌɪndeks] *subst.* number which gives the strength of an individual's serum reaction to bacteria *opsoniskt (fagocytärt) index*

opsonin ['ɒpsənɪn] *subst.* substance, usually an antibody, in blood which sticks to the surface of bacteria and helps to destroy them *opsonin*

optic ['ɒptɪk] *adj.* referring to the eye *or* to sight *optisk, syn-, synnervs-;* **optic chiasma** = structure where the optic nerves from each eye partially cross each other in the hypothalamus *chiasma opticum, synnervskorsningen;* **optic disc** *or* **optic papilla** = point on the retina where the optic nerve starts *papilla nervi optici, synnervspapillen;* **optic nerve** = second cranial nerve which transmits the sensation of sight from the eye to the brain ⇨ *illustration* EYE *nervus opticus, synnerven, 2:a kranialnerven;* **optic neuritis** = inflammation of the optic nerve, which makes objects appear blurred *optikusneurit, synnervsinflammation;* **optic radiations** = nerve tracts which take the optic impulses from the optic tracts to the visual cortex *synbanan;* **optic tracts** = nerve tracts which take the optic nerves from the optic chiasma to the optic radiations *synnervsbanorna*

optical ['ɒptɪk(ə)l] *adj.* referring to optics *optisk, syn-;* **optical illusion** = something which is seen wrongly so that it appears to be something else *optisk villa, synvilla*

optician [ɒp'tɪʃ(ə)n] *subst. optiker;* **dispensing optician** = person who fits and sells glasses but does not test eyes *optiker;* **ophthalmic optician** = qualified person who specializes in making glasses and in testing eyes and prescribing lenses *ung. legitimerad optiker* NOTE: in US English an **optician** is a technician who makes lenses and fits glasses, but cannot test patient's eyesight

> COMMENT: in the UK qualified ophthalmic opticians must be registered by the General Optical Council before they can practise

optics ['ɒptɪks] *subst.* study of light rays and sight *optik; see also* FIBRE OPTICS

optik ⇨ **optics**

optiker ⇨ **optician, ophthalmic**

optikusneurit ⇨ **retrobulbar neuritis**

optikuspapillit ⇨ **papillitis**

optisk ⇨ **optic, optical**

optometer [ɒp'tɒmɪtə] = REFRACTOMETER

optometri ⇨ **optometry**

optometrist [ɒp'tɒmətrɪst] *subst. mainly US* person who specializes in testing eyes and prescribing lenses *slags optiker*

optometry [ɒp'tɒmətri] *subst.* testing of eyes and prescribing of lenses to correct defects in sight *optometri, synmätning*

opåverkbar ⇨ **refractory**

OR [ˌəʊ'ɑː] *US* = OPERATING ROOM **an OR nurse**

oral ['ɔːr(ə)l] *adj.* referring to the mouth *oral, peroral, mun-;* **oral cavity** = the mouth *cavum oris, munhålan;* **oral contraceptive** = contraceptive pill which is swallowed *oralt preventivmedel, p-piller;* **oral medication** = medicine which is taken by swallowing *peroralt läkemedel;* **oral thermometer** = thermometer which is put into the mouth to take a patient's temperature *muntermometer*

orally ['ɔːr(ə)li] *adv.* (medicine taken) by the mouth *oralt, peroralt, genom munnen;* **the lotion cannot be taken orally** *compare* PARENTERAL

oralt ⇨ **orally**

orbicularis [ɔːˌbɪkju'leərɪs] *adj.* circular muscle in the face *ringmuskel (i ansiktet);* **orbicularis oculi** = muscle which opens and closes the eye *musculus orbicularis oculi, ögats ringmuskel;* **orbicularis oris** = muscle which closes the lips tight *musculis orbicularis oris*

orbit ['ɔːbɪt] *subst.* eye socket *or* hollow bony depression in the front of the skull in which each eye and lacrimal gland are situated ⇨ *illustration* SKULL *orbita, ögonhålan*

orbita ⇨ **orbit, socket**

orbital ['ɔːbɪt(ə)l] *adj.* referring to the orbit *orbital, ögonhåle-*

orchi- ['ɔːkɪ, ˌ--] *prefix* referring to the testes *orki(o)-, orkid(o)-, testikel-*

orchidalgia [ˌɔːkɪ'dældʒə] *subst.* neuralgic-type pain in a testis *orki(d)algi, testikelsmärta*

orchidectomy [ˌɔːkɪˈdektəmi] *subst.* surgical removal of a testis *orkidektomi, testikelexcision*

orchidopexy [ˈɔːkɪdəʊˌpeksi] *or* **orchiopexy** [ˌɔːkiəʊˈpeksi] *subst.* surgical operation to place an undescended testis in the scrotum *orki(d)opexi, orkido(r)rafi*

orchidotomy [ˌɔːkɪˈdɒtəmi] *subst.* surgical operation to make a cut into a testis *orkidotomi*

orchis [ˈɔːkɪs] *subst.* testis *orchis, testis, testikel*

orchitis [ɔːˈkaɪtɪs] *subst.* inflammation of the testes, characterized by hypertrophy, pain and a sensation of weight *orkit, testikelinflammation*

ordblindhet ➪ **alexia, dyslexia**

orderly [ˈɔːdəli] *subst.* person who does general work *person som utför allmänna göromål;* **hospital orderly** = person who does heavy work in a hospital, such as wheeling patients into the operating theatre, moving equipment about, etc. *ung. sjukvårdsbiträde, ung. vaktmästare, ung. "bärare"*

ordination ➪ **prescription**

ordinera ➪ **prescribe**

ordna ➪ **arrange, fix**

ordnande ➪ **arrangement**

ordning ➪ **arrangement**

ordning(sföljd) ➪ **sequence**

oregelbunden ➪ **irregular**

oregelbundenhet ➪ **arrhythmia**

oren ➪ **dirty, impure**

orenlighet ➪ **dirt, impurities**

organ [ˈɔːgən] *subst.* part of the body which is distinct from other parts and has a particular function (such as the liver *or* an eye *or* the ovaries, etc.) *organ;* **organ of Corti** *or* **spiral organ** = membrane in the cochlea which takes sounds and converts them into impulses sent to the brain along the auditory nerve *organon spirale, Cortis organ, Cortiska organet, hörselorganet;* **organ transplant** = transplanting of an organ from one person to another *organtransplantation*

organic [ɔːˈgænɪk] *adj.* **(a)** referring to organs in the body *organisk, kroppslig;* **organic disorder** = disorder caused by changes in body tissue *or* in an organ *organisk (kroppslig) sjukdom* **(b)** (i) (substance) which comes from an animal *or* plant *organisk;* (ii) (food) which has been cultivated naturally, without any chemical fertilizers *or* pesticides *alternativodlad*

organically [ɔːˈgænɪk(ə)li] *adv.* (food) grown using natural fertilizers and not chemicals *organiskt*

organisk ➪ **organic**

organiska syror ➪ **acid**

organiskt ➪ **organically**

organism [ˈɔːgənɪz(ə)m] *subst.* any single living plant, animal, bacterium or fungus *organism*

organoterapi ➪ **organotherapy**

organotherapy [ˌɔːgənəʊˈθerəpi] *subst.* treatment of a disease by using an extract from the organ of an animal (such as using liver extract to treat anaemia) *organoterapi*

organtransplantation ➪ **organ**

orgasm [ˈɔːgæz(ə)m] *subst.* climax of the sexual act, when a person experiences a moment of great excitement *orgasm, sexuell utlösning*

oriental sore [ˌɔːriˈent(ə)l ˌsɔː] *or* **Leishmaniasis** [ˌliːʃməˈna(ɪ)əsɪs] *subst.* skin disease of tropical countries caused by the parasite Leishmania *leishmaniasis cutanae, orientböld, aleppoböld*

orientböld ➪ **Baghdad boil, Delhi boil, oriental sore**

orifice [ˈɒrəfɪs] *subst.* opening *orificium, öppning, mynning;* **cardiac orifice** = opening where the oesophagus joins the stomach *övre magmunnen, öppningen där matstrupen övergår i magsäcken;* **ileocaecal orifice** = opening where the small intestine joins the large intestine *caecalporten, öppningen där tunntarmen övergår i tjocktarmen;* **pyloric orifice** = opening where the stomach joins the duodenum *pylorus, nedre magmunnen, magporten*

origin [ˈɒrɪdʒɪn] *subst.* place where a muscle is attached *or* where the branch of a nerve *or* blood vessel begins *ursprung, källa*

original [ə'rɪdʒ(ə)n(ə)l] *adj.* as in the first place *ursprunglig;* **the surgeon was able to move the organ back to its original position**

originate [ə'rɪdʒəneɪt] *vb.* to start (in a place) *uppstå, härröra;* to begin *or* to make something begin *börja;* **the treatment originated in China; drugs which originated in the tropics**

oriktig ⇨ **incorrect**

oris ['ɔ:rɪs] *see* CANCRUM ORIS, ORBICULARIS ORIS

ork ⇨ **energy**

orkidektomi ⇨ **orchidectomy**

orkidotomi ⇨ **orchidotomy**

orkit ⇨ **orchitis**

ormbett ⇨ **snake**

ormserum ⇨ **antivenene**

ornithine ['ɔ:nɪθaɪn] *subst.* amino acid produced by the liver *ornit(h)in*

ornithosis [ˌɔ:nɪ'θəʊsɪs] *subst.* disease of birds which can be passed to humans as a form of pneumonia *ornit(h)os; see also* PSITTACOSIS

oro ⇨ **anxiety, distress, nervousness**

orolig ⇨ **anxious, nervous, nervy, restless**

oropharynx ['ɔ:rəʊˌfærɪŋ(k)s] *subst.* part of the pharynx below the soft palate at the back of the mouth *orofarynx*

orsak ⇨ **agent, reason**

ortho- ['ɔ:θə(ʊ), ˌ--] *prefix* meaning correct *or* straight *orto-*

orthodiagraph [ˌɔ:θə(ʊ)'da(ɪ)əgrɑ:f] *subst.* X-ray photograph of an organ taken using only a thin stream of X-rays which allows accurate measurements of the organ to be made *ortodiagrafi*

orthodontic [ˌɔ:θə(ʊ)'dɒntɪk] *adj.* which corrects badly formed teeth *or* referring to orthodontics *som avser el. hör till tandreglering;* **he had to undergo a course of orthodontic treatment**

orthodontics [ˌɔ:θə(ʊ)'dɒntɪks] *or US* **orthodontia** [ˌɔ:θə(ʊ)'dɒnʃə] *subst.* branch of dentistry which deals with correcting badly placed teeth *ortodonti, tandreglering*

orthodontist [ˌɔ:θə(ʊ)'dɒntɪst] *subst.* dental surgeon who specializes in correcting badly placed teeth *ortodontist*

orthopaedic [ˌɔ:θə'pi:dɪk] *adj.* which corrects badly formed bones *or* joints *ortopedisk;* referring to *or* used in orthopaedics *ortopedisk;* **orthopaedic hospital** = hospital which specializes in operations to correct badly formed joints *or* bones *ortopediskt sjukhus;* **orthopaedic surgeon** = surgeon who specializes in orthopaedics *ortoped*

orthopaedics [ˌɔ:θə'pi:dɪks] *subst.* branch of surgery dealing with abnormalities, diseases and injuries of the locomotor system *ortopedi*

orthopaedist [ˌɔ:θə'pi:dɪst] *subst.* surgeon who specializes in orthopaedics *ortoped*

orthopnoea [ˌɔ:θəp'nɪə] *subst.* condition where the patient has great difficulty in breathing while lying down *ortopné, andfåddhet (i vila); see also* DYSPNOEA

orthopnoeic [ˌɔ:θəp'ni:ɪk] *adj.* referring to orthopnoea *ortopnoisk*

orthopsychiatry [ˌɔ:θəʊsaɪ'ka(ɪ)ətri] *subst.* science and treatment of behavioural and personality disorders *läran om och behandlingen av beteende- och personlighetsstörningar*

orthoptics [ɔ:'θɒptɪks] *subst.* methods used to treat squints *ortoptik, skelningskorrigering*

orthoptist [ɔ:'θɒptɪst] *subst.* eye specialist working in an eye hospital, who treats squints and other disorders of eye movement *ortoptist*

orthosis [ɔ:'θəʊsɪs] *subst.* device which is fitted to the outside of the body to support a weakness *or* correct a deformity (such as a surgical collar, leg braces, etc.) *ortos* NOTE: plural is **orthoses**

orthostatic [ˌɔ:θə'stætɪk] *adj.* referring to the position of the body when standing up straight *ortostatisk;* **orthostatic hypotension** = common condition where the blood pressure drops when someone stands up suddenly, causing dizziness *ortostatism*

orthotist ['ɔ:θətɪst] *subst.* qualified person who fits orthoses *person som prövar ut ortopediska hjälpmedel*

orto- ⇨ **ortho-**

ortodiagrafi ⇨ **orthodiagraph**

ortodonti ⇨ **orthodontia**

ortodontist ⇨ **orthodontist**

Ortolani's sign [ˌɔːtəˈlɑːnɪz ˌsaɪn] *subst.* test for congenital dislocation of the hip, where the hip makes a clicking noise if the joint is rotated *Ortolanis fenomen (knäpp), slags tecken på höftledsluxation*

ortoped ⇨ **orthopaedic, orthopaedist**

ortopedi ⇨ **orthopaedics**

ortopedisk ⇨ **orthopaedic, orthopaedic, surgical**

ortopedisk sko ⇨ **shoe**

ortopediskt ⇨ **surgically**

ortopné ⇨ **orthopnoea**

ortopnoisk ⇨ **orthopnoeic**

ortoptik ⇨ **orthoptics**

ortoptist ⇨ **orthoptist**

ortos ⇨ **orthosis**

ortostatisk ⇨ **orthostatic**

ortostatism ⇨ **orthostatic**

ortosömn ⇨ **slow-wave sleep**

orörlig ⇨ **immobile, immovable, motionless, quiescent**

os [ɒs] *Latin noun* **(a)** bone *os, ben, skelettben* NOTE: plural is **ossa** **(b)** mouth *os, munnen* NOTE: plural is **ora**

oscilloskop ⇨ **monitor**

osculum [ˈɒskjʊləm] *subst.* small opening *or* pore *por, liten öppning (mynning)*

-osis [ˈəʊsɪs] *suffix* referring to disease *-os, -sjukdom*

oskadlig ⇨ **harmless**

oskarp ⇨ **blurred**

oskuld ⇨ **virgin, virginity**

oskyldig ⇨ **innocent**

oskärpa ⇨ **blurring of vision**

Osler's nodes [ˈɒsləz ˌnəʊdz] *subst.* tender swellings at the ends of fingers and toes in patients suffering from subacute bacterial endocarditis *Oslerknutor*

osmidros ⇨ **bromhidrosis**

osmoreceptor [ˌɒzməʊrɪˈseptə] *subst.* cell in the hypothalamus which checks the level of osmotic pressure in the blood and regulates the amount of water in the blood *osmoreceptor*

osmosis [ɒzˈməʊsɪs] *subst.* movement of solvent from one part of the body through a semipermeable membrane to another part where there is a higher concentration of molecules *osmos*

osmotic pressure [ɒzˌmɒtɪk ˈpreʃə] *subst.* pressure required to stop the flow of the solvent through a membrane *osmotiskt tryck*

osmält ⇨ **undigested**

osseous [ˈɒsiəs] *adj.* bony *or* referring to bones *osseus, ben-;* **osseous labyrinth** = hard part of the temporal bone surrounding the inner ear *labyrinthus osseus, benlabyrinten*

osseus ⇨ **osseous**

ossicle [ˈɒsɪk(ə)l] *subst.* small bone *ossiculum, litet ben;* **auditory ossicles** = three little bones (the malleus, the incus and the stapes) in the middle ear *ossicula auditus, hörselbenen*

COMMENT: the auditory ossicles pick up the vibrations from the eardrum and transmit them through the oval window to the cochlea in the inner ear. The three bones are articulated together; the stapes is attached to the membrane of the oval window, and the malleus to the eardrum, and the incus lies between the other two

ossiculum ⇨ **ossicle**

ossification [ˌɒsɪfɪˈkeɪʃ(ə)n] *or* **osteogenesis** [ˌɒstiəʊˈdʒenəsɪs] *subst.* formation of bone *ossifikation, osteogenes, benbildning, förbening*

ossifikation ⇨ **ossification, osteogenesis**

ossium [ˈɒsiəm] *see* FRAGILITAS

ost- [ɒst] *or* **osteo-** [ˈɒstiəʊ, ˌ--] *prefix* referring to bone *ost(o)-, oste(o)-, ben-*

ostadig ⇨ **unsteady**

osteitis [ˌɒstiˈaɪtɪs] *subst.* inflammation of a bone due to injury *or* infection *ost(e)it, beninflammation;* **osteitis deformans** *or* **Paget's disease** = disease which gradually softens bones in the spine, legs and skull, so that they become curved *osteitis deformans, Pagets bensjukdom;* **osteitis fibrosis cystica** = generalized weakness of bones, associated with formation of cysts, where bone tissue is replaced by fibrous tissue, caused by excessive activity of the thyroid gland (the localized form is osteitis fibrosis localista) *osteodystrophia fibrosa (cystica) generalizata, von Recklinghausens sjukdom*

osteoarthritis [ˌɒstɪəʊɑːˈθraɪtɪs] *or* **osteoarthrosis** [ˌɒstiəʊɑːˈθrəʊsɪs] *subst.* chronic degenerative arthritic disease of middle-aged and elderly people, where the joints are inflamed and become stiff and painful *osteoartrit, artros*

osteoarthropathy [ˌɒstiəʊɑːˈθrɒpəθi] *subst.* disease of the bone and cartilage at a joint, particularly the ankles, knees or wrists, associated with carcinoma of the bronchi *osteoartropati*

osteoarthrosis [ˌɒstiəʊɑːˈθrəʊsɪs] *subst.* = OSTEOARTHRITIS

osteoarthrotomy [ˌɒstiəʊɑːˈθrɒtəmi] *subst.* surgical removal of the articular end of a bone *operativt avlägsnande av ben som ingår i led*

osteoartrit ⇨ **osteoarthritis**

osteoartropati ⇨ **osteoarthropathy**

osteoblast [ˈɒstiəʊblæst] *subst.* cell in an embryo which forms bone *osteoblast*

osteochondritis [ˌɒstiəʊkənˈdraɪtɪs] *subst.* degeneration of epiphyses *osteokondrit;* **osteochondritis dissecans** = painful condition where pieces of articular cartilage become detached from the joint surface *osteochondritis dissecans, avlossning av benbrosk*

osteochondroma [ˌɒstiəʊkənˈdrəʊmə] *subst.* tumour containing both bony and cartilaginous cells *osteokondrom, ben-brosktumör*

osteoclasia [ˌɒstiəʊˈkleɪziə] *or* **osteoclasis** [ˌɒstiˈɒkləsɪs] *subst.* (i) destruction of bone tissue by osteoclasts *benvävsupplösning orsakad av jätteceller;* (ii) surgical operation to fracture or refracture bone to correct a deformity *osteoklasi, operativt ingrepp där ben mekaniskt bryts sönder*

osteoclast [ˈɒstiəʊklæst] *subst.* (i) cell which destroys bone *osteoklast, benresorberande jättecell;* (ii) surgical instrument for breaking bones *osteoklast, slags kirurgiskt instrument*

osteoclastoma [ˌɒstiəʊklæˈstəʊmə] *subst.* usually benign tumour occurring at the ends of long bones *osteoklastom, jättecellstumör*

osteocyt ⇨ **osteocyte**

osteocyte [ˈɒstiəʊsaɪt] *subst.* bone cell *osteocyt*

osteodystrofi ⇨ **osteodystrophia**

osteodystrophia [ˌɒstiəʊdɪˈstrəʊfiə] *or* **osteodystrophy** [ˌɒstiəʊˈdɪstrəfi] *subst.* bone disease, especially one caused by disorder of the metabolism *osteodystrofi*

osteofoni ⇨ **conduction**

osteofyt ⇨ **osteophyte**

osteogenes ⇨ **ossification, osteogenesis**

osteogenesis [ˌɒstiəʊˈdʒenəsɪs] *subst.* formation of bone *osteogenes, ossifikation, benbildning, förbening;* **osteogenesis imperfecta** *or* **fragilitas ossium** = congenital condition where bones are brittle and break easily due to abnormal bone formation *osteogenesis imperfecta*

osteogenic [ˌɒstiəʊˈdʒenɪk] *adj.* made of bone tissue *or* starting from bone tissue *osteogen*

osteoklasi ⇨ **osteoclasia**

osteoklast ⇨ **osteoclast**

osteoklastom ⇨ **osteoclastoma**

osteokondrit ⇨ **osteochondritis**

osteokondrom ⇨ **osteochondroma**

osteology [ˌɒstiˈɒlədʒi] *subst.* study of bones and their structure *osteologi, benlära*

osteolysis [ˌɒstiˈɒləsɪs] *subst.* (i) destruction of bone tissue by osteoclasts *osteolys, benvävsupplösning orsakad av jätteceller;* (ii) removal of bone calcium *osteolys, urkalkning av benväv*

osteolytic [ˌɒstiəʊˈlɪtɪk] *adj.* referring to osteolysis *osteolytisk*

osteoma [ˌɒstiˈəʊmə] *subst.* benign tumour in a bone *osteom, benvävssvulst*

osteomalacia [ˌɒstiəʊməˈleɪʃiə] *subst.* condition in adults, where the bones become soft because of lack of calcium and vitamin D *osteomalaci, osteomalaki, benvävsuppmjukning, urkalkning av benväv*

osteomalaki ⇨ **osteomalacia**

osteomyelitis [ˌɒstiəʊma(ɪ)əˈlaɪtɪs] *subst.* inflammation of the interior of bone, especially the marrow spaces *osteomyelit, benmärgsinflammation, benröta*

osteon [ˈɒstiɒn] *subst.* = HAVERSIAN SYSTEM

osteopath [ˈɒstiəpæθ] *subst.* person who practises osteopathy *osteopat*

osteopathy [ˌɒstiˈɒpəθi] *subst.* (i) way of treating diseases and disorders by massage and manipulation of bones and joints *osteopati, slags behandling av ben och leder;* (ii) any disease of bone *osteopati, bensjukdom*

osteopetrosis [ˌɒstiəʊpəˈtrəʊsɪs] *or* **marble bone disease** [ˈmɑːb(ə)lbəʊn dɪˌziːz] *subst.* disease where bones become condensed *osteopetros, Albers-Schönbergs sjukdom, marmorbensjuka*

osteophony [ˌɒstiˈɒfəni] *see* CONDUCTION

osteophyte [ˈɒstiəʊfaɪt] *subst.* bony growth *osteofyt, artrofyt, godartat benutskott*

osteoplasty [ˈɒstiəʊˌplæsti] *subst.* plastic surgery on bones *osteoplastik*

osteoporosis [ˌɒstiəʊpɔːˈrəʊsɪs] *subst.* condition where the bones become thin, porous and brittle, because of lack of calcium and lack of physical exercise *osteoporos, benskörhet*

osteosarcoma [ˌɔːstiəʊsɑːˈkəʊmə] *subst.* malignant tumour of bone cells *osteosarkom*

osteosclerosis [ˌɒstiəʊskləˈrəʊsɪs] *subst.* condition where the bony spaces become hardened as a result of chronic inflammation *osteoskleros, benförhårdning, benförtätning*

osteotome [ˈɒstiəʊtəʊm] *subst.* type of chisel used by surgeons to cut bone *osteotom*

osteotomy [ˌɒstiˈɒtəmi] *subst.* surgical operation to cut a bone, especially to relieve pain in a joint *osteotomi*

osteril ⇨ **non-sterile, unsterilized**

ostium [ˈɒstiəm] *subst.* opening into a passage *ostium, öppning, mynning*

ostomy [ˈɒstəmi] *subst. (informal)* colostomy *or* ileostomy *stomi*

-ostomy [ˈɒstəmi] *suffix* referring to an operation to make an opening *-stomi*

osund ⇨ **morbid, unhealthy**

osynlig ⇨ **invisible**

OT [ˌəʊˈtiː] = OCCUPATIONAL THERAPIST

ot- [əʊˈt] *or* **oto-** [ˈəʊtə(ʊ), ˌ--] *prefix* referring to the ear *ot(o)-, aur-, öron-*

otalgi ⇨ **earache, otalgia**

otalgia [əʊˈtældʒə] *subst.* earache *or* pain in the ear *otalgi, örsprång, ont i öronen*

OTC [ˌəʊtiːˈsiː] *abbreviation* "over the counter": (drug) which can be bought freely at the chemist's shop, and does not need a prescription *inte receptbelagd*

otic [ˈəʊtɪk] *adj.* referring to the ear *oticus, öron-*

otikodini ⇨ **Ménière's disease**

otillräcklig ⇨ **inadequate**

otillräknelig ⇨ **non compos mentis**

otitis [ə(ʊ)ˈtaɪtɪs] *subst.* inflammation of the ear *otit, öroninflammation;* **otitis externa** *or* **external otitis** = any inflammation of the external auditory meatus to the eardrum *otitis externa, yttre öroninflammation;* **otitis interna** *or* **labyrinthitis** = inflammation of the inner ear *otitis interna (labyrinthiaca), inre öroninflammation;* **otitis media** *or* **tympanitis** = inflammation of the middle ear *otitis media, inflammation i mellanörat, örsprång;* **secretory otitis media** *or* **glue ear** = condition where fluid forms behind the eardrum and causes deafness *otosalpingit, adhesiv otit, sekretorisk inflammation i mellanörat; see also* PANOTITIS

otolaryngologist [ˌəʊtə(ʊ)ˌlærɪŋˈgɒlədʒɪst] *subst.* doctor who specializes in treatment of diseases of the ear and throat *otolaryngolog, specialist på öron- och halssjukdomar*

otolaryngology [ˌəʊtə(ʊ)ˌlærɪŋˈgɒlədʒi] *subst.* study of diseases of the ear and throat *otolaryngologi*

otolith [ˈəʊtə(ʊ)lɪθ] *subst.* (i) stone which forms in the inner ear *öronsten;* (ii) tiny piece of calcium carbonate attached to the hair cells in the saccule and utricle of the inner ear *otolit, statolit, hörselsten, öronsten;* **otolith organs** = two pairs of sensory organs (the saccule and the utricle) in the inner ear which pass information to the brain about the position of the head *balansorganets hinnsäckar sacculus och utriculus*

otolog ⇨ **otologist**

otologi ⇨ **otology**

otologist [əʊˈtɒlədʒɪst] *subst.* doctor who specializes in the study of the ear *otolog, öronspecialist*

otology [əʊˈtɒlədʒi] *subst.* scientific study of the ear and its diseases *otologi*

otomycosis [ˌəʊtə(ʊ)maɪˈkəʊsɪs] *subst.* infection of the external auditory meatus by a fungus *otomykos*

otomykos ⇨ **otomycosis**

otoplasty [ˈəʊtə(ʊ)ˌplæsti] *subst.* plastic surgery of the external ear to repair damage *or* deformity *plastikoperation av ytterörat*

otorhinolaryngologist [ˌəʊtə(ʊ)ˌraɪnəʊˌlærɪŋˈgɒlədʒɪst] *or* **ENT specialist** [ˌiːenˈtiː ˌspeʃəlɪst] *subst.* doctor who specializes in the study of the ear, nose and throat *otorinolaryngolog, specialist på öron-, näs- och halssjukdomar*

otorhinolaryngology (ENT) [ˌəʊtə(ʊ)ˌraɪnəʊˌlærɪŋˈgɒlədʒi (ˌiːenˈtiː)] *subst.* study of the ear, nose and throat *otorinolaryngologi*

otorinolaryngologi ⇨ **otorhinolaryngology (ENT)**

otorrhagia [ˌəʊtəˈreɪdʒə] *subst.* bleeding from the external ear *oto(r)ragi, öronblödning*

otorrhoea [ˌəʊtə(ʊ)ˈrɪə] *subst.* discharge of pus from the ear *oto(r)ré, öronflytning*

otosalpingit ⇨ **otitis**

otosalpinx ⇨ **Eustachian tube**

otosclerosis [ˌəʊtə(ʊ)skləˈrəʊsɪs] *subst.* condition where the ossicles in the middle ear become thicker, the stapes becomes fixed to the oval window, and the patient becomes deaf *otoskleros*

otoscope [ˈəʊtə(ʊ)skəʊp] = AURISCOPE

otoskleros ⇨ **otosclerosis**

otoskop ⇨ **auriscope**

otvättad ⇨ **unwashed**

outbildad ⇨ **unqualified**

outbreak [ˈaʊtbreɪk] *subst.* series of cases of a disease which start suddenly *utbrott;* **there is an outbreak of typhoid fever** *or* **a typhoid outbreak in the town**

outer [ˈaʊtə] *adj.* (part) which is outside *yttre, ytter-, utvändig;* **outer ear** *or* **pinna** = part of the ear on the outside of the head, with a channel leading into the eardrum *pinna, autris externa, ytterörat;* **outer pleura** = membrane attached to the diaphragm and covering the chest cavity *pleura parietalis (costalis), lungsäckens yttre blad*
NOTE: opposite is **inner**

outlet [ˈaʊtlet] *subst.* opening *or* channel through which something can go out *öppning, mynning;* **thoracic outlet** = large opening at the base of the thorax *apertura thoracis inferior, nedre toraxaperturen (toraxöppningen)*

out of hours [ˌaʊt əv ˈa(ʊ)əz] *adv.* not during the normal opening hours of a doctor's surgery *akut, under stängningstid;* **there is a special telephone number if you need to call the doctor out of hours**

outpatient [ˈaʊtˌpeɪʃ(ə)nt] *subst.* patient living at home, who comes to the hospital for treatment *poliklinisk patient;* **she goes for treatment as an outpatient; Outpatient** *or* **Outpatients' Department** = department of a hospital, which deals with outpatients *poliklinik;* **he cut his hand badly in the accident, and the police took him to the Outpatients' Department to have it dressed; 25 patients were selected from the Outpatient Department for testing** *see also* INPATIENT

outreach [ˈaʊtriːtʃ] *subst.* services provided for patients *or* the public outside a hospital *or* clinic *or* local government department *tjänster som tillhandahålls utanför sjukhuset etc.*

outvecklad ⇨ **embryonic, immature, rudimentary**

ov- ['əʊv, ˌ-] *or* **ovar-** ['əʊvər, ˌ--, əʊ'veər, -ˌ-] *prefix* referring to the ovaries *ovari(o)-, ovarial-, oofor(o)-, äggstocks-*

ova ['əʊvə] *see* OVUM

ovalocytos ⇨ **elliptocytosis**

oval window ['əʊv(ə)l ˌwɪndəʊ] *or* **fenestra ovalis** [fɪˌnestrə əʊ'veɪlɪs] *subst.* oval opening between the middle ear and the inner ear ⇨ *illustration* EAR *fenestra ovalis (vestibuli), ovala fönstret;* **foramen ovale** = opening between the two parts of the heart in a fetus *foramen ovale (cordis)*

ovanlig ⇨ **exceptional, rare**

ovaralgia [ˌəʊvə'rældʒə] *or* **ovarialgia** [əʊˌveəri'ældʒə] *subst.* pain in the ovaries *ovar(i)algi*

ovarial- ⇨ **oopho-, ov-, ovarian**

ovarialcykel ⇨ **cycle**

ovarialcysta ⇨ **ovarian**

ovarialsmärta ⇨ **oophoralgia**

ovarian [əʊ'veəriən] *adj.* referring to the ovaries *ovari(o)-, ovarial-, oofor(o)-, äggstocks-;* **ovarian cyst** = cyst which develops in the ovaries *ovarialcysta, äggstockscysta;* **ovarian follicle** *or* **Graafian follicle** = cell which contains an ovum *folliculus ovarii (oophori), Graafs (graafsk) follikel, äggblåsa*

ovariectomy [əʊˌveəri'ektəmi] *or* **oophorectomy** [ˌəʊəfə'rektəmi] *subst.* surgical removal of an ovary *ovariektomi, ooforektomi*

ovariektomi ⇨ **oophorectomy, ovariectomy**

ovariocele [əʊ'veəriəʊˌsi:(ə)l] *subst.* hernia of an ovary *ovariocele*

ovariosalpingektomi ⇨ **oophorosalpingectomy**

ovariotomy [əʊˌveəri'ɒtəmi] *subst.* surgical removal of an ovary *or* a tumour in an ovary *ovariotomi, ooforotomi, ooforektomi*

ovarit ⇨ **oophoritis, ovaritis**

ovaritis [ˌəʊvə'raɪtɪs] *or* **oophoritis** [ˌəʊəfə'raɪtɪs] *subst.* inflammation of an ovary or both ovaries *ovarit, ooforit, äggstocksinflammation*

ovary ['əʊv(ə)ri] *subst.* one of two organs in a woman, which produce ova *or* egg cells and secrete the female hormone oestrogen ⇨ *illustration* UROGENITAL SYSTEM (female) *ovarium, oophoron, äggstock*
NOTE: for other terms referring to ovaries, see words beginning with **oophor-**

over- ['əʊvə, ˌ--] *prefix* too much *över-*

overbite ['əʊvəbaɪt] *subst.* normal formation of the teeth, where the top incisors come down over and in front of the bottom incisors when the jaws are closed *överbett i vertikal riktning*

overcome [ˌəʊvə'kʌm] *vb.* **(a)** to fight something and win *besegra, övervinna;* **she overcame her disabilities and now leads a normal life (b)** to make someone lose consciousness *orsaka medvetslöshet hos;* **two people were overcome by smoke in the fire**
NOTE: **overcoming - overcame - has overcome**

overcompensate [ˌəʊvə'kɒmpənseɪt] *vb.* to try to cover the effects of a handicap by making too strenuous efforts *överkompensera*

overdose ['əʊvədəʊs] *subst.* dose (of a drug) which is larger than normal *överdos, överdosering;* **she went into a coma after an overdose of heroin** *or* **after a heroin overdose**

overdo (things) [ˌəʊvə'du: (ˌθɪŋz)] *vb. informal* to work too hard *or* to do too much exercises *överdriva, överanstränga (sig);* **he has been overdoing things and has to rest; she overdid it, working until 9 o'clock every evening** NOTE: **overdoing - overdid - overdone**

overeating [ˌəʊvə'ri:tɪŋ] *subst.* eating too much food **overeat** *äta för mycket, föräta (sig)*

overexertion [ˌəʊv(ə)rɪg'zɜ:ʃ(ə)n] *subst.* doing too much physical work *or* taking too much exercise *överansträngning*

overgrow [ˌəʊvə'grəʊ] *vb.* to grow over a tissue *växa över*

overgrowth ['əʊvəgrəʊθ] *subst.* growth of tissue over another tissue *överväxt*

overjet ['əʊvədʒet] *subst.* space which separates the top incisors from the bottom incisors when the jaws are closed *överbett i horisontell riktning*

overksam ⇨ **inactive, quiescent**

overksamhet ⇨ **inactivity**

overlap [ˌəʊvəˈlæp] *vb. (of bandages, etc.)* to lie partly on top of another *överlappa, delvis täcka över (varandra), gå omlott med*

overproduction [ˌəʊvəprəˈdʌkʃ(ə)n] *subst.* producing too much *överproduktion;* **the condition is caused by overproduction of thyroxine by the thyroid gland**

oversew [ˈəʊvəsəʊ] *vb.* to sew a patch of tissue over a perforation *suturera (sy över) perforation*
NOTE: **oversewing - oversewed - oversewn**

overweight [ˈəʊvəweɪt] *adj.* too fat and heavy *överviktig;* **he is several kilos overweight for his age and height**

overwork [ˌəʊvəˈwɜːk] **1** *subst.* doing too much work *överansträngning;* **he collapsed from overwork 2** *vb.* to work too much *or* to make something work too much *överanstränga (sig);* **he has been overworking his heart**

overwrought [ˌəʊvəˈrɔːt] *adj.* very tense and nervous *överspänd;* **he is rather overwrought because of troubles at work**

oviduct [ˈəʊvidʌkt] = FALLOPIAN TUBE

ovulate [ˈɒvjuleɪt] *vb.* to release a mature ovum into a Fallopian tube *ha ägglossning*

ovulation [ˌɒvjuˈleɪʃ(ə)n] *subst.* release of an ovum from the mature ovarian follicle into the Fallopian tube *ovulation, ägglossning*

ovum [ˈəʊvəm] *subst.* female egg cell *ovum, ägg, äggcell*
NOTE: the plural is **ova**. Note that for other terms referring to ova, see words beginning with **oo-**

ovälkommen ⇨ **unwanted**

oxeltand ⇨ **molar**

oxidase [ˈɒksɪdeɪz] *subst.* enzyme which encourages oxidation by removing hydrogen *oxidas; see also* MONOAMINE

oxidation [ˌɒksɪˈdeɪʃ(ə)n] *subst.* action of making oxides by combining with oxygen or removing hydrogen *oxidation*

> COMMENT: carbon compounds form oxides when metabolised with oxygen in the body, producing carbon dioxide

oxide [ˈɒksaɪd] *subst.* compound formed with oxygen *oxid;* **zinc oxide** = compound of zinc and oxygen, used in creams and lotions *zinkoxid*

oxihemoglobin ⇨ **oxyhaemoglobin**

oxycefali ⇨ **oxycephaly**

oxycephalic [ˌɒksɪkəˈfælɪk, ˌɒksɪsəˈfælɪk] *adj.* referring to oxycephaly *som avser el. hör till oxycefali*

oxycephaly [ˌɒksɪˈkef(ə)li] *or* **turricephaly** [ˌtʌrɪˈkef(ə)li] *subst.* condition where the skull is deformed into a point, with exophthalmos and defective sight *oxycefali*

oxygen [ˈɒksɪdʒ(ə)n] *subst.* chemical element, a common colourless gas which is present in the air and essential to human life *oxygen, syre, syrgas, O;* **oxygen cylinder** = heavy metal tube which contains oxygen and is connected to a patient's oxygen mask *syrgastub;* **oxygen mask** = mask connected to a supply of oxygen, which can be put over the face to help a patient with breathing difficulties *syrgasmask;* **oxygen tent** = type of cover put over a patient so that he can breathe in oxygen *syrgastält* NOTE: chemical symbol is **O**

> COMMENT: oxygen is absorbed into the bloodstream through the lungs and is carried to the tissues along the arteries; it is essential to normal metabolism and given to patients with breathing difficulties

oxygenate [ˈɒksɪdʒəneɪt] *vb.* to treat (blood) with oxygen *syrsätta;* **oxygenated** *or* **arterial blood** = blood which has received oxygen in the lungs and is being carried to the tissues along the arteries (it is brighter red than venous deoxygenated blood) *syrsatt (arteriellt) blod*

oxygenation [ˌɒksɪdʒəˈneɪʃ(ə)n] *subst.* becoming filled with oxygen *syrsättning;* **blood is carried along the pulmonary artery to the lungs for oxygenation**

oxygenator [ˌɒksɪdʒəˈneɪtə] *subst.* machine which puts oxygen into the blood, used as an artificial lung in surgery *slags ventilator*

oxyhaemoglobin [ˌɒksɪˌhiːməˈgləʊbɪn] *subst.* compound of haemoglobin and oxygen, which is the way oxygen is carried in arterial blood from the lungs to the tissues *oxyhemoglobin, oxihemoglobin; see also* HAEMOGLOBIN

oxyhemoglobin ⇨ **oxyhaemoglobin**

oxyntic cell [ɒk'sɪntɪk ˌsel] *or* **parietal cell** [pə'ra(ɪ)ət(ə)l ˌsel] *subst.* cell in the gastric gland which secretes hydrochloric acid *parietalcell*

oxytocin [ˌɒksɪ'təʊsɪn] *subst.* hormone secreted by the pituitary gland, which controls the contractions of the uterus and encourages the flow of milk *oxytocin, ocytocin*

COMMENT: an extract of oxytocin is used as an injection to start contractions of the uterus

oxyuriasis [ˌɒksɪju'raɪəsɪs] = ENTEROBIASIS

Oxyuris [ˌɒksɪ'jəʊrɪs] = ENTEROBIUS

ozaena [əʊ'zi:nə] *subst.* (i) disease of the nose, where the nasal passage is blocked and mucus forms, giving off an unpleasant smell *oz(a)ena, stinknäsa;* (ii) any unpleasant discharge from the nose *all slags obehaglig utsöndring från näsan*

oönskad ⇨ **unwanted**

oönskad graviditet ⇨ **pregnancy**

Pp

P *chemical symbol for* phosphorus *P, fosfor*

pacemaker ['peɪsˌmeɪkə] *subst.* **(a)** sinoatrial node *or* SA node *or* node in the heart which regulates the heartbeat *pacemaker, sinusknutan;* **ectopic pacemaker** = abnormal focus of the heart muscle which takes the place of the SA node *ektopiskt fokus* **(b)** **(cardiac) pacemaker** = electronic device implanted on a patient's heart, or which a patient wears attached to his chest, which stimulates and regulates the heartbeat *(konstgjord) pacemaker;* **the patient was fitted with a pacemaker; endocardial pacemaker** = pacemaker attached to the lining of the heart *pacemaker (vanligen) fästad vid hjärtats innerhinna;* **epicardial pacemaker** = pacemaker attached to the surface of the ventricle *pacemaker fästad vid hjärtkammarens utsida*

COMMENT: an electrode is usually attached to the epicardium and linked to the device which can be implanted in various positions in the chest

pachy- ['pæki, ˌ--] *prefix* meaning thickening *paky-*

pachydactyly [ˌpæki'dæktɪli] *subst.* condition where the fingers and toes become thicker than normal *pakydaktyli*

pachydermia [ˌpæki'dɜ:miə] *or* **pachyderma** [ˌpɜ:ki'dɜ:mə] *subst.* condition where the skin becomes thicker than normal *pakydermi, hudförtjockning*

pachymeningitis [ˌpækiˌmenɪn'dʒaɪtɪs] *subst.* inflammation of the dura mater *pakymeningit*

pachymeninx [ˌpæki'mi:nɪŋks] *or* **dura mater** ['djʊərəˌmeɪtə] *subst.* thicker outer layer covering the brain and spinal cord *dura mater, pakymeninx, hårda hjärnhinnan*

pachysomia [ˌpæki'səʊmiə] *subst.* condition where soft tissues of the body become abnormally thick *pakysomi*

pacifier ['pæsɪfa(ɪ)ə] *subst. US* rubber teat given to a baby to suck, to prevent it crying *napp, tröstnapp*
NOTE: GB English is **dummy**

pacing [peɪsɪŋ] *subst.* surgical operation to implant *or* attach a cardiac pacemaker *inläggning av pacemaker*

Pacinian corpuscle [pə'sɪniən ˌkɔ:pʌs(ə)l] *see* CORPUSCLE

pack [pæk] **1** *subst.* **(a)** (i) tampon of gauze *or* cotton wool, used to fill an orifice such as the nose *or* vagina *tampong, tamponad;* (ii) wet material folded tightly, used to press on the body *slags tryckförband;* (iii) treatment where a blanket or sheet is used to wrap round the patient's body *inpackning;* **cold pack** *or* **hot pack** = cold *or* hot wet cloth put on a patient's body to reduce *or* increase his body temperature *kallt (varmt) omslag;* **ice pack** = cold compress made of lumps of ice wrapped in a cloth, and pressed on a swelling *or* bruise to reduce the pain *slags kallt omslag* **(b)** box *or* bag of goods for sale *kartong, förpackning;* **a pack of sticking plaster; she bought a sterile dressing pack; the cough tablets are sold in packs of fifty 2** *vb.* **(a)** to fill an orifice with a tampon (of cotton wool) *tamponera;* **the ear was packed with cotton wool to absorb the discharge (b)** to put things in cases *or* boxes *packa;* **the transplant organ arrived at the hospital packed in ice; packed cell volume (haematocrit)** = volume of red blood cells in a patient's blood shown against the total volume of blood *erytrocytvolymfraktion, EVF, hematokrit*

packning ⇨ **plombage**

pack up [ˌpæk 'ʌp] *vb. (informal)* to stop working *packa ihop, paja, lägga av;* **his heart simply packed up under the strain**

pad [pæd] *subst.* (i) soft absorbent material, and placed on part of the body to protect it *kompress, förband, omslag, dyna;* (ii) thickening of part of the skin *hudförhårdnad;* **she wrapped a pad of soft cotton wool round the sore**

paed- ['ped, ˌ-, 'pi:d, ˌ-] *or* **paedo-** ['pi:dəʊ, ˌ--] *prefix* referring to children *paed(o)-, ped(o)-, barn-* NOTE: words beginning with **paed-** can also be written **ped-**

paediatric [ˌpi:di'ætrɪk] *adj.* referring to the treatment of the diseases of children *pediatrisk;* **a new paediatric hospital has been opened; parents can visit children in the paediatric wards at any time**

paediatrician [ˌpi:diə'trɪʃ(ə)n] *subst.* doctor who specializes in the treatment of diseases of children *pediat(rik)er, barnläkare*

paediatrics [ˌpi:di'ætrɪks] *subst.* study of children, their development and diseases *pediatri(k); compare* GERIATRICS

Paget's disease ['pædʒəts dɪˌzi:z] *subst.* **(a)** osteitis deformans *or* disease which gradually softens and thickens the bones in the spine, skull and legs, so that they become curved *osteitis deformans, Pagets bensjukdom* **(b)** form of breast cancer which starts as an itchy rash round the nipple *Pagets sjukdom i bröstvårtan*

pain [peɪn] *subst.* feeling which a person has when hurt *dolor, smärta, värk, plågor;* **she had pains in her legs after playing tennis; the doctor gave him an injection to relieve the pain; she is suffering from back pain; to be in great pain** = to have very sharp pains which are difficult to bear *ha mycket ont;* **abdominal pain** = pain in the abdomen, caused by indigestion or serious disorder *buksmärta;* **chest pains** = pains in the chest which may be caused by heart disease *bröstsmärtor;* **labour pains** = pains felt at regular intervals by a woman as the muscles of the uterus contract during childbirth *värkar, förlossningsvärkar;* **throbbing pain** = pain which continues in repeated short attacks *dunkande smärta;* **referred pain** = SYNALGIA; **pain pathway** = series of linking nerve fibres and neurones which carry impulses of pain from the site to the sensory cortex *nervbana för smärtimpulser;* **pain receptor** = nerve ending which is sensitive to pain *smärtreceptor;* **pain threshold** = point at which a person finds it impossible to bear pain without crying *smärttröskel* NOTE: pain can be used in the plural to show that it recurs: **she has pains in her left leg**

> COMMENT: pain is carried by the sensory nerves to the central nervous system; from the site it travels up the spinal column to the medulla and through a series of neurones to the sensory cortex. Pain is the method by which a person knows that part of the body is damaged *or* infected, though the pain is not always felt in the affected part (see synalgia)

painful ['peɪnf(ə)l] *adj.* which hurts *smärtsam, plågsam;* **she has a painful skin disease; his foot is so painful he can hardly walk; your eye looks very red - is it very painful?**

pain killer ['peɪn ˌkɪlə] *or* **pain-killing drug** ['peɪnkɪlɪŋ ˌdrʌg] *or* **pain-relieving drug** ['peɪnrɪˌli:vɪŋ drʌg] *or* **analgesic** [ˌæn(ə)l'dʒi:zɪk] *subst.* drug which stops a patient feeling pain *analgetikum, smärtstillande medel*

painless ['peɪnləs] *adj.* which does not hurt *or* which gives no pain *smärtfri;* **a painless method of removing warts**

paint [peɪnt] **1** *subst.* coloured antiseptic *or* analgesic *or* astringent liquid which is put on the surface of the body *färgad vätska som appliceras utvärtes* **2** *vb.* to cover (a wound) with an antiseptic *or* analgesic *or* astringent liquid or lotion *applicera vätska utvärtes;* **she painted the rash with calamine**

painter's colic ['peɪntəz ˌkɒlɪk] *subst.* form of lead poisoning caused by working with paint *slags blykolik*

paky- ⇨ **pachy-**

pakydaktyli ⇨ **pachydactyly**

pakydermi ⇨ **pachydermia**

pakymeningit ⇨ **pachymeningitis**

pakymeninx ⇨ **pachymeninx**

pakysomi ⇨ **pachysomia**

palate ['pælət] *subst.* roof of the mouth and floor of the nasal cavity (formed of the hard and soft palates) *palatum, gommen;* **cleft palate** = congenital defect, where there is a fissure in the hard palate allowing the mouth and nasal cavities to be linked, caused when the two bones forming the palate have not fused together properly *palatum fissum,* *gomklyvning, gomspalt, kluven gom;* **hard palate** = front part of the palate between the upper teeth, made of the horizontal parts of the palatine bone and processes of the maxillae *palatum durum, hårda gommen;* **soft palate** = back part of the palate leading to the uvula ⇨ *illustration* THROAT *palatum molle, mjuka gommen*

palatine ['pælətaɪn] *adj.* referring to the palate *som avser el. hör till gommen;* **palatine arches** = folds of tissue between the soft palate and the pharynx *arcus palatoglossus och arcus palatopharyngeus, gombågarna;* **palate bones** *or* **palatine bones** = two bones which form part of the hard palate, the orbits of the eyes and the cavity behind the nose *os palatum, gombenet;* **palatine tonsil** *or* **tonsil** = lymphoid tissue at the back of the throat, between the soft palate, the tongue and the pharynx *tonsilla palatina, gomtonsill, gommandel, mandel*

palato- ['pælətə(ʊ), ˌ---] *prefix* referring to the palate *palato-, gom-*

palatoglossal arch [ˌpælətə(ʊ)'glɒs(ə)l ˌɑːtʃ] *subst.* fold between the soft palate and the tongue, anterior to the tonsil *arcus palatoglossus, främre gombågen*

palatopharyngeal arch [ˌpælətə(ʊ)ˌfærɪn'dʒɪəl ˌɑːtʃ] *subst.* fold between the soft palate and the pharynx, posterior to the tonsil *arcus palatopharyngeus, bakre gombågen*

palatoplastik ⇨ **palatoplasty**

palatoplasty ['pælətə(ʊ)ˌplæsti] *subst.* plastic surgery of the roof of the mouth, such as to repair a cleft palate *palatoplastik*

palatoplegia [ˌpælətə(ʊ)'pliːdʒə] *subst.* paralysis of the soft palate *palatoplegi, gomförlamning*

palatorrhaphy [ˌpælə'tɔːrəfi] *or* **staphylorrhaphy** [ˌstæfi'lɔːrəfi] *or* **uraniscorrhaphy** [ˌjʊərəni'skɔːrəfi] *subst.* surgical operation to suture and close a cleft palate *palato(r)rafi, stafylo(r)rafi, urano(r)rafi*

pale [peɪ(ə)l] *adj.* light coloured *or* white *blek;* **after her illness she looked pale and tired; with his pale complexion and dark rings round his eyes, he did not look at all well; to turn pale** = to become white in the face, because the flow of blood is reduced *blekna, bli blek;* **some people turn pale at the sight of blood**

paleness ['pe(ɪ)lnəs] *or* **pallor** ['pælə] *subst.* being pale *blekhet*

pali- ['pælɪ, ˌ--] *or* **palin-** ['pælɪn, ˌ--] *prefix* which repeats *pali(n)-*

palilalia [ˌpælɪ'leɪliə] *subst.* speech defect where the patient repeats words *slags taldefekt, ekolali*

palindrom ⇨ **palindromic**

palindromic [ˌpælɪn'drəʊmɪk] *adj.* (disease) which recurs *palindrom, recidiverande, återkommande*

palliative ['pæliətɪv] *subst. & adj.* treatment *or* drug which relieves the symptoms, but does nothing to cure the disease which causes the symptoms (a pain killer can reduce the pain in a tooth, but will not cure the caries which causes the pain) *palliativum, lindrande medel, palliativ, lindrande*

> QUOTE coronary artery bypass grafting is a palliative procedure aimed at the relief of persistent angina pectoris
> **British Journal of Hospital Medicine**

pallor ['pælə] *subst.* paleness *or* being pale *pallor, blekhet*

palm [pɑːm] *subst.* soft inside part of the hand *palma, handflatan*

palmar ['pælmə] *adj.* referring to the palm *palmar-, handflate-;* **palmar arch** = one of two arches in the palm formed by two arteries which link together *arcus palmaris, handflatebågen, hålhandsbågen;* **palmar interosseus** = deep muscle between the bones in the hand *djupt liggande muskel mellan handens ben;* **palmar region** = area of skin around the palm *handflatans hudområde*
NOTE: in the hand **palmar** is the opposite of **dorsal**

palpable ['pælpəb(ə)l] *adj.* which can be felt when touched *kännbar, förnimbar;* which can be examined with the hand *palpabel*

> QUOTE mammography is the most effective technique available for the detection of occult (non-palpable) breast cancer. It has been estimated that mammography can detect a carcinoma two years before it becomes palpable
> **Southern Medical Journal**

palpation [pæl'peɪʃ(ə)n] *subst.* examination of part of the body by feeling it with the hand *palpation;* **breast palpation** = feeling a breast to see if a lump is present which might indicate breast cancer *bröstpalpation;* **digital palpation** = pressing part of the body with the fingers *palpation med hjälp av fingrarna*

palpebra ['pælpibrə] *subst.* eyelid *palpebra, ögonlocket* NOTE: plural is **palpebrae**

palpebral ['pælpibrəl] *adj.* referring to the eyelids *palpebral, ögonlocks-*

palpitate ['pælpɪteɪt] *vb.* to beat rapidly *or* to throb *or* to flutter *banka (bulta, klappa, slå) snabbt*

palpitation [ˌpælpɪ'teɪʃ(ə)n] *subst.* awareness that the heart is beating abnormally, caused by stress *or* by a disease *palpitation, hjärtklappning*

palsied ['pɔːlzid] *adj.* suffering from palsy *förlamad;* **cerebral palsied children**

palsy ['pɔːlzi] *subst.* paralysis *pares, förlamning;* **cerebral palsy** = disorder of the brain affecting spastics, due to brain damage which has occurred before birth or due to lack of oxygen during birth *cerebral pares, CP;* **Erb's palsy** = condition where an arm is paralysed because of birth injuries to the brachial plexus *Erbs förlamning, Ducenne-Erbs förlamning; see also* BELL'S PALSY

paludism ['pæljudɪz(ə)m] = MALARIA

pan- [pæn] *or* **pant-** ['pænt, ,-] *or* **panto-** ['pæntəʊ, ,--] *prefix* meaning generalized *or* affecting everything *pan(to)-, total*

panacea [ˌpænə'sɪə] *subst.* medicine which is supposed to cure everything *panacé, patentmedicin, universalmedicin*

panaritium ⇨ **whitlow**

panarthritis [ˌpænɑː'θraɪtɪs] *subst.* inflammation of all the tissues of a joint *or* of all the joints in the body *panartrit*

pancarditis [ˌpænkɑːdaɪtɪs] *subst.* inflammation of all the tissues in the heart, i.e. the heart muscle, the endocardium and the pericardium *pankardit, total kardit*

pancreas ['pæŋkriəs] *subst.* gland which lies across the back of the body between the kidneys *pankreas, bukspottkörteln*

> COMMENT: the pancreas has two functions: the first is to secrete the pancreatic juice which goes into the duodenum and digests proteins and carbohydrates; the second function is to produce the hormone insulin which regulates the use of sugar by the body. This hormone is secreted into the bloodstream by the islets of Langerhans which are all around the pancreas

pancreatectomy [ˌpæŋkriə'tektəmi] *subst.* surgical removal of all *or* part of the pancreas *pankreatektomi;* **partial pancreatectomy** = removal of part of the pancreas *partiell pankreatektomi;* **subtotal pancreatectomy** = removal of most of the pancreas *subtotal pankreatektomi;* **total pancreatectomy** *or* **Whipple's operation** = removal of the whole pancreas together with part of the duodenum *total pankreatektomi*

pancreatic [ˌpæŋkri'ætɪk] *adj.* referring to the pancreas *pankreatisk, bukspotts-;* **benign pancreatic disease** = chronic pancreatitis *kronisk pankreatit;* **pancreatic duct** = duct leading through the pancreas to the duodenum *ductus pancreaticus;* **pancreatic fibrosis** = CYSTIC FIBROSIS; **pancreatic juice** *or* **pancreatic secretion** = digestive juice formed of enzymes produced by the pancreas which digests fats and carbohydrates *pankreassaft, bukspott*

pancreatin ['pæŋkriətɪn] *subst.* substance made from enzymes secreted by the pancreas and used to treat a patient whose pancreas does not produce pancreatic enzymes *pankreatin*

pancreatitis [ˌpæŋkriə'taɪtɪs] *subst.* inflammation of the pancreas *pankreatit, bukspottkörtelinflammation;* **acute pancreatitis** = inflammation after pancreatic enzymes have escaped into the pancreas, causing symptoms of acute abdominal pain *akut pankreatit;* **chronic pancreatitis** = chronic inflammation, after repeated attacks of acute pancreatitis, where the gland becomes calcified *kronisk pankreatit;* **relapsing pancreatitis** = form of pancreatitis where the symptoms recur, but in a less painful form *recidiverande pankreatit*

pancreatomy [ˌpæŋkri'ætəmi] *or* **pancreatotomy** [ˌpæŋkriə'tɒtəmi] *subst.* surgical operation to open the pancreatic duct *pankreatotomi*

pancytopenia [ˌpænsaɪtə'piːniə] *subst.* condition where the numbers of red and white blood cells and blood platelets are all reduced together *pancytopeni, panhemato(cyto)peni*

pandemic [pæn'demɪk] *subst. & adj.* epidemic disease which affects many parts of the world *pandemisk; compare* ENDEMIC, EPIDEMIC

pang [pæŋ] *subst.* sudden sharp pain (especially in the intestine) *plötslig smärta;* **after not eating for a day, he suffered pangs of hunger**

panhysterectomy [ˌpænhɪstəˈrektmi] *subst.* surgical removal of all the womb and the cervix *panhysterektomi*

panhysterektomi ⇨ **panhysterectomy**

panic [ˈpænɪk] **1** *subst.* sudden great fear which cannot be stopped *panik, skräck;* **he was in a panic as he sat in the consultant's waiting room; panic attack** = sudden attack of panic *anfall av panik (skräck)* **2** *vb.* to be suddenly afraid *gripas av (råka i) panik, bli skräckslagen;* **he panicked when the surgeon told him he might have to have an operation**

pankardit ⇨ **pancarditis**

pankreas ⇨ **pancreas**

pankreassaft ⇨ **pancreatic**

pankreatektomi ⇨ **pancreatectomy**

pankreatin ⇨ **pancreatin**

pankreatisk ⇨ **pancreatic**

pankreatit ⇨ **pancreatitis**

pankreatotomi ⇨ **pancreatomy**

pann- ⇨ **frontal**

pannan ⇨ **brow, forehead**

pannbenet ⇨ **frontal**

panniculitis [pəˌnɪkjuˈlaɪtɪs] *subst.* inflammation of the panniculus adiposus, producing tender swellings on the thighs and breasts *pannikulit*

panniculus [peˈnɪkjʊləs] *subst.* layer of membranous tissue *panniculus;* **panniculus adiposus** = fatty layer of tissue underneath the skin *panniculus adiposus, underhudsfettväv*

pannikulit ⇨ **panniculitis**

pannloben ⇨ **frontal**

pannus [ˈpænəs] *subst.* growth on the cornea containing tiny blood vessels *pannus*

panophthalmia [ˌpænɒfˈθælmiə] *or* **panophthalmitis** [ˌpænɒfθælˈmaɪtɪs] *subst.* inflammation of the whole of the eye *panoftalmi(t)*

panosteitis [ˌpænˌɒstiˈaɪtɪs] *or* **panostitis** [ˌpænɒˈstaɪtɪs] *subst.* inflammation of all of a bone *panosteit*

panotitis [ˌpænəʊˈtaɪtɪs] *subst.* inflammation affecting all of the ear, but especially the middle ear *panotit*

panproctocolectomy [pænˌprɒktəkəˈlektəmi] *subst.* surgical removal of the whole of the rectum and the colon *panproktokolektomi*

pansarhjärta ⇨ **constrictive**

pant [pænt] *vb.* to take short breaths because of overexertion *or* to gasp for breath *flåsa, flämta, kippa efter andan;* **he was panting when he reached the top of the stairs**

pantotensyra ⇨ **pantothenic acid**

pantothenic acid [ˌpæntəˌθenɪk ˈæsɪd] *subst.* vitamin of the vitamin B complex, found in liver, yeast and eggs *pantot(h)en(ol), pantotensyra*

pantotropic [ˌpæntəˈtrɒpɪk] *or* **pantropic** [pænˈtrɒpɪk] *adj.* (virus) which attacks many different parts of the body *som angriper många olika organ*

Papanicolaou test [ˌpæpəˌnɪkəˈleɪuː ˌtest] *or* **Pap test** [ˈpæp ˌtest] *or* **Pap smear** [ˈpæp ˌsmɪə] *subst.* method of staining smears from various body secretions to test for malignancy, such as testing a cervical smear sample to see if cancer is present *Papanicolaouprov, Papsmear, Paptest, vaginalsmear, vaginalutstryk*

papegojsjuka ⇨ **psittacosis**

papel ⇨ **papule**

papilla [pəˈpɪlə] *subst.* small swelling which protrudes above the normal surface level *papill;* **the upper surface of the tongue is covered with papillae; hair papilla** = part of the skin containing capillaries which feed blood to the hair *papilla pili, hårpapill;* **optic papilla** *or* **optic disc** = point on the retina where the optic nerve starts ⇨ *illustration* TONGUE *papilla nervi potici, synnervspapillen; see also* CIRCUMVALLATE, FILIFORM, FUNGIFORM, VALLATE NOTE: plural is **papillae**

papillary [pəˈpɪlərɪ] *adj.* referring to papillae *papillar, papillär, vårtliknande*

papillitis [ˌpæpɪˈlaɪtɪs] *subst.* inflammation of the optic disc at the back of the eye *papillitis optica, optikuspapillit*

papilloedema [ˌpæpɪləʊˈdiːmə] *subst.* oedema of the optic disc at the back of the eye *papillödem, staspapill*

papilloma [ˌpæpɪˈləʊmə] *subst.* benign tumour on the skin *or* mucous membrane *papillom*

papillomatosis [ˌpæpɪˌləʊməˈtəʊsɪs] *subst.* (i) being affected with papillomata *angrepp av papillom;* (ii) formation of papillomata *papillombildning*

papillombildning ⇨ **papillomatosis**

papillär ⇨ **papillary**

papillödem ⇨ **papilloedema**

papovavirus [pəˈpəʊvəˌvaɪ(ə)rəs] *subst.* family of viruses which start tumours, some of which are malignant, and some of which, like warts, are benign *papovavirus*

Pap test [ˈpæp ˌtest] *or* **Pap smear** [ˈpæp ˌsmɪə] *see* PAPANICOLAOU TEST

papular [ˈpæpjʊlə] *adj.* referring to a papule *papulös*

papule [ˈpæpjuːl] *subst.* small coloured spot raised above the surface of the skin as part of a rash *papel, blemma, knottra* NOTE: a flat spot is a **macule**

papulopustular [ˌpæpjʊləˈpʌstjʊlə] *adj.* (rash) with both papules and pustules *(utslag) med både papler och pustler*

papulosquamous [ˌpæpjʊləˈskweɪməs] *adj.* (rash) with papules and a scaly skin *(utslag) med både papler och skvamös (fjällande) hud*

papulös ⇨ **papular**

para- [ˈpærə, ˌ--] *prefix* meaning (i) similar to *or* near *para-, bi-;* (ii) changed *or* beyond *para-, falsk*

-para ⇨ **parous**

paracentes ⇨ **paracentesis, tapping, tympanotomy**

paracentesis [ˌpærəsenˈtiːsɪs] *subst.* draining of fluid from a cavity inside the body, using a hollow needle, either for diagnostic purposes or because the fluid is harmful *paracentes, tappning*

paracetamol [ˌpærəˈsiːtəmɒl] *subst.* pain-killing drug *paracetamol*

paracolpitis [ˌpærəkɒlˈpaɪtɪs] = PERICOLPITIS

paracusis [ˌpærəˈkjuːsɪs] *or* **paracousia** [ˌpærəˈkuːsiə] *subst.* disorder of hearing *parakusi, Willis fenomen*

paradental ⇨ **periodontal**

paradentit ⇨ **periodontitis**

paradentium ⇨ **periodontal, periodontium**

paradoxical breathing [ˌpærəˈdɒksɪk(ə)l ˌbriːðɪŋ] *or* **respiration** [ˌrespəˈreɪʃ(ə)n] *subst.* condition of a patient with broken ribs, where the chest appears to move in when the patient breathes in, and appears to move out when he breathes out *paradox andning*

paradoxus [ˌpærəˈdɒksəs] *see* PULSUS

paraesthesia [ˌpæriːsˈθiːziə] *subst.* numbness and tingling feeling, like pins and needles *parestesi* NOTE: plural is **paraesthesiae**

> QUOTE the sensory symptoms are paraesthesiae which may spread up the arm over the course of about 20 minutes
> **British Journal of Hospital Medicine**

parafasi ⇨ **paraphasia**

paraffin [ˈpærəfɪn] *subst.* oil produced from petroleum, forming the base of some ointments, and also used for heating and light *paraffin, fotogen;* **liquid paraffin** = oil used as a laxative *paraffinum liquidum, flytande paraffin, paraffinolja;* **paraffin gauze** = gauze covered with solid paraffin, used as a dressing *paraffinkompress, salvkompress*

paraffinkompress ⇨ **paraffin**

paraffinolja ⇨ **paraffin**

parafimos ⇨ **paraphimosis**

parafreni ⇨ **paraphrenia**

parageusia [ˌpærəˈgjuːsiə] *subst.* (i) disorder of the sense of taste *parageusi, rubbning i smaksinnet;* (ii) unpleasant taste in the mouth *obehaglig smak*

paragonimiasis [ˌpærəˌgɒnəˈmaɪəsɪs] *or* **endemic haemoptysis** [ɪnˈdemɪk ˌhiːmɒpˈtaɪsɪs] *subst.* tropical disease where the patient's lungs are infested with a fluke and he coughs up blood *slags tropisk masksjukdom där patienten hostar upp blod*

paragraf ⇨ **section**

paraguard stretcher ['pærəgɑːd ˌstretʃə] *see* STRETCHER

para ihop ⇨ **match**

para-influenza virus [ˌpærəˌɪnflu'enzə ˌva(ɪ)ərəs] *subst.* virus which causes upper respiratory tract infection (in its structure it is identical to paramyxoviruses and the measles virus) *parainfluensavirus*

parakusi ⇨ **paracusis**

paralyse ['pærəlaɪz] *vb.* to weaken (muscles) so that they cannot function *paralysera, förlama;* **his arm was paralysed after the stroke; she is paralysed from the waist down**

paralysie générale ⇨ **paralysis**

paralysis [pə'ræləsɪs] *subst.* condition where the muscles of part of the body become weak and cannot be moved because the motor nerves have been damaged *paralys, förlamning;* **the condition causes paralysis of the lower limbs; he suffered temporary paralysis of the right arm; bulbar paralysis** = form of motor neurone disease which affects the muscles of the mouth, jaw and throat *paralysis bulbaris, bulbärparalys;* **facial paralysis** = BELL'S PALSY; **infantile paralysis** = POLIOMYELITIS; **paralysis agitans** = PARKINSON'S DISEASE; **general paralysis of the insane (GPI)** = very serious condition marking the final stages of syphilis *dementia paralytica, paralysie générale;* **spastic paralysis** *or* **cerebral palsy** = disorder of the brain affecting spastics, caused by brain damage before birth or lack of oxygen at birth *cerebral pares, CP; see also* DIPLEGIA, HEMIPLEGIA, MONOPLEGIA, PARAPLEGIA, QUADRIPLEGIA

> COMMENT: paralysis can have many causes: the commonest are injuries to *or* diseases of the brain or the spinal column

paralytic [ˌpærə'lɪtɪk] *adj.* referring to paralysis *paralytisk, förlamad;* (person) who is paralysed *förlamad person;* **paralytic ileus** = obstruction in the ileum caused by paralysis of the muscles of the intestine *paralytisk ileus*

paralytica [ˌpærə'lɪtɪkə] *see* DEMENTIA PARALYTICA

paralytisk ⇨ **paralytic**

paralytisk ileus ⇨ **adynamic ileus**

paramedian [ˌpærə'miːdiən] *adj.* near the midline of the body *paramedian*

paramedic [ˌpærə'medɪk] *subst.* person in a profession linked to that of nurse, doctor or surgeon *person med paramedicinskt yrke*

paramedical [ˌpærə'medɪk(ə)l] *adj.* referring to services linked to those given by nurses, doctors and surgeons *paramedicinsk*
NOTE: paramedic is used to refer to all types of services and staff, from therapists and hygienists, to ambulancemen and radiographers, but does not include doctors, nurses or midwives

paramedicinsk ⇨ **paramedical**

paramesonephric duct [ˌpærəˌmesə'nefrɪk ˌdʌkt] *or* **Müllerian duct** [mʊ'lɪəriən ˌdʌkt] *subst.* one of the two ducts in an embryo which develop into the uterus and Fallopian tubes *Müllers (müllersk) gång*

parameter [pə'ræmɪtə] *subst.* measurement of something (such as blood pressure) which may be an important factor in treating the condition which the patient is suffering from *parameter, storhet*

parametriet ⇨ **parametrium**

parametritis [ˌpærəmɪ'traɪtɪs] *subst.* inflammation of the parametrium *parametrit*

parametrium [ˌpærə'miːtriəm] *subst.* connective tissue around the womb *parametriet*

paramnesia [ˌpæræm'niːziə] *subst.* disorder of the memory where the patient remembers events which have not happened *paramnesi*

paramyxovirus [ˌpærəˌmɪksəʊ'vaɪ(ə)rəs] *subst.* one of a group of viruses, which cause mumps, measles and other infectious diseases *paramyxovirus*

paranasal [ˌpærə'neɪz(ə)l] *adj.* by the side of the nose *paranasalis, vid näsan;* **paranasal sinus** = one of the four sinuses in the skull near the nose **paranasal sinuses** *sinus paranasales, bihålorna*

> COMMENT: the four pairs of paranasal sinuses are the frontal, maxillary, ethmoidal, and sphenoidal

paranoia [ˌpærə'nɔɪə] *subst.* mental disorder where the patient has fixed delusions, usually that he is being persecuted *or* attacked *paranoia*

paranoiac [ˌpærəˈnɔɪæk] *subst.* person suffering from paranoia *paranoiker*

paranoid [ˈpærənɔɪd] *adj.* suffering from a fixed delusion *paranoid;* **paranoid schizophrenia** = form of schizophrenia where the patient believes he is being persecuted *schizophrenia paranoides, paranoid schizofreni*

paranoiker ⇨ **paranoiac**

paraparesis [ˌpærəpəˈriːsɪs] *subst.* incomplete paralysis of the legs *parapares*

paraphasia [ˌpærəˈfeɪziə] *subst.* speech defect where the patient uses a wrong sound in the place of the correct word or phrase *parafasi*

paraphimosis [ˌpærəfaɪˈməʊsɪs] *subst.* (i) condition where the foreskin is tight and has to be removed by circumcision *parafimos, spansk krage;* (ii) spasm of the eye muscle in infants, leading to congestion and oedema of the eyelids *slags kramp i ögonmuskel hos spädbarn*

paraphrenia [ˌpærəˈfriːniə] *subst.* paranoid psychosis, where the patient has delusions and the personality disintegrates *parafreni*

paraplegia [ˌpærəˈpliːdʒə] *subst.* paralysis which affects the lower part of the body and the legs, usually caused by an injury to the spinal cord *paraplegi, dubbelsidig förlamning;* **spastic paraplegia** = paraplegia caused by disturbed nutrition of the cortex in elderly people *spastisk paraplegi*

paraplegic [ˌpærəˈpliːdʒɪk] *subst. & adj.* (person) suffering from paraplegia *paraplegiker, paraplegisk*

paraplegiker ⇨ **paraplegic**

paraplegisk ⇨ **paraplegic**

parapsoriasis [ˌpærəsəˈraɪəsɪs] *subst.* group of skin diseases with scales, similar to psoriasis *parapsoriasis, "falsk psoriasis"*

parasitangrepp ⇨ **infestation**

parasite [ˈpærəsaɪt] *subst.* plant *or* animal which lives on or inside another organism and draws nourishment from that organism *parasit*

> COMMENT: the commonest parasites affecting humans are lice on the skin, and various types of worms in the intestines. Many diseases (such as malaria and amoebic dysentery) are caused by infestation with parasites

parasiterande ⇨ **parasitic**

parasitic [ˌpærəˈsɪtɪk] *adj.* referring to parasites *parasitär, parasiterande;* **parasitic cyst** = cyst produced by a parasite, usually in the liver *cysta bildad av parasit(er)*

parasiticide [ˌpærəˈsaɪtəsaɪd] *subst. & adj.* (substance) which kills parasites *parasiticid, (medel) som dödar parasiter*

parasitology [ˌpærəsɪˈtɒlədʒi] *subst.* scientific study of parasites *parasitologi*

parasitär ⇨ **parasitic**

parasuicide [ˌpærəˈsuːɪsaɪd] *subst.* act where the patient tries to kill himself, but without really intending to do so, rather as a way of drawing attention to his psychological condition *självmordsförsök (utan egentlig avsikt att begå självmord)*

parasympathetic nervous system [ˌpærəˌsɪmpəˈθetɪk ˌnɜːvəs ˌsɪstəm] *subst.* one of two systems in the autonomic nervous system *parasympatiska nervsystemet*

> COMMENT: the parasympathetic nervous system originates in some of the cranial and sacral nerves. It acts in opposition to the sympathetic nervous system, slowing down the action of the heart, reducing blood pressure, and increasing the rate of digestion

parathormon ⇨ **parathormone, parathyroid (gland)**

parathormone [ˌpærəˈθɔːməʊn] *subst.* parathyroid hormone *or* hormone secreted by the parathryoid glands which regulates the level of calcium in blood plasma *parathormon, paratyreoideahormon, bisköldkörtelhormon*

parathyroidectomy [ˌpærəˌθaɪrɔɪˈdektəmi] *subst.* surgical removal of a parathyroid gland *paratyreoidektomi*

parathyroid (gland) [ˌpærəˈθaɪ(ə)rɔɪd (ˌglænd)] *subst. & adj.* one of four glands in the neck, near the thyroid gland, which secrete parathyroid hormones *glandula parathyreoidea, paratyreoidea-, bisköldkörtel(-);* **parathyroid hormones** = hormones secreted by the parathyroid gland which regulate the level of calcium in blood plasma *parathormon, paratyreoideahormon, bisköldkörtelhormon*

paratyfus ⇨ **paratyphoid (fever)**

paratyfusvaccin ⇨ **TAB vaccine**

paratyphoid (fever) [ˌpærə'taɪfɔɪd (ˌfiːvə)] *subst.* infectious disease which has similar symptoms to typhoid and is caused by bacteria transmitted by humans or animals *paratyfoid (feber), tidigare paratyfus*

COMMENT: there are three forms of paratyphoid fever, known by the letters A, B, and C. They are caused by three types of bacterium, *Salmonella paratyphi* A, B, and C. TAB injections give immunity against paratyphoid A and B, but not against C

paratyreoidea- ⇨ **parathyroid (gland)**

paratyreoideahormon ⇨ **parathormone, parathyroid (gland)**

paratyreoidektomi ⇨ **parathyroidectomy**

paravertebral [ˌpærə'vɜːtɪbr(ə)l] *adj.* near the vertebrae *or* beside the spinal column *paravertebral;* **paravertebral injection** = injection of local anaesthetic into the back near the vertebrae *paravertebral injektion*

parenchyma [pə'reŋkɪmə] *subst.* tissues which contain the working cells of an organ as opposed to the stoma or supporting tissue *parenkym*

parenkym ⇨ **parenchyma**

parenkymikterus ⇨ **hepatocellular, jaundice**

parent ['peər(ə)nt] *subst.* mother or father *förälder;* **single parent family** = family which consists of a child or children and only one parent (because of death, divorce or separation) *familj med ensamförälder;* **parent cell** *or* **mother cell** = original cell which splits into daughter cells by mitosis *modercell*

QUOTE in most paediatric wards today open visiting is the norm, with parent care much in evidence. Parents who are resident in the hospital also need time spent with them

Nursing Times

parenteral [pæ'rent(ə)r(ə)l] *adj.* (drug) which is not given orally, and so not by way of the digestive tract, but given in the form of injections *or* suppositories *parenteral*

parenthood ['peər(ə)nthʊd] *subst.* state of being a parent *föräldraskap;* **planned parenthood** = situation where two people plan to have a certain number of children and take contraceptives to limit the number of children in the family *familjeplanering*

pares ⇨ **palsy, paresis**

paresis [pə'riːsɪs] *subst.* partial paralysis *pares, (lättare) förlamning*

parestesi ⇨ **paraesthesia**

paresthesia [ˌpæriːs'θiːziə] = PARAESTHESIA

parfymerad ⇨ **scented**

paries ['peəriˌiːz] *subst.* (i) superficial parts of a structure of organ *ytlig del av organ;* (ii) wall of a cavity *paries, skiljevägg, vägg*
NOTE: plural is **parietes**

parietal [pə'ra(ɪ)ət(ə)l] *adj.* referring to the wall of a cavity *or* any organ *parietal(-);* **parietal bones** *or* **parietals** = two bones which form the sides of the skull *ossa parietalia, parietalloben, hjässbenen;* **parietal cell** = OXYNTIC CELL; **parietal lobe** = middle lobe of the cerebral hemisphere, which is associated with language and other mental processes, and also contains the postcentral gyrus *lobus parietalis, parietalloben, hjässloben;* **parietal pericardium** = outer layer of the serous pericardium not in direct contact with the heart muscle, which lies inside and is attached to the fibrous pericardium *hjärtsäckens yttre blad;* **parietal peritoneum** = part of the peritoneum which lines the abdominal cavity and covers the abdominal viscera *peritoneum parietale, bukhinnans yttre blad, väggbukhinnan;* **parietal pleura** = membrane attached to the diaphragm, and covering the chest cavity and lungs *pleura parietalis (costalis), lungsäckens yttre blad*

parietalcell ⇨ **oxyntic cell**

parietalloben ⇨ **parietal**

Paris ['pærɪs] *see* PLASTER

parkinsonism ['pɑːkɪns(ə)nɪz(ə)m] *or* **Parkinson's disease** ['pɑːkɪns(ə)nz dɪˌziːz] *subst.* slow progressive disorder affecting elderly people *parkinsonism, Parkinsons sjukdom*

COMMENT: Parkinson's disease affects the parts of brain which control movement. The symptoms include trembling of the limbs, a shuffling walk and difficulty in speech. Some cases can be improved by treatment with levodopa

parodental ⇨ **periodontal**

parodontit ⇨ **periodontitis**

parodontium ⇨ **periodontal, periodontium**

parodontolog ⇨ **periodontist**

paronychia [ˌpærəˈnɪkiə] *subst.* inflammation near the nail which forms pus, caused by an infection in the fleshy part of the tip of a finger *paronyki, nagelböld; see also* WHITLOW

paronyki ⇨ **ingrowing toenail, paronychia**

parosmia [pəˈrɒzmiə] *subst.* disorder of the sense of smell *parosmi*

parotid [pəˈrɒtɪd] *adj. & subst.* near the ear *belägen nära örat;* **parotid glands** *or* **parotids** = glands which produce saliva, situated in the neck behind the joint of the jaw and ear ⇨ *illustration* THROAT **parotid gland** *(glandula) parotis, öronspottkörtel*

parotit, epidemisk ⇨ **mumps**

parotitis [ˌpærəˈtaɪtɪs] *subst.* inflammation of the parotid glands *parotit*

> COMMENT: mumps is the commonest form of parotitis, where the parotid gland becomes swollen and the sides of the face become fat

parous [ˈpeərəs] *adj.* (woman) who has given birth to one or more children *-para, (kvinna) som fött ett el. flera barn*

paroxysm [ˈpærəksɪz(ə)m] *subst.* (i) sudden movement of the muscles *paroxysm;* (ii) sudden appearance of symptoms of the disease *paroxysm, häftigt sjukdomsanfall;* (iii) sudden attack of coughing *or* sneezing *paroxysm, plötslig (häftig) hostattack el. nysning;* **he suffered paroxysms of coughing during the night**

paroxysmal [ˌpærəkˈsɪzm(ə)l] *adj.* referring to a paroxysm *paroxysmal, som uppträder anfallsvis;* similar to a paroxysm *paroxysmliknande;* **paroxysmal dyspnoea** = attack of breathlessness at night, caused by heart failure *paroxysmal dyspné;* **paroxysmal tachycardia** = sudden attack of rapid heartbeats *paroxysmal takykardi*

parrot disease [ˈpærət dɪˌziːz] = PSITTACOSIS

pars [pɑːz] *Latin word meaning* part *pars, del*

part [pɑːt] *subst.* piece *or* one of the sections which make up a whole organ *or* body *del, kroppsdel, organ;* **spare part surgery** = surgery where parts of the body (such as bones or joints) are replaced by artificial pieces *reservdelskirurgi*

partial [ˈpɑːʃ(ə)l] *adj.* not complete *or* affecting only part of something *partiell, delvis, ofullständig;* **he only made a partial recovery; partial amnesia** = being unable to remember certain facts, such as the names of people *partiell (ofullständig) minnesförlust;* **partial deafness** = being able to hear some sounds but not all *(partiell) hörselnedsättning;* **partial gastrectomy** *or* **partial mastectomy** = operations to remove part of the stomach *or* part of a breast *partiell gastrektomi (mastektomi);* **partial vision** = being able to see only a part of the total field of vision *or* not being able to see anything very clearly *begränsad syn(förmåga)*

partially [ˈpɑːʃ(ə)li] *adv.* not completely *partiellt, delvis, ofullständigt;* **he is partially paralysed in this right side; the partially sighted** = people who have only partial vision *personer med nedsatt syn*

particle [ˈpɑːtɪk(ə)l] *subst.* very small piece of matter *partikel*

particulate [pɑːˈtɪkjʊlət] *adj.* (i) referring to particles *som avser el. hör till partiklar;* (ii) made up of separate particles *uppbyggd av enskilda partiklar*

partiell ⇨ **incomplete, partial**

partiellt ⇨ **partially**

partikel ⇨ **particle**

partly [ˈpɑːtli] *adv.* not completely *delvis;* **she is partly paralysed**

parturient [pɑːˈtjʊəriənt] *adj.* (i) referring to childbirth *som avser el. hör till nedkomst (barnsbörd);* (ii) (woman) who is in labour *födande*

parturition [ˌpɑːtju(ə)ˈrɪʃ(ə)n] *subst.* childbirth *nedkomst, barnsbörd*

Paschen bodies [ˈpæʃken bɒdɪz] *subst pl.* particles which occur in the skin lesions of smallpox patients *slags partiklar i huden vid smittkoppor*

pass [pɑːs] *vb.* to allow faeces *or* urine to come out of the body *kasta (vatten), tömma (blåsan, tarmen), utsöndra;* **he passed blood in his bowel movement; she had pains when**

she passed water; he passed a small stone in his urine

passage ['pæsɪdʒ] *subst.* (i) long narrow channel inside the body *passage, gång, kanal;* (ii) moving from one place to another *vandring, spridning, överföring;* (iii) evacuation of the bowels *avföring, tarmtömning;* (iv) introduction of an instrument into a cavity *införande av instrument i hålrum;* **air passage** = tube which takes air to the lungs *luftväg;* **anal passage** *or* **back passage** = the anus *anus, ändtarmsmynningen*

pass away [ˌpɑːs ə'weɪ] *or* **pass on** [ˌpɑːs 'ɒn] *vb.* to die *gå bort, dö*

passiv ⇨ **dormant, passive**

passive ['pæsɪv] *adj.* not active *passiv;* **passive immunity** = immunity which is acquired by a baby in the womb *or* by a patient through an injection with an antitoxin *passiv immunitet;* **passive movement** = movement of a joint by a doctor *or* therapist, not by the patient himself *passiv rörelse*

pass on [ˌpɑːs 'ɒn] *vb.* to give to someone *föra vidare, sprida;* **haemophilia is passed on by a woman to her sons; the disease was quickly passed on by carriers to the rest of the population**

pass out [ˌpɑːs 'aʊt] *vb.* to faint *tuppa av, svimma;* **when we told her her father was ill, she passed out**

past [pɑːst] *adj.* (time) which has passed *förfluten;* **past history** = records of earlier illnesses *sjukdomshistoria, anamnes;* **he has no past history of renal disease**

pasta ⇨ **paste**

paste [peɪst] *subst.* medicinal ointment which is quite solid *pasta, kräm*

Pasteurella [ˌpæstə'relə] *subst.* genus of parasitic bacteria, one of which causes the plague *Pasteurella, slags stavformiga bakterier*

pasteurization [ˌpæst(ə)raɪ'zeɪʃ(ə)n] *subst.* heating of food *or* food products to destroy bacteria *pasteurisering, pastörisering*

pasteurize ['pæstəraɪz] *vb.* to kill bacteria in food by heating it *pasteurisera, pastörisera;* **the government is telling people to drink only pasteurized milk**

COMMENT: there are two types of Pasteur vaccine: simple vaccine containing a fixed virus, grown in rabbit brain, and duck embryo vaccine which is grown in the yolk sacs of fertile eggs. Pasteurization is carried out by heating food for a short time at a lower temperature than that used for sterilization: the two methods used are heating to 72°C for fifteen seconds (the high temperature short time method) *or* to 65° for half an hour, and then cooling rapidly. This has the effect of killing tuberculosis bacteria

Pasteur's vaccine [pæ'stɜːz ˌvæksiːn] *subst.* vaccine used for immunization after exposure *slags rabiesvaccin*

pastill ⇨ **lozenge, pastille**

pastille ['pæst(ə)l] *subst.* (i) sweet jelly with medication in it, which can be sucked to relieve a sore throat *pastill, tablett;* (ii) small paper disc covered with barium platinocyanide, which changes colour when exposed to radiation *slags liten pappersskiva med bariumförening*

pastörisera ⇨ **pasteurize**

pastörisering ⇨ **pasteurization**

pat [pæt] *vb.* to hit lightly *klappa;* **she patted the baby on the back to make it burp**

patch test ['pætʃ ˌtest] *subst.* test for allergies *or* tuberculosis, where a piece of plaster containing an allergic substance *or* tuberculin is stuck to the skin to see if there is a reaction *lapprov, lapptest; compare* MANTOUX TEST

patella [pə'telə] *or* **kneecap** ['niːkæp] *subst.* small bone in front of the knee joint *patella, knäskålen*

patellar [pə'telə] *subst.* referring to the kneecap *patellar, knä-;* **patellar reflex** *or* **knee jerk** = jerk made as a reflex action by the knee, when the legs are crossed and the patellar tendon is tapped sharply *patellarreflex;* **patellar tendon** = tendon just below the kneecap *patellarsenan*

patellarreflex ⇨ **patellar**

patellarsenan ⇨ **patellar**

patellectomy [ˌpætə'lektəmi] *subst.* surgical operation to remove the kneecap *patellektomi*

patellektomi ⇨ **patellectomy**

patency ['peɪt(ə)nsi] *subst.* being open *öppenhet;* **they carried out an examination to determine the patency of the Fallopian**

tubes; a salpingostomy was performed to restore the patency of the Fallopian tube

patent ['peɪt(ə)nt] *adj.* **(a)** open *öppen, öppetstående;* exposed *öppen;* **the presence of a pulse shows that the main blood vessels from the heart to the site of the pulse are patent; patent ductus arteriosus** = congenital condition where the ductus arteriosus does not close, allowing blood into the circulation without having passed through the lungs *ductus arteriosus persistens, medfödd öppetstående förbindelse mellan vänstra lungartären och stora kroppspulsådern* **(b) patent medicine** = medicinal preparation with special ingredients which is made and sold under a trade name *patentmedicin*

patentmedicin ⇨ **panacea, patent**

path- ['pæθ] *or* **patho-** ['pæθə(ʊ), ˌ--] *prefix* referring to disease *pat(o)-, sjukdoms-*

pathogen ['pæθədʒ(ə)n] *subst.* germ *or* microorganism which causes a disease *patogen (sjukdomsframkallande) mikroorganism*

pathogenesis [ˌpæθə'dʒenəsɪs] *subst.* origin *or* production *or* development of a morbid *or* diseased condition *patogenes*

pathogenetic [ˌpæθə(ʊ)dʒə'netɪk] *adj.* referring to pathogenesis *patogen, sjukdomsframkallande*

pathogenic [ˌpæθə'dʒenɪk] *adj.* which can cause *or* produce a disease *patogen, sjukdomsframkallande*

pathogenicity [ˌpæθə(ʊ)dʒə'nɪsəti] *subst.* ability of a pathogen to cause a disease *förmåga att orsaka sjukdom*

pathognomonic [ˌpæθəgnəʊ'mɒnɪk] *adj.* (symptom) which is typical and characteristic, and which indicates that a patient has a particular disease *patognom(on)isk*

pathological [ˌpæθə'lɒdʒɪk(ə)l] *adj.* referring to a disease *or* which is caused by a disease; which indicates a disease *patologisk, sjuklig;* **pathological fracture** = fracture of a diseased bone *patologisk fraktur*

pathologist [pə'θɒlədʒɪst] *subst.* **(a)** doctor who specializes in the study of diseases and the changes in the body caused by disease *patolog* **(b)** doctor who examines dead bodies to find out the cause of death *obducent*

pathology [pə'θɒlədʒi] *subst.* study of diseases and the changes in structure and function which diseases cause in the body *patologi;* **clinical pathology** = study of disease as applied to treatment of patients *klinisk patologi;* **pathology report** = report on tests carried out to find the cause of a disease *ung. remissvar från patologen*

pathway ['pɑːθweɪ] *subst.* series of linked neurones along which nerve impulses travel *bana, nervbana;* **final common pathway** = linked neurones which take all impulses from the central nervous system to a muscle *nedre motorneuron;* **motor pathway** = series of motor neurones leading from the brain to the muscles *motorisk bana*

-pathy [pəθi] *suffix* (i) diseased *-sjuk;* (ii) meaning a disease *-pati, -sjukdom*

patient ['peɪʃ(ə)nt] **1** *adj.* being able to wait a long time without getting annoyed *tålig, tålmodig;* **you will have to be patient if you are waiting for treatment - the doctor is late with his appointments 2** *subst.* person who is in hospital *or* who is being treated by a doctor *patient;* **the patients are all asleep in their beds; the doctor is taking the patient's temperature; private patient** = paying who is paying for treatment, and who is not being treated under the National Health Service *privatpatient*

patient ⇨ **subject**

patiently ['peɪʃ(ə)ntli] *adv.* without getting annoyed *tåligt, tålmodigt;* **they waited patiently for two hours before the consultant could see them**

patientövervakning ⇨ **monitoring**

pat(o)- ⇨ **path-**

patogen ⇨ **pathogenetic, pathogenic**

patogenes ⇨ **pathogenesis**

patolog ⇨ **pathologist**

patologi ⇨ **morbid, pathology**

patologisk ⇨ **morbid, pathological**

patulous ['pætjʊləs] *adj.* stretched open *or* patent *vidöppen, utspänd*

Paul-Bunnell reaction [ˌpɔːlbə'nel rɪˌækʃ(ə)n] *or* **Paul-Bunnell test** [ˌpɔːlbə'nel ˌtest] *subst.* blood test to see if a patient has glandular fever, where the patient's blood is tested against a solution containing glandular fever bacilli *Paul-Bunnells reaktion (test)*

Paul's tube ['pɔ:lz ˌtju:b] *subst.* glass tube used to remove the contents of the bowel after an opening has been made between the intestine and the abdominal wall *slags glasrör använt under operation*

paus ⇨ **rest**

pavement epithelium ['peɪvmənt ˌepɪ'θi:liəm] *or* **squamous epithelium** ['skweɪməs ˌepɪ'θi:liəm] *subst.* a simple type of epithelium with flattened cells like scales, forming the lining of the serous membrane of the pericardium, the peritoneum and the pleura *enskiktat skivepitel*

pay bed ['peɪ bed] *subst.* bed (usually in a separate room) in a National Health Service hospital for which a patient pays separately *betald sängplats (oftast i eget rum)*

Pb *chemical symbol for* lead *Pb, bly*

PBI test [ˌpi:bi:'aɪ ˌtest] = PROTEIN-BOUND IODINE TEST

PBJ ⇨ **protein-bound iodine**

p.c. [ˌpi:'si:] *abbreviation for the Latin phrase* "post cibium": after food (written on prescriptions) *post cibium, efter måltid*

PCC [ˌpi:si:'si:] = PROFESSIONAL CONDUCT COMMITTEE

PD ⇨ **peritoneal**

peang ⇨ **forceps**

pearl [pɜ:l] *see* BOHN

Pearson bed ['pɪəs(ə)n bed] *subst.* type of bed with a Balkan frame, used for patients with fractures *slags säng med ortopediska anordningar*

peau d'orange [ˌpəʊ dɒ'rɑ:nʒ] *French phrase meaning* "orange peel": thickened skin with many little depressions caused by lymphoedema which forms over a breast tumour or in elephantiasis *peau d'orange, apelsinhud (som tecken på underliggande sjukdom)*

pecten ['pektɪn] *subst.* (i) middle section of the wall of the anal passage *analpekten;* (ii) hard ridge on the pubis *pecten ossis pubis, blygdbenskammen*

pectineal [pek'tɪniəl] *adj.* (i) referring to the pecten of the pubis *som avser el. hör till blygdbenskammen;* (ii) (structure) with ridges like a comb *kamliknande*

pectoral ['pektər(ə)l] **1** *subst.* **(a)** therapeutic substance which has a good effect on respiratory disease *läkemedel mot andningsbesvär* **(b)** = PECTORAL MUSCLE **2** *adj.* referring to the chest *pektoral, bröst-, bröstkorgs-;* **pectoral girdle** *or* **shoulder girdle** = shoulder bones (the scapulae and clavicles) to which the upper arm bones are attached *skuldergördeln;* **pectoral muscle** *or* **chest muscle** = one of two muscles which lie across the chest and control movements of the shoulder and arm *musculus pectoralis, bröstmuskeln*

pectoralis [ˌpektə'reɪlɪs] *subst.* chest muscle *bröstmuskel;* **pectoralis major** = large chest muscle which pulls the arm forward or rotates it *musculus pectoralis major, stora bröstmuskeln;* **pectoralis minor** = small chest muscle which allows the shoulder to be depressed *musculus pectoralis minor, mindre bröstmuskeln*

pectoris ['pekt(ə)rɪs] *see* ANGINA

pectus ['pektəs] *subst.* anterior part of the chest *pectus, bröstet, bröstkorgen;* **pectus excavatum** = FUNNEL CHEST

ped- ['ped, ˌ-, 'pi:d, ˌ-] *or* **pedo-** ['pi:də(ʊ), ˌ--] *suffix* referring to children *paed(o)-, ped(o)-, barn-*

pediatrician [ˌpi:diə'trɪʃ(ə)n] *subst.* doctor who specializes in the treatment of children *pediat(rik)er, barnläkare; compare* GERIATRICS

pediatrics [ˌpi:di'ætrɪks] *subst.* study of children and their diseases *pediatri(k)*

pediatrisk ⇨ **paediatric**

pedicle ['pedɪk(ə)l] *subst.* (i) long thin piece of skin which attaches a skin graft to the place where it was growing originally *lambå;* (ii) piece of tissue which connects a tumour to healthy tissue *"skaft" på tumör;* (iii) bridge which connects the lamina of a vertebra to the body *pediculus arcus vertebrae, ryggkotebågens främre del*

pediculosis [pɪˌdɪkju'ləʊsɪs] *subst.* skin disease caused by being infested with lice *pedikulos, nedlusning*

Pediculus [pɪ'dɪkjʊləs] *subst.* louse *or* little insect which lives on humans and sucks blood *pediculus, lus;* **Pediculus capitis** = head louse *Pediculus capitis, huvudlus;* **Pediculus corporis** = body louse *Pediculus corporis, kroppslus, klädlus;* **Pediculus pubis** = pubic louse *Pediculus (Phthirius) pubis, flatlus*
NOTE: plural is **Pediculi**

pedikulos ⇨ **pediculosis**

pediodontia [ˌpidiəˈdɒnʃə] *subst.* study of children's teeth *pedodontologi*

pediodontist [ˌpi:diəˈdɒntɪst] *subst.* dentist who specializes in the treatment of children's teeth *barntandläkare*

pedodontologi ⇨ **pediodontia**

peduncle [pɪˈdʌŋk(ə)l] *subst.* stem *or* stalk *skänkel, stjälk;* **cerebellar peduncle** = bands of tissue supporting the nerve fibres which enter or leave the cerebellum *pedunculus cerebellaris, lillhjärnsskänkel, lillhjärnsstjälk;* **cerebral peduncles** = nerve fibres connecting the cerebral hemispheres to the midbrain ⇨ *illustration* BRAIN *pedunculi cerebri, hjärnskänklarna, hjärnstjälkarna*

peel [pi:l] *vb.* to take the skin off a fruit or vegetable *skala; (of skin)* to come off in pieces *fjälla, flagna;* **after getting sunburnt his skin began to peel**

PEEP [ˌpi:i:i:ˈpi:] = POSITIVE END-EXPIRATORY PRESSURE

pekfingret ⇨ **forefinger, index finger**

pektoral ⇨ **pectoral**

pektoralfremitus ⇨ **vocal**

pelarliknande ⇨ **columnar**

Pel-Ebstein fever [pelˈebstaɪn ˌfi:və] *subst.* fever (associated with Hodgkin's disease) which recurs regularly *regelbundet uppträdande feber (vid Hodgkins sjukdom)*

pellagra [pəˈlægrə] *subst.* disease caused by deficiency of nicotinic acid, riboflavine and pyridoxine from the vitamin B complex, where patches of skin become inflamed, and the patient has anorexia, nausea and diarrhoea *pellagra, B_3-avitaminos*

> COMMENT: in some cases the patient's mental faculties can be affected, with depression, headaches and numbness of the extremities. Treatment is by improving the patient's diet

Pellegrini-Stieda's disease [ˌpeləˌgri:niˈsti:dəz dɪˌzi:z] *subst.* disease where an injury to a knee causes the ligament to become calcified *slags förkalkning av ligament efter knäskada*

pellet [ˈpelɪt] *subst.* pill of steroid hormone, usually either oestrogen or testosterone *pellet, piller, särskilt om hormontablett*

pellicle [ˈpelɪk(ə)l] *subst.* thin layer of skin tissue *membran, tunn hinna*

pellucida [pɪˈlu:sɪdə] *see* ZONA

pelvic [ˈpelvɪk] *adj.* referring to the pelvis *pelvi-, bäcken-;* **pelvic brim** = line on the ilium which separates the false pelvis from the true pelvis *linea terminalis, linje mellan lilla och stora bäckenet;* **pelvic cavity** = space below the abdominal cavity above the pelvis *cavum pelvis, bäckenhålan;* **pelvic floor** = lower part of the space beneath the pelvic girdle formed of muscle *bäckenbotten;* **pelvic fracture** = fracture of the pelvis *bäckenfraktur;* **pelvic girdle** *or* **hip girdle** = ring formed by the two hip bones to which the thigh bones are attached *bäckengördeln, bäckenringen*

pelvimeter [pelˈvɪmɪtə] *subst.* instrument to measure the diameter and capacity of the pelvis *pelvimeter*

pelvimetri ⇨ **pelvimetry**

pelvimetry [pelˈvɪmətri] *subst.* measuring the pelvis, especially to see if the internal ring is wide enough for a baby to pass through in childbirth *pelvimetri, bäckenmätning*

pelvis [ˈpelvɪs] *subst.* **(a)** (i) group of bones and cartilage which form a ring and connect the thigh bones to the spine *pelvis, bukbäckenet, bäckenet;* (ii) the internal space inside the pelvic girdle *bäckenet* **(b) renal pelvis** *or* **pelvis of the kidney** = main central tube leading into the kidney from where the ureter joins it ⇨ *illustration* KIDNEY *pelvis renalis, njurbäckenet* NOTE: the plural is **pelves** *or* **pelvises.** Note also that for terms referring to the renal pelvis, see words beginning with **pyel-** or **pyelo-**

> COMMENT: the pelvis is a bowl-shaped ring, formed of the two hip bones, with the sacrum and the coccyx at the back. The hip bones are each in three sections: the ilium, the ischium and the pubis and are linked in front by the pubic symphysis. The pelvic girdle is shaped in a different way in men and women, the internal space being wider in women. The top part of the pelvis, which does not form a complete ring, is called the "false pelvis"; the lower part is the "true pelvis".

pelvospondylit ⇨ **spondylitis**

pemfigoid ⇨ **pemphigoid**

pemfigus ⇨ **pemphigus, pompholyx**

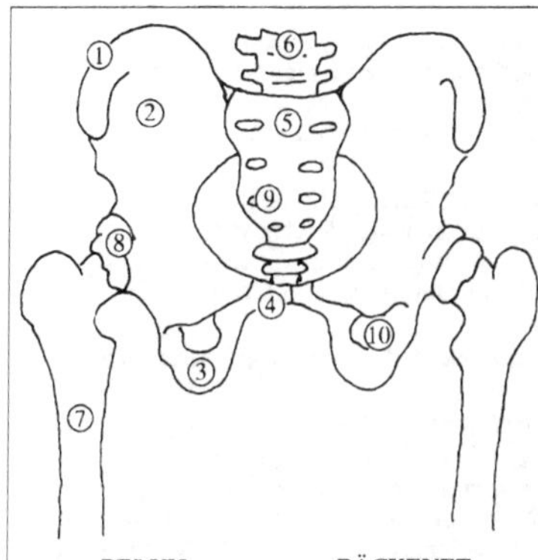

PELVIS (anterior view)

1. iliac crest
2. ilium
3. ischium
4. pubis
5. sacrum
6. vertebral column
7. femur
8. hip joint
9. sacral foramen
10. obturator foramen

BÄCKENET (framifrån)

1. höftbenskammen
2. höftbenet, tarmbenet
3. sittbenet
4. blygdbenet
5. korsbenet
6. kotpelaren, ryggraden
7. lårbenet
8. höftleden
9. foramen sacrale
10. foramen obturatum

pemphigoid ['pemfɪgɔɪd] *adj. & subst.* (skin disease) which is similar to pemphigus *pemfigoid*

pemphigus ['pemfɪgəs] *subst.* rare disease where large blisters form inside the skin *pemfigus*

penetrate ['penətreɪt] *vb.* to go through something *or* to go into something *penetrera, genomtränga, tränga in i;* **the end of the broken bone has penetrated the liver; the ulcer burst, penetrating the wall of the duodenum**

penetration [,penə'treɪʃ(ə)n] *subst.* act of penetrating *penetration, genomträngande, inträngande;* **the penetration of the vagina by the penis; penetration of an ovum by a spermatozoon**

penetrera ⇨ **penetrate**

-penia [pi:niə] *suffix* meaning lack *or* not enough of something *-peni, -brist;* **cytopenia** = lack of cellular elements in the blood *cytopeni*

penicillin [,penə'sɪlɪn] *subst.* common antibiotic produced from a fungus *penicillin*

> COMMENT: penicillin is effective against many microbial diseases, but some people can be allergic to it, and this fact should be noted on medical record cards

Penicillium [,penə'sɪliəm] *subst.* fungus from which penicillin is derived *Penicillium (notatum)*

penile ['pi:naɪ(ə)l] *adj.* referring to the penis *penil, penis-;* **penile urethra** = tube in the penis through which urine and semen pass *mannens urinrör*

penis ['pi:nɪs] *subst.* male genital organ, which also passes urine ⇨ *illustration* UROGENITAL SYSTEM (male) *penis, manslemmen; see also* KRAUROSIS

> COMMENT: the penis is a mass of tissue containing the urethra. When stimulated the tissue of the penis fills with blood and becomes erect

pension ⇨ **retirement**

pensioneras ⇨ **retire**

pensionering ⇨ **retirement**

pensionär ⇨ **elderly**

pentose ['pentəʊz] *subst.* sugar containing five carbon atoms *pentos*

pentosuria [,pentə'ʃʊəriə] *subst.* abnormal condition where pentose is present in the urine *pentosuri*

pep [pep] *vb. (informal)* to give (someone) a feeling of well-being *pigga upp;* **that pep up** *uppiggande;* **these pills will pep you up**

pep pill ['pep pɪl] = AMPHETAMINE

pepsin ['pepsɪn] *subst.* enzyme in the stomach which breaks down the proteins in food into peptones *pepsin*

pepsinogen [pep'sɪnədʒ(ə)n] *subst.* secretion from the gastric gland which is the inactive form of pepsin *pepsinogen*

peptic ['peptɪk] *adj.* referring to digestion *or* to the digestive system *peptisk;* **peptic ulcer** = benign ulcer in the duodenum *or* in the stomach *ulcus pepticum, peptiskt magsår*

peptidase ['peptɪdeɪz] *subst.* enzyme which breaks down proteins in the intestine into amino acids *peptidas*

peptide ['peptaɪd] *subst.* compound formed of two or more amino acids *peptid*

peptisk ⇨ **peptic**

peptone ['peptəʊn] *subst.* substance produced by the action of pepsins on proteins in food *pepton*

peptonuria [ˌpeptə'njʊəriə] *subst.* abnormal condition where peptones are present in the urine *peptonuri*

per [pɜː, pə] *prep.* out of *or* for each *per, på, för varje;* **ten per thousand** = ten out of every thousand *tio per tusen;* **the number of cases of cervical cancer per thousand patients tested**

per cent [pe'sent] *adv. & subst.* out of each hundred *procent;* **fifty per cent (50%) of the tests were positive; seventy-five per cent (75%) of hospital cases remain in hospital for less than four days** NOTE:
NOTE: **per cent** is written **%** when used with figures

percentage [pə'sentɪdʒ] *subst.* quantity shown as a part of one hundred *procent(tal);* **what is the percentage of long-stay patients in the hospital?**

perception [pə'sepʃ(ə)n] *subst.* impression formed in the brain as a result of information about the outside world which is passed back by the senses *perception, varseblivning, sinnesförnimmelse*

perceptive deafness [peˌseptɪv 'defnəs] *subst.* deafness caused by a disorder of the auditory nerves *or* the brain centres which receive nerve impulses *perceptiv (sensorineural) dövhet (hörselnedsättning)*

percussion [pə'kʌʃ(ə)n] *subst.* test (usually on the heart and lungs) in which the doctor taps part of the patient's body and listens to the sound produced *perkussion*

percutaneous [ˌpɜːkju'teɪniəs] *adj.* through the skin *perkutan*

per diem [pə 'diːem] *Latin phrase meaning* "per day" (written on prescriptions) *per diem, om dagen*

perennial [pə'reniəl] *adj.* which continues all the time, for a period of years *ständig, varaktig;* **she suffers from perennial bronchial asthma**

perfekt ⇨ **ideal**

perfekt minne ⇨ **recall**

perforate ['pɜːfəreɪt] *vb.* to make a hole through something *perforera, genomborra, få att brista;* **the ulcer perforated the duodenum; perforated eardrum** = eardrum with a hole in it *perforerad trumhinna;* **perforated ulcer** = ulcer which has made a hole in the wall of the intestine *ulcus perforatum, brustet magsår*

perforation [ˌpɜːfə'reɪʃ(ə)n] *subst.* hole through the whole thickness of a tissue *or* membrane (such as a hole in the intestine or in the eardrum) *perforation, genombrott*

perforera ⇨ **perforate, puncture**

perform [pə'fɔːm] *vb.* **(a)** to do (an operation) *utföra;* **a team of three surgeons performed the heart transplant operation** **(b)** to work *arbeta, fungera;* **the new heart has performed very well; the kidneys are not performing as well as they should**

performance [pə'fɔːməns] *subst.* way in which something works *uppförande, prestation(sförmåga);* **the doctors are not satisfied with the performance of the transplanted heart**

perfusion [pə'fjuːʒ(ə)n] *subst.* passing of a liquid through vessels *or* an organ *or* tissue, especially the flow of blood into lung tissue *perfusion;* **hypothermic perfusion** = method of preserving donor organs by introducing a preserving solution and then storing the organ at a low temperature *organgenomströmning med kyld vätska*

peri- ['peri, ˌ--] *prefix* meaning near *or* around *or* enclosing *peri-*

periadenitis [ˌperiədɪ'naɪtɪs] *subst.* inflammation of tissue round a gland *periadenit*

perianal [ˌperi'eɪn(ə)l] *adj.* around the anus *perianal;* **perianal haematoma** = small painful swelling outside the anus caused by forcing a bowel movement *perianalt hematom*

periarteritis [ˌperiɑːtə'raɪtɪs] *subst.* inflammation of the outer coat of an artery and the tissue round it *periarterit;* **periarteritis nodosa** *or* **polyarteritis nodosa** = collagen disease, where the walls of the arteries become inflamed, causing asthma, high blood pressure and kidney failure *periarteritis (polyarteritis) nodosa*

periarthritis [ˌperiɑː'θraɪtɪs] *subst.* inflammation of the tissue round a joint *periartrit;* **chronic periarthritis** *or* **scapulohumeral arthritis** = inflammation of tissues round the shoulder joint *periarthritis humero-scapularis*

pericard- [ˌperi'kɑːd, ˌ-ˌ-] *prefix* referring to the pericardium *perikard(io)-, hjärtsäcks-*

pericardectomy [ˌperikɑː'dektəmi] *or* **pericardiectomy** [ˌperiˌkɑːdi'ektəmi] *subst.* surgical removal of the pericardium *perikardektomi*

pericardial [ˌperi'kɑːdiəl] *adj.* referring to the pericardium *perikardisk, perikardiell, perikard-, hjärtsäcks-;* **pericardial effusion** = fluid which forms in the pericardial sac during pericarditis *perikardexsudat, utgjutning i hjärtsäcken;* **pericardial friction** = rubbing together of the two parts of the pericardium in pericarditis *perikardisk (perikardiell) gnidning, gnidning vid hjärtsäcksinflammation;* **pericardial sac** *or* **serous pericardium** = the inner part of the pericardium forming a sac which contains fluid to prevent the two parts of the pericardium rubbing together *perikardiet, hjärtsäcken*

pericardiocentesis [ˌperiˌkɑːdiəʊsen'tiːsɪs] *subst.* puncture of the pericardium to remove fluid *perikardiocentes, perikardpunktion*

pericardiorrhaphy [ˌperiˌkɑːdi'ɔːrəfi] *subst.* surgical operation to repair a wound in the pericardium *perikard(r)rafi*

pericardiostomy [ˌperiˌkɑːdi'ɒstəmi] *subst.* surgical operation to open the pericardium through the thoracic wall to drain off fluid *perikardiostomi*

pericarditis [ˌperikɑː'daɪtɪs] *subst.* inflammation of the pericardium *perikardit, hjärtsäcksinflammation;* **acute pericarditis** = sudden attack of fever and pains in the chest, caused by the two parts of the pericardium rubbing together *akut perikardit;* **chronic pericarditis** *or* **constrictive pericarditis** = condition where the pericardium becomes thickened and prevents the heart from functioning normally *pericarditis constrictiva, konstriktiv perikardit, pansarhjärta*

pericardium [ˌperi'kɑːdiəm] *subst.* membrane which surrounds and supports the heart *perikardiet, hjärtsäcken;* **fibrous pericardium** = outer part of the pericardium which surrounds the heart and is attached to the main blood vessels *hjärtsäckens yttersida;* **parietal pericardium** = outer layer of serous pericardium attached to the fibrous pericardium *hjärtsäckens yttre blad;* **serous pericardium** *or* **pericardial sac** = the inner part of the pericardium, forming a double sac which contains fluid to prevent the two parts of the pericardium from rubbing together *perikardiet, hjärtsäcken;* **visceral pericardium** = inner layer of serous pericardium, attached to the wall of the heart *epikardiet, hjärtsäckens inre blad*

pericardotomy [ˌperikɑː'dɒtəmi] *or* **pericardiotomy** [ˌperiˌkɑːdi'ɒtəmi] *subst.* surgical operation to open the pericardium *perikardiotomi*

perichondritis [ˌperikɒn'draɪtɪs] *subst.* inflammation of cartilage, especially in the outer ear *perikondrit*

perichondrium [ˌperi'kɒndriəm] *subst.* fibrous connective tissue which covers cartilage *perichondrium, broskhinna*

pericolpitis [ˌperikɒl'paɪtɪs] *or* **paracolpitis** [ˌpærəkɒl'paɪtɪs] *subst.* inflammation of the connective tissue round the vagina *perikolpit*

pericranium [ˌperɪ'kreɪniəm] *subst.* connective tissue which covers the surface of the skull *perikraniet, skallbenens yttre periost*

pericystitis [ˌperisi'staɪtɪs] *subst.* inflammation of the structures round the bladder, usually caused by infection in the uterus *pericystit*

perifer ⇨ **peripheral**

perifert motstånd ⇨ **resistance**

periflebit ⇨ **periphlebitis**

perifolliculitis [ˌperifəˌlɪkju'laɪtɪs] *subst.* inflammation of the skin round hair follicles *perifollikulit*

perihepatitis [ˌperiˌhepə'taɪtɪs] *subst.* inflammation of the membrane round the liver *perihepatit*

perikard- ⇨ **pericardial**

perikardektomi ⇨ **pericardectomy**

perikardexsudat ⇨ **pericardial**

perikardiell ⇨ **pericardial**

perikardiet ⇨ **pericardial, pericardium**

perikardiocentes ⇨ **pericardiocentesis**

perikardiostomi ⇨ **pericardiostomy**

perikardiotomi ⇨ **pericardotomy**

perikardisk ⇨ **pericardial**

perikardit ➪ **pericarditis**

perikardit, konstriktiv ➪ **pericarditis, Pick's disease**

perikardpunktion ➪ **pericardiocentesis**

perikolpit ➪ **pericolpitis**

perikondrit ➪ **perichondritis**

perikraniet ➪ **pericranium**

perilymph ['perilɪmf] *subst.* fluid found in the labyrinth of the inner ear *perilymfa*

perimeter [pə'rɪmɪtə] *subst.* instrument to measure the field of vision *perimeter*

perimeter ➪ **scotometer**

perimetri ➪ **perimetry**

perimetriet ➪ **perimetrium**

perimetritis [,perimə'traɪtɪs] *subst.* inflammation of the perimetrium *perimetrit*

perimetrium [,peri'mi:triəm] *subst.* membrane round the uterus *tunica serosa uteri, perimetriet*

perimetry [pə'rɪmətri] *subst.* measurement of the field of vision *perimetri*

perimysium [,peri'maɪsiəm] *subst.* sheath which surrounds a bundle of muscle fibres *perimysium*

perinatal [,perɪ'neɪt(ə)l] *adj.* referring to the period before and after childbirth *perinatal;* **perinatal mortality rate** = number of babies born dead *or* who die during the period immediately after childbirth, shown per thousand babies born *perinatal mortalitet (dödlighet)*

perineal [,perɪ'ni:əl] *adj.* referring to the perineum *perineal, perine(o)-, bäckenbotten-;* **perineal body** = mass of muscle and fibres between the anus and the vagina or prostate *området mellan anus och vagina el. blåshalskörteln;* **perineal muscles** = muscles which lie in the perineum *bäckenbottenmuskulaturen*

perinealsnitt ➪ **episiotomy**

perinefrit ➪ **perinephritis**

perinefritisk ➪ **perinephric**

perineoplasty [,peri'ni:ə,plæsti] *subst.* surgical operation to repair the perineum by grafting tissue *perineoplastik*

perineorrhaphy [,perini'ɔ:rəfi] *subst.* surgical operation to stitch up a perineum which has torn during childbirth *perineo(r)rafi*

perinephric [,peri'nefrɪk] *adj.* around the kidney *perinefritisk*

perinephritis [,perinɪ'fraɪtɪs] *subst.* inflammation of tissue round the kidney, which spreads from an infected kidney *perinefrit*

perineum [,perɪ'ni:əm] *subst.* skin and tissue between the opening of the urethra and the anus *perineum, bäckenbotten*

perineurium [,peri'njʊəriəm] *subst.* connective tissue which surrounds bundles of nerve fibres *perineurium*

period ['pɪəriəd] *subst.* **(a)** length of time *(tids)period;* **the patient regained consciousness after a short period of time; she is allowed out of bed for two periods each day; safe period** = time during the menstrual cycle when conception is not likely to occur (used as a method of contraception) *säker period; see also* RHYTHM METHOD **(b)** menstruation *or* bleeding which occurs in a woman each month as the lining of the uterus bleeds because no fertilized egg is present *menstruation, mens, reglering, månadsblödning;* **she always has heavy periods; some women experience abdominal pain during their periods; she has bleeding between periods**

period ➪ **cycle, term**

periodic [,pɪəri'ɒdɪk] *adj.* which occurs from time to time *periodisk, regelbundet återkommande;* **he has periodic attacks of migraine; she has to go to the clinic for periodic checkups; periodic fever** = disease of the kidneys, common in Mediterranean countries *familjär mediterran feber, periodisk feber;* **periodic paralysis** = recurrent attacks of weakness where the level of potassium in the blood is low *återkommande förlamningstillstånd pga låg kaliumnivå i blodet*

periodicity [,pɪəriə'dɪsəti] *subst.* timing of recurrent attacks of a disease *periodicitet*

periodisk ➪ **cyclical, periodic**

periodontal [,periə(ʊ)'dɒnt(ə)l] *or* **periodontic** [,periə(ʊ)'dɒntɪk] *adj.* referring to the area around the teeth *periodontal, parodental, paradental;*

periodontal disease = PERIODONTITIS; **periodontal membrane** *or* **periodontal ligament** = membrane which attaches a tooth to the bone of the jaw ⇨ *illustration* TOOTH *periodontium, parodontium, paradentium, tandrothinnan*

periodontia [ˌperiə(ʊ)'dɒnʃə] *subst.* study of diseases of the periodontal membrane *läran om tandrothinnans sjukdomar*

periodontist [ˌperiə(ʊ)'dɒntɪst] *subst.* dentist who specializes in the treatment of gum diseases *parodontolog*

periodontitis [ˌperiə(ʊ)dɒn'taɪtɪs] *subst.* infection of the periodontal membrane leading to pyorrhoea, and usually resulting in the teeth falling out *periodontit, parodontit, paradentit, tandlossning(ssjukdom)*

periodontium [ˌperiəʊ'dɒnʃiəm] *subst.* periodontal membrane, but also used to refer to the gums and bone around a tooth *periodontium, parodontium, paradentium, tandrothinnan*

periodontium ⇨ **periodontal**

perionychia [ˌperiəʊ'nɪkiə] *or* **perionyxis** [ˌperiəʊ'nɪksɪs] *subst.* painful swelling round a fingernail *perionyxi*

perionyxi ⇨ **perionychia**

periosteal [ˌperi'ɒstiəl] *adj.* referring to the periosteum *periost(e)al;* attached to the periosteum *periost(e)al*

periosteotome [ˌperi'ɒstiəʊtəʊm] *subst.* surgical instrument used to cut the periosteum *kirurgiskt instrument som används för att skära upp benhinnan*

periosteum [ˌperi'ɒstiəm] *subst.* dense layer of connective tissue around a bone ⇨ *illustration* BONE STRUCTURE *periost, (yttre) benhinnan*

periostitis [ˌperiə'staɪtɪs] *subst.* inflammation of the periosteum *periost(e)it, benhinneinflammation*

peripheral [pə'rɪf(ə)r(ə)l] *adj.* at the edge *perifer, yttre;* **peripheral nerves** = pairs of motor and sensory nerves which branch out from the brain and spinal cord *perifera nerver;* **peripheral nervous system (PNS)** = all the nerves in different parts of the body which are linked and governed by the central nervous system *perifera nervsystemet, PNS;* **peripheral vasodilator** = chemical substance which acts to widen the blood vessels in the arms and legs and so improves bad circulation *perifer vasodila(ta)tor, perifert verkande kärl(ut)vidgande medel*

periphlebitis [ˌperɪflə'baɪtɪs] *subst.* (i) inflammation of the outer coat of a vein *periflebit;* (ii) inflammation of the connective tissue round a vein *inflammation i vävnaderna kring ven*

perisalpingitis [ˌperiˌsælpɪn'dʒaɪtɪs] *subst.* inflammation of the peritoneum and other parts round a Fallopian tube *perisalpingit*

perisplenitis [ˌperisplə'naɪtɪs] *subst.* inflammation of the peritoneum and other parts round the spleen *perisplenit*

peristalsis [ˌperɪ'stælsɪs] *subst.* movement (like waves) produced by alternate contraction and relaxation of muscles along an organ such as the intestine *or* oesophagus, which pushes the contents of the organ along it automatically *peristaltik; compare* ANTIPERISTALSIS

peristaltic [ˌperɪ'stæltɪk] *adj.* occurring in waves, as in peristalsis *peristaltisk*

peristaltik ⇨ **peristalsis**

peristaltik, avsaknad av ⇨ **aperistalsis**

peritendinit ⇨ **peritendinitis, tenosynovitis**

peritendinitis [ˌperiˌtendi'naɪtɪs] *subst.* painful inflammation of the sheath round a tendon *peritendinit, ten(d)osynovit, senskideinflammation*

peritomy [pə'rɪtəmi] *subst.* (i) surgical operation on the eye, where the conjunctiva is cut in a circle round the cornea *peritomi;* (ii) circumcision *omskärelse*

peritoneal [ˌperitə'nɪəl] *adj.* referring or belonging to the peritoneum *peritoneal, bukhinne-;* **peritoneal cavity** = space between the layers of the peritoneum, containing the major organs of the abdomen *cavum peritonei (peritoneale), peritonealhålan;* **peritoneal dialysis** = removing waste matter from a patient's blood by introducing fluid into the peritoneum which then acts as a filter (as opposed to haemodialysis) *peritonealdialys, PD*

peritonealdialys ⇨ **peritoneal**

peritonealhålan ⇨ **peritoneal**

peritoneoscope [ˌperiˈtəʊniəskəʊp] = LAPAROSCOPE

peritoneoscopy [ˌperitəʊniˈɒskəpi] = LAPAROSCOPY

peritoneum [ˌperɪtə(ʊ)ˈniːəm] *subst.* membrane which lines the abdominal cavity and covers the organs in it *peritoneum, bukhinnan;* **parietal peritoneum** = part of the peritoneum which lines the inner abdominal wall *peritoneum parietale, bukhinnans yttre blad, väggbukhinnan;* **visceral peritoneum** = part of the peritoneum which covers the organs in the abdominal cavity *peritoneum viscerale, inälvsbukhinnan*

peritonitis [ˌperɪtə(ʊ)ˈnaɪtɪs] *subst.* inflammation of the peritoneum as a result of bacterial infection *peritonit, bukhinneinflammation;* **primary peritonitis** = peritonitis caused by direct infection from the blood *or* the lymph *bukhinneinflammation orsakad av infektion genom blod el. lymfa;* **secondary peritonitis** = peritonitis caused by infection from an adjoining tissue, such as the rupturing of the appendix *bukhinneinflammation orsakad av infektion från intilliggande vävnad*

> COMMENT: peritonitis is a serious condition and can have many causes. Its effect is to stop the peristalsis of the intestine so making it impossible for the patient to eat and digest

peritonsillar [ˌperɪˈtɒnsɪlə] *adj.* around the tonsils *peritonsillar, peritonsillär;* **peritonsillar abscess** = QUINSY

peritrichous [pəˈrɪtrɪkəs] *adj.* (bacteria) where the surface of the cell is covered with flagella *flagelltäckt*

periumbilical [ˌperiʌmˈbɪlɪk(ə)l] *adj.* around the navel *omkring naveln*

periureteritis [ˌperiˌjʊəritəˈraɪtɪs] *subst.* inflammation of the tissue round a ureter, usually caused by inflammation of the ureter itself *periuretrit*

periurethral [ˌperiju(ə)ˈriːərəl] *adj.* around the urethra *periuretral*

perkussion ⇨ **percussion**

perkussionshammare ⇨ **plessor, plexor**

perkutan ⇨ **percutaneous**

perleche [pəˈleʃ] *subst.* (i) cracks in dry skin at the corners of the mouth, often caused by riboflavine deficiency *perleche, angulär cheilit (cheilos), munvinkelragad;* (ii) candidiasis *candidainfektion, monoliasis, torsk, muntorsk*

permanent [ˈpɜːm(ə)nənt] *adj.* which exists always *permanent, bestående, ständig;* **the accident left him with a permanent disability; permanent teeth** = teeth in an adult, which replace the child's milk teeth during late childhood *permanenta tänderna*

> COMMENT: the permanent teeth consist of eight incisors, four canines, eight premolars and twelve molars, the last four molars (one on each side of the upper and lower jaw) being called the wisdom teeth

permanent ⇨ **permanently, second**

permanently [ˈpɜːm(ə)nəntli] *adv.* always *or* for ever *permanent, bestående, ständigt;* **he was permanently disabled in the accident**

permeability [ˌpɜːmiəˈbɪləti] *subst. (of a membrane)* ability to allow fluid containing chemical substances to pass through *permeabilitet, genomsläpplighet*

permeable membrane [ˈpɜːmiəb(ə)l ˌmembreɪn] *subst.* membrane which can allow substances in fluids to pass through it *permeabelt (genomsläppligt) membran, permeabel (genomsläpplig) hinna*

pernicious [pəˈnɪʃəs] *adj.* harmful *or* dangerous (disease) *or* abnormally severe (disease) which is likely to end in death *perniciös, elakartad, farlig;* **pernicious anaemia** *or* **Addison's anaemia** = disease where an inability to absorb vitamin B_{12} prevents the production of red blood cells and damages the spinal cord *perniciös anemi, Addisonanemi*

perniciös ⇨ **pernicious**

pernio [ˈpɜːniəʊ] *subst. pernio, frostknöl, köldknöl, kylknöl;* **erythema pernio** *or* **chilblain** = condition where the skin of the fingers, toes, nose or ears reacts to cold by becoming red, swollen and itchy *frosterytem, frostskada, kylskada*

perniosis [ˌpɜːniˈəʊsɪs] *subst.* any condition caused by cold which affects blood vessels in the skin *köldpåverkan på hudens blodkärl*

pero- [ˌperə(ʊ)] *prefix* meaning deformed *or* defective *pero-*

peromelia [ˌperə(ʊ)'mi:liə] *subst.* congenital deformity of the limbs *medfött tillstånd med missbildade extremiteter*

peroneal [ˌperə(ʊ)'ni:əl] *adj.* referring to the outside of the leg *peroneal, vadbens-;* **peroneal muscle** *or* **peroneus** = one of three muscles (brevis, longus, tertius) on the outside of the lower leg which make the leg turn outwards *musculus peroneus, peroneusmuskeln, vadmuskeln*

peroneusmuskeln ⇨ **peroneal**

peroral [pə'rɔ:rəl] *adj.* through the mouth *peroral, genom munnen*

peroral ⇨ **oral**

peroralt ⇨ **orally**

per primam ⇨ **first**

persecute ['pɜ:sɪkju:t] *vb.* to make someone suffer all the time *förfölja;* **in paranoia, the patient feels he is being persecuted**

persecution [ˌpɜ:sɪ'kju:ʃ(ə)n] *subst.* being made to suffer *förföljelse;* **he suffers from persecution mania**

perseveration [pəˌsəvə'reɪʃ(ə)n] *subst.* repeating actions *or* words without any stimulus *perseveration, perseverans*

persist [pə'sɪst] *vb.* to continue for some time *fortsätta, bestå;* **the weakness in the right arm persisted for two weeks**

persistent [pə'sɪst(ə)nt] *adj.* which continues for some time *ihållande, envis, bestående;* **she suffered from a persistent cough; treatment aimed at the relief of persistent angina**

person ['pɜ:s(ə)n] *subst.* man *or* woman *person, människa, individ*

person ⇨ **person, human, subject**

personal ['pɜ:s(ə)n(ə)l] *adj.* (i) referring to a person *personlig;* (ii) belonging to a person *personlig, privat;* **only certain senior members of staff can consult the personal records of the patients**

personal ⇨ **personnel, staff**

personality [ˌpɜ:sə'nælәti] *subst.* way in which one person is mentally different from another *personlighet;* **personality disorder** = disorder which affects the way a person behaves, especially in relation to other people *personlighetsstörning, personlighetsrubbning*

> QUOTE Alzheimer's disease is a progressive disorder which sees a gradual decline in intellectual functioning and deterioration of personality and physical coordination and activity
>
> **Nursing Times**

personlig ⇨ **personal, private, subjective**

personlighet ⇨ **personality**

personlighetsklyvning ⇨ **dissociation, schizoid**

personlighetsrubbning ⇨ **personality**

personlighetsstörning ⇨ **personality**

personnel [ˌpɜ:sə'nel] *subst.* members of staff *personal;* **all hospital personnel must be immunized against hepatitis; only senior personnel can inspect the patients' medical records** NOTE: **personnel** is singular

perspiration [ˌpɜ:spə'reɪʃ(ə)n] *subst.* (i) action of sweating *or* of producing moisture through the sweat glands *perspiration, transpiration, svettning;* (ii) sweat *or* moisture produced by the sweat glands *svett;* **perspiration broke out on his forehead; sensible perspiration** = drops of sweat which can be seen on the skin, secreted by the sweat glands *perspiratio sensibilis, märkbar svettning*

> COMMENT: perspiration is formed in the sweat glands under the epidermis and cools the body as the moisture evaporates from the skin. Sweat contains salt, and in hot countries it may be necessary to take salt tablets to replace the salt lost through perspiration

perspire [pə'spa(ɪ)ə] *vb.* to sweat *or* to produce moisture through the sweat glands *perspirera, transpirera, svettas;* **after the game of tennis he was perspiring**

Perthes' disease ['pɜ:ti:z dɪˌzi:z] *or* **Perthes' hip** ['pɜ:ti:z ˌhɪp] *subst.* disease (found in young boys) where the upper end of the femur degenerates and does not develop normally, sometimes resulting in a permanent limp *(Legg-Calvé-)Perthes sjukdom, osteochondritis deformans juvenilis, coxa plana*

pertussis [pə'tʌsɪs] = WHOOPING COUGH

perversion [pə'vɜ:ʃ(ə)n] *subst.* abnormal sexual behaviour *perversion, sexuell avvikelse*

pes [pes] *subst.* foot *pes, foten;* **pes cavus** = CLAW FOOT; **pes planus** = FLAT FOOT

pessar ⇨ **diaphragm, Dutch cap, pessary**

pessary ['pes(ə)ri] *subst.* **(a)** vaginal suppository *or* drug in soluble material which is pushed into the vagina and absorbed into the blood there *vagitorium* **(b)** contraceptive device worn inside the vagina to prevent spermatozoa entering *pessar, slidpessar* **(c)** device like a ring, which is put into the vagina as treatment for prolapse of the womb *prolapsring, framfallsring*

pest [pest] *subst.* animal which carries disease *or* attacks plants and animals and harms or kills them *skadedjur, skadeinsekt;* **a spray to remove insect pests**

pest ⇨ **plague**

pesticid ⇨ **pesticide**

pesticide ['pestɪsaɪd] *subst.* substance which kills pests *pesticid*

peta ⇨ **pick**

petechia [pe'ti:kiə] *subst.* small red spot, where blood has entered the skin **petechiae** *petekier, blödande hudutslag*
NOTE: the plural is **petechiae**

petekier ⇨ **petechia**

petit mal [pəˌtɪt 'mæl] *subst.* less severe form of epilepsy, where loss of consciousness attacks last only a few seconds and the patient appears simply to be thinking deeply *petit mal, epilepsia minora*

petri dish ['peɪtri ˌdɪʃ] *subst.* small glass *or* plastic dish with a lid, in which a culture is grown *petriskål*

petrosal [pə'trəʊs(ə)l] *adj.* referring to the petrous part of the temporal bone *petrosal, klippbens-*

petrositis [ˌpetrə(ʊ)'saɪtɪs] *subst.* inflammation of the petrous part of the temporal bone *petrosit*

petrous ['petrəs] *adj.* (i) like stone *stenliknande, stenhård;* (ii) petrosal *petrosal, klippbens-;* **petrous bone** = part of the temporal bone which forms the base of the skull and the inner and middle ears *pars petrosa (ossis temporalis), klippbenet*

-pexy [peksi] *suffix* referring to fixation of an organ by surgery *-pexi, -fixering*

Peyer's patches ['paɪəz ˌpætʃɪz] *subst.* patches of lymphoid tissue on the mucous membrane of the small intestine *folliculi lymphatici aggregati, Peyers plaques (plack)*

Peyronie's disease [ˌpærə'ni:z dɪˌzi:z] *subst.* condition where hard fibre develops in the penis which becomes painful when erect (associated with Dupuytren's contracture) *induratio penis plastica, slags sjukdom i penis*

pH [ˌpi:'eɪtʃ] *subst.* concentration of hydrogen ions in a solution, which determines its acidity *pH;* **pH factor** = factor which indicates acidity or alkalinity *pH-värde, surhetsgrad;* **pH test** = test to see how acid or alkaline a solution is *undersökning av pH*

> COMMENT: the pH factor is shown as a number; pH 7 is neutral

phaco- ['fækə(ʊ), ˌ--] *or* **phako-** ['fækə(ʊ), ˌ--] *prefix* referring to the lens of the eye *phak(o)-, fak(o)-, lins-*

phaeochromocytoma [ˌfi:əʊˌkrəʊməʊsaɪ'təʊmə] *subst.* tumour of the adrenal glands which affects the secretion of hormones such as adrenaline, which in turn results in hypertension and hyperglycaemia *feokromocytom*

phag- ['fæg, ˌ-] *or* **phago-** ['fægə(ʊ), ˌ--] *prefix* referring to eating *fag(o)-*

-phage [feɪdʒ] *suffix* which eats *-fag*

-phagia ['feɪdʒə] *suffix* referring to eating *-fagi*

phagocyte ['fægə(ʊ)saɪt] *subst.* cell, especially a white blood cell, which can surround and destroy other cells, such as bacteria cells *fagocyt*

phagocytic [ˌfægə(ʊ)'saɪtɪk] *adj.* (i) referring to phagocytes *fagocytisk, fagocytär;* (ii) which destroys cells *fagocyterande;* **monocytes become phagocytic during infection**

phagocytosis [ˌfægə(ʊ)saɪ'təʊsɪs] *subst.* destruction of bacteria cells and foreign bodies by phagocytes *fagocytos*

phako- [ˌfækə(ʊ)] *or* **phaco-** [ˌfækə(ʊ)] *prefix* referring to the lens of the eye *phak(o)-, fak(o)-, lins-*

phalangeal [fə'lændʒiəl] *adj.* referring to the phalanges *falangeal*

phalanges [fə'lændʒi:z] *plural of* PHALANX

phalangitis [ˌfælən'dʒaɪtɪs] *subst.* inflammation of the fingers or toes caused by infection of tissue *inflammation i fingrar el. tår*

phalanx ['fælæŋ(k)s] *subst.* bone in a finger or toe ⇨ *illustration* HAND, FOOT *phalanx, falang, ett av fingrarnas el. tårnas rörben*

> COMMENT: the fingers and toes have three phalanges each, except the thumb and big toe, which have only two

phalloplasty ['fælə(ʊ)plæsti] *subst.* surgical operation to repair a damaged *or* deformed penis *falloplastik*

phallus ['fæləs] *subst.* penis *or* male genital organ *phallos, fallos, penis, manslemmen*

phantom ['fæntəm] *subst. & adj.* **(a)** model of the whole body *or* part of the body, used to practise or demonstrate surgical operations *modell av hela el. del av kroppen* **(b)** ghost *or* something which is not there but seems to be there *spöke, inbillning;* **phantom limb** = condition where a patient seems to feel sensations in a limb which has been amputated *fantomsensation;* **phantom pregnancy** = PSEUDOCYESIS; **phantom tumour** = condition where a swelling occurs which imitates a swelling caused by the tumour *slags tumörliknande svullnad*

pharmaceutical [ˌfɑ:mə'su:tɪk(ə)l] **1** *adj.* referring to pharmacy *or* drugs *farmaceutisk;* **the Pharmaceutical Society** = professional association for pharmacists in Great Britain *facklig sammanslutning för farmaceuter i Storbritannien* **2** *subst.* **pharmaceuticals** = drugs *läkemedel*

pharmacist ['fɑ:məsɪst] *subst.* trained person who is qualified to prepare medicines according to the instructions on a doctor's prescription *apotekare, farmaceut;* **community pharmacist** *or* **retail pharmacist** = person who makes medicines and sells them in a chemist's shop *apotekare, farmaceut*

> COMMENT: qualified pharmacists must be registered by the Pharmaceutical Society of Great Britain before they can practise

pharmaco- ['fɑ:məkə(ʊ), ˌ---] *prefix* referring to drugs *farmak(o)-, läkemedels-*

pharmacological [ˌfɑ:məkə'lɒdʒɪk(ə)l] *adj.* referring to pharmacology *farmakologisk*

pharmacologist [ˌfɑ:mə'kɒlədʒɪst] *subst.* doctor who specializes in the study of drugs *farmakolog*

pharmacology [ˌfɑ:mə'kɒlədʒi] *subst.* study of drugs *or* medicines, and their actions, properties and characteristics *farmakologi*

pharmacopoeia [ˌfɑ:məkə'pi:ə] *subst.* official list of drugs, their methods of preparation, dosages and the ways in which they should be used *farmakopé, ung. FASS*

> COMMENT: the British Pharmocopoeia is the official list of drugs used in the United Kingdom. The drugs listed in it have the letters BP after their name. In the USA the official list is the United States Pharmacopoeia, or USP

pharmacy ['fɑ:məsi] *subst.* **(a)** study of making and dispensing of drugs *farmaci, läran om läkemedelsberedning;* **the six pharmacy students are taking their diploma examinations this year; he has a qualification in pharmacy (b)** shop *or* department in a hospital where drugs are prepared *apotek*

Pharmacy Act ['fɑ:məsi ˌækt] *or* **Poisons Act** ['pɔɪz(ə)nz ˌækt] *subst.* one of several Acts of the British Parliament (Pharmacy and Poisons Act 1933, Misuse of Drugs Act 1971, Poisons Act 1972) which regulate the making *or* prescribing *or* selling of drugs *ung. läkemedelsförordning*

pharyng- ['færɪn(d)ʒ, ˌ--] *or* **pharyngo-** [fə'rɪŋgə(ʊ), -ˌ--] *prefix* referring to the pharynx *faryng(o)-, svalg-*

pharyngeal [ˌfær(ə)n'dʒi:əl] *adj.* referring to the pharynx *faryngeal, farynx-, svalg-;* **pharyngeal pouch** *or* **visceral pouch** = one of the pouches in the side of the throat of an embryo *gälficka;* **pharyngeal tonsil** = adenoidal tonsil *or* lymphoid tissue at the back of the throat where the passages from the nose join the pharynx *tonsilla pharyngea, farynxtonsillen, svalgtonsillen, svalgmandeln*

pharyngectomy [ˌfærɪn'dʒektəmi] *subst.* surgical removal of part of the pharynx, especially in cases of cancer of the pharynx *faryngektomi*

pharyngismus [ˌfærɪn'dʒɪzməs] *or* **pharyngism** ['færɪndʒɪz(ə)m] *subst.* spasm which contracts the muscles of the pharynx *faryngism, svalgkramp*

pharyngitis [ˌfærɪn'dʒaɪtɪs] *subst.* inflammation of the pharynx *faryngit, svalginflammation*

pharyngocele [fə'rɪŋgə(ʊ),siː(ə)l] *subst.* (i) cyst which opens off the pharynx *cysta som öppnar sig mot svalget;* (ii) hernia of part of the pharynx *faryngocele*

pharyngolaryngeal [fə'rɪŋgə(ʊ)lə'rɪndʒ(ə)l] *adj.* referring to the pharynx and the larynx *som avser el. hör till både svalget och struphuvudet*

pharyngoscope [fə'rɪŋgə(ʊ)skəʊp] *subst.* instrument with a light attached, used by a doctor to examine the pharynx *laryngoskop*

pharyngotympanic tube [fə,rɪŋgə(ʊ)tɪm'pænɪk ,tjuːb] *or* **Eustachian tube** [juː'steɪʃ(ə)n ,tjuːb] *subst.* one of two tubes which connect the back of the throat to the middle ear *tuba auditiva, otosalpinx, eustachiska röret, örontrumpeten*

pharynx ['færɪŋ(k)s] *subst.* muscular passage leading from the back of the mouth to the oesophagus *farynx, svalget*

> COMMENT: the nasal cavity (or nasopharynx) leads to back of the mouth (or oropharynx) and then into the pharynx proper, which in turn becomes the oesophagus when it reaches the sixth cervical vertebra. The pharynx is the channel both for air and food; the trachea (or windpipe) leads off it before it joins the oesophagus. The upper part of the pharynx (the nasopharynx) connects with the middle ear through the Eustachian tubes. When air pressure in the middle ear is not equal to that outside (as when going up or down in a plane), the tube becomes blocked and pressure can be reduced by swallowing into the pharynx

phase [feɪz] *subst.* stage *or* period of development *stadium, skede, fas;* **if the cancer is diagnosed in its early phase, the chances of complete cure are much greater**

phenobarbitone [,fiːnə(ʊ)'bɑːbɪtəʊn] *subst.* barbiturate drug, used as a sedative *fenobarbital*

phenol ['fiːnɒl] *or* **carbolic acid** [kɑː,bɒlɪk 'æsɪd] *subst.* strong disinfectant used for external use *fenol, karbol(syra)*

phenotype ['fiːnə(ʊ)taɪp] *subst.* the particular characteristics of an organism *fenotyp; compare* GENOTYPE

> QUOTE all cancers may be reduced to fundamental mechanisms based on cancer risk genes or oncogenes. An oncogene is a gene that encodes a protein that contributes to the malignant phenotype of the cell
>
> **British Medical Journal**

phenylalanine [,fiːnɪ'læləniːn] *subst.* essential amino acid *fenylalanin*

phenylketonuria [,fiːnɪl,kiːtə(ʊ)'njʊəriə] *subst.* hereditary defect which affects the way in which the body breaks down phenylalanine, which in turn concentrates toxic metabolites in the nervous system causing brain damage *fenylketonuri, Föllings sjukdom*

> COMMENT: to have phenylketonuria, a child has to inherit the gene from both parents. The condition can be treated by giving the child a special diet

phial ['faɪ(ə)l] *subst.* small medicine bottle *liten medicinflaska*

-philia ['fɪliə] *suffix* meaning attraction *or* liking for something *-fili*

philtrum [fɪltrəm] *subst.* (i) groove in the centre of the top lip *philtrum nasi, "snorrännan";* (ii) drug believed to stimulate sexual desire *philtrum, afrodisiakum*

phimosis [faɪ'məʊsɪs] *subst.* condition where the foreskin is tight and has to be removed by circumcision *fimos, förhudsförträngning*

phleb- [,fleb, flɪ'b] *or* **phlebo-** ['fliːbə(ʊ), ,--, 'flebə(ʊ), ,--, flɪ'bɒ] *prefix* referring to a vein *fleb(o)-, ven-*

phlebectomy [flɪ'bektəmi] *subst.* surgical removal of a vein *or* part of a vein *flebektomi*

phlebitis [flɪ'baɪtɪs] *subst.* inflammation of a vein *flebit*

phlebogram ['flebə(ʊ)græm] *or* **venogram** ['viːnə(ʊ)græm] *subst.* X-ray picture of a vein *flebogram*

phlebography [flɪ'bɒgrəfi] *or* **venography** [vɪ'nɒgrəfi] *subst.* X-ray examination of a vein using a radio-opaque dye so that the vein will show up on the film *flebografi, venografi*

phlebolith ['flebə(ʊ)lɪθ] *subst.* stone which forms in a vein as a result of an old thrombus becoming calcified *flebolit, vensten*

phlebothrombosis [,flebə(ʊ)θrɒm'bəʊsɪs] *subst.* blood clot in a deep vein in the legs or pelvis, which can easily detach and form an embolus in a lung *flebotrombos, ventrombos*

phlebotomy [flɪ'bɒtəmi] *or* **venesection** [,venɪ'sekʃ(ə)n] *subst.*

operation where a vein is cut so that blood can be removed (as when taking blood from a donor) *flebotomi, venesektion, åderlåtning*

phlegm [ˌflem] *or* **sputum** ['spju:təm] *subst.* mucus found in an inflamed nose, throat or lung and coughed up by the patient *sputum, slem, upphostning;* **she was coughing up phlegm into her handkerchief**

phlegmasia alba dolens [fleg'meɪziə ˌælbə 'dəʊləns] *or* **milk leg** ['mɪlk leg] *subst.* condition which affects women after childbirth, where a leg becomes pale and inflamed as a result of lymphatic obstruction *phlegmasia alba dolens*

phlyctenule [flɪk'tenju:l] *subst.* (i) tiny blister on the cornea *or* conjunctiva *flykten;* **phlyctenules** *ögonskrofler;* (ii) any small blister *liten blåsa*

phobia ['fəʊbiə] *subst.* fear *fobi;* **he has a phobia about** *or* **of dogs; fear of snakes is one of the commonest phobias**

-phobia ['fəʊbiə] *suffix* meaning neurotic fear of something *-fobi, -skräck;* **agoraphobia** = fear of open spaces *agorafobi, torgskräck;* **claustrophobia** = fear of enclosed spaces *klaustrofobi, cellskräck*

phobic ['fəʊbɪk] *adj.* referring to a phobia *fobisk;* **phobic anxiety** = state of worry caused by a phobia *fobisk ångest*

-phobic ['fəʊbɪk] *suffix* person who has a phobia of something *-fobiker;* **agoraphobic** = person who is afraid of open spaces *agorafobiker*

phocomelia [ˌfəʊkə(ʊ)'mi:liə] *or* **phocomely** [fəʊ'kɒməli] *subst.* (i) congenital condition where the upper part of the limbs do not develop, leaving the hands or feet directly attached to the body *fokomeli;* (ii) congenital condition in which the legs develop normally, but the arms are absent or underdeveloped *fokomeli*

phon- ['fəʊn, ˌ-] *or* **phono-** ['fəʊnə(ʊ), ˌ--] *prefix* referring to sound *or* voice *fon(o)-*

phonocardiogram [ˌfəʊnə(ʊ)'kɑ:diə(ʊ)græm] *subst.* chart of the sounds made by the heart *fonokardiogram*

phonocardiography [ˌfəʊnə(ʊ)ˌkɑ:di'ɒgrəfi] *subst.* recording the sounds made by the heart *fonokardiografi*

phosphataemia [ˌfɒsfə'ti:miə] *subst.* presence of excess phosphates (such as calcium *or* sodium) in the blood *överskott på t.ex. natrium el. kalium i blodet*

phosphatase ['fɒsfəteɪz] *subst.* group of enzymes which are important in the cycle of muscle contraction and calcification of bones *fosfatas*

phosphate ['fɒsfeɪt] *subst.* salt of phosphoric acid, used in tonics *fosfat*

phosphaturia [ˌfɒsfə'tjʊəriə] *subst.* condition where excess phosphates are present in the urine *fosfaturi*

> COMMENT: the urine becomes cloudy, which can indicate stones in the bladder or kidney

phospholipid [ˌfɒsfə(ʊ)'lɪpɪd] *subst.* compound with fatty acids, which is one of the main components of membranous tissue *fosfatid, tidigare fosfolipid*

phosphonecrosis [ˌfɒsfə(ʊ)ne'krəʊsɪs] *subst.* necrotic condition affecting the kidneys, liver and bones, usually seen in people who work with phosphorus *fosfornekros*

phosphorescent [ˌfɒsfə'res(ə)nt] *adj.* which shines without producing heat *fosforescerande, självlysande*

phosphoric acid [fɒsˌfɒrɪk 'æsɪd] *subst.* acid which forms phosphates *fosforsyra*

phosphorus ['fɒsf(ə)rəs] *subst.* toxic chemical element which is present in minute quantities in bones and nerve tissue; it causes burns if it touches the skin, and can poison if swallowed *fosfor, P* NOTE: the chemical symbol is **P**

phossy jaw ['fɒsi dʒɔ:] *subst.* disintegration of the bones of the lower jaw, caused by inhaling phosphorus fumes *fosfornekros i käkbenet*

phot- [fɒt, fəʊ't] *or* **photo-** ['fəʊtə(ʊ), ˌ--, fə'tɒ] *prefix* referring to light *foto-, ljus-*

photalgia [fəʊ'tældʒə] *subst.* (i) pain in the eye caused by bright light *oftalmalgi, ögonsmärtor;* (ii) severe photophobia *allvarlig fotofobi (sjuklig rädsla för ljus)*

photocoagulation [ˌfəʊtəʊkəʊˌægju'leɪʃ(ə)n] *subst.* process where tissue coagulates from the heat caused by light *fotokoagulation*

> COMMENT: photocoagulation is used to treat a detached retina

photodermatosis [ˌfəʊtəʊˌdɜːmə'təʊsɪs] *subst.* lesion of the skin after exposure to bright light *fotodermatit, fotoallergi*

photogenic [ˌfəʊtə(ʊ)'dʒenɪk] *adj.* (i) which is produced by the action of light *ljusalstrad;* (ii) which produces light *fotogen, ljusalstrande*

photograph ['fəʊtəgrɑːf] **1** *subst.* picture taken with a camera, which uses the chemical action of light on sensitive film *foto(grafi);* **an X-ray photograph of the patient's chest 2** *vb.* to take a picture with a camera *fotografera*

photography [fə'tɒgrəfi] *subst.* taking pictures with a camera *fotografering;* **the discovery of X-ray photography has meant that internal disorders can be more easily diagnosed**

photophobia [ˌfəʊtə(ʊ)'fəʊbiə] *subst.* (i) condition where the eyes become sensitive to light and conjunctivitis may be caused (it can be associated with measles and some other infectious diseases) *ljuskänslighet;* (ii) morbid fear of light *fotofobi, ljusskygghet*

photophthalmia [ˌfəʊtəf'θælmiə] *subst.* inflammation of the eye caused by bright light, as in snow blindness *ophtalmia actinica*

photopic vision [fəʊˌtɒpɪk 'vɪʒ(ə)n] *subst.* vision which is adapted to bright light (as in daylight) by using the cones in the retina instead of the rods, as in scotopic vision *ljusadapterat seende, dagseende; see also* LIGHT ADAPTATION

photoreceptor neurone [ˌfəʊtəʊrɪ'septə ˌnjʊərəʊn] *subst.* rod or cone in the retina, which is sensitive to light or colour *fotoreceptor*

photoretinitis [ˌfəʊtəʊˌreti'naɪtɪs] *or* **sun blindness** ['sʌn blaɪndnəs] *subst.* damaged retina caused by looking at the sun *ophtalmia actinica, solblindhet*

photosensitive [ˌfəʊtə(ʊ)'sensətɪv] *adj.* (skin *or* lens) which is sensitive to light *or* which is stimulated by light *ljuskänslig*

photosensitivity [ˌfəʊtəʊˌsensə'tɪvəti] *subst.* being sensitive to light *ljuskänslighet*

phototherapy [ˌfəʊtəʊ'θerəpi] *subst.* treatment of jaundice and vitamin D deficiency, which involves exposing a patient to rays of ultraviolet light *fototerapi*

photuria [fəʊ'tjʊəriə] *subst.* phosphorescent urine *fosforescerande urin*

phren- ['fren, ˌ-] *or* **phreno-** ['frenə(ʊ), ˌ--] *prefix* referring to (i) the brain *fren(o)-;* (ii) the phrenic nerve *fren(o)-, mellangärdes-*

phrenemphraxis [ˌfrenem'fræksɪs] *subst.* surgical operation to crush the phrenic nerve in order to paralyse the diaphragm *frenemfraxis*

-phrenia ['friːniə] *suffix* meaning disorder of the mind *-freni*

phrenic ['frenɪk] *adj.* (i) referring to the diaphragm *mellangärdes-;* (ii) referring to the mind *or* intellect *själs-;* **phrenic nerve** = pair of nerves which controls the muscles in the diaphragm *nervus phrenicus;* **phrenic avulsion** *see* AVULSION

phrenicectomy [ˌfrenɪ'sektəmi] *subst.* surgical removal of all *or* part of the phrenic nerve *frenektomi*

phreniclasia [ˌfrenɪ'kleɪziə] *subst.* operation to clamp the phrenic nerve *operation för att klämma ihop nervus phrenicus*

phrenicotomy [ˌfrenɪ'kɒtəmi] *subst.* operation to divide the phrenic nerve *frenikotomi*

phthiriasis [θə'raɪəsɪs] *subst.* infestation with the crab louse *ftiriasis, nedlusning*

Phthirius pubis ['θaɪərəs ˌpjuːbɪs] *subst.* pubic louse *or* crab louse *or* louse which infests the pubic region *Pediculus (Phthirius) pubis, flatlus*

phthisis ['θaɪsɪs] *subst.* (i) old term for tuberculosis *ftis, lungsot;* (ii) any wasting disease of the body *tvinsot*

pH-värde ⇨ **pH**

phycomycosis [ˌfaɪkə(ʊ)maɪ'kəʊsɪs] *subst.* acute infection of the lungs, central nervous system and other organs by a fungus *slags akut svampinfektion*

physi- ['fɪzi, ˌ--] *or* **physio-** ['fɪziə(ʊ), ˌ--] *prefix* referring to (i) physiology *fysio-;* (ii) physical *fysisk, kroppslig*

physic ['fɪzɪk] *subst.* old term for medicine *läkekonst, läkarvetenskap*

physical ['fɪzɪk(ə)l] **1** *adj.* referring to the body, as opposed to the mind *fysisk, fysikalisk, kroppslig;* **physical dependence** = state where a person is addicted to a drug such as heroin and suffers physical effects if he stops taking the drug *fysiskt beroende;* **physical education**

= teaching of sports and exercises in school *gymnastik, skolgymnastik;* **physical examination** = examination of a patient's body to see if he is healthy *läkarundersökning;* **physical medicine** = branch of medicine which deals with physical disabilities *or* with treatment of disorders after they have been diagnosed *fysikalisk medicin;* **physical sign** = symptom which can be seen on the patient's body *or* which can be produced by percussion and palpitation *symtom, fysikaliskt tecken;* **physical therapy** = treatment of disorders by heat *or* by massage *or* by exercise and other physical means *fysikalisk terapi, fysioterapi, sjukgymnastik* **2** *subst.* physical examination *läkarundersökning;* **he has to pass a physical before being accepted by the police force**

physically ['fɪzɪk(ə)li] *adv.* referring to the body *fysiskt, kroppsligt;* **physically he is very weak, but his mind is still alert**

physician [fɪ'zɪʃ(ə)n] *subst.* registered doctor who is not a surgeon *läkare, medicinare*
NOTE: in GB English, physician refers to a specialist doctor, though not usually a surgeon, while in US English it is used for any qualified doctor

physio ['fɪziəʊ] *subst. informal* (i) session of physiotherapy treatment *ett enskilt tillfälle av sjukgymnastik;* (ii) physiotherapist *sjukgymnast*

physiological [ˌfɪziə'lɒdʒɪk(ə)l] *adj.* referring to physiology *or* to the normal functions of the body *fysiologisk;* **physiological saline** *or* **solution** = any solution used to keep cells *or* tissue alive *fysiologisk (koksalt)lösning*

physiologist [ˌfɪzɪ'ɒlədʒɪst] *subst.* scientist who specializes in the study of the functions of living organisms *fysiolog*

physiology [ˌfɪzɪ'ɒlədʒi] *subst.* **human physiology** study of the human body and its normal functions *(människans) fysiologi*

physiotherapist [ˌfɪzɪə(ʊ)'θerəpɪst] *subst.* trained specialist who gives physiotherapy *sjukgymnast*

physiotherapy [ˌfɪzɪə(ʊ)'θerəpi] *subst.* treatment of a disorder or condition by exercise *or* massage *or* heat treatment *or* infrared lamps, etc., to restore strength, to restore function after a disease or injury, to correct a deformity *fysikalisk terapi, fysioterapi, sjukgymnastik;* **physiotherapy clinic** = clinic where patients can have physiotherapy *ung. sjukgymnastikavdelning*

phyt- ['faɪt] *or* **phyto-** ['faɪtə(ʊ), ˌ--] *prefix* referring to plants *or* coming from plants *fyt(o)-*

pia mater [ˌpa(ɪ)ə 'meɪtə] *subst.* delicate inner layer of the meninges, the membrane which covers the brain and spinal cord *pia mater, mjuka hjärnhinnan*

pian [piː'ɑːn] = YAWS

pica ['paɪkə] *subst.* desire to eat things (such as wood *or* paper) which are not food, often found in pregnant women and small children *pica*

pick [pɪk] *vb.* to take away small pieces of something with the fingers *or* with a tool *plocka, peta;* **she picked the pieces of glass out of the wound with tweezers; to pick one's nose** = to take pieces of mucus out of the nostrils *peta näsan;* **to pick one's teeth with a pin** = to take away pieces of food which are stuck between the teeth *peta tänderna*

Pick's disease ['pɪks dɪˌziːz] *subst.* **(a)** rare condition, where a disorder of the lipoid metabolism causes retarded mental development, anaemia, loss of weight and swelling of the spleen and liver *Picks sjukdom, pseudoleverscirros* **(b)** constrictive pericarditis *konstriktiv perikardit*

pick up [ˌpɪk 'ʌp] *vb. (informal)* **(a)** to catch a disease *få, ådra sig;* **he must have picked up the disease when he was travelling in Africa (b)** to get stronger *or* better *krya på sig, hämta sig, bli bättre;* **he was ill for months, but he's picking up now**

picornavirus [piːˌkɔːnə'vaɪ(ə)rəs] *subst.* virus containing RNA, such as enteroviruses and rhinoviruses *picornavirus*

PID [ˌpiːaɪˌdiː] = PROLAPSED INTERVERTEBRAL DISC

pigeon chest ['pɪdʒ(ə)n ˌtʃest] *subst.* deformity of the chest, where the breastbone sticks out *pectus gallinaceum (anserium, carinatum), hönsbröst, gåsbröst, kölbröst*

pigeon toes [ˌpɪdʒ(ə)n ˌtəʊz] *subst.* condition where the feet turn towards the inside when a person is standing upright *slags inåtgång med tårna*

pigg ⇨ **alert, fit**

pigga upp ⇨ **pep**

pigment ['pɪgmənt] *subst.* (i) substance which gives colour to part of the body such as blood *or* the skin *or* hair *pigment, färgämne;* (ii) (in pharmacy) a paint *färgämne (för tabletter);* **bile pigment** = yellow colouring matter in bile *gallfärgämne;* **blood pigment** = HAEMOGLOBIN

COMMENT: the body contains several substances which control colour: melanin gives dark colour to the skin and hair; bilirubin gives yellow colour to bile and urine; haemoglobin in the blood gives the skin a pink colour; carotene can give a reddish-yellow colour to the skin if the patient eats too many tomatoes or carrots. Some pigment cells can carry oxygen and are called "respiratory pigments"

pigmentation [ˌpɪgmenˈteɪʃ(ə)n] *subst.* colouring of the body, especially that produced by deposits of pigment *pigmentering*

pigmented [pɪgˈmentɪd] *adj.* coloured *or* showing an abnormal colour *pigmenterad;* **pigmented epithelium** *or* **pigmented layer** = coloured tissue at the back of the retina *pigmentepitel*

pigmentepitel ➪ **pigmented**

pigmenterad ➪ **pigmented**

pigmentering ➪ **pigmentation**

piles [paɪ(ə)lz] = HAEMORRHOIDS

pill [pɪl] *subst.* small hard round ball of drug which is to be swallowed whole *piller, tablett;* **he has to take the pills twice a day; the doctor put her on a course of vitamin pills; the pill** = oral contraceptive *p-piller;* **she's on the pill** = she is taking a regular course of contraceptive pills *hon tar p-piller*

piller ➪ **pellet, pill**

pillertrillarrörelse ➪ **pill-rolling**

pillow [ˈpɪləʊ] *subst.* soft cushion on a bed which the head lies on when the patient is lying down *kudde, huvudkudde;* **the nurse gave her an extra pillow to keep her head raised**

pill-rolling [ˈpɪlˌrəʊlɪŋ] *subst.* nervous action of the fingers, in which the patient seems to be rolling a very small object, associated with Parkinson's disease *pillertrillarrörelse*

pilo- [ˈpaɪlə(ʊ), ˌ--] *prefix* referring to hair *pilo-, hår-*

pilomotor nerve [ˌpaɪləˈməʊtə ˌnɜːv] *subst.* nerve which supplies the arrector pili muscles attached to hair follicles *pilomotorisk nerv*

pilonidal cyst [ˌpaɪləˌnaɪd(ə)l ˈsɪst] *subst.* cyst containing hair, usually found at the bottom of the spine near the buttocks *pilonidalcysta, hårsäckscysta*

pilonidalcysta ➪ **pilonidal cyst, pilonidal sinus**

pilonidal sinus [ˌpaɪləˌnaɪd(ə)l ˈsaɪnəs] *subst.* small depression with hairs at the base of the spine *pilonidalcysta*

pilosebaceous [ˌpaɪləsəˈbeɪʃəs] *adj.* referring to the hair follicles and the glands attached to them *som avser el. hör till hudens hårsäckar och talgkörtlar*

pilosis [paɪˈləʊsɪs] *or* **pilosism** [ˈpaɪləsɪz(ə)m] *subst.* condition where someone has an abnormal amount of hair or where hair is present in an abnormal place *pilos(ism)*

pilsömmen ➪ **sagittal**

pilus [ˈpaɪləs] *subst.* (i) one hair *pilus, hår(strå);* (ii) hair-like process on the surface of a bacterium *hårliknande utskott på bakterie; see also* ARRECTOR PILI

pimple [ˈpɪmp(ə)l] *subst.* papule *or* pustule (small swelling on the skin, containing pus) *finne, kvissla, blemma;* **he had pimples on his neck; is that red pimple painful?; goose pimples** = reaction of the skin to cold *or* fear, where the skin forms many little bumps *cutis anserina, dermatospasm, horripilatio, gåshud, hönshud*

pimply [ˈpɪmpli] *adj.* covered with pimples *finnig*

pin [pɪn] **1** *subst.* **(a)** small sharp piece of metal for attaching things together *nål;* **the nurse fastened the bandage with a pin; safety pin** = special type of bent pin with a guard which protects the point, used for attaching nappies or bandages *säkerhetsnål* **(b)** metal nail used to attach broken bones *stift;* **he has had a pin inserted in his hip** **2** *vb.* to attach with a pin *nåla ihop, fästa med nål, förena med stift;* **she pinned the bandages carefully to stop them slipping; the bone had fractured in several places and needed pinning**

pincett ➪ **forceps, tweezers**

pinch [pɪn(t)ʃ] **1** *subst.* (i) squeezing the thumb and first finger together *nyp(ning);* (ii) quantity of something which can be held between the thumb and first finger *nypa;* **she put a pinch of salt into the water 2** *vb.* **(a)** to squeeze something tightly between the thumb and first finger *nypa* **(b)** to squeeze *klämma;* **she developed a sore on her ankle where her shoe pinched**

pineal (body) ['pɪniəl (bɒdi)] *or* **pineal gland** ['pɪniəl glænd] *subst.* small cone-shaped gland near the midbrain which produces melatonin and is believed to be associated with the circadian rhythm ⇨ *illustration* BRAIN *corpus pineale, epifysen, övre hjärnbihanget, tallkottkörteln*

pinguecula [pɪŋ'gwekjʊlə] *or* **pinguicula** [pɪŋ'gwɪkjʊlə] *subst.* condition affecting old people, where the conjunctiva in the eyes has small yellow growths near the edge of the cornea, usually on the nasal side *pinguecula, ögonspringefläck*

pink [pɪŋk] *adj.* of a colour like very pale red *rosa, skär;* **pink disease** *or* **erythroedema** *or* **acrodynia** = children's disease where the child's hands, feet and face swell and become pink, with a fever and loss of appetite, caused by an allergy to mercury *pink disease, erythroedema, akrodyni;* **pink eye** *or* **epidemic conjunctivitis** = inflammation of the conjunctiva, where the eyelids become swollen and sticky and discharge pus, common in schools and other institutions, caused by the Koch-Weeks bacillus *smittsam konjunktivit*

pinna ['pɪnə] *or* **outer ear** [,aʊtər 'ɪə] *subst.* part of the ear which is outside the head, connected by a passage to the eardrum ⇨ *illustration* EAR *pinna, auris externa, ytterörat*

"pinne" ⇨ **Steinmann's pin**

pinocytosis [,paɪnəʊsaɪ'təʊsɪs] *subst.* process by which a cell surrounds and takes in fluid *pinocytos*

pins and needles [,pɪnz ən 'ni:d(ə)lz] *subst.* non-medical term for an unpleasant tingling feeling, caused when a nerve is irritated, as when a limb has become numb after the circulation has been blocked for a short time *myrkrypning, känsla när kroppsdel "somnat"*

pint [paɪnt] *subst.* measure of liquids (= about .56 of a litre) *slags vätskemått, c 0,56 l i Storbritannien, c 0,47 l i USA;* **he was given six pints of blood in blood transfusions during the operation**

pinta ['pɪntə] *subst.* skin disease of the tropical regions of America, caused by a spirochaete **Treponema**

> COMMENT: the skin on the hands and feet swells and loses its colour

pinworm ['pɪnwɜ:m] *subst. US* threadworm *or* thin nematode worm **Enterobius vermicularis** which infests the large intestine *Enterobius vermicularis, springmask*

pipa ⇨ **wheeze**

pipande ⇨ **sibilant, wheezy**

pipette [pɪ'pet] *subst.* thin glass tube used in the laboratory for taking or measuring samples of liquid *pipett*

pipmugg ⇨ **feeding**

piriform fossae ['pɪrɪfɔ:m ,fɒsi:] *subst pl.* two hollows at the sides of the upper end of the larynx *recessus piriformis*

pisiform (bone) ['pɪsɪfɔ:m (bəʊn)] *subst.* one of the eight small carpal bones in the wrist ⇨ *illustration* HAND *os pisiforme, ärtbenet*

piskmask ⇨ **whipworm**

pisksnärtskada ⇨ **whiplash injury**

pit [pɪt] *subst.* hollow place on a surface *grop;* **the pit of the stomach** *or* **epigastrium** = part of the upper abdomen between the rib cage above the navel *epigastriet, maggropen; see also* ARMPIT

pitcher's elbow ['pɪtʃəz ,elbəʊ] *US* = TENNIS ELBOW

pithiatism [pɪ'θaɪətɪz(ə)m] *subst.* way of influencing the patient's mind by persuading him of something, as when the doctor treats a condition by telling the patient that he is in fact well *pitiatism*

pitiatism ⇨ **pithiatism**

pitted ['pɪtɪd] *adj.* covered with small hollows *gropig, ärrig, ojämn;* **his skin was pitted by acne**

pitting ['pɪtɪŋ] *subst.* formation of hollows in the skin *gropbildning*

pituitary body [pɪ'tju:ɪt(ə)ri bɒdɪ] *or* **pituitary gland** [pɪ'tju:ɪt(ə)ri glænd] *or* **hypophysis cerebri** [haɪ'pɒfəsɪs 'serəbraɪ] *subst.* main endocrine gland in the body ⇨ *illustration* BRAIN *glandula pituitaria (hypophysis), hypophysis cerebri, hypofysen;* **pituitary fossa** *or* **sella turcica** ▪ hollow in the upper surface of the sphenoid bone in which the pituitary gland sits *sella turcica, turksadeln*

COMMENT: the pituitary gland is about the size of a pea, and hangs down from the base of the brain, inside the sphenoid bone, on a stalk which attaches it to the hypothalamus. The front lobe of the gland (the adenohypophysis) secretes several hormones (TSH, ACTH) which stimulate the adrenal and thyroid glands, or which stimulate the production of sex hormones, melanin and milk. The posterior lobe of the pituitary gland (the neurohypophysis) secretes the antidiuretic hormone and oxytocin. The pituitary gland is the most important gland in the body because the hormones it secretes control the functioning of the other glands

pituitrin [pɪ'tju:ɪtrɪn] *subst.* hormone secreted by the pituitary gland *hypofyshormon*

pityriasis [ˌpɪtɪ'ra(ɪ)əsɪs] *subst.* any skin disease where the skin develops thin scales *pityriasis;* **pityriasis alba** = disease of children with flat white patches on the cheeks *pityriasis alba (sicca);* **pityriasis capitis** = dandruff *or* condition where pieces of dead skin form on the scalp and fall out when the hair is combed *pityriasis capitis, torr seborré, mjäll;* **pityriasis rosea** = mild irritating rash affecting young people, which appears especially in the early part of the year and has no known cause *pityriasis rosea;* **pityriasis rubra** = serious, sometimes fatal, skin disease where the skin turns dark red and is covered with white scales *slags allvarlig hudsjukdom*

pivot ['pɪvət] **1** *subst.* stem used to attach an artificial crown to the root of a tooth *stift* **2** *vb.* to rest and turn on a point *svänga (vrida sig) kring;* **the atlas bone pivots on the second vertebra; pivot joint** *or* **trochoid joint** = joint where a bone can rotate freely *articulatio trochoidea, rotationsled, vridled*

placebo [plə'si:bəʊ] *subst.* tablet which appears to be a drug, but has no medicinal substance in it *placebo, blindtablett*

COMMENT: placebos may be given to patients who have imaginary illnesses; placebos can also help in treating real disorders by stimulating the patient's psychological will to be cured. Placebos are also used on control groups in tests of new drugs (a placebo-controlled study)

placenta [plə'sentə] *subst.* tissue which grows inside the uterus during pregnancy and links the baby to the mother *placenta, moderkakan;* **placenta praevia** = condition where the fertilized egg becomes implanted in the lower part of the uterus, which means that the placenta may become detached during childbirth and cause brain damage to the baby *placenta praevia;* **battledore placenta** = placenta where the umbilical cord is attached at the edge and not the centre *placenta där navelsträngen utgår från kanten och inte från mitten*

COMMENT: the vascular system of the fetus is not directly connected to that of the mother. The placenta allows an exchange of oxygen and nutrients to be passed from the mother to the fetus to which she is linked by the umbilical cord. It stops functioning when the baby breathes for the first time and is then passed out of the womb as the afterbirth

placenta- ⇨ **placental**

placentainsufficiens ⇨ **placental**

placental [plə'sent(ə)l] *adj.* referring to the placenta *placentar, placenta-;* **placental insufficiency** = condition where the placenta does not provide the fetus with the necessary oxygen and nutrients *placentainsufficiens*

placentar ⇨ **placental**

placentography [ˌplæsən'tɒgrəfi] *subst.* X-ray examination of the placenta of a pregnant woman after a radio-opaque dye has been injected *placentografi*

placera ⇨ **position, site**

placerad ⇨ **situated**

Placido's disc [plə'saɪdəʊz ˌdɪsk] *or* **keratoscope** ['kerətəskəʊp] *subst.* instrument for examining the cornea to see if it has an abnormal curvature *Placidos skiva, keratoskop, ceratoskop, astigmatoskop*

plack ⇨ **dental, plaque**

plagiocephaly [ˌpleɪdʒiə'kef(ə)li] *subst.* condition where a person has a distorted head *plagiocefali, snedskallighet*

plague [pleɪg] *subst.* infectious disease which occurs in epidemics where many people are killed *pest;* **bubonic plague** = fatal disease caused by **Pasteurella pestis** in the lymph system transmitted to humans by fleas from rats *pestis bubonica, bubonpest, böldpest, digerdöden;* **pneumonic plague** = form of bubonic plague where mainly the lungs are affected *lungpest;* **septicaemic plague** = form of bubonic plague where the symptoms are generalized *pest med generella symtom som blodförgiftning;* **the hospitals cannot cope**

with all the plague victims; thousands of people are dying of plague

> COMMENT: bubonic plague was the Black Death of the Middle Ages; its symptoms are fever, delirium, prostration, rigor and swellings on the lymph nodes

plan [plæn] **1** *subst.* arrangement of how something should be done *plan;* **care plan** = plan drawn up by the nursing staff for the treatment of an individual patient *omvårdnadsplan, vårdplan* **2** *vb.* to arrange how something is going to be done *planera;* **they are planning to have a family** = they expect to have children and so are not taking contraceptives *de tänker skaffa sig barn*

> QUOTE one issue has arisen - the amount of time and effort which nurses need to put into the writing of detailed care plans. Few would now dispute the need for clear, concise nursing plans to guide nursing practice, provide educational tools and give an accurate legal record
>
> **Nursing Times**

plan ⇨ **flat, plane**

plane [pleɪn] *subst.* flat surface, especially that of the body seen from a certain angle *plan, plan yta; see* CORONAL, MEDIAN, SAGITTAL

planera ⇨ **arrange, plan**

planned parenthood [ˌplænd ˈpeər(ə)nthʊd] *subst.* situation where two people plan to have a certain number of children, and take contraceptives to control the number of children in the family *familjeplanering*

planning [ˈplænɪŋ] *subst.* arranging how something should be done *planering;* **family planning** = using contraceptives to control the number of children in a family *familjeplanering;* **family planning clinic** = clinic which gives advice on contraception *familjeplaneringsklinik*

planta [plæntə] *subst.* the sole of the foot *planta (pedis), fotsulan*

plantar [ˈplæntə] *adj.* referring to the sole of the foot *plantar, fot-, fotsule-;* **plantar arch** = curved part of the sole of the foot running along the length of the foot *hålfoten, fotvalvet;* **deep plantar arch** = curved artery crossing the sole of the foot *arcus plantaris, hålfotsbågen;* **plantar flexion** = bending of the toes downwards *plantarflexion;* **plantar reflex** *or* **plantar response** = normal downward movement of the toes when the sole of the foot is stroked in Babinski test *plantarreflex, Babinskis reflex;* **plantar region** = the sole of the foot *fotsulan;* **plantar surface** = the skin of the sole of the foot *fotsulans hud;* **plantar wart** = wart on the sole of the foot *verruca plantaris, fotvårta*

plantarflexion ⇨ **plantar**

plantarreflex ⇨ **plantar, Babinski reflex**

planus [ˈpleɪnəs] *see* LICHEN, PES

plaque [plæk] *subst.* flat area *plaque, plack;* **bacterial plaque** = hard smooth bacterial deposit on teeth *plack, tandbeläggning;* **atherosclerotic plaque** = deposit on the walls of arteries *aterosklerotiskt plack*

-plasia [ˈpleɪziə] *suffix* which develops *or* grows *-plasi*

plasm- [ˈplæz(ə)m, ˌ-] *or* **plasmo-** [ˈplæzməʊ, ˌ--] *prefix* referring to blood plasma *plasma-*

plasma [ˈplæzmə] *subst.* (i) yellow watery liquid which makes up the main part of blood *plasma, blodplasma;* (ii) lymph with no corpuscles *lymfa, lymfvätska;* (iii) cytoplasm *cytoplasma;* **the accident victim was given plasma; plasma cell** = lymphocyte which produces a certain type of antibody *plasmacell;* **plasma protein** = protein in plasma (such as albumin, gamma globulin and fibrinogen) *plasmaprotein* NOTE: no plural

> COMMENT: if blood does not clot it separates into blood corpuscles and plasma, which is formed of water and proteins, including the clotting agent fibrinogen. If blood clots, the corpuscles separate from serum, which is a watery liquid similar to plasma, but not containing fibrinogen. Dried plasma can be kept for a long time, and is used, after water has been added, for transfusions

plasmacell ⇨ **plasma**

plasmacytoma [ˌplæzməsaɪˈtəʊmə] *subst.* malignant tumour of plasma cells, normally found in lymph nodes *or* bone marrow *slags malign tumör*

plasmaferes ⇨ **plasmapheresis**

plasmapheresis [ˌplæzməfəˈriːsɪs] *subst.* operation to take blood from a patient, then to separate the red blood cells from the plasma, and to return the red blood cells suspended in a saline solution to the patient through a transfusion *plasmaferes*

plasmaprotein ⇨ **plasma**

plasmin ['plæzmɪn] *or* **fibrinolysin** [ˌfaɪbrɪ'nɒləsɪn] *subst.* enzyme which digests fibrin *plasmin, fibrinolysin*

plasminogen [plæz'mɪnədʒ(ə)n] *subst.* substance in blood plasma which becomes activated and forms plasmin *plasminogen*

Plasmodium [plæz'məʊdiəm] *subst.* type of parasite which infests red blood cells and causes malaria *Plasmodium*

plasmolysis [plæz'mɒlɪsɪs] *subst.* contraction of a cell protoplasm by dehydration, where the surrounding cell wall becomes smaller *plasmolys*

plast ⇨ **plastic**

plaster ['plɑːstə] *subst.* **(a)** white powder which is mixed with water and used to make a solid support to cover a broken limb *gips;* **after his accident he had his leg in plaster for two months; plaster cast** = hard support made of bandage soaked in liquid plaster of Paris which is allowed to harden, and is used to wrap round a fracture to prevent the limb moving while the bones are healing *gips(förband);* **plaster of Paris** = fine white plaster used to make plaster casts *gips;* **frog plaster** = plaster cast made to keep the legs in the correct position after an operation to correct a dislocated hip *slags gipsförband vid höftledsluxation* **(b) sticking plaster** = adhesive plaster *or* sticky tape used to cover a small wound *or* to attach a pad of dressing to the skin *plåster, häftplåster, häfta;* **put a plaster on your cut**

plastic ['plæstɪk] **1** *subst.* artificial material made from petroleum, and used to make many objects, including replacement organs *plast* **2** *adj.* which can be made in different shapes *plastisk, formbar, plastik-;* **plastic lymph** *or* **inflammatory lymph** = yellow liquid produced by an inflamed wound and which helps the healing process *pus, var, lymfvätska som bildas vid inflammation;* **plastic surgery** = surgery which repairs defective *or* deformed parts of the body *plastikkirurgi, rekonstruktiv kirurgi;* **plastic surgeon** = surgeon who specializes in plastic surgery *plastikkirurg*

> COMMENT: plastic surgery is especially impotant in treating accident victims or people who have suffered burns. It is also used to correct congenital deformities such as a cleft palate. When the objecty is simply to improve the patient's appearance, it is usually referred to as "cosmetic surgery"

plastik- ⇨ **plastic**

-plastik ⇨ **-plasty**

plastikkirurg ⇨ **plastic**

plastikkirurgi ⇨ **plastic, reconstructive surgery**

plastisk ⇨ **plastic**

-plasty [plæsti] *suffix* referring to plastic surgery *-plastik*

plate [pleɪt] *subst.* **(a)** flat round piece of china for putting food on *fat, tallrik;* **the nurses brought round sandwiches on a plate for lunch; pass your dirty plates to the person at the end of the table (b)** (i) flat sheet of metal *or* bone, etc. *platta, plåt;* (ii) flat piece of metal attached to a fractured bone to hold the broken parts together *platta;* **the surgeon inserted a plate in her skull; cribriform plate** = top part of the ethmoid bone which forms the roof of the nasal cavity and part of the top of the eye sockets *lamina cribrosa, silbensplattan;* **dental plate** = prosthesis made to the shape of the mouth, which holds artificial teeth *lösgom, tandprotes*

platelet [pleɪtlɪt] *or* **thrombocyte** ['θrɒmbəʊsaɪt] *subst.* little blood cell which encourages the coagulation of blood *trombocyt, blodplätt, blodplatta*

platonyki ⇨ **koilonychia**

plats ⇨ **locus, position, site, space**

platt ⇨ **flat**

platt- ⇨ **platy-**

platta ⇨ **plate**

plattfot ⇨ **arch, flat**

plattmask ⇨ **flatworm**

platy- ['plæti, ˌ--] *prefix* meaning flat *platy-, platt-*

platysma [plə'tɪzmə] *subst.* flat muscle running from the collar bone to the lower jaw *platysma*

-plegi ⇨ **-plegia**

-plegia ['pliːdʒə] *suffix* meaning paralysis *-plegi, -förlamning*

pleio- ['plaɪə(ʊ), ˌ--] *or* **pleo-** ['pliːə(ʊ), ˌ--] *prefix* meaning too many *plei(o)-, pleo-*

pleocytosis [ˌpliːə(ʊ)saɪ'təʊsɪs] *subst.* condition where there are an abnormal number of leucocytes in the cerebrospinal fluid *pleocytos*

pleoptics [pli:'ɒptɪks] *subst.* treatment to help the partially sighted *pleoptisk behandling*

plessor ['plesə] *or* **plexor** ['pleksə] *subst.* little hammer with a rubber tip, used by doctors to tap tendons to test for reflexes or for percussion of the chest *perkussionshammare*

plethora ['pleθ(ə)rə] *subst.* old term meaning too much blood in the body *plethora, blodfullhet*

plethoric [ple'θɒrɪk] *adj.* (appearance) due to dilatation of superficial blood vessels *pletorisk, blodfull*

plethysmography [ˌpleθɪz'mɒgrəfi] *subst.* method of recording the changes in the volume of organs, mainly used to measure blood flow in the limbs *pletysmografi*

pletorisk ⇨ **plethoric**

pletysmografi ⇨ **plethysmography**

pleur- ['plʊər, ˌ-] *or* **pleuro-** ['plʊərə(ʊ), ˌ--] *prefix* referring to the pleura *pleur(o)-, lungsäcks-*

pleura ['plʊərə] *subst.* one of two membranes lining the chest cavity and covering each lung *pleura, lungsäcken;* **parietal pleura** *or* **outer pleura** = membrane attached to the diaphragm and covering the chest cavity *pleura parietalis (costalis), lungsäckens yttre blad;* **visceral pleura** *or* **inner pleura** = membrane attached to the surface of the lung ⇨ *illustration* LUNGS *pleura visceralis (pulmonalis), lungsäckens inre blad* NOTE: plural is **pleurae**

pleuracentesis [ˌplʊərəsen'ti:sɪs] *see* PLEUROCENTESIS

pleuraexsudat ⇨ **pleural**

pleurahålan ⇨ **pleural**

pleural ['plʊər(ə)l] *adj.* referring to the pleura *pleural, pleura-, lungsäcks-;* **pleural cavity** = space between the inner and outer pleura *cavum pleurae, pleurahålan;* **pleural effusion** = excess fluid formed in the pleural sac *pleuraexsudat, utgjutning i lungsäcken;* **pleural fluid** = fluid which forms between the layers of the pleura in pleurisy *pleuravätska;* **pleural membrane** = PLEURA

pleuralgi ⇨ **pleurodynia**

pleurapunktion ⇨ **pleurocentesis, thoracentesis, thoracocentesis**

pleuravätska ⇨ **fluid, pleural**

pleurectomy [plʊə'rektəmi] *subst.* surgical removal of part of the pleura which has been thickened or made stiff by chronic empyema *dekortikering*

pleurisy ['plʊərɪsi] *subst.* inflammation of the pleura, usually caused by pneumonia *pleurit, lungsäcksinflammation;* **diaphragmatic pleurisy** = inflammation of the outer pleura only *inflammation enbart i lungsäckens yttre blad, vätska i lungsäcken*

> COMMENT: the symptoms of pleurisy are coughing, fever, and sharp pains when breathing, caused by the two layers of pleura rubbing together

pleurit ⇨ **pleurisy**

pleuritis [plʊə'raɪtɪs] = PLEURISY

pleur(o)- ⇨ **pleur-**

pleurocele ['plʊərə(ʊ)ˌsi:(ə)l] *subst.* (i) condition where part of the lung *or* pleura is herniated *lung- el. lungsäcksbråck;* (ii) fluid in the pleural cavity *utgjutning i pleurahålan*

pleurocentes ⇨ **pleurocentesis, thoracentesis, thoracocentesis**

pleurocentesis [ˌplʊərə(ʊ)sen'ti:sɪs] *or* **pleuracentesis** [ˌplʊərəsen'ti:sɪs] *subst.* operation where a hollow needle is put into the pleura to drain liquid *pleurocentes, pleurapunktion, torakocentes*

pleurodesis [plʊə'rɒdɪsɪs] *subst.* treatment for a collapsed lung, where the inner and outer pleura are stuck together *pleurodes*

pleurodynia [ˌplʊərə(ʊ)'dɪniə] *subst.* pain in the muscles between the ribs, due to rheumatic inflammation *pleurodyni, pleuralgi;* **epidemic pleurodynia** *or* **Bornholm disease** = virus disease affecting the intestinal muscles, with symptoms like influenza, (fever, headaches and pains in the chest) *pleurodynia (diaphragmatica) epidemica, bornholmssjuka*

pleuropneumonia [ˌplʊərə(ʊ)njʊ'məʊniə] *subst.* acute lobar pneumonia (the classic type of pneumonia) *pleuropneumoni*

plexor ['pleksə] *subst.* little hammer, used by doctors to tap tendons to test reflexes or in percussion of the chest *perkussionshammare*

plexus ['pleksəs] *subst.* network of nerves *or* blood vessels *or* lymphatics *plexus, nätverk;* **Auerbach's plexus** = group of nerve fibres in the intestine *plexus myentericus, Auerbachs plexus;* **brachial plexus** = group of nerves at the base of the neck, which lead to nerves in the arms and hands *plexus brachialis, armplexus, armflätan;* **cervical plexus** = group of nerves in front of the vertebrae in the neck, which lead to nerves supplying the skin and muscles of the neck, and also the phrenic nerve which controls the diaphragm *plexus cervicalis, halsplexus, halsflätan;* **choroid plexus (of the lateral ventricle)** = part of the pia mater, a network of small blood vessels in the ventricles of the brain which produce cerebrospinal fluid *plexus chorioideus;* **lumbar plexus** = point near the spine above the pelvis where several nerves supplying the thigh and abdomen are joined together *plexus lumbalis, ländplexus, ländflätan;* **sacral plexus** = group of nerves inside the pelvis near the sacrum which lead to nerves in the buttocks, back of the thigh and lower leg and foot *plexus sacralis, korsbensplexus, korsflätan;* **solar plexus** *or* **coeliac plexus** = network of nerves in the abdomen, behind the stomach *plexus solaris (coeliacus), solarplexus*

pliable ['pla(ɪ)əb(ə)l] *adj.* which can bend easily *böjlig*

plica ['plaɪkə] *subst.* fold *plica, veck*

plicate ['plaɪkeɪt] *adj.* folded *veckad*

plication [plaɪ'keɪʃ(ə)n] *subst.* (i) surgical operation to reduce the size of a muscle *or* a hollow organ by making folds in its walls and attaching them *slags operativt ingrepp där vävnad veckas;* (ii) the action of folding *veckning;* (iii) a fold *veck*

plocka ⇨ **pick**

plogbenet ⇨ **vomer**

plomb ⇨ **filling**

plombage [plɒm'bɑːʒ] *subst.* (i) packing bone cavities with antiseptic material *packning;* (ii) packing of the lung *or* pleural cavities with inert material *packning*

plombering ⇨ **filling**

plumbism ['plʌmbɪz(ə)m] *subst.* lead poisoning *blyförgiftning*

Plummer-Vinson syndrome [ˌplʌmə'vɪns(ə)n ˌsɪndrəʊm] *subst.* type of iron-deficiency anaemia, where the tongue and mouth become inflamed and the patient cannot swallow *dysphagia sideropenica, Plummer-Vinsons syndrom*

plunger ['plʌn(d)ʒə] *subst.* part of a hypodermic syringe which slides up and down inside the tube, either sucking liquid into the syringe or forcing the contents out *kolv*

pluripara ⇨ **multipara**

plåga ⇨ **bother, distress**

plågas ⇨ **suffer**

plågor ⇨ **dolor, pain**

plågsam ⇨ **painful, excruciating**

plåster ⇨ **adhesive, plaster**

plåt ⇨ **plate**

plötslig ⇨ **acute, sudden**

plötsligt ⇨ **sharply**

PM [ˌpiː'em] = POST MORTEM **what are the results of the PM?**

PMA [ˌpiːem'eɪ] = PROGRESSIVE MUSCULAR ATROPHY

PMT [ˌpiːem'tiː] = PREMENSTRUAL TENSION **she is being treated for PMT; the hospital has a special clinic for PMT sufferers**

-pnea [pniːə] *or* **-pnoea** [pniːə] *suffix* referring to breathing *-pné, -andning*

pneum- ['njuːm, ˌ-] *or* **pneumo-** ['njuːmə(ʊ), ˌ--] *prefix* referring to air *or* to the lungs *or* to breathing *pneum(o)-, pulm(on)-, luft-, lung-*

pneumatocefali ⇨ **pneumocephalus**

pneumatocele [nju'mætəʊsiː(ə)l] *subst.* (i) sac *or* tumour filled with gas *pneumatocele, luftbråck;* (ii) herniation of the lung *pneumocele, lungbråck*

pneumaturia [ˌnjuːmə'tjʊəriə] *subst.* passing air or gas in the urine *pneumaturi*

pneumocele ⇨ **pneumatocele**

pneumocephalus [ˌnjuːmə(ʊ)'kef(ə)ləs] *subst.* presence of air *or* gas in the brain *pneumatocefali*

pneumococcal [ˌnjuːmə(ʊ)'kɒk(ə)l] *adj.* referring to pneumococci *pneumokock-*

pneumococcus [ˌnju:mə(ʊ)ˈkɒkəs] *subst.* genus of bacteria which causes respiratory tract infections, including pneumonia *pneumokock* NOTE: plural is **pneumococci**

pneumoconiosis [ˌnju:məˌkəʊniˈəʊsɪs] *subst.* lung disease where fibrous tissue forms in the lungs because the patient has inhaled particles of stone *or* dust over a long period of time *pneumo(no)konios, dammlunga*

pneumoencefalografi ⇨ **encephalography, pneumoencephalography, ventriculography**

pneumoencephalography [ˌnju:məʊenˌkefəˈlɒgrəfi] *subst.* X-ray examination of the ventricles and spaces of the brain after air has been injected into the cerebrospinal fluid by lumbar puncture *pneumoencefalografi, ventrikulografi, encefalografi, luftskalle*

> COMMENT: the air takes the place of the cerebrospinal fluid and makes it easier to photograph the ventricles clearly

pneumogastric [ˌnju:mə(ʊ)ˈgæstrɪk] *adj.* referring to the lungs and the stomach *som avser el. hör till både lungorna och magsäcken;* **pneumogastric nerve** *or* **vagus nerve** = tenth cranial nerve, which controls swallowing and nerve fibres in the heart and chest *(nervus) vagus, 10:e kranialnerven*

pneumograph [ˈnju:mə(ʊ)grɑ:f] *subst.* instrument which records chest movements during breathing *slags instrument som registrerar bröstkorgens andningsrörelser*

pneumohaemothorax [ˌnju:məʊˌhi:məʊˈθɔ:ræks] *or* **haemopneumothorax** [ˌhi:məʊˌnju:mə(ʊ)ˈθɔ:ræks] *subst.* blood *or* air in the pleural cavity *hemopneumothorax*

pneumokock ⇨ **pneumococcus**

pneumokock- ⇨ **pneumococcal**

pneumomycosis [ˌnju:mə(ʊ)maɪˈkəʊsɪs] *subst.* infection of the lungs caused by a fungus *pneumomykos*

pneumon- [ˈnju:mən, ˌ--] *or* **pneumono-** [ˈnju:mənə(ʊ), ˌ---] *prefix* referring to the lungs *pneumon(o)-, pneum(o)-, pulm(on)-, lung-*

pneumonectomy [ˌnju:mə(ʊ)ˈnektəmi] *subst.* surgical removal of all *or* part of a lung *pneum(on)ektomi, pulm(on)ektomi*

pneumonia [njʊˈməʊniə] *subst.* inflammation of a lung, where the tiny alveoli of the lung become filled with fluid *pneumoni, lunginflammation;* **he developed pneumonia and had to be hospitalized; she died of pneumonia; bacterial pneumonia** = form of pneumonia caused by pneumococcus *bakteriell lunginflammation; see also* BRONCHOPNEUMONIA; **double pneumonia** *or* **bilateral pneumonia** = pneumonia in both lungs *dubbelsidig lunginflammation;* **hypostatic pneumonia** = pneumonia caused by fluid which accumulates in the posterior bases of the lungs of a bedridden patient *pneumonia hypostatica, hypostatisk lunginflammation;* **lobar pneumonia** = pneumonia which affects one or more lobes of the lung *pneumonia lobaris, lobär lunginflammation;* **viral** *or* **virus pneumonia** = type of inflammation of the lungs caused by a virus *pneumonia virogenes, viruspneumoni*

> COMMENT: the symptoms of pneumonia are shivering, pains in the chest, high temperature and sputum brought up by coughing

pneumonic plague [njuˈmɒnɪk ˌpleɪg] *subst.* form of bubonic plague which mainly affects the lungs *lungpest*

pneumonitis [ˌnju:mə(ʊ)ˈnaɪtɪs] *subst.* inflammation of the lungs *pneumonit, disseminerad interstitiell lunginflammation*

pneumoperitoneum [ˌnju:mə(ʊ)ˌperitəˈni:əm] *subst.* air in the peritoneal cavity *pneumoperitoneum, fri gas i bukhålan*

pneumoradiography [ˌnju:mə(ʊ)ˌreɪdiˈɒgrəfi] *subst.* X-ray examination of part of the body after air *or* a gas has been inserted to make the organs show more clearly *pneumoperitoneal röntgendiagnostik*

pneumothorax [ˌnju:mə(ʊ)ˈθɔ:ræks] *or* **collapsed lung** [kəˈlæpst ˌlʌŋ] *subst.* condition where air *or* gas is in the thorax *pneumot(h)orax;* **artificial pneumothorax** = former method of treating tuberculosis, where air was introduced between the layers of the pleura to make the lung collapse *artificiell (konstgjord) pneumotorax, "gasning";* **spontaneous pneumothorax** = pneumothorax caused by a rupture of an abnormal condition on the surface of the pleura *spontan pneumotorax;* **tension pneumothorax** = pneumothorax where rupture of the pleura forms an opening like a valve, through which air is forced during coughing but cannot escape *ventilpneumotorax;* **traumatic**

pneumothorax = pneumothorax which results from damage to the lung surface *or* wall of the chest, which allows air to leak into the space between the pleurae *traumatisk pneumotorax*

-pnoea [pniːə] *suffix* referring to breathing *-pné, -andning*

PNS [ˌpiːen'es] = PERIPHERAL NERVOUS SYSTEM

pock [pɒk] *subst.* (i) localized lesion on the skin, due to smallpox *or* chickenpox *koppa;* (ii) infective focus on the membrane of a fertile egg, caused by a virus *slags infektionshärd på fertilt ägg*

pocket ['pɒkɪt] *subst.* (i) small bag attached to the inside to a coat, etc. in which money, handkerchief, keys, etc., can be kept *ficka;* (ii) cavity in the body *ficka;* **pocket of infection** = place where an infection remains *infektionsficka*

pockmark ['pɒkmɑːk] *subst.* scar left by a pustule, as in smallpox *koppärr*

pockmarked ['pɒkmɑːkt] *adj.* (face) with scars from smallpox *koppärrig*

pod- [pɒ'd, pəʊ'd] *prefix* referring to the foot *pod-, fot-*

podagra [pɒ'dægrə] = GOUT

podalic version [pəʊ'dælɪk ˌvɜːʃ(ə)n] *subst.* turning of the fetus in the womb by the feet *vändning på fot*

podiatrist [pəʊ'da(ɪ)ətrɪst] *subst. US* person who specializes in the care of the foot and its diseases *fotvårdsspecialist*

podiatry [pəʊ'da(ɪ)ətri] *subst. US* study of minor diseases and disorders of the feet *läran om fötternas sjukdomar*

-poiesis [pɔɪ'iːsɪs] *suffix* which forms *-po(i)es, -bildning*

poikilo- ['pɔɪkɪlə(ʊ), ˌ---] *prefix* meaning irregular *or* varied *poikilo-*

poikilocyte ['pɔɪkɪlə(ʊ)saɪt] *subst.* abnormally large red blood cell with an irregular shape *poikilocyt*

poikilocytosis [ˌpɔɪkɪlə(ʊ)saɪ'təʊsɪs] *subst.* condition where poilkilocytes exist in the blood *poikilocytos*

poikilothermic [ˌpɔɪkɪlə(ʊ)'θɜːmɪk] *adj.* (animal) with cold blood *or* cold-blooded (animal) *kallblodig, växelvarm; compare* HOMOIOTHERMIC

COMMENT: the body temperature of cold-blooded animals changes with the outside temperature

point [pɔɪnt] *subst.* **(a)** sharp end *spets;* **surgical needles have to have very sharp points (b)** dot used to show the division between whole numbers and parts of numbers *punkt (motsvaras på svenska av komma)*
NOTE: **3.256**: say 'three point two five six'; **his temperature was 38.7**: say 'thirty-eight point seven' **(c)** mark in a series of numbers *punkt;* **what's the freezing point of water?**

pointed ['pɔɪntɪd] *adj.* with a sharp point *spetsig;* **a pointed rod**

poison ['pɔɪz(ə)n] **1** *subst.* substance which can kill *or* harm body tissues if eaten or drunk *gift;* **he died after someone put poison in his coffee; poisons must be kept locked up; poison ivy** *or* **poison oak** = American plants whose leaves can cause a painful rash if touched *giftek, giftsumak* **2** *vb.* to give someone a poison *or* a substance which can harm or kill *förgifta;* **the workers were poisoned by toxic fumes; the wound was poisoned by bacterial infection**

COMMENT: The commonest poisons, of which even a small amount can kill, are arsenic, cyanide and strychnine. Many common foods and drugs can be poisonous if taken in large doses. Common household materials such as bleach, glue and insecticides can also be poisonous. Some types of poisoning, such as Salmonella, can be passed to other people through lack of hygienic conditions

poisoning ['pɔɪz(ə)nɪŋ] *subst.* condition where a person is made ill *or* is killed by a poisonous substance *förgiftning;* **blood poisoning** = condition where bacteria are present in blood and cause illness *septikemi, sepsis, blodförgiftning;* **Salmonella poisoning** = poisoning by Salmonellae which develop in the intestines *matförgiftning med salmonellabakterier;* **staphylococcal poisoning** = poisoning by staphylococci in food *matförgiftning med stafylokocker*

poisonous ['pɔɪz(ə)nəs] *or* **toxic** ['tɒksɪk] *adj.* (substance) which is full of poison *or* which can kill or harm *giftig, toxisk;* **some mushrooms are good to eat and some are poisonous; poisonous gas** = gas which can kill *or* which can make someone ill *giftgas*

pojke ⇨ **boy**

pol ⇨ **pole**

polar ['pəʊlə] *adj.* with a pole *polar, polär;* **polar body** = small cell which is produced from an oocyte but does not develop into an ovum *liten cell som inte utvecklas till ägg*

pole [pəʊl] *subst.* (i) end of an axis *pol;* (ii) end of a rounded organ, such as the end of a lobe in the cerebral hemisphere *pol*

poli- ['pɒlɪ, ˌ--] *or* **polio-** ['pəʊliə(ʊ), ˌ--] *prefix* referring to grey matter in the nervous system *poli(o)-*

poliklinik ⇨ **outpatient**

polio ['pəʊliəʊ] *informal see* POLIOMYELITIS

polioencephalitis [ˌpəʊliəʊenˌkefə'laɪtɪs] *subst.* type of viral encephalitis, an inflammation of the grey matter in the brain caused by the same virus as poliomyelitis *polioencefalit, polio, barnförlamning*

polioencephalomyelitis [ˌpəʊliəʊenˌkefələʊˌma(ɪ)ə'laɪtɪs] *subst.* polioencephalitis which also affects the spinal cord *polioencefalomyelit*

poliomyelitis [ˌpəʊliə(ʊ)ma(ɪ)ə'laɪtɪs] *or* **polio** ['pəʊliəʊ] *or* **infantile paralysis** [ˌɪnf(ə)ntaɪ(ə)l pə'ræləsɪs] *subst.* infection of the anterior horn cells of the spinal cord caused by a virus which attacks the motor neurones and can lead to paralysis *paralysis infantilis, poliomyelit, polio, epidemisk barnförlamning;* **abortive poliomyelitis** = mild form of poliomyelitis which only affects the throat and intestines *abortiv poliomyelit;* **bulbar poliomyelitis** = poliomyelitis which affects a patient's breathing and swallowing *bulbär poliomyelit (paralys);* **nonparalytic poliomyelitis** = form of poliomyelitis similar to the abortive form but which also affects the muscles to a certain degree *polio utan förlamning;* **paralytic poliomyelitis** = poliomyelitis which affects the patient's muscles *polio med förlamning*

COMMENT: symptoms of poliomyelitis are paralysis of the limbs, fever and stiffness in the neck. The bulbar form may start with difficulty in swallowing. Poliomyelitis can be prevented by immunization and two vaccines are used: the Sabin vaccine is formed of live polio virus and is taken orally on a piece of sugar; Salk vaccine is given as an injection of dead virus

poliomyelitvirus ⇨ **poliovirus**

poliovirus [ˌpəʊliəʊ'vaɪ(ə)rəs] *subst.* virus which causes poliomyelitis *poliovirus, poliomyelitvirus*

Politzer bag ['pɒlɪtsə bæg] *subst.* rubber bag which is used to blow air into the middle ear to unblock a Eustachian tube *slags gummituta*

pollen ['pɒlən] *subst.* tiny cells from flowers which float in the air in spring and summer, and which cause hay fever *pollen;* **pollen count** = figure which shows the amount of pollen in a sample of air *pollenräkning, pollenrapport*

pollenrapport ⇨ **pollen**

pollenräkning ⇨ **pollen**

pollex ['pɒleks] *subst.* thumb *pollex, tummen*
NOTE: the plural is **pollices**

pollinosis [ˌpɒlə'nəʊsɪs] = HAY FEVER

pollutant [pə'lu:t(ə)nt] *subst.* substance which pollutes *förorening*

pollute [pə'lu:t] *vb.* to make the air *or* a river *or* the sea dirty, especially with industrial waste *förorena, smutsa (smitta) ned*

pollution [pə'lu:ʃ(ə)n] *subst.* making dirty *förorening, nedsmutsning, miljöförstöring;* **atmospheric pollution** = pollution of the air *luftförorening*

pollution ⇨ **emission**

poly- ['pɒli, ˌ--] *prefix* meaning many *or* much *or* touching many organs *poly-*

polyarteritis nodosa [ˌpɒliˌɑ:tə'raɪtɪs nə'dəʊsə] *or* **periarteritis nodosa** [ˌperiˌɑ:tə'raɪtɪs nə'dəʊsə] *subst.* collagen disease where the walls of the arteries in various parts of the body become inflamed, leading to asthma, high blood pressure and kidney failure *polyarteritis (periarteritis) nodosa*

polyarthritis [ˌpɒliɑ:'θraɪtɪs] *subst.* inflammation of several joints, such as rheumatoid arthritis *polyartrit*

polyartrit ⇨ **polyarthritis**

polycystitis [ˌpɒlisɪ'staɪtɪs] *subst.* congenital disease where several cysts form in the kidney at the same time *ren cysticus, cystnjure*

polycytemi ⇨ **polycythaemia**

polycythaemia [ˌpɒlisaɪˈθiːmiə] *subst.* blood disease where the number of red blood cells increases, often due to difficulties which the patient has in breathing *polycytemi;* **polycythaemia vera** *or* **erythraemia** = blood disease where the number of red blood cells increases, together with an increase in the number of white blood cells, making the blood thicker and slowing its flow *polycythaemia (rubra) vera, eryt(h)remi*

polydactylism [ˌpɒliˈdæktɪlɪz(ə)m] *or* **hyperdactylism** [ˌhaɪpəˈdæktɪlɪz(ə)m] *subst.* condition where a person has more than five fingers or toes *polydaktyli, hyperdaktyli*

polydipsia [ˌpɒliˈdɪpsiə] *subst.* condition (often caused by diabetes insipidus) where the patient is abnormally thirsty *polydipsi*

polyfagi ⇨ **polyphagia**

polyfarmaci ⇨ **polypharmacy**

polyfarmakoterapi ⇨ **polypharmacy**

polygraph [ˈpɒligrɑːf] *subst.* instrument which records the pulse in several parts of the body at the same time *slags instrument för pulsregistrering*

polymorfkärnig ⇨ **neutrophil**

polymorfonukleär ⇨ **neutrophil**

polymorph [ˈpɒlimɔːf] *or* **neutrophil** [ˈnjuːtrəfil] *subst.* type of leucocyte *or* white blood cell with an irregular nucleus *polymorfkärnig (polymorfonukleär) leukocyt (vit blodkropp), neutrofil leukocyt*

polymyalgia rheumatica [ˌpɒlimaɪˈældʒə ruˌmætɪkə] *subst.* disease of elderly people where the patient has pain and stiffness in the shoulder and hip muscles making them weak and sensitive *polymyalgia rheumatica, reumatisk polymyalgi*

polyneuritis [ˌpɒlinju(ə)ˈraɪtɪs] *subst.* inflammation of many nerves *polyneurit*

polyneuropathy [ˌpɒlinju(ə)ˈrɒpəθi] *subst.* any disease which affects several nerves *polyneuropati*

polyopia [ˌpɒliˈəʊpiə] *or* **polyopsia** [ˌpɒliˈɒpsiə] *or* **polyopy** [ˈpɒliəʊpi] *subst.* condition where the patient sees several images of one object at the same time *polyop(s)i, dubbelseende; compare* DIPLOPIA

polyp [ˈpɒlɪp] *or* **polypus** [ˈpɒlɪpəs] *subst.* tumour, growing on a stalk in mucous membrane, which can be cauterized, often found in the nose, mouth or throat *polyp*
NOTE: plural of **polypus** is **polypi**

polypeptide [ˌpɒliˈpeptaɪd] *subst.* type of protein formed of linked amino acids *polypeptid*

polyper (bakom näsan) ⇨ **adenoids, polyp**

polyphagia [ˌpɒliˈfeɪdʒə] *subst.* (i) condition where a patient eats too much *polyfagi, frosseri;* (ii) morbid desire for every kind of food *polyfagi, sjukligt matbegär*

polypharmacy [ˌpɒliˈfɑːməsi] *subst.* prescribing several drugs to be taken at the same time *polyfarmaci, polyfarmakoterapi*

polyploid [ˈpɒliplɔɪd] *adj.* (cell) where there are more than three sets of the haploid number of chromosomes *polyploid; compare* DIPLOID, HAPLOID

polyposis [ˌpɒliˈpəʊsɪs] *subst.* condition where many polyps form in the mucous membrane of the colon *polypos*

polypus [ˈpɒlɪpəs] = POLYP

polyradiculitis [ˌpɒliræˌdɪkjuˈlaɪtɪs] *subst.* disease of the nervous system which affects the roots of the nerves *polyradikulit*

polysaccharide [ˌpɒliˈsækəraɪd] *subst.* type of carbohydrate *polysackarid*

polyserositis [ˌpɒliˌsɪərəʊˈsaɪtɪs] *subst.* inflammation of the membranes lining the abdomen, chest and joints and exudation of serous fluid *polyserosit*

polyspermi ⇨ **polyspermia, spermatorrhoea**

polyspermia [ˌpɒliˈspɜːmiə] *or* **polyspermism** [ˌpɒliˈspɜːmɪz(ə)m] *or* **polyspermy** [ˌpɒliˈspɜːmi] *subst.* (i) excessive seminal secretion *polyspermi, spermatorré, även ofrivillig sädesavgång;* (ii) fertilization of one ovum by several spermatozoa *polyspermi*

polyunsaturated fat [ˌpɒliʌnˈsætʃəreɪtɪd ˌfæt] *subst.* fatty acid capable of absorbing more hydrogen (typical of vegetable and fish oils) *fleromättat fett*

polyuria [ˌpɒliˈjʊəriə] *subst.* condition where a patient passes a large quantity of urine, usually as a result of diabetes insipidus *polyuri*

polär ⇨ **polar**

pompholyx ['pɒmfɒlɪks] *subst.* (i) type of eczema with many irritating little blisters on the hands and feet *pompholyx;* (ii) morbid skin condition with bulbous swellings *hudsjukdom med blåsor, blåsdermatos, pemfigus*

pons [pɒnz] *subst.* (i) tissue which joins parts of an organ *brygga, bro;* (ii) part of the hindbrain, formed of fibres which continue the medulla oblongata ⇨ *illustration* BRAIN *pons (Varolii), commissura cerebelli, hjärnbryggan*

pontine ['pɒntaɪn] *subst.* referring to a pons *pontin;* **pontine cistern** = subarachnoid space in front of the pons, containing the basilar artery *cisterna pontis*

poor [pʊə] *adj.* not very good *dålig, klen, svag;* **he's in poor health; she suffers from poor circulation**

poorly ['pʊəli] *adj. (informal)* not very well *dålig, klen, svag;* **her mother has been quite poorly recently; he felt poorly and stayed in bed**

POP [ˌpi:əʊ'pi:] = PROGESTERONE ONLY PILL

popeyes ['pɒpˌaɪz] *subst. US* protruding eyes *utstående ögon*

popliteal [ˌpɒplɪ'ti:əl] *adj.* referring to the back of the knee *knävecks-;* **popliteal artery** = artery which branches from the femoral artery behind the knee and leads into the tibial arteries *arteria poplitea, knävecksartären;* **popliteal fossa** *or* **popliteal space** = space behind the knee between the hamstring and the calf muscle *fossa poplitea, knävecksgropen, knävecket*

popliteus [ˌpɒp'lɪtiəs] *or* **popliteal muscle** [ˌpɒplɪ'ti:əl ˌmʌs(ə)l] *subst.* muscle at the back of the knee *musculus popliteus, knävecksmuskeln*

population [ˌpɒpju'leɪʃ(ə)n] *subst.* **(a)** number of people living in a country *or* town *population, befolkning;* **population statistics show that the birth rate is slowing down; the government has decided to screen the whole population of the area (b)** number of patients in hospital *de intagna (på sjukhus);* **the hospital population in the area has fallen below ten thousand**

por ⇨ **osculum, pore**

pore [pɔ:] *subst.* (i) tiny hole in the skin through which the sweat passes *por;* (ii) small communicating passage between cavities ⇨ *illustration* SKIN & SENSORY RECEPTORS *öppning, mynning*

porencephaly [ˌpɔ:ren'kef(ə)li] *or* **porencephalia** [ˌpɔ:renkə'feɪliə] *or* **porencephalus** [ˌpɔ:ren'kef(ə)ləs] *subst.* abnormal cysts in the cerebral cortex, as a result of defective development *porencefali*

porfyri ⇨ **porphyria**

porfyrin ⇨ **porphyrin**

porfyrinuri ⇨ **porphyrinuria**

pormask ⇨ **blackhead**

porous ['pɔ:rəs] *adj.* (i) containing pores *porös;* (ii) (tissue) which allows fluid to pass through *genomsläpplig för vätska;* **porous bone surrounds the Eustachian tubes**

porphyria [ˌpɔ:'fɪriə] *subst.* hereditary disease affecting the metabolism of porphyrin pigments *porfyri*

> COMMENT: porphyria causes abdominal pains and attacks of mental confusion. The skin becomes sensitive to light and the urine becomes coloured and turns dark brown when exposed to the light

porphyrin ['pɔ:f(ə)rɪn] *subst.* family of biological pigments (the commonest is protoporphyrin IX) *porfyrin*

porphyrinuria [ˌpɔ:fɪrɪ'njʊəriə] *subst.* presence of excess porphyrins in the urine, a sign of porphyria or of metal poisoning *porfyrinuri*

porta ['pɔ:tə] *subst.* opening which allows blood vessels to pass into an organ *porta, port;* **porta hepatis** = opening in the liver through which the hepatic artery, hepatic duct and portal vein pass *porta hepatis, leverporten*

porta- ⇨ **portal**

portable ['pɔ:təb(ə)l] *adj.* which can be carried *bärbar, flyttbar, lös;* **he keeps a portable first aid kit in his car; the ambulance team carried a portable blood testing unit**

porta-cavaanastomos ⇨ **portocaval**

porta-cavashunt ⇨ **portocaval**

portal ['pɔ:t(ə)l] *adj.* referring to a porta, especially the portal system *or* the portal vein *portal, porta-;* **portal hypertension** = high pressure in the portal vein, caused by cirrhosis of the liver or a clot in the vein, causing internal bleeding *portal hypertension; see also* BANTI'S SYNDROME; **portal pyaemia** = infection of the portal vein in the liver, giving abscesses *slags infektion av portådern;* **portal system** = group of veins which have capillaries at both ends and do not go to the heart, such as the portal vein *portasystemet;* **portal vein** = vein which takes blood from the stomach, pancreas, gall bladder, intestines and spleen to the liver *vena portae, portvenen, portådern*

portasystemet ⇨ **portal**

porter ['pɔːtə] *subst.* person who does general work in a hospital, such as wheeling a patient's trolley into the operating theatre, moving heavy equipment, etc. *vaktmästare, "bärare"*

portocaval [ˌpɔːtəʊ'keɪv(ə)l] *adj.* linking the portal vein to the inferior vena cava *som förbinder portådern med nedre hålvenen;* **portocaval anastomosis** = surgical operation to join the portal vein to the inferior vena cava *porta-cavaanastomos;* **portocaval shunt** = artificial passage made between the portal vein and the inferior vena cava to relieve portal hypertension *porta-cavashunt*

porto-systemic encephalopathy [ˌpɔːtəʊsɪˌstiːmɪk enˌkefə'lɒpəθi] *subst.* mental disorder and coma caused by liver disorder due to portal hypertension *encefalopati pga högt tryck i portådern*
NOTE: for terms referring to the portal vein see words beginning with **pyl-** or **pyle-**

portvenen ⇨ **portal**

portvens- ⇨ **pyl-**

port wine stain ['pɔːt waɪn ˌsteɪn] *subst.* naevus *or* purple birthmark *naevus flammeus (vasculosus), eldsmärke*

portådern ⇨ **portal**

porös ⇨ **porous, spongy**

position [pə'zɪʃ(ə)n] **1** *subst.* **(a)** place (where something is) *position, plats, läge;* **the exact position of the tumour is located by an X-ray (b)** the way a patient stands *or* sits *or* lies *ställning, kroppsläge;* **genupectoral position** = kneeling with the chest on the floor *knäbröstläge;* **lithotomy position** = lying on the back with the hips and knees bent *litotomiläge, gynekologläge;* **recovery position** *or* **semiprone position** = lying face downwards, with one knee and one arm bent forwards, and the face turned to one side *framstupa sidoläge; see also* TRENDELENBURG'S **2** *vb.* to place in a certain position *placera;* **the fetus is correctly positioned in the uterus**

positive ['pɒzətɪv] *adj.* which indicates the answer "yes" *or* which shows the presence of something *positiv;* **her cervical smear was positive** *or* **she gave a positive test for cervical cancer; positive end-expiratory pressure (PEEP)** = forcing the patient to breathe through a mask in cases where fluid has collected in the lungs *positivt ändexspiratoriskt tryck, PEEP;* **positive feedback** = situation where the result of a process stimulates the process which caused it *positiv feedback;* **positive pressure ventilation (PPV)** = forcing air into the lungs to encourage the lungs to expand *övertrycksventilation;* **positive pressure respirator** = machine which forces air into a patient's lungs through a tube inserted in the mouth *respirator för övertrycksventilation*

positively ['pɒzətɪvli] *adv.* in a positive way *positivt;* **she reacted positively to the test**

positivt ⇨ **positively**

posology [pə(ʊ)'sɒlədʒi] *subst.* study of doses of medicine *posologi*

posseting ['pɒsɪtɪŋ] *subst. (in babies)* bringing up small quantities of curdled milk into the mouth after feeding *uppstötning av koagulerad mjölk efter amning*

Possum ['pɒs(ə)m] *subst.* device using electronic switches which helps a severely paralysed patient to work a machine such as a telephone or typewriter *slags elektroniskt hjälpmedel för handikappade*
NOTE: the name is derived from the first letters of **Patient-Operated Selector Mechanism**

post- ['pəʊst, ˌ-] *prefix* meaning after *or* later *post-, efter-, bakre*

postcentral gyrus [ˌpəʊst'sentr(ə)l ˌdʒaɪ(ə)rəs] *subst.* sensory area of the cerebral cortex, which receives impulses from receptor cells and senses pain, heat, touch, etc. *gyrus postcentralis, bakre hjärnvindlingen*

post-cibal [ˌpəʊst'saɪb(ə)l] *adj.* after having eaten food *postcibal, postprandial, efter måltid*

postconcussional [ˌpəʊstkən'kʌʃ(ə)n(ə)l] *adj.* (symptoms) which follow after a patient has had concussion *efter hjärnskakning*

post-epileptic [ˌpəʊstˌepɪˈleptɪk] *adj.* after an epileptic fit *efter epileptiskt anfall*

posterior [pɒˈstɪəriə] *adj.* at the back *posterior, bakre;* **the cerebellum is posterior to the medulla oblongata; posterior chamber (of the eye)** = part of the aqueous chamber which is behind the iris *camera posterior bulbi, bakre ögonkammaren;* **posterior synechia** = condition of the eye where the iris sticks to the anterior surface of the lens *bakre syneki*

posteriorly [pɒˈstɪəriəli] *adv.* behind *bakom;* **an artery leads to a posteriorly placed organ; rectal biopsy specimens are best taken posteriorly**
NOTE: the opposite is **anterior**

postganglionic [ˌpəʊstˌgæŋliˈɒnɪk] *adj.* placed after a ganglion *postganglionär;* **postganglionic fibre** = axon of a nerve cell which starts in a ganglion and extends beyond the ganglion *postganglionär tråd, axon;* **postganglionic neurone** = neurone which starts in a ganglion and ends in a gland *or* unstriated muscle *postganglionärt neuron, postganglionär nervcell*

posthepatic [ˌpəʊsthɪˈpætɪk] *adj.* after the liver *retrohepatisk;* **posthepatic bilirubin** = bilirubin which enters the plasma after being treated by the liver *plasmabilirubin efter passagen genom levern;* **posthepatic jaundice** *or* **obstructive jaundice** = jaundice caused by an obstruction in the bile ducts *icterus obstructivus, obstruktionsikterus, stasikterus, mekanisk ikterus*

post herpetic neuralgia [ˌpəʊst həˈpetɪk njuˌ(ə)ˈrældʒə] *subst.* pains felt after an attack of shingles *smärta efter bältros(anfall)*

posthitis [pɒsˈθaɪtɪs] *subst.* inflammation of the foreskin *postit*

posthumous [ˈpɒstjʊməs] *adj.* after death *postum;* **posthumous birth** = (i) birth of a baby after the death of the father *födelse efter faderns död;* (ii) birth of a baby by Caesarean section after the mother has died *födelse med hjälp av kejsarsnitt efter moderns död*

post-irradiation [ˌpəʊstˌɪriˈdeɪʃ(ə)n] *adj.* (pain *or* disorder) caused by X-rays *efter strålning (röntgen)*

postmature baby [ˌpəʊstməˈtʃʊə ˌbeɪbi] *subst.* baby born more than nine months after conception *postmaturt barn, överburet barn*

postmaturity [ˌpəʊstməˈtʃʊərəti] *subst.* pregnancy which lasts longer than nine months *postmaturitet, överburenhet*

postmenopausal [ˌpəʊstˌmenəʊˈpɔːz(ə)l] *adj.* after the menopause *postmenopausal;* **she experienced some postmenopausal bleeding**

post mortem [ˌpəʊst ˈmɔːtəm] *subst.* examination of a dead body by a pathologist to find out the cause of death *obduktion;* **the post mortem (examination) showed that he had been poisoned**

postnasal [ˌpəʊstˈneɪz(ə)l] *subst.* behind the nose *postnasal, bakom näsan;* **postnasal drip** = condition where mucus from the nose runs down into the throat and is swallowed *tillstånd då snuvan rinner bakåt ned i svalget*

postnatal [ˌpəʊstˈneɪt(ə)l] *adj.* after the birth of a child *postnatal, efter födelsen (förlossningen);* **postnatal depression** = depression which sometimes affects a woman after childbirth *postnatal depression*

postnecrotic cirrhosis [ˌpəʊstneˈkrɒtɪk səˈrəʊsɪs] *subst.* cirrhosis of the liver caused by viral hepatitis *postnekrotisk cirros*

postoperativ blödning ⇨ **reactive**

postoperative [ˌpəʊstˈɒp(ə)rətɪv] *adj.* after an operation *postoperativ;* **the patient has suffered postoperative nausea and vomiting; occlusion may appear as postoperative angina pectoris; the second postoperative day** = the second day after an operation *andra dagen efter operationen;* **postoperative pain** = pain felt by a patient after an operation *postoperativ smärta*

postpartum [ˌpəʊstˈpɑːtəm] *or* **postnatal** [ˌpəʊstˈneɪt(ə)l] *adj.* after the birth of a child *postpartum, p.p., postnatal, efter förlossningen (födelsen);* **postpartum haemorrhage (PPH)** = heavy bleeding after childbirth *kraftig blödning efter förlossningen*

postprandial [ˌpəʊstˈprændiəl] *adj.* after eating a meal *postprandial, postcibal, efter måltid*

post-primary tuberculosis [ˌpəʊstˈpraɪməri tjuˌbɜːkjuˈləʊsɪs] *subst.* reappearance of tuberculosis in a patient who has been infected with it before *postprimär (sekundär) tuberkulos*

postsynaptic [ˌpəʊstsɪˈnæptɪk] *adj.* after a synapse *postsynaptisk;* **postsynaptic axon =**

nerve leaving one side of a synapse *postsynaptiskt axon*

postum ⇨ **posthumous**

postural ['pɒstʃ(ə)r(ə)l] *adj.* referring to posture *postural, hållnings-, kroppsställnings-;* **a study of postural disorders; postural drainage** = removing matter from infected lungs by making the patient lie down with his head lower than his feet, so that he can cough more easily *dränagebehandling*

posture ['pɒstʃə] *subst.* way of standing *or* sitting *postura, hållning, kroppsställning;* **bad posture can cause pain in the back; she has to do exercises to correct her bad posture** *or* **she has to do posture exercises** NOTE: no plural

postviral [ˌpəʊst'vaɪ(ə)r(ə)l] *adj.* after a virus *postviral;* **postviral fatigue syndrome** = condition where the patient has weakness in the muscles and cannot work after having had a virus infection *(muskel)svaghet efter virusinfektion, kroniskt trötthetssyndrom, yuppie disease m.fl. namn*

potassium [pə'tæsiəm] *subst.* metallic element *kalium, K* NOTE: chemical symbol is **K**

potassium permanganate [pə'tæsiəm pə'mæŋgəneɪt] *subst.* purple-coloured poisonous salt, used as a disinfectant *kaliumpermanganat*

potträning ⇨ **toilet training**

Pott's disease ['pɒts dɪˌzi:z] *or* **Pott's caries** [ˌpɒts 'keərɪz] *subst.* tuberculosis of the spine, causing paralysis *Potts sjukdom (puckel)*

Pott's fracture [ˌpɒts 'fræktʃə] *subst.* fracture of the lower end of the fibula together with displacement of the ankle and foot outwards *Potts fraktur*

pouch [paʊtʃ] *subst.* small sack *or* pocket attached to an organ *säck, ficka, pung;* **brachial pouch** = pouch on the the side of the neck of an embryo *gälspringan*

poultice ['pəʊltɪs] *or* **fomentation** [ˌfəʊmen'teɪʃ(ə)n] *subst.* compress made of hot water and flour paste *or* other substances which is pressed on to an infected part to draw out pus *or* to relieve pain *or* to encourage the circulation *foment, grötomslag, varmt omslag*

pound [paʊnd] *subst.* measure of weight (about 450 grams) *slags viktmått (i Storbritannien c 454 gram);* **the baby weighed only four pounds at birth**
NOTE: with numbers **pound** is usually written **lb; the baby weighs 6lb**

Poupart's ligament [pu'pɑ:ts ˌlɪgəmənt] *or* **inguinal ligament** ['ɪŋgwɪn(ə)l ˌlɪgəmənt] *subst.* ligament in the groin, running from the spine to the pubis *ligamentum inguinale, Pouparts ligament, ljumskbandet*

powder ['paʊdə] *subst.* medicine like fine dry dust made from particles of drugs *pulver, puder;* **he took a powder to help his indigestion** *or* **he took an indigestion powder**

powdered ['paʊdəd] *adj.* crushed so that it forms a fine dry dust *pulveriserad, i pulverform;* **the medicine is available in tablets or in powdered form**

pox [pɒks] *subst.* (i) old name for syphilis *tidigare syfilis;* (ii) disease with eruption of vesicles *or* pustules *sjukdom med vesikler el. pustler*

poxvirus [pɒks'vaɪ(ə)rəs] *subst.* any of a group of viruses, such as those which cause cowpox and smallpox *poxvirus*

> QUOTE Molluscum contagiosum is a harmless skin infection caused by a poxvirus that affects mainly children and young adults
> **British Medical Journal**

p.p. ⇨ **postpartum**

PPD [ˌpi:pi:'di:] = PURIFIED PROTEIN DERIVATIVE

PPH [ˌpi:pi:'eɪtʃ] = POSTPARTUM HAEMORRHAGE

p-piller ⇨ **oral, pill**

PPV [ˌpi:pi:'vi:] = POSITIVE PRESSURE VENTILATION

p.r. [ˌpi:'ɑ:] *abbreviation for Latin phrase* "per rectum": examination by the rectum *per rektum, PR, p.r.*

practice ['præktɪs] *subst.* **(a)** patients of a doctor *or* dentist *läkares el. tandläkares patienter;* work of a doctor *or* dentist *praktik, mottagning;* **he has been in practice for six years; after qualifying he joined his father's practice; general practice** = doctor's practice where patients from an area are treated for all types of disease *allmän praktik;* **he left the hospital and went into general practice; she is in general practice in the North of London** *or* **she has a general practice in**

North London; group practice = medical practice where several doctors *or* dentists share the same office building and support services *ung. läkargrupp med gemensam praktik, läkarhus;* **practice leaflet** = leaflet produced by the doctors in a practice, giving details of the telephone numbers, hours when the surgery is open, etc. *reklamblad för läkarpraktik;* **practice nurse** = nurse employed by a clinic *or* doctor's practice who can give advice to patients *sjuksköterska med rådgivande funktion, ung. mottagningssköterska* **(b)** actual working *praktiken;* **it's a good idea, but will it work in practice?**

> QUOTE practice nurses play a major role in the care of patients with chronic disease and they undertake many preventive procedures. Patients presenting with symtoms of urinary tract infection were recruited in a general practice survey
> **Journal of the Royal College of General Practitioners**

practise ['præktɪs] *vb.* to work as a doctor *praktisera, utöva, vara verksam (som);* **he practises in North London; she practises homeopathy; a doctor must be registered before he can practise**

practitioner [præk'tɪʃ(ə)nə] *subst.* doctor *or* qualified person who practises *praktiker, praktiserande läkare;* **general practitioner (GP)** = doctor who treats many patients in an area for all types of illness and does not specialize *allmänpraktiker, allmänpraktiserande läkare;* **nurse practitioner** = (i) nurse employed by a clinic *or* doctor's practice who can give advice to patients *sjuksköterska med rådgivande funktion, ung. mottagningssköterska;* (ii); *US* trained nurse who has not been licensed *sjuksköterska som saknar legitimation;* **ophthalmic practitioner** = qualified person who specializes in testing eyes and prescribing lenses *ung. legitimerad optiker*

praecox ['pri:kɒks] *see* DEMENTIA, EJACULATIO

praevia ['pri:viə] *see* PLACENTA

praktik ⇨ **practice**

praktiken ⇨ **practice**

praktiker ⇨ **practitioner**

pre- ['pri:, ,-, prɪ'] *prefix* meaning before *or* in front of *pre-, för(e)-, främre;* **pre-anaesthetic round** = examination of patients by the surgeon before they are anaesthetized *premedicineringsrond*

precancer [,pri:'kænsə] *subst.* growth *or* cell which is not malignant but which may become cancerous *förstadium till cancer*

precancerous [,pri:'kæns(ə)rəs] *adj.* (growth) which is not malignant now, but which can become cancerous later *precancerös*

precaution [prɪ'kɔ:ʃ(ə)n] *subst.* action taken before something happens *försiktighetsåtgärd, säkerhetsåtgärd;* **she took the tablets as a precaution against seasickness; to take safety precautions** = to do things which will make yourself safe *vidta försiktighetsåtgärder (säkerhetsåtgärder)*

precede [prɪ'si:d] *vb.* to happen before *or* earlier *föregå;* **the attack was preceded by a sudden rise in body temperature**

precentral gyrus [,pri:'sentr(ə)l dʒaɪ(ə)rəs] *subst.* motor area of the cerebral cortex *gyrus precentralis, främre hjärnvindlingen*

precipitate 1 [prɪ'sɪpɪtət, prɪ'sɪpɪteɪt] *subst.* substance which is precipitated during a chemical reaction *precipitat, fällning, utfällning* **2** [prɪ'sɪpɪteɪt] *vb.* **(a)** to make a substance separate from a chemical compound and fall to the bottom of a liquid during a chemical reaction *fälla (ut);* **casein is precipitated when milk comes into contact with an acid (b)** to make something start suddenly *plötsligt framkalla, påskynda*

> QUOTE it has been established that myocardial infarction and sudden coronary death are precipitated in the majority of patients by thrombus formation in the coronary arteries
> **British Journal of Hospital Medicine**

precipitation [prɪ,sɪpɪ'teɪʃ(ə)n] *subst.* action of forming a precipitate *fällning, utfällning*

precipitin [prɪ'sɪpɪtɪn] *subst.* antibody which reacts to an antigen and forms a precipitate, used in many diagnostic tests *precipitin*

precis ⇨ **exact, precise**

precise [prɪ'saɪs] *adj.* very exact *or* correct *precis, exakt, noggrann;* **the instrument can give precise measurements of changes in heartbeat**

preclinical [,pri:'klɪnɪk(ə)l] *adj.* **(a)** before diagnosis *preklinisk, före diagnosen;* **the preclinical stage of an infection (b)** first part of a medical course, before the students are allowed to examine real patients *preklinisk, ung. före med. kand.*; **a preclinical student**

precocious [prɪ'kəʊʃəs] *adj.* more physically *or* mentally developed than is normal for a certain age *brådmogen, lillgammal*

precocity [prɪ'kɒsəti] *subst.* being precocious *brådmogenhet*

precordial [ˌpriː'kɔːdiəl] *adj.* referring to the precordium *prekordial, bröst-*

precordium [ˌpriː'kɔːdiəm] *subst.* part of the thorax over the heart *prekordiet, hjärttrakten*

precursor [prɪ'kɜːsə] *subst.* substance *or* cell from which another substance *or* cell is developed *föregångare, förelöpare*

predict [prɪ'dɪkt] *vb.* to say what will happen in the future *förutsäga, förutspå*; **doctors are predicting a rise in cases of whooping cough**

prediction [prɪ'dɪkʃ(ə)n] *subst.* saying what you expect will happen in the future *förutsägelse*; **the Health Ministry's prediction of a rise in cases of hepatitis B**

predictive [prɪ'dɪktɪv] *adj.* which predicts *som förutsäger (förutspår)*; **the predictive value of a test** = the accuracy of the test in predicting a medical condition *ett provs förmåga att förutsäga ngt*

predigested food [ˌpriːdaɪ'dʒestɪd ˌfuːd] *subst.* food which has undergone predigestion *föda där matspjälkningsprocessen satts igång, "lättsmält" mat*

predigestion [ˌpriːdaɪ'dʒestʃ(ə)n] *subst.* artificial starting of the digestive process before food is eaten *konstgjord igångsättning av matspjälkningsprocessen hos föda*

predisposed to [ˌpriːdɪ'spəʊzd tʊ] *adj.* with a tendency to *predisponerad (mottaglig, med anlag) för*; **all the members of the family are predisposed to vascular diseases**

predisposition [ˌpriːˌdɪspə'zɪʃ(ə)n] *subst.* tendency *disposition, mottaglighet, anlag*; **she has a predisposition to obesity**

predominant [prɪ'dɒmɪnənt] *adj.* which is more powerful than others *dominant, dominerande, övervägande, förhärskande*

pre-eclampsia [ˌpriːɪ'klæmpsiə] *subst.* condition of pregnant women towards the end of the pregnancy, which may lead to eclampsia *preeklampsi*; **early onset pre-eclampsia** = pre-eclampsia which appears before 37 weeks' gestation *tidigt insättande preeklampsi*

> COMMENT: symptoms are high blood pressure, oedema and protein in the urine

preemie ['priːmi] *subst. US informal* premature infant *prematurt barn*

prefrontal [ˌpriː'frʌnt(ə)l] *adj.* in the front part of the frontal lobe *prefrontal, i främre delen av pannloben*; **prefrontal leucotomy** = operation to divide some of the white matter in the prefrontal lobe, formerly used as a treatment for schizophrenia *prefrontal lobotomi*; **prefrontal lobe** = part of the brain in the front part of each hemisphere, in front of the frontal lobe, which is concerned with memory and learning *främre delen av pannloben*

preganglionic [ˌpriːˌæŋglɪ'ɒnɪk] *adj.* near to and in front of a ganglion *preganglionär*; **preganglionic fibre** = nerve fibre which ends in a ganglion where it is linked in a synapse to a postganglionic fibre *preganglionär tråd*; **preganglionic neurone** = neurone which ends in a ganglion *preganglionärt neuron, preganglionär nervcell*

pregnancy ['pregnənsi] *subst.* (i) time between conception and childbirth when a woman is carrying the unborn child in her womb *graviditetstid*; (ii) condition of being pregnant *gestation, graviditet, havandeskap, grossess*; **extrauterine** *or* **ectopic pregnancy** = pregnancy where the embryo develops outside the uterus, usually in one of the Fallopian tubes *X, extrauterin (ektopisk) graviditet, utomkvedshavandeskap*; **multiple pregnancy** = pregnancy where the mother is going to give birth to more than one child *flerbördsgraviditet*; **phantom pregnancy** *or* **pseudocyesis** = psychological condition where a woman has all the symptoms of pregnancy without being pregnant *skengraviditet*; **unwanted pregnancy** = condition where a woman becomes pregnant without wanting to have a child *oönskad graviditet*; **pregnancy-associated hypertension** = high blood pressure which is associated with pregnancy *högt blodtryck i samband med graviditet*; **pregnancy test** = test to see if a woman is pregnant or not *graviditetstest*

pregnant ['pregnənt] *adj.* (woman) with an unborn child in her uterus *gravid, havande*; **she is six months pregnant**

prehepatic [ˌpriːhɪ'pætɪk] *adj.* before the liver *prehepatisk, före levern*; **prehepatic bilirubin** = bilirubin in plasma before it passes through the liver *plasmabilirubin före* *passagen genom levern;* **prehepatic jaundice** = jaundice which occurs because of haemolysis before the blood reaches the liver *icterus haemolyticus, hemolytisk ikterus*

preklinisk ⇨ **preclinical**

prekordial ⇨ **precordial**

prekordiet ⇨ **precordium**

preliminär ⇨ **provisional**

preliminärt ⇨ **provisionally**

prematur ⇨ **premature, preterm**

premature ['premətʃə] *adj.* early *or* before the normal time *prematur, förtidig, underburen;* **the baby was born five weeks premature; premature baby** = baby born earlier than 37 weeks from conception, or weighing less than 2.5 kilos, but capable of independent life *prematurt (för tidigt fött, underburet) barn;* **premature beat** *or* **ectopic beat** = abnormal extra beat of the heart which can be caused by caffeine or other stimulants *ektopiskt hjärtslag, för tidigt utlöst hjärtslag;* **premature birth** = birth of a baby earlier than 37 weeks from conception *partus praematurus, för tidig födelse (förlossning), förtidsbörd;* **premature ejaculation** = situation where a man ejaculates too early during sexual intercourse *ejaculatio praecox, förtidig sädesavgång;* **premature labour** = starting to give birth earlier than 37 weeks from conception *prematura värkar;* **after the accident she went into premature labour**

> COMMENT: babies can survive even if born several weeks premature. Even babies weighing less than one kilo at birth can survive in an incubator, and develop normally

prematurely ['premətʃəli] *adv.* early *or* before the normal time *för tidigt, i förtid;* **the baby was born two weeks prematurely; a large number of people die prematurely from ischaemic heart disease**

prematuritet ⇨ **prematurity**

prematurity [ˌpremə'tʃʊərəti] *subst.* situation where something occurs early, before the normal time *prematuritet, underburenhet, underutveckling*

prematurt barn ⇨ **preemie**

premed [ˌpriː'med] *subst. informal* stage of being given premedication *premedicinering,* **the patient is in premed**

premedication [ˌpriːˌmedɪ'keɪʃ(ə)n] *subst.* drug (such as a sedative) given to a patient before an operation begins to block the parasympathetic nervous system and prevent vomiting during the operation *premedicinering*

premedicinering ⇨ **premed, premedication, pre-op**

premedicineringsrond ⇨ **pre-**

premenstrual [ˌpriː'menstru(ə)l] *adj.* before menstruation *premenstruell;* **premenstrual tension (PMT)** = nervous stress experienced by a woman during the period before menstruation starts *premenstruell spänning*

premolar [ˌpriː'məʊlə] *subst.* tooth with two points, situated between the canines and the first proper molar ⇨ *illustration* TEETH *dens premolaris, premolar, främre kindtand*

prenatal [ˌpriː'neɪt(ə)l] *adj.* before birth *prenatal, antenatal, foster-;* **prenatal diagnosis** *or* **antenatal diagnosis** = medical examination of a pregnant woman to see if the fetus is developing normally *prenataldiagnostik, fosterdiagnostik*

prenataldiagnostik ⇨ **prenatal**

pre-op [ˌpriː'ɒp] *abbreviation* PREOPERATIVE

preoperative [ˌpriː'ɒp(ə)rətɪv] *adj.* before a surgical operation *preop(erativ);* **preoperative medication** = drug (such as a sedative) given to a patient before an operation begins *premedicinering*

prep [prep] *subst. & vb. informal* getting a patient ready before an operation *operationsförberedelser, förbereda för operation;* **the prep is finished, so the patient can be taken to the operating theatre; has the patient been prepped?**

preparat ⇨ **preparation, section, slice, specimen**

preparation [ˌprepə'reɪʃ(ə)n] *subst.* **(a)** act of preparing a patient before an operation *operationsförberedelser* **(b)** medicine *or* liquid containing a drug *preparat, läkemedel, medel;* **he was given a preparation containing an antihistamine**

preparatnamn ⇨ **n.p.**

prepare [prɪ'peə] *vb.* to get something ready *förbereda, göra i ordning;* to make something *bereda;* **he prepared a soothing linctus; six rooms in the hospital were**

prepared for the accident victims; the nurses were preparing the patient for the operation

prepatellar bursitis [ˌpriːpəˌtelə bəˈsaɪtɪs] *or* **housemaid's knee** [ˈhaʊsmeɪdz ˌniː] *subst.* condition where the fluid sac at the knee becomes inflamed, caused by kneeling on hard surfaces *bursitis prepatellaris, skurgummeknä*

prepubertal [ˌpriːˈpjuːbət(ə)l] *adj.* referring to the period before puberty *prepubertal*

prepuce [ˈpriːpjuːs] *or* **foreskin** [ˈfɔːskɪn] *subst.* skin covering the top of the penis, which can be removed by circumcision *preputiet, förhuden*

preputiet ⇨ **prepuce**

presby- [ˈprezbi, ˌ--] *or* **presbyo-** [ˈprezbiə(ʊ), ˌ--] *prefix* referring to old age *presby(o)-, ålders-*

presbyakusi ⇨ **presbycousis**

presbycousis [ˌprezbiˈkuːsɪs] *subst.* condition where an old person's hearing fails gradually, due to degeneration of the internal ear *presbyakusi*

presbyopia [ˌprezbiˈəʊpiə] *subst.* condition where an old person's sight fails gradually, due to hardening of the lens *presbyopi, ålderssynthet*

prescribe [prɪsˈkraɪb] *vb.* to give instructions for a patient to get a certain dosage of a drug *or* a certain form of therapeutic treatment *ordinera, föreskriva;* **the doctor prescribed a course of antibiotics**

prescription [prɪˈskrɪpʃ(ə)n] *subst.* order written by a doctor to a pharmacist asking for a drug to be prepared and given or sold to a patient *ordination, recept, föreskrift*

presence [ˈprez(ə)ns] *subst.* being there *närvaro;* **tests showed the presence of sugar in the urine**

presenile [ˌpriːˈsiːnaɪ(ə)l] *adj.* (i) prematurely old *presenil;* (ii) (condition) which affects people of early or middle age, but has characteristics of old age *presenil;* **presenile dementia** = form of mental degeneration affecting adults before old age (as in Alzheimer's disease) *presenil demens*

presenility [ˌpriːsəˈnɪləti] *subst.* ageing of the body *or* brain before the normal time, with the patient showing symptoms which are normally associated with old people *för tidigt åldrande*

present 1 [prɪˈzent] *vb.* **(a)** to show *or* to be present *visa, förete, finnas;* **the patient presented with severe chest pains; the doctors' first task is to relieve the presenting symptoms; the condition may also present in a baby (b)** *(in obstetrics)* to appear (in the vaginal channel) *bjuda sig, vara föregående;* **the presenting part** = the part of the fetus which appears first *föregående fosterdel* **2** [ˈprez(ə)nt] *adj.* which is there *närvarande, aktuell, förhandenvarande;* **all the symptoms of the disease are present**

> QUOTE 26 patients were selected from the outpatient department on grounds of disabling breathlessness present for at least five years
> **Lancet**

> QUOTE chlamydia in the male commonly presents a urethritis characterized by dysuria
> **Journal of American College Health**

> QUOTE sickle cell chest syndrome is a common complication of sickle cell disease, presenting with chest pain, fever and leucocytosis
> **British Medical Journal**

> QUOTE a 24 year-old woman presents with an influenza-like illness of five days' duration
> **British Journal of Hospital Medicine**

> QUOTE the presenting symptoms of Crohn's disease may be extremely variable
> **New Zealand Medical Journal**

presentation [ˌprez(ə)nˈteɪʃ(ə)n] *subst.* way in which a baby will be born, i.e. the part of the baby's body which will appear first in the vaginal channel *bjudning, fosterbjudning;* **breech presentation** = position of the baby in the womb, where the buttocks will appear first *sätesbjudning;* **cephalic presentation** = normal presentation, where the baby's head will appear first *kronbjudning, hjässbjudning, huvudbjudning;* **face presentation** = position of the baby in the womb, where the face will appear first *ansiktsbjudning;* **transverse presentation** = position of the baby in the womb, where the baby's side will appear first *tvärläge*

presentera ⇨ **introduce**

preservation [ˌprezəˈveɪʃ(ə)n] *subst.* keeping of tissue sample *or* donor organ in good condition *bevarande (i gott tillstånd), konservering, fixering*

preserve [prɪˈzɜːv] *vb.* to keep *or* to stop (tissue sample) from rotting *bevara (i gott tillstånd), konservera, fixera*

press [pres] *vb.* to push *or* to squeeze *trycka, klämma;* **the tumour is pressing against a nerve**

pressor ['presə] *adj.* (nerve) which increases the action of part of the body *som avser el. hör till pressorreceptor;* (substance) which raises blood pressure *som avser el. hör till pressorsubstans*

pressure ['preʃə] *subst.* (i) action of squeezing *or* of forcing *tryck, klämning;* (ii) force of something on its surroundings *tryck;* (iii) mental *or* physical stress caused by external events *stress;* **blood pressure** = force of the blood as it is being pumped round the body *blodtryck;* **diastolic pressure** = low point of blood pressure during the diastole *diastoliskt (blod)tryck;* **osmotic pressure** = pressure by which a fluid goes through a membrane into another part of the body *osmotiskt tryck;* **pulse pressure** = difference between the diastolic and systolic pressure *pulstryck, pulsamplitud;* **systolic pressure** = high point of blood pressure during the systole *systoliskt (blod)tryck;* **pressure area** = area of the body where a bone is near the surface of the skin, so that if the skin is pressed the circulation will be cut off *område där trycksår lätt uppstår;* **pressure point** = place where an artery crosses over a bone, so that the blood can be cut off by pressing with the finger *punkt där artär passerar ben och blodflödet lätt kan stoppas;* **pressure sore** = ulcer which forms on the skin at a pressure area *or* where something presses on it *dekubitus, trycksår, liggsår*

prestation(sförmåga) ⇨ **performance**

presynaptic [ˌpriːsɪ'næptɪk] *adj.* before a synapse *presynaptisk;* **presynaptic axon** = nerve leading to one side of a synapse *presynaptiskt axon*

presystole [ˌpriː'sɪst(ə)li] *subst.* period before systole in the cycle of heartbeats *presystole*

preterm [ˌpriː'tɜːm] *adj.* premature (delivery) *prematur, för tidig*

prevalence ['prev(ə)ləns] *subst.* percentage *or* number of cases of a disease in a certain place at a certain time *prevalens, förekomst, utbredning;* **the prevalence of malaria in some tropical countries; the prevalence of cases of malnutrition in large towns; a high prevalence of renal disease**

prevalent ['prev(ə)lənt] *adj.* common (in comparison to something) *allmän(t förekommande), utbredd;* **the disease is prevalent in some African countries; a condition which is more prevalent in the cold winter months**

prevent [prɪ'vent] *vb.* to stop something happening *förhindra, förebygga;* **the treatment is given to prevent the patient's condition from getting worse; doctors are trying to prevent the spread of the outbreak of legionnaires' disease** NOTE: you prevent something **from** happening or simply **prevent something happening**

prevention [prɪ'venʃ(ə)n] *subst.* stopping something happening *profylax, förebyggande, förhindrande;* **accident prevention** = taking steps to prevent accidents happening *olycksförebyggande åtgärder*

preventiv- ⇨ **contraceptive**

preventive [prɪ'ventɪv] *adj.* which prevents *preventiv, profylaktisk, förebyggande;* **preventive medicine** = medical action to prevent a disease from occurring *preventiv (förebyggande) medicin (hälsovård), profylax;* **preventive measure** = step taken to prevent a disease from occurring *preventiv (profylaktisk, förebyggande) åtgärd*

> COMMENT: preventive measures include immunization, vaccination and quarantine

preventivmedel ⇨ **contraception, contraceptive**

preventivmedel, oralt ⇨ **oral**

prevertebral [ˌpriː'vɜːtɪbr(ə)l] *adj.* in front of the spinal column *or* a vertebra *prevertebral*

priapism ['pra(ɪ)əpɪz(ə)m] *subst.* erection of the penis without sexual stimulus, caused by a blood clot in the tissue of the penis *or* injury to the spinal cord *or* stone in the urinary bladder *priapism, erectio dolorosa*

prick [prɪk] *vb.* to make a small hole with a sharp point *punktera, sticka (hål i);* **the nurse pricked the patient's finger to take a blood sample; she pricked her finger on the syringe and the spot became infected**

prick ⇨ **mark, punctum, spot**

prickle cell ['prɪk(ə)l ˌsel] *subst.* cell with many processes connecting it to other cells, found in the inner layer of the epidermis *taggcell*

prickly heat [ˌprɪkli 'hiːt] = MILIARIA

primary ['praɪməri] *adj.* **(a)** (condition) which is first, and leads to another (the secondary condition) *primär(-), första-, ursprunglig;* **primary complex** = first lymph node to be infected by tuberculosis *primärkomplex;* **primary haemorrhage** = bleeding which occurs immediately after an injury has been suffered *primärblödning;* **primary tubercle** = first infected spot where tuberculosis starts in a lung *primärkomplex;* **primary tuberculosis** = infection of a patient with tuberculosis for the first time *primär tuberkulos; see also* AMENORRHOEA **(b)** which is most important *primär, främst, viktigast;* **primary colour** = main colour in the spectrum (red, yellow, blue) from which other colours are formed *grundfärg;* **primary health care** *or* **primary medical care** = treatment provided by a general practitioner *primärvård; compare* SECONDARY

> QUOTE among primary health care services, 1.5% of all GP consultations are due to coronary heart disease
> **Health Services Journal**

> QUOTE primary care is largely concerned with clinical management of individual patients, while community medicine tends to view the whole population as its patient
> **Journal of the Royal College of General Practitioners**

primigravida [,praɪmɪ'grævɪdə] *or* **unigravida** [,juːnɪ'grævɪdə] *subst.* woman who is pregnant for the first time *primigravida*

primipara [praɪ'mɪp(ə)rə] *or* **unipara** [ju'nɪp(ə)rə] *subst.* woman who has given birth to one child *primipara, förstföderska*

primordial [praɪ'mɔːdiəl] *adj.* in the very first stage of development *primordial, ursprunglig;* **primary follicle** = first stage of development of an ovarian follicle *primärfollikel*

primordialägg ⇨ **oogonium**

primär ⇨ **primary**

primärblödning ⇨ **primary**

primärfollikel ⇨ **primordial**

primärhärd ⇨ **tubercle**

primärkomplex ⇨ **primary, tubercle**

primärläkning ⇨ **first**

primärmedaljong ⇨ **herald patch**

primärvård ⇨ **primary**

princip ⇨ **principle**

principle ['prɪnsəp(ə)l] *subst.* rule *or* theory *princip, grundsats;* **active principle** = main ingredient of a drug which makes it have the required effect on a patient *aktiv beståndsdel*

privat ⇨ **personal, private, privately**

private ['praɪvət] *adj.* (i) belonging to one person, not to the public *privat, personlig;* (ii) which is paid for by a person *privat;* **he runs a private clinic for alcoholics; she is in private practice as an orthopaedic consultant; private patient** = patient who is paying for his treatment, not having it done through the National Health Service *privatpatient;* **private practice** = services of a doctor *or* surgeon *or* dentist which are paid for by the patients themselves (or by a medical insurance), but not by the National Health Service *privatpraktik*

privately ['praɪvətli] *adv.* paid by the patient, not by the National Health Service *privat;* **she decided to have the operation done privately**
NOTE: the opposite is **on the National Health**

privatpatient ⇨ **private**

privatpraktik ⇨ **private**

privatsjukhus ⇨ **hospital**

privatägd ⇨ **proprietary**

p.r.n. [,piːɑːr'en] *abbreviation for the Latin phrase* "pro re nata": as and when required (written on a prescription) *vid behov, v.b.*

pro- ['prəʊ, ,-] *prefix* meaning before *or* in front of *pro-, för(e)-, framför*

probang ['prəʊbæŋ] *subst.* surgical instrument, like a long rod with a brush at one end, formerly used to test and find strictures in the oesophagus and to push foreign bodies into the stomach *slags kirurgiskt instrument för att sondera matstrupen*

probe [prəʊb] **1** *subst.* (i) instrument used to explore inside a cavity *or* wound *sond;* (ii) device inserted into a medium to obtain information *sond;* **laser probe** = metal probe which is inserted into the body, then heated by a laser beam, used to burn through blocked arteries *lasersond;* **ultrasonic** *or* **ultrasound probe** = instrument which locates organs *or* tissues inside the body, using ultrasound *ultraljudssond* **2** *vb.* to investigate the inside of something *sondera;* **the surgeon probed the wound with a scalpel**

problem ['prɒbləm] *subst.* **(a)** something which is difficult to find an answer to *problem;* **scientists are trying to find a solution to the problem of drug-related disease; problem child** = child who is difficult to control *problembarn* **(b)** medical disorder, usually an addiction *problem, besvär;* **he has an alcohol problem** *or* **a drugs problem** = he is addicted to alcohol *or* drugs *han har alkoholproblem (narkotikaproblem), han missbrukar sprit (narkotika);* **problem drinking** = alcoholism which has a bad effect on a person's behaviour or work *alkoholproblem*

problembarn ⇨ **problem**

procedure [prə(ʊ)'siːdʒə] *subst.* (i) type of treatment *behandlingsmetod, förfarande;* (ii) treatment given at one time *behandling;* **the hospital has developed some new procedures for treating Parkinson's disease; we are hoping to increase the number of procedures carried out per day**

> QUOTE disposable items now available for medical and nursing procedures range from cheap syringes to expensive cardiac pacemakers
> **Nursing Times**

> QUOTE the electromyograms and CT scans were done as outpatient procedures
> **Southern Medical Journal**

procent ⇨ **per cent**

process ['prəʊses] **1** *subst.* **(a)** projecting part of the body *utskott, utsprång;* **articulating process** = piece of bone which sticks out of the neural arch in a vertebra and articulates with the next vertebra *processus articularis, ledutskott;* **ciliary processes** = series of ridges behind the iris to which the lens of the eye is attached ⇨ *illustration* EYE *fliktiga utskott på ciliarkroppen;* **mastoid process** = part of the temporal bone which protrudes at the side of the head behind the ear ⇨ *illustration* SKULL *processus mastoideus, vårtutskottet;* **transverse process** = part of a vertebra which protrudes at the side *processus transversus, tvärutskott;* **xiphoid process** = bottom part of the breastbone which is originally cartilage but becomes bone by middle age *processus xiphoideus (ensiformis), svärdsutskottet* **(b)** technical *or* scientific action *process, metod;* **a new process for testing serum samples has been developed in the research laboratory (c) nursing process** = standard method of treatment carried out by nurses, and the documents which go with it *omvårdnad(sprocess)* **2** *vb.* to examine *or* to test samples *undersöka, pröva, testa;* **the blood samples are being processed by the laboratory**

> QUOTE the nursing process serves to divide overall patient care into that part performed by nurses and that performed by the other professions
> **Nursing Times**

> QUOTE all relevant sections of the nurses' care plan and nursing process records had been left blank
> **Nursing Times**

procidentia [ˌprəʊsɪ'denʃ(i)ə] *subst.* movement of an organ downwards *framfall;* **uterine procidentia** = condition where the womb has passed through the vagina *prolapsus uteri, meproptos, livmoderframfall*

proct- ['prɒkt, ˌ-] *or* **procto-** ['prɒktə(ʊ), ˌ--] *prefix* referring to the anus *or* rectum *prokt(o)-, rekt(o)-, ändtarms-*

proctalgia [prɒk'tældʒə] *subst.* pain in the lower rectum *or* anus, caused by neuralgia *proktalgi;* **proctalgia fugax** = condition where the patient suffers sudden pains in the rectum during the night, usually relieved by eating or drinking *proctalgia fugax*

proctatresia [ˌprɒktə'triːziə] *or* **imperforate anus** [ɪm'pɜːfəreɪt ˌeɪnəs] *subst.* condition where the anus does not have an opening *atresia ani, anus imperforatus, proktatresi*

proctectasia [ˌprɒktek'teɪziə] *subst.* condition where the rectum *or* anus is dilated because of continued constipation *proktektasi*

proctectomy [prɒk'tektəmi] *subst.* surgical removal of the rectum *proktektomi*

proctitis [prɒk'taɪtɪs] *subst.* inflammation of the rectum *proktit, ändtarmsinflammation*

proctocele ['prɒktə(ʊ)siː(ə)l] *subst.* **vaginal proctocele** = condition associated with prolapse of the womb, where the rectum protrudes into the vagina *vaginalt proktocele*

proctoclysis [prɒk'tɒkləsɪs] *subst.* introduction of a lot of fluid into the rectum slowly *klysma, lavemang*

proctocolectomy [ˌprɒktəʊkɒ'lektəmi] *subst.* surgical removal of the rectum and the colon *proktokolektomi*

proctocolitis [ˌprɒktə(ʊ)kə'laɪtɪs] *subst.* inflammation of the rectum and part of the colon *proktokolit*

proctodynia [ˌprɒktə(ʊ)'dɪniə] *subst* sensation of pain in the anus *proktodyni*

proctology [prɒk'tɒlədʒi] *subst.* scientific study of the rectum and anus and their associated diseases *proktologi*

proctorrhaphy [prɒk'tɔːrəfi] *subst.* surgical operation to stitch up a tear in the rectum *or* anus *prokto(r)rafi*

proctoscope ['prɒktəskəʊp] *subst.* surgical instrument consisting of a long tube with a light in the end, used to examine the rectum *proktoskop*

proctoscopy [prɒk'tɒskəpi] *subst.* examination of the rectum using a proctoscope *proktoskopi*

proctosigmoiditis [ˌprɒktəʊˌsɪgmɔɪ'daɪtɪs] *subst.* inflammation of the rectum and the sigmoid colon *proktosigmoidit*

proctotomy [prɒk'tɒtəmi] *subst.* (i) surgical operation to divide a structure of the rectum *or* anus *proktotomi;* (ii) opening of an imperforate anus *öppnande vid proktatresi*

prodromal [prəʊ'drəʊm(ə)l] *adj.* (time) between when the first symptoms of a disease appear, and the appearance of the major effect, such as a fever *or* rash *prodromal;* **prodromal rash** = early rash *or* rash which appears as a symptom of a disease before the major rash *hudutslag som prodromalsymtom*

prodromalsymtom ⇨ **prodromal, prodrome**

prodrome ['prəʊdrəʊm] *or* **prodroma** [prəʊ'drəʊmə] *subst.* early symptom of an attack of a disease *prodrom, prodromalsymtom*

> QUOTE in classic migraine a prodrome is followed by an aura, then a headache, and finally a recovery phase. The prodrome may not be recognised
> **British Journal of Hospital Medicine**

produce [prə'djuːs] *vb.* to make *framkalla, alstra, bilda;* **the drug produces a sensation of dizziness; doctors are worried by the side-effects produced by the new pain killer**

product ['prɒdʌkt] *subst.* (i) thing which is produced *produkt;* (ii) result *or* effect of a process *resultat, alster;* **pharmaceutical products** = medicines *or* pills *or* lozenges *or* creams which are sold in chemists' shops *farmaceutiska produkter (preparat)*

proenzyme [prəʊ'enzaɪm] *or* **zymogen** ['zaɪməʊdʒ(ə)n] *subst.* first mature form of an enzyme, before it develops into an active enzyme *proenzym, zymogen*

profas ⇨ **prophase**

profession [prə'feʃ(ə)n] *subst.* (i) type of job for which special training is needed *profession, yrke;* (ii) all people working in a specialized type of employment for which they have been trained *yrkeskår;* **the medical profession** = all doctors *den medicinska yrkeskåren, läkarna;* **he's a doctor by profession** = his job is being a doctor *han är läkare till yrket*

professional [prə'feʃ(ə)n(ə)l] *adj.* referring to a profession *professionell, yrkes-;* **professional body** = organization which acts for all the members of a profession *fackförbund, yrkesförening;* **Professional Conduct Committee (PCC)** = committee of the General Medical Council which decides on cases of professional misconduct *slags medicinsk ansvarsnämnd;* **professional misconduct** = action which is thought to be wrong by the body which regulates a profession (such as an action by a doctor which is considered wrong by the General Medical Council) *olämpligt el. olagligt agerande av en yrkesman, tjänstefel*

profound [prə'faʊnd] *adj.* deep *or* serious *djup(gående), allvarlig;* **a profound abnormality of the immune system**

profunda [prə'fʌndə] *adj.* (blood vessels) which lie deep in tissues *djupt liggande*

profuse [prə'fjuːs] *adj.* very large quantity *ymnig, riklig;* **fever accompanied by profuse sweating; pains with profuse internal bleeding**

profylaktikum ⇨ **prophylactic**

profylaktisk ⇨ **preventive, prophylactic**

profylax ⇨ **prevention, preventive, prophylaxis**

progeria [prəʊ'dʒɪəriə] *or* **Hutchinson-Gilford syndrome** [ˌhʌtʃɪns(ə)n'gɪlfəd ˌsɪndrəʊm] *subst.* premature senility *progeri, Hutchinsons syndrom*

progesterone [prə(ʊ)'dʒestərəʊn] *subst.* hormone produced in the second part of the menstrual cycle by the corpus luteum and which stimulates the formation of the placenta if an ovum is fertilized (it is also produced by the placenta itself) *progesteron*

progestogen [prə(ʊ)'dʒestədʒ(ə)n] *subst.* any substance which has the same effect as progesterone *progestogen*

COMMENT: because natural progesterones prevent ovulation during pregnancy, synthetically produced progestogens are used to make contraceptive pills

prognathic jaw [prɒg'næθɪk ˌdʒɔː] *subst.* jaw which protrudes further than the other *prognati(sm), framskjutande käke*

prognathism ['prɒgnəθɪz(ə)m] *subst.* condition where one jaw (especially the lower) or both jaws protrude *prognati(sm), särskilt underbett*

prognosis [prəg'nəʊsɪs] *subst.* opinion of how a disease *or* disorder will develop *prognos; compare* DIAGNOSIS

prognostic [prəg'nɒstɪk] *adj.* referring to prognosis *prognostisk;* **prognostic test** = test to decide how a disease will develop *or* how long a patient will survive an operation *prognostiskt test (prov)*

programme ['prəʊgræm] *subst.* series of medical treatments given in a set way at set times *behandlingsserie;* **the doctor prescribed a programme of injections; she took a programme of steroid treatment**

progress 1 ['prəʊgres] *subst.* development *or* way in which a person is becoming well *framsteg, förbättring, utveckling;* **the doctors seem pleased that she has made such good progress since her operation 2** [prə(ʊ)'gres] *vb.* to develop *or* to continue to do well *göra framsteg, förbättras, utvecklas;* **the patient is progressing well; the doctor asked how the patient was progressing**

progression [prə(ʊ)'greʃ(ə)n] *subst.* development *progression, utveckling, fortskridande;* **progression of a disease** = way in which a disease develops *sjukdoms utveckling*

progressive [prə(ʊ)'gresɪv] *adj.* which develops all the time *progressiv, fortskridande, tilltagande;* **Alzheimer's disease is a progressive disorder which sees a gradual decline in intellectual functioning; progressive deafness** = condition where the patient becomes more and more deaf *tilltagande hörselnedsättning;* **progressive muscular atrophy** = any form of muscular dystrophy, with progressive weakening of the muscles, particularly in the pelvic and shoulder girdles *progressiv muskelatrofi, tilltagande muskelförtvining*

progressively [prə(ʊ)'gresɪvli] *adv.* more and more *progressivt, tilltagande;* **he became progressively more disabled**

proinsulin [prəʊ'ɪnsʊlɪn] *subst.* substance produced by the pancreas, then converted to insulin *proinsulin*

project [prə'dʒekt] *vb.* to protrude *or* to stick out *skjuta ut (fram)*

projection [prə'dʒekʃ(ə)n] *subst.* **(a)** piece of a part which protrudes *utsprång, utskott, utskjutande del;* **projection tract** = fibres connecting the cerebral cortex with the lower parts of the brain and spinal cord *projektionsbana* **(b)** *(in psychology)* mental action, where the patient blames another person for his own faults *projektion, projicering*

projektionsbana ⇨ **projection**

projicerad smärta ⇨ **synalgia**

projicering ⇨ **projection**

proktalgi ⇨ **proctalgia**

proktatresi ⇨ **proctatresia**

proktektasi ⇨ **proctectasia**

proktektomi ⇨ **proctectomy**

proktit ⇨ **proctitis**

prokt(o)- ⇨ **proct-**

proktocele ⇨ **rectocele**

proktodyni ⇨ **proctodynia**

proktokolektomi ⇨ **proctocolectomy**

proktokolit ⇨ **proctocolitis**

proktologi ⇨ **proctology**

proktosigmoidektomi ⇨ **rectosigmoidectomy**

proktosigmoidit ⇨ **proctosigmoiditis**

proktoskop ⇨ **proctoscope**

proktoskopi ⇨ **proctoscopy**

proktotomi ⇨ **proctotomy**

prolactin [prəʊ'læktɪn] *or* **lactogenic hormone** [ˌlæktəʊ'dʒenɪk ˌhɔːməʊn] *subst.* hormone secreted by the pituitary gland which stimulates the production of milk *prolaktin, mammotropin, laktationshormon*

prolaps ⇨ **prolapse, ptosis**

prolapse ['prəʊlæps] *subst.* condition where an organ has moved downwards out of its normal position *ptos, prolaps, framfall;* **rectal prolapse** *or* **prolapse of the rectum** = condition where mucous membrane of the rectum moves downwards and passes through the anus *prolapsus recti, rektalprolaps;* **prolapsed intervertebral disc (PID)** *or* **slipped disc** = condition where an intervertebral disc becomes displaced *or* where the soft centre of a disc passes through the hard cartilage of the exterior and presses onto a nerve *hernia disci intervertebralis, diskprolaps, diskbråck;* **prolapsed womb** *or* **prolapse of the uterus** = UTERINE PROLAPSE

prolapsring ⇨ **pessary**

proliferate [prə(ʊ)'lɪfəreɪt] *vb.* to produce many similar cells or parts, and so grow *föröka sig genom celldelning*

proliferation [prə(ʊ)ˌlɪfə'reɪʃ(ə)n] *subst.* process of proliferating *proliferation, spridning, utbredning, tillväxt*

proliferationsfas ⇨ **proliferative**

proliferative [prə(ʊ)'lɪf(ə)rətɪv] *adj.* which multiplies *proliferativ;* **proliferative phase** = period when a disease is spreading fast *proliferationsfas, tillväxtperiod*

proline ['prəʊlɪn] *subst.* amino acid found in proteins, especially in collagen *prolin*

prolong [prə(ʊ)'lɒŋ] *vb.* to make longer *förlänga;* **the treatment prolonged her life by three years**

prolonged [prə(ʊ)'lɒŋd] *adj.* very long *långvarig;* **she had to undergo a prolonged course of radiation treatment**

prominence ['prɒmɪnəns] *subst.* projection *or* part of the body which stands out *utsprång, utskott, utskjutande del;* **the laryngeal prominence** = the Adam's apple *prominentia laryngea, pomum Adami, adamsäpplet*

prominent ['prɒmɪnənt] *adj.* which stands out *or* which is very visible *framträdande, iögonfallande, utstående;* **she had a prominent scar on her neck which she wanted to have removed**

promontory ['prɒmənt(ə)ri] *subst.* projection *or* section of an organ (especially the middle ear and sacrum) which stands out above the rest *promontorium, utskjutande del*

promote [prə'məʊt] *vb.* to help something take place *befrämja, gynna;* **the drug is used to promote blood clotting**

pronate ['prəʊneɪt] *vb.* (i) to lie face downwards *ligga på magen;* (ii) to turn the hand so that palm faces downwards *pronera*

pronation [prəʊ'neɪʃ(ə)n] *subst.* turning the hand round so that the palm faces downwards *pronation*

pronator [prəʊ'neɪtə] *subst.* muscle which makes the hand turn face downwards *(musculus) pronator*

prone [prəʊn] *adj.* (i) lying face downwards *framstupa, på magen;* (ii) (arm) with the palm facing downwards *pronerad*
NOTE: the opposite is **supination, supine**

pronera ⇨ **pronate**

pronerad ⇨ **prone**

pronounced [prə'naʊnst] *adj.* very obvious *or* marked *uttalad, framträdande, markerad;* **she has a pronounced limp**

propagate ['prɒpəgeɪt] *vb.* to multiply *propagera, utbreda, fortplanta, föröka, sprida*

propagation [ˌprɒpə'geɪʃ(ə)n] *subst.* increasing *or* causing something to spread *propagation, utbredning, fortplantning, förökning, spridning*

propagera ⇨ **propagate**

properdin ['prəʊpədɪn] *subst.* protein in blood plasma which can destroy Gram-negative bacteria and neutralize viruses when acting together with magnesium *properdin*

prophase ['prəʊfeɪz] *subst.* first stage of mitosis when the chromosomes are visible as long thin double threads *profas*

prophylactic [ˌprɒfə'læktɪk] *subst. & adj.* (substance) which helps to prevent the development of a disease *profylaktikum, profylaktisk, förebyggande (medel)*

> QUOTE most pacemakers are inserted prophylactically for either atrioventricular block or sick sinus syndrome
> **British Journal of Hospital Medicine**

prophylaxis [ˌprɒfə'læksɪs] *subst.* (i) prevention of disease *profylax;* (ii) preventive treatment *profylax, förebyggande behandling (åtgärd)*

proportion [prə'pɔːʃ(ə)n] *subst.* quantity of something, especially as compared to the whole *proportion;* **a high proportion of cancers can be treated by surgery; the proportion of outpatients to inpatients is increasing**

> QUOTE the target cells for adult myeloid leukaemia are located in the bone marrow, and there is now evidence that a substantial proportion of childhood leukaemias also arise in bone marrow
> **British Medical Journal**

propp ⇨ **obturator, occlusion**

proprietary [prə'pra(ɪ)ət(ə)ri] *adj.* which belongs to a commercial company *privatägd;* **proprietary drug** = drug which is sold under a trade name *farmaceutisk specialitet, varumärke;* **proprietary name** = trade name for a drug *preparatnamn (skilt från generiskt namn, se generic)*

proprioception [ˌprəʊpriə'sepʃ(ə)n] *subst.* reaction of nerves to body movements and relation of information about movements to the brain *proprioception*

proprioceptive [ˌprəʊpriə'septɪv] *adj.* referring to sensory impulses from the joints, muscles and tendons, which relate information about body movements to the brain *proprioceptiv*

proprioceptor [ˌprəʊpriə'septə] *subst.* end of a sensory nerve which reacts to stimuli from muscles and tendons as they move *proprioceptor*

proptosis [prɒp'təʊsɪs] *subst.* forward displacement of the eyeball *proptos*

prosencephalon ⇨ **forebrain**

prosop- ['prɒsəp, ˌ--] *or* **prosopo-** ['prɒsəpə(ʊ), ˌ---] *prefix* referring to the face *prosop(o)-, ansikts-*

prostaglandins [ˌprɒstə'glændɪnz] *subst. pl.* fatty acids present in many parts of the body, which are associated with the sensation of pain and have an effect on the nervous system, blood pressure and in particular the uterus at menstruation *prostaglandiner*

prostata- ⇨ **prostatic**

prostatahypertrofi ⇨ **prostatic**

prostatamassage ⇨ **prostatic**

prostatectomy [ˌprɒstə'tektəmi] *subst.* surgical removal of all *or* part of the prostate gland *prostatektomi;* **retropubic prostatectomy** = prostatectomy where the operation is performed through the membrane surrounding the prostate gland *retropubisk prostatektomi;* **transurethral prostatectomy** *or* **transurethral resection** = prostatectomy where the operation is performed through the urethra *transuretral prostatektomi (resektion), TUR;* **transvesical prostatectomy** = prostatectomy where the operation is performed through the bladder *transvesikal prostatektomi; see also* HARRIS'S OPERATION

prostate (gland) ['prɒsteɪt (ˌglænd)] *subst.* gland in men which produces a secretion in which sperm cells float *prostata, blåshalskörteln;* **he has prostate trouble** = he is suffering from prostatitis *or* he has an enlarged prostate gland ⇨ *illustration* UROGENITAL SYSTEM (MALE) *han har prostatabesvär*

> COMMENT: the prostate gland lies under the bladder and surrounds the urethra (the tube leading from the bladder to the penis). It secretes a fluid containing enzymes. As a man grows older, the prostate gland tends to enlarge and constrict the point at which the urethra leaves the bladder, making it difficult to pass urine

prostatektomi ⇨ **prostatectomy**

prostatic [prɒ'stætɪk] *adj.* referring to the prostate gland; belonging to the prostate gland *prostata-, blåshalskörtel-;* **prostatic hypertrophy** = enlargement of the prostate gland *prostatahypertrofi;* **prostatic massage** = removing fluid from the prostate gland through the rectum *prostatamassage;* **prostatic urethra** = section of the urethra which passes through the prostate *pars prostatica, den del av urinröret som ligger i blåshalskörteln;* **prostatic utricle** = sac branching from the prostatic urethra *utriculus prostaticus*

prostatitis [ˌprɒstə'taɪtɪs] *subst.* inflammation of the prostate gland *prostatit, blåshalskörtelinflammation*

prostatocystitis [prɒˌsteɪtəʊsɪ'staɪtɪs] *subst.* inflammation of the prostatic part of the urethra and the bladder *prostatocystit*

prostatorrhoea [ˌprɒstətə'rɪə] *subst.* discharge of fluid from the prostate gland *prostatorré*

prostetisk ⇨ **prosthetic**

prosthesis [prɒs'θiːsɪs] *subst.* device which is attached to the body to take the place

of a part which is missing (such as an artificial leg *or* glass eye, etc.) *protes;* **dental prosthesis** = one or more false teeth *protes, tandprotes*
NOTE: plural is **prostheses**

prosthetic [prɒs'θetɪk] *adj.* (artificial limb) which replaces a part of the body which has been amputated *or* removed *prostetisk, protes-;* **he was fitted with a prosthetic hand**

prosthetics [prɒs'θetɪks] *subst.* study and making of prostheses *protetik*

prosthetist [prɒs'θətɪst] *subst.* qualified person who fits prostheses *protesutprovare*

prostration [prɒs'treɪʃ(ə)n] *subst.* extreme tiredness of body *or* mind *prostration, fullständig utmattning*

protamine ['prəʊtəmi:n] *subst.* simple protein found in fish, used with insulin to slow down the insulin absorption rate *protamin*

protanopia [,prəʊtə'nəʊpiə] = DALTONISM

protease ['prəʊtieɪz] *or* **proteolytic enzyme** [,prəʊtiə(ʊ)'lɪtɪk ,enzaɪm] *subst.* digestive enzyme which breaks down protein in food by splitting the peptide link *proteas*

protect [prə'tekt] *vb.* to keep something safe from harm *skydda;* **the population must be protected against the spread of the virus**

protection [prə'tekʃ(ə)n] *subst.* thing which protects *skydd;* **children are vaccinated as a protection against disease**

protective [prə'tektɪv] *adj.* which protects *protektiv, skyddande;* **protective cap** = condom *or* rubber sheath put over the penis before intercourse as a contraceptive or as a protection against venereal disease *kondom*

protein ['prəʊti:n] *subst.* nitrogen compound which is present in and is an essential part of all living cells in the body, formed by the condensation of amino acids *protein, äggviteämne;* **protein balance** = situation when the nitrogen intake in protein is equal to the excretion rate (in the urine) *proteinbalans;* **protein deficiency** = lack of enough proteins in the diet *proteinbrist*

> COMMENT: proteins are necessary for growth and repair of the body's tissue; they are mainly formed of carbon, nitrogen and oxygen in various combinations as amino acids. Certain foods (such as beans, meat, eggs, fish and milk) are rich in protein

proteinbalans ⇨ **protein**

protein-bound iodine ['prəʊti:n,baʊnd 'aɪədi:n] *subst.* compound of thyroxine and iodine *proteinbunden jod, PBJ;* **protein-bound iodine test (PBI test)** = test to measure if the thyroid gland is producing adequate quantities of thyroxine *mätning av mängden PBJ i blodet*

proteinbrist ⇨ **protein**

proteinspjälkande ⇨ **proteolytic**

proteinuri ⇨ **globulinuria, proteinuria**

proteinuria [,prəʊti'njʊəriə] *subst.* proteins in the urine *proteinuri*

protektiv ⇨ **protective**

proteolysis [,prəʊti'ɒləsɪs] *subst.* breaking down of proteins in food by proteolytic enzymes *proteolys*

proteolytic [,prəʊtiə(ʊ)'lɪtɪk] *adj.* referring to proteolysis *proteolytisk, proteinspjälkande;* **proteolytic enzyme** = PROTEASE

protes ⇨ **prosthesis**

protes- ⇨ **prosthetic**

protesutprovare ⇨ **prosthetist**

protetik ⇨ **prosthetics**

Proteus ['prəʊtju:s] *subst.* genus of bacteria commonly found in the intestines *Proteus, slags tarmbakterie*

prothrombin [,prəʊ'θrɒmbɪn] *subst.* Factor II *or* protein in blood which helps blood to coagulate and which needs vitamin K to be effective *protrombin, koagulationsfaktor II;* **prothrombin time** = time taken (in Quick's test) for clotting to take place *koaguleringstid vid Quicks test*

proto- ['prəʊtə(ʊ), ,--] *prefix* meaning first *or* at the beginning *prot(o)-*

protokoll ⇨ **record**

protokollföra ⇨ **record**

protopathic [,prəʊtəʊ'pæθɪk] *adj.* (i) referring to nerves which are able to sense only strong sensations *som avser el. hör till nerver som endast reagerar på starka stimuli;* (ii) referring to a first symptom *or* lesion *protopatisk, idiopatisk;* (iii) referring to the first sign of partially restored function in an injured nerve *som avser el. hör till första* *tecknet på återvunnen funktion hos skadad nerv; see also* EPICRITIC

protoplasm ['prəʊtə(ʊ)plæz(ə)m] *subst.* substance like a jelly which makes up the largest part of each cell *protoplasma*

protoplasmic [,prəʊtə(ʊ)'plæzmɪk] *adj.* referring to protoplasm *som avse el. hör till protoplasma*

protoporphyrin IX [,prəʊtəʊ'pɔ:f(ə)rɪn ,naɪn] *subst.* commonest form of porphyrin, found in haemoglobin and chlorophyll *protoporfyrin (IX)*

Protozoa [,prəʊtə(ʊ)'zəʊə] *subst pl.* tiny simple organisms with a single cell *protozoer, urdjur* NOTE: the singular is **protozoon**

COMMENT: parasitic Protozoa can cause several diseases, such as amoebiasis, malaria and other tropical diseases

protozoan [,prəʊtə(ʊ)'zəʊən] *adj.* referring to the Protozoa *protozoisk*

protrombin ⇨ **prothrombin**

protrude [prə'tru:d] *vb.* to stick out *sticka fram (ut), skjuta fram (ut);* **protruding** *utstående;* **she wears a brace to correct her protruding teeth; protruding eyes are associated with some forms of goitre**

protuberance [prə'tju:b(ə)r(ə)ns] *subst.* rounded part of the body which projects above the rest *protuberans, utsprång*

proud flesh [,praʊd 'fleʃ] *subst.* new vessels and young fibrous tissue which form when a wound *or* incision *or* lesion is healing *granulationsvävnad, svallkött*

prov ⇨ **sample, specimen, test**

prova ⇨ **test**

provfrukost ⇨ **test meal**

provide [prə'vaɪd] *vb.* to supply *or* to give *tillhandahålla, ge, ombesörja;* **a balanced diet should provide the necessary protein required by the body; a dentist's surgery should provide adequate room for patients to wait in; the hospital provides an ambulance service to the whole area**

provision [prə'vɪʒ(ə)n] *subst.* act of providing *tillhandahållande, ombesörjande;* **the provision of aftercare facilities for patients recently discharged from hospital**

provisional [prə'vɪʒ(ə)n(ə)l] *adj.* temporary *or* which may be changed *provisorisk, tillfällig, preliminär;* **the hospital has given me a provisional date for the operation; the paramedical team attached sticks to the broken leg to act as provisional splints**

provisionally [prə'vɪʒ(ə)n(ə)li] *adv.* in a temporary way *or* not certainly *provisoriskt, tillfälligt, preliminärt;* **she has provisionally accepted the offer of a bed in the hospital**

provisorisk ⇨ **provisional, temporary**

provisoriskt ⇨ **provisionally**

provocera (fram) ⇨ **provoke**

provoke [prə'vəʊk] *vb.* to stimulate *or* make something happen *provocera (fram), framkalla, utlösa, vålla;* **the medication provoked a sudden rise in body temperature; the fit was provoked by the shock of the accident**

provrör ⇨ **test tube**

provrörsbarn ⇨ **test tube**

provrörsbefruktning ⇨ **in vitro**

proximal ['prɒksɪm(ə)l] *adj.* near the midline *or* the central part of the body *proximal, närmare belägen;* **proximal convoluted tubule** = part of the kidney filtering system, between the loop of Henle and the glomerulus *proximala tubulus*
NOTE: the opposite is **distal**

prurigo [pru(ə)'raɪgəʊ] *subst.* itchy eruption of papules *prurigo;* **Besnier's prurigo** = irritating form of prurigo on the backs of the knees and the insides of the elbows *Besniers prurigo*

pruritus [pru(ə)'raɪtəs] *subst.* irritation of the skin which makes a patient want to scratch *pruritus, klåda;* **pruritus ani** = itching round the anal orifice *pruritus anus, ändtarmsklåda;* **pruritus vulvae** = itching round the vulva *pruritus vulvae*

prussic acid [,prʌsɪk 'æsɪd] = CYANIDE

pröva ⇨ **process**

pseduomeningit ⇨ **meningism**

pseud- ['sju:d, ,-] *or* **pseudo-** ['sju:də(ʊ), ,--] *prefix* meaning false *or* similar to something, but not the same *pseud(o)-, falsk, sken-*

pseudoangina [ˌsjuːdəʊæn'dʒaɪnə] *subst.* pain in the chest, caused by worry but not indicating heart disease *pseudoangina*

pseudoarthrosis [ˌsjuːdəʊɑː'θrəʊsɪs] *subst.* false joint, as when the two broken ends of a fractured bone do not bind together but heal separately *pseud(o)artros, falsk led*

pseudobursa ⇨ **bunion**

pseudocoxalgia [ˌsjuːdə(ʊ)kɒk'sældʒə] *or* **Legg-Calvé-Perthes disease** [ˌlegkʌlˌveɪ'pɜːtiːz dɪˌziːz] *subst.* degeneration of the upper end of the femur (in young boys) which prevents the femur from growing properly and can result in a permanent limp *osteochondritis deformans juvenilis, coxa plana, (Legg-Calvé-)Perthes sjukdom*

pseudocrisis [ˌsjuːdəʊ'kraɪsɪs] *subst.* sudden fall in the temperature of the patient with fever, but which does not mark the end of the fever *pseudokris*

pseudocroup [ˌsjuːdəʊ'kruːp] *subst.* (i) laryngismus stridulus *laryngismus stridulosa, pseudokrupp, falsk krupp;* (ii) form of asthma, where contractions take place in the larynx *slags astma med kramp i struphuvudet, slags virusinfektion, ofta parainfluenza (jfr croup)*

pseudocyesis [ˌsjuːdəʊsaɪ'iːsɪs] *or* **phantom pregnancy** ['fæntəm ˌpregnənsi] *subst.* condition where a woman has the physical symptoms of pregnancy, but is not pregnant *skengraviditet*

pseudocyst ['sjuːdəʊsɪst] *subst.* (i) false cyst *falsk cysta;* (ii) space which fills with fluid in an organ, but without the walls which would form a cyst, as a result of softening *or* necrosis of the tissue *slags vätskefyllt hålrum i vävnad*

pseudodementia [ˌsjuːdəʊdɪ'menʃ(i)ə] *subst.* condition of extreme apathy found in hysterical people (where their behaviour corresponds to what they imagine to be insanity, though they show no signs of true dementia) *pseudodemens*

pseudohypertrophic muscular dystrophy [ˌsjuːdəʊˌhaɪpəˌtrɒfɪk ˌmʌskjʊlə 'dɪstrəfi] *subst.* Duchenne muscular dystrophy *or* hereditary disease affecting the muscles, which swell and become weak, beginning in early childhood *muskeldystrofi med pseudohypertrofi, Duchenne-Griesingers sjukdom*

pseudohypertrophy [ˌsjuːdəʊhaɪ'pɜːtrəfi] *subst.* overgrowth of fatty *or* fibrous tissue in a part *or* organ, which results in the part *or* organ being enlarged *pseudohypertrofi*

pseudokris ⇨ **pseudocrisis**

pseudokrupp ⇨ **pseudocroup**

pseudoleverscirros ⇨ **Pick's disease**

pseudomyxoma [ˌsjuːdəʊmɪk'səʊmə] *subst.* tumour rich in mucus *pseudomyxom*

pseudoplegia [ˌsjuːdəʊ'pliːdʒə] *or* **pseudoparalysis** [ˌsjuːdəʊpə'ræləsɪs] *subst.* (i) loss of muscular power in the limbs, but without true paralysis *förlust av muskelkraft i lemmarna;* (ii) paralysis caused by hysteria *hysterisk förlamning*

pseudopolyposis [ˌsjuːdəʊˌpɒli'pəʊsɪs] *subst.* condition where polyps are found in many places in the intestine, usually resulting from an earlier infection *slags tarmpolypos*

psilosis [saɪ'ləʊsɪs] *or* **sprue** [spruː] *subst.* disease of the small intestine, which prevents the patient from absorbing food properly *sprue*

NOTE: the condition is often found in the tropics, and results in diarrhoea and loss of weight

psittacosis [ˌsɪtə'kəʊsɪs] *or* **parrot disaese** ['pærət dɪˌziːz] *subst.* disease of parrots which can be transmitted to humans *psittakos, papegojsjuka*

> COMMENT: the disease is similar to typhoid fever, but atypical pneumonia is present; symptoms include fever, diarrhoea and distension of the abdomen

psoasarkaden ⇨ **arcuate**

psoas major [ˌsəʊæs 'meɪdʒə] *subst.* muscle in the groin which flexes the hip *musculus psoas major, stora ländmuskeln;* **psoas minor** = small muscle, similar to the psoas major, but which is not always present *musculus psoas minor*

psoriasis [sə'ra(ɪ)əsɪs] *subst.* common inflammatory skin disease where red patches of skin are covered with white scales *psoriasis*

psoriasisartrit ⇨ **psoriatic**

"psoriasis, falsk" ⇨ **parapsoriasis**

psoriatic [ˌsɔːri'ætɪk] *adj.* referring to psoriasis *psoriatisk;* **psoriatic arthritis =** form of psoriasis which is associated with arthritis *psoriasis arthropathica, psoriasisartrit*

psych- ['saɪk, ˌ-] *or* **psycho-** ['saɪkəʊ, ˌ--] *prefix* referring to the mind *psyk(o)-, mental-*

psychasthenia [ˌsaɪkæs'θiːniə] *subst.* (i) any psychoneurosis, except hysteria *psykoneuros, neuros;* (ii) psychoneurosis characterized by fears and phobias *psykasteni*

psyche ['saɪki] *subst.* the mind *psyket, själen, förståndet, intellektet, medvetandet*

psychedelic [ˌsaɪkə'delɪk] *adj.* (drug, such as LSD) which expands a person's consciousness *psykedelisk*

psychiatric [ˌsaɪki'ætrɪk] *adj.* referring to psychiatry *psykiatrisk;* **he is undergoing psychiatric treatment; psychiatric hospital =** hospital which specializes in the treatment of patients with mental disorders *psykiatriskt sjukhus, mentalsjukhus*

psychiatrist [saɪ'ka(ɪ)ətrɪst] *subst.* doctor who specializes in the diagnosis and treatment of mental disorders and behaviour *psykiat(rik)er*

psychiatry [saɪ'ka(ɪ)ətri] *subst.* branch of medicine concerned with diagnosis and treatment of mental disorders and behaviour *psykiatri*

psychoanalysis [ˌsaɪkəʊə'næləsɪs] *subst.* treatment of mental disorder, where a specialist talks to the patient and analyses with him his condition and the past events which have caused it *psykoanalys*

psychoanalyst [ˌsaɪkəʊ'æn(ə)lɪst] *subst.* doctor who is trained in psychoanalysis *psykoanalytiker*

psychogenic [ˌsaɪkə(ʊ)'dʒenɪk] *or* **psychogenetic** [ˌsaɪkə(ʊ)dʒə'netɪk] *or* **psychogenous** [saɪ'kɒdʒənəs] *adj.* (illness) which starts in the mind, rather than in a physical state *psykogen*

psychogeriatrics [ˌsaɪkəʊˌdʒeri'ætrɪks] *adj.* study of the mental disorders of old people *läran om mentala störningar hos åldringar*

psychological [ˌsaɪkə'lɒdʒɪk(ə)l] *adj.* referring to psychology *psykologisk;* caused by a mental state *psykisk, mental;* **psychological dependence =** state where a person is addicted to a drug (such as cannabis) but does not suffer physical effects if he stops taking it *psykiskt beroende*

psychologically [ˌsaɪkə'lɒdʒɪk(ə)li] *adv.* in a way which is caused by a mental state *psykologiskt, psykiskt, mentalt;* **she is psychologically incapable of making decisions; he is psychologically addicted to tobacco**

psychologist [saɪ'kɒlədʒɪst] *subst.* doctor who specializes in the study of the mind and mental processes *psykolog;* **clinical psychologist =** psychologist who studies and treats sick patients in hospital *klinisk psykolog;* **educational psychologist =** psychologist who studies the problems of education *ung. skolpsykolog*

psychology [saɪ'kɒlədʒi] *subst.* study of the mind and mental processes *psykologi*

psychometrics [ˌsaɪkə(ʊ)'metrɪks] *subst.* way of measuring intelligence and personality where the result is shown as a number on a scale *psykometri, psykologiska mätningar (mätmetoder)*

psychomotor [saɪkə(ʊ)'məʊtə] *adj.* referring to muscle movements caused by mental activity *psykomotorisk;* **psychomotor disturbance =** muscles movements (such as twitching) caused by mental disorder *psykomotorisk störning;* **psychomotor epilepsy =** epilepsy in which fits are characterized by blurring of consciousness and accompanied by coordinated but wrong movements *epilepsia psychomotorica, epilepsia (regioni) lobi temporalis;* **psychomotor retardation =** slowing of thought and action *psykomotorisk hämning*

psychoneurosis [ˌsaɪkə(ʊ)nju(ə)'rəʊsɪs] *or* **neurosis** [nju(ə)'rəʊsɪs] *subst.* any of a group of mental disorders in which a patient has a faulty response to the stresses of life *psykoneuros, neuros*

psychopath ['saɪkə(ʊ)pæθ] *subst.* person whose behaviour is abnormal and may be violent and antisocial *psykopat*

psychopathic [ˌsaɪkə(ʊ)'pæθɪk] *adj.* referring to psychopathy *psykopatisk*

psychopathological [ˌsaɪkəʊˌpæθə'lɒdʒɪk(ə)l] *adj.* referring to psychopathology *psykopatologisk*

psychopathology [ˌsaɪkə(ʊ)pə'θɒlədʒi] *subst.* branch of medicine concerned with the pathology of mental disorders and diseases *psykopatologi*

psychopathy [saɪ'kɒpəθi] *subst.* any disease of the mind *mentalsjukdom, sinnessjukdom, mental (psykisk) störning*

psychopharmacology [ˌsaɪkəʊˌfɑːmə'kɒlədʒi] *subst.* study of the actions and applications of drugs which have a powerful effect on the mind and behaviour *psykofarmakologi*

psychophysiological [ˌsaɪkəʊˌfɪziə'lɒdʒɪk(ə)l] *adj.* referring to psychophysiology *psykofysiologisk*

psychophysiology [ˌsaɪkəʊˌfɪzi'ɒlədʒi] *subst.* physiology of the mind and its functions *psykofysiologi*

psychosis [saɪ'kəʊsɪs] *subst.* general term for any serious mental disorder where the patient shows lack of insight *psykos*

psychosomatic [ˌsaɪkə(ʊ)sə(ʊ)'mætɪk] *adj.* referring to the relationship between body and mind *psykosomatisk*

> COMMENT: many physical disorders, such as duodenal ulcers or high blood pressure, can be caused by mental conditions like worry or stress, and are termed psychosomatic

psychosurgery [ˌsaɪkəʊ'sɜːdʒ(ə)ri] *subst.* brain surgery, used as a treatment for psychological disorders *psykokirurgi, psykiatrisk kirurgi*

psychosurgical [ˌsaɪkəʊ'sɜːdʒik(ə)l] *adj.* referring to psychosurgery *psykokirurgisk*

psychotherapeutic [ˌsaɪkə(ʊ)ˌθerə'pjuːtɪk] *adj.* referring to psychotherapy *psykoterapeutisk*

psychotherapist [ˌsaɪkə(ʊ)'θerəpɪst] *subst.* person trained to give psychotherapy *psykoterapeut*

psychotherapy [ˌsaɪkə(ʊ)'θerəpi] *subst.* treatment of mental disorders by psychological methods, as when a psychotherapist talks to the patient and encourages him to talk about his problems *psykoterapi; see also* THERAPY

psychotic [saɪ'kɒtɪk] *adj.* (i) referring to psychosis *psykotisk;* (ii) characterized by mental disorder *mentalt (psykiskt) störd*

psychotropic [ˌsaɪkə(ʊ)'trɒpɪk] *adj.* (drug) which affects a patient's mood (such as a stimulant or a sedative) *psykotrop(isk)*

psykasteni ⇨ **psychasthenia**

psykedelisk ⇨ **psychedelic**

psykiatri ⇨ **psychiatry**

psykiatrisk ⇨ **mental, psychiatric**

psykisk ⇨ **mental, psychological**

psykiskt ⇨ **mentally, psychologically**

psykiskt utvecklingsstörd ⇨ **subnormal**

psyk(o)- ⇨ **psych-**

psykoanalys ⇨ **psychoanalysis**

psykoanalytiker ⇨ **psychoanalyst**

psykofarmakologi ⇨ **psychopharmacology**

psykofysiologi ⇨ **psychophysiology**

psykofysiologisk ⇨ **psychophysiological**

psykogen ⇨ **psychogenic**

psykokirurgi ⇨ **psychosurgery**

psykokirurgisk ⇨ **psychosurgical**

psykolog ⇨ **psychologist**

psykologi ⇨ **psychology**

psykologisk ⇨ **psychological**

psykologiskt ⇨ **psychologically**

psykometri ⇨ **psychometrics**

psykomotorisk ⇨ **psychomotor**

psykoneuros ⇨ **psychasthenia, psychoneurosis**

psykopat ⇨ **psychopath**

psykopatologi ⇨ **psychopathology**

psykopatologisk ⇨ **psychopathic, psychopathological**

psykos ⇨ **psychosis**

psykosomatisk ⇨ **psychosomatic**

psykoterapeut ⇨ **psychotherapist**

psykoterapeutisk ⇨ **psychotherapeutic**

psykoterapi ⇨ **psychotherapy**

psykotisk ⇨ **psychotic**

pterion ['tɪərɪɒn] *subst.* point on the side of the skull where the frontal, temporal parietal and sphenoid bones meet *pterion*

pterygium [tə'rɪdʒəm] *subst.* triangular growth of conjunctiva which covers part of the cornea, with its apex towards the pupil *pterygium*

pterygo- ['terɪgə(ʊ), ˌ---] *suffix* referring to the pterygoid process *pterygo-*

pterygoid process ['terɪgɔɪd ˌprəʊses] *subst.* one of two projecting parts on the sphenoid bone *processus pterygoideus, vingutskottet på kilbenet;* **pterygoid plate** = small flat bony projection on the pterygoid process *yta på vingutskottet;* **pterygoid plexus** = group of veins and sinuses which join together behind the cheek *plexus pterygoideus*

pterygomandibular [ˌterɪgə(ʊ)mæn'dɪbjʊlə] *adj.* referring to the pterygoid process and the mandible *pterygomandibular, pterygomandibulär*

pterygopalatine fossa [ˌterɪgə(ʊ)'pælətɪn ˌfɒsə] *subst.* space between the pterygoid process and the upper jaw *fossa pterygo-palatina*

ptomaine ['təʊmeɪn] *subst.* group of nitrogenous substances produced in rotting food, which gives the food a special smell *ptomain(er)*
NOTE: **ptomaine poisoning** was the term formerly used to refer to any form of food poisoning

ptos ⇨ **prolapse, ptosis**

ptosis ['təʊsɪs] *subst.* (i) prolapse of an organ *ptos, prolaps, framfall;* (ii) drooping of the upper eyelid, which makes the eye stay half closed *ptosis palpebrae*

-ptosis ['təʊsɪs] *suffix* meaning prolapse *or* fallen position of an organ *-ptos, -prolaps, -framfall*

ptyal- ['ta(ɪ)əl, ˌ-] *or* **ptyalo-** ['ta(ɪ)ələʊ, ˌ---] *prefix* referring to the saliva *ptyal(o)-, sial(o)-, saliv-, spott-*

ptyalagoga ⇨ **sialagogue**

ptyalin ['ta(ɪ)əlɪn] *subst.* enzyme in saliva which cleanses the mouth and converts starch into sugar *ptyalin*

ptyalism ['ta(ɪ)əlɪz(ə)m] *subst.* production of an excessive amount of saliva *ptyalism, ptyalorré, sialism, sialorré*

ptyalith ['ta(ɪ)əlɪθ] *or* **sialolith** [saɪ'æləʊlɪθ] *subst.* stone in the salivary gland *ptyalolit, sialolit, salivsten, spottsten*

ptyalography [ˌta(ɪ)ə'lɒgrəfi] *or* **sialography** [ˌsa(ɪ)ə'lɒgrəfi] *subst.* X-ray examination of the ducts of the salivary gland *sialografi*

ptyalolit ⇨ **ptyalith, sialolith, salivary**

ptyalorré ⇨ **ptyalism, sialorrhoea**

pubertal ['pju:bət(ə)l] *or* **puberal** ['pju:b(ə)r(ə)l] *adj.* referring to puberty *pubertal, pubertets-*

pubertet ⇨ **puberty**

pubertets- ⇨ **pubertal**

puberty ['pju:bəti] *subst.* physical and psychological changes which take place when childhood ends and adolescence and sexual maturity begin and the sex glands become active *pubertet, könsmognad*

> COMMENT: puberty starts at about the age of 10 in girls, and slightly later in boys

pubes ['pju:bi:z] *subst.* part of the body just above the groin, where the pubic bones are found *pubes, blygden*

pubesbehåring ⇨ **pubic**

pubic ['pju:bɪk] *adj.* referring to the area near the genitals *pubisk, blygd-, blygdbens-;* **pubic bone** = pubis *or* bone in front of the pelvis *(os) pubis, blygdbenet;* **pubic hair** = tough hair growing in the genital region *pubesbehåring, blygdhår;* **pubic louse** *or* **Phthirius** = louse which infests the pubic regions *Phthirius (Pediculus) pubis, flatlus;* **pubic symphysis** = piece of cartilage which joins the two sections of the pubic bone *symphysis pubica (ossis pubis), symfysen, blygdbensfogen*

> COMMENT: in a pregnant woman, the pubic symphysis stretches to allow the pelvic girdle to expand so that there is room for the baby to pass through

pubis ['pju:bɪs] *subst.* bone forming the front part of the pelvis *(os) pubis, blygdbenet*
NOTE: the plural is **pubes**

puckel ⇨ **gibbosity, kyphos**

puckelrygg ⇨ **hunchback, kyphosis**

pudendal [pju'dend(ə)l] *adj.* referring to the pudendum *pudendal, blygd-;* **pudendal block** = operation to anaesthetize the pudendum during childbirth *pudendusblockad*

pudendum [pju'dendəm] *subst.* external genital organ of a woman *pudendum, blygden*
NOTE: the plural is **pudenda**

pudendusblockad ⇨ **pudendal**

puder ⇨ **powder, pulvis**

puerpera [pju'ɜ:p(ə)rə] *subst.* woman who has recently given birth *or* is giving birth, and whose womb is still distended *puerpera, barnaföderska, barnsängskvinna*

puerperal [pju'ɜ:p(ə)r(ə)l] *or* **puerperous** [pju'ɜ:p(ə)rəs] *adj.* (i) referring to the puerperium *puerperal, barnsängs-;* (ii) referring to childbirth *puerperal, barnsbörds-;* (iii) which occurs after childbirth *puerperal, som inträffar efter förlossningen;* **puerperal fever** = form of septicaemia, which was formerly common in mothers immediately after childbirth and caused many deaths *puerperalfeber, puerperalsepsis, barnsängsfeber*

puerperalfeber ⇨ **puerperal**

puerperalism [pju'ɜ:p(ə)rəlɪz(ə)m] *subst.* illness of a baby or its mother resulting from *or* associated with childbirth *sjukdom hos mor el. barn under barnsängstiden*

puerperalsepsis ⇨ **puerperal**

puerperiet ⇨ **puerperium**

puerperium [ˌpju:ə'pɪəriəm] *subst.* period of about six weeks which follows immediately after the birth of a child, during which the mother's sexual organs recover from childbirth *puerperiet, barnsängstiden*

puke [pju:k] *vb. (informal)* to vomit *or* to be sick *kräkas, spy*

Pulex ['pju:leks] *subst.* genus of human fleas *Pules (irritans), människoloppa, loppa*

pull [pʊl] *vb.* to strain *or* to make a muscle move in a wrong direction *sträcka;* **he pulled a muscle in his back**

pulley ['pʊli] *subst.* device with rings through which wires *or* cords pass, used in traction to make wires tense *trissa, talja, block*

pull through [ˌpʊl 'θru:] *vb. informal* to recover from a serious illness *klara sig, återhämta sig;* **the doctor says she is strong and should pull through**

pull together [ˌpʊl tə'geðə] *vb.* **to pull yourself together** = to become calmer *ta sig samman, lugna sig;* **although he was very angry he soon pulled himself together**

pulmo- ['pʌlmə(ʊ), ˌ--] *or* **pulmon-** ['pʌlmən, ˌ--] *or* **pulmono-** ['pʌlmənəʊ, ˌ---] *prefix* referring to the lungs *pulm(on)-, pneum(o)-, lung-*

pulmonal ⇨ **pulmonary**

pulmonale [ˌpʌlmə'neɪli] *see* COR PULMONALE

pulmonalisartärerna ⇨ **pulmonary**

pulmonalisinsufficiens ⇨ **pulmonary**

pulmonalisklaff ⇨ **pulmonary**

pulmonalisstenos ⇨ **pulmonary**

pulmonalisven ⇨ **pulmonary**

pulmonary ['pʌlmən(ə)ri] *adj.* referring to the lungs *pulmonal, pulmonell, lung-;* **pulmonary arteries** = arteries which take deoxygenated blood from the heart to the lungs for oxygenation ⇨ *illustration* HEART *arteria pulmonalis dextra resp. sinistra, pulmonalisartärerna, lungpulsådrorna;* **pulmonary circulation** = circulation of blood from the heart through the pulmonary arteries to the lungs for oxygenation and back to the heart through the pulmonary veins *lungkretsloppet, lilla kretsloppet;* **pulmonary embolism** = blockage of a pulmonary artery by a blood clot *lungemboli;* **pulmonary hypertension** = high blood pressure in the blood vessels supplying blood to the lungs *pulmonell hypertension;* **pulmonary insufficiency** *or* **incompetence** = dilatation of the main pulmonary artery and stretching of the valve ring, due to pulmonary hypertension *pulmonalisinsufficiens;* **pulmonary oedema** = collection of fluid in the lungs, as occurs in left-sided heart failure *oedema pulmonum, lungödem;* **pulmonary stenosis** = condition where the opening of the right ventricle becomes narrow *stenosis pulmonalis, pulmonalisstenos;* **pulmonary valve** = valve at the opening of the pulmonary artery *valva trunci pulmonalis,* *pulmonalisklaff;* **pulmonary vein** = vein which takes oxygenated blood from the lungs to the atrium of the heart *vena pulmonalis, pulmonalisven, lungven*

pulmonectomy [ˌpʌlmə(ʊ)'nektəmi] *or* **pneumonectomy** [ˌnjuːmə(ʊ)'nektəmi] *subst.* surgical removal of a lung *or* part of a lung *pulm(on)ektomi, pneum(on)ektomi*

pulmonell ⇨ **pulmonary**

pulp [pʌlp] *subst.* soft tissue, especially when surrounded by hard tissue such as the inside of a tooth *pulpa, tandpulpa, märg;* **pulp cavity** = centre of a tooth containing soft tissue *cavum dentis, pulpahåla, pulpakammare*

pulpa ⇨ **dental, pulp**

pulpahåla ⇨ **cavity, pulp**

pulpakammare ⇨ **cavity, pulp**

pulpy ['pʌlpi] *adj.* made of pulp *pulpös;* **the pulpy tissue inside a tooth**

pulpös ⇨ **pulpy**

puls ⇨ **pulse**

puls- ⇨ **sphygmo-**

pulsamplitud ⇨ **pulse**

pulsation [pʌl'seɪʃ(ə)n] *subst.* action of beating regularly, such as the visible pulse which can be seen under the skin in some parts of the body *pulsation*

pulse [pʌls] *subst.* **(a)** (i) any regular recurring variation in quantity *puls;* (ii) pressure wave which can be felt in an artery each time the heart beats to pump blood *puls, pulsslag;* **to take someone's pulse** = to place fingers on an artery to feel the pulse and count the number of beats per minute *ta pulsen på ngn;* **has the patient's pulse been taken? her pulse is very irregular; carotid pulse** = pulse in the carotid artery at the side of the neck *carotispuls;* **radial pulse** = main pulse in the wrist, taken near the outer edge of the forearm, just above the wrist *radialispuls;* **ulnar pulse** = secondary pulse in the wrist, taken near the inner edge of the forearm *ulnarispuls;* **pulse point** = place on the body where the pulse can be taken *tryckpunkt;* **pulse pressure** = difference between the diastolic and systolic pressure *pulstryck, pulsamplitud; see also* CORRIGAN **(b)** *(food)* **pulses** = beans and peas *baljfrukter;* **pulses provide a large amount of protein**

pulseless ['pʌlsləs] *adj.* (patient) who has no pulse because the heart is beating very weakly *pulslös*

pulsfrekvens ⇨ **rate**

pulslös ⇨ **pulseless**

pulsslag ⇨ **pulse**

pulstryck ⇨ **pulse**

pulsus ['pʌlsəs] *subst.* the pulse *pulsen;* **pulsus alternans** = pulse with a beat which is alternately strong and weak *pulsus alternans;* **pulsus bigeminus** = double pulse, with an extra ectopic beat *pulsus bigeminus, tvåslagspuls;* **pulsus paradoxus** = condition where there is a sharp fall in the pulse when a patient breathes in *pulsus paradoxus*

> COMMENT: the normal, adult pulse is about 72 beats per minute, but it is higher in children. The pulse is normally taken by placing the fingers on the patient's wrist, at the point where the radial artery passes through the depression just below the thumb

pulsåder ⇨ **artery**

pulsåder- ⇨ **arterial, arterio-**

pulsåderbråck ⇨ **aneurysm**

pulver ⇨ **powder, pulvis**

pulveriserad ⇨ **powdered**

pulvis ['pʌlvɪs] *subst.* powder *pulvis, pulver, puder*

pump [pʌmp] **1** *subst.* machine which forces liquids *or* air into or out of something *pump;* **stomach pump** = instrument for sucking out the contents of a patient's stomach, especially if he has just swallowed a poison *magpump* **2** *vb.* to force liquid *or* air along a tube *pumpa;* **the heart pumps blood round the body; the nurses tried to pump the poison out of the stomach**

punch drunk syndrome [ˌpʌn(t)ʃ 'drʌŋk ˌsɪndrəʊm] *subst.* condition of a patient (usually a boxer) who has been hit on the head many times, and develops impaired mental faculties, trembling limbs and speech disorders *punch-drunk-syndrom*

punctum ['pʌŋ(k)təm] *subst.* point *punkt, prick;* **puncta lacrimalia** = small openings at the corners of the eyes through which tears drain into the nose *puncta lacrimalia, tårpunkterna*

NOTE: plural is **puncta**

puncture ['pʌŋ(k)tʃə] **1** *subst.* (i) neat hole made by a sharp instrument *stick, instick;* (ii) making a hole in an organ *or* swelling to take a sample of the contents *or* to remove fluid *punktur, punktion, instick;* **lumbar puncture** *or* **spinal puncture** = surgical operation to remove a sample of cerebrospinal fluid by inserting a hollow needle into the lower part of the spinal canal *lumbalpunktion, spinalpunktion* (NOTE: US English is also **spinal tap**) **sternal puncture** = surgical operation to remove a sample of bone marrow from the breastbone for testing *sternalpunktion;* **puncture wound** = wound made by a sharp instrument which makes a hole in the tissue *vulnus ictum (punctum), sticksår* **2** *vb.* to make a hole in tissue with a sharp instrument *punktera, perforera, sticka hål på*

pundnäsa ⇨ **rhinophyma**

pung ⇨ **pouch**

pungen ⇨ **scrotum**

pungåderbråck ⇨ **varicocele**

punkt ⇨ **point, punctum**

punktera ⇨ **prick, puncture**

punktion ⇨ **puncture**

punktur ⇨ **puncture**

pupil ['pju:p(ə)l, -pɪl] *subst.* central opening in the iris of the eye, through which light enters the eye ⇨ *illustration* EYE *pupilla, pupillen*

pupillar ⇨ **pupillary**

pupillary ['pju:p(ə)l(ə)ri] *adj.* referring to the pupil *pupillar, pupillär;* **pupillary reaction** *or* **light reflex** = reflex where the pupil changes size according to the amount of light going into the eye *pupill(ar)reaktion, pupillreflex, ljusreflex*

pupilldilatation ⇨ **dilatation, mydriasis**

pupillen ⇨ **pupil**

pupillförminskning ⇨ **miosis**

pupillförträngning ⇨ **miosis**

pupillreflex ⇨ **pupillary**

pupillsammandragande medel ⇨ **miotic**

pupillsfinktern ⇨ **sphincter (muscle)**

pupillvidgande medel ⇨ **mydriatic**

pupillvidgning ⇨ **dilatation, mydriasis**

pupillär ⇨ **pupillary**

pure [pjʊə] *adj.* very clean *or* not mixed with other substances *ren, oblandad;* **pure alcohol** *or* **alcohol BP** = alcohol with 5% water *95% sprit*

purgans ⇨ **purgative**

purgation [pɜ:'geɪʃ(ə)n] *subst.* using a drug to make a bowel movement *laxering*

purgative ['pɜ:gətɪv] *or* **laxative** ['læksətɪv] *subst. & adj.* (medicine) which causes evacuation of the bowels *purgans, laxermedel, avföringsmedel, laxerande, purgerande, avförande*

purge [pɜ:dʒ] *vb.* to induce evacuation of a patient's bowels *purgera, laxera (kraftigt)*

purgerande ⇨ **cathartic, purgative**

purify ['pjʊərɪfaɪ] *vb.* to make pure *rena;* **purified protein derivative (PPD)** = pure form of tuberculin, used in tuberculin tests *pure protein derivative, PPD, Mantoux prov, tuberkulinprov*

Purkinje cells [pə'kɪndʒi ˌselz] *subst. pl.* neurones in the cerebellar cortex *Purkinjes celler*

Purkinje fibres [pə'kɪndʒi ˌfaɪb(ə)z] *subst. pl.* bundle of fibres which form the atrioventricular bundle and pass from the AV node to the septum *Purkinjes muskeltrådar, purkinjetrådar*

Purkinje shift [pə'kɪndʒi ˌʃɪft] *subst.* change which takes place in the eye when darkness falls, when the eye starts using the rods instead of the cones *övergång till mörkerseende*

purkinjetrådar ⇨ **Purkinje fibres**

purpura ['pɜ:pjʊrə] *subst.* purple colouring on the skin, similar to a bruise, caused by blood disease and not by trauma *purpura, hudblödningar;* **Henoch's purpura** = blood disorder of children, where the skin becomes purple and bleeding takes place in the intestine *Henoch-Schönleins purpura, purpura allergica (nervosa, rheumatica);* **Schönlein's purpura** = blood disorder of children, where the skin becomes purple and the joints are swollen and painful *Henoch-Schönleins purpura, purpura allergica (nervosa, rheumatica)*

pursestring ['pɜːsˌstrɪŋ] *see* SHIRODKAR

purulent ['pjʊərʊlənt] *or* **suppurating** ['sʌpjʊ(ə)reɪtɪŋ] *adj.* containing *or* producing pus *purulent, varig*

pus [pʌs] *subst.* yellow liquid composed of blood serum, pieces of dead tissue, white blood cells and the remains of bacteria, formed by the body in reaction to infection *pus, var*
NOTE: for terms referring to pus see words beginning with **py-** or **pyo-**

pustel ⇨ **pustule**

pustular ['pʌstjʊlə] *adj.* (i) covered with *or* composed of pustules *pustulös;* (ii) referring to pustules *pustulös*

pustule ['pʌstjuːl] *subst.* small pimple filled with pus *pustel*

pustulös ⇨ **pustular**

putrefaction [ˌpjuːtrɪ'fækʃ(ə)n] *subst.* decompositon of organic substances by bacteria, making an unpleasant smell *putrefaktion, putrescens, förruttnelse*

putrefy ['pjuːtrɪfaɪ] *vb.* to rot *or* to decompose *ruttna*

putrescens ⇨ **putrefaction**

p.v. [ˌpiː'viː] *abbreviation for the Latin phrase* "per vaginam": by examination of the vagina *per vaginam, genom slidan*

py- ['paɪ, ˌ-] *or* **pyo-** ['paɪə(ʊ), ˌ--] *prefix* referring to pus *py(o)-, var-*

pyaemia [paɪ'iːmiə] *subst.* invasion of blood with bacteria, which then multiply and form many little abscesses in various parts of the body *pyemi, allmän blodförgiftning*

pyarthrosis [ˌpaɪɑː'θrəʊsɪs] *subst.* acute suppurative arthritis *or* condition where a joint becomes infected with pyogenic organisms and fills with pus *pyartros, varig ledgångsinflammation*

pyel- ['pa(ɪ)əl, ˌ--] *or* **pyelo-** ['pa(ɪ)ələ(ʊ), ˌ---] *prefix* referring to the pelvis of the kidney *or* renal pelvis *pyel(o)-, njurbäcken(s)-*

pyelitis [ˌpa(ɪ)ə'laɪtɪs] *subst.* inflammation of the central part of the kidney *pyelit, njurbäckensinflammation*

pyelocystitis [ˌpa(ɪ)ələ(ʊ)sɪ'staɪtɪs] *subst.* inflammation of the pelvis of the ureter and the urinary bladder *pyelocystit*

pyelogram ['pa(ɪ)ələ(ʊ)græm] *subst.* X-ray photograph of a kidney and the urinary tract *urografi;* **intravenous pyelogram** = X-ray photograph of a kidney using intravenous pyelography *urografi*

pyelography [ˌpa(ɪ)ə'lɒgrəfi] *subst.* X-ray examination of a kidney after introduction of a contrast medium *urografi;* **intravenous pyelography** = X-ray examination of a kidney after opaque liquid has been injected intravenously into the body and taken by the blood into the kidneys *urografi;* **retrograde pyelography** = X-ray examination of the kidney where a catheter is passed into the kidney and the opaque liquid is injected directly into it *retrograd pyelografi*

pyelolithotomy [ˌpa(ɪ)ələ(ʊ)lɪ'θɒtəmi] *subst.* surgical removal of a stone from the pelvis of the ureter *pyelolitotomi*

pyelonephritis [ˌpa(ɪ)ələ(ʊ)nɪ'fraɪtɪs] *subst.* inflammation of the kidney and the pelvis of the ureter *pyelonefrit, nefropyelit*

pyeloplasty ['pa(ɪ)ələ(ʊ)plæsti] *subst.* any surgical operation on the pelvis of the ureter *kirurgiskt ingrepp i njurbäckenet*

pyelotomy [ˌpa(ɪ)ə'lɒtəmi] *subst.* surgical operation to make an opening in the pelvis of the ureter *pyelotomi*

pyemia [paɪ'iːmiə] = PYAEMIA

pyknolepsy [ˌpɪknə(ʊ)'lepsi] *subst.* former name for a type of frequent attack of petit mal epilepsy, affecting children *pyknolepsi, petit mal*

pyl- ['paɪl, ˌ-] *or* **pyle-** ['paɪli, ˌ--] *prefix* referring to the portal vein *pyl(e)-, portvens-*

pylephlebitis [ˌpaɪliflə'baɪtɪs] *subst.* thrombosis of the portal vein *pyleflebit*

pylethrombosis [ˌpaɪliθrɒm'bəʊsɪs] *subst.* condition where blood clots are present in the portal vein or any of its branches *pyletrombos*

pylor- [paɪˌlɔːr] *or* **pyloro** [paɪˈlɔːrə(ʊ), -ˌ--] *prefix* referring to the pylorus *pylor(o)-, pylorus-, magports-*

pylorectomy [ˌpaɪlə(ʊ)ˈrektəmi] *subst.* surgical removal of the pylorus and the antrum of the stomach *pylorektomi*

pyloric [paɪˈlɒrɪk] *adj.* referring to the pylorus *pylorus-, magports-;* **pyloric antrum** = space at the bottom of the stomach before the pyloric sphincter *antrum pyloricum (ventriculi);* **pyloric orifice** = opening where the stomach joins the duodenum *pylorus, nedre magmunnen, magporten;* **pyloric sphincter** = muscle which surrounds the pylorus, makes it contract and separates it from the duodenum *(musculus) sphincter pylori, pylorussfinktern;* **pyloric stenosis** = blockage of the pylorus, which prevents food from passing from the stomach into the duodenum *stenosis pylori, pylorusstenos*

pyloroplasty [paɪˈlɔːrə(ʊ)plæsti] *subst.* surgical operation make the pylorus larger, sometimes combined with treatment for peptic ulcers *pyloroplastik*

pylorospasm [paɪˈlɔːrə(ʊ)spæz(ə)m] *subst.* muscle spasm which closes the pylorus so that food cannot pass through into the duodenum *pylorospasm*

pylorotomy [ˌpaɪlə(ʊ)ˈrɒtəmi] *or* **Ramstedt's operation** [ˈrɑːmstets ˌɒpəˈreɪʃ(ə)n] *subst.* surgical operation to cut into the muscle surrounding the pylorus to relieve pyloric stenosis *slags kirurgiskt ingrepp vid pylorusstenos*

pylorus [paɪˈlɔːrəs] *subst.* opening at the bottom of the stomach leading into the duodenum *pylorus, nedre magmunnen, magporten*

pylorus- ▷ **pylor-, pyloric**

pylorussfinktern ▷ **pyloric**

pylorusstenos ▷ **pyloric**

pyo- [ˈpaɪə(ʊ), ˌ--] *prefix* referring to pus *py(o)-, var-*

pyocele [ˈpaɪə(ʊ)siː(ə)l] *subst.* enlargement of a tube *or* cavity due to accumulation of pus *pyocele*

pyocolpos [ˌpaɪə(ʊ)ˈkɒlpəs] *subst.* accumulation of pus in the vagina *pyokolpos*

pyoderma [ˌpaɪə(ʊ)ˈdɜːmə] *subst.* eruption of pus in the skin *pyodermi, pyodermatos, pyogen dermatos*

pyogenic [ˌpaɪə(ʊ)ˈdʒenɪk] *adj.* which produces *or* forms pus *pyogen, varbildande*

pyokolpos ▷ **pyocolpos**

pyometra [ˌpaɪə(ʊ)ˈmiːtrə] *subst.* accumulation of pus in the uterus *pyometra*

pyomyositis [ˌpaɪə(ʊ)ˌmaɪə(ʊ)ˈsaɪtɪs] *subst.* inflammation of a muscle caused by staphylococci *or* streptococci *muskelinflammation orsakad av stafylo- el. streptokocker*

pyonephrosis [ˌpaɪə(ʊ)nɪˈfrəʊsɪs] *subst.* distension of the kidney with pus *pyonefros*

pyopericarditis [ˌpaɪə(ʊ)ˌperikɑːˈdaɪtɪs] *subst.* bacterial pericarditis *or* inflammation of the pericardium due to infection with staphylococci *or* streptococci *or* pneumococci *pyopericarditis*

pyorrhoea [ˌpa(ɪ)əˈrɪə] *subst.* discharge of pus *pyorré, varflöde;* **pyorrhoea alveolaris** = suppuration from the supporting tissues round the teeth *pyorrhoea alveolaris, alveolarpyorré*

pyosalpinx [ˌpaɪə(ʊ)ˈsælpɪŋks] *subst.* inflammation and formation of pus in a Fallopian tube *pyosalpinx*

pyosis [paɪˈəʊsɪs] *subst.* formation of pus *or* suppuration *suppuration, varbildning*

pyothorax [ˌpaɪə(ʊ)ˈθɔːræks] = EMPYEMA

pyr- [paɪ(ə)r] *or* **pyro-** [ˈpaɪ(ə)rə(ʊ), ˌ--] *prefix* referring to burning *or* fever *pyr(o)-, feber-*

pyramid [ˈpɪrəmɪd] *subst.* cone-shaped part of the body, especially a cone-shaped projection on the surface of the medulla oblongata *or* in the medulla of the kidney ▷ *illustration* KIDNEY *pyramid*

pyramid- ▷ **pyramidal**

pyramidal [pɪˈræmɪd(ə)l] *adj.* referring to a pyramid *pyramidal, pyramid-;* **pyramidal cell** = cone-shaped cell in the cerebral cortex *pyramidcell;* **pyramidal tracts** = tracts in the brain and spinal cord which carry the motor neurone fibres from the cerebral cortex *pyramidbanorna*

pyramidbana ▷ **tract**

pyramidbanorna ▷ **cerebrospinal, pyramidal**

pyramidcell ⇨ **pyramidal**

pyrexia [paɪ(ə)'reksiə] *or* **fever** ['fi:və] *subst.* rise in the body temperature *or* sickness when the temperature of the body is higher than normal *pyrexi, feber*

pyridoxine [ˌpɪri'dɒksɪn] = VITAMIN B_6

pyrodruvsyra ⇨ **pyruvic acid**

pyrogen ['paɪ(ə)rə(ʊ)dʒen] *subst.* substance which causes a fever *pyrogen, pyrotoxin, feberframkallande ämne*

pyrogenic [ˌpaɪ(ə)rə(ʊ)'dʒenɪk] *adj.* which causes a fever *pyrogen, feberframkallande*

pyrosis [paɪ(ə)'rəʊsɪs] = HEARTBURN

pyrotoxin ⇨ **pyrogen**

pyruvic acid [ˌpaɪ(ə)ˌru:vɪk 'æsɪd] *subst.* substance formed from muscle glycogen when it is broken down to release energy *acidum puruvicum, pyrodruvsyra*

pyuria [paɪ'jʊəriə] *subst.* pus in the urine *pyuri*

påfresta ⇨ **strain**

påfrestande ⇨ **strenuous**

påfrestning ⇨ **strain, stress, wear and tear**

påse ⇨ **bag**

påskynda ⇨ **hurry, precipitate**

påssjuka ⇨ **mumps**

påstrykare ⇨ **applicator**

påträffas ⇨ **occur**

påverka ⇨ **affect, influence**

påverkan ⇨ **influence**

påverkbarhet ⇨ **responsiveness**

pärlsvulst ⇨ **cholesteatoma**

Qq

q.d.s. [ˌkju:di:'es] *or* **q.i.d.** [ˌkju:aɪ'di:] *abbreviation for Latin phrase* "quater in die sumendus": four times a day (written on prescriptions) *quater in dies, fyra gånger om dagen (dagligen)*

Q fever ['kju: ˌfi:və] *subst.* infectious rickettsial disease of sheep and cows caused by **Coxiella burnetti** transmitted to humans *Q-feber*

> COMMENT: Q fever mainly affects farm workers and workers in the meat industry. The symptoms are fever, cough and headaches

q.s. [ˌkju:'es] *abbreviation for the Latin phrase* "quantum sufficiat": as much as necessary (written on prescriptions) *quantum satis, (så mycket som är) tillräckligt*

quad [kwɒd] = QUADRUPLET

quadrant ['kwɒdr(ə)nt] *subst.* quarter of a circle *kvadrant*

quadrantanopia [ˌkwɒdr(ə)ntə'nəʊpiə] *subst.* blindness in a quarter of the field of vision *kvadrantanopsi, kvadranthemi(an)opsi*

quadrate lobe ['kwɒdreɪt ˌləʊb] *subst.* lobe on the lower side of the liver *lobus quadratus*

quadratus [kwɒ'dreɪtəs] *subst.* any muscle with four sides *fyrkantig muskel;* **quadratus femoris** = muscle at the top of the femur, that rotates the thigh *musculus quadratus femoris, fyrkantiga lårmuskeln*

quadri- ['kwɒdrɪ, ˌ--] *prefix* referring to four *quadri-, fyr-*

quadriceps femoris [ˌkwɒdrɪseps 'femɒrɪs] *subst.* large muscle in the front of the thigh, which extends to the leg *musculus quadriceps femoris, knästräckarmuskeln*

> COMMENT: the quadriceps femoris is divided into four parts: the rectus femoris, vastus lateralis, vastus medialis, and the vastus intermedius. It is the sensory receptors in the quadriceps which react to give a knee jerk when the patellar tendon is tapped

quadriplegia [ˌkwɒdrɪˈpliːdʒə] *subst.* paralysis of all four limbs: both arms and both legs *quadriplegi*

quadriplegic [ˌkwɒdriˈpledʒɪk] *subst. & adj.* (person) paralysed in all four arms and legs *quadriplegiker, quadriplegisk*

quadriplegiker ⇨ **quadriplegic**

quadriplegisk ⇨ **quadriplegic**

quadruple [ˈkwɒdrʊp(ə)l] *adj.* four times *or* in four parts *fyrdubbel, fyrfaldig;* **quadruple vaccine** = vaccine which immunizes against four diseases: diphtheria, whooping cough, poliomyelitis, and tetanus *vaccin som samtidigt skyddar mot difteri, kikhosta, polio och stelkramp*

quadruplet [ˈkwɒdrʊplət] *or* **quad** [kwɒd] *subst.* one of four babies born to a mother at the same time *fyrling;* **she had quadruptlets** *or* **quads** *see also* QUINTUPLET, SEXTUPLET, TRIPLET, TWIN

qualification [ˌkwɒlɪfɪˈkeɪʃ(ə)n] *subst.* being qualified *kvalifikation, merit, utbildning, examen, kompetens, behörighet;* **she has a qualification in pharmacy; are his qualifications recognized in Great Britain?**

qualify [ˈkwɒlɪfaɪ] *vb.* to pass a course of study and be accepted as being able to practise *kvalificera (meritera) sig, uppfylla kraven (villkoren), avlägga examen, skaffa sig behörighet (kompetens);* **he qualified as a doctor two years ago**

quarantine [ˈkwɒr(ə)ntiːn] **1** *subst.* period (originally forty days) when an animal *or* person *or* ship just arrived in a country has to be kept separate in case a serious disease may be carried, to allow the disease time to develop *karantän;* **the animals were put in quarantine on arrival at the port; a ship in quarantine shows a yellow flag called the quarantine flag 2** *vb.* to put a person *or* animal in quarantine *sätta ngn (ngt) i karantän*

> COMMENT: animals coming into Great Britain are quarantined for six months because of the danger of rabies. People who are suspected of having an infectious disease can be kept in quarantine for a period which varies according to the incubation period of the disease. The main diseases concerned are cholera, yellow fever and typhus

quartan fever [ˈkwɔːt(ə)n fiːvə] *subst.* infectious disease *or* form of malaria caused by **Plasmodium malariae** where the fever returns every four days *(febris) quartana, vartredjedagsfeber, vartredjedagsfrossa, kvartärmalaria; see also* TERTIAN

Queckenstedt test [ˈkwekənsted ˌtest] *subst.* test done during a lumbar puncture where pressure is applied to the jugular veins, to see if the cerebrospinal fluid is flowing correctly *Quenckenstedts test*

quickening [ˈkwɪk(ə)nɪŋ] *subst.* first sign of life in an unborn baby, usually after about four months of pregnancy, when the mother can feel it moving in her uterus *första fosterrörelserna, första "sparkarna"*

Quick test [ˈkwɪk ˌtest] *subst.* test to identify the clotting factors in a blood sample *Quicks test*

quiescent [kwɪˈes(ə)nt] *adj.* inactive *orörlig, overksam;* (disease) with symptoms reduced either by treatment *or* in the normal course of the disease *tyst, slumrande, inaktiv*

quin [kwɪn] = QUINTUPLET

Quinckeödem ⇨ **angioneurotic oedema**

quinidine [ˈkwɪnɪdiːn] *subst.* drug similar to quinine, used to treat tachycardia *kinidin*

quinine [kwɪˈniːn] *subst.* alkaloid drug made from the bark of a South American tree (the cinchona) *kinin;* **quinine poisoning =** illness caused by taking too much quinine *kininförgiftning*

quininism [ˈkwɪniːnɪz(ə)m] *or* **quinism** [ˈkwɪnɪz(ə)m] *subst.* quinine poisoning *kininförgiftning*

> COMMENT: quinine was formerly used to treat the fever symptoms of malaria, but is not often used now because of its side-effects. Symptoms of quinine poisoning are dizziness and noises in the head. Small amounts of quinine have a tonic effect and are used in tonic water

quinsy [ˈkwɪnzi] *or* **peritonsillar abscess** [ˌperiˈtɒnsɪlər ˌæbses] *subst.* acute throat inflammation with an abscess round a tonsil *peritonsillarabscess, peritonsillär abscess, halsböld*

quintuplet [ˈkwɪntjʊplət] *or* **quin** [kwɪn] *subst.* one of five babies born to a mother at the same time *femling; see also* QUADRUPLET, SEXTUPLET, TRIPLET, TWIN

quotidian [kwə(ʊ)'tɪdiən] *adj.* recurring daily *daglig;* **quotidian fever** = violent form of malaria where the fever returns at daily or even shorter intervals *febris quotidianan, varjedagsfeber, varjedagsfrossa*

quotient ['kwəʊʃ(ə)nt] *subst.* result when one number is divided by another *kvot;* **intelligence quotient (IQ)** = ratio of the result of an intelligence test shown as a relationship of the mental age to the actual age of the person tested (the average being 100) *intelligenskvot, IQ, IK;* **respiratory quotient** = ratio of the amount of carbon dioxide passed from the blood into the lungs to the amount of oxygen absorbed into the blood from the air *respiratorisk kvot, RQ*

Rr

R symbol for roentgen *R, röntgen*

R/ abbreviation for the Latin word "recipe": prescription *recipe, Rec, tag!*

RA ⇨ **arthritis, rheumatoid**

Ra *chemical symbol for* radium *Ra, radium*

rabbit fever ['ræbɪt fi:və] = TULARAEMIA

rabdovirus ⇨ **rhabdovirus**

rabid ['ræbɪd] *adj.* referring to rabies *or* suffering from rabies *som avser el. hör till rabies;* **he was bitten by a rabid dog; rabid encephalitis** = fatal encephalitis resulting from the bite of a rabid animal *encefalit (hjärninflammation) pga rabies*

rabies ['reɪbi:z] *or* **hydrophobia** [ˌhaɪdrə(ʊ)'fəʊbiə] *subst.* frequently fatal viral disease transmitted to humans by infected animals *rabies, hydrofobi, vattuskräck*

> COMMENT: rabies affects the mental balance, and the symptoms include difficulty in breathing or swallowing and an intense fear of water (hydrophobia) to the point of causing convulsions at the sight of water

rachi- ['reɪki, ˌ--] *or* **rachio-** ['reɪkiə(ʊ), ˌ--] *prefix* referring to the spine *raki(o)-, ryggrads-*

rachianaesthesia [ˌreɪkiˌænəs'θi:ziə] = SPINAL ANAESTHESIA

rachiotomy [ˌreɪki'ɒtəmi] *or* **laminectomy** [ˌlæmi'nektəmi] *subst.* surgical operation to cut through a vertebra in the spine to reach the spinal cord *raki(o)tomi, laminektomi*

rachis ['reɪkɪs] = BACKBONE

rachischisis [reɪ'kɪskɪsɪs] = SPINA BIFIDA

rachitic [rə'kɪtɪk] *adj.* (child) with rickets *rakitisk*

rachitis [rə'kaɪtɪs] = RICKETS

rad [ræd] *subst.* SI unit of radiation absorbed into the body *rad; see also* BECQUEREL
NOTE: **Gray** is now more often used

rad ⇨ **range, succession**

radial ['reɪdiəl] *adj.* (i) referring to something which branches *radial, radio-, strål(nings)-;* (ii) referring to the radius, one of the bones in the forearm *radial(-), radio-, radialis-, strålbens-;* **radial artery** = artery which branches from the brachial artery, running near the radius, from the elbow to the palm of the hand *arteria radialis, radialartären;* **radial nerve** = main motor nerve in the arm, running down the back of the upper arm and the outer side of the forearm *nervus radialis, radialnerven;* **radial pulse** = main pulse in the wrist, taken near the outer edge of the forearm, just above the wrist *radialispuls;* **radial recurrent** = artery in the arm which forms a loop beside the brachial artery *arteria recurrens radialis, bakåtgående slinga i radialartären;* **radial reflex** = jerk made by the forearm when the insertion in the radius of one of the muscles (the brachioradialis) is hit *radialisreflex*

radialartären ⇨ **radial**

radialis- ⇨ **radial, radio-**

radialispuls ⇨ **radial**

radialisreflex ⇨ **radial**

radialnerven ⇨ **radial**

radiate ['reɪdɪeɪt] *vb.* **(a)** to spread out in all directions from a central point *radiera, stråla ut;* **the pain radiates from the site of the infection (b)** to send out rays *radiera, bestråla, sända ut;* **heat radiates from the body**

radiation [ˌreɪdiˈeɪʃ(ə)n] *subst.* waves of energy which are given off by certain substances, especially radioactive substances *strålning, bestrålning;* **radiation burn** = burning of the skin caused by exposure to large amounts of radiation *strålskada;* **radiation enteritis** = enteritis caused by X-rays *tarminflammation pga radioaktiv bestrålning (röntgenbestrålning);* **radiation sickness** = illness caused by exposure to radiation from radioactive substances *strålsjuka, strålningssjukdom;* **radiation treatment** = RADIOTHERAPY *see also* OPTIC RADIATION, SENSORY RADIATION

COMMENT: prolonged exposure to many types of radiation can be harmful. Nuclear radiation is the most obvious, but exposure to X-rays (either as a patient being treated, or as a radiographer) can cause radiation sickness. First symptoms of the sickness are diarrhoea and vomiting, but radiation can also be followed by skins burns and loss of hair. Massive exposure to radiation can kill quickly, and any person exposed to radiation is more likely to develop certain types of cancer than other members of the population

radical [ˈrædɪk(ə)l] *adj.* (i) very serious *or* which deals with the root of a problem *radikal, ursprunglig;* (ii) (operation) which removes the whole of a part *or* of an organ and its lymph system, along with other tissue *radikal, genomgripande;* **radical mastectomy** = surgical removal of a breast and the lymph nodes and muscles associated with it *radikal mastektomi;* **radical treatment** = treatment which aims at complete eradication of a disease *radikal behandling*

radicle [ˈrædɪk(ə)l] *subst.* (i) a small root *or* vein *radikulit, liten rot (ven);* (ii) tiny fibre which forms the root of a nerve *radikulit, nervrot*

radicular [rəˈdɪkjʊlə] *adj.* referring to a radicle *radikul-*

radiculitis [rəˌdɪkjʊˈlaɪtɪs] *subst.* inflammation of a radicle of a cranial *or* spinal nerve *radikulit; see also* POLYRADICULITIS

radiera ⇨ **radiate**

radik- ⇨ **rhiz-**

radikal ⇨ **radical**

radikul- ⇨ **radicular**

radikulit ⇨ **radicle, radiculitis**

radio- [ˈreɪdiəʊ, ˌ--] *prefix* referring to (i) radiation *radio-, röntgen-, strål(nings)-;* (ii) radioactive substances *radioaktiv;* (iii) the radius in the arm *radialis-, radio-, strålbens-*

radio- ⇨ **radial, radio-**

radioactive [ˌreɪdiəʊˈæktɪv] *adj.* (substance) which gives off energy in the form of radiation which can pass through other substances *radioaktiv*

COMMENT: the commonest radioactive substances are radium and uranium. Other substances can be made radioactive for medical purposes. Radioactive iodine is used to treat conditions such as thyrotoxicosis

radioactivity [ˌreɪdiəʊækˈtɪvəti] *subst.* giving off energy in the form of radiation *radioaktivitet*

radioaktiv ⇨ **radio-, radioactive**

radioaktivitet ⇨ **radioactivity**

radiobiologist [ˌreɪdiəʊbaɪˈɒlədʒɪst] *subst.* doctor who specializes in radiobiology *radiobiolog, strålbiolog*

radiobiology [ˌreɪdiəʊbaɪˈɒlədʒi] *subst.* scientific study of radiation and its effects on living things *radiobiologi*

radiocarpal joint [ˌreɪdiəʊˈkɑːp(ə)l ˌdʒɔɪnt] *subst.* wrist joint *or* joint where the radius articulates with the scaphoid (one of the carpal bones) *articulatio radio-carpea, radiokarpalleden*

radiodermatitis [ˌreɪdiəʊˌdɜːməˈtaɪtɪs] *subst.* inflammation of the skin after exposure to radiation *radiodermatit*

radiofarmakon ⇨ **radiopharmaceutical**

radiografi ⇨ **radiography, teleradiography**

radiogram ⇨ **radiograph, roentgenogram**

radiograph [ˈreɪdiə(ʊ)grɑːf] *subst.* X-ray photograph *radiogram, röntgenbild*

radiographer [ˌreɪdiˈɒgrəfə] *subst.* (i) person specially trained to operate a machine to take X-ray photographs *or* radiographs (diagnostic radiographer) *röntgenassistent;* (ii) person specially trained to use X-rays *or* radioactive isotopes in treatment of patients (therapeutic radiographer) *röntgenassistent*

radiography [ˌreɪdiˈɒɡrəfi] *subst.* examining the internal parts of a patient by taking X-ray photographs *radiografi, röntgenografi, röntgenfotografering*

radioimmunoassay [ˌreɪdiəʊˌɪmjuːnəʊˈæseɪ] *subst.* process of finding out if antibodies are present by injecting radioactive tracers into the bloodstream *radioimmunoassay, RIA*

radioisotop ⇨ **radioisotope**

radioisotope [ˌreɪdiəʊˈaɪsətəʊp] *subst.* isotope of a chemical element which has been made radioactive *radioisotop, radioaktiv isotop*

COMMENT: radioisotopes are used in medicine to provide radiation for radiation treatment. Radioisotopes of iodine are used to investigate thyroid activity

radiokarpalleden ⇨ **radiocarpal joint**

radiologi ⇨ **radiology, roentgenology**

radiologist [ˌreɪdɪˈɒlədʒɪst] *subst.* doctor who specializes in radiology *radiolog, röntgenolog, röntgenläkare*

radiology [ˌreɪdiˈɒlədʒi] *subst.* use of radiation to diagnose disorders (as in the use of X-rays or radioactive tracers) *or* to treat diseases such as cancer *radiologi, röntgenologi*

radio-opaque [ˌreɪdiəʊəʊˈpeɪk] *adj.* (substance) which absorbs all or most of a radiation *radiopak, röntgentät*

COMMENT: radio-opaque substances appear dark on X-rays and are used to make it easier to have clear radiographs of certain organs

radiopak ⇨ **radio-opaque**

radiopharmaceutical [ˌreɪdiəʊˌfɑːməˈsuːtɪk(ə)l] *subst.* radioisotope used in medical diagnosis *or* treatment *radiofarmakon*

radio pill [ˈreɪdiəʊ pɪl] *subst.* tablet with a tiny radio transmitter *tablett med radiosändare*

COMMENT: the patient swallows the pill and as it passes through the body it gives off information about the digestive system

radioscopy [ˌreɪdiˈɒskəpi] *subst.* examining an X-ray photograph on a fluorescent screen *radioskopi, fluoroskopi, röntgengenomlysning, genomlysning*

radiosensitive [ˌreɪdiəʊˈsensətɪv] *adj.* (cancer cell) which is sensitive to radiation and can be treated by radiotherapy *strålkänslig*

radioskopi ⇨ **fluoroscopy, radioscopy**

radioterapi ⇨ **irradiation, radiotherapy**

radiotherapy [ˌreɪdiəʊˈθerəpi] *subst.* treating a disease by exposing the affected part to radioactive rays such as X-rays *or* gamma rays *radioterapi, strålbehandling*

COMMENT: many forms of cancer can be treated by directing radiation at the diseased part of the body

radium [ˈreɪdiəm] *subst.* radioactive metallic element *radium, Ra*
NOTE: chemical symbol is **Ra**

radius [ˈreɪdiəs] *subst.* the shorter and outer of the two bones in the forearm between the elbow and the wrist (the other bone is the ulna) ⇨ *illustration* HAND, SKELETON *radius, strålbenet*

radix [ˈreɪdɪks] *or* **root** [ruːt] *subst.* (i) point from which a part of the body grows *radix, rot;* (ii) part of a tooth which is connected to a socket in the jaw *radix, tandrot*

radon [ˈreɪdɒn] *subst.* radioactive gas, formed from radium, and used in capsules (known as radon seeds) to treat cancers inside the body *radon, Rn*
NOTE: chemical symbol is **Rn**

rafe ⇨ **raphe**

ragader ⇨ **rhagades**

ragla ⇨ **stagger**

raise [reɪz] *vb.* **(a)** to lift *lyfta, höja;* **lie with your legs raised above the level of your head (b)** to increase *öka, höja;* **anaemia causes a raised level of white blood cells in the body**

rak ⇨ **erect, rectus, straight, upright**

raka (sig) ⇨ **shave**

raki(o)- ⇨ **rachi-, rhachio-**

rakischis ⇨ **spina bifida**

rakit ⇨ **rickets**

rakitisk ⇨ **rachitic**

rakning ⇨ **shave**

rale [rɑːl] = CREPITATION

ram ⇨ **frame**

ramla (omkull) ⇨ **fall**

Ramstedt's operation [ˈrɑːmstets ˌɒpəˈreɪʃ(ə)n] = PYLOROTOMY

ramus [ˈreɪməs] *subst.* **(a)** branch of a nerve *or* artery *or* vein *ramus, gren* **(b)** the ascending part on each side of the mandible *ramus mandibulae, underkäksgrenen*
NOTE: plural is **rami**

rand ⇨ **border, limbus, ridge, weal**

range [reɪn(d)ʒ] *subst.* (i) series of different but similar things *rad, räcka;* (ii) difference between lowest and highest values in a series of data *räckvidd, omfång;* **the drug offers protection against a wide range of diseases; doctors have a range of drugs which can be used to treat arthritis**

ranula [ˈrænjʊlə] *subst.* small cyst under the tongue, on the floor of the mouth, which forms when a salivary duct is blocked *ranula, retentionscysta (under tungan), spottkörtelcysta*

Ranvier [rɑːnvɪˈeɪ] *see* NODE

rapa ⇨ **belch, burp, wind**

raphe [ˈreɪfi] *subst.* long thin fold which looks like a seam, along a midline such as on the dorsal face of the tongue *rafe, söm, sammanväxningslinje*

rapid [ˈræpɪd] *adj.* fast *hastig, snabb;* **rapid eye movement (REM) sleep** = phase of normal sleep with fast movements of the eyeballs which occur at intervals *REM-sömn*
NOTE: During REM sleep, a person dreams, breathes lightly and has a raised blood pressure and an increased rate of heartbeat. The eyes may be half-open, and the sleeper may make facial movements

rap(ning) ⇨ **belch, burp**

rapport ⇨ **report**

rapportera ⇨ **notify, report**

rare [reə] *adj.* not common *or* (disease) of which there are very few cases *ovanlig, sällsynt;* **he is suffering from a rare blood disorder; AO is not a rare blood group**

rarefaction [ˌreərɪˈfækʃ(ə)n] *subst.* condition where bone tissue becomes more porous and less dense because of lack of calcium *rarefaktion, rarefikation, benvävsförtunning*

rarefaktion ⇨ **rarefaction**

rarefikation ⇨ **rarefaction**

rarefy [ˈreərɪfaɪ] *vb.* (of bones) to become less dense *förtunnas*

raseri ⇨ **furor**

raserianfall ⇨ **tantrum**

rash [ræʃ] *subst.* mass of small spots which stays on the skin for a period of time, and then disappears *utslag, hudutslag;* **to break out in a rash** = to have a rash which starts suddenly *plötsligt få utslag;* **she had a high temperature and then broke out in a rash; nappy** *or* *US* **diaper rash** = sore red skin on a baby's buttocks and groin, caused by long contact with ammonia in a wet nappy *blöjdermatit, blöjeksem*

> COMMENT: many common diseases such as chickenpox and measles have a special rash as their main symptom. Rashes can be very irritating, but the itching can be relieved by bathing in calamine lotion

rashygien ⇨ **eugenics**

rasp ⇨ **raspatory**

raspatory [ˈræspət(ə)ri] *subst.* surgical instrument like a file, which is used to scrape the surface of a bone *raspatorium, rasp, skavjärn*

rassel ⇨ **crepitation**

rast ⇨ **rest**

rastlös ⇨ **agitated, restless**

rat-bite fever [ˈrætbaɪt ˌfiːvə] *subst.* fever developing after having been bitten by a rat, caused by either of two bacteria, **Spirillum minus** or **Actinomyces muris,** transmitted to humans from rats *sodoku, råttbettsfeber, råttbettssjuka*

rate [reɪt] *subst.* **(a)** amount *or* proportion of something compared to something else *tal;* **birth rate** = number of children born per 1000 of population *nativitet, födelsetal;* **fertility rate** = number of births per year calculated per 1000 females aged between 15 and 44 *fertilitetstal, fruktsamhetstal* **(b)** number of times something happens *frekvens, hastighet;*

the heart was beating at a rate of only 59 per minute; heart rate = number of times the heart beats per minute *hjärtfrekvens;* **pulse rate** = number of times the pulse beats per minute *puls, pulsfrekvens*

COMMENT: pulse rate is the heart rate felt at various parts of the body

ratio ['reɪʃiəʊ] *subst.* number which shows a proportion *or* which is the result of one number divided by another *kvot;* **an IQ is the ratio of the person's mental age to his chronological age**

Rauwolfia [rɔː'wʊlfiə] *subst.* tranquillizing drug extracted from a plant **Rauwolfia serpentina** sometimes used to treat high blood pressure *Rauwolfia (serpertina); see also* RESERPINE

raw [rɔː] *adj.* **(a)** not cooked *rå* **(b)** (i) sensitive (skin) *öm;* (ii) (skin) scraped *or* partly removed *hudlös, oläkt;* **the scab came off leaving the raw wound exposed to the air**

ray [reɪ] *subst.* line of light *or* radiation *or* heat *stråle;* **infrared rays** = long invisible rays, below the visible red end of the spectrum, used to warm body tissue *infraröda strålar, infraröd strålning;* **ultraviolet rays (UV rays)** = short invisible rays beyond the violet end of the spectrum, which form the element in sunlight which tans the skin *ultravioletta strålar, UV-strålning, UV-ljus; see also* X-RAY

Raynaud's disease [reɪ'nəʊz dɪˌziːz] *or* **dead man's fingers** [ˌded mænz 'fɪŋgəz] *subst.* condition where the fingers and toes become cold, white and numb at temperatures that would not affect a normal person *acrocyanosis chronica anaesthetica, Raynauds fenomen (sjukdom, syndrom), vasospasm*

RBC [ˌɑːbiː'siː] = RED BLOOD CELL

RCGP [ˌɑːsiːdʒiː'piː] = ROYAL COLLEGE OF GENERAL PRACTITIONERS

RCN [ˌɑːsiː'en] = ROYAL COLLEGE OF NURSING

RCOG [ˌɑːsiːəʊ'dʒiː] = ROYAL COLLEGE OF OBSTETRICIANS AND GYNAECOLOGISTS

RCP [ˌɑːsiː'piː] = ROYAL COLLEGE OF PHYSICIANS

reabsorb [ˌriːəb'sɔːb] *vb.* to absorb again *resorbera, återuppsuga, återuppta;* **glucose is reabsorbed by the tubules in the kidney**

reabsorption [ˌriːəb'sɔːpʃ(ə)n] *subst.* process of being reabsorbed *resorption, återuppsugning, återupptag;* **some substances which are filtered into the tubules of the kidney, then pass into the bloodstream by tubular reabsorption**

reach [riːtʃ] **1** *subst.* distance which one can stretch a hand; distance which one can travel easily *räckhåll;* **medicines should be kept out of the reach of children; the hospital is in easy reach of the railway station 2** *vb.* to arrive at a point *nå (fram till);* **infection has reached the lungs**

react [ri'ækt] *vb.* **(a) to react to something** = to act because of something else *or* to act in response to something *reagera för ngt;* **the tissues reacted to the cortisone injection; the patient reacted badly to the penicillin; she reacted positively to the Widal test (b)** *(of a chemical substance)* **to react with something** = to change because of the presence of another substance *reagera med ngt*

reaction [ri'ækʃ(ə)n] *subst.* **(a)** (i) action which takes place because of something which has happened earlier *reaktion, svar;* (ii) effect produced by a stimulus *respons, reaktion, svar;* **a rash appeared as a reaction to the penicillin injection; the patient suffers from an allergic reaction to oranges (b)** particular response of a patient to a test *reaktion, svar;* **Wassermann reaction** = reaction to a blood test for syphilis *Wassermanns reaktion, WR*

reactivate [ri'æktɪveɪt] *vb.* to make active again *reaktivera;* **his general physical weakness has reactivated the dormant virus**

reactive [ri'æktɪv] *or* **reactionary** [ri'ækʃ(ə)n(ə)ri] *adj.* which takes place because of a reaction *reaktiv;* **reactionary haemorrhage** = bleeding which follows an operation *postoperativ blödning;* **reactive hyperaemia** = congestion of blood vessels after an occlusion has been removed *reaktiv hyperemi*

reading ['riːdɪŋ] *subst.* note taken of figures, especially of degrees on a scale *avläsning, gradtal, värde;* **the sphygmomanometer gave a diastolic reading of 70**

reagent [ri'eɪdʒ(ə)nt] *subst.* chemical substance which reacts with another substance (especially when used to detect the presence of the second substance) *reagens*

reagera för ngt ⇨ **react**

reagin ['rɪədʒɪn] *subst.* antibody which reacts against an allergen *reagin*

reaktion ⇨ **reaction, response**

reaktiv ⇨ **reactive**

reaktivera ⇨ **reactivate**

reappear [ˌriːəˈpɪə] *vb.* to appear again *åter visa sig (dyka upp, synas)*

reappearance [ˌriːəˈpɪər(ə)ns] *subst.* appearing again *återuppträdande;* **the reappearance of the symptoms after a period of several months**

reason [ˈriːz(ə)n] *subst.* **(a)** thing which explains why something happens *skäl, anledning, orsak;* **what was the reason for the sudden drop in the patient's pulse rate?** **(b)** being mentally stable *förstånd, förnuft;* **her reason was beginning to fail**

reassurance [ˌriːəˈʃʊər(ə)ns] *subst.* act of reassuring *uppmuntran, försäkran, tröst*

reassure [ˌriːəˈʃɔː] *vb.* to make someone sure *or* to give someone hope *uppmuntra, inge tillförsikt (lugn), försäkra, trösta;* **the doctor reassured her that the drug had no unpleasant side-effects; he reassured the old lady that she should be able to walk again in a few weeks**

rebore [ˈriːbɔː] *subst. informal* endarterectomy *or* surgical operation to remove the lining of a blocked artery *sotning*

rebuild [ˌriːˈbɪld] *vb.* to build up again bone which has been destroyed *återuppbygga;* **she has had a rebuilding operation on the pelvis**

recalcitrant [rɪˈkælsɪtr(ə)nt] *adj.* (condition) which does not respond to treatment *ihållande, ihärdig, envis*

recall [rɪˈkɔːl] **1** *subst.* act of remembering something from the past *hågkomst, minne;* **total recall** = being able to remember something in complete detail *perfekt minne* **2** *vb.* to remember something which happened in the past *komma ihåg, minnas*

receive [rɪˈsiːv] *vb.* to get something (especially a transplanted organ) *motta, få;* **she received six pints of blood in a transfusion; he received a new kidney from his brother**

recept ⇨ **formula, prescription**

receptaculum [ˌriːsepˈtækjʊləm] *subst.* part of a tube which is expanded to form a sac *receptaculum, behållare*

receptbelagd ⇨ **ethical**

receptbelagd, inte ⇨ **OTC**

receptor (cell) [rɪˈseptə (ˌsel)] *subst.* nerve ending which senses a change in the surrounding environment *or* in the body (such as cold *or* pressure *or* pain) and reacts to it by sending an impulse to the central nervous system *receptorcell; see also* ADRENERGIC, CHEMORECEPTOR, EXTEROCEPTOR, INTEROCEPTOR, THERMORECEPTOR, VISCERORECEPTOR

recess [rɪˈses] *subst.* hollow part in an organ *recess, ficka*

recessive [rɪˈsesɪv] *adj. & subst.* (trait) which is weaker than and hidden by a dominant gene *recessiv, vikande*

> COMMENT: since each physical characteristic is governed by two genes, if one is dominant and the other recessive, the resulting trait will be that of the dominant gene. Traits governed by recessive genes will appear if both genes are recessive

recidiv ⇨ **recrudescence, recurrence, relapse**

recidivera ⇨ **relapse**

recidiverande ⇨ **palindromic, recrudescent**

recipient [rɪˈsɪpiənt] *subst.* person who receives something, such as a transplant *or* a blood transfusion from a donor *recipient, mottagare*

> QUOTE bone marrow has to be carefully matched with the recipient or graft-versus-host disease will ensue
>
> **Hospital Update**

Recklinghausen [ˈreklɪŋˌhaʊzən] *see* VON RECKLINGHAUSEN

recognize [ˈrekəgnaɪz] *vb.* **(a)** to sense something (as to see a person *or* to taste a food) and remember it from an earlier sensing *känna igen;* **she did not recognize her mother** **(b)** to approve of something officially *erkänna;* **the diploma is recognized by the Department of Health**

recommend [ˌrekəˈmend] *vb.* to suggest that it would be a good thing if someone did something *rekommendera, föreslå;* **the doctor recommended that she should stay in bed; I would recommend following a diet to try to lose some weight**

reconstructive surgery [ˌriːkənˈstrʌktɪv ˌsɜːdʒ(ə)ri] *subst.* plastic surgery *or* surgery which repairs defective *or* deformed parts of the body *rekonstruktiv kirurgi, plastikkirurgi*

reconvert [ˌriːkənˈvɜːt] *vb.* to convert back into an earlier form *återomvandla;* **the liver reconverts some of its stored glycogen into glucose**

record 1 [rɪˈkɔːd] *vb.* to note information *registrera, uppteckna, protokollföra;* **the chart records the variations in the patient's blood pressure; you must take the patient's temperature every hour and record it in this book 2** [ˈrekɔːd] *subst.* piece of information about something *registrering, uppteckning, protokoll;* **medical records =** information about a patient's medical history *journal*

COMMENT: patients are not usually allowed to see their medical records because the information in them is confidential to the doctor

recover [rɪˈkʌvə] *vb.* **(a)** to get better after an illness *or* operation *or* accident *tillfriskna, återhämta sig;* **she recovered from her concussion in a few days; it will take him weeks to recover from the accident** NOTE: you recover **from** an illness **(b)** to get back something which has been lost *återfå;* **will he ever recover the use of his legs? she recovered her eyesight after all the doctors thought she would be permanently blind**

recovery [rɪˈkʌvəri] *subst.* getting better after an illness *or* accident *or* operation *tillfrisknande, bättring, återhämtning;* **he is well on the way to recovery =** he is getting better *han är på bättringsvägen (håller på att tillfriskna);* **she made only a partial recovery =** she is better, but will never be completely well *hon har inte återhämtat sig helt (fullständigt);* **she has made a complete *or* splendid recovery =** she is completely well *hon har blivit helt frisk (har återhämtat sig fullständigt);* **recovery room =** room in a hospital where a patient who has had an operation is placed until the effects of the anaesthetic have worn off and he can be moved into an ordinary ward *uppvakningsrum;* **recovery position =** position where the patient lies faces downwards, with one knee and one arm bent forwards, and the face turned to one side *framstupa sidoläge*

COMMENT: called the recovery position because it is recommended for accident victims *or* people who are suddenly ill, while waiting for an ambulance to arrive. The position prevents the patient from swallowing and choking on blood *or* vomit

recrudescence [ˌriːkruːˈdes(ə)ns] *subst.* reappearance of symptoms (of a disease which seemed to have got better) *recidiv, återfall*

recrudescent [ˌriːkruːˈdes(ə)nt] *adj.* (symptom) which has reappeared *recidiverande, åter uppblossande (utbrytande)*

recruit [rɪˈkruːt] *vb.* to get people to join the staff *or* a group *rekrytera, värva, anställa;* **we are trying to recruit more nursing staff**

QUOTE patients presenting with symptoms of urinary tract infection were recruited in a general practice surgery
Journal of the Royal College of General Practitioners

rect- [ˈrekt] *or* **recto-** [ˈrektə(ʊ)] *prefix* referring to the rectum *rekt(o)-, prokt(o)-, ändtarms-*

rectal [ˈrekt(ə)l] *adj.* referring to the rectum *rektal, ändtarms-;* **rectal fissure =** crack in the wall of the anal canal *fissura ani, analfissur, rektalfissur;* **rectal prolapse =** condition where part of the rectum moves downwards and passes through the anus *prolapsus recti, rektalprolaps;* **rectal temperature =** temperature in the rectum, taken with a rectal thermometer *rektaltemp(eratur);* **rectal thermometer =** thermometer which is inserted into the patient's rectum to take the temperature *rektaltermometer;* **rectal triangle** *or* **anal triangle =** posterior part of the perineum *bakre delen av bäckenbotten*

rectally [ˈrekt(ə)li] *adv.* through the rectum *rektalt;* **the temperature was taken rectally**

rectocele [ˈrektəʊˌsiː(ə)l] *or* **proctocele** [ˈprɒktəʊˌsiː(ə)l] *subst.* condition associated with prolapse of the womb, where the rectum protrudes into the vagina *rektocele, proktocele, ändtarmsbråck*

rectopexy [ˈrektəʊˌpeksi] *subst.* surgical operation to attach a rectum which has prolapsed *rektopexi*

rectosigmoidectomy [ˌrektəʊˌsɪgmɔɪˈdektəmi] *subst.* surgical removal of the sigmoid colon and the rectum *proktosigmoidektomi*

rectovaginal examination [ˌrektəʊˈvædʒɪn(ə)l ɪgˌzæmɪˈneɪʃ(ə)n] *subst.* examination of the rectum and vagina *rektovaginal undersökning*

rectovesical [ˌrektəʊˈvesɪk(ə)l] *adj.* referring to the rectum and the bladder *rektovesikal*

rectum ['rektəm] *subst.* end part of the large intestine leading from the sigmoid colon to the anus ⇨ *illustration* DIGESTIVE SYSTEM, UROGENITAL TRACT *rektum, ändtarmen*
NOTE: for terms referring to the rectum see words beginning with **procto-**

rectus ['rektəs] *subst.* straight muscle *rak muskel;* **rectus abdominis** = long straight muscle which runs down the front of the abdomen *musculus rectus abdominis, raka bukmuskeln;* **rectus femoris** = flexor muscle in the front of the thigh, one of the four parts of the quadriceps femoris *musculus rectus femoris, del av knästräckarmuskeln* NOTE: plural is **recti**

> QUOTE there are four recti muscles and two oblique muscles in each eye, which coordinate the movement of the eyes and enable them to work as a pair
> **Nursing Times**

recumbent [rɪ'kʌmbənt] *adj.* lying down *liggande, vilande*

recuperate [rɪ'kju:pəreɪt] *vb.* to recover *or* to get better after an illness *or* accident *hämta sig, tillfriskna;* **he is recuperating after an attack of flu; she is going to stay with her mother while she recuperates**

recuperation [rɪ,kju:pə'reɪʃ(ə)n] *subst.* getting better after an illness *tillfrisknande, återhämtning, konvalescens;* **his recuperation will take several months**

recur [rɪ'kɜ:] *vb.* to return *återkomma;* **the headaches recurred frequently, but usually after the patient had eaten chocolate**

recurrence [rɪ'kʌr(ə)ns] *subst.* act of returning *rekurrens, recidiv, återfall;* **he had a recurrence of a fever which he had caught in the tropics**

recurrent [rɪ'kʌr(ə)nt] *adj.* **(a)** which occurs again *återkommande;* **recurrent abortion** = condition where a woman has abortions with one pregnancy after another *habituell abort;* **recurrent fever** = fever (like malaria) which returns at regular intervals *febris recurrens, återfallsfeber* **(b)** (vein *or* artery *or* nerve) which forms a loop *rekurrent, rekurrerande, tillbakalöpande;* **radial recurrent** = artery in the arm which forms a loop beside the brachial artery *arteria recurrens radialis, bakåtgående slinga i radialartären*

red [red] *adj. & subst.* (of) a colour like the colour of blood *röd, rödhet, röd färg;* **blood in an artery is bright red, but venous blood is darker; red blood cell (RBC)** *or* **erythrocyte** = blood cell which contains haemoglobin and carries oxygen *erytrocyt, röd blodkropp;* **red eye** = PINK EYE

Red Crescent [,red 'krez(ə)nt] *subst.* organization similar to the Red Cross, working in Muslim countries *Röda halvmånen*

Red Cross [,red 'krɒs] *subst.* international organization which provides mainly medical help, but also relief to victims of earthquakes, floods, etc., or to prisoners of war *Röda korset*

redig ⇨ **lucid**

redness ['rednəs] *subst.* being red *or* red colour *rödhet, röd färg, rodnad;* **the redness showed where the skin had reacted to the injection**

redskap ⇨ **instrument**

reduce [rɪ'dju:s] *vb.* **(a)** to make something smaller *or* lower *reducera, minska, sänka;* **they used ice packs to try to reduce the patient's temperature (b)** to put (a dislocated *or* a fractured bone, a displaced organ *or* part) back into its proper position, so that it can heal *reponera*

> QUOTE blood pressure control reduces the incidence of first stroke and aspirin appears to reduce the risk of stroke after transient ischaemic attacks by some 15%
> **British Journal of Hospital Medicine**

reducera ⇨ **cut, lessen, lower, reduce**

reducible [rɪ'dju:səb(ə)l] *adj.* (hernia) where the organ can be pushed back into place without an operation *reponibel, reponerbar*

reduction [rɪ'dʌkʃ(ə)n] *subst.* **(a)** making less *or* becoming less *reduktion, minskning, sänkning;* **they noted a reduction in body temperature (b)** putting (a hernia *or* dislocated joint *or* a broken bone) back into the correct position *reponering*

reduktion ⇨ **reduction**

reduktionsdelning ⇨ **meiosis**

re-emerge [,ri:ɪ'mɜ:dʒ] *vb.* to come out again *åter komma (träda) fram*

re-emergence [,ri:ɪ'mɜ:dʒ(ə)ns] *subst.* coming out again *återuppträdande*

refer [rɪ'fɜ:] *vb.* **(a)** to mention *or* to talk about something *referera, hänvisa;* **the doctor**

referred to the patient's history of sinus problems (b) to suggest that someone should consult something *referera, hänvisa, vända sig;* **for method of use, please refer to the manufacturer's instructions; the user is referred to the page giving the results of the tests (c)** to pass on information about a patient to someone else *remittera;* **she was referred to a gynaecologist; the GP referred the patient to a consultant** = he passed details about the patient's case to the consultant so that the consultant could examine him *den allmänpraktiserande läkaren remitterade patienten till en specialist* **(d)** to send to another place *förflytta;* **referred pain** = SYNALGIA

> QUOTE 27 adult patients admitted to hospital with acute abdominal pains were referred for study because their attending clinicians were uncertain whether to advise an urgent laparotomy
> **Lancet**

> QUOTE many patients from outside districts were referred to London hospitals by their GPs
> **Nursing Times**

referral [rɪ'fɜːr(ə)l] *subst.* sending a patient to a specialist *remittering, remiss;* **she asked for a referral to a gynaecologist**

> QUOTE he subsequently developed colicky abdominal pain and tenderness which caused his referral
> **British Journal of Hospital Medicine**

reflex ['riːfleks] *subst.* automatic reaction to something (such as a knee jerk) *reflex;* **accommodation reflex** = reaction of the pupil when the eye focuses on an object which is close *ackommodationsreflex;* **light reflex** = reaction of the pupil of the eye which changes size according to the amount of light going into the eye *pupill(ar)reaktion, pupillreflex, ljusreflex;* **reflex arc** = basic system of a reflex action, where a receptor is linked to a motor neurone which in turn is linked to an effector muscle *reflexbåge;* **reflex action** = automatic reaction to a stimulus (such as a sneeze) *autonom reflex; see also* PATELLAR, PLANTAR, RADIAL

reflexbåge ⇨ **reflex**

reflux ['riːflʌks] *subst.* flowing backwards (of a liquid) in the opposite direction to normal flow *reflux, regurgitation, återflöde;* **the valves in the veins prevent blood reflux; reflux oesophagitis** = inflammation of the oesophagus caused by regurgitation of acid juices from the stomach *inflammation i matstrupen pga regurgitation; see also* VESICOURETERIC

refract [rɪ'frækt] *vb.* to make light rays change direction as they go from one medium (such as air) to another (such as water) at an angle *bryta;* **the refracting media in the eye are the cornea, aqueous humour and vitreous humour**

refraction [rɪ'frækʃ(ə)n] *subst.* (i) change of direction of light rays as they enter a medium (such as the eye) *refraktion, ljusbrytning;* (ii) measuring the angle at which the light rays bend, as a test to see if someone needs to wear glasses *mätning av ögats brytningsindex*

refractometer [ˌriːfræk'tɒmɪtə] *or* **optometer** [ɒp'tɒmɪtə] *subst.* instrument which measures the refraction of the eye *refraktometer, optometer, brytningsmätare*

refractory [rɪ'frækt(ə)ri] *adj.* which it is difficult *or* impossible to treat *or* (condition) which does not respond to treatment *refraktär, okänslig, opåverkbar;* **refractory period** = short space of time after the ventricles of the heart have contracted, when they cannot contract again *refraktärperiod, refraktärfas*

refraktion ⇨ **refraction**

refraktionsanomali ⇨ **ametropia**

refraktometer ⇨ **refractometer**

refraktär ⇨ **refractory**

refraktärfas ⇨ **refractory**

refraktärperiod ⇨ **refractory**

refrigerate [rɪ'frɪdʒəreɪt] *vb.* to make something cold *kyla ned (av);* **the serum should be kept refrigerated**

refrigeration [rɪˌfrɪdʒə'reɪʃ(ə)n] *subst.* (i) making something cold *refrigeration, avkylning, nedkylning;* (ii) making part of the body very cold, to give the effect of an anaesthetic *refrigeration, nedkylning*

refrigerator [rɪ'frɪdʒəreɪtə] *subst.* machine which keeps things cold *kylskåp*

regain [rɪ'geɪn] *vb.* to get back something which was lost *återfå, återvinna;* **he has regained the use of his left arm; she went into a coma and never regained consciousness**

regelbunden ⇨ **regular**

regelbundet ⇨ **regularly**

regenerate [rɪ'dʒenəreɪt] *vb.* to grow again *regenerera, återbilda*

regeneration [rɪˌdʒenə'reɪʃ(ə)n] *subst.* growing again of tissue which has been destroyed *regeneration, återbildning*

regenerera ⇨ **regenerate**

regimen ['redʒɪmen] *subst.* fixed course of treatment (such as a course of drugs *or* a special diet) *regim, kur*

region ['ri:dʒ(ə)n] *subst.* area *or* part which is around something *region, område;* **she experienced itching in the anal region; the rash started in the region of the upper thigh; the plantar region is very sensitive**

regional ['ri:dʒ(ə)n(ə)l] *adj.* in *or* referring to a particular region *regional;* **Regional Health Authority (RHA)** = administrative unit in the National Health Service which is responsible for the planning of health services in a large part of the country *administrativ enhet inom National Health Service;* **regional ileitis** *or* **regional enteritis** *or* **Crohn's disease** *see* ILEITIS

register ['redʒɪstə] **1** *subst.* official list *register;* **the Medical Register** = list of doctors approved by the General Medical Council *register över legitimerade läkare i Storbritannien;* **the committee ordered his name to be struck off the register 2** *vb.* to write a name on an official list, especially to put your name on the official list of patients treated by a GP *or* dentist *or* on the list of patients suffering from a certain disease *registrera, ung. legitimera, skriva in (sig);* **she registered with her local GP; he is a registered heroin addict; they went to register the birth with the Registrar of Births, Marriages and Deaths; before registering with the GP, she asked if she could visit him; all practising doctors are registered with the General Medical Council; registered midwife** = qualified midwife who is registered to practise *legitimerad barnmorska;* **Registered Nurse (RN)** *or* **Registered General Nurse (RGN)** = nurses who have been registered by the UKCC *legitimerad sjuksköterska; see also note at* NURSE

registerkort ⇨ **card**

registrar [ˌredʒɪ'strɑ:] *subst.* **(a)** qualified doctor *or* surgeon in a hospital who supervises house officers *ung. specialistläkare, avdelningsläkare, biträdande överläkare* **(b)** person who registers something officially *registrator;* **Registrar of Births, Marriages and Deaths** = official who keeps the records of people who have been born, married or who have died in a certain area *ung. person ansvarig för folkbokföring*

registration [ˌredʒɪ'streɪʃ(ə)n] *subst.* act of registering *registrering, ung. legitimering;* **a doctor cannot practise without registration by the General Medical Council**

registrator ⇨ **registrar**

registrera ⇨ **record, register**

registrering ⇨ **record, registration**

reglera ⇨ **regulate**

reglering ⇨ **catamenia, menses, menstruation, period, regulation**

regnbågshinnan ⇨ **iris**

regnbågshinne- ⇨ **irid-**

regress [rɪ'gres] *vb.* to return to an earlier stage *or* condition *regress(ion), tillbakagång, återgång*

regress ⇨ **regress, retrogression**

regression [rɪ'greʃ(ə)n] *subst.* (i) stage where symptoms of a disease are disappearing and the patient is getting better *regress(ion), tillbakagång, återgång;* (ii) *(in psychiatry)* returning to a mental state which existed when the patient was younger *regression*

regression ⇨ **regression, retrogression**

regular ['regjʊlə] *adj.* which takes place again and again after the same period of time; which happens at the same time each day *regelbunden;* **he was advised to make regular visits to the dentist; she had her regular six-monthly checkup**

regularly ['regjʊləli] *adv.* happening repeatedly after the same period of time *regelbundet;* **the tablets must be taken regularly every evening; you should go to the dentist regularly**

regulate ['regjuleɪt] *vb.* to make something work (in a regular way) *reglera, styra;* **the heartbeat is regulated by the sinoatrial node**

regulation [ˌregju'leɪʃ(ə)n] *subst.* act of regulating *reglering, styrning;* **the regulation of the body's temperature**

regurgitate [rɪ'gɜ:dʒɪteɪt] *vb.* to bring into the mouth food which has been partly digested in the stomach *regurgitera, stöta upp*

regurgitation [rɪˌgɜ:dʒɪ'teɪʃ(ə)n] *subst.* flowing back in the opposite direction to the normal flow, especially bringing up partly digested food from the stomach into the mouth *regurgitation, reflux, återflöde;* **aortic regurgitation** = flow of blood backwards, caused by a defective heart valve *återflöde i aorta, aortainsufficiens*

regurgitera ⇨ **regurgitate**

rehabilitate [ˌri:ə'bɪlɪteɪt] *vb.* to make someone fit to work *or* to lead a normal life *rehabilitera, återanpassa*

rehabilitation [ˌri:əˌbɪlɪ'teɪʃ(ə)n] *subst.* making a patient fit to work *or* to lead a normal life again *rehabilitering, återanpassning*

rehabilitera ⇨ **rehabilitate, restore**

rehabilitering ⇨ **rehabilitation**

rehydration [ˌri:haɪ'dreɪʃ(ə)n] *subst.* giving water *or* liquid to a patient suffering from dehydration *rehydrering, återuppvätskning*

reinfect [ˌri:ɪn'fekt] *vb.* to infect again *åter infektera*

Reiter's syndrome ['raɪtəz ˌsɪndrəʊm] *or* **Reiter's disease** ['raɪtəz dɪˌzi:z] *subst.* illness which may be venereal, with arthritis, urethritis and conjunctivitis at the same time, affecting mainly men *uroartrit, Reiters syndrom (sjukdom)*

reject [rɪ'dʒekt] *vb.* not to accept *förkasta, stöta av (bort);* **the new heart was rejected by the body; they gave the patient drugs to prevent the transplant being rejected**

rejection [rɪ'dʒekʃ(ə)n] *subst.* act of rejecting tissue *rejektion, avstötning, bortstötning;* **the patient was given drugs to reduce the possibility of tissue rejection**

rejektion ⇨ **rejection**

rekommendera ⇨ **recommend**

rekrytera ⇨ **recruit**

rektal ⇨ **rectal**

rektalfissur ⇨ **fissure**

rektalprolaps ⇨ **rectal**

rektalt ⇨ **rectally**

rektaltemp(eratur) ⇨ **rectal**

rektaltermometer ⇨ **thermometer**

rekt(o)- ⇨ **rect-**

rektocele ⇨ **rectocele**

rektopexi ⇨ **rectopexy**

rektovesikal ⇨ **rectovesical**

rektum ⇨ **rectum**

rekurrens ⇨ **recurrence**

rekurrent ⇨ **recurrent**

rekurrerande ⇨ **recurrent**

relapse [rɪ'læps] **1** *subst. (of patient or disease)* becoming worse *or* reappearing (after seeming to be getting better) *relaps, recidiv, återfall* **2** *vb.* to become worse *or* to return *recidivera, återfalla;* **he relapsed into a coma; relapsing fever** = disease caused by a bacterium, where attacks of fever recur at regular intervals *slags återkommande feber orsakad av bakterie;* **relapsing pancreatitis** = form of pancreatitis where the symptoms recur, but in a milder form *recidiverande pankreatit*

relate [rɪ'leɪt] *vb.* to connect to *ha samband med, bero på;* **the disease is related to the weakness of the heart muscles**

-related [rɪ'leɪtɪd] *suffix* connected to *-beroende;* **drug-related diseases**

relationship [rɪ'leɪʃ(ə)nʃɪp] *subst.* way in which someone *or* something is connected to another *relation, förhållande, samband;* **the incidence of the disease has a close relationship to the environment; he became withdrawn and broke off all relationships with his family**

relax [rɪ'læks] *vb.* to become less tense *or* less strained *relaxera, slappna av, slappa;* **he was given a drug to relax the muscles; after a hard day in the clinic the nurses like to relax by playing tennis; the muscle should be fully relaxed**

relaxant [rɪ'læks(ə)nt] *adj.* (substance) which relieves strain *relaxerande, avslappande;* **muscle relaxant** = drug which reduces contractions in muscles *muskelrelaxans, muskelrelaxerande (muskelavslappande) medel*

relaxation [ˌriːlækˈseɪʃ(ə)n] *subst.* (i) reducing strain in a muscle *relaxation, avslappning;* (ii) reducing stress in a person *avslappning, avkoppling;* **relaxation therapy** = treatment of a patient where he is encouraged to relax his muscles to reduce stress *avslappningsterapi*

relaxative [rɪˈlæksətɪv] *subst. US* drug which reduces stress *sedativ(um), lugnande medel*

relaxin [rɪˈlæksɪn] *subst.* hormone which may be secreted by the placenta to make the cervix relax and open fully in the final stages of pregnancy before childbirth *relaxin*

release [rɪˈliːs] **1** *subst.* allowing something to go out *frisättning;* **the slow release of the drug into the bloodstream 2** *vb.* to let something out *or* to let something go free *frisätta, frigöra;* **hormones are released into the body by glands; release hormones** = hormones secreted by the hypothalamus which make the pituitary gland release certain hormones *releasing factors, hypofysiotropiner*

relief [rɪˈliːf] *subst.* making better *or* easier *lättnad, lindring;* **the drug provides rapid relief for patients with bronchial spasms**

> QUOTE complete relief of angina is experienced by 85% of patients subjected to coronary artery bypass surgery
>
> **British Journal of Hospital Medicine**

relieve [rɪˈliːv] *vb.* to make better *or* to make easier *lätta, lindra;* **nasal congestion can be relieved by antihistamines; the patient was given an injection of morphine to relieve the pain; the condition is relieved by applying cold compresses**

> QUOTE replacement of the metacarpophalangeal joint is mainly undertaken to relieve pain, deformity and immobility due to rheumatoid arthritis
>
> **Nursing Times**

REM [rem] = RAPID EYE MOVEMENT

remedial [rɪˈmiːdiəl] *adj.* which cures *botande, läkande*

remedy [ˈremədi] *subst.* cure *or* drug which will cure *botemedel, läkemedel, kur;* **honey and glycerine is an old remedy for sore throats**

remember [rɪˈmembə] *vb.* to bring back into the mind something which has been seen *or* heard before *minnas, komma ihåg;* **he remembers nothing** *or* **he can't remember anything about the accident**

remiss ⇨ **referral**

remission [rɪˈmɪʃ(ə)n] *subst.* period when an illness *or* fever is less severe *remission, lättnad, förbättring*

re. mist. [ˈriː ˈmɪst] *abbreviation for the Latin phrase* "repetatur mistura": repeat the same mixture (written on a prescription) *repetatur mistura, upprepa!*

remittent fever [rɪˈmɪt(ə)nt ˌfiːvə] *subst.* fever which goes down for a period each day, like typhoid fever *febris remittens, återkommande feber*

remittera ⇨ **refer**

remittering ⇨ **referral**

removal [rɪˈmuːv(ə)l] *subst.* action of removing *avlägsnande, borttagande;* **an appendicectomy is the surgical removal of an appendix**

remove [rɪˈmuːv] *vb.* to take away *avlägsna, ta bort;* **he will have an operation to remove an ingrowing toenail**

remsa ⇨ **strip, tape**

ren ⇨ **blank, clean, fresh, pure, sanitary**

ren- [ren] *or* **reni-** [ˈreni, ˌ--] *or* **reno-** [ˈriːnəʊ, ˌ--] *prefix* referring to the kidneys *ren(o)-, nefr(o)-, njur-*

rena ⇨ **purify**

renal [ˈriːn(ə)l] *adj.* referring to the kidneys *renal, njur-;* **renal arteries** = pair of arteries running from the abdominal aorta to the kidneys *arteriae renales, njurartärerna;* **renal calculus** = stone in the kidney *calculus renalis, njursten;* **renal capsule** = fibrous tissue surrounding a kidney *njurens bindvävskapsel;* **renal colic** = sudden pain caused by kidney stones in the ureter *colica renalis, njurkolik, ofta njurstensanfall;* **renal corpuscle** = part of a nephron in the cortex of a kidney *corpusculum renis, Malpighis kropp;* **renal cortex** = outer covering of the kidney, immediately beneath the capsule *cortex renis, njurbarken;* **renal hypertension** = high blood pressure linked to kidney disease *renal hypertoni;* **renal pelvis** = upper and wider part of the ureter leading from the kidney where urine is collected before passing down the ureter into the bladder *pelvis renalis, njurbäckenet;* **renal rickets** = form of rickets caused by kidneys which do not function properly *rakit pga njursjukdom;* **renal sinus** = cavity in which the renal pelvis and other tubes leading into the kidney fit *njurhilus;* **renal tubule** *or* **uriniferous tubule** = tiny tube which is part of a nephron **renal tubules** *tubuli renales, njurkanalerna*

rengöra ➪ **clean, cleanse**

rengöringsmedel ➪ **cleanser, detergent**

renin ['ri:nɪn] *subst.* enzyme secreted by the kidney to prevent loss of sodium, and which also affects blood pressure *renin*

renlighet ➪ **cleanliness, hygiene**

rennin ['renɪn] *subst.* enzyme which makes milk coagulate in the stomach, so as to slow down the passage of the milk through the digestive system *rennin*

renodla ➪ **isolate**

renography [ri:'nɒgrəfi] *subst.* examination of a kidney after injection of a radioactive substance, using a gamma camera *renografi*

rensa ➪ **clear**

reovirus [ˌri:əʊ'vaɪ(ə)rəs] *subst.* virus which affects both the intestine and the respiratory system, but does not cause serious illness *reovirus; compare* ECHOVIRUS

rep [rep] *abbreviation of Latin word* "repetatur": repeat (a prescription) *repetatur, upprepa!*

repa ➪ **scratch**

repair [rɪ'peə] *vb.* to mend *or* to make something good again *reparera, laga;* **surgeons operated to repair a defective heart valve**

reparera ➪ **mend, repair**

repa sig ➪ **improve**

repeat [rɪ'pi:t] *vb.* to say *or* do something again *upprepa;* **the course of treatment was repeated after two months; repeat prescription** = prescription which is exactly the same as the previous one, and is often given without examination of the patient by the doctor, and sometimes over the telephone *förnyat (telefon)recept*

repel [rɪ'pel] *vb.* to make something go away *repellera, stöta bort;* **if you spread this cream on your skin it will repel insects**

replace [rɪ'pleɪs] *vb.* (i) to put back *sätta (ställa, lägga) tillbaka;* (ii) to exchange one part for another *substituera, ersätta;* **an operation to replace a prolapsed uterus; the surgeons replaced the diseased hip with a metal one**

replacement [rɪ'pleɪsmənt] *subst.* operation to replace part of the body with an artificial part *ersättning, utbyte, substitution;* **replacement transfusion** *or* **exchange transfusion** = treatment for leukaemia *or* erythroblastosis where almost all the abnormal blood is removed from the body and replaced by normal blood *utbytestransfusion;* **hip replacement** = surgical operation to replace a defective *or* arthritic hip with an artificial one *höftledsplastik*

replication [ˌreplɪ'keɪʃ(ə)n] *subst.* process in the division of a cell, where the DNA makes copies of itself *replikation*

reponera ➪ **reduce, set**

reponerbar ➪ **reducible**

reponering ➪ **reduction**

reponibel ➪ **reducible**

report [rɪ'pɔ:t] **1** *subst.* official note stating what action has been taken *or* what treatment given *or* what results have come from a test, etc. *journal, rapport, anmälan;* **the patient's report card has to be filled in by the nurse; the inspector's report on the hospital kitchens is good 2** *vb.* to make an official report about something *rapportera, anmäla;* **the patient reported her doctor to the FPC for misconduct; occupational diseases** *or* **serious accidents at work must be reported to the local officials; reportable diseases** = diseases (such as asbestosis *or* hepatitis *or* anthrax) which may be caused by working conditions or may infect other workers and must be reported to the District Health Authority *ung. arbetssjukdomar för vilka anmälningsplikt råder*

reposition ➪ **taxis**

repositor [rɪ'pɒzɪtə] *subst.* surgical instrument used to push a prolapsed organ back into its normal position *repositor*

representant ➪ **agent**

repress [rɪ'pres] *vb.* to hide in the back of the mind feelings *or* thoughts which may be unpleasant *or* painful *tränga bort*

repression [rɪ'preʃ(ə)n] *subst. (in psychiatry)* hiding feelings *or* thoughts which might be unpleasant *bortträngning*

reproduce [ˌriːprə'djuːs] *vb.* **(a)** to produce children; *(of bacteria, etc.)* to produce new cells *reproducera sig, fortplanta sig, föröka sig* **(b)** to do a test again in exactly the same way *upprepa*

reproduction [ˌriːprə'dʌkʃ(ə)n] *subst.* process of making children *or* derived cells, etc *reproduktion, fortplantning, förökning;* **organs of reproduction** = REPRODUCTIVE ORGANS

reproductive [ˌriːprə'dʌktɪv] *adj.* referring to reproduction *reproduktiv, fortplantnings-, köns-;* **reproductive organs** = parts of the bodies of men and women which are involved in the conception and development of a fetus *reproduktionsorgan, fortplantningsorgan, könsorgan, genitalia, genitalorgan;* **reproductive system** = arrangement of organs and ducts in the bodies of men and women which produces spermatozoa and ova *reproduktionsorganen, fortplantningsapparaten;* **reproductive tract** = series of tubes and ducts which carry spermatozoa and ova from one part of the body to another *gångkanalerna i fortplantningsapparaten (reproduktionsorganen)*

COMMENT: in the human male, the testes form the spermatozoa, which pass through the vasa efferentia and the vasa deferentia where they receive liquid from the seminal vesicles, then out of the body through the urethra and penis on ejaculation; in the female, ova are produced by the ovaries, and pass through the Fallopian tubes where they are fertilized by spermatozoa from the male. The fertilized ovum moves down into the uterus where it develops into an embryo

reproduktionsorgan ➪ **reproductive, sex**

require [rɪ'kwa(ɪ)ə] *vb.* to need *kräva, begära, behöva;* **his condition may require surgery; is it a condition which requires immediate treatment?; required effect** = effect which a drug is expected to have *önskad effekt;* **if the drug does not produce the required effect, the dose should be increased**

requirement [rɪ'kwa(ɪ)əmənt] *subst.* something which is necessary *behov, krav;* **one of the requirements of the position is a qualification in pharmacy**

RES [ˌɑːiː'es] = RETICULOENDOTHELIAL SYSTEM

resa sig (upp) ➪ **stand up**

research [rɪ'sɜːtʃ] **1** *subst.* scientific study which investigates something new *forskning;* **he is the director of a medical research unit; she is doing research into finding a cure for leprosy; research workers** *or* **research teams are trying to find a vaccine against AIDS; the Medical Research Council (MRC)** = government body which organizes and pays for medical research *medicinskt forskningsråd i Storbritannien* **2** *vb.* to carry out scientific study *forska;* **he is researching the origins of cancer**

resecera ➪ **resect**

resect [rɪ'sekt] *vb.* to remove part of the body by surgery *resecera, resekera, skära bort, avlägsna (kirurgiskt)*

resection [rɪ'sekʃ(ə)n] *subst.* surgical removal of part of an organ *resektion, bortskärande, (kirurgiskt) avlägsnande;* **submucous resection** = removal of bent cartilage from the nasal septum *kirurgiskt avlägsnande under slemhinna, t.ex. av brosk i näsan;* **transurethral resection (TUR)** *or* **resection of the prostate** = surgical removal of the prostate gland through the urethra *transuretral prostatektomi (resektion), TUR*

resectoscope [rɪ'sektəskəʊp] *subst.* surgical instrument used to carry out a transurethral resection *resektoskop*

resekera ➪ **resect**

resektion ➪ **resection**

resektoskop ➪ **resectoscope**

reserpine ['resəpiːn] *subst.* tranquillizing drug derived from Rauwolfia, used in the treatment of high blood pressure and nervous tension *reserpin*

reserv- ➪ **auxiliary, spare**

reservdelskirurgi ➪ **spare**

reservoar ➪ **cistern**

reset [ˌriː'set] *vb.* to break a badly set bone and set it again correctly *bryta upp, reponera och åter fixera;* **his arm had to be reset**

resident ['rezɪd(ə)nt] *subst. & adj.* **(a)** (person) who lives in a place *(person) som bor på ett ställe;* **all the residents of the old people's home were tested for food**

poisoning; resident doctor *or* **nurse** = doctor *or* nurse who lives in a certain building (such as an old people's home) *läkare (sjuksköterska) som bor på sjukhuset etc.* **(b)** *US* qualified doctor who is employed by a hospital and sometimes lives in the hospital *ung. FV-läkare, ung. ST-läkare; compare* INTERN

residential [ˌrezɪ'denʃ(ə)l] *adj.* living in a hospital *or* at home *boende, inneliggande;* **residential care** = care of patients either in a hospital or at home (but not as outpatients) *patientvård på sjukhus etc.*

residual [rɪ'zɪdju(ə)l] *adj.* remaining *or* which is left behind *residual, kvarbliven, återstående;* **residual urine** = urine left in the bladder after a person has passed as much water as possible *residualurin, resturin;* **residual air** *or* **residual volume** = air left in the lungs after a person has breathed out as much air as possible *residualluft, residualvolym, restluft*

residualluft ⇨ **residual**

residualurin ⇨ **residual**

residualvolym ⇨ **residual**

resin ['rezɪn] *subst.* sticky juice which comes from some types of tree *resina, kåda, harts*

resist [rɪ'zɪst] *vb.* to be strong enough to fight against a disease *or* to avoid being killed *or* attacked by a disease *tåla, vara motståndskraftig (göra motstånd) mot;* **a healthy body can resist some infections**

resistance [rɪ'zɪst(ə)ns] *subst.* **(a)** (i) ability of a person not to get a disease *motståndskraft;* (ii) ability of a germ not to be affected by antibiotics *resistens, okänslighet;* **the bacteria have developed a resistance to certain antibiotics; after living in the tropics his resistance to colds was low** **(b)** opposition to force *motstånd;* **peripheral resistance** = ability of the peripheral blood vessels to slow down the flow of blood inside them *perifert motstånd*

resistant [rɪ'zɪst(ə)nt] *adj.* able not to be affected by something *resistent, motståndskraftig, okänslig;* **the bacteria are resistant to some antibiotics; resistant strain** = strain of bacterium which is not affected by antibiotics *resistent bakteriestam*

resistens ⇨ **mass, resistance**

resistent ⇨ **resistant**

resolution [ˌrezə'lu:ʃ(ə)n] *subst.* (i) amount of detail which can be seen in a microscope *resolution, upplösning;* (ii) point in the development of a disease where the inflammation begins to disappear *resolution, upplösning*

resolve [rɪ'zɒlv] *vb. (of inflammation)* to begin to disappear *börja försvinna, upplösas*

> QUOTE valve fluttering disappears as the pneumothorax resolves. Always confirm resolution with a physical examination and X-ray
>
> **American Journal of Nursing**

resonance ['rez(ə)n(ə)ns] *subst.* sound made by a hollow part of the body when hit *resonans, genklang*

resonans ⇨ **resonance**

resorbera ⇨ **dissolve, reabsorb**

resorption [rɪ'sɔ:pʃ(ə)n] *subst.* absorbing again of a substance already produced back into the body *resorption, återuppsugning, återupptag*

resorption ⇨ **reabsorption**

respiration [ˌrespə'reɪʃ(ə)n] *subst.* action of breathing *respiration, ventilation, andning;* **artificial respiration** = way of reviving someone who has stopped breathing (as by mouth-to-mouth resuscitation) *artificiell respiration, konstgjord andning;* **assisted respiration** = breathing with the help of a machine *assisterad andning (ventilation);* **controlled respiration** = control of a patient's breathing by an anaesthetist during an operation, if normal breathing has stopped *kontrollerad andning (ventilation);* **external respiration** = part of respiration concerned with oxygen in the air being exchanged in the lungs for carbon dioxide from the blood *yttre respiration;* **internal respiration** = part of respiration concerned with the passage of oxygen from the blood to the tissues, and the passage of carbon dioxide from the tissues to the blood *inre respiration;* **respiration rate** = number of times a person breathes per minute *andningsfrekvens*

> COMMENT: respiration includes two stages: breathing in (inhalation) and breathing out (exhalation). Air is taken into the respiratory system through the nose or mouth, and goes down into the lungs through the pharynx, larynx, and windpipe. In the lungs, the bronchi take the air to the alveoli (air sacs) where oxygen in the air is passed to the bloodstream in exchange for waste carbon dioxide which is then breathed out

respiration ⇨ **breathing, respiration, ventilation**

respirations- ⇨ **respiratory**

respirationscentrum ⇨ **respiratory**

respirationsinsufficiens ⇨ **respiratory**

respirationssystemet ⇨ **respiratory**

respirator ['respəreɪtə] *or* **ventilator** ['ventɪleɪtə] *subst.* **(a)** machine which gives artificial respiration *respirator, ventilator;* **cuirass respirator** = type of iron lung, where the patient's limbs are not enclosed *slags respirator;* **Drinker respirator** *or* **iron lung** = machine which encloses all a patient's body, except the head, and in which air pressure is increased and decreased in turn, so forcing the patient to breathe *slags respirator, järnlunga;* **positive pressure respirator** = machine which forces air into a patient's lungs through a tube inserted in the mouth *or* in the trachea (after a tracheostomy), and then let out by releasing pressure *respirator för övertrycksventilation;* **the patient was put on a respirator** = the patient was attached to a machine which forced him to breathe *patienten lades i respirator* **(b)** mask worn to prevent someone breathing gas *or* fumes *andningsmask*

respiratorisk ⇨ **respiratory**

respiratory [rɪ'spɪrət(ə)ri] *adj.* referring to breathing *respiratorisk, respirations-, andnings-;* **respiratory bronchiole** = end part of a bronchiole in the lung, which joins the alveoli *(innersta delarna av) bronkiolerna (bronchiole);* **respiratory centre** = nerve centre in the brain which regulates the breathing *respirationscentrum, andningscentrum;* **respiratory distress syndrome** *or* **hyaline membrane disease** = condition of newborn babies, where the lungs do not expand properly, due to lack of surfactant (the condition is common among premature babies) *idiopatiskt respiratoriskt distress-syndrom, IRDS, syndrome membranarum hyalinarum, hyalina membran;* **respiratory failure** = failure of the lungs to oxygenate the blood correctly *respirationsinsufficiens, andningsinsufficiens;* **respiratory illness** = illness which affects the patient's breathing *lungsjukdom;* **upper respiratory infection** = infection in the upper part of the respiratory system *övre luftvägsinfektion, ÖLI, "förkylning";* **respiratory pigment** = blood pigment which can carry oxygen collected in the lungs and release it in tissues *hemoglobin, Hb;* **respiratory quotient (RQ)** = ratio of the amount of carbon dioxide taken into the alveoli of the lungs from the blood to the amount the oxygen which the alveoli take from the air *respiratorisk kvot, RQ;* **respiratory syncytial virus (RSV)** = virus which causes infections of the nose and throat in adults but serious bronchiolitis in children *respiratory syncytial virus, RS-virus;* **respiratory system** = series of organs and passages which take air into the lungs, and exchange oxygen for carbon dioxide *respirationssystemet, andningsapparaten*

respond [rɪ'spɒnd] *vb.* to react to something *or* to begin to get better because of a treatment *svara på, reagera (vara känslig) för;* **the cancer is not responding to drugs; she is responding to treatment**

> QUOTE many severely confused patients, particularly those in advanced stages of Alzheimer's disease, do not respond to verbal communication
> **Nursing Times**

respons ⇨ **reaction, response**

response [rɪ'spɒns] *subst.* reaction by an organ *or* tissue *or* a person to an external stimulus *respons, reaktion, svar;* **immune response** = reaction of a body which rejects a transplant *immunitetsreaktion*

> QUOTE anaemia may be due to insufficient erythrocyte production, in which case the reticulocyte count will be low, or to haemolysis or haemorrhage, in which cases there should be a reticulocyte response
> **Southern Medical Journal**

responsible [rɪ'spɒnsəb(ə)l] *adj.* which is the cause of something *ansvarig;* **to be responsible for** *vara orsak (skyldig, skuld) till;* **the allergen which is responsible for the patient's reaction; this is one of several factors which can be responsible for high blood pressure**

responsiveness [rɪ'spɒnsɪvnəs] *subst.* being able to respond to other people *or* to sensations *mottaglighet, påverkbarhet*

rest [rest] **1** *subst.* lying down *or* being calm *vila, lugn, ro, rast, paus;* **what you need is a good night's rest; I had a few minutes' rest and then I started work again; the doctor prescribed a month's total rest** **2** *vb.* to lie down *or* to be calm *vila (sig);* **don't disturb your mother - she's resting**

restless ['restləs] *adj.* not still *or* not calm *rastlös, orolig;* **the children are restless in the heat; she had a few hours' restless sleep**

restluft ⇨ **residual**

restore [rɪ'stɔː] *vb.* to give back *rehabilitera, återställa;* **she needs vitamins to restore her strength; the physiotherapy should restore the strength of the muscles; a salpingostomy was performed to restore the patency of the Fallopian tube**

restrict [rɪ'strɪkt] *vb.* (i) to make less *or* smaller *minska;* (ii) to set limits to something *hämma, begränsa, inskränka;* **the blood supply is restricted by the tight bandage; the doctor suggested she should restrict her intake of alcohol**

restrictive [rɪ'strɪktɪv] *adj.* which restricts *or* which makes smaller *restriktiv, hämmande, begränsande, inskränkande*

restriktiv ⇨ **restrictive**

resturin ⇨ **residual**

result [rɪ'zʌlt] **1** *subst.* figures at the end of a calculation *or* at the end of a test *resultat;* **what was the result of the test? the doctor told the patient the result of the pregnancy test; the result of the operation will not be known for some weeks 2** *vb.* to happen because of something *vara (bli) följden;* **the cancer resulted from exposure to radiation at work; his illness resulted in his being away from work for several weeks**

resultat ⇨ **product, result**

resuscitate [rɪ'sʌsɪteɪt] *vb.* to make someone who appears to be dead start breathing again, and to restart the circulation of blood *återuppliva*

resuscitation [rɪˌsʌsɪ'teɪʃ(ə)n] *subst.* reviving someone who seems to be dead, by making him breathe again and restarting the heart *återupplivning;* **cardiopulmonary resuscitation (CPR)** = method of reviving someone where stimulation is applied to both heart and lungs *hjärtlungräddning*

COMMENT: the commonest methods of resuscitation are artificial respiration and cardiac massage

reta ⇨ **excite, irritate**

retain [rɪ'teɪn] *vb.* to keep *or* to hold *behålla, hålla (kvar);* **he was incontinent and unable to retain urine in his bladder** *see also* RETENTION

retard [rɪ'tɑːd] *vb.* to make something slower *or* to slow down the action of a drug *försena, hämma,* **the drug will retard the onset of the fever; the injections retard the effect of the anaesthetic**

retardation [ˌriːtɑː'deɪʃ(ə)n] *subst.* making slower *retardation, försening, hämning;* **mental retardation** = condition where a person's mind has not developed as fully as normal, so that he is not as advanced mentally as others of the same age *mental (psykisk, intellektuell) utvecklingsstörning, efterblivenhet;* **psychomotor retardation** = slowing of movement and speech, caused by depression *psykomotorisk hämning*

retarded [rɪ'tɑːdɪd] *adj.* (person) who has not developed mentally as far as others of the same age *retarderad, utvecklingsstörd;* **a school for retarded children; by the age of four, he was showing signs of being mentally retarded**

retbar ⇨ **irritable**

retbarhet ⇨ **irritability**

retch [retʃ, riːtʃ] *vb.* to try to vomit without bringing any food up from the stomach *försöka kräkas*

retching ['retʃɪŋ, 'riːtʃɪŋ] *subst.* attempting to vomit without being able to do so *kräkningsförsök*

rete ['riːtiː] *subst.* structure, formed like a net, made up of tissue fibres *or* nerve fibres *or* blood vessels *rete, nät;* **rete testis** = network of channels in the testis which take the sperm to the epididymis *rete testis; see also* RETICULAR

NOTE: the plural is **retia**

retention [rɪ'tenʃ(ə)n] *subst.* holding back (such as holding back urine in the bladder) *retention, kvarhållande;* **retention cyst** = cyst which is formed when a duct from a gland is blocked *retentionscysta;* **retention of urine** = condition where passing urine is difficult *or* impossible because the urethra is blocked *or* because the prostate gland is enlarged *ischuri, urinretention, urinstämma*

retentionscysta ⇨ **retention**

reticular [rɪ'tɪkjʊlə] *adj.* made like a net *or* (fibres) which criss-cross or branch *retikulär;* **reticular fibres** *or* **reticular tissue** = fibres in connective tissue which support organs *or* blood vessels, etc. *retikulära fibrer, retikeltrådar, retikulär bindväv*

reticulin [rɪ'tɪkjʊliːn] *subst.* fibrous protein which is one of the most important components of reticular fibres *retikulin*

reticulocyte [rɪ'tɪkjʊləʊsaɪt] *subst.* red blood cell which has not yet fully developed *retikulocyt*

reticulocytosis [rɪˌtɪkjʊləʊsaɪ'təʊsɪs] *subst.* condition where the number of reticulocytes in the blood increases abnormally *aretikulocytos*

reticuloendothelial system (RES) [rɪˌtɪkjʊləʊˌendəʊ'əiːliəl ˌsɪstəm (ˌɑːriː'es)] *subst.* series of phagocytic cells in the body (found especially in bone marrow, lymph nodes, liver and spleen) which attack and destroy bacteria and form antibodies *retikuloendoteliala systemet, RES;* **reticuloendothelial cell** = phagocytic cell in the RES *fagocyt i retikuloendoteliala systemet (RES)*

reticuloendotheliosis [rɪˌtɪkjʊləʊˌendəʊˌəiːli'əʊsɪs] *subst.* condition where cells in the RES grow large and form swellings in bone marrow *or* destroy bones *retikuloendotelios*

reticulosis [rɪˌtɪkjʊ'ləʊsɪs] *subst.* any of several conditions where cells in the reticuloendothelial system grow large and form usually malignant tumours *retikulos*

reticulum [rɪ'tɪkjʊləm] *subst.* series of small fibres *or* tubes forming a network *retikel, litet nät;* **endoplasmic reticulum (ER)** = network in the cytoplasm of a cell *reticulum endoplasmaticum, endoplasmatiskt retikel;* **sarcoplasmic reticulum** = network in the cytoplasm of striated muscle fibres *reticulum sarcoplasmaticum, sarkoplasmatiskt retikel*

retikel ⇨ **reticulum**

retikeltrådar ⇨ **reticular**

retikulin ⇨ **reticulin**

retikulocyt ⇨ **reticulocyte**

retikuloendotelios ⇨ **reticuloendotheliosis**

retikulos ⇨ **reticulosis**

retikulär ⇨ **reticular**

retina ['retɪnə] *subst.* inside layer of the eye which is sensitive to light *retina, näthinnan;* **detached retina** = RETINAL DETACHMENT ⇨ *illustration* EYE

retinaculum [retɪ'nækjuləm] *subst.* band of tissue which holds a structure in place, as found in the wrist and ankle over the flexor tendons *retinaculum, bindvävssträng*

retinal ['retɪn(ə)l] *adj.* referring to the retina *retinal, näthinne-;* **retinal artery** = sole artery of the retina (it accompanies the optic nerve) *arteria centralis retinae;* **retinal detachment** = condition where the retina is partly detached from the choroid *ablatio (amotio, solutio) retinae, näthinneavlossning*

retinerad ⇨ **impacted**

retinitis [ˌretɪ'naɪtɪs] *subst.* inflammation of the retina *retinit, näthinneinflammation;* **retinitis pigmentosa** = hereditary condition where inflammation of the retina can result in blindness *retinitis pigmentosa*

retinoblastoma [ˌretɪnəʊblæ'stəʊmə] *subst.* rare tumour in the retina, affecting infants *retinoblastom*

retinol ['retɪnɒl] *subst.* vitamin A *or* vitamin (found in liver, vegetables, eggs and cod liver oil) which is essential for good vision *retinol, A-vitamin*

retinopathy [ˌretɪ'nɒpəθi] *subst.* any disease of the retina *retinopati;* **diabetic retinopathy** = defect in vision linked to diabetes *retinopathia diabetica, diabetesretinopati*

retinoscope ['retɪnəskəʊp] *subst.* instrument with various lenses, used to measure the refraction of the eye *retinoskop, skiaskop*

> COMMENT: light enters the eye through the pupil and strikes the retina. Light-sensitive cells in the retina (cones and rods) convert the light to nervous impulses; the optic nerve sends these impulses to the brain which interprets them as images. The point where the optic nerve joins the retina has no light-sensitive cells, and is known as the blind spot

retire [rɪ'ta(ɪ)ə] *vb.* to stop work at a certain age *pensioneras;* **most men retire at 65, but women only go on working until they are 60; although she has retired, she still does voluntary work at the clinic**

retirement [rɪ'ta(ɪ)əmənt] *subst.* act of retiring *pensionering;* being retired *pension;* **the retirement age for men is 65**

retledningssystemet ⇨ **conducting system**

retledningstråd ⇨ **conduction**

retlig ⇨ **fretful, irritable**

retmedel ⇨ **irritant**

retning ⇨ **excitement, irritation, stimulus**

retraction [rɪ'trækʃ(ə)n] *subst.* moving backwards *or* becoming shorter *retraktion, indragning, förkortning;* **there is retraction of the overlying skin; retraction ring** *or* **Bandl's ring** = groove round the womb, separating the upper and lower parts of the uterus, which, in obstructed labour, prevents the baby from moving forward normally into the cervical canal *slags förlossningshinder*

retractor [rɪ'træktə] *subst.* surgical instrument which pulls and holds back the edge of the incision in an operation *hake, sårhake*

retraktion ⇨ **retraction**

retro- ['retrə(ʊ), ˌ--] *prefix* meaning at the back *or* behind *retro-, bakåt-, tillbaka-, åter-*

retrobulbar neuritis [ˌretrəʊ'bʌlbə nju(ə)ˌraɪtɪs] *or* **optic neuritis** ['ɒptɪk nju(ə)ˌraɪtɪs] *subst.* inflammation of the optic nerve which makes objects appear blurred *neuritis optica retrobulbaris, optikusneurit, synnervsinflammation*

retrobulbär ⇨ **retro-ocular**

retrofaryngeal ⇨ **retropharyngeal**

retroflexion [ˌretrə(ʊ)'flekʃ(ə)n] *subst.* being bent backwards *retroflexion, bakåtböjning;* **uterine retroflexion** *or* **retroflexion of the uterus** = condition where the uterus bends backwards away from its normal position *retroflexio uteri, retroflexion (bakåtknickning) av livmodern*

retrograde ['retrə(ʊ)greɪd] *adj.* going backwards *retrograd, bakåtgående;* **retrograde pyelography** = X-ray examination of the kidney where a catheter is passed into the kidney through the ureter, and the opaque liquid is injected directly into it *retrograd pyelografi*

retrogression [ˌretrə(ʊ)'greʃ(ə)n] *subst.* returning to an earlier state *regress, regression, tillbakagång, återgång*

retrohepatisk ⇨ **posthepatic**

retrolental fibroplasia [ˌretrəʊ'lent(ə)l ˌfaɪbrəʊ'pleɪzɪə] *subst.* condition where fibrous tissue develops behind the lens of the eye, resulting in blindness *retrolental fibroplasi*

> COMMENT: the condition is likely in premature babies if they are treated with large amounts of oxygen immediately after birth

retro-ocular [ˌretrəʊ'ɒkjʊlə] *adj.* at the back of the eye *retrookulär, retrobulbär*

retrookulär ⇨ **retro-ocular**

retroperitoneal [ˌretrəʊˌperitəʊ'ni:əl] *adj.* at the back of the peritoneum *retroperitoneal*

retropharyngeal [ˌretrəʊˌfær(ə)n'dʒi:əl] *adj.* at the back of the pharynx *retrofaryngeal*

retropubic [ˌretrə(ʊ)'pju:bɪk] *adj.* at the back of the pubis *retropubisk;* **retropubic prostatectomy** = removal of the prostate gland which is carried out through a suprapubic incision and by cutting the membrane which surrounds the gland *retropubisk prostatektomi*

retrospection [ˌretrə(ʊ)'spekʃ(ə)n] *subst.* recalling what happened in the past *återblick, tillbakablickande*

retroversion [ˌretrə(ʊ)'vɜ:ʃ(ə)n] *subst.* sloping backwards *retroversion, bakåtvridning, bakåtlutning;* **uterine retroversion** *or* **retroversion of the uterus** = condition where the uterus slopes backwards away from its normal position *retroversion (bakåtlutning) av livmodern*

retroverted uterus [ˌretrəʊˌvɜ:tɪd 'ju:t(ə)rəs] *subst.* uterus which slopes backwards from the normal position *retroverterad (bakåtlutad) livmoder*

retroverterad livmoder ⇨ **tipped womb**

reumatisk ⇨ **rheumatic**

reumatism ⇨ **rheumatism**

reumatoid ⇨ **rheumatoid**

reumatolog ⇨ **rheumatologist**

reumatologi ⇨ **rheumatology**

reva ⇨ **tear**

revben ⇨ **rib**

revbens- ⇨ **cost-, costal**

revbensbrosk ⇨ **costal**

revbenshöjare ⇨ **scalenus**

reveal [rɪ'vi:l] *vb* to show *avslöja, uppenbara, visa;* **digital palpation revealed a growth in the breast**

revive [rɪ'vaɪv] *vb.* to bring back to life *or* to consciousness *återuppliva;* **they tried to revive him with artificial respiration; she collapsed on the floor and had to be revived by the nurse**

revorm ⇨ **lichen, ringworm, tinea**

Reye's syndrome ['raɪz ˌsɪndrəʊm] *subst.* encephalopathy affecting young children who have had a viral infection *slags encefalit hos barn*

RGN [ˌɑ:dʒi:'en] = REGISTERED GENERAL NURSE

Rh *abbreviation for* rhesus *Rh, rhesus*

RHA [ˌɑ:reɪtʃ'eɪ] = REGIONAL HEALTH AUTHORITY

rhabdovirus ['ræbdə(ʊ)ˌvaɪ(ə)rəs] *subst.* any of a group of viruses containing RNA, one of which causes rabies *rabdovirus*

rhachio- ['reɪkiə(ʊ), ˌ--] *prefix* referring to the spine *raki(o)-, ryggrads-*

rhagades ['rægədi:z] *subst.* fissures *or* long thin scars in the skin round the nose, mouth or anus, seen in syphilis *ragader, sårsprickor*

rhesus factor ['ri:səs ˌfæktə] *or* **Rh factor** [ˌɑ:r'eɪtʃ ˌfæktə] *subst.* antigen in red blood cells, which is an element in blood grouping *rhesusfaktor, Rh-faktor;* **rhesus baby** = baby with erythroblastosis fetalis *barn som lider av erythroblastosis fetalis (neonatorum);* **Rh-negative** = (person) who does not have the rhesus factor in his blood *Rh-negativ, Rh -;* **Rh-positive** = (person) who has the rhesus factor in his blood *Rh-positiv, Rh*

> COMMENT: the rhesus factor is important in blood grouping, because, although most people are Rh-positive, a Rh-negative patient should not receive a Rh-positive blood transfusion as this will cause the formation of permanent antibodies. If a Rh-negative mother has a child by a Rh-positive father, the baby will inherit Rh-positive blood, which may then pass into the mother's circulation at childbirth and cause antibodies to form. This can be prevented by an injection of anti D immunoglobulin immediately after the birth of the first Rh-positive child and any subsequent Rh-positive children. If a Rh-negative mother has formed antibodies to Rh-positive blood in the past, these antibodies will affect the blood of the fetus and may cause erythroblastosis fetalis

rheumatic [ru'mætɪk] *adj.* referring to rheumatism *reumatisk;* **rheumatic fever** *or* **acute rheumatism** = collagen disease of young people and children, caused by haemolytic streptococci, where the joints and also the valves and lining of the heart become inflamed *reumatisk feber*

> COMMENT: rheumatic fever often follows another streptococcal infection such as a strep throat *or* tonsillitis. Symptoms are high fever, pains in the joints, which become red, formation of nodules on the ends of bones, and difficulty in breathing. Although recovery can be complete, rheumatic fever can recur and damage the heart permanently

rheumatism ['ru:mətɪz(ə)m] *subst.* general term for pains and stiffness in the joints and muscles *reumatism;* **she has rheumatism in her hips; he has a history of rheumatism; she complained of rheumatism in her knees; muscular rheumatism** = pains in muscles *or* joints, usually caused by fibrositis *or* inflammation of the muscles *or* osteoarthritis *rheumatismus musculorum, muskelreumatism; see also* RHEUMATOID ARTHRITIS, RHEUMATIC FEVER, OSTEOARTHRITIS

rheumatoid ['ru:mətɔɪd] *adj.* similar to rheumatism *reumatoid;* **rheumatoid arthritis** = general painful disabling collagen disease affecting any joint, but especially the hands, feet and hips, making them swollen and inflamed *reumatoid artrit, RA, kronisk ledgångsreumatism;* **rheumatoid erosion** = erosion of bone and cartilage in the joints caused by rheumatoid arthritis *ledförslitning p.g.a. reumatisk värk*

> QUOTE rheumatoid arthritis is a chronic inflammatory disease which can affect many systems of the body, but mainly the joints. 70% of sufferers develop the condition in the metacarpophalangeal joints
>
> **Nursing Times**

rheumatologist [ˌru:mə'tɒlədʒɪst] *subst.* doctor who specializes in rheumatology *reumatolog*

rheumatology [ˌru:mə'tɒlədʒi] *subst.* branch of medicine dealing with rheumatic disease of muscles and joints *reumatologi*

Rh factor [ˌɑ:r'eɪtʃ ˌfæktə] *see* RHESUS FACTOR

Rh-faktor ⇨ **rhesus factor**

rhin- [raɪn] *or* **rhino-** ['raɪnə(ʊ), ˌ--] *prefix* referring to the nose *rin(o)-, nas(o)-, näs-*

rhinitis [raɪ'naɪtɪs] *subst.* inflammation of the mucous membrane in the nose, which makes the nose run, caused by a virus infection (cold) *or* an allergic reaction to dust *or* flowers, etc. *rinit, snuva;* **acute rhinitis** = common cold *or* a virus infection which causes inflammation of the mucous membrane in the nose and throat *akut rinit;* **allergic rhinitis** = HAY FEVER; **chronic catarrhal rhinitis** = chronic form of inflammation of the nose where excess mucus is secreted by the mucous membrane *hösnuva*

rhinology [raɪ'nɒlədʒi] *subst.* branch of medicine dealing with diseases of the nose and the nasal passage *rinologi*

rhinomycosis [ˌraɪnəʊmaɪ'kəʊsɪs] *subst.* infection of the nasal passages by a fungus *svampinfektion i näsan*

rhinophyma [ˌraɪnəʊ'faɪmə] *subst.* condition caused by rosacea, where the nose becomes permanently red and swollen *rinophyma, kopparnäsa, pundnäsa*

rhinoplasty ['raɪnəʊˌplæsti] *subst.* plastic surgery to correct the appearance of the nose *rinoplastik*

rhinorrhoea [ˌraɪnəʊ'rɪə] *subst.* watery discharge from the nose *rinorré*

rhinoscopy [raɪ'nɒskəpi] *subst.* examination of the inside of the nose *rinoskopi*

rhinosporidiosis [ˌraɪnəʊspɒˌrɪdi'əʊsɪs] *subst.* infection of the nose, eyes, larynx and genital organs by a fungus Rhinosporidium seeberi *rinosporidios*

rhinovirus [ˌraɪnəʊ'vaɪ(ə)rəs] *subst.* group of viruses containing RNA, which cause infection of the nose, including the virus which causes the common cold *rhinovirus*

rhiz- [raɪz] *or* **rhizo-** ['raɪzə(ʊ), ˌ--] *prefix* referring to a root *rhiz(o)-, riz(o)-, radik-, rot-*

rhizotomy [raɪ'zɒtəmi] *subst.* surgical operation to cut *or* divide the roots of a nerve to relieve severe pain *rizotomi*

Rh-negativ ⇨ **rhesus factor**

rhodopsin [rəʊ'dɒpsɪn] *or* **visual purple** [ˌvɪʒu(ə)l 'pɜːp(ə)l] *subst.* light-sensitive purple pigment in the rods of the retina, which makes it possible to see in dim light *rodopsin, synpurpur*

rhombencephalon [ˌrɒmben'kef(ə)lɒn] *or* **hindbrain** ['haɪndbreɪn] *subst.* part of the brain which contains the cerebellum, the medulla oblongata and the pons *rombencefalon, ruthjärnan, bakhjärnan*

rhomboid ['rɒmbɔɪd] *subst.* one of two muscles in the top part of the back which move the shoulder blades *musculus rhomboideus*

rhonchus ['rɒŋkəs] *subst.* abnormal sound in the chest, heard through a stethoscope, caused by a partial blockage in the bronchi **rhonchi** *rhonchi, ronki*
NOTE: the plural is **rhonchi**

Rh-positiv ⇨ **rhesus factor**

rhythm ['rɪð(ə)m] *subst.* regular movement *or* beat *rytm; see also* CIRCADIAN; **rhythm method** = method of birth control where sexual intercourse should take place only during the safe periods *or* when conception is least likely to occur, that is at the beginning and at the end of the menstrual cycle *preventivmetod som bygger på s k säkra perioder*

> COMMENT: this method is not as safe as other methods of contraception because the time when ovulation takes place cannot be accurately calculated if a woman does not have regular periods

rhythmic ['rɪðmɪk] *adj.* regular *or* with a repeated rhythm *rytmisk*

RIA ⇨ **radioimmunoassay**

rib [rɪb] *subst.* one of twenty-four curved bones which protect the chest *revben;* **cervical rib** = extra rib sometimes found attached to the cervical vertebrae *costa cervicalis, halsrevben;* **false ribs** = the bottom five ribs on each side which are not directly attached to the breastbone *de fem understa paren revben;* **floating ribs** = two lowest false ribs on each side, which are not attached to the breastbone *costae fluctuans, de två understa paren revben;* **true ribs** = top seven pairs of ribs *costae verae, äkta revbenen;* **rib cage** = the ribs and the space enclosed by them *bröstkorgen* NOTE: for other terms referring to the ribs see words beginning with **cost-**

> COMMENT: the rib cage is formed of twelve pairs of curved bones. The top seven pairs (the true ribs) are joined to the breastbone in front by costal cartilage; the other five pairs of ribs (the false ribs) are not attached to the breastbone, though the 8th, 9th and 10th pairs are each attached to the rib above. The bottom two pairs, which are not attached to the breastbone at all, are called the floating ribs

riboflavine [ˌraɪbəʊ'fleɪvɪn] = VITAMIN B_{12}

ribonuclease [ˌraɪbəʊ'nju:klieɪz] *subst.* enzyme which breaks down RNA *ribonukleas*

ribonucleic acid (RNA) [ˌraɪbəʊnju'kli:ɪk 'æsɪd (ˌɑ:ren'eɪ)] *subst.* one of the nucleic acids in the nucleus of all living cells, which takes coded information form DNA and translates it into specific enzymes and proteins *ribonukleinsyra, RNA; see also* DNA

ribonukleas ⇨ **ribonuclease**

ribonukleinsyra ⇨ **ribonucleic acid (RNA)**

ribose ['raɪbəʊs] *subst.* type of sugar found in RNA *ribos*

ribosomal [ˌraɪbə(ʊ)'səʊm(ə)l] *adj.* referring to ribosomes *som avser el. hör till ribosom(er)*

ribosome ['raɪbə(ʊ)səʊm] *subst.* tiny particle in a cell, containing RNA and protein, where protein is synthesized *ribosom*

rice [raɪs] *subst.* common food plant, grown in hot countries, of which the whitish grains are eaten *ris(gryn)*

ricewater stools ['raɪswɔ:tə ˌstu:lz] *subst. pl.* typical watery stools, passed by patients suffering from cholera *vattnig diarré*

rich [rɪtʃ] *adj.* **(a) rich in** = having a lot of something *rik på, -rik;* **green vegetables are rich in minerals; the doctor has prescribed a diet which is rich in protein** *or* **a protein-rich diet (b)** (food) which has high calorific value *fet, kraftig, mäktig*

> QUOTE the sublingual region has a rich blood supply derived from the carotid artery
> **Nursing Times**

ricin ['raɪsɪn] *subst.* highly toxic albumin found in the seeds of the castor oil *ricin*

ricinolja ⇨ **castor oil**

rickets ['rɪkɪts] *or* **rachitis** [rə'kaɪtɪs] *subst.* disease of children, where the bones are soft and do not develop properly because of lack of vitamin D *rakit, engelska sjukan;* **renal rickets** = form of rickets caused by poor kidney function *rakit pga njursjukdom*

COMMENT: initial treatment for rickets in children is a vitamin-rich diet, together with exposure to sunshine which causes vitamin D to form in the skin

Rickettsia [rɪ'ketsiə] *subst.* genus of microorganisms which causes several diseases including Q fever and typhus *Rickettsia*

rickettsial [rɪ'ketsiəl] *adj.* referring to Rickettsia *som avser el. hör till Rickettsia;* **rickettsial pox** = disease found in North America, caused by **Rickettsia akari** passed to humans by bites from mites which live on mice *fläcktyfus, fläckfeber*

rid [rɪd] *vb.* **to get rid of something** = to make something go away *göra sig av med ngt;* **to be rid of something** = not to have something unpleasant any more *bli kvitt (av med) ngt, slippa ngt;* **he can't get rid of his cold - he's had it for weeks; I'm very glad to be rid of my flu**

ridge [rɪdʒ] *subst.* long raised part on the surface of a bone *or* organ *rygg, kant, rand*

right [raɪt] **1** *adj. & adv. & subst.* not left *or* referring to the side of the body which usually has the stronger hand (which most people use to write with) *höger;* **my right arm is stronger than my left; he writes with his right hand 2** *subst.* what the law says a person is bound to have *rätt(ighet);* **the patient has no right to inspect his medical records; you always have the right to ask for a second opinion**

right-hand [ˌraɪt'hænd] *adj.* on the right side *höger;* **the stethoscope is in the right-hand drawer of the desk**

right-handed [ˌraɪt'hændɪd] *adj.* using the right hand more often than the left *högerhänt;* **he's right-handed; most people are right-handed**

rigid ['rɪdʒɪd] *adj.* stiff *or* not moving *rigid, styv, stel*

rigidity [rɪ'dʒɪdəti] *subst.* being rigid *or* bent *or* not able to be moved *rigiditet, styvhet, stelhet; see also* SPASTICITY

rigor ['rɪgə] *subst.* attack of shivering, often with fever *rigor, stelhet;* **rigor mortis** = condition where the muscles of a dead body become stiff a few hours after death and then become relaxed again *rigor mortis, likstelhet*

COMMENT: rigor mortis starts about eight hours after death, and begins to disappear several hours later; environment and temperature play a large part in the timing

riklig ⇨ **profuse**

riktig ➪ **accurate, exact**

riktigt ➪ **accurately**

rima ['raɪmə] *subst.* narrow crack *or* cleft *rima, spricka, springa;* **rima glottidis** = space between the vocal cords *rima glottidis, röstspringan, ljudspringan*

ring [rɪŋ] *subst.* circle of tissue; tissue *or* muscle shaped like a circle *ring, cirkel;* **ring finger** *or* **third finger** = the finger between the little finger and the middle finger *ringfingret*

ringa ➪ **call**

ringbrosket ➪ **cricoid cartilage**

ringfingret ➪ **ring**

ringformad ➪ **annular**

ringing in the ear [ˌrɪŋɪŋ ɪn ði 'ɪə] *see* TINNITUS

ringmuskel ➪ **orbicularis, sphincter (muscle)**

ringorm ➪ **ringworm, tinea**

ringworm ['rɪŋwɜːm] *subst.* any of various infections of the skin by a fungus, in which the infection spreads out in a circle from a central point (ringworm is very contagious and difficult to get rid of) *tinea, ringorm, revorm; see also* TINEA

rinit ➪ **rhinitis**

rinna ➪ **flow, run**

Rinne's test ['rɪnɪz ˌtest] *subst.* hearing test *Rinnes prov*

> COMMENT: a tuning fork is hit and its handle placed near the ear (to test for air conduction) and then on the mastoid process (to test for bone conduction). It is then possible to determine the type of lesion which exists by finding if the sound is heard for a longer period by air *or* by bone conduction

rin(o)- ➪ **rhin-**

rinologi ➪ **rhinology**

rinophyma ➪ **rhinophyma**

rinoplastik ➪ **rhinoplasty**

rinorré ➪ **rhinorrhoea**

rinoskopi ➪ **rhinoscopy**

rinosporidios ➪ **rhinosporidiosis**

rinse out [ˌrɪns 'aʊt] *vb.* to wash the inside of something to make it clean *skölja ur (ren);* **she rinsed out the measuring jar; rinse your mouth out with mouthwash**

ripple bed ['rɪp(ə)l ˌbed] *subst.* type of bed with an air-filled mattress divided into sections, in which the pressure is continuously being changed so that the patient's body can be massaged and bedsores can be avoided *cirkulationssäng, säng med dekubitusmadrass*

rise [raɪz] *vb.* to go up *stiga, gå upp, tillta, öka(s);* **his temperature rose sharply**
NOTE: **rises - rising - rose - has risen**

risk [rɪsk] **1** *subst.* possible harm *or* possibility of something happening *risk, fara;* **there is a risk of a cholera epidemic; there is no risk of the disease spreading to other members of the family; businessmen are particularly at risk of having a heart attack; children at risk** = children who are more likely to be harmed *or* to catch a disease *barn i riskzonen; see also* HIGH-RISK, LOW-RISK
2 *vb.* to do something which may possibly harm *or* have bad results *riskera;* **if the patient is not moved to an isolation ward, all the patients and staff in the hospital risk catching the disease**

> QUOTE adenomatous polyps are a risk factor for carcinoma of the stomach
> **Nursing Times**

> QUOTE three quarters of patients aged 35 - 64 on GPs' lists have at least one major risk factor: high cholesterol, high blood pressure or addiction to tobacco
> **Health Services Journal**

risk ➪ **danger; safely**

riskera ➪ **risk**

riskfri ➪ **safe**

rispa ➪ **scratch, tear**

rispning ➪ **scarification**

risus sardonicus ['raɪsəs sɑː'dɒnɪkəs] *subst.* twisted smile which is a symptom of tetanus *risus sardonicus, sardoniskt leende*

riva ➪ **scratch**

river blindness ['rɪvə blaɪndnəs] *subst.* blindness caused by larvae getting into the eye in cases of onchocerciasis *blindhet pga onchocerciasis (slags tropisk masksjukdom)*

rivsår ⇨ **lacerated, laceration**

riz(o)- ⇨ **rhiz-**

rizotomi ⇨ **rhizotomy**

RM [ˌɑːr'em] = REGISTERED MIDWIFE

RMN [ˌɑːrem'en] = REGISTERED MENTAL NURSE

RN [ˌɑːr'en] = REGISTERED NURSE

Rn *chemical symbol for* radon *Rn, radon*

RNA [ˌɑːren'eɪ] = RIBONUCLEIC ACID; **messenger RNA** = type of RNA which transmits information from DNA to form enzymes and proteins *messenger-RNA, budbärar-RNA*

RNMH [ˌɑːrenem'eɪtʃ] = REGISTERED NURSE FOR THE MENTALLY HANDICAPPED

ro ⇨ **rest**

rock ⇨ **gown, jacket**

Rocky Mountain spotted fever [ˌrɒki ˌmaʊntɪn 'spɒtɪd ˌfiːvə] *subst.* type of typhus caused by **Rickettsia rickettsii,** transmitted to humans by ticks *slags fläckfeber*

rod [rɒd] *subst.* **(a)** long thin round stick *stav;* **some bacteria are shaped like rods** *or* **are rod-shaped (b)** one of two types of light-sensitive cell in the retina of the eye *stav; see also* CONE

> COMMENT: rods are sensitive to poor light. They contain rhodopsin *or* visual purple, which produces the nervous impulse which the rod transmits to the optic nerve

rodent ulcer [ˌrəʊd(ə)nt 'ʌlsə] *or* **basal cell carcinoma** [ˌbeɪs(ə)l 'sel ˌkɑːsɪˌnəʊmə] *subst.* malignant tumour on the face *ulcus rodens, hudkarcinom, basalcellscancer, basaliom*

> COMMENT: rodent ulcers are different from some other types of cancer in that they do not spread to other parts of the body and do not metastasize, but remain on the face, usually near the mouth or eyes. Rodent ulcer is rare before middle age

rodna ⇨ **blush, flush**

rodnad ⇨ **blush, flare, flush, flushed, redness, rubor**

rodnadsframkallande (ämne) ⇨ **rubefacient**

rodopsin ⇨ **rhodopsin**

roentgen ['rɒntgən] *subst.* unit which measures the amount of exposure to X-rays *or* gamma rays *röntgen;* **roentgen rays** = X-rays *or* gamma rays which can pass through tissue and leave an image on a photographic film *röntgenstrålar, röntgenstrålning*

roentgenogram [rɒnt'genəgræm, 'rɒntgenəgræm] *subst.* X-ray photograph *röntgenogram, radiogram, röntgenbild*

roentgenology [ˌrɒntgə'nɒlədʒi] *subst.* study of X-rays and their use in medicine *röntgenologi, radiologi*

roller bandage ['rəʊlə ˌbændɪdʒ] *subst.* bandage in the form of a long strip of cloth which is rolled up from one or both ends *(rullad) binda*

rombencefalon ⇨ **rhombencephalon**

Romberg's sign ['rɒmbɜːgz ˌsaɪn] *subst.* symptom of a sensory disorder in the position sense *Rombergs prov (symtom, tecken)*

> COMMENT: if a patient cannot stand upright when his eyes are closed, this shows that nerves in the lower limbs which transmit position sense to the brain are damaged

rond ⇨ **round**

rongeur [rɔ̃'gɜːr] *subst.* strong surgical instrument like a pair of pliers, used for cutting bone *gougetång*

ronki ⇨ **rhonchus**

roof [ruːf] *subst.* top part of the mouth *or* other cavity *tak, gommen*

root [ruːt] *or* **radix** ['reɪdɪks] *subst.* (i) origin *or* point from which a part of the body grows *radix, rot;* (ii) part of a tooth which is connected to a socket in the jaw *radix, tandrot;* **root canal** = canal in the root of a tooth through which the nerves and blood vessels pass ⇨ *illustration* TOOTH *rotkanalen*

Rorschach test ['rɔːʃɑːk ˌtest] *or* **ink blot test** ['ɪŋk blɒt ˌtest] *subst.* test used in psychological diagnosis, where the patient is shown a series of blots of ink on paper, and is asked to say what each blot reminds him of.

The answers give information about the patient's psychological state *Rorschachtest*

rosa ⇨ **pink**

rosacea [rəʊ'zeɪʃə] *subst.* common skin disease affecting the face, and especially the nose, which becomes red because of enlarged blood vessels; the cause is not known *(acne) rosacea*

rosea ['rəʊziə] *see* PITYRIASIS

rosenådern ⇨ **saphenous nerve**

roseola [rə(ʊ)'ziːələ] *subst.* any disease with a light red rash *roseol;* **roseola infantum** *or* **exanthem subitum** = sudden infection of small children, with fever, swelling of the lymph glands and a rash *roseola infantum, spädbarnsroseol, exanthema subitum, sjätte sjukdomen, tredagarsfeber*

ros(feber) ⇨ **erysipelas**

rossla ⇨ **wheeze**

rosslande andning ⇨ **stertor, wheezing**

rosslig ⇨ **wheezy**

rostral ['rɒstr(ə)l] *adj.* like the beak of a bird *rostral, näbbliknande*

rostrum ['rɒstrəm] *subst.* projecting part of a bone *or* structure shaped like a beak *rostrum, näbb*
NOTE: plural is **rostra**

rot [rɒt] *vb.* to decay *or* to become putrefied *ruttna;* **the flesh was rotting round the wound as gangrene set in; the fingers can rot away in leprosy**

rot ⇨ **hilum, radix, root**

rot- ⇨ **hilar, rhiz-**

rotate [rəʊ'teɪt] *vb.* to move in a circle *rotera, vrida (sig) runt*

rotation [rəʊ'teɪʃ(ə)n] *subst.* moving in a circle *rotation, (rund)vridning;* **lateral and medial rotation** = turning part of the body to the side *or* towards the midline *vridning av kroppsdel åt sidan (mot mitten)*

rotationsled ⇨ **pivot**

rotator [rəʊ'teɪtə] *subst.* muscle which makes a limb rotate *rotator*

rotavirus ['rəʊtəˌvaɪ(ə)rəs] *subst.* any of a group of viruses associated with gastroenteritis in children *Rotavirus*

> QUOTE rotavirus is now widely accepted as an important cause of childhood diarrhoea in many different parts of the world
> **East African Medical Journal**

rotera ⇨ **rotate**

Rothera's test ['rɒðərəz ˌtest] *subst.* test to see if acetone is present in urine, a sign of ketosis which is a complication of diabetes mellitus *Rhoteras prov*

Roth spot ['rəʊt ˌspɒt] *subst.* pale spot which sometimes occurs on the retina of a person suffering from leukaemia or some other diseases *slags fläck på näthinnan (oftast vid endokardit)*

rotkanalen ⇨ **root**

rots ⇨ **glanders**

rotunda [rə(ʊ)'tʌndə] *see* FENESTRA

rough [rʌf] *adj.* not smooth *ojämn, skrovlig, knottrig, sträv;* **she put cream on her hands which were rough from heavy work**

roughage ['rʌfɪdʒ] *or* **dietary fibre** ['da(ɪ)ət(ə)ri ˌfaɪbə] *subst.* fibrous matter in food, which cannot be digested *fibrer, kostfibrer*

> COMMENT: roughage is found in cereals, nuts, fruit and some green vegetables. It is believed to be necessary to help digestion and avoid developing constipation, obesity and appendicitis

rouleau [ruː'ləʊ] *subst.* roll of red blood cells which have stuck together like a column of coins *myntrulle(bildning)*
NOTE: the plural is **rouleaux**

round [raʊnd] **1** *adj.* shaped like a circle *rund, cirkel-;* **round ligament** = band of ligament which stretches from the uterus to the labia *ligamentum teres uteri;* **round window** *or* **fenestra rotunda** = round opening between the middle ear and the inner ear *fenestra rotunda (cochleae), runda fönstret* **2** *subst.* regular visit *rond;* **to do the rounds of the wards** = to visit various wards in a hospital and talk to the nurses and check on patients, progress *or* condition *gå ronden på avdelningarna;* **a health visitor's rounds** = regular series of visits made by a health visitor *ung. rond av distriktssköterska (distriksbarnmorska, sjuksköterska från mödra- el. barnavårdscentral)*

roundworm ['raʊn(d)wɜːm] *subst.* any of several common types of parasitic worms with round bodies, such as hookworms (as opposed to flatworms) *nematod, rundmask, trådmask*

Rovsing's sign ['rɒvsɪŋs ˌsaɪn] *subst.* pain in the right iliac fossa when the left iliac fossa is pressed *Rovsings symtom*

COMMENT: a sign of acute appendicitis

Royal College of Nursing [ˌrɔɪ(ə)l ˌkɒlɪdʒ əv 'nɜːsɪŋ] *subst.* professional association which represents nurses *facklig sammanslutning av sjuksköterskor i Storbritannien*

RQ [ˌɑː'kjuː] = RESPIRATORY QUOTIENT

-(r)rafi ⇨ **-rrhaphy**

-(r)ré ⇨ **-rrhoea**

-(r)rexi ⇨ **-rrhexis**

-rrhagia ['reɪdʒə] *or* **-rrhage** [rɪdʒ] *suffix* referring to abnormal flow *or* discharge of blood *-(r)ragi, -blödning*

-rrhaphy ['rəfi] *suffix* referring to surgical sewing *or* suturing *-(r)rafi, -sutur, -söm*

-rrhexis ['reksɪs] *suffix* referring to splitting *or* rupture *-(r)rexi, -ruptur, -bristning*

-rrhoea ['rɪə] *suffix* referring to an abnormal flow *or* discharge of fluid from an organ *-(r)ré, -flöde*

RSCN [ˌɑːressiː'en] = REGISTERED SICK CHILDREN'S NURSE

RSV [ˌɑːres'viː] = RESPIRATORY SYNCYTIAL VIRUS

RS-virus ⇨ **respiratory**

rub [rʌb] **1** *subst.* lotion used to rub on the skin *liniment;* **the ointment is used as a rub 2** *vb.* to move something (especially the hands) backwards and forwards over a surface *frottera, gnugga, gnida;* **she rubbed her leg after she knocked it against the table; he rubbed his hands to make the circulation return**

rubbad ⇨ **disordered**

rubber ['rʌbə] *subst.* material which we can be stretched and compressed, made from the thick white liquid (latex) from a tropical tree *gummi; US kondom;* **rubber sheet =** waterproof sheet put on hospital beds *or* on the bed of a child who suffers from bedwetting, to protect the mattress *gummiduk*

rubbing alcohol ['rʌbɪŋ ˌælkəhɒl] *subst. US* ethyl alcohol, used as a disinfectant *or* for rubbing on the the skin *ryggsprit*
NOTE: GB English is **surgical spirit**

rubbning ⇨ **derangement, disorder, disturbance, upset**

rubefacient [ˌruːbi'feɪʃ(ə)nt] *adj. & subst.* (substance) which makes the skin warm, and pink or red *rodnadsframkallande (ämne)*

rubella [ru'belə] = GERMAN MEASLES

rubeola [ru'biːələ] = MEASLES

Rubin's test ['ruːbɪnz ˌtest] *subst.* test to see if the Fallopian tubes are free from obstruction *hysterosalpingografi, HSG, slags undersökning av passagen i äggledarna*

rub into ['rʌb ɪntʊ] *vb.* to make an ointment go into the skin by rubbing *frottera (gnugga, gnida) in;* **rub the liniment gently into the skin**

rubor ['ruːbə] *subst.* redness (of the skin *or* tissue) *rubor, rodnad*

rubra ['ruːbrə] *see* = PITYRIASIS

rudimentary [ˌruːdɪ'ment(ə)ri] *adj.* which exists in a small form *or* which has not developed fully *rudimentär, outvecklad;* **the child was born with rudimentary arms**

rudimentär ⇨ **rudimentary, vestigial**

Ruffini corpuscles [ru'fiːnɪ ˌkɔːpʌs(ə)l] *or* **Ruffini nerve endings** [ru'fiːnɪ ˌnɜːv ˌendɪŋz] *see* CORPUSCLE

ruga ['ruːgə] *subst.* fold *or* ridge (especially in mucous membrane such as the lining of the stomach) *ruga, veck*
NOTE: plural is **rugae**

rulla ⇨ **wheel**

rullbord ⇨ **trolley**

rullstol ⇨ **invalid, wheelchair**

rum ⇨ **ward; chamber; space**

rumbling ['rʌmblɪŋ] *subst.* noise in the intestine caused by gas bubbles *knorr(ande), kurr(ande)*

run [rʌn] *vb. (of the nose)* to drip with liquid secreted from the mucous membrane in the nasal passage *rinna, droppa;* **his nose is running; if your nose is running, blow it on a handkerchief; one of the symptoms of a cold is a running nose**

rund ⇨ **round**

rundmask ⇨ **nematode, roundworm**

R-unit ['ɑ:ju:nɪt] = ROENTGEN UNIT

ruptur ⇨ **rupture, tear**

-ruptur ⇨ **-rrhexis**

rupture ['rʌptʃə] **1** *subst.* **(a)** breaking *or* tearing (of an organ such as the appendix) *ruptur, bristning* **(b)** hernia *or* condition where the muscles *or* wall round an organ become weak and the organ bulges through the wall *bråck* **2** *vb.* to break *or* tear *rupturera, brista, spricka;* **ruptured spleen** = spleen which has been torn by piercing *or* by a blow *rupterad (brusten) mjälte*

Russell traction ['rʌs(ə)l ˌtrækʃ(ə)n] *subst.* type of traction with weights and slings used to straighten a femur which has been fractured *slags sträck*

ruthjärnan ⇨ **rhombencephalon**

ruttna ⇨ **decay, decompose, putrefy, rot**

ryckig ⇨ **jerky, spasmodic, spastic**

ryckning ⇨ **spasm, twitching**

rygg ⇨ **back; dorsum, ridge**

rygg- ⇨ **dorsal, dorsi-**

ryggkota ⇨ **spondyl, vertebra**

ryggkote- ⇨ **vertebral**

ryggkoteartärerna ⇨ **vertebral**

ryggkotehålet ⇨ **vertebral**

ryggkoteutskott ⇨ **spinous process**

ryggkotsbåge ⇨ **neural**

rygglåge, i ⇨ **supine**

ryggmusklerna ⇨ **back**

ryggmärgen ⇨ **spinal**

ryggmärgs- ⇨ **myel-, spinal, spino-**

ryggmärgsbråck ⇨ **myelocele**

ryggmärgshinne- ⇨ **mening-, meningeal**

ryggmärgshinnebråck ⇨ **meningocele**

ryggmärgsinflammation ⇨ **myelitis**

ryggmärgstvinsot ⇨ **tabes**

ryggmärgsuppmjukning ⇨ **myelomalacia**

ryggraden ⇨ **backbone, spinal, spine, vertebral**

ryggrads- ⇨ **rachi-, rhachio-, spinal, spino-**

ryggradsinflammation ⇨ **spondylitis**

ryggradskanalen ⇨ **spinal**

ryggskott ⇨ **lumbago**

ryggsprit ⇨ **rubbing alcohol, surgical**

ryggsträckarmuskeln ⇨ **erector spinae**

ryggvärk ⇨ **back, backache**

Ryle's tube ['raɪlz ˌtju:b] *subst.* thin tube which is passed into a patient's stomach through either the nose *or* mouth, used to pump out the contents of the stomach *or* to introduce a barium meal in the stomach *slags ventrikelsond (magsond)*

rymd ⇨ **capacity**

rynka ⇨ **wrinkle**

rynkig ⇨ **wrinkled, shrivel**

rysa ⇨ **shiver**

rytm ⇨ **rhythm**

rytmisk ⇨ **rhythmic**

rytmrubbning ⇨ **dysrhythmia**

råd ⇨ **advice, suggestion**

råda ⇨ **advise**

rådfråga ⇨ **consult**

rådgivning ⇨ counselling

råmjölk ⇨ colostrum

råttbettsfeber ⇨ rat-bite fever, sodokosis

räcka ⇨ hand

räckhåll ⇨ reach

räckvidd ⇨ range

rädd ⇨ frightened

rädda ⇨ save

rädsla ⇨ fear

räta (ut) ⇨ straighten

rätta till ⇨ correct

rättelse ⇨ correction

rättsmedicin ⇨ forensic medicine

röd ⇨ red

röda hund ⇨ German measles

Röda korset ⇨ cross

röd benmärg ⇨ myeloid

rödblindhet ⇨ Daltonism

rödbrusigt ansikte ⇨ congested

rödhet ⇨ red, redness

rödsot ⇨ dysentery

rök ⇨ fumes, smoke

röka ⇨ smoke

rökare ⇨ smoker

rökfri ⇨ smokeless

rökhosta ⇨ smoker

rökning ⇨ fumigation

röntga ⇨ X-ray

röntgen ⇨ R, roentgen, X-ray

röntgen- ⇨ radio-

röntgenassistent ⇨ radiographer

röntgenbild ⇨ radiograph, roentgenogram, X-ray

röntgenfotografera ⇨ X-ray

röntgengenomlysning ⇨ fluoroscopy, imaging, radioscopy

röntgenkontrast(medel) ⇨ opaque

röntgenläkare ⇨ radiologist

röntgenografi ⇨ radiography

röntgenogram ⇨ roentgenogram

röntgenolog ⇨ radiologist

röntgenologi ⇨ radiology, roentgenology

röntgenstrålning ⇨ roentgen, X-ray

röntgentät ⇨ radio-opaque

rör ⇨ conduit, duct, ductus, meatus, tube

rörelse ⇨ motion, movement

rörelseförmåga ⇨ locomotion

rörelse, passiv ⇨ passive

rörelsesjuka ⇨ motion

rörelsesvårigheter ⇨ dyskinesia

rörformig ⇨ tubular

rörlig ⇨ mobile, motile

rörlighet ⇨ mobility, motility

rörlig njure ⇨ nephroptosis

rörsocker ⇨ sucrose

röst ⇨ voice

röst- ⇨ vocal

röstspringan ⇨ rima

Ss

Sabin vaccine ['seɪbɪn ˌvæksiːn] *subst.* vaccine against poliomyelitis *Sabin-vaccin, oralt (levande) poliovaccin; compare* SALK

COMMENT: the Sabin vaccine is given orally, and consists of weak live polio virus

sac [sæk] *subst.* part of the body shaped like a bag *säck;* **amniotic sac** = thin sac which covers an unborn baby in the womb, containing the amniotic fluid *amnionsäcken;* **hernial sac** = membranous sac of peritoneum where an organ has pushed through a cavity in the body *bråcksäck;* **pericardial sac** = the serous pericardium *perikardiet, hjärtsäcken*

sacchar- ['sækə, ˌ--] *or* **saccharo-** ['sækərə(ʊ), ˌ---] *prefix* referring to sugar *sackar(o)-, socker-*

saccharide ['sækəraɪd] *subst.* form of carbohydrate *sackarid*

saccharin ['sæk(ə)rɪn] *subst.* sweet substance, used in place of sugar because although it is nearly 500 times sweeter than sugar it contains no carbohydrates *sackarin*

saccule ['sækjuːl] *or* **sacculus** ['sækjuləs] *subst.* smaller of two sacs in the vestibule of the inner ear which is part of the mechanism which relates information about the position of the head in space *sacculus (labyrinthi membranacei)*

Sachs sjukdom ⇨ **Tay-Sachs disease**

sackaras ⇨ **invertase, sucrase**

sackarid ⇨ **saccharide**

sackarin ⇨ **saccharin**

sackar(o)- ⇨ **sacchar-**

sackaromykos ⇨ **blastomycosis**

sackaros ⇨ **sucrose**

sacral ['seɪkr(ə)l] *adj.* referring to the sacrum *sakral(-), korsbens-, kors-;* **sacral foramina** = openings *or* holes in the sacrum through which pass the sacral nerves ⇨ *illustration* PELVIS *foramina sacralia;* **sacral nerves** = nerves which branch from the spinal cord in the sacrum *nervi sacrales, sakralnerverna, korsnerverna;* **sacral plexus** = plexus *or* group of nerves inside the pelvis near the sacrum, which supply nerves in the buttocks, back of the thigh and lower leg, foot and the urogenital area *plexus sacralis, korsbensplexus, korsflätan;* **sacral vertebrae** = five vertebrae in the lower part of the spine which are fused together to form the sacrum *vertebrae sacrales, sakralkotorna, korsbenskotorna, korskotorna*

sacralization [ˌsækrəlaɪ'zeɪʃ(ə)n] *subst.* abnormal condition where the lowest lumbar vertebra fuses with the sacrum *sakralisation*

sacro- ['seɪkrə(ʊ), ˌ--] *prefix* referring to the sacrum *sakr(o)-, korsbens-*

sacrococcygeal [ˌseɪkrə(ʊ)kɒk'siːdʒiəl] *adj.* referring to the sacrum and the coccyx *sakrococcygeus*

sacroiliac [ˌseɪkrə(ʊ)'ɪliæk] *adj.* referring to the sacrum and the ilium *sakroiliakal;* **sacroiliac joint** = joint where the sacrum joins the ilium *articulatio sacroiliaca, sacroiliacaleden*

sacroiliitis [ˌseɪkrə(ʊ)ˌɪli'aɪtɪs] *subst.* inflammation of the sacroiliac joint *sakroiliit*

sacrotuberous ligament [ˌseɪkrə(ʊ)'tjuːb(ə)rəs ˌlɪgəmənt] *subst.* large ligament between the iliac spine, the sacrum, the coccyx and the ischial tuberosity *ligamentum sacrotuberale*

sacrum ['seɪkrəm] *subst.* flat triangular bone, between the lumbar vertebrae and the coccyx with which it articulates, formed of five sacral vertebrae fused together *sacrum, sakrum, korsbenet;* it also articulates with the hip bones ⇨ *illustration* PELVIS, VERTEBRAL COLUMN

saddle joint ['sæd(ə)l ˌdʒɔɪnt] *subst.* synovial joint where one element is concave and the other convex, like the joint between the thumb and the wrist *articulatio sella, sadelled*

saddle-nose ['sæd(ə)lnəʊz] *subst.* deep bridge of the nose, normally a sign of injury but sometimes a sign of tertiary syphilis *sadelnäsa*

sadelled ⇨ **saddle joint**

sadelnäsa ⇨ **saddle-nose**

sadism ['seɪdɪz(ə)m] *subst.* abnormal sexual condition, where a person finds sexual pleasure in hurting others *sadism*

sadist ['seɪdɪst] *subst.* person whose sexual urge is linked to sadism *sadist*

sadistic [sə'dɪstɪk] *adj.* referring to sadism *sadistisk; compare* MASOCHISM

safe [seɪf] *adj.* not likely to hurt or cause damage *ofarlig, riskfri, säker;* **medicines should be kept in a place which is safe from children; this antibiotic is safe to be used on very small babies; it is a safe pain killer, with no harmful side-effects; it is not safe to take the drug and also drink alcohol; safe dose** = amount of a drug which can be taken without causing harm to the patient *säker dos, maximaldos;* **safe period** = time during the menstrual cycle, when conception is not likely to occur, and sexual intercourse can take place (used as a method of contraception) *säker period*
NOTE: **safe - safer - safest**

safely ['seɪfli] *adv.* without danger *or* without being hurt *säkert, utan fara, utan risk;* **you can safely take six tablets a day without any risk of side-effects**

safety ['seɪfti] *subst.* being safe *or* without danger *säkerhet;* **to take safety precautions** = to do certain things which make your actions or condition safe *vidta säkerhetsåtgärder (försiktighetsåtgärder);* **safety belt** = belt which is worn in a car or a plane to help to stop a passenger being hurt if there is an accident *säkerhetsbälte, bilbälte;* **safety pin** = special type of bent pin with a guard which covers the point, used for attaching nappies *or* bandages *säkerhetsnål*

saft ⇨ **juice, succus**

sagittal ['sædʒɪt(ə)l] *adj.* which goes from the front of the body to the back, dividing it into right and left *sagittal;* **sagittal plane** *or* **median plane** = division of the body along the midline, at right angles to the coronal plane. diving the body into right and left parts *sagittalplan, medianplanet;* **sagittal section** = any section *or* cut through the body, going from the front to the back along the length of the body *sagittalsnitt;* **sagittal suture** = joint along the top of the head where the two parietal bones are fused *sutura sagittalis, pilsömmen*

sagittalplan ⇨ **sagittal**

sagittalsnitt ⇨ **sagittal**

sagrada(extrakt) ⇨ **cascara (sagrada)**

sakkunnig ⇨ **expert**

sakral(-) ⇨ **sacral**

sakralisation ⇨ **sacralization**

sakralkotorna ⇨ **sacral**

sakralnerverna ⇨ **sacral**

sakr(o)- ⇨ **sacro-**

sakrococcygeus ⇨ **sacrococcygeal**

sakroiliakal ⇨ **sacroiliac**

sakroiliit ⇨ **sacroiliitis**

sakrum ⇨ **sacrum**

sal ⇨ **ward**

salaamkramp ⇨ **spasmus nutans**

salicylate [sə'lɪsɪleɪt] *or* **acetylsalicylic acid** [ˌæsɪˌtaɪ(ə)lˌsælɪˌsɪlɪk 'æsɪd] *subst.* pain-killing substance, derived from salicylic acid, used in the treatment of rheumatism, headaches and minor pains *salicylat, (acetyl)salicylsyra*

salicylic acid [ˌsælɪˌsɪlɪk 'æsɪd] *subst.* white antiseptic substance, which destroys bacteria and fungi and which is used in ointments to treat corns, warts and other skin disorders *acidum salicylicum, salicylsyra*

salicylsyra ⇨ **salicylic acid**

saline ['seɪlaɪn] **1** *adj.* referring to salt *salinisk, salt-, salthaltig;* **the patient was given a saline transfusion; she is on a saline drip; saline drip** = drip containing a saline solution *saltlösning (elektrolytlösning) för infusion;* **saline solution** = salt solution, made of distilled water and sodium chloride, which is introduced into the body intravenously through a drip *saltlösning, elektrolytlösning* **2** *subst.* saline solution *saltlösning, elektrolytlösning*

saliv ⇨ **saliva**

saliv- ⇨ **ptyal-, salivary, sial-**

saliva [sə'laɪvə] *subst.* fluid in the mouth, secreted by the salivary glands, which starts the process of digesting food *saliv, spott*

COMMENT: saliva is a mixture of a large quantity of water and a small amount of mucus, secreted by the salivary glands. Saliva acts to keep the mouth and throat moist, allowing food to be swallowed easily. It also contains the enzyme ptyalin, which begins the digestive process of converting starch into sugar while food is still in the mouth. Because of this association with food, the salivary glands produce saliva automatically when food is seen, smelt or even simply talked about. The salivary glands are situated under the tongue (the sublingual glands), beneath the lower jaw (the submandibular glands) and in the neck at the back of the lower jaw joint (the parotid glands)

salivary ['sælɪv(ə)ri, sə'laɪv(ə)ri] *adj.* referring to saliva *saliv-, spott-;* **salivary calculus** = stone which forms in a salivary gland *glandulus salivalis (salivaris), ptyalolit, sialolit, salivsten, spottsten;* **salivary glands** = glands which secrete saliva *glandulae salivarae (salivales, salivares), spottkörtlarna, salivkörtlarna*

salivate ['sælɪveɪt] *vb.* to produce saliva *avsöndra saliv (spott)*

salivation [ˌsælɪ'veɪʃ(ə)n] *subst.* production of saliva *salivation, salivavsöndring, spottavsöndring* NOTE: for terms referring to saliva, see words beginning with **ptyal-, sial-**

salivavsöndring ➪ **salivation**

salivkörtlarna ➪ **salivary**

salivsten ➪ **salivary, sialolith**

Salk vaccine ['sɑːk ˌvæksiːn] *subst.* vaccine against poliomyelitis *Salk-vaccin, avdödat poliovaccin (som ges med spruta); compare* SABIN

COMMENT: the Salk vaccine consists of dead polio virus and is given by injection

Salmonella [ˌsælmə'nelə] *subst.* genus of bacteria which are in the intestines, which are pathogenic, are usually acquired by eating contaminated food, and cause typhoid or paratyphoid fever, gastroenteritis or food poisoning *Salmonella;* **five people were taken to hospital with Salmonella poisoning** NOTE: plural is **Salmonellae**

salmonellosis [ˌsælmənə'ləʊsɪs] *subst.* food poisoning caused by **Salmonella** in the digestive system *salmonellos*

salping- ['sælpɪndʒ, ˌ--] *or* **salpingo-** [ˌsælpɪŋ'gɒ, sælˌpɪŋgəʊ] *prefix* referring to a tube (i) the Fallopian tubes *salping(o)-, tubar(-), tubär, äggledar-;* (ii) the auditory meatus *salping(o)-, örontrumpets-*

salpingectomy [ˌsælpɪn'dʒektəmi] *subst.* surgical operation to remove *or* cut a Fallopian tube (used as a method of contraception) *salpingektomi*

salpingitis [ˌsælpɪn'dʒaɪtɪs] *subst.* inflammation, usually of a Fallopian tube *salpingit, äggledarinflammation*

salpingography [ˌsælpɪŋ'gɒgrəfi] *subst.* X-ray examination of the Fallopian tubes *salpingografi*

salpingooforektomi ➪ **oophorosalpingectomy**

salpingo-oophoritis [sælˌpɪŋgəʊˌəʊˌɒfə'raɪtɪs] *or* **salpingo-oothecitis** [sælˌpɪŋgəʊəʊˌɒɵɪ'saɪtɪs] *subst.* inflammation of a Fallopian tube and the ovary connected to it *salpingooforit, ooforosalpingit*

salpingo-oophorocele [sælˌpɪŋgəʊˌəʊ'ɒfərəʊsiː(ə)l] *or* **salpingo-oothecocele** [sælˌpɪŋgəʊˌəʊɒ'ɵiːkəʊsiː(ə)l] *subst.* hernia where a Fallopian tube and its ovary pass through a weak point in surrounding tissue *bråck av ovarium och äggledare*

salpingostomi ➪ **salpingostomy**

salpingostomy [ˌsælpɪŋ'gɒstəmi] *subst.* surgical operation to open up a blocked Fallopian tube *salpingostomi, tubarplastik*

salpingovariektomi ➪ **oophorosalpingectomy**

salpinx ['sælpɪŋks] = FALLOPIAN TUBE

salt [sɔːlt, sɒlt] **1** *subst.* **(a) common salt =** sodium chloride, a white powder used to make food, especially meat, fish and vegetables, taste better *salt, koksalt, natriumklorid;* **salt depletion** = loss of salt from the body, by sweating or vomiting, which causes cramp and other problems *saltförlust, saltbrist;* **a patient with heart failure is put on a salt-restricted diet; he should reduce his intake of salt (b)** chemical compound formed from an acid and a metal *salt;* **bile salts** = alkaline salts in the bile *gallsalter;* **Epsom salts** = sulphate of magnesium *or* white powder used as a laxative when dissolved in water *magnesiumsulfat* NOTE: the plural is not used for meaning (a) **2**

adj. tasting of salt *salt;* **sea water is salt; sweat tastes salt**

COMMENT: salt forms a necessary part of diet, as it replaces salt lost in sweating and helps to control the water balance in the body. It also improves the working of the muscles and nerves. Most diets contain more salt than each person actually needs, and although it has not been proved to be harmful, it is generally wise to cut down on salt consumption. Salt is one of the four tastes, the others being sweet, sour and bitter

salt- ➪ **saline**

saltbalans ➪ **sodium**

saltbrist ➪ **salt**

saltfattig kost ➪ **diet**

saltförlust ➪ **salt**

salthaltig ➪ **saline**

saltlösning ➪ **saline**

saltsyra ➪ **hydrochloric acid**

salva ➪ **cream, ointment, salve, unguent, unguentum**

salve [sælv, sɑːv] *subst.* ointment *unguentum, salva;* **lip salve** = ointment, usually sold as a soft stick, used to rub on lips to prevent them cracking *läppsalva, cerat*

salvkompress ➪ **paraffin**

samband ➪ **relationship**

samhälle ➪ **community**

samhälls- ➪ **social**

samhällsfarlig ➪ **antisocial**

samlag ➪ **intercourse, sex, sexual, coition, copulation**

samlas ➪ **collect, gather**

samling ➪ **collection**

samlingsrör ➪ **collecting duct**

sammanbitning ➪ **occlusion**

sammanbrott ➪ **collapse**

sammandragande ➪ **constrictive, styptic**

sammandragen ➪ **tense**

sammandragning ➪ **constriction, contraction; systole**

sammansatt ➪ **complex**

sammanslutning ➪ **association**

sammansmält ➪ **synostosis**

sammansmältning ➪ **fusion**

sammansättning ➪ **composition, compound**

sammanväxning ➪ **adhesion, symphysis, synechia, union**

sammanväxningslinje ➪ **raphe**

sammanväxt ➪ **synechia, synostosis**

samordna ➪ **coordinate**

samordning ➪ **coordination**

sample [ˈsɑːmp(ə)l] *subst.* small quantity of something used for testing *sampel, stickprov, prov;* **blood samples were taken from all the staff in the hospital; the doctor asked her to provide a urine sample**

samtycke ➪ **consent**

samverkan ➪ **coordination, synergism, synergy**

sanatorium [ˌsænəˈtɔːrɪəm] *subst.* institution (like a hospital) which treats certain types of disorder, such as tuberculosis, or offers special treatment such as hot baths, massage, etc. *sanatorium, kuranstalt*
NOTE: plural is **sanatoria, sanatoriums**

sandflea [ˈsændfliː] *or* **jigger** [ˈdʒɪgə] *subst.* tropical insect which enters the skin between the toes and digs under the skin, causing intense irritation *sandloppa*

sandflugefeber ➪ **sandfly fever**

sandfly fever [ˈsændflaɪ ˌfiːvə] *subst.* virus infection like influenza, which is transmitted by the bite of the sandfly **Phlebotomus papatasii** and is common in the Middle East *sandflugefeber*

sandloppa ➪ **sandflea**

sanguineous [sæŋˈgwɪnɪəs] *adj.* referring to blood *or* containing blood *blod-, blodfull*

sanies ['seɪnɪˌi:z] *subst.* discharge from a sore *or* wound which has an unpleasant smell *sanies, var*

sanitary ['sænət(ə)ri] *adj.* (i) clean *ren;* (ii) referring to hygiene *or* to health *sanitär, hälsovårds-, hygienisk;* **sanitary napkin** *or* **sanitary towel** = wad of absorbent cotton placed over the vulva to absorb the menstrual flow *dambinda*

sanitation [ˌsænɪ'teɪʃ(ə)n] *subst.* being hygienic (especially referring to public hygiene) *sanitet, hygien;* **poor sanitation in crowded conditions can result in the spread of disease**

sanitet ⇨ **sanitation**

sanitär ⇨ **sanitary**

sann ⇨ **true**

SA node [ˌes'eɪ ˌnəʊd] *or* **S - A node** [ˌes'eɪ ˌnəʊd] = SINOATRIAL NODE

saphenous nerve [sə'fi:nəs ˌnɜ:v] *subst.* branch of the femoral nerve which connects with the sensory nerves in the skin of the lower leg *nervus saphenus;* **saphenous opening** = hole in the fascia of the thigh through which the saphenous vein passes *hiatus saphenus;* **saphenous vein** *or* **saphena** = one of two veins which take blood from the foot up the leg *vena saphena (magna), rosenådern*

> COMMENT: the long (internal) saphenous vein, the longest vein in the body, runs from the foot up the inside of the leg and joins the femoral vein. The short (posterior) saphenous vein runs up the back of the lower leg and joins the popliteal vein

sapraemia [sæ'pri:miə] *subst.* blood poisoning by saprophytes *sapremi*

saprofil ⇨ **saprophytic**

saprofyt ⇨ **saprophyte**

saprofytisk ⇨ **saprophytic**

saprofytär ⇨ **saprophytic**

saprophyte ['sæprəfaɪt] *subst.* microorganism which lives on dead *or* decaying tissue *saprofyt*

saprophytic [ˌsæprə(ʊ)'fɪtɪk] *adj.* (organism) which lives on dead *or* decaying tissue *saprofytisk, saprofytär, saprofil*

sarc- ['sɑ:k, ˌ-] *or* **sarco-** ['sɑ:kə(ʊ), ˌ--] *prefix* referring to (i) flesh *sark(o)-;* (ii) muscle *sark(o)-*

sarcoid ['sɑ:kɔɪd] *subst. & adj.* (tumour) which is like a sarcoma *sarkoid, sarkomliknande (bildning)*

sarcoidosis [ˌsɑ:kɔɪ'dəʊsɪs] *or* **Boeck's disease** ['beks dɪˌzi:z] *subst.* disease causing enlargement of the lymph nodes, where small nodules *or* granulomas form in certain tissues, especially in the lungs *or* liver and other parts of the body *sarkoidos, (Besnier-)Boecks sarkoid*

> COMMENT: the Kveim test confirms the presence of sarcoidosis

sarcolemma [ˌsɑ:kə(ʊ)'lemə] *subst.* membrane surrounding a muscle fibre *sarkolemma*

sarcoma [sɑ:'kəʊmə] *subst.* cancer of connective tissue, such as bone, muscle or cartilage *sarkom*

sarcomatosis [ˌsɑ:kəʊmə'təʊsɪs] *subst.* condition where a sarcoma has spread through the bloodstream to many parts of the body *sarkomatos*

sarcomatous [sɑ:'kɒmətəs] *adj.* referring to a sarcoma *sarkomatös, sarkom-*

sarcomere ['sɑ:kə(ʊ)ˌmɪə] *subst.* filament in myofibril *(myo)filament i myofibrill*

sarcoplasm ['sɑ:kə(ʊ)plæz(ə)m] *or* **myoplasm** ['maɪəʊplæz(ə)m] *subst.* semi-liquid cytoplasm in muscle membrane *sarkoplasma*

sarcoplasmic [ˌsɑ:kəʊ'plæzmɪk] *adj.* referring to sarcoplasm *sarkoplasmatisk;* **sarcoplasmic reticulum** = network in the cytoplasm of striated muscle fibres *reticulum sarcoplasmaticum, sarkoplasmatiskt retikel*

sarcoptes [sɑ:'kɒpti:z] *subst.* type of mite which causes scabies *Sarcoptes scabei, skabbdjuret*

sardonicus [sɑ:'dɒnɪkəs] *see* RISUS

sark(o)- ⇨ **sarc-**

sarkoid ⇨ **sarcoid**

sarkoidos ⇨ **sarcoidosis**

sarkolemma ⇨ **sarcolemma**

sarkom ⇨ **sarcoma**

sarkom- ⇨ **sarcomatous**

sarkomatos ⇨ **sarcomatosis**

sarkomatös ⇨ **sarcomatous**

sarkoplasma ⇨ **myoplasm, sarcoplasm**

sarkoplasmatisk ⇨ **sarcoplasmic**

sartorius [sɑː'tɔːriəs] *subst.* very long muscle (the longest muscle) which runs from the anterior iliac spine, across the thigh down to the tibia *musculus sartorius, skräddarmuskeln*

saturated fat ['sætʃəreɪtɪd ˌfæt] *subst.* fat which has the largest amount of hydrogen possible *mättat fett*

> COMMENT: animal fats such as butter and fat meat are saturated fatty acids. It is known that increasing the amount of unsaturated and polyunsaturated fats (mainly vegetable fats and oils, and fish oil), and reducing saturated fats in the food intake helps reduce the level of cholesterol in the blood, and so lessens the risk of atherosclerosis

saturnism ['sætənɪz(ə)m] *subst.* lead poisoning *saturnism, blyförgiftning*

satyriasis [ˌsætə'ra(ɪ)əsɪs] *subst.* abnormal sexual urge in a man *satyriasis, satyromani*
NOTE: in a woman, called **nymphomania**

save [seɪv] *vb.* to rescue someone *or* to stop someone from being hurt or killed *or* to stop something from being damaged *rädda;* **the doctors saved the little boy from dying of cancer; the surgeons were unable to save the sight of their patient; the surgeons saved her life** = they stopped the patient from dying *kirurgerna räddade livet på henne*

saw [sɔː] **1** *subst.* tool with a long metal blade with teeth along its edge, used for cutting *såg* **2** *vb.* to cut with a saw *såga*
NOTE: **saws - sawing - sawed - has sawn**

sax ⇨ **scissors**

saxgång ⇨ **scissors**

Sayre's jacket ['seɪəz ˌdʒækɪt] *subst.* plaster cast which supports the spine when vertebrae have been deformed by tuberculosis or spinal disease *slags gipsvagga (gipskorsett)*

s.c. [ˌes'siː] = SUB CUTANEOUS

scab [skæb] *subst.* crust of dry blood which forms over a wound and protects it *sårskorpa, skorpa*

scabicide ['skeɪbɪsaɪd] *subst. & adj.* (solution) which kills mites *(medel) mot skabb*

scabies ['skeɪbiːz] *subst.* very irritating infection of the skin caused by a mite which lives under the skin *scabies, skabb*

scala ['skɑːlə] *subst.* spiral canal in the cochlea *scala (tympani resp. ventibuli)*

> COMMENT: the cochlea is formed of three spiral canals: the scala vestibuli which is filled with perilymph and connects with the oval window; the scala media which is filled with endolymph and transmits vibrations from the scala vestibuli through the basilar membrane to the scala tympani, which in turn transmits the sound vibrations to the round window

scald [skɔːld] **1** *subst.* burn made by a very hot liquid *or* steam *skållskada* **2** *vb.* to burn with a very hot liquid *skålla*

scale [skeɪl] **1** *subst.* **(a)** flake of dead tissue (as dead skin in dandruff) *fjäll, flaga* **(b)** **scales** = machine for weighing *våg;* **the nurses weighed the baby on the scales** **2** *vb.* to scrape teeth to remove plaque *skrapa bort (tandsten)*

scalenus [ˌskeɪ'liːnəs] *or* **scalene** ['skeɪliːn] *subst.* one of a group of muscles in the neck which bend the neck forwards and sideways, and also help expand the lungs in deep breathing *(musculus) scalenus, revbenshöjare;* **scalenus syndrome** = pain in an arm, caused by the scalenus anterior muscle pressing the subclavian artery and the brachial plexus against the vertebrae *scalenussyndrom*

scalenussyndrom ⇨ **scalenus, thoracic**

scale off [ˌskeɪl 'ɒf] *vb.* to fall off in scales *fjälla, flaga*

scaler ['skeɪlə] *subst.* surgical instrument for scaling teeth *instrument att ta bort tandsten med*

scalp [skælp] *subst.* thick skin and muscle (with the hair) which covers the skull *skalpen, huvudsvålen, hårbottnen;* **scalp wound** = wound in the scalp *sår i hårbottnen*

scalpel ['skælp(ə)l] *subst.* small sharp pointed knife used in surgery *skalpell, operationskniv*

scaly ['skeɪli] *adj.* covered in scales *fjällig, flagnande;* **the pustules harden and become scaly**

scan [skæn] **1** *subst.* making a three-dimensional picture of part of the body on a screen, using information supplied by X-rays directed by a computer *scanning, scintigrafi;* **CAT scan** = scan where a narrow X-ray beam is controlled by a computer and photographs from different angles a thin section of the body *or* of an organ; the results are fed into the computer which analyses them and produces a picture of a slice of the body or of an organ *datortomografi, DT, skiktröntgen* **2** *vb.* to examine part of the body, using computer-interpreted X-rays, and create a picture of the part on a screen *avsöka (granska) med hjälp av scanning (scintigrafi)*

scanner ['skænə] *subst.* **(a)** machine which scans a part of the body *scintigraf;* **a brain scanner** *or* **a body scanner** = machines which scan only the brain *or* all the body *scintigraf för huvud resp. kropp* **(b)** (i) person who examines a test slide *granskare;* (ii) person who operates a scanning machine *person som sköter scintigraf*

scanning speech ['skænɪŋ spiːtʃ] *subst.* defect in speaking, where each sound is spoken separately and given equal stress *slags talfel med skanderande sätt att tala*

scaphocephalic [ˌskæfəʊsə'fælɪk] *adj.* having a long narrow skull *skafocefal*

scaphocephaly [ˌskæfəʊ'kef(ə)li] *subst.* condition where the skull is abnormally long and narrow *skafocefali, båtskallighet*

scaphoid (bone) ['skæfɔɪd (bəʊn)] *subst.* one of the carpal bones in the wrist *os scaphoideum, handlovens båtben*

scaphoiditis [ˌskæfəʊ'daɪtɪs] *subst.* degeneration of the navicular bone in children *skafoidit, Köhlers sjukdom*

scapula ['skæpjʊlə] *subst.* shoulder blade *or* one of two large flat bones covering the top part of the back *scapula, skulderbladet* NOTE: plural is **scapulae**

scapular ['skæpjʊlə] *adj.* referring to the shoulder blade *skapular, skapulär*

scapulohumeral [ˌskæpjuləʊ'hjuːm(ə)r(ə)l] *adj.* referring to the scapula and humerus *som avser el. hör till både skulderbladet och överarmsbenet;* **scapulohumeral arthritis** = PERIARTHRITIS

scar [skɑː] **1** *subst.* cicatrix *or* mark left on the skin after a wound *or* surgical incision has healed *ärr;* **he still has the scar of his appendicectomy; scar tissue** = fibrous tissue which forms a scar *ärrvävnad* **2** *vb.* to leave a scar on the skin *bilda ärr;* **the burns have scarred him for life; plastic surgeons have tried to repair the scarred arm; patients were given special clothes to reduce hypertrophic scarring**

scarification [ˌskærɪfɪ'keɪʃ(ə)n] *subst.* scratching *or* making minute cuts on the surface of the skin (as for smallpox vaccination) *skarifikation, koppning, rispning*

scarlatina [ˌskɑːlə'tiːnə] *or* **scarlet fever** [ˌskɑːlət 'fiːvə] *subst.* infectious disease with a fever, sore throat and red rash, caused by a haemolytic streptococcus *scarlatina, scharlakansfeber*

> COMMENT: scarlet fever can sometimes have serious complications if the kidneys are infected

Scarpa's triangle ['skɑːpɑːz ˌtraɪæŋg(ə)l] *or* **femoral triangle** ['fem(ə)r(ə)l ˌtraɪæŋg(ə)l] *subst.* slight hollow in the groin; it contains the femoral vessels and nerve *trigonum femorale, Scarpas triangel*

scat- [skæt] *or* **scato-** ['skætə(ʊ), ˌ--, skæ'tɒ] *prefix* referring to the faeces *skat(o)-, fekal-, exkrement-*

scatole ['skætəʊl] *subst.* substance in faeces, formed in the intestine, which causes a strong smell *starkt illaluktande ämne i avföringen*

SCD [ˌessiː'diː] = SICKLE CELL DISEASE

> QUOTE even children with the milder forms of SCD have an increased frequency of pneumococcal infection
>
> **Lancet**

scent [sent] *subst.* (i) pleasant smell *vällukt;* (ii) cosmetic substance which has a pleasant smell *parfym;* (iii) smell given off by a substance which stimulates the sense of smell *lukt, doft;* **the scent of flowers makes me sneeze**

scented ['sentɪd] *adj.* with a strong pleasant smell *parfymerad;* **he is allergic to scented soap**

schanker ⇨ **chancre**

schanker, lymfogranulomatös ⇨ **lymphogranuloma inguinale**

scharlakansfeber ⇨ **scarlatina**

scharnerled ⇨ **ginglymus, hinge joint**

schema ['ski:mə] *see* BODY SCHEMA

Scheuermann's disease ['ʃɔɪəmənz dɪˌzi:z] *subst.* inflammation of the bones and cartilage in the spine, usually affecting adolescents *Scheuermanns sjukdom*

Schick test ['ʃɪk ˌtest] *subst.* test to see if a person is immune to diphtheria *Schicks reaktion*

> COMMENT: in this test, a small amount of diphtheria toxin is injected, and if the point of injection becomes inflamed it shows the patient is not immune to the disease (= positive reaction)

Schilling test ['ʃɪlɪŋ ˌtest] *subst.* test to see if a patient can absorb vitamin B_{12} through the intestines, to determine cases of pernicious anaemia *Schillings test, Schillingtest*

-schisis ['skaɪsɪs] *suffix* referring to a fissure *or* split *-klyvning, -spricka, -spalt*

schisto- ['sɪstə(ʊ), ˌ--] *or* **schizo-** ['skɪtsə(ʊ), ˌ--] *prefix* referring to something which is split *schisto-, schizo-*

Schistosoma [ˌʃɪstə(ʊ)'səʊmə] *or* **schistosome** ['ʃɪstə(ʊ)səʊm] = BILHARZIA

schistosomiasis [ˌʃɪstə(ʊ)səʊ'maɪəsɪs] = BILHARZIASIS

schiz- ['skɪts, ˌ-] *or* **schizo-** ['skɪtsə(ʊ), ˌ--] *prefix* referring to something which is split *schisto-, schizo-*

schizofren ⇨ **schizoid**

schizofreni ⇨ **dementia, schizophrenia**

schizoid ['skɪtsɔɪd] **1** *adj.* referring to schizophrenia *schizofren;* **schizoid personality** *or* **split personality** = disorder where the patient is cold towards other people, thinks mainly about himself and behaves in an odd way *schizoid personlighet, personlighetsklyvning* **2** *subst.* person suffering from a less severe form of schizophrenia *schizoid person*

schizophrenia [ˌskɪtsə(ʊ)'fri:niə] *subst.* mental disorder where the patient withdraws from contact with other people, has delusions and seems to lose contact with the real world *schizofreni;* **catatonic schizophrenia** *see* CATATONIC

schizophrenic [ˌskɪtsə(ʊ)'frenɪk] *subst. & adj.* (person) suffering from schizophrenia *schizofren (person)*

Schlatter's disease ['ʃlætəz dɪˌzi:z] *subst.* inflammation in the bones and cartilage at the top of the tibia *(Osgood-)Schlatters sjukdom*

Schlemm's canal ['ʃlemz kəˌnæl] *subst.* circular canal in the sclera of the eye, which drains the aqueous humour *sinus venosus sclerae, Schlemms kanal*

school [sku:l] *subst.* **(a)** place where children are taught *skola;* **school health service** = special service, part of the Local Health Authority, which looks after the health of children in school *skolhälsovård* **(b)** specialized section of a university *fakultet;* **medical school** = section of a university which teaches medicine *medicinsk fakultet;* **he is at medical school; she is taking a course at the School of Dentistry**

Schwann cells ['ʃvɒn selz] *subst. pl.* cells which form the myelin sheath round a nerve fibre ⇨ *illustration* NEURONE *Schwanns (schwannska) celler*

schwannoma [ʃvɒ'nəʊmə] *or* **neurofibroma** [ˌnju(ə)rəʊfaɪ'brəʊmə] *subst.* benign tumour of a peripheral nerve *schwannom, schwannogliom*

Schwartze's operation ['ʃvɔ:tsɪz ˌɒpə'reɪʃ(ə)n] *subst.* the original surgical operation to drain fluid and remove infected tissue from the mastoid process *slags mastoidektomi (uppmejsling av vårtutskottet bakom örat)*

Schönlein's purpura ['ʃɜ:nlaɪnz ˌpɜ:p(ə)rə] *see* PURPURA

sciatic [saɪ'ætɪk] *adj.* referring to (i) the hip *höft-;* (ii) the sciatic nerve *ischias-;* **sciatic nerve** = one of two main nerves which run from the sacral plexus into the thighs, dividing into a series of nerves in the lower legs and feet; it is the largest nerve in the body *nervus ischiadicus, ischiasnerven*

sciatica [saɪ'ætɪkə] *subst.* pain along the sciatic nerve, usually at the back of the thighs and legs *ischias, ischialgi*

> COMMENT: sciatica can be caused by a slipped disc which presses on a spinal nerve, or can simply be caused by straining a muscle in the back

science ['sa(ɪ)əns] *subst.* study based on looking at and noting facts, especially facts arranged into a system *vetenskap, naturvetenskap*

scientific [ˌsa(ɪ)ən'tɪfɪk] *adj.* referring to science *vetenskaplig, naturvetenskaplig;* **he carried out scientific experiments**

scientist ['sa(ɪ)əntɪst] *subst.* person who specializes in scientific studies *vetenskapsman, naturvetenskapsman, forskare*

scintigraf ⇨ **scanner**

scintigrafi ⇨ **scan**

scintigram ['sɪntɪgræm] *subst.* recording radiation from radioactive isotopes injected into the body *scintigram*

scintillascope [sɪn'tɪləskəʊp] *subst.* instrument which produces a scintigram *scintillationsdetektor*

scintillationsdetektor ⇨ **scintillascope**

scintillator ['sɪntɪleɪtə] *subst.* substance which produces a flash of light when struck by radiation *scintvätska*

scintiscan ['sɪntɪskæn] *subst.* scintigram which shows the variations in radiation from one part of the body to another *scintundersökning*

scintundersökning ⇨ **scintiscan**

scintvätska ⇨ **scintillator**

scirrhous ['sɪrəs] *adj.* hard (tumour) *skirrös*

scirrhus ['sɪrəs] *subst.* hard malignant tumour (especially in the breast) *scirrhus, skirr*

scissors ['sɪzəz] *subst pl.* instrument for cutting, made of two blades and two handles *sax;* **scissor legs** = deformed legs, where one leg is permanently crossed over in front of the other *missbildade ben som ger saxgång*
NOTE: say "a pair of scissors" when referring to one instrument

scler- [sklɪə] *or* **sclero-** ['sklɪərə(ʊ), ˌ--] *prefix* (i) meaning hard *or* thick *skler(o)-;* referring to (ii) sclera *skler(o)-, senhinne-;* (iii) sclerosis *skler(o)-*

sclera ['sklɪərə] *or* **sclerotic (coat)** [sklə'rɒtɪk (ˌkəʊt)] *subst.* hard white outer covering of the eyeball ⇨ *illustration* EYE *tunica albuginea oculi, sclera, sklera, senhinnan, ögonvitan*

COMMENT: the front part of the sclera is the transparent cornea, through which the light enters the eye. The conjunctiva, or inner skin of the eyelids, connects with the sclera and covers the front of the eyeball

sclera ⇨ **albuginea, sclerotic**

scleral ['sklɪər(ə)l] *adj.* referring to the sclera *skleral, senhinne-;* **scleral lens** = large contact lens which covers most of the front of the eye *slags kontaktlins*

scleritis [sklə'raɪtɪs] *subst.* inflammation of the sclera *sklerit, senhinneinflammation*

scleroderma [ˌsklɪərə(ʊ)'dɜːmə] *subst.* collagen disease which thickens connective tissue and produces a hard thick skin *skleroderma, sklerodermi*

scleroma [sklə'rəʊmə] *subst.* patch of hard skin *or* hard mucous membrane *sklerom, slemhinneförhårdning*

scleromalacia (perforans) [ˌsklɪərəʊmə'leɪʃiə (pəˌfɔːrəns)] *subst.* condition of the sclera in which holes appear *skleromalaci*

sclerosing [sklə'rəʊsɪŋ] *adj.* which becomes hard *or* which makes tissue hard *skleroserande;* **sclerosant agent** *or* **sclerosing agent** *or* **sclerosing solution** = irritating liquid injected into tissue to harden it *skleroserande medel*

sclerosis [sklə'rəʊsɪs] *subst.* hardening of tissue *skleros, cirros, induration;* **multiple sclerosis** *or* **disseminated sclerosis** = nervous disease which gets progressively worse, where patches of the fibres of the central nervous system lose their myelin, causing numbness in the limbs and progressive weakness and paralysis *sclerosis disseminata, multiple skleros, MS; see also* ATHEROSCLEROSIS, ARTERIOSCLEROSIS, GEHRIG'S DISEASE

sclerotherapy [ˌsklɪərəʊ'θerəpi] *subst.* treatment of a varicose vein by injecting a sclerosing agent into the vein, and so encouraging the blood in the vein to clot *skleroterapi*

sclerotic [sklɪə'rɒtɪk] **1** *adj.* referring to sclerosis; suffering from sclerosis *sklerotisk* **2** *subst.* hard white covering of the eyeball *sclera, senhinnan, ögonvitan*

sclerotome ['sklɪərə(ʊ)təʊm] *subst.* sharp knife used in sclerotomy *sklerotom*

sclerotomy [sklə'rɒtəmi] *subst.* surgical operation to cut into the sclera *sklerotomi*

scolex ['skəʊleks] *subst.* head of a tapeworm, with hooks which attach it to the wall of the intestine *skolex, bandmaskens huvud*

scoliosis [ˌskəʊli'əʊsɪs] *subst.* condition where the spine curves sideways *skolios*

scoop stretcher ['sku:p ˌstretʃə] *subst.* type of stretcher formed of two jointed sections which can slide under a patient and lock together *bår av teleskoptyp som kan föras under patienten och låsas*

-scope [skəʊp] *suffix* referring to an instrument for examining by sight *-skop*

scorbutic [skɔ:'bju:tɪk] *adj.* referring to scurvy *skorbutisk, skörbjuggs-; see note at* SCURVY

scorbutus [skɔ:'bju:təs] *or* **scurvy** ['skɜ:vi] *subst.* disease caused by lack of vitamin C *or* ascorbic acid which is found in fruit and vegetables *skorbut, skörbjugg*

scoto- ['skəʊtə(ʊ), ˌ--] *prefix* meaning dark *skoto-, mörker-*

scotoma [skɒ'təʊmə] *subst.* small area in the field of vision where the patient cannot see *skotom*

scotometer [skə(ʊ)'tɒmɪtə] *subst.* instrument used to measure areas of defective vision *perimeter*

scotopia [skə(ʊ)'təʊpiə] *subst.* the power of the eye to adapt to poor lighting conditions and darkness *skotopi, mörkeradaptation*

scotopic [skə(ʊ)'tɒpɪk] *adj.* referring to scotopia *skotopisk, mörker-;* **scotopic vision =** vision in the dark and in dim light (the rods of the retina are used instead of the cones which are used for photopic vision) *skotopiskt seende, mörkerseende; see* DARK ADAPTATION

scrape [skreɪp] *vb.* to remove the surface of something by moving a sharp knife across it *skrapa (av)*

scratch [skrætʃ] **1** *subst.* slight wound on the skin made when a sharp point is pulled across it *skråma, rispa, repa;* **she had scratches on her legs and arms; wash the dirt out of that scratch in case it gets infected 2** *vb.* to harm the skin by moving a sharp point across it *klösa, riva, rispa, repa;* **the cat scratched the girl's face; be careful not to scratch yourself on the wire**

scream [skri:m] **1** *subst.* loud sharp cry *skrik, tjut;* **you could hear the screams of the people in the burning building 2** *vb.* to make a loud sharp cry *skrika, tjuta;* **she screamed when a man suddenly opened the door**

screen [skri:n] **1** *subst.* **(a)** light wall, sometimes with a curtain, which can be moved about and put round a bed to shield the patient *skärm, skiljevägg* **(b)** screening *screening, massundersökning* **2** *vb.* to examine large numbers of people to test them for a disease *massundersöka;* **the population of the village was screened for meningitis**

> QUOTE in the UK the main screen is carried out by health visitors at 6 - 10 months. With adequately staffed and trained community services, this method of screening can be extremely effective
> **Lancet**

screening ['skri:nɪŋ] *subst.* testing large numbers of people to see if any has a certain type of disease *screening, massundersökning*

> QUOTE GPs are increasingly requesting blood screening for patients concerned about HIV
> **Journal of the Royal College of General Practitioners**

scrofula ['skrɒfjʊlə] *subst.* form of tuberculosis in the lymph nodes in the neck, formerly caused by unpasteurized milk, but now rare *skrofulos, skrofelsjuka, skrofler*

scrofuloderma [ˌskrɒfjʊləʊ'dɜ:mə] *subst.* form of tuberculosis of the skin, forming ulcers, and secondary to tuberculous infection of an underlying lymph gland *or* structure *slags hudturberkulos*

scrofulous ['skrɒfjʊləs] *adj.* suffering from scrofula *skrofulös, skrofelsjuk*

scrotal ['skrəʊt(ə)l] *adj.* referring to the scrotum *skrotal, pung-*

scrotum ['skrəʊtəm] *subst.* bag of skin hanging from behind the penis, containing the testes, epididymides and part of the spermatic cord ⇨ *illustration* UROGENITAL SYSTEM (male) *scrotum, skrotum, pungen*

scrub nurse ['skrʌb ˌnɜ:s] *subst.* nurse who cleans the operation site on a patient's body before an operation *operationssköterska (som tvättar operationsområdet före operationen)*

scrub typhus ['skrʌb ˌtaɪfəs] *or* **tsutsugamushi disease** [ˌtsuːtsuːgə'mʊʃi dɪˌziːz] *subst.* severe form of typhus caused by Rickettsia bacteria, passed to humans by mites, found in South East Asia *tsutsugamushifeber*

scrub up [ˌskrʌb 'ʌp] *vb. (of surgeon or theatre nurse)* to wash the hands and arms carefully before an operation *steriltvätta sig, tvätta sig (före operation)*

scurf [skɜːf] *or* **dandruff** ['dændrʌf] *or* **pityriasis capitis** [ˌpɪtɪ'raɪəsɪs ˌkæpətɪs] *subst.* pieces of dead skin which form on the scalp and fall out when the hair is combed *pityriasis capitis, torr seborré, mjäll*

scurvy ['skɜːvi] *or* **scorbutus** [skɔː'bjuːtəs] *subst.* disease caused by lack of vitamin C *or* ascorbic acid which is found in fruit and vegetables *skorbut, skörbjugg*

> COMMENT: scurvy causes general weakness and anaemia, with bleeding from the gums, joints, and under the skin. In severe cases, the teeth drop out. Treatment consists of vitamin C tablets and a change of diet to include more fruit and vegetables

scybalum ['sɪbələm] *subst.* very hard faeces *skybalum, hårt exkrement*

sea [siː] *subst.* area of salt water which covers a large part of the earth *hav;* **when the sea is rough he is often sick**

seasick ['siːsɪk] *adj.* suffering from travel sickness on a ship *sjösjuk;* **as soon as the ferry started to move she felt seasick**

seasickness ['siːsɪknəs] *or* **travel sickness** ['træv(ə)lsɪknəs;] *or* **motion sickness** ['məʊʃ(ə)nsɪknəs] *subst.* illness, with nausea, vomiting and sometimes headache, caused by the movement of a ship *kinetos, sjösjuka;* **take some seasickness tablets if you are going on a long journey**

sebaceous [sə'beɪʃəs] *adj.* (i) referring to sebum *talgig, talg-;* (ii) which produces oil *fettavsöndrande;* **sebaceous cyst** = cyst which forms when a sebaceous gland is blocked *steatom, aterom, talg(körtel)cysta;* **sebaceous gland** = gland in the skin which secretes sebum at the base of each hair follicle ⇨ *illustration* SKIN & SENSORY RECEPTORS *glandula sebacea, talgkörtel*

seborré ⇨ **seborrhoea**

seborré, torr ⇨ **dandruff**

seborrhoea [ˌsebə'riːə] *subst.* excessive secretion of sebum by the sebaceous glands, common in young people at puberty, and sometimes linked to seborrhoeic dermatitis *seborré*

seborrhoeic [ˌsebə'riːɪk] *adj.* (i) caused by seborrhoea *seborroisk;* (ii) with an oily secretion *med fettavsöndring;* **seborrhoeic dermatitis** *or* **seborrhoeic eczema** = type of eczema where scales form on the skin *seborroisk dermatit, seborroiskt eksem;* **seborrhoeic rash** = rash where the skin surface is oily *utslag pga fet hy*

seborroisk ⇨ **seborrhoeic**

sebum ['siːbəm] *subst.* oily substance secreted by a sebaceous gland, which makes the skin smooth; it also protects the skin against bacteria and the body against rapid evaporation of water *sebum, talg*

second ['sek(ə)nd] **1** *subst.* unit of time equal to 1/60 of a minute *sekund* **2** *adj.* coming after the first *andra, sekundär, permanent;* **second intention** = healing of an infected wound *or* ulcer, which takes place slowly and leaves a prominent scar *sanatio per secundam intentionem, sekundärläkning;* **second molars** = molars at the back of the jaw, before the wisdom teeth, erupting at about 12 years of age *dentes multicuspidati, permanenta molarerna (oxeltänderna, kindtänderna)*

secondary ['sek(ə)nd(ə)ri] **1** *adj.* (i) which comes after the first *andra;* (ii) (condition) which develops from another condition (the primary condition) *sekundär(-);* **he was showing symptoms of secondary syphilis; secondary amenorrhoea** *see* AMENORRHOEA; **secondary bronchi** = air passages which supply a lobe of the lung *lobbronkerna;* **secondary haemorrhage** = haemorrhage which occurs some time after an injury, usually due to infection of the wound *sekundärblödning;* **secondary medical care** = specialized treatment provided by a hospital *specialistvård på sjukhus;* **secondary prevention** = ways (such as screening tests) of avoiding a serious disease by detecting it early *allmänprevention;* **secondary sexual characteristics** = sexual characteristics (such as pubic hair *or* breasts) which develop after puberty *sekundära könskaraktärer* **2** *subst.* malignant tumour which metastasized from another malignant tumour *metastas, sekundärtumör; see also* PRIMARY

secrete [sɪ'kriːt] *vb. (of a gland)* to produce a substance (such as hormone *or* oil *or* enzyme) *avsöndra, utsöndra*

secretin [sɪˈkriːtɪn] *subst.* hormone secreted by the duodenum, which encourages the production of pancreatic juice *sekretin*

secretion [sɪˈkriːʃ(ə)n] *subst.* **(a)** process by which a substance is produced by a gland *sekretion, avsöndring, utsöndring;* **the pituitary gland stimulates the secretion of hormones by the adrenal gland (b)** substance produced by a gland *sekret;* **sex hormones are bodily secretions**

secretor [sɪˈkriːtə] *subst.* person who secretes ABO blood group substances into mucous fluids in the body (such as the semen, the saliva) *sekretor*

secretory [sɪˈkriːt(ə)ri] *adj.* referring to *or* accompanied by *or* producing a secretion *sekretorisk*

section [ˈsekʃ(ə)n] *subst.* **(a)** part of something *sektion, del, stycke;* **the middle section of the aorta (b)** (i) action of cutting tissue *sektion, snitt, insnitt;* (ii) cut made in tissue *sektion, snitt, insnitt;* **Caesarean section** = surgical operation to deliver a baby by cutting through the abdominal wall into the uterus *sectio caesarea, kejsarsnitt* **(c)** slice of tissue cut for examination under a microscope *preparat, snitt* **(d)** part of a document, such as an Act of Parliament *paragraf, avsnitt;* **she was admitted under section 5 of the Mental Health Act**

sedate [sɪˈdeɪt] *vb.* to calm (a patient) by giving a drug which acts on the nervous system and relieves stress *or* pain, and in larger doses makes a patient sleep *sedera, ge lugnande medel;* **elderly or confused patients may need to be sedated to prevent them wandering**

sedation [sɪˈdeɪʃ(ə)n] *subst.* calming a patient with a sedative *sedering;* **under sedation** = having been given a sedative *som sederats (fått lugnande medel);* **he was still under sedation, and could not be seen by the police**

sedative [ˈsedətɪv] *subst. & adj.* (drug) which acts on the nervous system to help a patient sleep *or* to relieve stress *sedativ(um), lugnande (medel);* **she was prescribed sedatives by the doctor**

sedativum ⇨ **depressant, tranquillizer**

sedentary [ˈsednt(ə)ri] *adj.* sitting *sittande, stillasittande;* **sedentary occupations** = jobs where the workers sit down for most of the time *yrken med mycket stillasittande*

> QUOTE changes in lifestyle factors have been related to the decline in mortality from ischaemic heart disease. In many studies a sedentary lifestyle has been reported as a risk factor for ischaemic heart disease
> **Journal of the American Medical Association**

sedera ⇨ **sedate**

sedering ⇨ **sedation**

sediment [ˈsedɪmənt] *subst.* solid particles, usually insoluble, which fall to the bottom of a liquid *sediment, fällning, avlagring, bottensats*

sedimentation [ˌsedɪmenˈteɪʃ(ə)n] *subst.* action of solid particles falling to the bottom of a liquid *sedimentering, fällning, avlagring;* **erythrocyte sedimentation rate (ESR)** = test to show how fast erythrocytes settle in a sample of blood plasma *sedimentation rate, SR, blodsänkningsreaktion, sänkan*

seende ⇨ **eyesight, sighted, vision**

-seende ⇨ **-opia**

seg ⇨ **tough, viscid**

segment [ˈsegmənt] *subst.* part of an organ *or* piece of tissue which is clearly separate from other parts *segment*

segmental [segˈment(ə)l] *adj.* formed of segments *segmentell, segment-;* **segmental ablation** = surgical removal of part of a nail as treatment for an ingrowing toenail *operativt avlägsnande av del av nagel; see also* BRONCHI

segmentation [ˌsegmenˈteɪʃ(ə)n] *subst.* movement of separate segments of the wall of the intestine to mix digestive juice with the food before it is passed along by the action of peristalsis *segmentell kontraktion av tunntarmen*

segmentbronkerna ⇨ **bronchi, tertiary**

segmented [segˈmentɪd] *adj.* formed of segments *segmenterad*

segmentell ⇨ **segmental**

segmenterad ⇨ **segmented**

seizure [ˈsiːʒə] *subst.* fit *or* convulsion *or* sudden contraction of the muscles, especially in a heart attack *or* stroke *or* epileptic fit *attack, anfall*

sekret ➪ **secretion**

sekretin ➪ **secretin**

sekretion ➪ **secretion**

sekretor ➪ **secretor**

sekretorisk ➪ **secretory**

sektion ➪ **section**

sekund ➪ **second**

sekundär ➪ **second**

sekundär(-) ➪ **secondary**

sekundärblödning ➪ **secondary**

sekundärläkning ➪ **second**

sekundärtumör ➪ **metastasis, secondary**

sekvens ➪ **sequence**

sekvensbestämma ➪ **sequence**

sekvester ➪ **sequestrum**

sekvestrotomi ➪ **sequestrectomy**

select [sɪ'lekt] *vb.* to make a choice *or* to choose some things, but not others *välja, utse;* **the committee is meeting to select the company which will supply kitchen equipment for the hospital service; she was selected to go on a midwifery course**

selection [sɪ'lekʃ(ə)n] *subst.* act of choosing some things, but not others *selektion, val, urval, uttagning;* **the candidates for the post have to go through a selection process; the selection of suitable donor for a bone marrow transplant; genetic selection** = choosing only the best examples of a genus for reproduction *genetiskt urval*

selective [sɪ'lektɪv] *adj.* which choose only certain things, and not others *selektiv, urvals-*

selektion ➪ **selection**

selektiv ➪ **selective**

selenium [sɪ'li:niəm] *subst.* non-metallic trace element *selen*
NOTE: the chemical symbol is **Se**

self- ['self, ˌ-] *prefix* referring to oneself *själv-, egen-*

self-admitted [ˌselfəd'mɪtɪd] *adj.* (patient) who has admitted himself to hospital without being sent by a doctor *som inte kommer på remiss*

self-care [ˌself'keə] *subst.* looking after yourself properly, so that you remain healthy *egenvård*

self-defence [ˌselfdɪ'fens] *subst.* defending yourself when someone is attacking you *självförsvar*

sella turcica [ˌselə 'tɜ:sɪkə] *subst.* pituitary fossa *or* hollow in the upper surface of the sphenoid bone in which the pituitary gland sits *sella turcica, turksadeln*

semeiology [ˌsi:maɪ'ɒlədʒi] = SYMPTOMATOLOGY

semen ['si:mən] *subst.* thick pale fluid containing spermatozoa, produced by the testes and seminal vesicles, and ejaculated from the penis *semen, säd(esvätska), sperma*

semi- ['semi, ˌ--] *prefix* meaning half *semi-, halv-*

semicircular [ˌsemi'sɜ:kjʊlə] *adj.* shaped like half a circle *semicirkulär, halvcirkelformig;* **semicircular canals** = three canals in the inner ear filled with fluid and which regulate the sense of balance ➪ *illustration* EAR *canales semicirculares, båggångarna;* **semicircular ducts** = ducts inside the canals in the inner ear *ductus semicurculares, halvcirkelformiga gångarna*

COMMENT: the three semicircular canals are on different planes. When a person's head moves (as when he bends down), the fluid in the canals moves and this movement is communicated to the brain through the vestibular section of the auditory nerve

semi-conscious [ˌsemi'kɒnʃəs] *adj.* half conscious *or* only partly aware of what is going on *halvt vid medvetande;* **she was semi-conscious for most of the operation**

semi-liquid [ˌsemi'lɪkwɪd] *adj.* half solid and half liquid *halvfast*

semilunar [ˌsemi'lu:nə] *adj.* shaped like half a moon *semilunar, halvmånformig;* **semilunar cartilage** *or* **meniscus** = one of two pads of cartilage (lateral meniscus and medial meniscus) between the femur and the tibia in the knee *menisk;* **semilunar cartilages** *cartilagines seminlunares, semilunarbrosken, meniskerna;* **semilunar valves** = two valves in the heart, the pulmonary and the aortic valve, through which blood flows out of the ventricles *valvulae semilunares, semilunarklaffarna, fickklaffarna*

semilunarbrosken ⇨ **semilunar, meniscus**

semilunarklaffarna ⇨ **semilunar, valve**

seminal ['semɪn(ə)l] *adj.* referring to semen *seminal, sädes-;* **seminal fluid** = fluid part of semen, formed in the epididymis and seminal vesicles *sädesvätska;* **seminal vesicles** = two glands near the prostate gland which secrete fluid into the vas deferens ⇨ *illustration* UROGENITAL SYSTEM (male) *vesiculae seminales, sädesblåsorna*

seminiferous tubule [ˌsemiˈnɪf(ə)rəs ˌtjuːbjuːl] *subst.* tubule in the testis which carries semen **seminiferous tubules** *tubuli seminiferi, sädeskanalerna*

seminoma [ˌsemiˈnəʊmə] *subst.* malignant tumour in the testis *seminom*

semiologi ⇨ **symptomatology**

semiotik ⇨ **symptomatology**

semipermeable membrane [ˌsemiˈpɜːmiəb(ə)l ˌmembreɪn] *subst.* membrane which allows some substances in liquid solution to pass through, but not others *semipermeabelt membran, semipermeabel hinna*

semiprone [ˌsemiˈprəʊn] *adj.* (position) where the patient lies face down, with one leg and one arm bent forwards, and the face turned to one side *framstupa*

semi-solid [ˌsemiˈsɒlɪd] *adj.* halfway between solid and liquid *halvfast*

SEN [ˌesiːˈen] = STATE ENROLLED NURSE

sen- ⇨ **tendinous, teno-**

sena ⇨ **sinew, tendon**

senescence [sɪˈnes(ə)ns] *subst.* the ageing process *senescens, åldrande*

senescent [sɪˈnes(ə)nt] *adj.* becoming old *åldrande*

Sengstaken tube [ˈseŋzteɪkən ˌtjuːb] *subst.* tube with a balloon, which is passed through the mouth into the oesophagus to stop oesophageal bleeding *Sengstakentub, Sengstakensond*

senhinna ⇨ **aponeurosis**

senhinnan ⇨ **albuginea, sclera, sclerotic**

senhinne- ⇨ **scler-, scleral**

senhinneinflammation ⇨ **scleritis**

senile [ˈsiːnaɪ(ə)l] *adj.* (i) referring to old age *or* to the infirmities of old age *senil, ålders-, ålderdoms-;* (ii) (person) whose mental faculties have become weak because of age *senil;* **senile cataract** = cataract which occurs in an elderly person *catarrhacta senilis, ålder(dom)sstarr;* **senile dementia** = form of mental degeneration sometimes affecting old people *senil demens, senilitet*

senilis [səˈnaɪlɪs] *see* ARCUS

senilitet ⇨ **dementia, senile, senility**

senility [səˈnɪləti] *subst.* weakening of the mental and physical faculties in an old person *senilitet, ålderdomssvaghet*

seninflammation ⇨ **tendinitis, tenonitis**

senior [ˈsiːniə] *adj. & subst.* (person) who has a more important position than others *överordnad, över-;* **he is the senior anaesthetist in the hospital; senior members of staff are allowed to consult the staff records**

senknut ⇨ **ganglion**

senna [ˈsenə] *subst.* laxative made from the dried fruit and leaves of a tropical tree *senna*

sensation [senˈseɪʃ(ə)n] *subst.* feeling *or* information about something which has been sensed by a sensory nerve and is passed to the brain *sensation, sinnesförnimmelse*

sense [sens] **1** *subst.* one of the five faculties by which a person notices things in the outside world (sight, hearing, smell, taste and touch) *sinne;* **when he had a cold, he lost his sense of smell; blind people develop an acute sense of touch; sense organ** = organ (such as the nose, the skin) in which there are various sensory nerves and which can detect environmental stimuli (such as scent, heat and pain) and transmit information about them to the central nervous system *sinnesorgan* **2** *vb.* to notice something *känna, märka, uppfatta;* **teeth can sense changes in temperature**

sensibilisera ⇨ **sensitize**

sensibilisering ⇨ **sensitization**

sensibility [ˌsensəˈbɪləti] *subst.* being able to detect and interpret sensations *sensibilitet, känslighet*

sensible [ˈsensəb(ə)l] *adj.* which can be detected by the senses *sensibel, sinnes-, känsel-;* **sensible perspiration** = drops of sweat which can be seen on the skin *perspiratio sensibilis, märkbar svettning*

sensitive [ˈsensətɪv] *adj.* able to respond to a stimulus coming from outside *sensitiv, känslig, mottaglig*

sensitivitetsträningsgrupp ⇨ **encounter group**

sensitivity [ˌsensəˈtɪvəti] *subst.* (i) being able to respond to an outside stimulus *sensitivitet, känslighet, mottaglighet;* (ii) rate of positive responses in a test, from persons with a specific disease (a high rate of sensitivity means a low rate of false negatives) *känslighet (hos prov)* NOTE: compare with **specificity**

sensitization [ˌsensətaɪˈzeɪʃ(ə)n] *subst.* (i) making a person sensitive *sensibilisering;* (ii) abnormal reaction to an allergen *or* to a drug, caused by the presence of antibodies which were created when the patient was exposed to the drug *or* allergen in the past *överkänslighet*

sensitize [ˈsensətaɪz] *vb.* to make someone sensitive to a drug or allergen *sensibilisera, göra känslig (överkänslig);* **sensitized person** = person who is allergic to a drug *or* who reacts badly to a drug *sensibiliserad (överkänslig) person;* **sensitizing agent** = substance which, by acting as an antigen, makes the body form antibodies *sensibiliserande medel*

sensiträningsgrupp ⇨ **encounter group**

senskida ⇨ **tendon**

senskideinflammation ⇨ **tendovaginitis, tenosynovitis, tenovaginitis**

sensorineural deafness [ˌsensərɪˌnjuː(ə)r(ə)l ˈdefnəs] *or* **perceptive deafness** [pəˌseptɪv ˈdefnəs] *subst.* deafness caused by a disorder in the auditory nerves *or* the brain centres which receive impulses from the nerves *perceptiv (sensorineural) dövhet (hörselnedsättning)*

sensorisk ⇨ **sensory**

sensory [ˈsens(ə)ri] *subst.* referring to the detection of sensations by nerve cells *sensorisk, sinnes-;* **sensory cortex** = term which was formerly used to refer to the area of the cerebral cortex which receives information from nerves in all parts of the body *sensoriska (hjärn)barken;* **sensory deprivation** = condition where a person becomes confused because of lacking sensations *sensorisk deprivation;* **sensory nerve** = afferent nerve which transmits impulses relating to a sensation (such as a taste *or* a smell) to the brain *sensorisk nerv, afferent (inåtledande) nerv;* **sensory neurone** = nerve cell which transmits impulses relating to sensations from the receptor to the central nervous system *sensoriskt neuron, sensorisk nervcell;* **sensory receptor** = nerve ending *or* special cell which senses a change in the surrounding environment (such as cold *or* pressure) and reacts to it by sending out an impulse through the nervous system ⇨ *illustration* SKIN & SENSORY RECEPTORS *sensorisk receptor*

sensutur ⇨ **tenorrhaphy**

sensöm ⇨ **tenorrhaphy**

separate [ˈsepəreɪt] *vb.* to move two things apart *or* to divide *separera, särskilja, skilja åt;* **the surgeons believe it may be possible to separate the Siamese twins; the retina has become separated from the back of the eye**

separation [ˌsepəˈreɪʃ(ə)n] *subst.* act of separating *or* dividing *separation, särskiljande, avlossning*

separera ⇨ **separate**

sepsis [ˈsepsɪs] *subst.* presence of bacteria and their toxins in the body (usually following the infection of a wound), which kill tissue and produce pus *septikemi, sepsis, blodförgiftning*

sept- [ˈsept, ˌ-] *or* **septi-** [ˈseptɪ, ˌ--] *prefix* referring to sepsis *sept(i)-, septisk*

septa- [ˈseptə, ˌ--] *prefix* referring to a septum *sept(o)-, septum-*

septal [ˈsept(ə)l] *adj.* referring to a septum *septal, septum-;* **(atrial** *or* **ventricular) septal defect** = congenital defect where a hole exists in the wall between the two atria *or* the two ventricles of the heart which allows blood to flow abnormally through the heart and lungs *defectus septi, septumdefekt*

septate [ˈsepteɪt] *adj.* divided by a septum *delad av septum (skiljevägg)*

septic [ˈseptɪk] *adj.* referring to *or* produced by sepsis *septisk*

septicaemia [ˌseptɪ'si:miə] *or* **blood poisoning** ['blʌd pɔɪz(ə)nɪŋ] *subst.* condition where bacteria or their toxins are present in the blood, multiply rapidly and destroy tissue *septikemi, sepsis, blodförgiftning*

septicaemic [ˌseptɪ'si:mɪk] *adj.* caused by septicaemia *or* associated with septicaemia *septikemisk; see also* PLAGUE

septikemi ➪ **sepsis, septicaemia**

septikemisk ➪ **septicaemic**

septisk ➪ **sept-, septic**

septo- ['septəʊ, ˌ--] *prefix* referring to a septum *sept(o)-, septum-*

sept(o)- ➪ **septa-, septo-**

septum ['septəm] *subst.* wall between two parts of an organ (as between two parts of the heart *or* between the two sides of the nose) ➪ *illustration* HEART *septum, skiljevägg;* **interatrial septum** = membrane between the right and left atria in the heart *septum interatriale;* **interventricular septum** = membrane between the right and left ventricles in the heart *septum interventriculare;* **nasal septum** = wall of cartilage between the two nostrils and the two parts of the nasal cavity *septum nasi, nässkiljeväggen;* **septum defect** = condition where a hole exists in a septum (usually the septum of the heart) *defectus septi, septumdefekt*
NOTE: the plural is **septa**

septum- ➪ **septa-, septal, septo-**

septumdefekt ➪ **septal, septum**

sequelae [sɪ'kwi:li:] *subst. pl.* disease *or* conditions which follow on from an earlier disease *sequela, svit(er), följdtillstånd;* **Kaposi's sarcoma can be a sequela of AIDS; biochemical and hormonal sequelae of the eating disorders**
NOTE: singular is **sequela, sequel**

sequence ['si:kwəns] **1** *subst.* series of things, numbers, etc., which follow each other in order *sekvens, serie, ordning(sföljd)* **2** *vb.* to put in order *ordna (i ordningsföljd), sekvensbestämma;* **to sequence amino acids** = to show how amino acids are linked together in chains to form protein *sekvensbestämma aminosyror*

sequestrectomy [ˌsi:kwe'strektəmi] *subst.* surgical removal of a sequestrum *sekvestrotomi*

sequestrum [sɪ'kwestrəm] *subst.* piece of dead bone which is separated from whole bone *sekvester*

ser- [ser] *or* **sero-** ['sɪərəʊ, ˌ--] *prefix* referring to (i) blood serum *ser(o)-, serum-, blodserum-;* (ii) serous membrane *ser(o)-*

sera ['sɪərə] *see* SERUM

serie ➪ **course, sequence, succession**

serine ['serɪn] *subst.* an amino acid in protein *serin*

serious ['sɪəriəs] *adj.* very bad *allvarlig, svår;* **he's had a serious illness; there was a serious accident on the motorway; there is a serious shortage of plasma**

seriously ['sɪəriəsli] *adv.* in a serious way *allvarligt, svårt;* **she is seriously ill**

serological [ˌsɪərəʊ'lɒdʒɪk(ə)l] *adj.* referring to serology *serologisk;* **serological type** = SEROTYPE

serology [sɪ'rɒlədʒi] *subst.* scientific study of serums *serologi*

seronegative [ˌsɪərəʊ'negətɪv] *adj.* (person) who gives a negative reaction to a serological test *seronegativ*

seropositive [ˌsɪərəʊ'pɒzətɪv] *adj.* (person) who gives a positive reaction to a serological test *seropositiv*

seropus [ˌsɪərəʊ'pʌs] *subst.* mixture of serum and pus *blandning av blodserum och var*

serosa [sɪ'rəʊsə] *subst.* serous membrane *or* membrane which lines an internal cavity which has no contact with air (such as the peritoneum) *(tunica) serosa, serös hinna, seröst membran*

serositis [ˌsɪərəʊ'saɪtɪs] *subst.* inflammation of serous membrane *serosit*

serotherapy [ˌsɪərəʊ'θerəpi] *subst.* treatment of a disease using serum from immune individuals or immunized animals *serumterapi, serumbehandling, serumprofylax*

serotonin [ˌsɪərəʊ'təʊnɪn] *subst.* compound (5-hydroxytryptamine) which exists mainly in blood platelets and is released after tissue is injured *serotonin*

serotyp ➪ **serotype**

serotypa ➪ **serotype**

serotype ['sɪərəʊtaɪp] *or* **serological type** [ˌsɪərəʊ'lɒdʒɪk(ə)l ˌtaɪp] **1** *subst.* (i) category of microorganisms *or* bacteria that have some antigens in common *serotyp;* (ii) series of common antigens which exists in microorganisms and bacteria *serotyp* **2** to group microorganisms and bacteria according to their antigens *serotypa, typa mikroorganismer med hjälp av antiserum*

serous ['sɪərəs] *adj.* referring to serum *or* producing serum *or* like serum *serös;* **serous membrane** *or* **serosa** = membrane which lines an internal cavity which has no contact with air (such as the peritoneum and pleura) and covers the organs in the cavity (such as the heart and lungs) *(tunica) serosa, serös hinna, seröst membran*

serpens ['sɜːpens] *see* ERYTHEMA

serpiginous [sə'pɪdʒɪnəs] *adj.* (i) (ulcer *or* eruption) which creeps across the skin *serpiginös, krypande;* (ii) (wound *or* ulcer) with a wavy edge *med ojämn (vågig) kant*

serrated [sə'reɪtɪd] *adj.* (wound) with a zigzag *or* saw-like edge *sågtandad, tandad*

serration [sə'reɪʃ(ə)n] *subst.* one of the points in a zigzag *or* serrated edge *udd (spets) på tandad kant*

Sertoli cells [sə'təʊli ˌselz] *subst. pl.* cells which support the seminiferous tubules in the testis *Sertolis celler*

serum ['sɪərəm] *subst.* **(a) blood serum** = yellowish liquid which separates from (whole) blood when the blood clots *blodserum, serum;* **serum albumin** = major protein in plasma *serumalbumin* **(b) antitoxic serum** = immunizing agent formed of serum taken from an animal which has developed antibodies to a disease and used to protect a patient from that disease *antitoxiskt serum;* **snake bite serum** = ANTIVENENE; **serum hepatitis** = HEPATITIS B; **serum sickness** = anaphylactic shock *or* allergic reaction to a serum injection *serumsjuka; see also* ANTISERUM NOTE: plural is **sera, serums**

COMMENT: blood serum is plasma without the clotting agents. It contains salt and small quantities of albumin, fats and sugars; its main component is water. Serum used in serum therapy is taken from specially treated animals; in rare cases this can cause an allergic reaction in a patient

serum- ⇨ **ser-**

serumalbumin ⇨ **serum**

serumbehandling ⇨ **serotherapy**

serumbilirubin ⇨ **bilirubin**

serumhepatit ⇨ **hepatitis**

serumjärnbrist ⇨ **deficiency, sideropenia**

serumprofylax ⇨ **serotherapy**

serumsjuka ⇨ **serum**

serumterapi ⇨ **serotherapy**

service ['sɜːvɪs] *subst.* group of people working together *service, tjänst, förvaltning;* **the National Health Service** = British medical system, including all doctors, nurses, dentists, hospitals, clinics, etc., which provide free or cheap treatment to patients *allmänna hälso- och sjukvården (i Storbritannien), ung. offentlig sjukvård*

servicehus ⇨ **sheltered accommodation**

serös ⇨ **serous**

sesamoid bone ['sesəmɔɪd bəʊn] *subst.* any small bony nodule in a tendon, the largest being the kneecap *os sesamoideum, sesamben*

sessile ['sesaɪ(ə)l] *adj.* anything which has no stem (often applied to a tumour) *sessil, fastsittande, inte stjälkad*

session ['seʃ(ə)n] *subst.* visit of a patient to a therapist for treatment *besök, behandling(stillfälle);* **she has two sessions a week of physiotherapy; the evening session had to be cancelled because the therapist was ill**

set [set] *vb.* **(a)** to put the parts of a broken bone back into their proper places and keep the bone fixed until it has mended *reponera och fixera;* **the doctor set his broken arm (b)** *(of a broken bone)* to mend *or* to form a solid bone again *fixera sig;* **his arm has set very quickly; her broken wrist is setting very well** *see also* RESET

settle ['set(ə)l] *vb. (of a sediment)* to fall to the bottom of a liquid *(av)sätta sig, sjunka till botten; (of a parasite)* to attach itself *or* to stay in a part of the body *sätta sig, slå sig ner;* **the fluke settles in the liver**

sever ['sevə] *vb.* to cut off *avskilja, skilja, hugga (slita, klippa, skära) av;* **his hand was severed at the wrist; surgeons tried to sew the severed finger back onto the patient's hand**

severe [sɪ'vɪə] *adj.* very bad *svår, allvarlig;* **the patient is suffering from severe bleeding; a severe outbreak of whooping cough occurred during the winter; she is suffering from severe vitamin D deficiency**

severely [sɪ'vɪəli] *adv.* very badly *svårt, allvarligt;* **severely handicapped children need special care; her breathing was severely affected**

> QUOTE many severely confused patients, particularly those in advanced stages of Alzheimer's disease, do not respond to verbal communication
> **Nursing Times**

severity [sɪ'verəti] *subst.* degree to which something is bad *allvar, svårighetsgrad;* **treatment depends on the severity of the attack**

sex [seks] *subst.* one of two groups (male and female) into which animals and plants can be divided *kön;* **the sex of a baby can be identified before birth; the relative numbers of the two sexes in the population are not equal, more males being born than females; sex act** = act of sexual intercourse *coitus, könsumgänge, samlag;* **sex organs** = organs which are associated with reproduction and sexual intercourse (such as the testes and penis in men, and the ovaries, Fallopian tubes, vagina and vulva in women) *könsorgan, genitalia, genitalorgan, fortplantningsorgan, reproduktionsorgan;* **sex chromatin** *or* **Barr body** = chromatin found only in female cells, which can be used to identify the sex of a baby before birth *sexkromatin, könskromatin, kromatinfläck*

sex chromosome ['seks ˌkrəʊməʊsəʊm] *subst.* chromosome which determines if a person is male or female *gonosom, könskromosom*

> COMMENT: out of the twenty-three pairs of chromosomes in each human cell, two are sex chromosomes which are known as X and Y. Females have a pair of X chromosomes and males have a pair consisting of one X and one Y chromosome. The sex of a baby is determined by the father's sperm. While the mother's ovum only carries X chromosomes, the father's sperm can carry either an X or a Y chromosome. If the ovum is fertilized by a sperm carrying an X chromosome, the embryo will contain the XX pair and so be female

sex hormone ['seks ˌhɔːməʊn] *subst.* hormone secreted by the testis *or* ovaries, which regulates sexual development and reproductive functions *sexualhormon, könshormon*

> COMMENT: the male sex hormone is androgen, and the female hormones are oestrogen and progesterone

sexkromatin ⇨ **sex**

sexling ⇨ **sextuplet**

sex-linked [ˌseks'lɪŋ(k)t] *adj.* (i) (genes) which are linked to X chromosomes *könsbunden;* (ii) (characteristics, such as colour-blindness) which are transmitted through the X chromosomes *könsbunden*

sexology [seks'ɒlədʒi] *subst.* study of sex and sexual behaviour *sexologi*

sextuplet ['sekstjʊplət] *subst.* one of six babies born to a mother at the same time *sexling; see also* QUADRUPLET, QUINTUPLET, TRIPLET, TWIN

sexual ['sekʃu(ə)l] *adj.* referring to sex *sexuell, sexual-, köns-;* **sexual act** *or* **sexual intercourse** *or* **coitus** = action of inserting the man's erect penis into the woman's vagina, and releasing spermatozoa from the penis by ejaculation, which may fertilize ova from the woman's ovaries *coitus, könsumgänge, samlag*

sexualhormon ⇨ **sex hormone**

sexually transmitted disease (STD) ['sekʃu(ə)li trænsˌmɪtɪd dɪ'ziːz (ˌestiː'diː)] *subst.* any of several diseases which are transmitted from an infected person to another person during sexual intercourse *sexuellt överförd sjukdom, STD, könssjukdom, venerisk sjukdom, VS*

> COMMENT: among the commonest STDs are non-specific urethritis, genital herpes, hepatitis B and gonorrhoea; AIDS is also a sexually transmitted disease

sexuell ⇨ **sexual**

sexuell avvikelse ⇨ **perversion**

sexuellt överförd sjukdom ⇨ **sexually transmitted disease (STD), social, venereal disease (VD)**

sexuell utlösning ⇨ **orgasm**

sfeno- ⇨ **spheno-**

sfinkter ⇨ **sphincter (muscle)**

sfinkterektomi ⇨ **iridectomy, sphincterectomy**

sfinkteroplastik ⇨ **sphincteroplasty**

sfinkterotomi ⇨ **sphincterotomy**

sfygmo- ⇨ **sphygmo-**

sfygmograf ⇨ **sphygmocardiograph**

sfärocyt ⇨ **spherocyte**

sfärocytos ⇨ **spherocytosis**

shaft [ʃɑːft] *subst.* long central section of a long bone *diafys, skaft*

shake [ʃeɪk] *vb.* to move *or* make something move with short quick movements *skaka, darra*

sharp [ʃɑːp] *adj.* **(a)** which cuts easily *skarp, vass;* **a surgeon's knife has to be kept sharp (b)** acute (pain) (as opposed to dull pain) *skarp, häftig;* **she felt a sharp pain in her shoulder**

sharply ['ʃɑːpli] *adv.* suddenly *plötsligt, tvärt;* **his condition deteriorated sharply during the night**

shave [ʃeɪv] **1** *subst.* cutting off hair with a razor *rakning* **2** *vb.* to cut off hair with a razor *raka (sig);* **he cut himself while shaving; the nurse shaved the area where the surgeon was going to make the incision**

sheath [ʃiːθ] *subst.* **(a)** layer of tissue which surrounds a muscle *or* a bundle of nerve fibres *skida, slida* **(b) (contraceptive) sheath** = condom *or* rubber covering put over the penis before sexual intercourse as a protection against infection and also as a contraceptive *kondom*

shed [ʃed] *vb.* to lose (blood *or* tissue) *förlora, tappa, avstöta;* **the lining of the uterus is shed at each menstrual period; he was given a transfusion because he had shed a lot of blood**
NOTE: **shedding - has shed**

sheet [ʃiːt] *subst.* large piece of cloth which is put on a bed *lakan;* **the sheets must be changed each day; the soiled sheets were sent to the hospital laundry** *see also* DRAW-SHEET

shelf operation ['ʃelf ˌɒpəˌreɪʃ(ə)n] *subst.* surgical operation to treat congenital dislocation of the hip in children, where bone tissue is grafted onto the acetabulum *operation vid kongenital höftsledsluxation*

sheltered accommodation [ˌʃeltəd əˌkɒmə'deɪʃ(ə)n] *or* **sheltered housing** [ˌʃeltəd 'haʊzɪŋ] *subst.* rooms *or* small flats provided for elderly people, with a resident supervisor or nurse *ung. servicehus för äldre*

shift [ʃɪft] *subst.* **(a)** way of working, where one group of workers work for a period and are then replaced by another group; period of time worked by a group of workers *skift;* **she is working on the night shift; the day shift comes on duty at 6.30 in the morning (b)** movement *förändring, förskjutning;* **Purkinje shift** = change in colour sensitivity which takes place in the eye in low light, when the eye starts using the rods in the retina because the light is too weak to stimulate the cones *övergång till mörkerseende*

Shigella [ʃɪ'gelə] *subst.* genus of bacteria which causes dysentery *Shigella*

shigellosis [ˌʃɪge'ləʊsɪs] *subst.* infestation of the digestive tract with **Shigella,** causing bacillary dysentery *shigellos*

shin bone ['ʃɪn bəʊn] *subst.* the tibia *tibia, skenbenet, smalbenet;* **shin splints** = extremely sharp pains in the front of the leg, felt by athletes *smärtsam muskelsvullnad i underbenet pga träning*

shingles ['ʃɪŋg(ə)lz] = HERPES ZOSTER

Shirodkar's operation [ʃɪ'rɒdkɑːz ˌɒpəˌreɪʃ(ə)n] *or* **Shirodkar pursestring** [ʃɪ'rɒdkɑː ˌpɜːsstrɪŋ] *subst.* surgical operation to narrow the cervix of the womb in a woman who suffers from habitual abortion, to prevent another miscarriage, the suture being removed before labour starts *cerclage enligt Shirodkar (med tobakspungssutur)*

shiver ['ʃɪvə] *vb.* to shake all over the body, because of cold or because of a fever *darra, skaka, rysa*

shivering ['ʃɪv(ə)rɪŋ] *subst.* involuntary rapid contraction and relaxation of the muscles which helps to keep them warm *darrning, skakning, frossa*

shock [ʃɒk] **1** *subst.* **(a)** weakness caused by illness *or* injury, which suddenly reduces the blood pressure *chock;* **the patient went into shock; several of the passengers were treated for shock; a patient in shock should be kept warm and lying down, until plasma or blood transfusions can be given; shock syndrome** = group of symptoms (pale face, cold skin, high blood pressure, rapid and irregular pulse) which show that a patient is in a state of shock *chocksyndrom;* **neurogenic shock** = state of shock caused by bad news *or* an unpleasant surprise *neurogen chock;* **traumatic shock** = state of shock caused by

an injury which leads to loss of blood *traumatisk chock; see also* ANAPHYLACTIC
NOTE: you say that someone is **in shock, in a state of shock** or **went into shock (b) electric shock** = sudden pain caused by the passage of an electric current through the body *elektrisk chock;* **shock therapy** *or* **shock treatment** = method of treating some mental disorders by giving the patient an electric shock to induce an epileptic convulsion *chockbehandling, elbehandling, ECT, elchock* **2** *vb.* to give someone an unpleasant surprise, and so put him in a state of shock *chockera, chocka;* **she was still shocked several hours after the accident**

shoe [ʃu:] *subst.* piece of clothing made of leather or hard material which is worn on the foot *sko;* **surgical shoe** = specially made shoe to support *or* correct a deformed foot *ortopedisk sko*

short [ʃɔ:t] *adj.* lacking *or* with not enough of something **be short of** *ha ont om (knappt med, brist på), vara utan;* **after running up the stairs he was short of breath**

shortness of breath [ˌʃɔ:tnəs əv ˈbreθ] *subst.* panting *or* being unable to breathe quickly enough to supply oxygen needed *andfåddhet*

shortsighted [ˌʃɔ:tˈsaɪtɪd] = MYOPIC

shortsightedness [ˌʃɔ:tˈsaɪtɪdnəs] = MYOPIA

shot [ʃɒt] *subst. informal* injection *injektion, spruta;* **the doctor gave him a tetanus shot; he needed a shot of morphine to relieve the pain**

shoulder [ˈʃəʊldə] *subst.* joint where the top of the arm joins the main part of the body *skuldra, axel;* **he dislocated his shoulder; she was complaining of pains in her left shoulder** *or* **of shoulder pains; shoulder blade** *or* **scapula** = one of two large triangular flat bones covering the top part of the back *scapula, skulderbladet;* **shoulder girdle** *or* **pectoral girdle** = the shoulder bones (scapulae and clavicles) to which the arm bones are attached *skuldergördeln;* **shoulder joint** = ball and socket joint which allows the arm to rotate and move in any direction *articulatio humeri, skulderleden, axelleden;* **shoulder lift** = way of carrying a heavy patient where the upper part of his body rests on the shoulders of two carriers *australiensiskt lyft;* **frozen shoulder** = stiffness and pain in the shoulder, after injury *or* after the shoulder has been immobile for some time, when it may be caused by inflammation of the membranes of the shoulder joint with deposits forming in the tendons *periarthritis humeroscapularis, frozen shoulder*

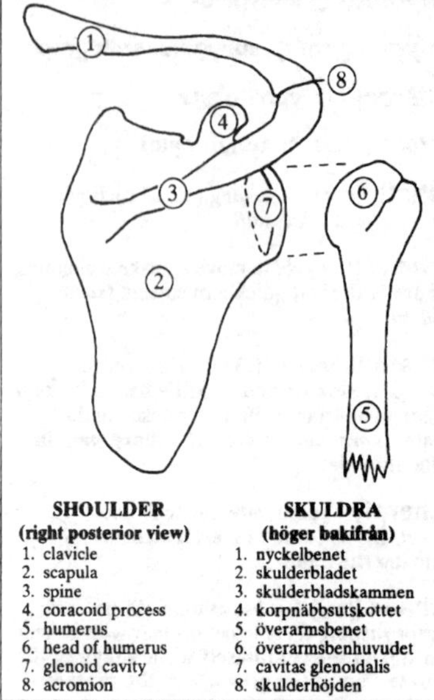

SHOULDER (right posterior view)
1. clavicle
2. scapula
3. spine
4. coracoid process
5. humerus
6. head of humerus
7. glenoid cavity
8. acromion

SKULDRA (höger bakifrån)
1. nyckelbenet
2. skulderbladet
3. skulderbladskammen
4. korpnäbbsutskottet
5. överarmsbenet
6. överarmsbenhuvudet
7. cavitas glenoidalis
8. skulderhöjden

show [ʃəʊ] *subst.* first discharge of blood at the beginning of childbirth *teckningsblödning*

shrivel [ˈʃrɪv(ə)l] *vb.* to become dry and wrinkled *skrumpna, bli rynkig*

shuffling walk [ˈʃʌflɪŋ ˌwɔ:k] *or* **shuffling gait** [ˈʃʌflɪŋ ˌgeɪt] *subst.* way of walking (as in Parkinson's disease) where the feet are not lifted off the ground *släpande gång, hasande gång*

shunt [ʃʌnt] **1** *subst.* (i) passing of blood through a channel which is not the usual one *shuntning;* (ii) channel which links two different blood vessels and carries blood from one to the other *shunt;* **portocaval shunt** = artificial passage made between the portal vein and the inferior vena cava to relieve pressure on the liver *porta-cavashunt;* **right-left shunt** = defect in the heart, allowing blood to flow from the pulmonary artery to the aorta *höger-vänstershunt* **2** *vb. (of blood)* to pass through a channel which is not the normal one *shunta;* **as much as 5% of venous blood can be shunted unoxygenated back to the arteries**

shunting [ˈʃʌntɪŋ] *subst.* condition where some of the deoxygenated blood in the lungs does not come into contact with air, and full gas exchange does not take place *shuntning*

shuntning ⇨ **shunt, shunting**

SI [ˌes'aɪ] *abbreviation for* Système International, the international system of metric measurements *SI(-systemet);* **SI units =** international system of units for measuring physical properties (such as weight *or* speed *or* light, etc.) *SI-enheter; see also table in supplement*

sial- ['saɪəl, ˌ--] *or* **sialo-** ['saɪələʊ, ˌ---] *prefix* meaning (i) saliva *sial(o)-, ptyal(o)-, saliv-, spott-;* (ii) a salivary gland *sial(o)-, ptyal(o)-, spottkörtel-*

sialadenitis [ˌsaɪəlˌædɪ'naɪtɪs] *or* **sialodenitis** [ˌsaɪələʊˌædɪ'naɪtɪs] *or* **sialitis** [ˌsaɪə'laɪtɪs] *subst.* inflammation of a salivary gland *sial(o)adenit, spottkörtelinflammation*

sialagogue [saɪ'æləgɒg] *or* **sialogogue** [saɪ'æləgɒg] *subst.* substance which increases the production of saliva *sialagoga, ptyalagoga, salivbefrämjande medel*

sialism ⇨ **ptyalism, sialorrhoea**

sialografi ⇨ **ptyalography, sialography**

sialography [ˌsaɪə'lɒgrəfi] *or* **ptyalography** [ˌtaɪə'lɒgrəfi] *subst.* X-ray examination of a salivary gland *sialografi*

sialolit ⇨ **salivary, sialolith**

sialolith [saɪ'æləʊlɪθ] *or* **ptyalith** ['taɪəlɪθ] *subst.* stone in a salivary gland *sialolit, ptyalolit, salivsten, spottsten*

sialorrhoea [ˌsaɪələʊ'rɪə] *subst.* production of an excessive amount of saliva *sialism, sialorré, ptyalism, ptyalorré*

Siamese twins [ˌsaɪəmiːz 'twɪnz] *or* **conjoined twins** [kən'dʒɔɪnd ˌtwɪns] *subst. pl.* twins who are joined together at birth *siamesiska tvillingar*

> COMMENT: Siamese twins are always identical twins, and can be joined at the head, chest or hip. In some cases Siamese twins can be separated by surgery, but this is not possible if they share a single important organ, such as the heart

sib [sɪb] = SIBLING

sibilant ['sɪbɪlənt] *adj. (applied to a rale)* whistling (sound) *sibilant, väsande, pipande*

sibling ['sɪblɪŋ] *subst.* brother *or* sister *syskon*

siccasyndrom ⇨ **Sjögren's syndrome**

sick [sɪk] *adj.* **(a)** ill *or* not well *sjuk;* **he was sick for two weeks; she's off sick from work; to report sick =** to say officially that you are ill and cannot work *sjukanmäla sig* **(b)** wanting to vomit *or* having a condition where food is brought up from the stomach into the mouth *illamående;* **the patient got up this morning and felt sick; he was given something to make him sick; the little boy ate too much and was sick all over the floor; she had a sick feeling** *or* **she felt sick =** she felt that she wanted to vomit *hon kände sig illamående (ville kräkas)*

sickbay ['sɪkbeɪ] *subst.* room where patients can visit a doctor for treatment in a factory *or* on a ship *sjukvårdsavdelning, sjukvårdshytt, läkarmottagning*

sickbed ['sɪkbed] *subst.* bed where a person is lying sick *sjuksäng;* **she sat for hours beside her daughter's sickbed**

sicken for ['sɪk(ə)n fɔː] *vb. (informal)* to begin to have an illness *or* to feel the first symptoms of an illness *börja bli sjuk (insjukna) i;* **she's looking pale - she must be sickening for something**

sickle cell ['sɪk(ə)l ˌsel] *or* **drepanocyte** ['drepənəʊsaɪt] *subst.* abnormal red blood cell shaped like a sickle, due to an abnormal haemoglobin (HbS), which can cause blockage of capillaries *drepanocyt, sickle-cell;* **sickle-cell disease (SCD) =** disease caused by sickle cells in the blood *sickle-cell disease;* **sickle-cell anaemia** *or* **drepanocytosis =** hereditary condition where the patient develops sickle cells which block the circulation, causing anaemia and pains in the joints and abdomen *drepanocytos, sicklecellsanemi;* **sickle-cell chest syndrome =** common complication of sickle-cell disease, with chest pain, fever and leucocytosis *sicklecellsyndrom med bröstsmärtor och feber*

> COMMENT: sickle-cell anaemia is a hereditary condition which is mainly found in Africa and the West Indies

> QUOTE children with sickle-cell anaemia are susceptible to severe bacterial infection. Even children with the milder forms of sickle-cell disease have an increased frequency of pneumococcal infection
>
> **Lancet**

sicklist ['sɪklɪst] *subst.* list of people (children in a school *or* workers in a factory) who are sick *lista med sjukanmälda;* **we have five members of staff on the sicklist**

sickly ['sɪkli] *adj. (usually of children)* always slightly ill *or* never completely well; weak *or* subject to frequent sickness *sjuklig;* **he was a sickly child, but now is a strong and healthy man**

sickness ['sɪknəs] *or* **illness** ['ɪlnəs] *subst.* **(a)** not being well *sjukdom;* **there is a lot of sickness in the winter months; many children are staying away from school because of sickness (b)** feeling of wanting to vomit *illamående*

sickroom ['sɪkru:m] *subst.* bedroom where someone is ill *sjukrum, sjuksal;* **visitors are not allowed into the sickroom**

sida ⇨ **side**

side [saɪd] *subst.* (i) part of the body between the hips and the shoulder *sidan;* (ii) part of an object which is not the front, back, top or bottom *sida;* **she was lying on her side; the nurse wheeled the trolley to the side of the bed; side rails** = rails at the side of a bed which can be lifted to prevent a patient falling out *sänggrindar; see also* BEDSIDE

side-effect ['saɪdɪˌfekt] *subst.* effect produced by a drug *or* treatment which is not the main effect intended *sidoeffekt, biverkning;* **one of the side-effects of chemotherapy is that the patient's hair falls out; doctors do not recommend using the drug for long periods because of the unpleasant side-effects; the drug is being withdrawn because of its side-effects**

> QUOTE the treatment is not without possible side-effects, some of which can be particularly serious. The side-effects may include middle ear discomfort, claustrophobia, increased risk of epilepsy
>
> **New Zealand Medical Journal**

sidero- ['saɪdərə(ʊ), ˌ---] *prefix* referring to iron *sidero-, järn-*

sideropeni ⇨ **deficiency, sideropenia**

sideropenia [ˌsaɪdərəʊ'pi:niə] *subst.* lack of iron in the blood probably caused by insufficient iron in diet *sideropeni, serumjärnbrist, järnbristanemi*

siderophilin [ˌsaɪdə'rɒfəlɪn] *or* **transferrin** [træns'fɜ:rɪn] *subst.* substance found in the blood, which carries iron in the bloodstream *transferrin*

siderosis [ˌsaɪdə'rəʊsɪs] *subst.* (i) condition where iron deposits form in tissue *sideros;* (ii) inflammation of the lungs caused by inhaling dust containing iron *sideros*

sido- ⇨ **lateral**

sidobild ⇨ **lateral**

sidoeffekt ⇨ **side-effect**

SIDS [ˌesaɪdi:'es] *US* = SUDDEN INFANT DEATH SYNDROME

SI-enheter ⇨ **SI**

siffra ⇨ **digit**

sight [saɪt] *subst.* one of the five senses, the ability to see *syn(sinnet);* **his sight is beginning to fail; surgeons are fighting to save her sight; he lost his sight** = he became blind *han förlorade synen (blev blind)*

sighted ['saɪtɪd] *adj.* (person) who can see *seende;* **the sighted** = people who can see *de seende;* **he is partially sighted and uses a white stick**

sigmoid ['sɪgmɔɪd] *or* **sigmoid colon** ['sɪgmɔɪd ˌkəʊlən] *or* **sigmoid flexure** ['sɪgmɔɪd ˌflekʃə] *subst.* fourth section of the colon which joins the rectum ⇨ *illustration* DIGESTIVE SYSTEM *(colon) sigmoideum, sigmaformade delen av tjocktarmen*

sigmoidectomy [ˌsɪgmɔɪ'dektəmi] *subst.* surgical operation to remove the sigmoid colon *sigmoidektomi*

sigmoidoscope [sɪg'mɔɪdəskəʊp] *subst.* surgical instrument with a light at the end which can be passed into the rectum so that the sigmoid colon can be examined *sigmoidoskop*

sigmoidostomy [ˌsɪgmɔɪ'dɒstəmi] *subst.* surgical operation to bring the sigmoid colon out through a hole in the abdominal wall *sigmoidostomi*

sign [saɪn] **1** *subst.* **(a)** movement *or* mark *or* colouring *or* change which has a meaning and can be recognized by a doctor as indicating a condition *tecken* NOTE: a change in function which is also noticed by the patient is a **symptom (b) sign language** = signs made with the fingers and hands, used to indicate words when talking to a deaf and dumb person, or when such a person wants to communicate *teckenspråk* **2** *vb.* to write one's name on a form, cheque, etc. or at the end of a letter *signera, underteckna;* **the doctor signed the death certificate**

signalsubstans ⇨ **neurosecretion, neurotransmitter**

signature ['sɪgnətʃə] *subst.* name which someone writes when he signs *signatur, namnteckning, underskrift;* **the chemist could not read the doctor's signature; her signature is easy to recognize**

signera ⇨ **sign**

sil ⇨ **filter**

silbenet ⇨ **ethmoid bone**

silbens- ⇨ **ethmoidal**

silbenscellerna ⇨ **ethmoidal**

silbensplattan ⇨ **cribriform plate**

silence ['saɪləns] *subst.* lack of noise *or* lack of speaking *tystnad;* **the crowd waited in silence**

silent ['saɪlənt] *adj.* **(a)** not making any noise *or* not talking *tyst* **(b)** not visible *or* showing no symptoms *tyst, subklinisk;* **genital herpes may be silent in women; graft occlusion is often silent with 80% of patients**

silicosis [ˌsɪlɪ'kəʊsɪs] *subst.* kind of pneumoconiosis *or* disease of the lungs caused by inhaling silica dust from mining *or* stone-crushing operations *silikos*

COMMENT: this is a serious disease which makes breathing difficult and can lead to emphysema and bronchitis

silning ⇨ **filtration**

silver ['sɪlvə] *subst.* white-coloured metallic element *silver, Ag* NOTE: chemical symbol is **Ag**

silvernitrat ⇨ **silver nitrate**

silver nitrate [ˌsɪlvə 'naɪtreɪt] *subst.* salt of silver, mixed with a cream or solution, used to disinfect burns, to kill warts, etc. *silvernitrat, lapis*

Silvester method [sɪl'vestə ˌmeθəd] *subst.* method of giving artificial respiration where the patient lies on his back and the first aider brings the patient's hands together on his chest and then moves them above the patient's head *metod för konstgjord andning; see also* HOLGER NIELSEN METHOD

Silvius ['sɪlviəs] *see* AQUEDUCT

Simmonds' disease ['sɪməndz dɪˌziːz] *subst.* condition of women where there is lack of activity in the pituitary gland, resulting in wasting of tissue, brittle bones and premature senility, due to postpartum haemorrhage *Simmonds kakexi (sjukdom)*

simple ['sɪmp(ə)l] *adj.* ordinary *or* not very complicated *enkel, okomplicerad;* **simple epithelium** = epithelium formed of a single layer of cells *enskiktat epitel;* **simple fracture** = fracture where the skin surface around the damaged bone has not been broken and the broken ends of the bone are close together *sluten fraktur, okomplicerad fraktur; see also* TACHYCARDIA

simplex ['sɪmpleks] *see* HERPES

simulera ⇨ **malingering**

sinew ['sɪnjuː] *subst.* ligament *or* tissue which holds together the bones at a joint; tendon *or* tissue which attaches a muscle to a bone *tendo, sena*

singultus [sɪŋ'gʌltəs] = HICCUP

sinne ⇨ **mind, sense**

sinnes- ⇨ **sensible, sensory**

sinnesförnimmelse ⇨ **perception, sensation**

sinnesförvirring ⇨ **aberration**

sinneslugn ⇨ **ataraxia, balance**

sinnesorgan ⇨ **sense**

sinnesrubbad ⇨ **deranged**

sinnesrörelse ⇨ **affection**

sinnessjuk ⇨ **insane**

sinnessjukdom ⇨ **insanity, psychopathy**

sinnesstämning ⇨ **mind, mood, temper**

sino- ['saɪnəʊ, ˌ--] *or* **sinu-** ['saɪnə, ˌ--] *prefix* referring to a sinus *sino-, sinus-*

sinoatrial node (SA node) [ˌsaɪnəʊ'eɪtriəl ˌnəʊd (ˌes'eɪ ˌnəʊd)] *subst.* node in the heart at the junction of the superior vena cava and the right atrium, which regulates the heartbeat *nodus sinu-atrialis, sinusknutan*

sinogram ['saɪnəʊgræm] *subst.* X-ray photograph of a sinus *bild vid sinusröntgen*

sinography [saɪ'nɒgrəfi] *subst.* examining a sinus by taking an X-ray photograph *sinusröntgen*

sinuatrial node [,saɪnə'eɪtriəl ,nəʊd] = SINOATRIAL NODE

sinuit ⇨ **sinusitis**

sinus ['saɪnəs] *subst.* (i) cavity inside the body, including the cavities inside the head behind the cheekbone, forehead and nose *sinus, hålrum, bihåla;* (ii) tract *or* passage which develops between an infected place where pus has gathered and the surface of the skin *fistel;* (iii) wide venous blood space *blodsinus, buktig (utvidgad) ven;* **he has had sinus trouble during the winter; the doctor diagnosed a sinus infection; carotid sinus** = expanded part attached to the carotid artery which monitors blood pressure in the skull *sinus caroticus, carotissinus;* **cavernous sinus** = one of two cavities in the skull behind the eyes, which form part of the venous drainage system *sinus cavernosus;* **coronary sinus** = vein which takes most of the venous blood from the heart muscles to the right atrium *sinus coronarius;* **ethmoidal sinuses** = air cells inside the ethmoid bone *sinus ethmoidei, silbenscellerna;* **frontal sinus** = one of two sinuses in the front of the face above the eyes and near the nose *sinus frontalis, pann(bens)hålan;* **maxillary sinus** = one of two sinuses behind the cheekbones in the upper jaw *antrum Highmori, sinus maxillaris, överkäkshålan;* **paranasal sinus** = one of the four pairs of sinuses in the skull near the nose (the frontal, maxillary, ethmoidal and sphenoidal) **paranasal sinuses** *sinus paranasales, bihålorna;* **renal sinus** = cavity in which the tubes leading into a kidney fit *njurhilus;* **sphenoidal sinus** = one of two sinuses behind the nasal passage *sinus sphenoidalis, kilbenshålan;* **sinus nerve** = nerve which branches from the glossopharyngeal nerve *ramus sinus carotici, gren av 9:e kranialnerven; see also* TACHYCARDIA

sinus- ⇨ **sino-**

sinusitis [,saɪnə'saɪtɪs] *or* **sinus trouble** ['saɪnəs ,trʌb(ə)l] *subst.* inflammation of the mucous membrane in the sinuses, especially the maxillary sinuses *sinusit, sinuit, bihåleinflammation;* **she has sinus trouble** = she has a disorder in her sinuses *hon har besvär med bihålorna*

sinusknutan ⇨ **pacemaker, sinoatrial node (SA node)**

sinusoid ['saɪnəsɔɪd] *subst.* specially shaped small blood vessel in the liver, adrenal glands and other organs *sinusoid*

sinusröntgen ⇨ **sinography**

sinustakykardi ⇨ **tachycardia**

sinus venosus ['saɪnəs və'nəʊsɪs] *subst.* cavity in the heart of an embryo, part of which develops into the coronary sinus, and part of which is absorbed into the right atrium *sinus venosus*

siphonage ['saɪfənɪdʒ] *subst.* removing liquid from one place to another, with a tube, as used to empty the stomach of its contents *sugning (tömning) av vätska med hjälp av sond (hävert)*

sippra ⇨ **ooze**

Sippy diet ['sɪpi ,da(ɪ)ət] *subst. US* alkaline diet of milk and dry biscuits, as a treatment for peptic ulcers *slags magsårsdiet*

sista ⇨ **final**

sista suck ⇨ **expiration**

sister ['sɪstə] *subst.* **(a)** female who has the same father and mother as another child *syster;* **he has three sisters; her sister works in a children's clinic (b)** senior nurse *(överordnad) sjuksköterska, ung. avdelningsföreståndare;* **sister in charge** *or* **ward sister** = senior nurse in charge of a hospital ward *avdelningsföreståndare;* **nursing sister** = sister with certain administrative duties *sjuksköterska med vissa administrativa uppgifter*

NOTE: sister can be used with names: **Sister Jones**

site [saɪt] **1** *subst.* position of something *or* place where something happened; place where an incision is to be made in an operation *plats, källa;* **the X-ray showed the site of the infection 2** *vb.* to put something *or* to be in a particular place *placera, lokalisera, vara belägen, ligga;* **the infection is sited in the right lung**

QUOTE arterial thrombi have a characteristic structure: platelets adhere at sites of endothelial damage and attract other platelets to form a dense aggregate
British Journal of Hospital Medicine

QUOTE the sublingual site is probably the most acceptable and convenient for taking temperature
Nursing Times

> QUOTE with the anaesthetist's permission, the scrub nurse and surgeon began the process of cleaning up the skin round the operation site
> **NATNews**

sittande ⇨ **sedentary**

sittbad(kar) ⇨ **hip, sitz bath**

sittbenet ⇨ **ischium**

sittbensknölen ⇨ **ischial**

situ ['saɪtuː] *see* CARCINOMA-IN-SITU

situated ['sɪtjueɪtɪd] *adj.* in a place *placerad, belägen, lokaliserad;* **the tumour is situated in the bowel; the atlas bone is situated above the axis**

sit up [ˌsɪt 'ʌp] *vb.* (i) to sit with your back straight *sitta (upp, rak, upprätt);* (ii) to move from a lying to a sitting position *sätta sig upp;* **the patient is sitting up in bed**

situs inversus viscerum ['saɪtəs ɪnˌvɜːsəs 'vɪsərəm] *subst.* abnormal congenital condition, where the organs are not on the normal side of the body (i.e. where the heart is on the right side and not the left) *situs inversus viscerum, transpositio viscerum, spegelvändning av de inre organens läge*

sitz bath ['sɪts bɑːθ] *subst.* small low bath where a patient can sit, but not lie down *sittbad(kar)*

sjudagarsfeber ⇨ **dengue**

sjuk ⇨ **ailing, bad, diseased, disordered, ill, invalid, morbid, sick, unwell**

-sjuk ⇨ **-pathy, sufferer**

sjukanmäla sig ⇨ **sick**

sjukavdelning ⇨ **infirmary**

sjukdom ⇨ **ailment, complaint, condition, disease, illness, sickness, trouble**

-sjukdom ⇨ **-iasis, -osis, -pathy**

sjukdoms- ⇨ **noso-, path-**

sjukdomsalstrande ⇨ **virulent**

sjukdomsanfall, häftigt ⇨ **paroxysm**

sjukdomsfall ⇨ **case**

sjukdomsfrekvens ⇨ **morbidity**

sjukdomshistoria ⇨ **history, past**

sjukdomslära ⇨ **nosology**

sjukdomsorsak ⇨ **aetiology**

sjukdomstecken ⇨ **symptom**

sjukförsäkring ⇨ **health, insurance**

sjukgymnast ⇨ **physio, physiotherapist**

sjukgymnastik ⇨ **physical, physiotherapy**

sjukhem ⇨ **nursing**

sjukhistoria ⇨ **history**

sjukhus ⇨ **hospital, infirmary**

sjukhusföreståndare ⇨ **matron**

sjukhuskurator ⇨ **almoner**

sjukhuspräst ⇨ **chaplain**

sjukhussjuka ⇨ **nosocomial**

sjukhussäng ⇨ **bed**

sjukintyg ⇨ **medical**

sjukjournal ⇨ **case**

sjuklig ⇨ **invalid, morbid, pathological, sickly**

sjuklighet ⇨ **ill health, morbidity**

sjukrum ⇨ **infirmary, sickroom**

sjuksköterska ⇨ **nurse, sister**

sjuksköterska, legitimerad ⇨ **register**

sjuksköterskestuderande ⇨ **student**

sjuksköterskeyrket ⇨ **nursing**

sjukstuga ⇨ **cottage hospital**

sjuksäng ⇨ **sickbed**

sjukvård, offentlig ⇨ **National Health Servioo (NHS)**

sjukvårdsavdelning ⇨ **sickbay**

sjukvårdsbiträde ➪ **auxiliary, orderly**

sjukvårdshytt ➪ **sickbay**

sjukvårdsstatistik ➪ **hospital**

sjunka ➪ **go down, settle**

själen ➪ **psyche**

själsförmögenheter ➪ **faculty**

själv- ➪ **auto-, self-**

självförsvar ➪ **self-defence**

självhäftande ➪ **adhesive**

självinfektion ➪ **autoinfection**

självlysande ➪ **phosphorescent**

självmord ➪ **suicide**

självmords- ➪ **suicidal**

självmordsförsök ➪ **suicide**

självstyrande ➪ **autonomic**

självständig ➪ **autonomic, independent**

självständighet ➪ **autonomy**

självständigt ➪ **independently**

sjätte sjukdomen ➪ **roseola**

Sjögren's syndrome ['ʃɜːgrenz ˌsɪndrəʊm] *subst.* chronic autoimmune disease where the lacrimal and salivary glands become infiltrated with lymphocytes and plasma cells, and the mouth and eyes become dry *Sjögrens syndrom, siccasyndrom*

sjösjuk ➪ **seasick**

sjösjuka ➪ **seasickness**

skabb ➪ **itch, scabies**

skabbdjuret ➪ **sarcoptes**

skada ➪ **damage, harm, hurt, injure, injury, lesion, trauma, wound**

skadedjur ➪ **pest**

skadlig ➪ **harmful, noxious**

skadliga rummet ➪ **dead**

skafocefal ➪ **scaphocephalic**

skafocefali ➪ **scaphocephaly**

skafoidit ➪ **Köhler's disease, scaphoiditis**

skaft ➪ **diaphysis, shaft**

skaka ➪ **shake, shiver, tremble, vibrate**

skakning ➪ **concussion, shivering, trembling, tremor, vibration**

skall- ➪ **cephalic, crani-, cranial**

skallben ➪ **cranial**

skallen ➪ **cranium, skull**

skallfraktur ➪ **skull**

skallig ➪ **bald**

skallighet ➪ **alopecia, baldness**

skallindex ➪ **cephalic**

skallröntgen ➪ **cephalogram**

skalltaket ➪ **calvaria**

skalpell ➪ **scalpel**

skalpen ➪ **epicranium, scalp**

skalpmuskeln ➪ **epicranius**

skanderande tal ➪ **staccato speech**

skapa ➪ **create**

skapulär ➪ **scapular**

skarifikation ➪ **scarification**

skarp ➪ **acute, keen, lancinating, sharp**

skat(o)- ➪ **scat-**

skatole ['skætəʊl] *or* **scatole** ['skætəʊl] *subst.* substance in faeces which causes a strong foul smell *starkt illaluktande ämne i avföringen*

skava ➪ **chafe**

skavjärn ➪ **raspatory**

skavsår ➪ **excoriation**

sked ➪ **spoon, spoonful**

skede ➪ **phase, stage**

skednaglar ➪ **koilonychia**

skela ➪ **squint**

skeletal ['skelɪt(ə)l] *adj.* referring to a skeleton *skelett-;* **skeletal muscle** *or* **voluntary muscle** = muscle which is attached to a bone, which makes a limb move *skelettmuskel, tvärstrimmig muskel*

skeleton ['skelɪt(ə)n] *subst.* all the bones which make up a body *skelett, benstomme;* **appendicular skeleton** = part of the skeleton, formed of the pelvic girdle, pectoral girdle and the bones of the arms and legs *de (hängande) delar av skelettet som fäster vid ryggraden;* **axial skeleton** = trunk *or* main part of the skeleton, formed of the spine, skull, ribs and breastbone *de delar av skelettet som består av skallen, ryggraden och revbenen*

skelett- ➪ **skeletal**

skelettmuskel ➪ **skeletal**

skelning ➪ **squint, strabismus**

skelningskorrigering ➪ **orthoptics**

skelögd ➪ **strabismal**

sken- ➪ **false, pseud-**

skena ➪ **brace, calliper, splint**

skenbenet ➪ **shin bone, tibia**

skenbens- ➪ **tibial, tibio-**

skenbensartärerna ➪ **tibial**

Skene's glands ['ski:nz ˌglændz] *subst.* small mucous glands in the urethra in women *små slemavsöndrande körtlar i kvinnans urinrör*

skengraviditet ➪ **pseudocyesis**

skepnad ➪ **form**

skia- ['skaɪə, ˌ--] *prefix* meaning shadow *skia-*

skiagram ['skaɪəgræm] *subst.* old term for X-ray photograph *tidigare radiogram (röntgenogram, röntgenbild)*

skiaskop ➪ **retinoscope**

skick ➪ **condition, state**

skida ➪ **sheath**

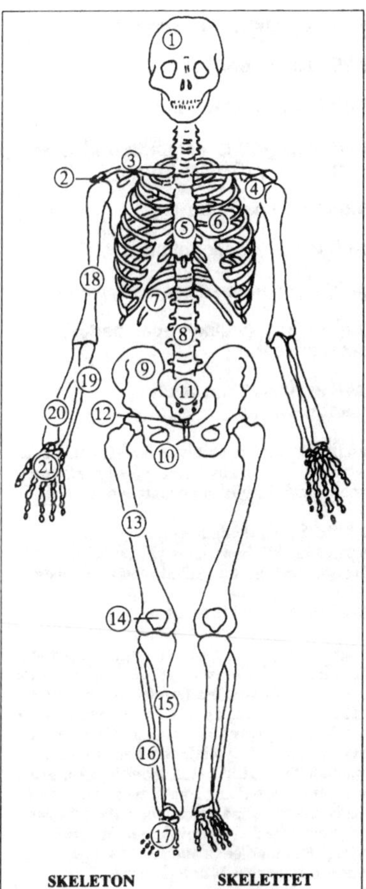

SKELETON	SKELETTET
1. skull	1. skallen
2. acromion	2. skulderhöjden
3. clavicle	3. nyckelbenet
4. scapula	4. skulderbladet
5. sternum	5. bröstbenet
6. rib	6. revben
7. floating rib	7. två understa revbenen
8. vertebral column	8. kotpelaren, ryggraden
9. ilium	9. höftbenet, tarmbenet
10. ischium	10. sittbenet
11. sacrum	11. korsbenet
12. coccyx	12. svansbenet
13. femur	13. lårbenet
14. patella	14. knäskålen
15. tibia	15. skenbenet
16. fibula	16. vadbenet
17. foot	17. foten
18. humerus	18. överarmsbenet
19. ulna	19. armbågsbenet
20. radius	20. strålbenet
21. hand	21. handen

skift ➪ **shift**

skikt ⇨ **coat, layer, stratum**

skiktad ⇨ **stratified**

skiktbild ⇨ **tomogram**

skiktröntgen ⇨ **computerized axial tomography (CAT), scan**

skildra ⇨ **describe**

skildring ⇨ **description**

skilja ⇨ **detach, dissociate, sever**

skiljevägg ⇨ **diaphragm, paries, screen, septum**

skiljeväggsliknande ⇨ **diaphragmatic**

skill [skɪl] *subst.* ability to do difficult work, which is acquired by training *färdighet;* **you need special skills to become a doctor**

skilled [skɪld] *adj.* having acquired a particular skill by training *yrkesutbildad, kvalificerad;* **he's a skilled plastic surgeon**

skillnad ⇨ **difference**

skin [skɪn] *subst.* tissue (the epidermis and dermis) which forms the outside surface of the body *cutis, huden;* **his skin turned brown in the sun; after the operation she had to have a skin graft; skin problems in adolescents may be caused by diet; she went to see a specialist about her skin trouble; skin graft** = layer of skin transplanted from one part of the body to cover an area where the skin has been destroyed *hudtransplantat, hudgraft*
NOTE: for other terms referring to skin see words beginning with **cut-** or **derm-**

COMMENT: the skin is the largest organ in the human body. It is formed of two layers: the epidermis is the outer layer, and includes the top layer of particles of dead skin which are continuously flaking off. Beneath the epidermis is the dermis, which is the main layer of living skin. Hairs and nails are produced by the skin, and pores in the skin secrete sweat from the sweat glands underneath the dermis. The skin is sensitive to touch and heat and cold, which are sensed by the nerve endings in the skin. The skin is a major source of vitamin D which it produces when exposed to sunlight

skinny ['skɪni] *adj. informal* very thin *mager*

skirr ⇨ **scirrhus**

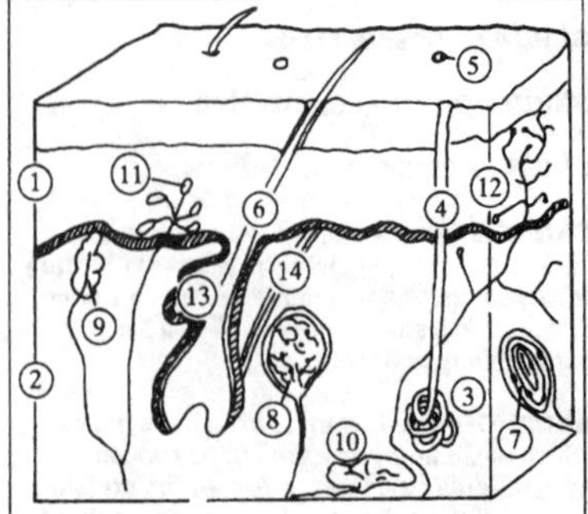

SKIN & SENSORY RECEPTORS	**HUDEN OCH SENSORISKA RECEPTORER**
1. epidermis	1. överhuden
2. dermis	2. läderhuden
3. sweat gland	3. svettkörtel
4. sweat duct	4. svettkörtelns utförsgång
5. pore	5. por
6. hair	6. hår
7. Pacinian corpuscle (pressure)	7. Pacinis känselkropp (tryck)
8. Meissner's corpuscle (touch)	8. Meissners känselkropp (beröring)
9. Krause corpuscle (cold)	9. Krauses känselkropp (kyla)
10. Ruffini corpuscle (heat)	10. Ruffinis känselkropp (värme)
11. Merkel's discs (touch)	11. Merkels känselkropp (beröring)
12. free nerve endings (pain)	12. fria nervändar (smärta)
13. sebaceous gland	13. talgkörtel
14. arrector pili	14. hårresarmuskel

skirrös ⇨ **scirrhous**

skiva ⇨ **disc**

skivepitel, enskiktat ⇨ **pavement epithelium**

skjorta ⇨ **gown**

skjuta ut (fram) ⇨ **project**

sklera ⇨ **albuginea, sclera**

skleral ⇨ **scleral**

sklerit ⇨ **episcleritis, scleritis**

sklerodaktyli ⇨ **acrosclerosis**

skleroderma ⇨ **scleroderma**

sklerodermi ⇨ **scleroderma**

sklerom ⇨ **scleroma**

skleromalaci ⇨ **scleromalacia (perforans)**

skleros ⇨ **induration, sclerosis**

skleroserande ⇨ **sclerosing**

skleroterapi ⇨ **sclerotherapy**

sklerotisk ⇨ **sclerotic**

sklerotom ⇨ **sclerotome**

sklerotomi ⇨ **sclerotomy**

skolex ⇨ **scolex**

skolgymnastik ⇨ **physical**

skolhälsovård ⇨ **school**

skolios ⇨ **curvature, scoliosis**

skolpsykolog ⇨ **psychologist**

skonkost ⇨ **bland**

skonsam ⇨ **bland**

-skop ⇨ **-scope**

skopolamin ⇨ **hyoscine**

skorbut ⇨ **scorbutus, scurvy**

skorbutisk ⇨ **scorbutic**

skorpa ⇨ **scab**

skorv ⇨ **cradle, favus**

skorvig ⇨ **furfuraceous**

skoto- ⇨ **scoto-**

skotom ⇨ **scotoma**

skotopi ⇨ **scotopia**

skotopisk ⇨ **scotopic**

skottskada ⇨ **wound**

skrapa ⇨ **chafe**

skrapa bort (tandsten) ⇨ **scale**

skrapning ⇨ **curettage, dilatation**

skratta ⇨ **laugh**

skrevet ⇨ **crotch**

skrik ⇨ **cry, scream**

skriva in (sig) ⇨ **register**

skriva ut ⇨ **discharge**

skrivkramp ⇨ **dysgraphia, writer's cramp**

skrofelsjuk ⇨ **scrofulous**

skrofelsjuka ⇨ **scrofula**

skrofler ⇨ **scrofula**

skrofulös ⇨ **scrofulous**

skrotal ⇨ **scrotal**

skrotum ⇨ **scrotum**

skrovlig ⇨ **hoarse, husky, rough**

skrubba ⇨ **chafe, graze**

skrubbsår ⇨ **abrasion, graze**

skrumplever ⇨ **cirrhosis of the liver, hobnail liver, Laennec's cirrhosis**

skrumpna ⇨ **shrivel**

skrumpning ⇨ **kraurosis**

skrumpnjure ⇨ **nephrosclerosis**

skråma ⇨ **graze, scratch**

skräck ⇨ **panic, -phobia**

skräddarmuskeln ⇨ **sartorius**

skrämma ⇨ **frighten**

skröplighet ⇨ **infirmity, weakness**

skulderbladet ⇨ **scapula, shoulder**

skulderbladskammen ⇨ **spine**

skuldergördeln ⇨ **girdle**

skulderhöjden ⇨ **acromion**

skulderleden ⇨ **glenohumeral, shoulder**

skuldra ⇨ **shoulder**

skull [skʌl] *subst.* bones which are fused *or* connected together to form the head *kranium, skallen;* **skull fracture** *or* **fracture of the skull** = condition where one of the bones in the skull has been fractured *skallfraktur* NOTE: for other terms referring to the skull see words beginning with **crani-**

COMMENT: the skull is formed of eight cranial bones which make up the head, and fourteen facial bones which form the face

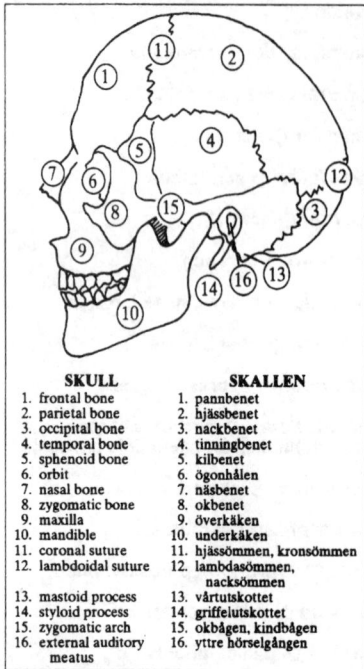

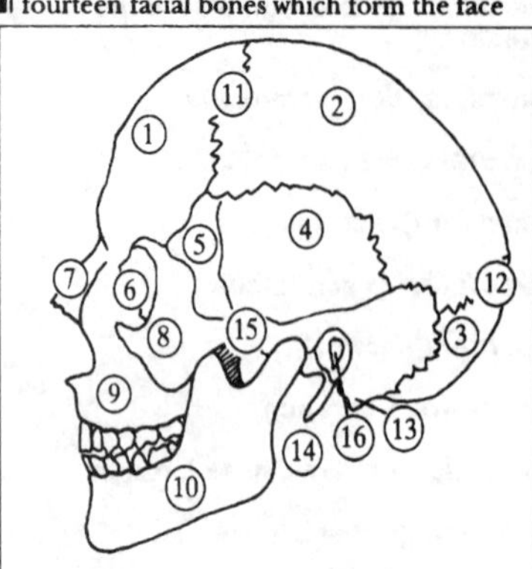

SKULL	SKALLEN
1. frontal bone	1. pannbenet
2. parietal bone	2. hjässbenet
3. occipital bone	3. nackbenet
4. temporal bone	4. tinningbenet
5. sphenoid bone	5. kilbenet
6. orbit	6. ögonhålen
7. nasal bone	7. näsbenet
8. zygomatic bone	8. okbenet
9. maxilla	9. överkäken
10. mandible	10. underkäken
11. coronal suture	11. hjässömmen, kronsömmen
12. lambdoidal suture	12. lambdasömmen, nacksömmen
13. mastoid process	13. vårtutskottet
14. styloid process	14. griffelutskottet
15. zygomatic arch	15. okbågen, kindbågen
16. external auditory meatus	16. yttre hörselgången

skurgummeknä ▷ **bursitis**

skvalpljud ▷ **succussion**

skvamös ▷ **squamous**

skybalum ▷ **scybalum**

skydd ▷ **barrier, cap, cover, covering, defence, protection**

skydda ▷ **cover, protect**

skyddande ▷ **protective**

skyddskräm ▷ **barrier**

skyddsympa ▷ **vaccinate**

skyddsympning ▷ **vaccination**

skymning ▷ **twilight**

skymt ▷ **occult**

skynda sig ▷ **hurry**

skyttegravsfot ▷ **immersion foot, trench fever**

skål ▷ **basin, bowl**

skåljärn ▷ **gouge**

skållskada ▷ **burn, scald**

skåp ▷ **cabinet**

skåra ▷ **incision, gash, slash**

skäggfinne ▷ **sycosis**

skäggsvamp ▷ **sycosis, tinea**

skäl ▷ **reason**

skälvning ▷ **thrill**

skänkel ▷ **crus, peduncle**

skära bort ▷ **resect**

skärm ▷ **screen**

skärpa ▷ **acuity**

skärsår ▷ **cut, incised, slash**

skärva ▷ **splinter**

sköld- ▷ **thyroid**

sköldbrosket ▷ **thyroid**

sköldbroskhornen ▷ **cornu**

sköldbrosks- ▷ **thyro-**

sköldkörtel- ▷ **thyro, thyroid**

sköldkörtelextrakt ▷ **thyroid**

sköldkörtelhormon ▷ **thyroid**

sköldkörtelinflammation ▷ **thyroiditis**

sköldkörteln ▷ **thyroid**

sköldkörtelsvullnad ▷ **thyrocele**

skölja ur (ren) ▷ **rinse out**

sköljkanna ▷ **douche, vaginal**

sköljning ▷ **douche, irrigation, lavage**

skör ▷ **brittle, delicate, fragile, frail**

skörbjugg ▷ **scorbutus**

skörbjuggs- ⇨ **scorbutic**

sköta ⇨ **attend, attend to, manage**

sköta om ⇨ **nurse**

sladdrig ⇨ **flabby, flaccid**

slag ⇨ **apoplexy, beat, ictus, knock, nature**

slaganfall ⇨ **apoplexy, cerebral, stroke**

slaggprodukt ⇨ **breakdown**

slagvolym ⇨ **stroke**

slang ⇨ **hose**

slank ⇨ **slim**

slapp ⇨ **flaccid, listless**

slapphet ⇨ **inertia, listlessness**

slappna av ⇨ **relax**

slash [slæʃ] **1** *subst.* long cut with a knife *långt skärsår, lång skåra, djupt hack;* **he had bruises on his face and slashes on his hands; the slash on her leg needs three stitches 2** *vb.* **(a)** to cut with a knife *or* sharp edge *skära (hugga, slitsa) upp;* **to slash one's wrists** = to try to kill oneself by cutting the blood vessels in the wrists *skära sig i handlederna* **(b)** to cut costs *or* spending sharply *skära ned (minska, reducera) kraftigt;* **the hospital building programme has been slashed**

SLE [ˌeselˈiː] = SYSTEMIC LUPUS ERYTHEMATOSUS

sleep [sliːp] **1** *subst.* resting (usually at night) when the eyes are closed and you are not conscious of what is happening *sömn;* **most people need eight hours' sleep each night; you need to get a good night's sleep if you have a lot of work to do tomorrow; he had a short sleep in the middle of the afternoon; to get to sleep** *or* **go to sleep** = to start sleeping *somna;* **don't make a noise, the baby is trying to go to sleep 2** *vb.* to be asleep *or* to rest with the eyes closed not knowing what is happening *sova;* **he always sleeps for eight hours each night; don't disturb him - he's trying to sleep** NOTE: **sleeps - sleeping - slept - has slept**

> COMMENT: sleep is a period when the body rests and rebuilds tissue, especially protein. Most adults need eight hours' sleep each night. Children require more (10 to 12 hours) but old people need less, possibly only four to six hours. Sleep forms a regular pattern of stages: during the first stage the person is still conscious of his surroundings, and will wake if he hears a noise; afterwards the sleeper goes into very deep sleep (slow-wave sleep), where the eyes are tightly closed, the pulse is regular and the sleeper breathes deeply. During this stage the pituitary gland produces the growth hormone somatotrophin. It is difficult to wake someone from deep sleep. This stage is followed by rapid eye movement sleep (REM sleep), where the sleeper's eyes are half open and move about, he makes facial movements, his blood pressure rises and he has dreams. After this stage he relapses into the first sleep stage again

sleeping pill [ˈsliːpɪŋ pɪl] *or* **sleeping tablet** [ˈsliːpɪŋ ˌtæblət] *subst.* drug (usually a barbiturate) which makes a person sleep *sömntablett, sömnpiller;* **she died of an overdose of sleeping tablets**

sleeping sickness [ˈsliːpɪŋ ˌsɪknəs] *or* **African trypanosomiasis** [ˈæfrɪk(ə)n traɪˌpænəʊsəʊˈmaɪəsɪs] *subst.* African disease, spread by the tsetse fly, where trypanosomes infest the blood *trypanos(omiasis), afrikansk sömnsjuka*

> COMMENT: symptoms are headaches, lethargy and long periods of sleep. The disease is fatal if not treated

sleeplessness [ˈsliːpləsnəs] *or* **insomnia** [ɪnˈsɒmniə] *subst.* being unable to sleep *insomni, sömnlöshet*

sleepwalker [ˈsliːpwɔːkə] = SOMNAMBULIST

sleepwalking [ˈsliːpwɔːkɪŋ] = SOMNAMBULISM

sleepy [ˈsliːpi] *adj.* feeling ready to go to sleep *sömnig;* **the children are very sleepy by 10 o'clock; sleepy sickness** *or* **lethargic encephalitis** = virus infection, a form of encephalitis which formerly occurred in epidemics *encephalitis epidemica (lethargica), sömnsjuka*
NOTE: **sleepy - sleepier - sleepiest** for other terms referring to sleep see words beginning with **hypn-, narco-**

slem ⇨ **mucus, phlegm, sputum**

slem- ⇨ **blenno-, muco-, mucous**

slemavsöndrande ⇨ **mucous**

slemcell ⇨ **mucous**

slemcysta ⇨ **mucocele**

slemfylld ⇨ **mucous**

slemhinna ⇨ **mucosa, mucous**

slemhinneförhårdning ⇨ **scleroma**

slemhinneinflammation ⇨ **catarrh**

slemhinnesvulst ⇨ **myxoma**

slemhinneutslag ⇨ **enanthema**

slemliknande ⇨ **mucoid**

slemlösande ⇨ **mucolytic**

slemlösande medel ⇨ **expectorant**

slemmig ⇨ **mucous**

slemsäck ⇨ **bursa**

slemsäcksinflammation ⇨ **bursitis**

slice [slaɪs] *subst.* thin flat piece of tissue which has been cut off *utsnitt, snitt, preparat;* **he examined the slice of brain tissue under the microscope**

slicka ⇨ **lick**

slid- ⇨ **colp-, vaginal, vagin(o)-**

slida ⇨ **sheath**

slidan ⇨ **vagina**

slide [slaɪd] **1** *subst.* piece of glass, on which a tissue sample is placed, to be examined under a microscope *objektglas* **2** *vb.* to move along smoothly *glida;* **the plunger slides up and down the syringe; sliding traction** = traction for a fracture of a femur, where weights are attached to pull the leg *slags glidsträck för behandling av lårbensbrott*

slidinflammation ⇨ **vaginitis**

slidpessar ⇨ **diaphragm, Dutch cap, pessary**

slidsköljning ⇨ **douche**

slidvalvet ⇨ **fornix**

slight [slaɪt] *adj.* not very serious *lätt, lindrig;* **he has a slight fever; she had a slight accident**
NOTE: **slight - slighter - slightest**

slim [slɪm] **1** *adj.* pleasantly thin *slank, smärt;* **she has become slim again after being pregnant 2** *vb.* to try to become thinner *or* to weight less *banta;* **he stopped eating bread when he was slimming; she is trying to slim before she goes on holiday; slimming diet** *or* **slimming food** = special diet *or* special food which is low in calories and which is supposed to stop a person getting fat *bantningsmat, bantningsdiet*

sling [slɪŋ] *subst.* triangular bandage attached round the neck, and wrapped round an injured arm to prevent it from moving *mitella;* **elevation sling** = sling tied round the neck, used to hold an injured hand or arm in a high position to prevent bleeding *mitella som håller armen i högläge*

slinga ⇨ **loop**

slipped disc [ˈslɪpt ˌdɪsk] *subst.* condition where a disc of cartilage separating two bones in the spine becomes displaced *or* where the soft centre of a disc passes through the hard cartilage outside and presses on a nerve *hernia disci intervertebralis, diskbråck, diskprolaps*

slitage ⇨ **wear and tear**

slitas ⇨ **wear**

slita sönder ⇨ **lancinate**

slitsår ⇨ **lacerated, laceration**

slough [slʌf] **1** *subst.* dead tissue (especially dead skin) which has separated from healthy tissue *dödkött, sårskorpa* **2** *vb.* to lose dead skin which falls off *ömsa skinn, förlora skorpa (dödkött)*

slow-wave sleep [ˈsləʊweɪv ˌsliːp] *subst.* period of sleep when the sleeper sleeps deeply and the eyes do not move *ortosömn*

> COMMENT: during slow-wave sleep, the pituitary gland secretes the hormone somatotrophin

slump ⇨ **accident**

slumra ⇨ **doze, drop off**

slumrande ⇨ **quiescent**

slut ⇨ **end, ending, termination, all over**

slut- ⇨ **final, terminal**

sluta ⇨ **end**

sluten fraktur ⇨ **simple**

slynga ⇨ **loop, snare**

slå ⇨ **beat, knock**

slå ut ⇨ **erupt**

släkt ⇨ **species**

släkt- ⇨ **generic**

släkt(ing) ⇨ **kin**

släktskap ⇨ **consanguinity**

"släng" ⇨ **bout**

släpande gång ⇨ **shuffling walk**

släppa sig (väder) ⇨ **wind**

slät ⇨ **smooth**

slö ⇨ **blunt; dozy, listless**

slöhet ⇨ **hebetude, listlessness, obtusion, torpor**

smak- ⇨ **gustatory**

smaka ⇨ **taste**

smaklök ⇨ **taste**

smak(sinnet) ⇨ **taste**

smal ⇨ **narrow, thin**

smalbenet ⇨ **shin bone**

small [smɔːl] *adj.* **(a)** not large *liten;* **his chest was covered with small red spots; she has a small cyst in the colon; small intestine** = section of the intestine from the stomach to the caecum, consisting of the duodenum, jejunum and ileum *tunntarmen;* **small stomach** = stomach which is reduced in size after an operation, making the patient unable to eat large meals *magsäck som minskats genom operation* **(b)** young *liten, ung;* **he had chickenpox when he was small; small children** = young children (between about 1 and 14 years of age) *barn mellan 1 och 14 år*

small of the back [ˌsmɔːl əv ðə ˈbæk] *subst.* middle part of the back between and below the shoulder blades *korsryggen, veka livet*

smallpox [ˈsmɔːlpɒks] *or* **variola** [vəˈra(ɪ)ələ] *subst.* formerly a very serious, usually fatal, contagious disease, caused by the poxvirus, with a severe rash, leaving masses of small scars on the skin *variola, smittkoppor*

> COMMENT: vaccination has proved effective in eradicating smallpox

smalna ⇨ **narrow**

smear [smɪə] *subst.* sample of soft tissue (such as blood *or* mucus) taken from a patient and spread over a glass slide to be examined under a microscope *smear(test), smearprov, utstryk;* **cervical smear** = test for cervical cancer, where cells taken from the mucus in the cervix of the uterus are examined *cervixsmear, utstryk från livmoderhalsen;* **smear test** = PAP TEST

smearprov ⇨ **smear**

smegma [ˈsmegmə] *subst.* oily secretion with an unpleasant smell, which collects on and under the foreskin of the penis *smegma*

smeka ⇨ **stroke**

smell [smel] **1** *subst.* one of the five senses *or* the sense which is felt through the nose *lukt(sinnet);* **dogs have a good sense of smell; the smell of flowers makes him sneeze 2** *vb.* **(a)** to notice the smell of something through the nose *känna lukten av;* **I can smell smoke; he can't smell anything because he's got a cold (b)** to produce a smell *lukta;* **it smells of gas in here** NOTE: **smells - smelling - smelled** *or* **smelt - has smelled** *or* **has smelt**

> COMMENT: the senses of smell and taste are closely connected, and together give the real taste of food. Smells are sensed by receptors in the nasal cavity which transmit impulses to the brain. When food is eaten, the smell is sensed at the same time as the taste is sensed by the taste buds, and most of what we think of as taste is in fact smell, which explains why food loses its taste when someone has a cold and a blocked nose

smelling salts [ˈsmelɪŋ sɔːlts] *subst. pl.* crystals of an ammonia compound, which give off a strong smell and can revive someone who has fainted *luktsalt*

smidig ⇨ **ductile, flexible**

Smith-Petersen nail [ˌsmɪθˈpiːtəs(ə)n ˌneɪl] *subst.* metal nail used to attach the fractured neck of a femur *slags spik använd vid lårbenshalsbrott (collumfraktur)*

smitta ⇨ **contagion, infection**

smittade föremål ⇨ **fomites**

smittande ⇨ **catching**

smittas av ⇨ **catch**

smittbärare ⇨ **carrier**

smittkoppor ⇨ **smallpox**

smittsam ⇨ **catching, contagious, infectious, infective**

smittsam gulsot ⇨ **jaundice**

smittsam sjukdom ⇨ **communicable disease**

smittskyddsvård ⇨ **barrier**

smittämne ⇨ **contagion, contaminant**

smog [smɒg] *subst.* pollution of the atmosphere in towns, caused by warm damp air combining with smoke and exhaust fumes from cars *smog*

smoke [sməʊk] **1** *subst.* white, grey or black product made of small particles, given off by something which is burning *rök;* **the room was full of cigarette smoke; several people died from inhaling toxic smoke 2** *vb.* to breathe in smoke from a cigarette, cigar, pipe, etc., which is held in the lips *röka;* **she was smoking a cigarette; he only smokes a pipe; doctors are trying to persuade people to stop smoking; smoking can injure your health**

COMMENT: the connection between smoking tobacco, especially cigarettes, and lung cancer has been proved to the satisfaction of the British government, which prints a health warning on all packets of cigarettes. Smoke from burning tobacco contains nicotine and other substances which stick in the lungs, and can in the long run cause cancer

QUOTE three quarters of patients aged 35-64 on GPs' lists have at least one major risk factor: high cholesterol, high blood pressure or addiction to tobacco. Of the three risk factors, smoking causes a quarter of heart disease deaths
Health Services Journal

smokeless ['sməʊkləs] *adj.* where there is no smoke *or* where smoke is not allowed *rökfri;* **smokeless** *or* **smoke-free area** = part of a public place (restaurant *or* aircraft, etc.) where smoking is not allowed *rökfritt område;* **smokeless fuel** = special fuel which does not make smoke when it is burnt *rökfritt bränsle;* **smokeless zone** = part of a town where open fires are not permitted *område där det är förbjudet att göra upp öppen eld*

smoker ['sməʊkə] *subst.* person who smokes cigarettes *rökare;* **smoker's cough** = dry asthmatic cough, often found in people who smoke large numbers of cigarettes *rökhosta*

smooth [smu:ð] **1** *adj.* flat *or* not rough *glatt, jämn, slät;* **smooth muscle** *or* **involuntary muscle** = muscle which moves without a person being aware of it, such as the muscle in the walls of the intestine which makes the intestine contract *glatt muskel; compare* STRIATED, VOLUNTARY MUSCLE
NOTE: **smooth - smoother - smoothest 2** *vb.* to make something smooth *jämna (släta) till;* **she smoothed down the sheets on the bed**

smuts ⇨ **dirt**

smutsa (ned) ⇨ **soil**

smutsig ⇨ **dirty**

småbarn ⇨ **infant**

smälta (mat) ⇨ **digest**

smärt ⇨ **slim**

smärta ⇨ **dolor, pain, pang, twinge**

smärtfri ⇨ **painless**

smärtfrihet ⇨ **analgesia**

smärtreceptor ⇨ **pain**

smärtsam ⇨ **painful**

smärtsam trängning ⇨ **tenesmus**

smärtstillande ⇨ **analgesic**

smärttröskel ⇨ **pain**

smörja ⇨ **lubricate**

smörjmedel ⇨ **lubricant**

snabb ⇨ **rapid**

snabb- ⇨ **crash**

snake [sneɪk] *subst.* long smooth animal with no legs which moves by sliding *orm;* **snake bite** = bite from a poisonous snake *ormbett*

snare [sneə] *subst.* surgical instrument made of a loop of wire, used to remove growths without the need of an incision *slynga;* **diathermy snare** = snare which is heated by electrodes and burns away tissue *diatermislynga*

snarka ➪ **snore**

snarkande ➪ **snoring, stertor**

snarkning ➪ **snore**

snava ➪ **trip**

sned ➪ **oblique**

snedfraktur ➪ **fracture, oblique**

snedskallighet ➪ **plagiocephaly**

snedtändning ➪ **trip**

sneeze [sniːz] **1** *subst.* reflex action to blow air suddenly out of the nose and mouth because of irritation in the nasal passages *nysning;* **she gave a loud sneeze 2** *vb.* to blow air suddenly out of the nose and mouth because of irritation in the nasal passages *nysa;* **the smell of flowers makes him sneeze; he was coughing and sneezing and decided to stay in bed**

> COMMENT: a sneeze sends out a spray of droplets of liquid, which, if infectious, can then infect anyone who happens to inhale them

sneezing fit ['sniːzɪŋ fɪt] *subst.* sudden attack when the patient sneezes many times *nysningsanfall*

Snellen chart ['snelən ˌtʃɑːt] *subst.* chart commonly used by opticians to test eyesight *slags ögontavla (med bokstäver);* **Snellen type** = different type sizes used on a Snellen chart *slags bokstäver använda på ögontavla*

> COMMENT: the Snellen chart has rows of letters, the top row being very large, and the bottom very small, with the result that the more rows a person can read, the better his eyesight

sniff [snɪf] **1** *subst.* breathing in air *or* smelling through the nose *inandning, snörvling, sniffning;* **they gave her a sniff of smelling salts to revive her 2** *vb.* to breathe in air *or* to smell through the nose *andas (dra) in (luft), snörvla, sniffa (lukta) (på), vädra;* **he was sniffing because he had a cold; she sniffed and said that she could smell smoke; he is coughing and sniffing and should be in bed**

sniffles ['snɪf(ə)lz] *subst. pl. (informal, used to children)* cold (when you sniff and sneeze) *snuva;* **don't go out into the cold when you have the sniffles**

sniffning ➪ **sniff**

sniffning (av lösningsmedel) ➪ **solvent**

snitt ➪ **cut, incision, section, slice**

-snitt ➪ **-tomy**

snor ➪ **snot**

snore [snɔː] **1** *subst.* loud noise produced in the nose and throat when asleep *snarkning* **2** *vb.* to make a loud noise in your nose and throat when you are asleep *snarka*

> COMMENT: a snore is produced by the vibration of the soft palate at the back of the mouth, and occurs when a sleeping person breathes through both mouth and nose

snoring ['snɔːrɪŋ] *subst.* making a series of snores *snarkande*

"snorrännan" ➪ **philtrum**

snot [snɒt] *subst. (informal)* mucus in the nose *snor*

snow [snəʊ] *subst.* water which falls as white flakes in cold weather *snö;* **snow blindness** = temporary painful blindness caused by bright sunlight shining on snow *ophthalmia nivalis, snöblindhet;* **carbon dioxide snow** = carbon dioxide which has been solidified at a very low temperature and is used in treating skin growths such as warts, or to preserve tissue samples *kolsyresnö, torris*

snubbla ➪ **trip**

snuffles ['snʌf(ə)lz] *subst. pl. (informal, used of small children)* breathing noisily through a nose which is blocked with mucus, which can sometimes be a sign of congenital syphilis *snörvlingar;* **have the snuffles** *vara täppt i näsan*

snuva ➪ **cold, rhinitis, sniffles**

snäckformig ➪ **spiral**

snäll ➪ **gentle**

snöblindhet ➪ **arc**

snörvla ➪ **sniff**

snörvling ➪ **sniff, snuffles**

soak [səʊk] *vb.* to put something in liquid, so that it absorbs some of it *blöta, lägga i blöt;*

use a compress made of cloth soaked in warm water

social ['səʊʃ(ə)l] *adj.* referring to society *or* to groups of people *social-, samhälls-; US* **social disease** = sexually transmitted disease *sexuellt överförd sjukdom, STD, könssjukdom, venerisk sjukdom, VS;* **social medicine** = medicine as applied to treatment of diseases which occur in certain social groups *socialmedicin;* **social security** = payments made by the government to people *or* families who need money *socialbidrag;* **social worker** = government official who works to improve living standards of groups (such as families) *socialarbetare, socialsekreterare*

socialarbetare ⇨ **social**

socialbidrag ⇨ **social, welfare**

socialdepartementet ⇨ **department**

socialförsäkring ⇨ **insurance**

socialmedicin ⇨ **community, social**

socialmedicinare ⇨ **community**

socialsekreterare ⇨ **social**

socker ⇨ **sugar**

socker- ⇨ **sacchar-**

sockerfri ⇨ **diabetic**

sockerhalt ⇨ **sugar**

sockersjuka ⇨ **diabetes**

socket ['sɒkɪt] *subst.* hollow part in a bone, into which another bone *or* organ fits *ledskål, ledpanna;* **the tip of the femur fits into a socket in the pelvis; ball and socket joint** *see* JOINT; **eye socket** *or* **orbit** = hollow bony depression in the front of the skull in which each eye is placed *orbita, ögonhålan*

soda ['səʊdə] *see* BICARBONATE

sodium ['səʊdiəm] *subst.* chemical element which is the basic substance in salt *natrium, Na;* **sodium balance** = balance maintained in the body between salt lost in sweat and urine and salt taken in from food, the balance is regulated by aldosterone *natriumbalans, saltbalans;* **sodium bicarbonate** = sodium salt used in cooking, also as a relief for indigestion and acidity *natriumbikarbonat;* **sodium chloride** = common salt *natriumklorid, koksalt, NaCl;* **sodium pump** = cellular process where sodium is immediately excreted from any cell which it enters and potassium is brought in *natrium(kalium)pumpen* NOTE: chemical symbol is **Na**

> COMMENT: salt is an essential mineral and exists in the extracellular fluid of the body. Sweat and tears also contain a high proportion of sodium chloride

sodokosis [ˌsəʊdəʊ'kəʊsɪs] *or* **sodoku** ['səʊdəʊku:] *subst.* form of rat-bite fever, but without swellings in the jaws *sodoku, råttbettsfeber, råttbettssjuka*

sodomy ['sɒdəmi] *subst.* anal sexual intercourse between men *sodomi, särskilt analsamlag mellan män*

soft [sɒft] *adj.* not hard *mjuk;* **soft palate** = back part of the palate, leading to the uvula *palatum molle, mjuka gommen;* **soft sore** *or* **soft chancre** *or* **chancroid** = infected sore in the groin caused by the venereal disease chancroid, but not a sign of syphilis *ulcus venereum simplex, ulcus molle, mjuk schanker* NOTE: **soft - softer - softest**

soften ['sɒf(ə)n] *vb.* to make *or* become soft *mjuka upp, lindra, mildra*

soil [sɔɪl] **1** *subst.* earth in which plants grow *jord* **2** *vb.* to make dirty *smutsa (ned), fläcka (ned);* **he soiled his sheets; soiled bedclothes are sent to the hospital laundry**

sol ⇨ **sun**

solarium [sə'leəriəm] *subst.* room where patients can lie under sun lamps *or* where patients can lie in the sun *solarium*

solar plexus [ˌsəʊlə 'pleksəs] *subst.* nerve network situated at the back of the abdomen between the adrenal glands *plexus solaris (coeliacus), solarplexus*

solbad ⇨ **heliotherapy, sunbathing**

solbehandling ⇨ **heliotherapy**

solblindhet ⇨ **blindness, photoretinitis**

solbränd ⇨ **sunburnt**

sole [səʊl] *subst.* part under the foot *fotsulan;* **the soles of the feet are very sensitive**

soleus ['səʊliəs] *subst.* flat muscle which goes down the calf of the leg *musculus soleus*

solglasögon ⇨ **sunglasses**

solid ['sɒlɪd] *adj.* hard *or* not liquid *solid, hel, fast;* **water turns solid when it freezes; solid food** *or* **solids** = food which is chewed and eaten, not drunk *fast föda;* **she is allowed some solid food** *or* **she is allowed to eat solids**

solidify [sə'lɪdɪfaɪ] *vb.* to become solid *stelna, övergå (överföra) till fast form;* **carbon dioxide solidifies at low temperatures**

solljus ⇨ **sunlight**

soln *abbreviation for* = SOLUTION

solsting ⇨ **sunstroke**

soluble ['sɒljʊb(ə)l] *adj.* which can dissolve *löslig, upplösbar;* **a tablet of soluble aspirin; soluble fibre** = fibre in vegetables, fruit and pulses and porridge oats, which is partly digested in the intestine and reduces the absorption of fats and sugar into the body, so lowering the level of cholesterol *lösliga fibrer*

solute ['sɒlju:t] *subst.* solid substance which is dissolved in a solvent to make a solution *(upp)löst ämne (substans)*

solution [sə'lu:ʃ(ə)n] *subst.* mixture of a solid substance dissolved in a liquid *solution, lösning;* **barium solution** = liquid solution containing barium sulphate which a patient drinks to increase the contrast of a stomach X-ray *bariumgröt, kontrast*

solvent ['sɒlv(ə)nt] *subst.* liquid in which a solid substance can be dissolved *lösningsmedel;* **solvent inhalation** *or* **solvent abuse** *or* **glue sniffing** = type of drug abuse where the addict inhales the toxic fumes given off by certain types of solvent *sniffning (av lösningsmedel)*

> QUOTE deaths among teenagers caused by solvent abuse have reached record levels
> **Health Visitor**

soma ['səʊmə] *subst.* the body (as opposed to the mind) *soma, kroppen*

somat- ['səʊmət, ,--] *or* **somato-** [səʊmətə(ʊ), ,---] *prefix* (i) referring to the body *somat(o)-, kropps-;* (ii) meaning somatic *somat(o)-, kropps-*

somatic [sə(ʊ)'mætɪk] *adj.* referring to the body (i) as opposed to the mind *somatisk, kroppslig;* (ii) as opposed to the intestines and inner organs *somatisk;* **somatic nerves** = sensory and motor nerves which control skeletal muscles *somatiska nerver; see also* PSYCHOSOMATIC

somatotrophic hormone [,səʊmətə'trɒfɪk ,hɔ:məʊn] *or* **somatotrophin** [,səʊmətə'trəʊfɪn] *subst.* growth hormone, secreted by the pituitary gland, which stimulates the growth of long bones *somatotropin, STH, (human) growth hormone, HGH, GH, tillväxthormon*

-some [səʊm] *suffix* referring to tiny cell bodies *-som*

somna ⇨ **fall asleep, sleep**

somnambul ⇨ **somnambulistic, somnambulist**

somnambulism [sɒm'næmbjulɪz(ə)m] *or* **sleepwalking** ['sli:pwɔ:kɪŋ] *subst.* condition affecting some people (especially children), where the person gets up and walks about while still asleep *somnambulism, sömngång*

somnambulist [sɒm'næmbjʊlɪst] *or* **sleepwalker** ['sli:pwɔ:kə] *subst.* person who walks in his sleep *somnambul, sömngångare*

somnambulistic [sɒm,næmbjʊ'lɪstɪk] *adj.* referring to sleepwalking *somnambul, sömngångar-*

somnolent ['sɒmnələnt] *adj.* sleepy *somnolent, sömnig*

somnolism ['sɒmnəlɪz(ə)m] *subst.* trance which is induced by hypnotism *trans orsakad av hypnos*

-somy [səʊmi] *suffix* referring to the presence of chromosomes *-somi*

son [sʌn] *subst.* male child of a parent *son;* **they have two sons and one daughter**

sond ⇨ **probe, sound**

sondera ⇨ **probe, sound**

sondmatning ⇨ **gavage**

sondotter ⇨ **granddaughter**

Sonne dysentery ['sɒnə ,dɪs(ə)ntri] *subst.* common form of mild dysentery in the UK, caused by Shigella sonnei *slags bacillär dysenteri*

sonogram ['səʊnəgræm] *subst.* chart produced using ultrasound waves to find where something is situated in the body *sonogram, registrering vid ultrasonografi (ultraljudsundersökning)*

sonoplacentography [ˌsəʊnəˌplæsən'tɒgrəfi] *subst.* use of ultrasound waves to find how the placenta is placed in a pregnant woman *ultraljudsundersökning av moderkakan*

sonotopography [ˌsəʊnətə'pɒgrəfi] *subst.* use of ultrasound waves to produce a sonogram *(ultra)sonografi, ultraljudsundersökning*

sonson ⇨ **grandson**

soothe [suːð] *vb.* to relieve pain *lindra, mildra, stilla;* **the calamine lotion will soothe the rash**

soothing ['suːðɪŋ] *adj.* which relieves pain *or* makes someone less tense *lindrande, lugnande;* **they played soothing music in the dentist's waiting room**

soporific [ˌsɒpə'rɪfɪk] *subst. & adj.* (drug) which makes a person go to sleep *hypnotiskt (medel), hypnotikum, sömnmedel*

sordes ['sɔːdiːz] *subst. pl.* dry deposits round the lips of a patient suffering from fever *krustor på läpparna hos febrig patient*

sore [sɔː] **1** *subst.* small wound on any part of the skin, usually with a discharge of pus *sår;* **cold sore** *or* **herpes simplex** = burning sore, usually on the lips *herpes simplex (labialis);* **running sore** = sore which is discharging pus *vätskande sår, varigt sår;* **soft sore** = infected sore in the groin, sign of a venereal disease *ulcus venerum simplex, ulcus molle, mjuk schanker; see also* BEDSORE **2** *adj.* rough and inflamed (skin) *öm;* painful (muscle); **sore throat** = condition where the mucous membrane in the throat is inflamed (sometimes because the patient has been talking too much, but usually because of an infection) *ont i halsen, halsont*

sort ⇨ **nature, strain**

s.o.s. [ˌesəʊ'es] *abbreviation for the Latin phrase* "si opus sit": if necessary (written on a prescription to show that the dose should be taken once) *si opus sit*

sota ⇨ **unblock**

sotning ⇨ **endarterectomy, rebore**

souffle ['suːf(ə)l] *subst.* soft breathing sound, heard through a stethoscope *blåsljud*

sound [saʊnd] **1** *subst.* **(a)** something which can be heard *ljud, ton;* **the doctor listened to the sounds of the patient's lungs; his breathing made a whistling sound (b)** long rod, used to examine *or* to dilate the inside of a cavity in the body *sond* **2** *adj.* strong and healthy *sund, frisk;* **he has a sound constitution; her heart is sound, but her lungs are congested 3** *vb.* **(a)** to make a noise *ljuda, låta;* **her lungs sound as if she had pneumonia (b)** to examine the inside of a cavity using a rod *sondera*

sour ['sa(ʊ)ə] *adj.* one of the basic tastes, not bitter, salt or sweet *sur*

source [sɔːs] *subst.* substance which produces something; place where something comes from *källa, ursprung, upphov;* **sugar is a source of energy; vegetables are important sources of vitamins; the source of the allergy has been identified; the medical team has isolated the source of the infection**

sova ⇨ **sleep**

sovande ⇨ **asleep**

soya ['sɔɪə] *subst.* plant which produces edible beans which have a high protein and fat content and very little starch *soja*

space [speɪs] *subst.* place *or* empty area between things *plats, utrymme, mellanrum, håla;* **an abscess formed in the space between the bone and the cartilage; write your name in the space at the top of the form; dead space** = breath in the last part of the inspiration which does not get further than the bronchial tubes *dead space, döda rummet, skadliga rummet*

-spalt ⇨ **-schisis**

spansk krage ⇨ **paraphimosis**

spara ⇨ **keep**

spara på ⇨ **conserve**

spare [speə] **1** *adj.* extra *or* which is only used in emergencies *extra, reserv-;* **we have no spare beds in the hospital at the moment; the doctor carries a spare set of instruments in his car; spare part surgery** = surgery where parts of the body (such as bones *or* joints) are replaced by artificial pieces *reservdelskirurgi* **2** *vb.* to be able to give *or* spend *avvara, undvara;* **can you spare the time to see the next patient? we have only one bed to spare at the moment**

sparganosis [ˌspɑːgə'nəʊsɪs] *subst.* condition caused by the larvae of the worm Sparganum under the skin (it is widespread in the Far East) *slags hudsjukdom orsakad av larv*

spark ⇨ **kick**

sparka ⇨ **kick**

"sparkarna", första ⇨ **quickening**

spasm ['spæz(ə)m] *subst.* sudden, usually painful, involuntary contraction of a muscle (as in cramp) *spasm, kramp, ryckning;* **the muscles in his leg went into spasm; she had painful spasms in her stomach; clonic spasms** = spasms which recur regularly; *(of a muscle) kloniska (muskel)kramper;* **to go into spasm** = to begin to contract *börja dra ihop sig (kontraheras)*

spasmo- ['spæzmə(ʊ), ˌ--] *prefix* referring to a spasm *spasmo-, kramp-*

spasmodic [spæz'mɒdɪk] *adj.* (i) which occurs in spasms *spastisk, krampartad, ryckig;* (ii) which happens from time to time *sporadisk*

spasmolytic [ˌspæzmə(ʊ)'lɪtɪk] *subst.* drug which relieves muscle spasms *spasmolytisk, kramplösande*

spasmus nutans ['spæzməs 'nju:təns] *subst.* condition where the patient nods his head and at the same time has spasms in the neck muscles and rapid movements of the eyes *spasmus nutans, nickningskramp, salaamkramp, infantil spasm*

spastic ['spæstɪk] **1** *adj.* (i) with spasms *or* sudden contractions of muscles *spastisk, krampartad, ryckig;* (ii) referring to cerebral palsy *spastisk;* **spastic colon** = MUCOUS COLITIS; **spastic diplegia** *or* **Little's disease** = congenital form of cerebral palsy which affects mainly the legs *diplegia spastica infantilis, Littles sjukdom;* **spastic gait** = way of walking where the legs are stiff and the feet not lifted off the ground *spastisk gång;* **spastic paralysis** *or* **cerebral palsy** = disorder of the brain affecting spastics, due to brain damage which has occurred before birth *cerebral pares, CP, spastisk förlamning;* **spastic paraplegia** = paralysis of one side of the body after a stroke *spastisk paraplegi* **2** *subst.* **a spastic** = patient suffering from cerebral palsy *en spastiker*

spasticity [spæ'stɪsəti] *subst.* condition where a limb resists passive movement *spasticitet; see also* RIGIDITY

spastisk ⇨ **spasmodic, spastic**

spastisk kolit ⇨ **mucous**

spatel ⇨ **depressor**

speak [spi:k] *vb.* to say words *or* to talk *tala;* **he is learning to speak again after a laryngectomy** NOTE: **speaks - speaking - spoke - has spoken**

speak up [ˌspi:k 'ʌp] *vb.* to speak louder *tala högre;* **speak up, please - I can't hear you!**

special ['speʃ(ə)l] *adj.* which refers to one particular thing *or* which is not ordinary *speciell, särskild, special-;* **he has been given a special diet to cure his allergy; she wore special shoes to correct a defect in her ankles; special care baby unit** = unit in a hospital which deals with premature babies *or* babies with serious disorders *ung. neonatalavdelning;* **special hospital** = hospital for dangerous mental patients *ung. mentalsjukhus;* **special school** = school for children who are handicapped *specialskola för handikappade (utvecklingsstörda)*

specialisering ⇨ **specialization**

specialist ['speʃ(ə)lɪst] *subst.* doctor who specializes in a certain branch of medicine *specialist;* **he is a heart specialist; she was referred to an ENT specialist**

specialistläkare ⇨ **consultancy, registrar**

specialitet ⇨ **specialization, specialty**

specialization [ˌspeʃ(ə)laɪ'zeɪʃ(ə)n, -ʃəlɪ'z-] *subst.* (i) act of specializing in a certain branch of medicine *specialisering;* (ii) particular branch of medicine which a doctor specializes in *specialitet*

specialize in ['speʃəlaɪz ɪn] *vb.* to study *or* to treat one particular disease *or* one particular type of patient *specialisera sig på (inom), bli specialist på (inom);* **he specializes in children with breathing problems; she decided to specialize in haematology**

specialty ['speʃ(ə)lti] *subst.* particular branch of medicine *specialitet*

speciell ⇨ **special**

species ['spi:ʃi:z] *subst.* division of a genus *or* group of living things which can interbreed *art, släkt*

specific [spə'sɪfɪk] **1** *adj.* particular *or* (disease) caused by one microbe *specifik, som orsakas av viss specifik mikroorganism;* **specific urethritis** = inflammation of the urethra caused by gonorrhoea *gonorroisk uretrit; see also* NON-SPECIFIC **2** *subst.*

drug which is used to treat a particular disease *specifikum, specifikt medel*

specificity [ˌspesɪˈfɪsəti] *subst.* rate of negative responses in a test from persons free from a disease (a high specificity means a low rate of false positives) *andel negativa svar från friska personer på ett prov; compare with* SENSITIVITY

specifikum ⇨ **specific**

specimen [ˈspesəmɪn] *subst.* (i) small quantity of something given for testing *specimen, prov, preparat;* (ii) one item out of a group *specimen, prov, exemplar;* **he was asked to bring a urine specimen; we keep specimens of diseased organs for students to examine**

spectacles [ˈspektək(ə)lz] *subst pl.* glasses which are worn in front of the eyes to help correct defects in vision *glasögon;* **the optician said he needed a new pair of spectacles; she was wearing a pair of spectacles with gold frames**

> COMMENT: spectacles can correct defects in the focusing of the eye, such as shortsightedness, longsightedness and astigmatism. Where different lenses are required for reading, an optician may prescribe two pairs of spectacles, one for normal use and the other reading glasses. Otherwise, spectacles can be fitted with a divided lens (bifocals)

spectrography [spekˈtrɒgrəfi] *subst.* recording of a spectrum on photographic film *spektrografi*

spectroscope [ˈspektrəskəʊp] *subst.* instrument used to analyse a spectrum *spektroskop*

spectrum [ˈspektrəm] *subst.* (i) range of colours (from red to violet) into which white light can be split (different substances in solution have different spectra) *(färg)spektrum;* (ii) range of diseases which an antibiotic can be used to treat *spektrum, bakteriespektrum*

> QUOTE narrow-spectrum compounds have a significant advantage over broad-spectrum ones in that they do not upset the body's normal flora to the same extent
>
> **British Journal of Hospital Medicine**

speculum [ˈspekjʊləm] *subst.* surgical instrument which is inserted into an opening in the body (such as the vagina) to keep it open, and allow a doctor to examine the inside *spekulum*
NOTE: plural is **specula, speculums**

speech [spiːtʃ] *subst.* making intelligible sounds with the vocal cords *tal, talförmåga;* **speech block** = temporary inability to speak, caused by the effect of nervous stress on the mental processes *talhämning, talblockering;* **speech impediment** = condition where a person cannot speak properly because of a deformed mouth or tongue *talfel, talrubbning;* **speech therapist** = qualified person who practises speech therapy *talpedagog, logoped;* **speech therapy** = treatment to cure a speech disorder such as stammering *talterapi, logopedisk behandling*

spegelvändning ⇨ **situs inversus viscerum**

spektrografi ⇨ **spectrography**

spektroskop ⇨ **spectroscope**

spektrum ⇨ **spectrum**

spekulum ⇨ **speculum**

spell [spel] *subst.* short period *attack, anfall;* **she has dizzy spells; he had two spells in hospital during the winter**

sperm [spɜːm] *subst.* spermatozoon *or* male sex cell *spermie, spermatozo, sädescell, sädeskropp;* **sperm bank** = place where sperm can be stored for use in artificial insemination *spermabank;* **sperm count** = calculation of the number of sperm in a quantity of semen *spermieräkning;* **sperm duct** *or* **vas deferens** = tube along which sperm pass from the epididymis to the prostate gland *(vas) ductus deferens, sädesledaren* NOTE: no plural for **sperm: there are millions of sperm in each ejaculation**

> COMMENT: a human spermatozoon is very small, and is formed of a head, neck and very long tail. A spermatozoon can swim by moving its tail from side to side. The sperm are formed in the testis and ejaculated through the penis. Each ejaculation may contain millions of sperm. Once a sperm has entered the female uterus, it remains viable for about three days

sperm- [ˈspɜːm, ˌ-] *or* **spermi(o)-** [ˈspɜːmiəʊ, ˌ--] *or* **spermo-** [ˈspɜːmə(ʊ), ˌ--] *prefix* referring to sperm and semen *sperm(o)-, spermi(o)-, spermat(o)-, sädes-*

sperma ⇨ **semen**

spermabank ⇨ **sperm**

spermat- [ˈspɜːmət, ˌ--] *or* **spermato-** [ˈspɜːmətə(ʊ), ˌ---] *prefix* referring to (i) sperm *spermat(o)-, sperm(o)-, spermi(o)-,* *sädes-;* (ii) the male reproductive system *spermat(o)-*

spermatic [spɜːˈmætɪk] *adj.* referring to sperm *spermatisk;* **spermatic artery** = artery which leads into the testes *arteria testicularis;* **spermatic cord** = cord running from the testis to the abdomen carrying the vas deferens, the blood vessels, nerves and lymphatics of the testis *funiculus spermaticus, sädessträngen*

spermatid [ˈspɜːmətɪd] *subst.* immature cell, formed from a spermatocyte, which becomes a spermatozoon *spermatid, spermid*

spermatisk ⇨ **spermatic**

spermatocele [ˈspɜːmətəsiː(ə)l] *subst.* cyst which forms in the scrotum *spermatocele*

spermatocyte [ˈspɜːmətə(ʊ)saɪt] *subst.* early stage in the development of a spermatozoon *spermatocyt, spermiocyt*

spermatogenesis [ˌspɜːmətə(ʊ)ˈdʒenəsɪs] *subst.* formation and development of spermatozoa in the testes *spermatogenes*

spermatogonium [ˌspɜːmətəˈgəʊniəm] *subst.* cell which forms a spermatocyte *spermatogonium, spermiogon*

spermatorré ⇨ **polyspermia, spermatorrhoea**

spermatorrhoea [ˌspɜːmətə(ʊ)ˈrɪə] *subst.* discharge of a large amount of semen frequently and without an orgasm *spermatorré, polyspermi, ofrivillig sädesavgång*

spermatozo ⇨ **sperm, spermatozoon**

spermatozoon [ˌspɜːmətəˈzəʊɒn] *or* **sperm** [spɜːm] *subst.* mature male sex cell, which is ejaculated from the penis and is capable of fertilizing an ovum *spermatozo, spermie, sädescell, sädeskropp* NOTE: plural is **spermatozoa**

spermaturi ⇨ **spermaturia**

spermaturia [ˌspɜːməˈtjʊəriə] *subst.* sperm in the urine *spermaturi*

spermicid ⇨ **spermicidal, spermicide**

spermicidal [ˌspɜːmɪˈsaɪd(ə)l] *adj.* which can kill sperm *spermicid, spermiedödande*

spermicide [ˈspɜːmɪsaɪd] *subst.* substance which kills sperm *spermicid, spermiedödande medel*

spermid ⇨ **spermatid**

spermie ⇨ **sperm, spermatozoon**

spermiedödande ⇨ **spermicidal**

spermieräkning ⇨ **sperm**

spermi(o)- ⇨ **sperm-, spermat-**

spermiocyt ⇨ **spermatocyte**

spermiogon ⇨ **spermatogonium**

sperm(o)- ⇨ **sperm-, spermat-**

spets ⇨ **point**

spetsig ⇨ **pointed**

spetälska ⇨ **leprosy**

spheno- [ˈsfiːnə(ʊ), ˌ--] *prefix* referring to the sphenoid bone *spheno-, sfeno-, kilbens-*

sphenoid bone [ˈsfiːnɔɪd ˌbəʊn] *subst.* one of two bones in the skull which form the side of the socket of the eye *os sphenoidale, kilbenet;* **sphenoid sinus** *or* **sphenoidal sinus** = one of the sinuses in the skull behind the nasal passage *sinus sphenoidalis, kilbenshålan;* **sphenopalatine ganglion** = ganglion in the pterygopalatine fossa associated with maxillary sinus *ganglion pterygopalatinum (sphenopalatinum)*

spherocyte [ˈsfɪərəʊsaɪt] *subst.* abnormal round red blood cell *sfärocyt*

spherocytosis [ˌsfɪərəʊsaɪˈtəʊsɪs] *subst.* condition where a patient has spherocytes in his blood, causing anaemia, enlarged spleen and gallstones, as in acholuric jaundice *sfärocytos*

sphincterectomy [ˌsfɪŋ(k)təˈrektəmi] *subst.* surgical operation to remove (i) a sphincter *operativt avlägsnande av sfinkter;* (ii) part of the edge of the iris in the eye *sfinkterektomi, iridektomi, korektomi*

sphincter (muscle) [ˈsfɪŋ(k)tə (ˌmʌs(ə)l)] *subst.* ring of muscle at the opening of a passage in the body, which can contract to close the passage *musculus sphincter, sfinkter, ringmuskel;* **anal sphincter** = ring of muscle which closes the anus *(musculus) sphincter ani, analsfinktern;* **pyloric sphincter** = muscle which surrounds the pylorus, makes it contract and separates it from the duodenum *(musculus) sphincter pylori, pylorussfinktern;* **sphincter pupillae muscle** = annular muscle in the iris which constricts the pupil *(musculus) sphincter pupillae, pupillsfinktern*

sphincteroplasty ['sfɪŋ(k)tərə,plæsti] *subst.* surgery to relieve a tightened sphincter *sfinkteroplastik*

sphincterotomy [,sfɪŋ(k)tə'rɒtəmi] *subst.* surgical operation to make an incision into a sphincter *sfinkterotomi*

sphyg [sfɪg] *subst. informal* = SPHYGMOMANOMETER

sphygmo- ['sfɪgmə(ʊ), ,--] *prefix* referring to the pulse *sfygmo-, puls-*

sphygmocardiograph [,sfɪgmə(ʊ)'kɑːdiə(ʊ)grɑːf] *subst.* device which records heartbeats and pulse rate *sfygmograf*

sphygmograph ['sfɪgmə(ʊ)grɑːf] *subst.* device which records the pulse *slags pulsmätare*

sphygmomanometer [,sfɪgməʊmə'nɒmɪtə] *subst.* instrument which measures blood pressure in the arteries *blodtrycksmätare*

COMMENT: the sphygmomanometer is a rubber sleeve connected to a scale with a column of mercury, allowing the nurse to take a reading; the rubber sleeve is usually wrapped round the arm and inflated until the blood flow is stopped; the blood pressure is determined by listening to the pulse with a stethoscope placed over an artery as the pressure in the rubber sleeve is slowly reduced, and by the reading on the scale

spica ['spaɪkə] *subst.* way of bandaging a joint where the bandage criss-crosses over itself like the figure 8 on the inside of the bend of the joint *förband med åttatalsturer*

spicule ['spɪkjuːl] *subst.* small splinter of bone *spicula, bentagg*

spina bifida [,spaɪnə 'bɪfɪdə] *or* **rachischisis** [reɪ'kɪskɪsɪs] *subst.* serious condition where the backbone and spinal cord has a gap in it, allowing the spinal cord to pass through *spina bifida, rakischis*

COMMENT: spina bifida takes two forms: a mild form, spina bifida occulta, where only the bone is affected, and there are no visible signs of the condition; and the serious spina bifida cystica where part of the meninges *or* spinal cord passes through the gap; it may result in paralysis of the legs, and mental retardation is often present where the condition is associated with hydrocephalus

spinal ['spaɪn(ə)l] *adj.* referring to the spine *spinal-, ryggrads-, ryggmärgs-;* **he has spinal problems; she suffered spinal injuries in the crash; spinal accessory nerve** = eleventh cranial nerve which supplies the muscles in the neck and shoulders *nervus accessorius, 11:e kranialnerven;* **spinal anaesthesia** = anaesthesia (subarachnoid *or* epidural) of one part of the body only, caused by injecting an anaesthetic into the space around the spinal cord *spinalanestesi, spinalbedövning;* **spinal block** = reduction of pain by giving a spinal anaesthetic *spinalblockad;* **spinal canal** *or* **vertebral canal** = hollow running down the back of the vertebrae, containing the spinal cord *canalis vertebralis, spinalkanalen, vertebralkanalen, ryggradskanalen;* **spinal column** = backbone *or* spine *or* vertebral column *columna spinalis (vertebralis), kotpelaren, ryggraden;* **spinal cord** = part of the central nervous system running from the medulla oblongata to the filum terminale; in the vertebral canal of the spine *medulla spinalis, ryggmärgen;* **spinal curvature** *or* **curvature of the spine** = abnormal bending of the spine *onormal krökning på ryggraden;* **spinal fusion** = surgical operation to join two vertebrae together to make the spine more rigid *fusionsoperation;* **spinal nerves** = 31 pairs of nerves which lead from the spinal cord *nervi spinales, spinalnerverna;* **spinal puncture** *or* **lumbar puncture** *or* *US* **spinal tap** = surgical operation to remove a sample of cerebrospinal fluid by inserting a hollow needle into the lower part of the spinal canal *spinalpunktion, lumbalpunktion*

NOTE: for terms referring to the spinal cord, see words beginning with **myel-, myelo-, rachi-, rachio-**

spinal- ⇨ **spinal, spino-**

spinalanestesi ⇨ **anaesthetic, spinal**

spinalbedövning ⇨ **anaesthetic, spinal**

spinalblockad ⇨ **spinal**

spinalblödning ⇨ **haematomyelia**

spinalganglion ⇨ **ganglion**

spinalkanalen ⇨ **spinal**

spinalnerverna ⇨ **spinal**

spinalpunktion ⇨ **spinal**

spinalutskott ⇨ **spinous process**

spindelfiber ⇨ **spindle**

spindelfingrar ⇨ **arachnodactyly**

spindelvävshinnan ⇨ **arachnoid mater**

spindle ['spɪnd(ə)l] *subst.* long thin structure *spindel (i maskin), slända, spole;* **spindle fibre** = one of the elements visible during cell division *spindelfiber;* **muscle spindles** = sensory receptors which lie along striated muscle fibres *muskelspolar*

spine [spaɪn] *subst.* (i) backbone *or* series of bones linked together to form a flexible column running from the pelvis to the skull *spina, ryggraden;* (ii) any sharp projecting part of a bone *kam, utskott, tagg;* **she injured her spine** *or* **she had spine injuries in the crash; spine of the scapula** = ridge on the posterior face of the scapula ⇨ *illustration* SHOULDER *spina scapulae, skulderbladskammen*

> COMMENT: the spine is made up of twenty-four ring-shaped vertebrae, with the sacrum and coccyx, separated by discs of cartilage. The hollow canal of the spine (the spinal canal) contains the spinal cord. See also note at VERTEBRA

spino- ['spaɪnə(ʊ), ˌ--] *prefix* referring to (i) the spine *spino-, spinal-, ryggrads-;* (ii) the spinal cord *spino-, spinal-, ryggmärgs-*

spinocerebellar tracts [ˌspaɪnəʊˌserə'belə ˌtrækts] *subst. pl.* nerve fibres in the spinal cord, taking impulses to the cerebellum *spinocerebellära banorna*

spinous process ['spaɪnəs ˌprəʊses] *subst.* projection on a vertebra *or* a bone, that looks like a spine ⇨ *illustration* VERTEBRAL COLUMN *processus spinosus, spinalutskott, ryggkoteutskott*

spiral ['spaɪ(ə)r(ə)l] *adj.* which runs in a continuous circle upwards *spiral-, snäckformig;* **spiral bandage** = bandage which is wrapped round a limb, each turn overlapping the one before *förband med överlappande turer (åttatalsturer);* **spiral ganglion** = ganglion in the eighth cranial nerve which supplies the organ of Corti *ganglion spirale, hörselnervsganglion;* **spiral organ** = ORGAN OF CORTI

spiral ⇨ **coil, intrauterine, loop**

spiral- ⇨ **spiral**

spiralleder ⇨ **joint**

Spirillum [spɪ'rɪləm] *subst.* one of the bacteria which cause rat-bite fever *Spirillum (se sodokosis)*

spirit ['spɪrɪt] *subst.* strong mixture of alcohol and water *sprit, alkohol;* **methylated spirit** = almost pure alcohol, with wood alcohol and colouring added *denaturerad sprit;* **surgical spirit** = ethyl alcohol with an additive giving it an unpleasant taste, used as a disinfectant *or* for cleansing the skin *tvättsprit, ryggsprit*

spiro- ['spaɪ(ə)rə(ʊ), ˌ--] *prefix* referring to (i) a spiral *spiro-;* (ii) the respiration *spiro-*

spirochaetaemia [ˌspaɪ(ə)rə(ʊ)kɪ'tiːmiə] *subst.* presence of spirochaetes in the blood *närvaro av spiroketer i blodet*

spirochaete ['spaɪ(ə)rə(ʊ)kiːt] *or US* **spirochete** ['spaɪ(ə)rə(ʊ)kiːt] *subst.* bacterium with a spiral shape, such as that which causes syphilis *spiroket*

spirogram ['spaɪ(ə)rə(ʊ)græm] *subst.* record of a patient's breathing made by a spirograph *spirogram*

spirograph ['spaɪ(ə)rə(ʊ)grɑːf] *subst.* device which records depth and rapidity of breathing *slags utrustning för lungfunktionstest*

spirography [spaɪ(ə)'rɒgrəfi] *subst.* recording of a patient's breathing by use of a spirograph *slags lungfunktionstest*

spiroket ⇨ **spirochete**

spirometer [ˌspaɪ(ə)'rɒmɪtə] *subst.* instrument which measures how much air a person inhales or exhales *spirometer*

spirometry [spaɪ(ə)'rɒmətri] *subst.* measurement of the vital capacity of the lungs by use of a spirometer *spirometri*

spit [spɪt] **1** *subst.* saliva which is sent out of the mouth *spott* **2** *vb.* to send liquid out of the mouth *spotta;* **rinse your mouth out and spit into the cup provided; he spat out the medicine**
NOTE: **spitting - spat - has spat**

Spitz-Holter valve [ˌspɪts'hɒltə ˌvælv] *subst.* valve with a one-way system, surgically placed in the skull, and used to drain fluid from the brain in hydrocephalus *Spitz-Holters shunt (ventil)*

spjäla ⇨ **brace, caliper, splint**

spjälkat hudtransplantat ⇨ **flap**

splanchnic ['splæŋknɪk] *adj.* referring to viscera *splankno-, inälvs-;* **splanchnic nerve** = any sympathetic nerve which supplies organs in the abdomen *nervus splanchnicus, inälvsnerv*

splanchnology [splæŋk'nɒlədʒi] *subst.* special study of the organs in the abdominal cavity *splanknologi*

splankno- ⇨ **splanchnic**

splanknologi ⇨ **splanchnology**

spleen [spli:n] *subst.* organ in the top part of the abdominal cavity behind the stomach and below the diaphragm ⇨ *illustration* DIGESTIVE SYSTEM *lien, mjälten*

COMMENT: the spleen, which is the largest endocrine (ductless) gland, appears to act to remove dead blood cells and fight infection, but its functions are not fully understood and an adult can live normally after his spleen has been removed

splen- [splə'n] *or* **spleno-** ['spli:nə(ʊ), ,--] *prefix* referring to the spleen *splen(o)-, mjält-*

splenectomy [sple'nektəmi] *subst.* surgical operation to remove the spleen *splenektomi*

splenic ['splenɪk] *adj.* referring to the spleen *lienal, mjält-;* **splenic anaemia** *or* **Banti's syndrome** = type of anaemia where the patient has portal hypertension and an enlarged spleen caused by cirrhosis of the liver *hepatolienal fibros, Bantis sjukdom (syndrom);* **splenic flexure** = bend in the colon, where the transverse colon joins the descending colon *flexura coli sinistra (coli lienalis)*

splenitis [splə'naɪtɪs] *subst.* inflammation of the spleen *splenit, mjältinflammation*

splenomegaly [,spli:nəʊ'meg(ə)li] *subst.* condition where the spleen is abnormally large, associated with several disorders including malaria and some cancers *splenomegali, mjältförstoring*

splenorenal anastomosis [,spli:nəʊ'ri:n(ə)l ə,næstə'məʊsɪs] *subst.* surgical operation to join the splenic vein to a renal vein, as a treatment for portal hypertension *splenorenal venanastomos*

splenovenography [,spli:nəʊvə'nɒgrəfi] *subst.* X-ray examination of the spleen and the veins which are connected to it *röntgenundersökning av mjälten och dess vener*

splint [splɪnt] *subst.* stiff support attached to a limb to prevent a broken bone from moving *spjäla, skena;* **he had to keep his arm in a splint for several weeks** *see also* BRAUN'S SPLINT, DENIS BROWNE SPLINT, FAIRBANKS' SPLINT, THOMAS'S SPLINT

splinter ['splɪntə] *subst.* tiny thin piece of wood *or* metal which gets under the skin and can be irritating and cause infection *flisa, skärva, sticka, splitter*

split [splɪt] *vb.* to divide *dela, klyva*

split-skin graft [,splɪt'skɪn ,grɑ:ft] *or* **Thiersch graft** ['tɪəʃ ,grɑ:ft] *subst.* type of skin graft where thin layers of skin are grafted over a wound *hudtransplantat för thierschning, slags delhudstransplantat*

splitter ⇨ **splinter**

splitterbrott ⇨ **comminuted fracture**

spole ⇨ **spindle**

spolformad ⇨ **fusiform**

spolmasken, vanliga ⇨ **Ascaris lumbricoides**

spolmaskinfektion ⇨ **ascariasis**

spolning ⇨ **irrigation**

spondyl ['spɒndɪl] *subst.* a vertebra *ryggkota, kota*

spondyl- ['spɒndɪl, ,--] *or* **spondylo-** ['spɒndɪlə(ʊ), ,---] *prefix* referring to the vertebrae *spondyl(o)-, kot-*

spondylitis [,spɒndɪ'laɪtɪs] *subst.* inflammation of the vertebrae *spondylit, ryggradsinflammation;* **ankylosing spondylitis** = condition with higher incidence in young men, where the vertebrae and sacroiliac joints are inflamed and become stiff *spondylarthritis ancylopo(i)etica, Bechterews sjukdom, pelvospondylit*

spondylolisthesis [,spɒndɪlə(ʊ)'lɪsθəsɪs] *subst.* condition where one of the lumbar vertebrae moves forward over the one beneath *spondylolistes, kotförskjutning*

spondylosis [ˌspɒndɪˈləʊsɪs] *subst.* stiffness in the spine and degenerative changes in the intervertebral discs, with osteoarthritis (it is common in older people) *spondylos*

sponge bath [ˈspʌn(d)ʒ bɑːθ] *subst.* washing a a patient in bed, using a sponge *or* damp cloth *helavtvättning;* **the nurse gave the old lady a sponge bath**

spongioblastoma [ˌspʌn(d)ʒiəʊblæˈstəʊmə] *subst.* = GLIOBLASTOMA

spongiosum [ˌspʌn(d)ʒɪˈəʊsəm] *see* CORPUS

spongiös ⇨ **spongy**

spongy [ˈspʌn(d)ʒi] *adj.* soft and full of holes like a sponge *spongiös, porös;* **spongy bone** = the soft inner core of a bone, containing the marrow *pars spongiosa, porös benvävnad, spongiöst ben*

spontaneous [spɒnˈteɪniəs] *adj.* which happens without any particular outside cause *spontan;* **spontaneous abortion** = MISCARRIAGE

spontan pneumotorax ⇨ **pneumothorax**

spoon [spuːn] *subst.* instrument with a long handle at one end and a small bowl at the other, used for taking liquid medicine *sked;* **a 5 ml spoon**

spoonful [ˈspuːnfʊl] *subst.* quantity which a spoon can hold *sked (som mått);* **take two 5 ml spoonfuls of the medicine twice a day**

sporadic [spəˈrædɪk] *adj.* (disease) where outbreaks occur as separate cases, not in epidemics *sporadisk, enstaka, spridd*

sporadisk ⇨ **spasmodic, sporadic**

spordjur ⇨ **Sporozoa**

spordödande ⇨ **sporicidal**

spore [spɔː] *subst.* reproductive body of certain bacteria which can survive in extremely hot or cold conditions for a long time *spor*

sporicidal [ˌspɔːrɪˈsaɪd(ə)l] *adj.* which kills spores *sporicid, spordödande*

sporicide [ˈspɔːrɪsaɪd] *subst.* substance which kills bacterial spores *spordödande medel*

sporotrichosis [ˌspɔːrə(ʊ)traɪˈkəʊsɪs] *subst.* fungus infection of the skin which causes abscesses *sporotrikos*

Sporozoa [ˌspɔːrəˈzəʊə] *subst.* type of parasitic Protozoa which includes Plasmodium, the cause of malaria *sporozo, spordjur*

sporra ⇨ **stimulate**

sporre ⇨ **spur**

spot [spɒt] *subst.* small round mark *or* pimple *fläck, prick, utslag;* **the disease is marked by red spots on the chest; he suddenly came out in spots on his chest; black spots (in front of the eyes)** = moving black dots seen when looking at something, more noticeable when a person is tired *or* run-down, more common in shortsighted people *mouches volantes, svarta fläckar (för ögonen);* **to break out in spots** *or* **to come out in spots** = to have a sudden rash *få utslag; see also* KOPLIK

spott ⇨ **saliva, spit**

spott- ⇨ **ptyal-, salivary, sial-**

spotta ⇨ **spit**

spottavsöndring ⇨ **salivation**

spotted fever [ˌspɒtɪd ˈfiːvə] *or* **meningococcal meningitis** [meˌnɪŋgəʊˈkɒk(ə)l ˌmenɪnˈdʒaɪtɪs] *subst.* commonest epidemic form of meningitis, caused by a bacterial infection, where the meninges become inflamed causing headaches and fever *meningitis cerebrospinalis (epidemica), epidemisk hjärnhinneinflammation; see also* ROCKY MOUNTAIN

spottkörtelcysta ⇨ **ranula**

spottkörtelinflammation ⇨ **sialadenitis**

spottkörtlarna ⇨ **salivary**

spottsten ⇨ **salivary, sialolith**

spotty [ˈspɒti] *adj.* covered with pimples *finnig*

sprain [spreɪn] **1** *subst.* condition where the ligaments in a joint are stretched or torn because of a sudden movement *vrickning, stukning, sträckning* **2** *vb.* to tear the ligaments in a joint with a sudden movement *vricka (stuka, sträcka) (sig);* **she sprained her wrist when she fell**

spray [spreɪ] **1** *subst.* **(a)** mass of tiny drops *spray, sprej;* **an aerosol sends out a liquid in a fine spray (b)** special liquid for spraying onto an infection *spray, sprej;* **throat spray** *or* **nasal spray 2** *vb.* to send out a liquid in fine drops *spraya, spreja, bespruta;* **they sprayed the room with disinfectant**

spray ➪ **aerosol, nebula, spray, vaporizer**

spray(flaska) ➪ **atomizer**

spread [spred] *vb.* to go out over a large area *sprida (sig);* **the infection spread right through the adult population; sneezing in a crowded bus can spread infection** NOTE: **spreads - spreading - spread - has spread**

> QUOTE spreading infection may give rise to cellulitis of the abdominal wall and abscess formation
>
> **Nursing Times**

sprej ➪ **aerosol, nebula, spray, vaporizer**

sprej(flaska) ➪ **atomizer**

Sprengel's deformity [ˌspreŋgəlz dɪˈfɔːməti] *or* **Sprengel's shoulder** [ˌspreŋgəlz ˈʃəʊldə] *subst.* congenitally deformed shoulder, where one scapula is smaller and higher than the other *Sprengels deformitet*

spricka ➪ **burst, crack, fissure, rima, rupture**

-spricka ➪ **-schisis**

sprickbildning ➪ **fissure**

sprickning ➪ **chapping**

sprida ➪ **pass on, propagate, transmit**

sprida (sig) ➪ **spread, suffuse**

spridd ➪ **disseminated, generalized, sporadic**

spridning ➪ **dissemination, passage, proliferation, propagation**

springmask ➪ **Enterobius, threadworm**

sprit ➪ **alcohol, spirit**

spritavtvättning ➪ **alcohol**

spritmissbruk ➪ **abuse, alcohol**

sprucken ➪ **chapped**

sprue [spruː] = PSILOSIS

spruta ➪ **hypodermic; shot**

spruta in ➪ **inject**

språngbenet ➪ **ankle, astragalus, talus**

språngbens- ➪ **talo-**

spräcka ➪ **crack**

spröd ➪ **brittle, delicate**

spud [spʌd] *subst.* needle used to get a piece of dust *or* other foreign body out of the eye *främmande-kroppsinstrument*

spur [spɜː] *subst.* sharp projecting part of a bone *sporre, utskott*

sputum [ˈspjuːtəm] *or* **phlegm** [flem] *subst.* mucus which is formed in the inflamed nose *or* throat *or* lungs and is coughed up *sputum, slem, upphostning;* **she was coughing up bloodstained sputum**

spy ➪ **puke, throw up, vomit**

spår ➪ **trace**

spårelement ➪ **trace, tracer**

spårämne ➪ **trace, tracer**

spädbarn ➪ **baby, infant, neonate**

spädbarns- ➪ **infantile**

spädbarnsdödlighet ➪ **infant, neonatal**

spädbarnsklinik ➪ **baby**

spädbarnsmisshandelssyndrom ➪ **battered baby**

spädbarnsroseol ➪ **roseola**

spädbarnsvård ➪ **baby**

spädning ➪ **dilution**

spänd ➪ **tense**

spänna (fast) ➪ **strap (up)**

spänna (ut) ➪ **stretch**

spänning ➪ **stress, tension**

spänning, premenstruell ⇨ **premenstrual**

spänningshuvudvärk ⇨ **tension**

spärr ⇨ **barrier**

spöke ⇨ **phantom**

squama ['skweɪmə] *subst.* thin piece of hard tissue, such as a thin flake of bone *or* scale on the skin *squama, fjäll* NOTE: plural is **squamae**

squamous ['skweɪməs] *adj.* thin and hard like a scale *skvamös, fjällig, fjälliknande;* **squamous bone** = part of the temporal bone which forms the side of the skull *squama temporalis;* **squamous epithelium** *or* **pavement epithelium** = epithelium with flat cells like scales which forms the lining of the pericardium, the peritoneum and the pleura *enskiktat skivepitel*

squint [skwɪnt] **1** *subst.* strabismus *or* condition where the eyes focus on different points *strabism, skelning, vindögdhet;* **convergent squint** = condition where one or both eyes look towards the nose *strabismus convergens (internus), konvergent strabism (skelning), inåtskelning;* **divergent squint** = condition where one or both eyes look away from the nose *strabismus divergens (externus), divergent strabism (skelning), utåtskelning* **2** *vb.* to have one eye or both eyes looking towards the nose *skela, vara vindögd;* **babies often appear to squint, but it is corrected as they grow older**

SR ⇨ **sedimentation**

SRN [ˌesɑː'en] = STATE REGISTERED NURSE

stab [stæb] **1** *subst.* **(a) stab wound** = deep wound made by the point of a knife *vulnus punctum, sticksår* **(b)** sharp pain *plötslig skarp smärta;* **he had a stab of pain in his right eye** **2** *vb.* to cut by pushing the point of a knife into the flesh *sticka, stöta, genomborra;* **he was stabbed in the chest**

stabbing ['stæbɪŋ] *adj.* (pain) in a series of short sharp stabs *stickande;* **he had stabbing pains in his chest**

stable ['steɪb(ə)l] *adj.* not changing *stabil;* **his condition is stable; stable angina** = angina which has not changed for a long time *stabilt tillstånd av angina pectoris*

staccato speech [stə'kɑːtəʊ ˌspiːtʃ] *subst.* abnormal way of speaking, with short pauses between each word *skanderande tal (som vid MS)*

Stacke's operation ['stækɪz ˌɒpəˌreɪʃ(ə)n] *subst.* surgical operation to remove the posterior and superior wall of the auditory meatus *Stackes operation*

stadium ⇨ **phase, stage, state**

stadium invasioni ['steɪdiəm ɪnˌveɪʃi'əʊni] *subst.* incubation period *or* period between catching an infectious disease and the appearance of the first symptoms of the disease *inkubationsstadium*

staff [stɑːf] *subst.* people who work in a hospital, clinic, doctor's surgery, etc. *personal;* **we have 25 full-time medical staff; the hospital is trying to recruit more nursing staff; the clinic has a staff of 100; staff midwife** = midwife who is on the permanent staff of a hospital *barnmorska vid sjukhus;* **staff nurse** = senior nurse who is employed full-time *(fast anställd) sjuksköterska vid sjukhus*
NOTE: when used as a subject, **staff** takes a plural verb: **a staff of 25** but **the ancillary staff work very hard**

stafylektomi ⇨ **staphylectomy**

stafylokock- ⇨ **staphylococcal**

stafylom ⇨ **staphyloma**

stage [steɪdʒ] *subst.* point in the development of a disease, which allows a decision to be taken about the treatment which should be given *stadium, skede;* **the disease has reached a critical stage; this is a symptom of the second stage of syphilis**

> QUOTE memory changes are associated with early stages of the disease in later stages, the patient is frequently incontinent, immobile and unable to communicate
> **Nursing Times**

stagger ['stægə] *vb.* to move from side to side while walking *or* to walk unsteadily *vackla, vingla, ragla, stappla*

stagnant loop syndrome [ˌstægnənt 'luːp ˌsɪndrəʊm] *see* LOOP

stain [steɪn] **1** *subst.* dye *or* substance used to give colour to tissues which are going to be examined under the microscope *fläck, färg(ämne), färgstoff* **2** *vb.* to treat a piece of tissue with a dye to increase contrast before it is examined under the microscope *färga*

staining ['steɪnɪŋ] *subst.* colouring of tissue *or* bacterial samples, etc., to make it possible to examine them and to identify them under the microscope *färgning*

stalk [stɔ:k] *subst.* stem *or* piece of tissue which attaches a growth to the main tissue *stjälk*

stam ⇨ **stem, strain**

stamkultur ⇨ **stock culture**

stamma ⇨ **stammer, stutter**

stammare ⇨ **stammerer**

stammer ['stæmə] **1** *subst.* speech defect, where the patient repeats parts of a word or the whole word several times *or* stops to try to pronounce a word *stamning;* **he has a bad stammer; she is taking therapy to try to correct her stammer 2** *vb.* to speak with a stammer *stamma*

stammerer ['stæmərə] *subst.* person who stammers *stammare*

stammering ['stæmərɪŋ] *or* **dysphemia** [dɪs'fi:miə] *subst.* difficulty in speaking, where the person repeats parts of a word or the whole word several times *or* stops to try to pronounce a word *stamning; see also* STUTTER

stamning ⇨ **stammer, stammering, stutter, stuttering**

stamp out [ˌstæmp 'aʊt] *vb.* to remove completely *utrota, göra (få) slut på;* **international organizations have succeeded in stamping out smallpox; the government is trying to stamp out waste in the hospital service**

standard ['stændəd] **1** *adj.* normal *standard-, normal(-);* **it is the standard practice to take the patient's temperature twice a day 2** *subst.* something which has been agreed upon and is used to measure other things by *standard, norm, måttstock;* **the standard of care in hospitals has increased over the last years; the report criticized the standards of hygiene in the clinic**

stand up [ˌstænd 'ʌp] *vb.* **(a)** to get up from being on a seat *resa sig (upp), ställa sig (stiga, stå) upp;* **he tried to stand up, but did not have the strength (b)** to hold yourself upright *stå (upprätt);* **she still stands up straight at the age of ninety-two**

stank ⇨ **fetor**

stanna ⇨ **stay, wait**

stapedectomy [ˌsteɪpi'dektəmi] *subst.* surgical operation to remove the stapes *stapedektomi*

stapediolysis [stəˌpi:dɪ'ɒləsɪs] *or* **stapedial mobilization** [stə'pi:diəl ˌməʊb(ə)laɪ'zeɪʃ(ə)n] *subst.* surgical operation to relieve deafness by detaching an immobile stapes from the fenestra ovalis *staped(i)olys, stapesmobilisering*

stapes ['steɪpi:z] *subst.* one of the three ossicles in the middle ear, shaped like a stirrup *stapes, stigbygeln;* **mobilization of the stapes** = STAPEDIOLYSIS ⇨ *illustration* EAR

> COMMENT: the stapes fills the fenestra ovalis, and is articulated with the incus, which in turn articulates with the malleus

stapesmobilisering ⇨ **mobilization, stapediolysis**

staphylectomy [ˌstæfɪ'lektəmi] *subst.* surgical operation to remove the uvula *stafylektomi*

staphylococcal [ˌstæfɪlə(ʊ)'kɒk(ə)l] *adj.* referring to Staphylococci *stafylokock-;* **staphylococcal poisoning** = poisoning by Staphylococci which have spread in food *matförgiftning med stafylokocker*

Staphylococcus [ˌstæfɪlə(ʊ)'kɒkəs] *subst.* bacterium which grows in a bunch like a bunch of grapes, and causes boils and food poisoning *Staphylococcus*
NOTE: plural is **Staphylococci**

staphyloma [ˌstæfɪ'ləʊmə] *subst.* swelling of the cornea or the white of the eye *stafylom*

staphylorrhaphy [ˌstæfɪ'lɔ:rəfi] = PALATORRHAPHY

staple ['steɪp(ə)l] *subst.* small piece of bent metal, used to attach tissues together *märla*

stapler ['steɪplə] *subst.* device used in surgery to attach tissues with staples, instead of suturing *apparat att fästa agraffer med*

stappla ⇨ **stagger**

starch [stɑ:tʃ] *subst.* usual form in which carbohydrates exist in food, especially in bread, rice and potatoes *stärkelse*

> COMMENT: starch is present in common foods, and is broken down by the digestive process into forms of sugar

starchy ['stɑːtʃi] *adj.* (food) which contains a lot of starch *stärkelsehaltig, stärkelserik;* **he eats too much starchy food**

stark ⇨ **heavy, tough, violent, virulent**

Starling's Law ['stɑːlɪŋz ˌlɔː] *subst.* law that the contraction of the ventricles is in proportion to the length of the ventricular muscle fibres at end of diastole *Starlings hjärtlag*

starr, grå ⇨ **cataract**

starr, grön ⇨ **glaucoma**

starroperation ⇨ **cataract**

starr, svart ⇨ **amaurosis**

starvation [stɑː'veɪʃ(ə)n] *subst.* having had very little *or* no food *svält;* **starvation diet** = diet which contains little nourishment, and is not enough to keep a person healthy *svältkost, svältkur*

starve [stɑːv] *vb.* to have little *or* no food or nourishment *svälta;* **the parents let the baby starve to death**

stasikterus ⇨ **jaundice**

stasis ['steɪsɪs] *subst.* stoppage *or* slowing in the flow of a liquid (such as blood in veins *or* food in the intestine) *stas, blodstockning*

-stasis ['steɪsɪs] *suffix* referring to stoppage in the flow of a liquid *-stas*

staspapill ⇨ **papilloedema**

stat. *abbreviation for the Latin word* "statim": immediately (written on prescriptions) *statim*

state [steɪt] *subst.* the condition of something *or* of a person *tillstånd, skick, stadium;* **his state of health is getting worse; the disease is in an advanced state**

statim ⇨ **stat.**

statistics [stə'tɪstɪks] *subst pl.* study of facts in the form of official figures *statistik;* **population statistics show that the birth rate is slowing down**

statolit ⇨ **otolith**

status ['steɪtəs] *Latin for* "state" *status, tillstånd;* **status asthmaticus** = attack of bronchial asthma which lasts for a long time and results in exhaustion and collapse *status asthmaticus;* **status epilepticus** = repeated and prolonged epileptic seizures without recovery of consciousness between them *status epilepticus;* **status lymphaticus** = condition where the glands in the lymphatic system are enlarged *status lymphaticus (thymolymphaticus, thymicus)*

> QUOTE the main indications being inadequate fluid and volume status and need for evaluation of patients with a history of severe heart disease
> **Southern Medical Journal**

> QUOTE the standard pulmonary artery catheters have four lumens from which to obtain information about the patient's haemodynamic status
> **RN Magazine**

stav ⇨ **rod**

stavbräm ⇨ **microvillus**

stay [steɪ] **1** *subst.* time which someone spends in a place *tid, vistelse;* **the patient is only in hospital for a short stay; long stay patient** = patient who will stay in hospital for a long time *långvårdspatient;* **long stay ward** = ward for patients who will stay in hospital for a long time *långvårdsavdelning* **2** *vb.* to stop in a place for some time *stanna, vistas, "ligga";* **she stayed in hospital for two weeks; he's ill with flu and has to stay in bed**

STD [ˌestiː'diː] = SEXUALLY TRANSMITTED DISEASE

steapsin [sti'æpsɪn] *subst.* enzyme produced by the pancreas, which breaks down fats in the intestine *steapsin, lipas*

stearic acid [stiˌærɪk 'æsɪd] *subst.* one of the fatty acids *stearinsyra*

stearré ⇨ **steatorrhoea**

steat- ['stiːət, ˌ--] *or* **steato-** ['stiːətə(ʊ), ˌ---] *prefix* referring to fat *steat(o)-, fett-, talg-*

steatoma [ˌstiːə'təʊmə] *subst.* sebaceous cyst *or* cyst in a blocked sebaceous gland *steatom, aterom, talg(körtel)cysta*

steatorrhoea [ˌstiːətə'rɪə] *subst.* condition where fat is passed in the faeces *steatorré, stearré*

steg ⇨ **step**

stegring ⇨ **elevation**

Stein-Leventhal syndrome [ˌstaɪn'levəntɑːl ˌsɪndrəʊm] *subst.* condition in young women, where menstruation becomes rare, or never takes place, together with growth of body hair, usually due to cysts in the ovaries *Stein-Leventhals syndrom*

Steinmann's pin ['staɪnmænz ˌpɪn] *subst.* pin for attaching traction wires to a fractured bone *"pinne"*

stel ⇨ **rigid, stiff**

stelhet ⇨ **akinesia, rigidity, rigor, stiffness**

stelkramp ⇨ **tetanus**

stelkramps- ⇨ **tetanic**

stellate ['steleɪt] *adj.* shaped like a star *stjärnformig;* **stellate fracture** = fracture of the kneecap, shaped like a star *fractura stellata, stjärnformad fraktur;* **stellate ganglion** = inferior cervical ganglion *or* group of nerve cells in the neck *ganglion stellatum*

Stellwag's sign ['stelvɑ:gz ˌsaɪn] *subst.* symptom of exophthalmic goitre, where the patient does not blink often, because the eyeball is protruding *Stellwags Basedowssyndrom*

stelna ⇨ **congeal, solidify**

steloperation av led ⇨ **arthrodesis**

stem [stem] *subst.* thin piece of tissue which attaches an organ *or* growth to the main tissue *stam, stjälk;* **brain stem** = lower part of the brain which connects the brain to the spinal cord *truncus cerebri, hjärnstammen*

sten ⇨ **calculus, stone**

sten- ⇨ **lith-**

stendöv ⇨ **stone deaf**

stenkrossning ⇨ **litholapaxy**

stenliknande ⇨ **petrous**

steno- ['stenəʊ, ˌ--] *prefix* meaning (i) narrow *steno-;* (ii) constricted *steno-*

stenos ⇨ **constriction, stenosis**

stenose [ste'nəʊs] *vb.* to make narrow *stenosera, förtränga;* **stenosed valve** = valve which has become narrow *or* constricted *stenoserad (förträngd) klaff;* **stenosing condition** = condition which makes a passage narrow *stenoserande (förträngande) förhållande*

stenosera ⇨ **stenose**

stenosis [ste'nəʊsɪs] *subst.* condition where a passage becomes narrow *stenos, förträngning;* **aortic stenosis** = condition where the aortic valve is narrow *stenosis aortae, aortastenos;* **mitral stenosis** = condition where the opening in the mitral valve becomes smaller because the cusps have fused (almost always the result of rheumatic endocarditis) *stenosis valvulae mitralis, mitralisstenos;* **pulmonary stenosis** = condition where the opening to the pulmonary artery in the right ventricle becomes narrow *stenosis pulmonalis, pulmonalisstenos*

stenostomia [ˌstenəʊ'stəʊmiə] *or* **stenostomy** [ste'nɒstəmi] *subst.* abnormal narrowing of an opening *stenostomi*

Stensen's duct ['stens(ə)nz ˌdʌkt] *subst.* duct which carries saliva from the parotid gland *ductus Stenonis, Stensens gång*

stensjukdom ⇨ **lithiasis**

stent [stent] *subst.* support of artificial material often inserted in a tube *or* vessel which has been sutured *slags stöd av konstgjort material som läggs in i t.ex. kärl som sutureras*

step [step] *subst.* movement of the foot and the leg as in walking *steg, fotsteg;* **he took two steps forward; the baby is taking his first steps**

step up [ˌstep 'ʌp] *vb. (informal)* to increase *öka(s);* **the doctor has stepped up the dosage**

sterco- ['stɜ:kə(ʊ), ˌ--] *prefix* referring to faeces *sterko-, fekal-, exkrement-*

stercobilin [ˌstɜ:kə(ʊ)'baɪlɪn] *subst.* brown pigment which colours the faeces *sterkobilin, urobilin*

stercobilinogen [ˌstɜ:kə(ʊ)baɪ'lɪnədʒen] *subst.* substance which is broken down from bilirubin and produces stercobilin *sterkobilinogen, urobilinogen*

stercolith ['stɜ:kə(ʊ)lɪθ] *subst.* hard ball of dried faeces in the bowel *sterkolit, fekalit, koprolit, fekalsten*

stercoraceous [ˌstɜ:kə(ʊ)'reɪʃəs] *adj.* made of faeces *sterkoral, fekal, exkrement-, avförings-;* similar to faeces *exkrementliknande, avföringsliknande etc.;* containing faeces *som innehåller exkrement (avföring etc.)*

stereognosis [ˌsteriɒgˈnəʊsɪs] *subst.* being able to tell the shape of an object in three dimensions by means of touch *stereognosi*

stereoscopic vision [ˌsteriəˈskɒpɪk ˌvɪʒ(ə)n] *subst.* being able to judge the distance and depth of an object by binocular vision *stereoskopiskt (tredimensionellt) seende, stereoseende, djupseende*

stereoseende ➪ **stereoscopic vision**

stereotaxy [ˌsteriəʊˈtæksi] *or* **stereotaxic surgery** [ˌsteriəʊˈtæksɪk ˌsɜːdʒ(ə)ri] *subst.* surgical procedure to identify a point in the interior of the brain, before an operation can begin, to locate exactly the area to be operated on *stereotaxi, stereotaktisk kirurgi*

stereotypy [ˈsteriə(ʊ)ˌtaɪpi] *subst.* repeating the same action *or* word again and again *stereotypi*

sterila handskar ➪ **surgical**

sterile [ˈsteraɪ(ə)l] *adj.* **(a)** with no microbes *or* infectious organisms *steril;* **she put a sterile dressing on the wound; he opened a pack of sterile dressings (b)** infertile *or* not able to produce children *steril, infertil, ofruktsam*

sterilisera ➪ **sterilize**

sterilisering ➪ **sterilization**

steriliseringsapparat ➪ **sterilizer**

sterilitet ➪ **infertility, sterility**

sterility [stəˈrɪləti] *subst.* (i) being free from germs *sterilitet;* (ii) infertility *or* being unable to produce children *sterilitet, infertilitet, ofruktsamhet*

sterilization [ˌster(ə)laɪˈzeɪʃ(ə)n] *subst.* (i) action of making instruments, etc., free from germs *sterilisering;* (ii) action of making a person sterile *sterilisering*

> COMMENT: sterilization of a woman can be done by removing the ovaries or cutting the Fallopian tubes; sterilization of a man is carried out by cutting the vas deferens (vasectomy)

sterilize [ˈsterəlaɪz] *vb.* **(a)** to make something sterile (by killing microbes *or* bacteria) *sterilisera;* **surgical instruments must be sterilized before use; not using sterilized needles can cause infection (b)** to make a person unable to have children *sterilisera*

sterilizer [ˈsterəlaɪzə] *subst.* machine for sterilizing surgical instruments by steam *or* boiling water, etc. *steriliseringsapparat*

steril rock ➪ **theatre**

sterilt förband ➪ **unmedicated dressing**

steriltvätta sig ➪ **scrub up**

sterko- ➪ **sterco-**

sterkobilin ➪ **stercobilin, urobilin**

sterkobilinogen ➪ **stercobilinogen, urobilinogen**

sterkolit ➪ **coprolith, stercolith**

sterkoral ➪ **faecal, stercoraceous**

sternal [ˈstɜːn(ə)l] *adj.* referring to the breastbone *sternal, bröstbens-;* **sternal angle** = ridge of bone where the manubrium articulates with the body of the sternum *angulus sterni;* **sternal puncture** = surgical operation to remove a sample of bone marrow from the breastbone for testing *sternalpunktion*

sternalpunktion ➪ **puncture, sternal**

Sternbergs sjukdom ➪ **Hodgkin's disease**

sternoclavicular angle [ˌstɜːnəʊkləˈvɪkjʊlə ˌæŋg(ə)l] *subst.* angle between the sternum and the clavicle *articulatio sternoclavicularis*

sternocleidomastoid muscle [ˌstɜːnəʊˌklaɪdəʊˈmæstɔɪd mʌs(ə)l] *subst.* muscle in the neck, running from the breastbone to the mastoid process *musculus sternocleidomastoideus*

sternocostal joint [ˌstɜːnəʊˈkɒst(ə)l ˌdʒɔɪnt] *subst.* joint where the breastbone joins a rib **sternocostal joints** *articulatios sternocostales*

sternohyoid muscle [ˌstɜːnəʊˈhaɪɔɪd ˌmʌs(ə)l] *subst.* muscle in the neck which runs from the breastbone into the hyoid bone *musculus sternohyoideus*

sternomastoid [ˌstɜːnəʊˈmæstɔɪd] *adj.* referring to the breastbone and the mastoid *sternomastoid;* **sternomastoid muscle** = STERNOCLEIDOMASTOID MUSCLE;

sternomastoid tumour = benign tumour which appears in the sternomastoid muscle in newborn babies *tumör i musculus sternocleidomastoideus hos nyfödda*

sternotomy [stɜː'nɒtəmi] *subst.* surgical operation to cut through the breastbone, so as to be able to operate on the heart *sternotomi*

sternum ['stɜːnəm] *or* **breastbone** ['brestbəʊn] *subst.* bone in the centre of the front of the chest *sternum, bröstbenet*

> COMMENT: the sternum runs from the neck to the bottom of the diaphragm. It is formed of the manubrium (the top section), the body of the sternum, and the xiphoid process. The upper seven pairs of ribs are attached to the sternum

sternutatory [ˌstɜːnju'teɪt(ə)ri] *subst.* substance which makes someone sneeze *sternutatorium, nysmedel*

steroid ['stɪərɔɪd] *subst.* any of several chemical compounds with characteristic ring systems, including the sex hormones, which affect the body and its functions *steroid*

> COMMENT: the word steroid is usually used to refer to corticosteroids. Synthetic steroids are used in steroid therapy, to treat arthritis, asthma and some blood disorders. They are also used by some athletes to improve their physical strength, but these are banned by athletic organizations and can have serious side-effects

sterol ['stiərɒl] *subst.* insoluble substance which belongs to the steroid alcohols such as cholesterol *sterol*

stertor ['stɜːtə] *subst.* noisy breathing sounds in an unconscious patient *stertor, rosslande andning, snarkande andning*

steth- ['steθ, ˌ-] *or* **stetho-** ['steθə, ˌ--] *prefix* referring to the chest *steto-*

stethograph ['steθəgrɑːf] *subst.* instrument which records breathing movements of the chest *instrument som registrerar bröstkorgens andningsrörelser*

stethography [ste'θɒgrəfi] *subst.* recording movements of the chest *registrering av bröstkorgens andningsrörelser*

stethometer [ste'θɒmɪtə] *subst.* instrument which records how far the chest expands when a person breathes in *instrument som mäter bröstkorgens utvidgning vid inandning*

stethoscope ['steθəskəʊp] *subst.* surgical instrument with two earpieces connected to a tube and a metal disc, used by doctors to listen to sounds made inside the body (such as the sound of the heart *or* lungs) *stetoskop;* **electronic stethoscope** = stethoscope with an amplifier which makes sounds louder *elektroniskt stetoskop*

steto- ⇨ **steth-**

stetoskop ⇨ **stethoscope**

Stevens-Johnson syndrome [ˌstiːv(ə)nz 'dʒɒns(ə)n ˌsɪndrəʊm] *subst.* severe form of erythema multiforme affecting the face and genitals, caused by an allergic reaction to drugs *Stevens-Johnsons syndrom*

STH ⇨ **growth, hormone, somatotrophic hormone**

stick [stɪk] *vb.* to attach *or* to fix together (as with glue) *fastna, klibba (hänga, sitta) fast, häfta (vid);* **in bad cases of conjunctivitis the eyelids can stick together**

stick ⇨ **bite, puncture, sting**

sticka ⇨ **splinter; stab, sting, tingle**

sticka (hål i) ⇨ **prick**

sticking plaster ['stɪkɪŋ plɑːstə] *subst.* adhesive plaster *or* tape used to cover a small wound or to attach a pad of dressing to the skin *plåster, häfta*

stickprov ⇨ **sample**

sticksår ⇨ **puncture, stab**

sticky ['stɪki] *adj.* which attached like glue *klibbig, kladdig;* **sticky eye** = condition in babies where the eyes remain closed because of conjunctivitis *igenklistrade ögonlock, varig inflammation i ögats bindehinna*

stiff [stɪf] *adj.* which cannot be bent *or* moved easily *stel, styv, oböjlig;* **my knee is stiff after playing football; stiff neck =** condition where moving the neck is painful, usually caused by a strained muscle *or* by sitting in cold draughts *nackstyvhet, stelhet i nacken*
NOTE: **stiff - stiffer - stiffest**

stiffly ['stɪfli] *adv.* in a stiff way *stelt;* **he is walking stiffly because of the pain in his hip**

stiffness ['stɪfnəs] *subst.* being stiff *stelhet, styvhet, oböjlighet;* **arthritis accompanied by stiffness in the joints**

stift ⇨ **dilator, pin, pivot, stylus**

stiga ⇨ **rise**

stiga upp ⇨ **get up**

stigbygeln ⇨ **stapes, stirrup**

stigma ['stɪgmə] *subst.* visible symptom which shows that a patient has a certain disease *stigma, kännetecken (synligt tecken) på sjukdom*
NOTE: plural is **stigmas, stigmata**

stilet [staɪ'let] *or* **stilette** [staɪ'let] *subst.* thin wire inside a catheter to make it rigid *troakar*

stilla ⇨ **soothe**

stillasittande ⇨ **sedentary**

stillbirth ['stɪlbɜːθ] *subst.* birth of a dead fetus, more than 28 weeks after conception *dödfödsel*

stillborn ['stɪlbɔːn] *adj.* (baby) born dead *dödfödd;* **her first child was stillborn**

stillestånd ⇨ **arrest, stoppage**

Still's disease ['stɪlz dɪˌziːz] *subst.* arthritis affecting children, similar to rheumatoid arthritis in adults *Stills sjukdom*

stimulant ['stɪmjʊlənt] *subst. & adj.* (substance) which makes part of the body function faster *stimulans, excitans, stimulerande (uppiggande) (medel);* **caffeine is a stimulant**

> COMMENT: natural stimulants include some hormones, and drugs such as digitalis which encourage a weak heart. Drinks such as tea and coffee contain stimulants

stimulate ['stɪmjuleɪt] *vb.* to make a person *or* organ react *or* respond *or* function *stimulera, sporra, pigga upp;* **the drug stimulates the heart; the therapy should stimulate the patient into attempting to walk unaided**

stimulation [ˌstɪmju'leɪʃ(ə)n] *subst.* action of stimulating *stimulering*

stimulera ⇨ **encourage, excite, stimulate**

stimulering ⇨ **stimulation**

stimulus ['stɪmjʊləs] *subst.* something (drug, impulse, etc.) which makes part of the body react *stimulus, retning* NOTE: plural is **stimuli**

sting [stɪŋ] **1** *subst.* piercing of the skin by an insect which passes a toxic substance into the bloodstream *stick, sting, bett* **2** *vb. (of an insect)* to make a hole in the skin and pass a toxic substance into the blood *sticka, stinga, bita*

> COMMENT: stings by some insects, such as the tsetse fly can transmit a bacterial infection to a patient. Other insects such as bees have toxic substances which they pass into the bloodstream of the victim, causing irritating swellings. Some people are particularly allergic to insect stings

sting ⇨ **bite, sting**

stinknäsa ⇨ **ozaena**

stirrup ['stɪrəp] *or* **stapes** ['steɪpiːz] *subst.* one of the three ossicles in the middle ear *stapes, stigbygeln*

stitch [stɪtʃ] **1** *subst.* **(a)** suture *or* small loop of thread or gut, used to attach the sides of a wound or incision to help it to heal *sutur, stygn;* **he had three stitches in his head; the doctor told her to come back in ten days' time to have the stitches taken out (b)** pain caused by cramp in the side of the body after running *håll;* **he had to stop running because he developed a stitch 2** *vb.* to attach with a suture *suturera, sy (fast);* **they tried to stitch back the finger which had been cut off in an accident**

stjälk ⇨ **peduncle, stalk, stem**

stjälkad, inte ⇨ **sessile**

stjärnformig ⇨ **stellate**

stjärten ⇨ **bottom**

ST-läkare ⇨ **resident**

stock culture ['stɒk ˌkʌltʃə] *subst.* basic culture of bacteria, from which other cultures can be taken *stamkultur*

Stokes-Adams syndrome [ˌstəʊks 'ædəmz ˌsɪndrəʊm] *subst.* loss of consciousness due to the stopping of the action of the heart because of asystole *or* fibrillation *Stokes-Adams syndrom, Adams-Stokes syndrom*

stolpiller ⇨ **suppository**

stoma ['stəʊmə] *subst.* (i) any opening into a cavity in the body *stoma, öppning;* (ii) the mouth *stoma, munnen;* (iii); *(informal)* colostomy *stomi* NOTE: the plural is **stomata**

stomach ['stʌmək] *subst.* **(a)** part of the body shaped like a bag, into which food passes after being swallowed and where the process of digestion continues *stomachus, ventrikeln, magsäcken;* **she complained of pains in the stomach** *or* **of stomach pains; he has had stomach trouble for some time; acid stomach** *see* ACIDITY; **stomach ache** = pain in the abdomen *or* stomach (caused by eating too much food *or* by an infection) *buksmärtor, magknip, ont i magen;* **stomach cramp** = sharp spasm of the stomach muscles *kramp i magen;* **stomach pump** = instrument for sucking out the contents of a patient's stomach, especially if he has just swallowed a poisonous substance *magpump;* **stomach tube** = tube passed into the stomach to wash it out or to take samples of the contents *magsond, ventrikelsond;* **stomach upset** = slight infection of the stomach *magbesvär, krångel med magen* **(b)** region of the abdomen *buken, magen;* **he had been kicked in the stomach**

COMMENT: the stomach is situated in the top of the abdomen, and on the left side of the body between the oesophagus and the duodenum. Food is partly broken down by hydrochloric acid and other gastric juices secreted by the walls of the stomach and is mixed and squeezed by the action of the muscles of the stomach, before being passed on into the duodenum. The stomach continues the digestive process started in the mouth, but few substances (except alcohol and honey) are actually absorbed into the bloodstream in the stomach

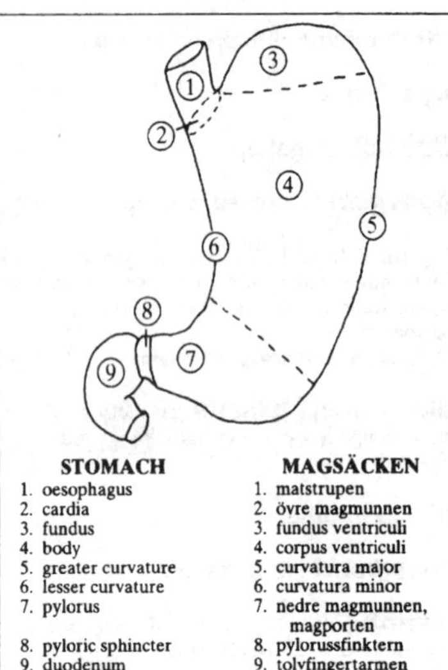

STOMACH	MAGSÄCKEN
1. oesophagus	1. matstrupen
2. cardia	2. övre magmunnen
3. fundus	3. fundus ventriculi
4. body	4. corpus ventriculi
5. greater curvature	5. curvatura major
6. lesser curvature	6. curvatura minor
7. pylorus	7. nedre magmunnen, magporten
8. pyloric sphincter	8. pylorussfinktern
9. duodenum	9. tolvfingertarmen

stomachic [stə'mækɪk] *subst.* substance which increases the appetite of a person by stimulating the secretion of gastric juice by the stomach *stomakikum, aptitbefordrande medel, aptitretande medel* NOTE: for other terms referring to the stomach, see words beginning with **gastr-**

stomakikum ⇨ **stomachic**

stomal ['stəʊm(ə)l] *adj.* referring to a stoma *som avser el. hör till stoma;* **stomal ulcer** = ulcer in the region of the jejunum *magsår i jejunum (tunntarmen)*

stomat- ['stəʊmət, ˌ--] *or* **stomato-** ['stəʊmətə, ˌ---] *prefix* referring to the mouth *stomat(o)-, mun-*

stomatitis [ˌstəʊmə'taɪtɪs] *subst.* inflammation of the inside of the mouth *stomatit, muninflammation*

stomatology [ˌstəʊmə'tɒlədʒi] *subst.* branch of medicine which studies diseases of the mouth *stomatologi*

stomi ⇨ **ostomy, stoma**

stomme ⇨ **body, frame, framework**

-stomy [stəmi] *or* **-ostomy** ['ɒstəmi] *suffix* meaning an operation to make an opening *-stomi*

stone [stəʊn] *subst.* **(a)** calculus *or* hard mass of calcium like a little piece of stone which forms inside the body *calculus, sten, konkrement; see also* GALLSTONE, KIDNEY STONE NOTE: for other terms referring to stones see words beginning or ending with **lith** **(b)** measure of weight (= 14 pounds or 6.35 kilograms) *slags viktmått (6,35 kg);* **he tried to lose weight and lost three stone; she weighs eight stone ten (i.e. 8 stone 10 pounds)** NOTE: no plural for (b): **'she weighs ten stone'**

stone deaf [ˌstəʊn'def] *adj.* totally deaf *totalt (helt, fullständigt) döv, stendöv*

stools [stu:lz] *or* **faeces** ['fi:si:z] *subst pl.* solid waste matter passed from the bowel through the anus *f(a)eces, fekalier, exkrement(er), avföring* NOTE: can also be used in the singular: **'he passed an abnormal stool'**

stop needle ['stɒp ni:d(ə)l] *subst.* needle with a ring round it, so that it can only be pushed a certain distance into the body *nål med (justerbar) stoppring för t.ex. benmärgspunktion*

stopp ⇨ **block, blockage, obstruction, stoppage**

stoppage ['stɒpɪdʒ] *subst.* act of stopping the function of an organ *stopp, avbrott, stillestånd;* **heart stoppage** = condition where the heart has stopped beating *hjärtstillestånd*

stor ⇨ **great, heavy, large, major, massive**

stora hjärnskäran ⇨ **cerebrum**

stora kroppspulsådern ⇨ **aorta**

stora lymfgången ⇨ **thoracic**

storhjärnan ⇨ **cerebrum**

storhjärnsbarken ⇨ **cerebral**

storhjärnshemisfär ⇨ **cerebral**

storrökare ⇨ **heavy**

stortån ⇨ **toe, hallux**

stove-in chest [ˌstəʊv'ɪn ˌtʃest] *subst.* result of an accident, where several ribs are broken and pushed towards the inside *intryckt bröstkorg*

strabismal [strə'bɪzm(ə)l] *adj.* cross-eyed *strabistisk, skelögd, vindögd*

strabismus [strə'bɪzməs] *or* **squint** [skwɪnt] *subst.* condition where the eyes focus on different points *strabism, skelning, vindögdhet;* **convergent strabismus** = condition where one or both eyes look towards the nose *strabismus convergens (internus), konvergent strabism (skelning), inåtskelning;* **divergent strabismus** = condition where one or both eyes look away from the nose *strabismus divergens (externus), divergent strabism (skelning), utåtskelning*

strabistisk ⇨ **cross-eyed, strabismal**

straight [streɪt] *adj.* (line) with no irregularities such as bends, curves or angles *rak*

straighten ['streɪt(ə)n] *vb.* to make straight *räta (ut);* **his arthritis is so bad that he cannot straighten his knees**

strain [streɪn] **1** *subst.* **(a)** condition where a muscle has been stretched *or* torn by a strong or sudden movement *sträckning;* **back strain** = condition where the muscles *or* ligaments in the back have been stretched *sträckning i ryggen* **(b)** group of microorganisms which are different from others of the same type *stam, sort;* **a new strain of influenza virus** **(c)** nervous tension and stress *stress, påfrestning, ansträngning, belastning;* **her work is causing her a lot of strain; he is suffering from nervous strain and needs to relax** **2** *vb.* to stretch a muscle too far *sträcka, påfresta, anstränga, belasta;* **he strained his back lifting the table; she had to leave the game with a strained calf muscle; the effort of running upstairs strained his heart**

stram led ⇨ **amphiarthrosis**

strangle ['stræŋg(ə)l] *vb.* to kill someone by squeezing his throat so that he cannot breathe or swallow *strypa, kväva*

strangulated ['stræŋgjuleɪtɪd] *adj.* (part of the body) caught in an opening in such a way that the circulation of blood is stopped *strypt, kvävd, tillsnörd, inklämd;* **strangulated hernia** = condition where part of the intestine is squeezed in a hernia and the supply of blood to it is cut *hernia incarcerata, inklämt bråck*

strangulation [ˌstræŋgju'leɪʃ(ə)n] *subst.* squeezing a passage in the body, especially the throat *strangulation, strypning, kvävning, inklämning*

strangury ['stræŋgjəri] *subst.* condition where very little urine is passed, although the patient wants to pass water, caused by a bladder disorder *or* by a stone in the urethra *stranguri, urinstämma*

strapats ⇨ **exposure**

strapping ['stræpɪŋ] *subst.* wide strong bandages *or* adhesive plaster used to bandage a large part of the body *häftförband*

strap (up) [stræp ('ʌp)] *vb.* to wrap a bandage round a limb tightly *or* to attach tightly *lägga stramt (åtsittande), spänna (fast);* **the nurses strapped up his stomach wound; the patient was strapped to the stretcher**

stratified ['strætɪfaɪd] *adj.* made of several layers *skiktad;* **stratified epithelium** = epithelium formed of several layers of cells *flerskiktat epitel*

stratum ['strɑːtəm] *subst.* layer of tissue forming the epidermis *stratum, skikt, lager*
NOTE: the plural is **strata**

> COMMENT: the main layers of the epidermis are: the Malpighian layer *or*

stratum germinativum which produces the cells that are pushed up to form the stratum lucidum *or* thin clear layer of dead and dying cells, and the stratum corneum *or* outside layer made of dead keratinized cells

strawberry mark ['strɔ:b(ə)ri mɑ:k] *subst.* naevus *or* red birthmark in children, which will disappear in later life *hemangiom*

streak [stri:k] *subst.* long thin line of a different colour *strimma*

strength [streŋθ] *subst.* being strong *styrka, kraft(er);* **after her illness she had no strength in her limbs; full strength solution** = solution which has not been diluted *outspädd lösning* NOTE: no plural

strengthen ['streŋθ(ə)n] *vb.* to make strong *(för)stärka, styrka*

strenuous ['strenjuəs] *adj.* (exercise) which involves using a lot of force *ansträngande, påfrestande, krävande;* **avoid doing any strenuous exercise for some time while the wound heals**

strep throat ['strep ˌθrəʊt] *subst.* *informal* infection of the throat by a streptococcus *streptokockinfektion i halsen, halsfluss*

strepto- ['streptə, ˌ--] *prefix* referring to organisms which grow in chains *strepto-*

streptobacillus ['streptəbə'sɪləs, ˌ---'--] *subst.* type of bacterium which forms a chain *streptobacill*

streptococcal [ˌstreptə'kɒk(ə)l] *adj.* (infection) caused by a streptococcus *streptokock-*

streptococcus [ˌstreptə'kɒkəs] *subst.* genus of bacteria which grows in long chains, and causes fevers such as scarlet fever, tonsillitis and rheumatic fever *streptococcus, streptokock* NOTE: plural is **streptococci**

streptodornase [ˌstreptə'dɔ:neɪs] *subst.* enzyme formed by streptococci which can make pus liquid *streptodornas*

streptokinase [ˌstreptə'kaɪneɪs] *subst.* enzyme formed by streptococci which can break down blood clots *streptokinas*

streptokock ▷ **streptococcus**

streptokock- ▷ **streptococcal**

streptolysin [strep'tɒləsɪn] *subst.* toxin produced by streptococci in rheumatic fever, which acts to destroy red blood cells *streptolysin*

Streptomyces [ˌstreptə'maɪsi:z] *subst.* genus of bacteria used to produce antibiotics *Streptomyces*

streptomycin [ˌstreptə'maɪsɪn] *subst.* antibiotic used against many types of infection, but especially tuberculosis *streptomycin*

stress [stres] *subst.* condition where an outside influence changes the working of the body, used especially of mental *or* emotional stress which can affect the hormone balance *stress, påfrestning, spänning;* **stress fracture** = fracture of a bone caused by excessive force, as in certain types of sport *stressfraktur, utmattningsfraktur;* **stress incontinence** = condition where the sufferer is not able to retain his urine when coughing *stressinkontinens*

stress ▷ **pressure, strain, stress**

stressfraktur ▷ **stress**

stressinkontinens ▷ **stress**

stretch [stretʃ] *vb.* to pull out *or* to make longer *sträcka, spänna (ut), tänja (töja) ut;* **stretch marks** = marks on the skin of the abdomen of a pregnant woman *or* of a woman who has recently given birth *striae (albicantes, gravidarum);* **stretch reflex** = reflex reaction of a muscle which contracts after being stretched *myotatisk reflex, sträckreflex*

stretcher ['stretʃə] *subst.* folding bed, with handles, on which an injured person can be carried by two people *bår;* **she was carried out of the restaurant on a stretcher; some of the accident victims could walk to the ambulances, but there were several stretcher cases; stretcher bearer** = person who helps to carry a stretcher *bårbärare;* **stretcher case** = person who is so ill that he has to be carried on a stretcher *patient som är så allvarligt sjuk att han/hon måste bäras på bår;* **stretcher party** = group of people who carry a stretcher and look after the patient on it *ung. ambulanspersonal;* **Furley stretcher** *or* **standard stretcher** = stretcher made of a folding frame with a canvas bed, with carrying poles at each side and small feet underneath *tygbår med små fötter;* **paraguard stretcher** *or* **Neil Robertson stretcher** = type of strong stretcher to which the injured person is attached, so that he can be carried upright (used for rescuing people from mountains *or* from tall buildings) *slags bår som används t.ex. vid olyckor i bergen;* **pole and canvas stretcher** = simple stretcher made of a piece of canvas and two poles which slide into tubes at the side of the canvas *(enklare) bår;* **scoop stretcher** = stretcher in two sections which slide under the patient and can lock together *bår av teleskoptyp som kan föras under patienten och låsas*

stria ['stra(ɪ)ə] *subst.* pale line on skin which is stretched (as in obese people) *stria, strimma;* **striae gravidarum** = lines on the skin of the abdomen of a pregnant woman *or* of a woman who has just given birth *striae (albicantes, gravidarum)* NOTE: plural is **striae**

striae ⇨ **stretch, stria**

striated [straɪ'eɪtɪd] *adj.* marked with pale lines *tvärstrimmig;* **striated muscle** = muscle which is attached to the bone which it moves *tvärstrimmig muskel; compare* SMOOTH

strict [strɪkt] *adj.* severe *or* which must not be changed *sträng, hård, strikt;* **she has to follow a strict diet; the doctor was strict with the patients who wanted to drink alcohol in the hospital**

stricture ['strɪktʃə] *subst.* narrowing of a passage in the body *striktur, förträngning;* **urethral stricture** = narrowing *or* blocking of the urethra by a growth *uretrostriktur, uretrostenos, urinrörsförträngning*

stridor ['straɪdɔː] *or* **stridulus** ['straɪdjʊləs] *subst.* sharp high sound made when air passes an obstruction in the larynx *stridor; see also* LARYNGISMUS

strikt ⇨ **strict**

striktur ⇨ **coarctation, stricture**

strimma ⇨ **streak, stria, weal**

strip [strɪp] **1** *subst.* long thin piece of material *or* tissue *remsa;* **the nurse bandaged the wound with strips of gauze; he grafted a strip of skin over the burn 2** *vb.* to take off (especially clothes) *ta av (sig), klä av (sig);* **the patients had to strip for the medical examination; to strip to the waist** = to take off the clothes on the top part of the body *klä av sig på överkroppen*

stroke [strəʊk] **1** *subst.* **(a)** sudden loss of consciousness caused by a cerebral haemorrhage or a blood clot in the brain *stroke, slag(anfall), hjärnblödning;* **he had a stroke and died; she was paralysed after a stroke; heat stroke** = condition where the patient becomes too hot and his body temperature rises abnormally *termoplegi, värmeslag;* **sunstroke** = serious condition caused by exposure to the sun *or* to hot conditions, where the patient becomes dizzy, has a fever, but does not perspire *insolation, solsting* **(b) stroke volume** = amount of blood pumped out the ventricle at each heartbeat *slagvolym* **2** *vb.* to touch softly with the fingers *smeka, stryka*

COMMENT: there are two causes of stroke: cerebral haemorrhage (haemorrhagic stroke), when an artery bursts and blood leaks into the brain, and cerebral thrombosis (occlusive stroke), where a blood clot blocks an artery

QUOTE stroke is the third most frequent cause of death in developed countries after ischaemic heart disease and cancer
British Journal of Hospital Medicine

QUOTE raised blood pressure may account for as many as 70% of all strokes. The risk of stroke rises with both systolic and diastolic blood pressure
British Journal of Hospital Medicine

stroma ['strəʊmə] *subst.* tissue which supports an organ, as opposed to parenchyma *or* functioning tissues in the organ *stroma, stödjevävnad, interstitiell bindväv*

Strongyloides [ˌstrɒndʒi'lɔɪdiːz] *subst.* parasitic worm which infests the intestines *Strongyloides*

strongyloidiasis [ˌstrɒndʒilɔɪ'daɪəsɪs] *subst.* being infested with **Strongyloides** which enters the skin and then travels to the lungs *strongyloidiasis*

structure ['strʌktʃə] *subst.* way in which an organ *or* muscle is formed *struktur, uppbyggnad*

struma ['struːmə] *subst.* goitre *struma*

strumaframkallande ⇨ **goitrogen**

strup- ⇨ **laryng-**

strupen ⇨ **throat**

struphuvudet ⇨ **larynx, voice box**

struphuvuds- ⇨ **laryng-, laryngeal**

struphuvudsförträngning ⇨ **laryngostenosis**

strupkatarr ⇨ **laryngitis**

struplocket ⇨ **epiglottis**

struplocksinflammation ⇨ **epiglottitis**

strychnine ['strɪkniːn] *subst.* poisonous alkaloid drug, made from the seeds of a tropical tree, and formerly used in small dose as a tonic *stryknin*

strypa ⇨ **strangle**

strypning ⇨ **strangulation**

strypsjuka, äkta ⇨ **croup**

stråk ⇨ **tract**

strålbehandling ⇨ **irradiation, radiotherapy**

strålbenet ⇨ **radius**

strålbens- ⇨ **radial, radio-**

strålbiolog ⇨ **radiobiologist**

stråle ⇨ **beam, ray**

strålknippe ⇨ **beam**

strålkänslig ⇨ **radiosensitive**

strålning ⇨ **irradiation, radiation**

strål(nings)- ⇨ **radial, radio-**

strålningssjukdom ⇨ **radiation**

strålsjuka ⇨ **radiation**

strålskada ⇨ **radiation**

strålsvampsjuka ⇨ **actinomycosis**

sträck ⇨ **traction**

sträcka ⇨ **pull, strain, stretch**

sträckmuskel ⇨ **extensor (muscle), tensor**

sträckning ⇨ **extension, sprain, strain**

sträckreflex ⇨ **myotactic, stretch**

sträng ⇨ **chorda, cord, fasciculus, funiculus; strict**

sträv ⇨ **rough**

ström ⇨ **flow**

student ['stju:d(ə)nt] *subst.* person who is studying at a college or university *student, studerande;* **all the medical students have to spend some time in hospital; student nurse** = person who is studying to become a nurse *sjuksköterskestuderande*

studera ⇨ **study**

studerande ⇨ **student**

studiegång ⇨ **course**

study ['stʌdi] **1** *subst.* examining something to learn about it *undersökning, granskning;* **he's making a study of diseases of small children; they have finished their study of the effects of the drug on pregnant women 2** *vb.* to examine something to learn about it *undersöka, granska, studera;* **he's studying pharmacy; doctors are studying the results of the screening programme**

stuffy ['stʌfi] *or* **stuffed up** [ˌstʌft 'ʌp] *adj.* (nose) which is blocked with mucus *täppt*

stuka ⇨ **distort, sprain, twist**

stukning ⇨ **distortion, sprain, twist**

stumhet ⇨ **dumbness, mutism**

stump [stʌmp] *subst.* short piece of a limb which is left after the rest has been amputated *stump, amputationsstump*

stunt [stʌnt] *vb.* to stop something growing *hämma (i växten el. utvecklingen);* **the children's development was stunted by disease**

stupe [stju:p] *subst.* wet medicated dressing used as a compress *våtvarmt omslag*

stupor ['stju:pə] *subst.* state of being semi-conscious *stupor, tillstånd med sänkt vakenhetsgrad;* **after the party several people were found lying on the floor in a stupor**

Sturge-Weber syndrome [ˌstɜ:dʒ'webə ˌsɪndrəʊm] *subst.* dark red mark on the skin above the eye, together with similar marks inside the brain, possibly causing epileptic fits *angiomatosis Sturge-Weber, Sturge-Webers sjukdom*

stutter ['stʌtə] **1** *subst.* speech defect where the patient repeats the sound at the beginning of a word several times *stamning;* **he is taking therapy to try to cure his stutter 2** *vb.* to speak with a stutter *stamma*

stuttering ['stʌt(ə)rɪŋ] *or* **dysphemia** [dɪs'fi:miə] *subst.* difficulty in speaking where the person repeats parts of words *or* stops to try to pronounce words *stamning*

St Vitus' dance [s(ə)nt 'vaɪtəs ˌdɑ:ns] *subst.* old name for Sydenham's chorea *Sydenhams chorea, chorea minor, danssjuka*

stycke ⇨ **section**

stye [staɪ] *or* **hordeolum** [hɔːˈdiːələm] *subst.* inflammation of the gland at the base of an eyelash *hordeolum, vagel*

stygn ⇨ **stitch**

stylo- [ˈstaɪləʊ, ˌ--] *prefix* referring to the styloid process *stylo-*

styloglossus [ˌstaɪləʊˈglɒsəs] *subst.* muscle which links the tongue to the styloid process *musculus styloglossus*

styloid [ˈstaɪlɔɪd] *adj.* pointed *styloid, griffelliknande;* **styloid process** = piece of bone which projects from the bottom of the temporal bone ⇨ *illustration* SKULL *processus styloideus (ossis temporalis), (tinningbenets) griffelliknande utskott*

stylus [ˈstaɪləs] *subst.* long thin instrument used for applying antiseptics *or* ointments onto the skin *stift*

styptic [ˈstɪptɪk] *adj. & subst.* (substance) which stops bleeding *styptikum, styptiskt (medel), adstringerande (medel), sammandragande (medel), blodstillande (medel);* **styptic pencil** = stick of alum, used to stop bleeding from small cuts *blodstillande stift*

styra ⇨ **control, direct, regulate**

styrelse ⇨ **authority, council**

styrka ⇨ **force, strength, virulence**

styrning ⇨ **control, regulation**

styv ⇨ **rigid, stiff**

styvhet ⇨ **rigidity, stiffness**

stånd ⇨ **erection**

stång ⇨ **support**

stå (upprätt) ⇨ **stand up**

städa ⇨ **clean**

städet ⇨ **anvil, incus**

ställföreträdande ⇨ **vicarious**

ställning ⇨ **position**

stäm- ⇨ **vocal**

stämbanden ⇨ **cord, ventricular**

stämbanden, falska ⇨ **vestibular**

stämbandsinflammation ⇨ **chorditis**

stämfremitus ⇨ **fremitus, vocal**

stämgaffel ⇨ **tuning fork**

stämma ⇨ **voice**

ständig ⇨ **constant, continual, continuous, perennial, permanent**

stänga ⇨ **lock, obstruct**

stärka ⇨ **improve**

stärkande medel ⇨ **tonic**

stärkelse ⇨ **starch**

stärkelse- ⇨ **farinaceous**

stärkelserik ⇨ **starchy**

stöd ⇨ **brace, support, sustentaculum**

stöd- ⇨ **sustentacular**

stödförband ⇨ **binder, suspensory**

stödja ⇨ **support, sustain**

stödjande ⇨ **supportive, suspensory**

stödjevävnad ⇨ **connective tissue, stroma**

stödstrumpor ⇨ **surgical**

störa ⇨ **disturb, interfere**

störd ⇨ **deranged, disordered, upset**

störning ⇨ **derangement, disorder, disturbance, interference, upset**

störning, mental ⇨ **psychopathy**

större ⇨ **greater, major**

störta ⇨ **crash**

störthjälm ⇨ **crash**

stöt ⇨ **bump, concussion, ictus, impulse**

stöta ⇨ **bump, stab**

stöta av (bort) ⇨ **reject, repel**

stötas bort, inte ⇨ **take**

stöta upp ⇨ **regurgitate**

sub- [sʌb-] *prefix* meaning underneath *sub-, under-*

subacute [ˌsʌbəˈkjuːt] *adj.* (condition) which is not acute but may become chronic *subakut;* **subacute bacterial endocarditis** = inflammation of the lining of the heart caused by bacteria *subakut bakteriell endokardit;* **subacute combined degeneration (of the spinal cord)** = condition (caused by vitamin B_{12} deficiency) where the sensory and motor nerves in the spinal cord become damaged and the patient has difficulty in moving

subakut ⇨ **subacute**

subarachnoid [ˌsʌbəˈræknɔɪd] *adj.* beneath the arachnoid membrane *subaraknoidal;* **subarachnoid haemorrhage** = bleeding into the cerebrospinal fluid of the subarachnoid space *subaraknoidalblödning;* **subarachnoid space** = space between the arachnoid membrane and the pia mater in the brain, containing cerebrospinal fluid *subaraknoidalrummet*

subaraknoidal ⇨ **subarachnoid**

subaraknoidalblödning ⇨ **subarachnoid**

subaraknoidalrummet ⇨ **subarachnoid**

subclavian [ˌsʌbˈkleɪviən] *adj.* underneath the clavicle *subklavikulär;* **subclavian artery** = one of two arteries branching from the aorta on the left, and from the innominate artery on the right, continuing into the brachial arteries and supplying blood to each arm *arteria subclavia, nyckelbensartären;* **subclavian veins** = veins which continue the axillary veins into the brachiocephalic vein; **subclavian vein** *(vena) subclavia, nyckelbensvenen*

subclinical [ˌsʌbˈklɪnɪk(ə)l] *adj.* (disease) which is present in the body, but which has not yet developed any symptoms *subklinisk*

subconscious [ˌsʌbˈkɒnʃəs] *adj. & subst.* (referring to) mental processes (such as the memory) of which people are not aware all the time, but which can affect their actions *omedveten, undermedveten;* **the subconscious** *det omedvetna (undermedvetna)*

subcortical [ˌsʌbˈkɔːtɪk(ə)l] *adj.* beneath a cortex *subkortikal*

subcostal [ˌsʌbˈkɒst(ə)l] *adj.* below the ribs *subkostal;* **subcostal plane** = imaginary horizontal line drawn across the front of the abdomen below the ribs *tänkt horisontellt plan genom kroppen under revbensbågen*

subculture [ˈsʌbˌkʌltʃə] *subst.* culture of bacteria which is taken from a stock culture *subkultur*

subculturing [ˌsʌbˈkʌltʃərɪŋ] *subst.* taking of a bacterial culture from a stock culture *tagande av bakteriekultur från stamkultur*

subcutaneous [ˌsʌbkjuˈteɪniəs] *adj.* under the skin *subkutan;* **subcutaneous injection** = injection made just under the skin (as to administer pain-killing drugs) *subkutan injektion;* **subcutaneous oedema** = fluid collecting under the skin, usually at the ankles *subkutant ödem;* **subcutaneous tissue** = fatty tissue under the skin *subkutan vävnad*

subdural [ˌsʌbˈdjʊər(ə)l] *adj.* between the dura mater and the arachnoid *subdural*

subduralhematom ⇨ **haematoma**

subfrenisk ⇨ **subphrenic**

subinvolution [ˌsʌbɪnvəˈluːʃ(ə)n] *subst.* condition where a part of the body does not go back to its former size and shape after having swollen *or* stretched (as in the case of the uterus after childbirth) *ofullständig återbildning*

subject [ˈsʌbdʒekt] *subst.* **(a)** patient *or* person suffering from a certain disease *patient, person;* **the hospital has developed a new treatment for arthritic subjects (b)** thing which is being studied *or* written about *ämne;* **the subject of the article is "Rh-negative babies"**

subjective [səbˈdʒektɪv] *adj.* referring to the person concerned *subjektiv, personlig;* **the psychiatrist gave a subjective opinion on the patient's problem**

subject to [ˈsʌbdʒekt tʊ] *adv.* likely to suffer from *utsatt för, med anlag (viss benägenhet) för, som lider (besväras) av;* **the patient is subject to fits; after returning from the tropics he was subject to attacks of malaria**

subjektiv ⇨ **subjective**

subklavikulär ⇨ **subclavian**

subklinisk ⇨ **silent, subclinical**

subkortikal ⇨ **subcortical**

subkostal ⇨ **subcostal**

subkultur ⇨ **subculture**

subkutan ⇨ **hypodermic, subcutaneous**

sublimate ['sʌblɪmət; 'sʌblɪmeɪt] **1** *subst.* deposit left when a vapour condenses *sublimat* **2** *vb.* to convert violent emotion into a certain action which is not antisocial *sublimera*

sublimation [ˌsʌblɪ'meɪʃ(ə)n] *subst.* doing a certain action as an unconscious way of showing violent emotions which would otherwise be expressed in antisocial behaviour *sublimering*

sublimera ⇨ **sublimate**

sublimering ⇨ **sublimation**

subliminal [ˌsʌb'lɪmɪn(ə)l] *adj.* (stimulus) which is too slight to be noticed by the senses *subliminal, omedveten, undermedveten*

sublingual [ˌsʌb'lɪŋgw(ə)l] *adj.* under the tongue *sublingual;* **sublingual gland** = salivary gland under the tongue ⇨ *illustration* THROAT *glandula sublingualis, undertungsspottkörteln*

> QUOTE the sublingual region has a rich blood supply derived from the carotid artery and indicates changes in central body temperature more rapidly than the rectum
>
> **Nursing Times**

subluxation [ˌsʌblʌk'seɪʃ(ə)n] *subst.* condition where a joint is partially dislocated *subluxation*

submandibular gland [ˌsʌbmæn'dɪbjʊlə ˌglænd] *or* **submaxillary gland** [sʌb'mæksɪl(ə)ri ˌglænd] *subst.* salivary gland on each side of the lower jaw ⇨ *illustration* THROAT *glandula submandibularis, underkäksspottkörteln*

submental [ˌsʌb'ment(ə)l] *adj.* under the chin *submental*

submucosa [ˌsʌbmju'kəʊsə] *subst.* tissue under mucous membrane *(tela) submucosa*

submucous [sʌb'mju:kəs] *adj.* under mucous membrane *submukös;* **submucous resection** = removal of a bent cartilage from the septum in the nose *kirurgiskt avlägsnande under slemhinna, t.ex. av brosk i näsan*

submukös ⇨ **submucous**

subnormal [ˌsʌb'nɔ:m(ə)l] *adj.* (patient) with a mind which has not developed fully *subnormal, psykiskt utvecklingsstörd;* **severely subnormal** = (patient) whose mind has not developed and is incapable of looking after himself *allvarligt psykiskt utvecklingsstörd*

subnormalitet ⇨ **subnormality**

subnormality [ˌsʌbnɔ:'mæləti] *subst.* condition where a patient's mind has not developed fully *subnormalitet, psykisk utvecklingsstörning, efterblivenhet*

suboccipital [ˌsʌbɒk'sɪpɪt(ə)l] *adj.* beneath the back of the head *suboccipital*

subphrenic [ˌsʌb'frenɪk] *adj.* under the diaphragm *subfrenisk;* **subphrenic abscess** = abscess which forms between the diaphragm and the liver *subfrenisk abscess*

subside [səb'saɪd] *vb.* to go down *or* to become less violent *avta, gå ned;* **after being given the antibiotics, his fever subsided**

substance ['sʌbst(ə)ns] *subst.* chemical material *substans, ämne;* **toxic substances released into the bloodstream; he became addicted to certain substances**

substans ⇨ **matter, substance**

substituera ⇨ **replace**

substitution [ˌsʌbstɪ'tju:ʃ(ə)n] *subst.* replacing one thing with another *substitution, ersättning, utbyte;* **substitution therapy** = treating a condition by using a different drug from the one used before *substitutionsterapi, ersättningsterapi*

substitutionsterapi ⇨ **substitution**

substrate ['sʌbstreɪt] *subst.* substance which is acted on by an enzyme *substrat*

> QUOTE insulin is a protein hormone and the body's major anabolic hormone, regulating the metabolism of all body fuels and substrates
>
> **Nursing 87**

subsultus [ˌsʌb'sʌltəs] *subst.* twitching of the muscles and tendons, caused by fever *subsultus (tendinum)*

subtertian fever [ˌsʌb'tɜ:ʃ(ə)n ˌfi:və] *subst.* type of malaria, where the fever is present most of the time *slags malaria*

subtotal [ˌsʌb'təʊt(ə)l] *adj.* (operation) to remove most of an organ *subtotal;* **subtotal**

gastrectomy = surgical removal of most of the stomach *subtotal gastrektomi;* **subtotal hysterectomy** = removal of the uterus, but not the cervix *subtotal hysterektomi;* **subtotal thyroidectomy** = removal of most of the thyroid gland *subtotal tyreoidektomi*

subungual [ˌsʌbˈʌŋgw(ə)l] *adj.* under a nail *subungual*

succeed [səkˈsiːd] *vb.* to do well *or* to do what one was trying to do *lyckas, ha framgång;* **scientists have succeeded in identifying the new influenza virus; they succeeded in stopping the flow of blood**

success [səkˈses] *subst.* **(a)** doing something well *or* doing what one was trying to do *framgång;* **they tried to isolate the virus but without success (b)** something which does well *framgång;* **the operation was a complete success**

successful [səkˈsesf(ə)l] *adj.* which works well *framgångsrik, lyckad;* **the operation was completely successful**

succession [səkˈseʃ(ə)n] *subst.* line of things, one after the other *följd, serie, rad;* **she had a succession of miscarriages**

successive [səkˈsesɪv] *adj.* (things) which follow one after the other *på varandra följande;* **she had a miscarriage with each successive pregnancy**

succus [ˈsʌkəs] *subst.* juice secreted by an organ *suc(c)us, saft;* **succus entericus** = juice formed of enzymes, produced in the intestine to help the digestive process *succus entericus, tarmsaft*

succussion [səˈkʌʃ(ə)n] *subst.* splashing sound made when there is a large amount of liquid inside a cavity in the body (as in the stomach) *skvalpljud*

suck [sʌk] *vb.* to pull liquid *or* air into the mouth *or* into a tube *suga;* **they applied the stomach pump to suck out the contents of the patient's stomach; the baby's sucking its thumb**

sucrase [ˈsuːkreɪz] *subst.* enzyme in the intestine which breaks down sucrose into glucose and fructose *sackaras*

sucrose [ˈsuːkrəʊs] *subst.* sugar found in plants, especially in sugar cane, beet and maple syrup (sucrose is formed of glucose and fructose) *sackaros, rörsocker*

suction [ˈsʌkʃ(ə)n] *subst.* action of sucking *suktion, sug(ning), aspiration;* **the dentist hooked a suction tube into the patient's mouth**

sudamen [sʊˈdeɪmən] *subst.* little blister caused by sweat *sudamen, svettblåsa*
NOTE: plural is **sudamina**

sudden [ˈsʌd(ə)n] *adj.* which happens quickly *plötslig;* **sudden death** = death without identifiable cause *or* not preceded by an illness *mors subita, plötslig död; US* **sudden infant death syndrome (SIDS)** *or* **crib death** = sudden death of a baby in bed, without any identifiable cause *plötslig spädbarnsdöd*

suddig ⇨ **blurred**

Sudeck's atrophy [ˈsuːdeks ˌætrəfi] *subst.* osteoporosis in the hand or foot *Sudecks atrofi*

sudor [ˈsuːdɔː] *subst.* sweat *sudor, transpiration, svett*

sudoriferum ⇨ **sudorific**

sudorific [ˌsuːdəˈrɪfɪk] *subst.* drug which makes a patient sweat *sudoriferum, svettdrivande medel*

suffer [ˈsʌfə] *vb.* **(a)** to have an illness for a long period of time *lida (av), drabbas (av);* **she suffers from headaches; he suffers from not being able to distinguish certain colours (b)** to feel pain *lida, plågas, ha ont;* **did she suffer much in her last illness? he did not suffer at all, and was conscious until he died**

sufferer [ˈsʌf(ə)rə] *subst.* person who has a certain disease *person som har viss sjukdom, -offer, -sjuk;* **a drug to help asthma sufferers** *or* **sufferers from asthma**

suffering [ˈsʌf(ə)rɪŋ] *subst.* feeling pain over a long period of time *lidande;* **the doctor gave him a morphine injection to relieve his suffering**

suffocate [ˈsʌfəkeɪt] *vb.* to make someone stop breathing by cutting off the supply of air to his nose and mouth *kväva(s)*

suffocation [ˌsʌfəˈkeɪʃ(ə)n] *subst.* making someone become unconscious by cutting off his supply of air *kvävning*

suffuse [səˈfjuːz] *vb.* to spread over something *sprida sig (över)*

suffusion [səˈfjuːʒ(ə)n] *subst.* spreading (of a red flush) over the skin *suffusion, utgjutning*

sug ⇨ **aspirator, suction**

suga ⇨ **suck**

sugar ['ʃʊgə] *subst.* any of several sweet carbohydrates *socker;* **blood sugar level** = amount of glucose in the blood *blodsockernivå, B-glukosnivå;* **sugar content** = percentage of sugar in a substance *or* food *sockerhalt;* **sugar intolerance** = diarrhoea caused by sugar which has not been absorbed *laktosintolerans, intolerans mot socker* NOTE: for other terms referring to sugar see words beginning with **glyc-**

> COMMENT: there are several natural forms of sugar: sucrose (in plants), lactose (in milk), fructose (in fruit), glucose and dextrose (in fruit and in body tissue). Edible sugar used in the home is a form of refined sucrose. All sugars are useful sources of energy, though excessive amounts of sugar can increase weight and cause tooth decay. Diabetes mellitus is a condition where the body is incapable of using sugar properly, causing high levels of sugar in blood and urine.

suga upp ⇨ **absorb**

suggest [sə'dʒest] *vb.* to mention an idea *föreslå, antyda;* **the doctor suggested that she should stop smoking**

suggestion [sə'dʒestʃ(ə)n] *subst.* **(a)** idea which has been mentioned *förslag, råd, antydan;* **the doctor didn't agree with the suggestion that the disease had been caught in the hospital (b)** *(in psychiatry)* making a person's ideas change, by suggesting different ideas which the patient can accept, such as that he is in fact cured *suggestion*

sugklocka ⇨ **vacuum extractor**

sugmask ⇨ **trematode**

suicidal [ˌsuːɪ'saɪd(ə)l] *adj.* (person) who wants to kill himself *suicidal, självmords-;* **he has suicidal tendencies**

suicide ['suːɪsaɪd] *subst.* act of killing oneself *suicid(ium), självmord;* **to commit suicide** = to kill yourself *begå självmord;* **after his wife died he committed suicide; attempted suicide** = trying to kill yourself, but not succeeding *självmordsförsök*

suktion ⇨ **suction**

sulcus ['sʌlkəs] *subst.* groove *or* fold (especially between the gyri in the brain) *sulcus, fåra;* **Harrison's sulcus** = hollow on either side of the chest which develops in children with lung problems *Harrisons fåra;* **lateral sulcus and central sulcus** = two grooves which divide a cerebral hemisphere into lobes *sulcus lateralis och sulcus centralis* NOTE: plural is **sulci**

sulfapreparat ⇨ **sulphonamide**

sulfat ⇨ **sulphate**

sulfonamid ⇨ **sulphonamide**

sulphate ['sʌlfeɪt] *subst.* salt of sulphuric acid *sulfat;* **barium sulphate** = salt of barium not soluble in water and which shows as opaque in X-ray photographs *bariumsulfat*

sulphonamide [sʌl'fɒnəmaɪd] *or* **sulpha drug** ['sʌlfə ˌdrʌg] *or* **sulpha compound** ['sʌlfə 'kɒmpaʊnd] *subst.* bacteriostatic drug used to treat bacterial infection, especially in the intestine and urinary system *sulfonamid, sulfapreparat*

sulphur ['sʌlfə] *subst.* yellow non-metallic chemical element which is contained in some amino acids and is used in creams to treat some skin disorders *svavel, S* NOTE: chemical symbol is **S.** Note also that words beginning **sulph-** are spelt **sulf-** in US English

sun [sʌn] *subst.* very hot star round which the earth travels and which gives light and heat *sol*

sunbathing ['sʌnbeɪðɪŋ] *subst.* lying in the sun to absorb sunlight *solbad*

sun blindness ['sʌnblaɪndnəs] = PHOTORETINITIS

sunburn ['sʌnbɜːn] *subst.* damage to the skin by excessive exposure to sunlight *solbränna, brännskada efter solbestrålning*

sunburnt ['sʌnbɜːnt] *adj.* (skin) made brown *or* red by exposure to sunlight *solbränd, brännskadad av solen*

sund ⇨ **sound**

sunglasses ['sʌnˌglɑːsɪz] *subst pl.* dark glasses which are worn to protect the eyes from the sun *solglasögon*

sunlight ['sʌnlaɪt] *subst.* light from the sun *solljus;* **he is allergic to strong sunlight**

> COMMENT: sunlight is essential to give the body vitamin D, but excessive exposure to sunlight will not simply turn the skin brown, but also may burn the surface of the skin so badly that it dies and pus forms beneath. Constant exposure to the sun can cause cancer of the skin

sunstroke ['sʌnstrəʊk] *subst.* serious condition caused by excessive exposure to the sun *or* to hot conditions, where the patient becomes dizzy, and has a high body temperature but does not perspire *insolation, solsting*

super- ['su:pə] *prefix* meaning (i) above *super-, över-;* (ii) extremely *super-, hyper-*

superaciditet ➪ **hyperchlorhydria**

superciliary [ˌsu:pə'sɪlɪəri] *adj.* referring to the eyebrows *superciliär*

superciliär ➪ **superciliary**

superego [ˌsu:p(ə)r'i:gəʊ] *subst. (in psychology)* part of the mind which is the conscience *or* which is concerned with right and wrong *överjaget*

superfecundation [ˌsu:pəˌfi:kən'deɪʃ(ə)n] *subst.* condition where two or more ova produced at the same time are fertilized by different males *superfekundation, överbefruktning*

superfekundation ➪ **superfecundation**

superfetation [ˌsu:pəfi:'teɪʃ(ə)n] *subst.* condition where an ovum is fertilized in a woman who is already pregnant *superfetation, överbefruktning*

superficial [ˌsu:pə'fɪʃ(ə)l] *adj.* on the surface *or* close to the surface *or* on the skin *ytlig;* **superficial burn** = burn on the skin surface *ytlig brännskada;* **superficial fascia** = membranous layers of connective tissue found just under the skin *fascia superficialis;* **superficial vein** = vein near the surface of the skin (as opposed to deep vein) *ytlig ven*

superinfection [ˌsu:pərɪn'fekʃ(ə)n] *subst.* second infection which affects the treatment of the first infection, because it is resistant to the drug used to treat the first *superinfektion*

superior [su:'pɪəriə] *adj. (of part of the body)* higher up than another part *superior, övre;* **superior vena cava** = branch of the large vein into the heart, carrying blood from the head and the top part of the body *vena cava superior, övre hålvenen*

NOTE: the opposite is **inferior, inferiority**

superiority [suˌpɪəri'ɒrəti] *subst.* being better than something *or* someone else *överlägsenhet;* **superiority complex** = condition where a person feels he is better in some way than others and pays little attention to them *överlägsenhetskomplex*

supernumerary [ˌsu:pə'nju:m(ə)r(ə)ri] *adj.* extra; *(of teeth, etc.)* one (or more than one) more than the usual number *supernumerär, övertalig*

> QUOTE allocation of supernumerary students to clinical areas is for their educational needs and not for service requirements
>
> **Nursing Times**

supervise ['su:pəvaɪz] *vb.* to manage *or* to organize something *övervaka, ha tillsyn (uppsyn) över, kontrollera;* **the administration of drugs has to be supervised by a qualified person; she has been appointed to supervise the transfer of patients to the new ward**

supervision [ˌsu:pə'vɪʒ(ə)n] *subst.* management *or* organization *övervakning, tillsyn, kontroll;* **elderly patients need constant supervision; the sheltered housing is under the supervision of a full-time nurse**

supervisor ['su:pəvaɪzə] *subst.* person who supervises *person som övervakar (kontrollerar, har tillsyn el. uppsyn över);* **the supervisor of hospital catering services**

supinate ['su:pɪneɪt] *vb.* to turn (the hand) so that the palm is upwards *supinera*

supination [ˌsu:pɪ'neɪʃ(ə)n] *subst.* turning the hand so that palm faces upwards *supination*

supinator ['su:pɪneɪtə] *subst.* muscle which turns the hand so that the palm faces upwards *musculus supinator*

supine ['su:paɪn] *adj.* (i) lying on the back *på rygg, i ryggläge, liggande;* (ii) with the palm of the hand facing upwards *supinerad*
NOTE: the opposite is **pronation, prone**

supinera ➪ **supinate**

supinerad ➪ **supine**

supp ➪ **suppository**

supply [sə'plaɪ] **1** *subst.* something which is provided *tillförsel, förråd, försörjning;* **the arteries provide a continuous supply of oxygenated blood to the tissues; the hospital service needs a constant supply of blood for transfusion; the government sent medical supplies to the disaster area** **2** *vb.* to provide *or* to give something which is needed *förse (med), tillföra, tillhandhålla;* **a balanced diet will supply the body with all the vitamins**

and trace elements it needs; the brachial artery supplies the arms and hands

support [sə'pɔ:t] **1** *subst.* **(a)** help to keep something in place *stöd;* **the bandage provides some support for the knee; he was so weak that he had to hold onto a chair for support (b)** handle *or* metal rail which a person can hold *stöd, stång, ledstång, sänggrind;* **there are supports at the side of the bed; the bath is provided with metal supports 2** *vb.* to hold something *or* to keep something in place *stödja;* **he wore a truss to support a hernia**

supportive [sə'pɔ:tɪv] *adj.* (person) who helps *or* comforts someone in trouble *stödjande, som fungerar som stöd (hjälp);* **her family were very supportive when she was in hospital; the local health authority has been very supportive of the hospital management**

suppository [sə'pɒzɪt(ə)ri] *subst.* piece of soluble material (such as glycerine jelly) containing a drug, which is placed in the rectum (to act as lubricant), or in the vagina (to treat disorders such as vaginitis) and is dissolved by the body's fluids *suppositorium, supp, stolpiller*

suppress [sə'pres] *vb.* to remove (a symptom) *or* to reduce the action of something completely *or* to stop (the release of a hormone) *undertrycka, dämpa, hämma;* **a course of treatment which suppresses the painful irritation; the drug suppresses the body's natural instinct to reject the transplanted tissue; the release of adrenaline from the adrenal cortex is suppressed**

suppression [sə'preʃ(ə)n] *subst.* act of suppressing *suppression, undertryckande, dämpning, hämning;* **the suppression of allergic responses; the suppression of a hormone**

suppurate ['sʌpju(ə)reɪt] *vb.* to form and discharge pus *suppurera, vara sig, varas, bli varig*

suppurating ['sʌpju(ə)reɪtɪŋ] *or* **purulent** ['pjʊərʊlənt] *adj.* containing *or* discharging pus *suppurativ, purulent, varig*

suppuration [ˌsʌpju(ə)'reɪʃ(ə)n] *subst.* formation and discharge of pus *suppuration, varbildning*

suppurativ ⇨ **suppurating**

suppurera ⇨ **suppurate**

supra- ['su:prə, ˌ--] *prefix* meaning above *or* over *supra-*

supraoptic nucleus [ˌsu:prə'ɒptɪk ˌnju:kliəs] *subst.* nucleus in the hypothalamus from which nerve fibres run to the posterior pituitary gland *nucleus supraopticus*

supraorbital [ˌsuprə'ɔ:bɪt(ə)l] *adj.* above the orbit of the eye *supraorbital;* **supraorbital ridge** = ridge of bone above the eye, covered by the eyebrow *benkanten under ögonbrynet*

suprapubic [ˌsu:prə'pju:bɪk] *adj.* above the pubic bone *suprapubisk*

suprarenal [ˌsu:prə'ri:n(ə)l] *adj.* above the kidney *suprarenal, binjure-;* **suprarenal area** = the area of the body above the kidney *området ovanför njurarna;* **suprarenal glands** *or* **suprarenals** *or* **adrenal glands** = two endocrine glands at the top of the kidneys, which secrete adrenaline and other hormones *glandulae suprarenales, binjurarna*

sur ⇨ **sour**

surface ['sɜ:fɪs] *subst.* top layer of something *yta, utsida;* **the surfaces of the two membranes may rub together**

surfactant [sɜ:'fækt(ə)nt] *subst.* substance in the alveoli of the lungs which keeps the surfaces of the lungs wet and prevents lung collapse *ytaktivt medel, ytspänningsnedsättande medel (substans)*

surgeon ['sɜ:dʒ(ə)n] *subst.* doctor who specializes in surgery *kirurg;* **eye surgeon** = surgeon who specializes in operations on eyes *ögonkirurg;* **heart surgeon** = surgeon who specializes in operations on hearts *hjärtkirurg;* **plastic surgeon** = surgeon who repairs defective *or* deformed parts of the body *plastikkirurg* NOTE: although surgeons are doctors, in the UK they are traditionally called "Mr" and not "Dr", so "Dr Smith" may be a GP, but "Mr Smith" is a surgeon

surgery ['sɜ:dʒ(ə)ri] *subst.* **(a)** treatment of a disease *or* disorder which requires an operation to cut into *or* to remove *or* to manipulate tissue *or* organs *or* parts *kirurgi, operation(er);* **the patient will need plastic surgery to remove the scars he received in the accident; the surgical ward is for patients waiting for surgery; two of our patients had to have surgery; exploratory surgery** = surgical operations in which the aim is to discover the cause of the patient's symptoms *or* the extent of the illness *explorativ kirurgi;* **major surgery** = surgical operations involving important organs in the body *större operation(er);* **plastic surgery** *or*

reconstructive surgery = surgery to repair defective *or* deformed parts of the body *plastikkirurgi, rekonstruktiv kirurgi;* **spare part surgery** = surgical operations where parts of the body (such as bones *or* joints) are replaced by artificial pieces *reservdelskirurgi; see also* CRYOSURGERY, MICROSURGERY **(b)** room where a doctor *or* dentist sees and examines patients *undersökningsrum, mottagning, operationssal;* **there are ten patients waiting in the surgery; surgery hours are from 8.30 in the morning to 6.00 at night**

surgical ['sɜːdʒɪk(ə)l] *adj.* (i) referring to surgery *kirurgisk, ortopedisk, operations-;* (ii) (disease) which can be treated by surgery *kirurgisk, ortopedisk, operations-;* **all surgical instruments must be sterilized; we manage to carry out six surgical operations in an hour; surgical care** = looking after patients who have had surgery *kirurgisk vård;* **surgical emphysema** = air bubbles in tissue, not in the lungs *emphysema subcutaneum, hudemfysem, kirurgiskt emfysem;* **surgical gloves** = thin plastic gloves worn by surgeons *operationshandskar, sterila handskar;* **surgical neck** = narrow part at the top of the humerus, where the arm can easily be broken *collum chirurgicum (humeri);* **surgical spirit** = ethyl alcohol with an additive which gives it an unpleasant taste, used as a disinfectant *or* for rubbing on the skin *tvättsprit, ryggsprit* (NOTE: the US English is **rubbing alcohol**) **surgical stockings** = strong elastic stockings worn to support a weak joint in the knee, or to hold varicose veins tightly *stödstrumpor;* **surgical ward** = ward in a hospital for patients who have to have operations *kirurgavdelning, kirurgisk (vård)avdelning*

surgically ['sɜːdʒɪk(ə)li] *adv.* using surgery *kirurgiskt, ortopediskt, med hjälp av operation;* **the growth can be treated surgically**

surhet ⇨ **acidity**

surhetsgrad ⇨ **acidity, pH**

sur mage ⇨ **acidosis**

surrogate ['sʌrəgət] *adj.* taking the place of *surrogat-, ersättnings-;* **surrogate mother** = (i) person who takes the place of a real mother *surrogatmor;* (ii) woman who has a child by AID for a couple where the wife cannot bear children, with the intention of handing the child over to them when it is born *surrogatmor*

surrogatmor ⇨ **surrogate**

surround [sə'raʊnd] *vb.* to be all around something *omge;* **the wound is several millimetres deep and the surrounding flesh is inflamed**

surroundings [sə'raʊndɪŋz] *subst. pl.* area round something *omgivning, miljö;* **the cottage hospital is set in pleasant surroundings**

survival [sə'vaɪv(ə)l] *subst.* continuing to live *överlevnad;* **the survival rate of newborn babies has begun to fall**

survive [sə'vaɪv] *vb.* to continue to live *överleva;* **he survived two attacks of pneumonia; they survived a night on the mountain without food; the baby only survived for two hours**

survivor [sə'vaɪvə] *subst.* person who survives *överlevande*

susceptibility [səˌseptə'bɪləti] *subst.* lack of resistance to a disease *mottaglighet, känslighet, ömtålighet*

> QUOTE low birthweight has been associated with increased susceptibility to infection
> **East African Medical Journal**

> QUOTE even children with the milder forms of sickle-cell disease have an increased frequency of pneumococcal infection. The reason for this susceptibility is a profound abnormality of the immune system
> **Lancet**

susceptible [sə'septəb(ə)l] *adj.* likely to catch (a disease) *mottaglig, känslig, ömtålig;* **she is susceptible to colds** *or* **to throat infections**

suspect 1 ['sʌspekt] *subst.* person who doctors believe may have a disease *misstänkt (person);* **they are screening all typhoid suspects 2** [səs'pekt] *vb.* to think that someone may have a disease *misstänka;* **he is a suspected diphtheria carrier; several cases of suspected meningitis have been reported**

> QUOTE those affected are being nursed in five isolation wards and about forty suspected sufferers are being barrier nursed in other wards
> **Nursing Times**

suspension [sə'spenʃ(ə)n] *subst.* liquid with solid particles in it *suspension, uppslamning*

suspensory [sə'spens(ə)ri] *adj.* which is hanging down *bärande, stödjande;* **suspensory bandage** = bandage to hold a part of the body which hangs *stödförband;* **suspensory**

ligament = ligament which holds a part of the body in position *ligamentum suspensorium, stödjande ligament*

sustain [sə'steɪn] *vb.* to keep *or* to support *stödja, hålla uppe*

sustentacular [ˌsʌstən'tækjʊlə] *adj.* referring to sustentaculum *stöd-*

sustentaculum [ˌsʌstən'tækjʊləm] *subst.* part of the body which supports another part *sustentaculum, stöd*

sutur ⇨ **stitch, suture**

-sutur ⇨ **-rrhaphy**

suture ['suːtʃə] **1** *subst.* **(a)** fixed joint where two bones are fused together, especially the bones in the skull ⇨ *illustration* SKULL *sutur, bensöm, benfog;* **coronal suture** = horizontal joint across the top of the skull between the parietal and frontal bones *sutura coronalis, hjässömmen, kronsömmen;* **lambdoidal suture** = horizontal joint across the back of the skull between the parietal and occipital bones *sutura lambdoides, lambdasömmen, nacksömmen;* **sagittal suture** = joint along the top of the head between the two parietal bones *sutura sagittalis, pilsömmen* **(b)** attaching the sides of an incision *or* wound with thread, so that healing can take place *sutur(ering)* **(c)** thread used for attaching the sides of a wound so that they can heal *sutur, tråd* **2** *vb.* to attach the sides of a wound *or* incision together with thread so that healing can take place *suturera, sy (fast)*

COMMENT: wounds are usually stitched using thread or catgut which is removed after a week or so. Sutures inside the body are made of soluble material which is gradually dissolved by body fluids

suturera ⇨ **stitch, suture**

svag ⇨ **faint, feeble, weak; poor, poorly**

sval ⇨ **cool**

svalg- ⇨ **pharyng-, pharyngeal**

svalget ⇨ **throat, fauces, pharynx**

svalginflammation ⇨ **pharyngitis**

svalgkramp ⇨ **pharyngismus**

svalgmandeln ⇨ **pharyngeal**

svalgringen, lymfatiska ⇨ **Waldeyer's ring**

svalgtonsillen ⇨ **pharyngeal**

svallkött ⇨ **proud flesh**

svamp ⇨ **fungus**

svamp- ⇨ **fungal, myc-**

svampförgiftning ⇨ **fungus**

svampliknande ⇨ **fungoid**

svampsjukdom ⇨ **fungus, mycosis**

svankrygg ⇨ **lordosis**

svans- ⇨ **caudal, coccy-**

svansbenet ⇨ **coccyx**

svansbens- ⇨ **coccy-**

svanskotorna ⇨ **coccygeal vertebrae**

svar ⇨ **answer, reaction, response**

svara ⇨ **answer**

svara på ⇨ **respond**

svart ⇨ **black**

svartvattenfeber ⇨ **blackwater fever**

svavel ⇨ **sulphur**

sveda ⇨ **burn**

svetsblände ⇨ **welder's flash**

svett ⇨ **perspiration, sweat**

svett- ⇨ **hidr-**

svettas ⇨ **perspire, sweat**

svettblåsa ⇨ **sudamen**

svettkörtel ⇨ **sweat**

svettkörtelinflammation ⇨ **hidradenitis**

svettutsöndring, nedsatt ⇨ **hypohidrosis**

svikt ⇨ **failure**

svimma ⇨ **faint, pass out**

svimning ⇨ **faint, fainting**

svimningsanfall ➪ **fainting**

svindel ➪ **dizziness, giddiness, vertigo**

svinkoppor ➪ **impetigo**

sviter ➪ **sequelae, after-effects**

svullen ➪ **tumid, turgid**

svullnad ➪ **intumescence, swelling, tumefaction, tumescence, tumor, turgescence, turgor**

svulst ➪ **bump, growth, horn, tuber, tumor**

svår ➪ **bad, difficult, hard, serious, severe, violent**

svårbehandlad ➪ **intractable**

svårighet ➪ **difficulty**

svårighetsgrad ➪ **severity**

svårt ➪ **seriously, severely**

svälja ➪ **swallow**

sväljning ➪ **deglutition, swallowing**

sväljningssmärta ➪ **odynophagia**

sväljningssvårigheter ➪ **dysphagia**

svälla ➪ **swell**

svälla ut ➪ **bulge**

svällkropp ➪ **corpus**

svält ➪ **malnutrition, starvation**

svälta ➪ **starve**

svältkost ➪ **starvation**

svältkur ➪ **starvation**

svärdsliknande ➪ **ensiform**

svärdsutskottet ➪ **ensiform, xiphisternum**

swab [swɒb] *subst.* cotton wool pad, often attached to a small stick, used to clean a wound *or* to apply ointment, etc. *tork, bomullstopp*

swallow ['swɒləʊ] *vb.* to make liquid *or* food (and sometimes air) go down from the mouth to the stomach *svälja;* **patients suffering from nosebleeds should try not to swallow the blood**

swallowing ['swɒləʊɪŋ] *or* **deglutition** [ˌdi:glu:'tɪʃ(ə)n] *subst.* action of passing food *or* liquids (sometimes also air) from the mouth into the oesophagus and down into the stomach *deglutition, sväljning; see also* AEROPHAGY

sweat [swet] **1** *subst.* sudor *or* perspiration *or* salt moisture produced by the sweat glands *sudor, transpiration, svett;* **sweat was running off the end of his nose; her hands were covered with sweat; sweat duct** = thin tube connecting the sweat gland with the surface of the skin **sweat ducts** *ductus sudoriferi, svettkörtlarnas utförsgångar;* **sweat gland** = gland which produces sweat, situated beneath the dermis and connected to the surface of the skin by a thin tube *glandula sudorifera, svettkörtel;* **sweat pore** = hole in the skin through which the sweat comes out ➪ *illustration* SKIN & SENSORY RECEPTORS *porus sudorifer, svettförande por* **2** *vb.* to perspire *or* to produce moisture through the sweat glands and onto the skin *svettas;* **after working in the fields he was sweating**

> COMMENT: sweat cools the body as the moisture evaporates from the skin. Sweat contains salt, and in hot countries it may be necessary to take salt tablets to replace the salt lost through the skin

sweet [swi:t] *adj.* one of the basic tastes, not bitter, sour or salt *söt;* **sugar is sweet, lemons are sour**

swell [swel] *vb.* to become larger *svälla, svullna (upp);* **the disease affects the lymph glands, making them swell; the doctor noticed that the patient had swollen glands in his neck; she finds her swollen ankles painful** NOTE: **swelling - swelled - has swollen**

swelling ['swelɪŋ] *subst.* condition where fluid accumulates in tissue, making the tissue become large *svullnad, bula;* **they applied a cold compress to try to reduce the swelling**

sycosis [saɪ'kəʊsɪs] *subst.* bacterial infection of hair follicles *sykos;* **sycosis barbae** *or* **barber's rash** = infection of hair follicles on the sides of the face and chin *sycosis barbae (vulgaris), skäggfinne, skäggsvamp*

Sydenham's chorea ['sɪdənhæmz kəʊ'rɪə] *see* CHOREA

sy (fast) ➪ **stitch, suture**

syfilid ⇨ **syphilide**

syfilis ⇨ **lues, pox, syphilis**

syfilissvulst ⇨ **gumma**

syfilitiker ⇨ **syphilitic**

syfilitisk ⇨ **syphilitic**

syfilitisk ryggmärgsförtvining ⇨ **tabes**

syfilom ⇨ **gumma**

sykos ⇨ **sycosis**

Sylvius ['sɪlviəs] *see* AQUEDUCT

symbiosis [ˌsɪmbɪ'əʊsɪs] *subst.* condition where two organisms exist together and help each other to survive *symbios*

symblepharon [sɪm'blef(ə)rɒn] *subst.* condition where the eyelid sticks to the eyeball *symblepharon*

symbol ['sɪmb(ə)l] *subst.* sign *or* letter which means something *symbol, tecken;* **chemical symbol** = letters which indicate a chemical substance *kemiskt tecken;* **Na is the symbol for sodium**

Syme's amputation ['saɪmz ˌæmpju'teɪʃ(ə)n] *subst.* surgical operation to amputate the foot above the ankle *Symes amputation*

symfys ⇨ **cartilaginous, symphysis**

symfysen ⇨ **interpubic joint**

symfyseotomi ⇨ **symphysiotomy**

sympathectomy [ˌsɪmpə'θektəmi] *subst.* surgical operation to cut part of the sympathetic nervous system, as a treatment of high blood pressure *sympatektomi*

sympathetic nervous system [ˌsɪmpə'θetɪk ˌnɜːvəs ˌsɪstəm] *subst.* part of the autonomic nervous system, which runs down the spinal column and connects with various important organs, such as the heart, the lungs, the sweat glands, etc. *sympatiska nervsystemet*

sympatholytic [ˌsɪmpəθəʊ'lɪtɪk] *subst.* drug which stops the sympathetic nervous system working *sympatikusdämpande medel*

sympathomimetic [ˌsɪmpəθəʊmɪ'metɪk] *adj.* (drug) which stimulates the activity of the sympathetic nervous system *sympatomimetisk*

sympatikusdämpande medel ⇨ **sympatholytic**

sympatiska nervsystemet ⇨ **sympathetic nervous system**

symphysiectomy [sɪmˌfɪzi'ektəmi] *subst.* surgical operation to remove part of the pubic symphysis to make childbirth easier *symfyseotomi (förut vid bäckenträngsel)*

symphysiotomy [sɪmˌfɪzi'ɒtəmi] *subst.* surgical operation to make an incision in the pubic symphysis to make the passage for a fetus wider *symfyseotomi*

symphysis ['sɪmfəsɪs] *subst.* point where two bones are joined by cartilage which makes the joint rigid *symfys, sammanväxning, fog;* **pubic symphysis** *or* **interpubic joint** = piece of cartilage which joins the two sections of the pubic bone *symphysis pubica (ossis pubis), (blygdbens)symfysen, blygdbensfogen;* **symphysis menti** = point in the front of the lower jaw where the two halves of the jaw are fused to form the chin *underkäkens symfys (fog)*

symptom ['sɪm(p)təm] *subst.* change in the way the body works *or* change in the body's appearance, which shows that a disease *or* disorder is present and is noticed by the patient himself *symtom, symptom, sjukdomstecken;* **the symptoms of hay fever are a running nose and eyes; a doctor must study the symptoms before making his diagnosis; the patient presented all the symptoms of rheumatic fever** NOTE: if a symptom is noticed only by the doctor, it is a **sign**

symptomatic [ˌsɪm(p)tə'mætɪk] *adj.* which is a symptom *sym(p)tomatisk, kännetecknande;* **the rash is symptomatic of measles**

symptomatology [sɪm(p)ˌtɒmə'tɒlədʒi] *or* **semeiology** [ˌsemi'ɒlədʒi] *subst.* branch of medicine concerned with the study of symptoms *sym(p)tomatologi, sym(p)tomlära, semiologi, semiotik*

symptomkomplex ⇨ **complex**

symtom ⇨ **manifestation, physical, symptom**

symtomfri ⇨ **asymptomatic**

symtomkomplex ⇨ **syndrome**

syn- ['sɪn, ˌ-] *prefix* meaning joint *or* fused *syn-*

syn- ⇨ **optic, optical, syn-, visual**

synalgia [sɪ'nældʒ(ɪ)ə] *or* **referred pain** [rɪ'fɜ:d ˌpeɪn] *subst.* pain which is felt in one part of the body, but is caused by a condition in another part (such as pain in the groin which can be a symptom of kidney stone and pain in the right shoulder which can indicate gall bladder infection) *synalgi, referred pain, överförd smärta, ung. projicerad smärta*

synaps ⇨ **synapse, synaptic**

synapse ['saɪnæps] **1** *subst.* point in the nervous system where the axons of neurones are in contact with the dendrites of other neurones *synaps* **2** *vb.* to link with a neurone *kopplas samman med nervcell*

synaptic [sɪn'æptɪk] *adj.* referring to a synapse *synaptisk;* **synaptic connection** = link between the dendrites of one neurone with another neurone *synaps*

synarthrosis [ˌsɪnɑ:'θrəʊsɪs] *subst.* joint (as in the skull) where the bones have fused together *synartros*

synas ⇨ **appear**

synaxel ⇨ **visual**

synbanan ⇨ **optic**

synbar ⇨ **noticeable**

syncentrum ⇨ **area, visual**

synchondrosis [ˌsɪnkɒn'drəʊsɪs] *subst.* joint, as in children, where the bones are linked by cartilage, before the cartilage has changed to bone *synkondros, broskfog*

synchysis ['sɪnkɪsɪs] *subst.* condition where the vitreous humour in the eye becomes soft *synchysis (corporis vitrel)*

syncope ['sɪŋkəpi] *or* **fainting fit** ['feɪntɪŋ fɪt] *subst.* becoming unconscious for a short time because of reduced flow of blood to the brain *syncope, synkope, svimning(sanfall)*

syncytium [sɪn'sɪʃiəm] *subst.* continuous length of tissue in muscle fibres *syncytium, cellförband;* **respiratory syncytial virus** = virus which causes infections of the nose and throat in children *respiratory syncytial virus, RS-virum*

syndactyly [sɪn'dæktɪli] *subst.* condition where two toes *or* fingers are joined together with tissue *syndaktyli(sm)*

syndesm- [ˌsɪndes'm] *or* **syndesmo-** [sɪn'desməʊ, -ˌ--] *prefix* referring to ligaments *syndesm(o)-, bindvävs-*

syndesmology [ˌsɪndes'mɒlədʒi] *subst.* branch of medicine which studies joints *syndesmologi, läran om ligament o.dyl.*

syndesmos ⇨ **fibrous, syndesmosis**

syndesmosis [ˌsɪndes'məʊsɪs] *subst.* joint where the bones are tightly linked by ligaments *syndesmos, bindvävsfog*

syndrom ⇨ **complex, syndrome**

syndrome ['sɪndrəʊm] *subst.* group of symptoms and other changes in the body's functions which, when taken together, show that a particular disease is present *syndrom, symtomkomplex*

synechia [sɪ'nekiə] *subst.* condition where the iris sticks to another part of the eye *synechi, syneki, sammanväxning, sammanväxt*

syneresis [sɪ'nɪərəsɪs] *subst.* releasing of fluid as in a blood clot when it becomes harder *avskiljande av vätska genom sammandragning*

synergism ['sɪnədʒɪz(ə)m] *subst. (of two things)* acting together in such a way that both are more effective *synergi(sm), samverkan*

synergist ['sɪnədʒɪst] *subst.* muscle *or* drug which acts with another and increases the effectiveness of both *synergist, samverkande faktor*

synergy ['sɪnədʒi] *subst.* working together, so that the combination is twice as effective *synergi(sm), samverkan*

synfält ⇨ **field, vision, visual**

synförmåga ⇨ **vision**

syn(förmågan) ⇨ **eyesight**

syngent transplantat ⇨ **syngraft**

syngraft ['sɪngrɑ:ft] *or* **isograft** ['aɪsəʊgrɑ:ft] *subst.* graft of tissue from an identical twin *syngent transplantat, isogent (isologt) transplantat*

synkondros ⇨ **cartilaginous, joint, synchondrosis**

synkope ➪ **fainting, syncope**

synkrets ➪ **vision, visual**

synlig ➪ **noticeable, visible**

synmätning ➪ **optometry**

synnerven ➪ **optic**

synnervs- ➪ **optic**

synnervsbanorna ➪ **optic**

synnervsinflammation ➪ **retrobulbar neuritis**

synnervskorsningen ➪ **centre, chiasm**

synnervspapillen ➪ **optic**

synoptophore [sɪ'nɒptəfɔː] *subst.* instrument used to correct a squint *synoptofor*

synostosis [ˌsɪnɒ'stəʊsɪs] *subst.* fusing of two bones together by forming new bone tissue *synostos, bensammansmältning;* **synostosed** = *(of bones)* fused together with bone tissue *sammanväxt, sammansmält*

synovectomy [ˌsɪnəʊ'vektəmi] *subst.* surgical operation to remove the synovial membrane of a joint *synovektomi*

synovia [saɪ'nəʊviə] *or* **synovial fluid** [saɪ'nəʊviəl ˌfluːɪd] *subst.* fluid secreted by a synovial membrane to lubricate a joint *synovia, synovialvätska, ledvätska*

synovial [saɪ'nəʊviəl] *adj.* referring to the synovium *synovial, led-;* **synovial cavity** = space inside a synovial joint *ledspalt, ledhåla;* **synovial fluid** = fluid secreted by a synovial membrane to lubricate a joint *synovia, synovialvätska, ledvätska;* **synovial joint** *or* **diarthrosis** = joint which can move freely in any direction *diart(h)ros;* **synovial membrane** *or* **synovium** = smooth membrane which forms the inner lining of the capsule covering a joint and secretes the fluid which lubricates the joint *synovialmembran, synovialhinna*

synovialhinna ➪ **synovial**

synovialmembran ➪ **synovial**

synovialsarkom ➪ **synovioma**

synovialvätska ➪ **synovia**

synovioma [sɪˌnəuvi'əʊmə] *subst.* tumour in a synovial membrane *synovi(al)om, synovialsarkom*

synovitis [ˌsaɪnə(ʊ)'vaɪtɪs] *subst.* inflammation of the synovial membrane *synovit*

synovium [sɪ'nəʊviəm] = SYNOVIAL MEMBRANE ➪ *illustration* JOINTS

> QUOTE 70% of rheumatoid arthritis sufferers develop the condition in the metacarpophalangeal joints. The synovium produces an excess of synovial fluid which is abnormal and becomes thickened
>
> **Nursing Times**

synpurpur ➪ **visual**

syn(sinnet) ➪ **sight, vision**

synskärpa ➪ **visual**

syntetisera ➪ **synthesize**

syntetisk ➪ **synthetic**

syntetiskt ➪ **synthetically**

synthesize ['sɪnθəsaɪz] *vb.* to make a chemical compound from its separate components *syntetisera, framställa;* **essential amino acids cannot be synthesized; the body cannot synthesize essential fatty acids and has to absorb them from food**

-syn(thet) ➪ **-opia**

synthetic [sɪn'θetɪk] *adj.* made by man *or* made artificially *syntetisk, artificiell, konstgjord*

synthetically [sɪn'θetɪk(ə)li] *adv.* made artificially *syntetiskt, artificiellt, konstgjort;* **synthetically produced hormones are used in hormone therapy**

synvilla ➪ **illusion**

syphilide ['sɪfɪlaɪd] *subst.* rash *or* open sore which is a symptom of the second stage of syphilis *syphiloderma, syfilid*

syphilis ['sɪf(ə)lɪs] *subst.* sexually transmitted disease caused by a spirochaete Treponema pallidum *syfilis, lues;* **congenital syphilis** = syphilis which is passed on from a mother to her unborn child *syphilis congenita (congenitalis, hereditaria), lues congenita (congenitalis, hereditaria), medfödd syfilis*

syphilitic [ˌsɪfə'lɪtɪk] *subst. & adj.* (person) suffering from syphilis *syfilitiker, syfilitisk*

COMMENT: syphilis is a serious sexually transmitted disease, but it is curable with penicillin injections if the treatment is started early. Syphilis has three stages: in the first (or primary) stage, a hard sore (chancre) appears on the genitals or sometimes on the mouth; in the second (or secondary) stage about two or three months later, a rash appears, with sores round the mouth and genitals. It is at this stage that the disease is particularly infectious. After this stage, symptoms disappear for a long time, sometimes many years. The disease reappears in the third (or tertiary) stage in many different forms: blindness, brain disorders, ruptured aorta, or general paralysis leading to insanity and death. The tests for syphilis are the Wassermann test and the less reliable Kahn test

syphiloderma ⇨ **syphilide**

syra ⇨ **acid**

syre ⇨ **oxygen**

syrefattigt blod ⇨ **deoxygenate**

syrgas ⇨ **oxygen**

syrgasmask ⇨ **oxygen**

syrgastub ⇨ **oxygen**

syrgastält ⇨ **oxygen**

syring- ['sɪrɪn(d)ʒ, ˌ--] *or* **syringo-** [sɪ'rɪŋgəʊ, -ˌ--] *prefix* referring to tubes, especially the central canal of the spinal cord *syring(o)-*

syringe [sɪ'rɪn(d)ʒ] *subst.* surgical instrument made of a tube with a plunger which slides down inside it, forcing the contents out through a needle (as in an injection) or slides up the tube, allowing a liquid to be sucked into it *spruta, injektionsspruta*

syringobulbia [sɪˌrɪŋgəʊ'bʌlbiə] *subst.* syringomyelia in the brain stem *syringobulbi, syringomyeli*

syringocystadenoma [sɪˌrɪŋgəʊˌsɪstədɪ'nəʊmə] *or* **syringoma** [ˌsɪrɪŋ'gəʊmə] *subst.* benign tumour in sweat glands and ducts *syringocystadenom*

syringomyelia [sɪˌrɪŋgəʊmaɪ'i:liə] *subst.* disease which forms cavities in the neck section of the spinal cord, affecting the nerves so that the patient loses his sense of touch and pain *syringomyeli*

syringomyelocele [sɪˌrɪŋgəʊ'maɪələʊsi:(ə)l] *subst.* severe form of spina bifida where the spinal cord pushes through a hole in the spine *syringo(myelo)cele*

syrinx ['sɪrɪŋ(k)s] = EUSTACHIAN TUBE

syrsätta ⇨ **oxygenate**

syrsättning ⇨ **oxygenation**

syskon ⇨ **sibling**

system ['sɪstəm] *subst.* **(a)** the body as a whole *kroppen, organismen;* **amputation of a limb gives a serious shock to the system (b)** arrangement of certain parts of the body so that they work together *system;* **the alimentary system** = system of organs and tracts which digest and break down food (including the alimentary canal, the salivary glands, the liver, etc.) *digestionssystemet, matspjälkningsapparaten;* **the cardiovascular system** = system of organs and blood vessels where the blood circulates round the body (including the heart, arteries and veins) *kardiovaskulära systemet, hjärt-kärlsystemet, cirkulationsapparaten;* **central nervous system** = the brain and spinal cord which link together all the nerves *centrala nervsystemet, CNS;* **respiratory system** = series of organs and passages which take air into the lungs and exchange oxygen for carbon dioxide *respirationssystemet, andningsapparaten;* **urinary system** = system of organs and ducts which separate waste liquids from blood and excrete them as urine (including the kidneys, bladder, ureters and urethra) *njurarna och urinvägarna; see also* AUTONOMIC, PARASYMPATHETIC, PERIPHERAL, SYMPATHETIC

system ⇨ **classification, system, tract**

system- ⇨ **systemic**

systematisera ⇨ **classify**

Système International [sɪ'stæm ˌɛ̃nte'nasjɒ'nal] *see* SI

systemic [sɪ'sti:mɪk] *adj.* referring to the whole body *systemisk, system-, kropps-;* **septicaemia is a systemic infection; systemic circulation** = circulation of blood around the whole body (except the lungs), starting with the aorta and returning through the venae cavae *stora kretsloppet;* **systemic lupus erythematosus (SLE)** = one of several collagen diseases, forms of lupus, where red patches form on the skin and spread throughout the body *systemisk lupus erythematosus (erythematodes), SLE, lupus erythematosus el. erythematodes (disseminatus), LED*

syster ⇨ **sister**

systole ['sɪst(ə)li] *subst.* phase in the beating of the heart when it contracts as it pumps blood out *systole, hjärtats sammandragning (kontraktionsfas);* **the heart is in systole** = the heart is contracting and pumping *hjärtat befinner sig i systole (kontraktionsfasen)* NOTE: often used without the: **"at systole the heart pumps blood into the arteries"**

systolic [sɪ'stɒlɪk] *adj.* referring to the systole *systolisk;* **systolic pressure** = blood pressure taken at the systole *systoliskt (blod)tryck; compare* DIASTOLE, DIASTOLIC

COMMENT: systolic pressure is always higher than diastolic

såg ⇨ **saw**

såga ⇨ **saw**

sågtandad ⇨ **serrated**

sår ⇨ **sore, trauma, ulcer, wound**

sår- ⇨ **ulcerative, ulcerous**

såra ⇨ **wound**

sårbar ⇨ **vulnerable**

sårbildning ⇨ **ulceration**

sårfeber ⇨ **traumatic**

sårhake ⇨ **retractor**

sårig ⇨ **ulcerated, ulcerative, ulcerous**

sårklämma ⇨ **clamp, clip**

sårliknande ⇨ **ulcerous**

sårskorpa ⇨ **scab, slough**

sårsprickor ⇨ **rhagades**

säck ⇨ **bag, pouch, sac**

sädes- ⇨ **seminal, sperm-, spermat-**

sädesavgång ⇨ **ejaculation**

sädesblåsorna ⇨ **seminal**

sädescell ⇨ **sperm, spermatozoon**

sädeskanalerna ⇨ **seminiferous tubule**

sädeskropp ⇨ **sperm, spermatozoon**

sädesledar- ⇨ **vas-, vaso-**

sädesledaren ⇨ **ductus, sperm, vas deferens**

sädessträngen ⇨ **spermatic**

sädesuttömning ⇨ **ejaculation**

sädesvätska ⇨ **semen, seminal**

säker ⇨ **safe**

säkerhetsbälte ⇨ **belt, safety**

säkerhetsnål ⇨ **safety**

säkerhetsåtgärd ⇨ **precaution**

säkert ⇨ **safely**

säkra perioder ⇨ **rhythm**

sällsynt ⇨ **exceptional, rare**

säng ⇨ **bed, hospital**

sängbunden ⇨ **bedridden**

sängbunden, inte ⇨ **ambulatory**

sängdags ⇨ **bedtime**

sänggrind ⇨ **support, side**

sängkläder ⇨ **bedclothes**

sängliggande ⇨ **bedridden**

sängplats ⇨ **hospital**

sängvätning ⇨ **bedwetting, enuresis**

sänka ⇨ **lower, reduce**

sänkan ⇨ **erythrocyte, sedimentation**

sänkas ⇨ **drop**

sänkning ⇨ **drop, reduction**

sänkt kroppstemperatur ⇨ **hypothermia**

särdrag ⇨ **characteristic**

särskild ⇨ **special**

särskilja ⇨ **differentiate, separate**

sätes- ⇨ **gluteal**

sätesbjudning ⇨ **breech**

sätesförlossning ⇨ **breech**

sätesmuskel ⇨ **gluteus**

sätesmusklerna ⇨ **gluteal**

sätet ⇨ **bottom, breech, buttocks**

sätt ⇨ **manner, method**

sätta igång ⇨ **trigger**

sätta ngt i halsen ⇨ **choke**

sökande ⇨ **candidate**

söm ⇨ **commissure, raphe; suture**

-söm ⇨ **-rrhaphy**

sömn ⇨ **sleep**

sömn- ⇨ **hypn-**

sömngivande ⇨ **hypnotic, narcotic**

sömngång ⇨ **somnambulism**

sömngångar- ⇨ **somnambulistic**

sömngångare ⇨ **somnambulist**

sömnig ⇨ **dozy, sleepy, somnolent**

sömnlöshet ⇨ **insomnia, sleeplessness, wakefulness**

sömnmedel ⇨ **soporific, sleeping pill**

sömnsjuk ⇨ **lethargic**

sömnsjuka ⇨ **encephalitis**

sömntablett ⇨ **sleeping pill**

sönderdela ⇨ **dissociate**

sönderdelning ⇨ **dissociation**

sönderfall ⇨ **decomposition, disintegration**

sönderriven ⇨ **lacerated**

sönderrivning ⇨ **laceration**

sönderslíten ⇨ **lacerated**

sönderslitning ⇨ **laceration**

söt ⇨ **sweet**

söva (ned) ⇨ **anaesthetize**

sövning ⇨ **anaesthesia, general**

Tt

T3 ⇨ **liothyronine, triiodothyronine**

T4 ⇨ **thyroxine**

Ta *chemical symbol for* tantalum *Ta, tantal*

ta ⇨ **take**

tabes ['teɪbi:z] *subst. pl.* wasting away *tabes, degeneration, förtvining;* **tabes dorsalis** *or* **locomotor ataxia** = disease of the nervous system, caused by advanced syphilis, where the patient loses his sense of feeling, the control of his bladder, the ability to coordinate movements of the legs, and suffers severe pains *tabes dorsalis, syfilitisk ryggmärgsförtvining, ryggmärgstvinsot;* **tabes mesenterica** = wasting of glands in the abdomen *tuberkulos i lymfkörtlar i buken*

tabetic [tə'betɪk] *adj.* which is wasting away *or* affected by tabes dorsalis *tabetisk*

table ['teɪb(ə)l] *subst.* piece of furniture with a flat top and legs, used to eat at *or* to work at *bord;* **operating table** = special flat table on which a patient lies while undergoing an operation *operationsbord*

tablet ['tæblət] *subst.* small flat round piece of dry drug which a patient swallows *tablett;* **a bottle of aspirin tablets; the soluble tablets dissolve in water; take two tablets three times a day**

tablett ⇨ **lozenge, pastille, pill, tablet**

taboparesis [ˌteɪbəʊpə'ri:sɪs] *subst.* final stage of syphilis where the patient has locomotor ataxia and general paralysis of the insane *tabopares, tabes dorsalis och paralysie générale*

TAB vaccine [ˌti:eɪ:'bi: ˌvæksi:n] *subst.* vaccine which immunizes against typhoid fever and paratyphoid A and B *tyfus/paratyfusvaccin, vaccin mot tyfoid liksom mot paratyfoid A och B;* **he was given a TAB injection; TAB injections give only temporary immunity against paratyphoid**

tachy- ['tæki, ˌ--] *prefix* meaning fast *tachy-, taky-*

tachycardia [ˌtækɪ'kɑːdiə] *subst.* rapid beating of the heart *takykardi;* **paroxysmal tachycardia** = sudden attack of rapid heartbeats *paroxysmal takykardi;* **sinus tachycardia** *or* **simple tachycardia** = rapid heartbeats caused by stimulation of the sinoatrial node *sinustakykardi*

tachyphrasia [ˌtæki'freɪziə] *subst.* rapid speaking, as in some mentally disturbed patients *takyfasi, takyfrasi*

tachyphyl(l)axis [ˌtækifi'læksɪs] *subst.* rapid decrease of the effect of a drug *takyfylaxi(s)*

tachypnoea [ˌtæki'pnɪə] *subst.* very fast breathing *takypné*

tactile ['tæktaɪ(ə)l] *adj.* which can be sensed by touch *taktil, känsel-;* **tactile anaesthesia** = loss of sensation of touch *förlust av beröringskänslan*

taenia ['tiːniə] *subst.* **(a)** long ribbon-like part of the body *taenia;* **taenia coli** = outer band of muscle running along the large intestine *taenia coli* **(b)** **Taenia** = genus of tapeworm *Taenia, slags bandmask* NOTE: plural is **taeniae, Taeniae**

> COMMENT: the various species of Taenia which affect humans are taken into the body from eating meat which has not been properly cooked. The most obvious symptom of tapeworm infestation is a sharply increased appetite, together with a loss of weight. The most serious infestation is with *Taenia solium,* found in pork, where the larvae develop in the body and can form hyatid cysts

taeniacide ['tiːniəsaɪd] *adj.* substance which kills tapeworms *bandmaskdödande ämne*

taeniafuge ['tiːniəfjuːdʒ] *subst.* substance which makes tapeworms leave the body *bandmaskfördrivande ämne*

taeniasis [tiː'naɪəsɪs] *subst.* infestation of the intestines with tapeworms *bandmaskangrepp i tarmarna*

tag! ⇨ **R/**

tagg ⇨ **spine**

taggcell ⇨ **prickle cell**

take [teɪk] **1** *subst.* **on the take** = on duty *i tjänst* **2** *vb.* **(a)** to swallow *or* to drink (a medicine) *ta, inta;* **she has to take her tablets three times a day; the medicine should be taken in a glass of water (b)** to do certain actions *ta;* **the dentist took an X-ray of his teeth; the patient has been allowed to take a bath (c)** *(of graft)* to be accepted by the body *accepteras, inte stötas bort;* **the skin graft hasn't taken; the kidney transplant took easily** NOTE: **takes - taking - took - has taken**

take after [ˌteɪk 'ɑːftə] *vb.* to be like (a parent) *likna, brås på;* **he takes after his father**

take care of [ˌteɪk 'keər əv] *vb.* to look after *or* to attend to (a patient) *ta hand om, vårda;* **the nurses will take care of the accident victims**

take off [ˌteɪk 'ɒf] *vb.* to remove (especially clothes) *ta av, klä av;* **the doctor asked him to take his shirt off** *or* **to take off his shirt**

takhinnan ⇨ **tectorial membrane**

taktil ⇨ **tactile**

taky- ⇨ **tachy-**

takyfasi ⇨ **tachyphrasia**

takyfrasi ⇨ **tachyphrasia**

takykardi ⇨ **tachycardia**

takypné ⇨ **tachypnoea**

tal ⇨ **digit, rate; speech**

tal- ⇨ **vocal**

tala ⇨ **speak**

talamus ⇨ **thalamus**

talamusstjälken ⇨ **thalamocortical tract**

talamusstrålningen ⇨ **thalamocortical tract**

talamussyndrom ⇨ **thalamic syndrome**

talblockering ⇨ **speech**

talc [tælk] *subst.* soft white powder used to dust on irritated skin *talk*

talcum powder ['tælkəm ˌpaudə] *subst.* scented talc *talkpuder*

talfel ▷ **speech**

talförmåga ▷ **speech**

talg ▷ **sebum**

talg- ▷ **sebaceous, steat-**

talgig ▷ **sebaceous**

talgkörtel ▷ **sebaceous**

talg(körtel)cysta ▷ **steatoma**

talhämning ▷ **speech**

talipes ['tælɪpi:z] *or* **club foot** ['klʌb fʊt] *subst.* congenitally deformed foot *talipes, klumpfot*

> COMMENT: the most usual form (talipes equinovarus) is where the person walks on the toes because the foot is permanently bent forward; in other forms, the foot either turns towards the inside (talipes varus) *or* towards the outside (talipes valgus) *or* upwards (talipes calcaneus) at the ankle, so that the patient cannot walk on the sole of the foot

talja ▷ **pulley**

talk ▷ **talc**

talkpuder ▷ **talcum powder**

tall [tɔ:l] *adj.* high, usually higher than other people *lång;* **he's the tallest in the family - he's taller than all his brothers; how tall is he? he's 5 foot 7 inches (5'7") tall** *or* **1.25 metres tall**
NOTE: **tall - taller - tallest**

tallkottkörteln ▷ **epiphysis, pineal (body)**

tallrik ▷ **plate**

talo- ['teɪləʊ, ˌ--] *prefix* referring to the ankle bone *talo-, språngbens-*

tal, osammanhängande ▷ **leresis**

talpedagog ▷ **speech**

talrubbning ▷ **dyslalia, speech**

talterapi ▷ **speech**

talus ['teɪləs] *subst.* ankle bone *or* top bone in the tarsus which articulates with the tibia and fibula in the leg, and with the calcaneus in the heel ▷ *illustration* FOOT *talus, språngbenet*

tampon ['tæmpɒn] *subst.* (i) wad of absorbent material put into a wound to soak up blood during an operation *bukduk, duk, tork;* (ii) type of sanitary towel *or* wad of absorbent material which is inserted into the vagina to absorb menstrual flow *tampong*

tamponad ▷ **pack, tamponade**

tamponade [ˌtæmpə'neɪd] *subst.* (i) putting a tampon into a wound *tamponad, tamponering;* (ii) abnormal pressure on part of the body *tamponad;* **cardiac tamponade** = pressure on the heart when the pericardial cavity fills with blood *hjärt(säcks)tamponad*

tampong ▷ **pack, tampon**

tan [tæn] *vb. (of skin)* to become brown (in sunlight) *bli solbränd;* **he tans easily; she is using a tanning lotion**

tand ▷ **tooth, dens**

tand- ▷ **dental, odont-**

tandad ▷ **serrated**

tandbeläggning ▷ **dental, plaque**

tandben ▷ **dentine**

tandborste ▷ **toothbrush**

tandbro ▷ **bridge**

tandbrygga ▷ **bridge**

tandböld ▷ **gumboil**

tandcement ▷ **cementum**

tandemalj ▷ **enamel**

tandfyllning ▷ **filling**

tandgarnityr ▷ **denture**

tandhals ▷ **neck**

tandhygien ▷ **hygiene**

tandhygienist ▷ **dental**

tandinflammation ▷ **odontitis**

tandkirurgi ▷ **dental**

tandkrona ▷ **crown**

tandkräm ▷ **dentifrice, toothpaste**

tandköttet ▷ **gingiva, gum**

tandköttsinflammation ⇨ **gingivitis, ulitis**

tandköttssvulst ⇨ **epulis**

tandlossning ⇨ **periodontitis**

tandläkarborr ⇨ **drill**

tandläkare ⇨ **dental, dentist**

tandläkarförbundet, brittiska ⇨ **British Dental Association (BDA)**

tandläkarmottagning ⇨ **dental**

tandläkarstol ⇨ **chair**

tandläkaryrket ⇨ **dentistry**

tandlös ⇨ **edentulous**

tandprotes ⇨ **denture, false, plate, prosthesis**

tandpulpa ⇨ **dental**

tandpulver ⇨ **dentifrice**

tandreglering ⇨ **orthodontia**

tandrot ⇨ **root, radix**

tandrothinnan ⇨ **periodontal, periodontium**

tandrotsspets ⇨ **apex**

tandröta ⇨ **caries**

tandsprickning ⇨ **teething**

tandsten ⇨ **tartar**

tandställning ⇨ **brace**

tandsvulst ⇨ **odontoma**

tandtekniker ⇨ **dental**

tandtråd ⇨ **dental**

tanduppsättning ⇨ **dentition**

tandvård ⇨ **dental**

tandvärk ⇨ **odontalgia, toothache**

tangent ⇨ **key**

tannin ['tænɪn] *or* **tannic acid** [ˌtænɪk 'æsɪd] *subst.* substance found in the bark of trees and in tea and other liquids, which stains brown *tannin, garvsyra*

tantalum ['tænt(ə)ləm] *subst.* rare metal, used to repair damaged bones *tantal, Ta;* **tantalum mesh** = type of net made of tantalum wire, used to repair cranial defects *slags tantalnät*
NOTE: chemical symbol is **Ta**

tantrum ['tæntrəm] *subst.* violent attack of bad behaviour, usually in a child, where the child breaks things *or* lies on the floor and screams *raserianfall, raseriutbrott*

tap [tæp] **1** *subst.* pipe with a handle which can be turned to make a liquid *or* gas come out of a container *kran* **2** *vb.* **(a)** to remove *or* drain liquid from part of the body *tappa, ta vätskeprov; see also* SPINAL **(b)** to hit lightly *knacka (lätt) på;* **the doctor tapped his chest with his finger**

tape [teɪp] *subst.* long thin flat piece of material *band, remsa;* **tape measure** *or* **measuring tape** = tape with marks on it showing centimetres or inches *måttband*

tapeworm ['teɪpwɜːm] *subst.* parasitic worm with a small head and long body like a ribbon *binnikemask, bandmask*

> COMMENT: tapeworms enter the intestine when a person eats raw meat or fish. The worms attach themselves with hooks to the side of the intestine and grow longer by adding sections to their bodies. Tapeworm larvae do not develop in humans, with the exception of the pork tapeworm, Taenia solium

tapotement [ˌtɑːpəʊtmɔː] *subst.* type of massage where the therapist taps the patient with his hands *tapotemang*

tapp ⇨ **cone**

tappa ⇨ **drain, shed, tap**

tapping ['tæpɪŋ] *or* **paracentesis** [ˌpærəsen'tiːsɪs] *subst.* removing liquid from part of the body using a hollow needle *paracentes, tappning*

tappning ⇨ **drainage, paracentesis, tapping**

tappningskateter ⇨ **catheter**

target ['tɑːgɪt] *subst.* place which is to be hit by something *mål;* **target cell** *or* **target organ** = (i) cell *or* organ which is affected by a drug *or* by a hormone *or* by a disease *target cell, målcell, organ som särskilt angrips etc.;* (ii) large red blood cell which shows a red spot in the middle when stained *target cell*

> QUOTE the target cells for adult myeloid leukaemia are located in the bone marrow
> **British Medical Journal**

tarm- ➪ **enter-, enteral, enteric, intestinal**

tarmanastomos ➪ **intestinal**

tarmarna ➪ **bowel, gut, intestine**

tarmbenet ➪ **hip, ilium**

tarmbråck ➪ **enterocele**

tarmflora ➪ **intestinal**

tarmframfall ➪ **enteroptosis**

tarminfektion ➪ **intestinal**

tarminflammation ➪ **enteric, enteritis**

tarmkäks- ➪ **mesenteric**

tarmkäxet ➪ **mesentery**

tarmludd ➪ **microvillus, villus**

tarmlymfa ➪ **chyle**

tarmobstruktion ➪ **intestinal**

tarmresektion ➪ **enterectomy**

tarmsaft ➪ **intestinal, succus**

tarmsjukdom ➪ **enteropathy**

tarmsten ➪ **enterolith**

tarmsutur ➪ **enterorrhaphy**

tarmtömning ➪ **bowel, defaecation, evacuation, motion, passage**

tarmvred ➪ **volvulus**

tarmvägg ➪ **intestinal**

tarsal ['tɑːs(ə)l] **1** *adj.* referring to the tarsus *tarsal, fotleds-, vrist-, ankel-;* **tarsal bones** = seven small bones in the ankle, including the talus (ankle bone) and calcaneus (heel bone) *ossa tarsi, tarsalbenen, fotledsbenen, vristbenen, ankelbenen;* **tarsal gland** = MEIBOMIAN GLAND **2** *subst.* **the tarsals** = seven small bones which form the ankle *ossa tarsi, tarsalbenen, fotledsbenen, vristbenen, ankelbenen*

tarsalbenen ➪ **tarsal**

tarsalgia [tɑː'sældʒə] *subst.* pain in the ankle *tarsalgi, vristsmärta etc.*

tarsectomy [tɑː'sektəmi] *subst.* surgical operation to remove (i) one of the tarsal bones in the ankle *tarsektomi;* (ii) the tarsus of the eyelid *tarsektomi*

tarsitis [tɑː'saɪtɪs] *subst.* inflammation of the edge of the eyelid *tarsit*

tars(o)- ['tɑːs(əʊ), ,--] *prefix* referring to (i) the ankle bones *tars(o)-, vrist-;* (ii) the edge of an eyelid *tars(o)-, ögonlocksrands-*

tarsorrhaphy [tɑː'sɒrəfi] *subst.* operation to join the two eyelids together to protect the eye after an operation *tarso(r)rafi, kanto(r)rafi, blefo(r)rafi*

tarsus ['tɑːsəs] *subst.* **(a)** the seven small bones of the ankle *tarsus pedis, fotleden, vristen, ankeln* **(b)** connective tissue which supports an eyelid ➪ *illustration* FOOT *tarsus palpebrae (palpebrarum), övre ögonlockets brosk* NOTE: plural is **tarsi**

> COMMENT: the seven bones of the tarsus are: calcaneus, cuboid, the three cuneiforms, navicular and talus

tartar ['tɑːtə] *subst.* hard deposit of calcium which forms on teeth, and has to be removed by scaling *tandsten*

taste [teɪst] **1** *subst.* one of the five senses, where food *or* substances in the mouth are noticed through the tongue *smak(sinnet);* **he doesn't like the taste of onions; he has a cold, so food seems to have lost all taste** *or* **seems to have no taste; taste bud** = tiny sensory receptor in the vallate and fungiform papillae of the tongue, and in part of the back of the mouth *caliculus gustatorius, smaklök* **2** *vb.* (i) to notice the taste of something with the tongue *smaka, känna smaken av (på);* (ii) to have a taste *smaka;* **you can taste the salt in this butter; this cake tastes of chocolate; he has a cold so he can't taste anything**

> COMMENT: the taste buds can tell the difference between salt, sour, bitter and sweet tastes. The buds on the tip of the tongue identify salt and sweet tastes, those on the sides of the tongue identify sour, and those at the back of the mouth the bitter tastes. Note that most of what we think of as taste is in fact smell, and this is why when someone has a cold and a blocked nose, food seems to lose its taste. The impulses from the taste buds are received by the taste cortex in the temporal lobe of the cerebral hemisphere

taurine ['tɔːriːn] *subst.* amino acid which forms bile salts *taurin*

taxis ['tæksɪs] *subst.* pushing *or* massaging dislocated bones or hernias to make them return to their normal position *taxis, reposition*

-taxis ['tæksɪs] *suffix* meaning manipulation *-taxis*

Tay-Sachs disease [ˌteɪ'sæks dɪˌziːz] *or* **amaurotic familial idiocy** [ˌæmɔː'rɒtɪk fəˌmɪliəl 'ɪdiəsi] *subst.* inherited form of mental abnormality, where the legs are paralysed and the child becomes blind and mentally retarded *gangliosidos, Tay-Sachs sjukdom, Sachs sjukdom*

TB [ˌtiː'biː] *abbreviation for* = TUBERCULOSIS **he is suffering from TB; she has been admitted to a TB sanatorium**

T bandage ['tiː ˌbændɪdʒ] *subst.* bandage shaped like the letter T, used for bandaging the area between the legs *T-binda, T-format förband*

tb(c)- ⇨ **tubercular**

TBI [ˌtiːbiː'aɪ] = TOTAL BODY IRRADIATION

T-binda ⇨ **T bandage**

T-cell ['tiːˌsel] *or* **T-lymphocyte** ['tiːˌlɪmfə(ʊ)saɪt] *subst.* lymphocyte produced by the thymus gland *T-cell, T-lymfocyt*

t.d.s. [ˌtiːdiː'es] *or* **TDS** [ˌtiːdiː'es] *abbreviation for the Latin phrase* "ter in diem sumendus": three times a day (written on prescriptions) *ter in diem sumendus, tre gånger dagligen*

tea [tiː] *subst.* (i) dried leaves of a plant used to make a hot drink *te(blad);* (ii) hot drink made by pouring hot water onto the dried leaves of a plant *te, infusion;* **herb tea** = hot drink made from the leaves of a herb *örtte;* **she drank a cup of peppermint tea**

teach [tiːtʃ] *vb.* (i) to give lessons *lära (ut), undervisa;* (ii) to show someone how to do something *lära (ut);* **Professor Smith teaches neurosurgery; she was taught first aid by her mother; teaching hospital** = hospital which is part of a medical school, where student doctors work and study as part of their training *undervisningssjukhus*
NOTE: **teaches - teaching - taught - has taught**

team [tiːm] *subst.* group of people who work together *team, lag;* **the heart-lung transplant was carried out by a team of surgeons**

tear [tɪə, teə] **1** *subst.* **(a)** salty excretion which forms in the lacrimal gland when a person cries *lacrima, tår;* **tears ran down her face; she burst into tears** = she suddenly started to cry *plötsligt började hon gråta, hon brast i gråt;* **tear gland** *or* **lacrimal gland** = gland which secretes tears *glandula lacrimalis, tårkörtel* NOTE: for other terms referring to tears see words beginning with **dacryo-, lacrim-, lacrym-** **(b)** a hole *or* a split in a tissue often due to over-stretching *reva, rispa, ruptur;* **an episiotomy was needed to avoid a tear in the perineal tissue** **2** *vb.* to make a hole *or* a split in a tissue by pulling or stretching too much *reva, rispa, slita sönder (av), ruptera;* **he tore a ligament in his ankle; they carried out an operation to repair a torn ligament**
NOTE: **tears - tearing - tore - has torn**

teat [tiːt] *subst.* rubber nipple on the end of a baby's feeding bottle *napp*

technician [tek'nɪʃ(ə)n] *subst.* qualified person who does practical work in a laboratory *or* scientific institution *tekniker;* **he is a laboratory technician in a laboratory attached to a teaching hospital; dental technician** = qualified person who makes false teeth, plates, etc. *tandtekniker*

technique [tek'niːk] *subst.* way of doing scientific *or* medical work *teknik, metod;* **a new technique for treating osteoarthritis; she is trying out a new laboratory technique**

> QUOTE few parts of the body are inaccessible to modern catheter techniques, which are all performed under local anaesthesia
> **British Medical Journal**

> QUOTE the technique used to treat aortic stenosis is similar to that for any cardiac catheterization
> **Journal of the American Medical Association**

> QUOTE cardiac resuscitation techniques used by over half the nurses in a recent study were described as "completely ineffective"
> **Nursing Times**

tecken ⇨ **sign, symbol**

tecken, fysikaliskt ⇨ **physical**

teckenspråk ⇨ **dactylology, deaf**

teckningsblödning ⇨ **show**

tectorial membrane [tek'tɔːriəl ˌmembreɪn] *subst.* membrane in the inner ear which contains the hair cells which transmit impulses to the auditory nerve *membrana tectoria (ductus cochlearis), takhinnan*

tectospinal tract [ˌtektəʊ'spaɪn(ə)l ˌtrækt] *subst.* tract which takes nerve impulses from the mesencephalon to the spinal cord *tractus tectospinalis*

teeth [ti:θ] *see* TOOTH

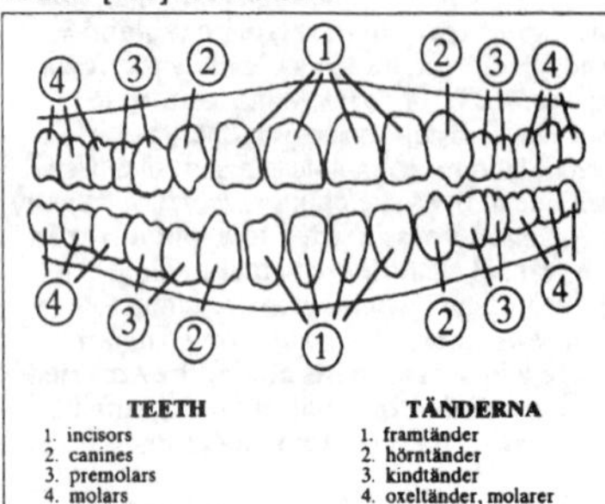

teething ['ti:ðɪŋ] *subst.* period when a baby's milk teeth are starting to erupt, and the baby is irritable *tandsprickning;* **he is awake at night because he is teething; she has teething trouble and won't eat**

tegmen ['tegmən] *subst.* covering for an organ *tegmen, hölje* NOTE: plural is **tegmina**

teknik ▷ **method, technique**

tekniker ▷ **technician**

tel- [tel, 'tel, ˌ-] *or* **tele-** ['telɪ, ˌ--] *prefix* meaning done at a distance *tel(e)-, fjärr-*

telangiectasis [telˌændʒi'ektəsɪs] *subst.* small dark red spots on the skin, formed by swollen capillaries *telangiektasi*

teleceptor ['telɪˌseptə] *subst.* sensory receptor which receives sensations from a distance *receptor som uppfångar signaler på avstånd*

telefonera ▷ **call**

telencephalon [ˌtelen'kef(ə)lɒn] *subst.* cerebrum *or* main part of the brain *telencefalon, ändhjärnan*

> COMMENT: the telencephalon is the largest part of the brain, formed of two cerebral hemispheres. It controls the main mental processes, including the memory

teleradiography [ˌtelɪˌreɪdi'ɒgrəfi] *subst.* radiography where the source of the X-rays is at a distance from the patient *radiografi där källan till röntgenstrålningen befinner sig på avstånd från patienten*

teleradiotherapy [ˌtelɪˌreɪdiəʊ'θerəpi] *subst.* radiotherapy, where the patient is some way away from the source of radiation *teleterapi, fjärrbestrålning*

teleterapi ▷ **teleradiotherapy**

telo- ['telə(ʊ), ˌ--] *prefix* meaning end *tel(o)-, änd-*

telophase ['teləʊfeɪz] *subst.* final stage of mitosis, the stage in cell division after anaphase *telofas*

temp ▷ **temperature**

temper ['tempə] *subst.* (usually bad) state of mind *humör, sinnesstämning;* **he's in a (bad) temper** = he is annoyed *han är på dåligt humör;* **he lost his temper** = he became very angry *han blev arg;* **temper tantrum** = violent attack of bad behaviour, usually in a child, where the child breaks things *or* lies on the floor and screams *vredesutbrott*

temperatur ▷ **temperature**

temperatur- ▷ **thermo-**

temperature ['temp(ə)rətʃə] *subst.* **(a)** heat of the body measured in degrees *temperatur, temp;* **the doctor asked the nurse what the patient's temperature was; his temperature was slightly above normal; the thermometer showed a temperature of 99°F; to take a patient's temperature** = to insert a thermometer in a patient's body to see what his body temperature is *ta tempen på en patient;* **they took his temperature every four hours; when her temperature was taken this morning, it was normal; central temperature** = temperature of the brain, thorax and abdomen, which is constant *kroppstemperatur;* **environmental temperature** = temperature of the air outside the body *yttertemperatur* **(b)** illness when your body is hotter than normal *feber;* **he's in bed with a temperature; her mother says she's got a temperature, and can't come to work**

> COMMENT: the normal average body temperature is about 37° Celsius or 98° Fahrenheit. This temperature may vary during the day, and can rise if a person has taken a hot bath or had a hot drink. If the environmental temperature is high, the body has to sweat to reduce the heat gained from the air around it. If the outside temperature is low, the body shivers, because rapid movement of the muscles

generates heat. A fever will cause the body temperature to rise sharply, to 40°C (103°F) or more. Hypothermia exists when the body temperature falls below about 35°C (95°F)

temperaturkurva ⇨ **chart, graph**

temple ['temp(ə)l] *subst.* flat part of the side of the head between the top of the ear and the eye *tinningen*

temporal ['temp(ə)r(ə)l] *adj.* referring to the temple *temporal(-), tinning-;* **temporal arteritis** = inflammation of the arteries in the temple *arteritis temporalis, temporalarterit;* **temporal fossa** = depression at the side of the temporal bone, above the zygomatic arch *fossa temporalis, tinninggropen;* **temporal lobe** = lobe above the ear in each cerebral hemisphere *lobus temporalis, temporalloben, tinningloben;* **temporal lobe epilepsy** = epilepsy due to a disorder of the temporal lobe and causing impaired memory, hallucinations and automatism *epilepsia psychomotorica, epilepsia (regionis) lobi temporalis*

temporal(-) ⇨ **temporal**

temporalarterit ⇨ **temporal**

temporal bone ['temp(ə)r(ə)l ˌbəʊn] *subst.* one the bones which form the sides and base of the cranium ⇨ *illustration* SKULL, EAR *os temporale, tinningbenet*

COMMENT: the temporal bone is in two parts: the petrous part forms the base of the skull and the inner and middle ears, while the squamous part forms the side of the skull. The lower back part of the temporal bone is the mastoid process, while the part between the ear and the cheek is the zygomatic arch

temporalis (muscle) [ˌtempə'reɪlɪs (ˌmʌs(ə)l)] *subst.* flat muscle running down the side of the head from the temporal bone to the coronoid process, which makes the jaw move up and down *musculus temporalis*

temporalloben ⇨ **temporal**

temporallobs- ⇨ **temporo-**

temporary ['temp(ə)r(ə)ri] *adj.* which is not permanent *or* which is not final *temporär, tillfällig, provisorisk;* **the dentist gave him a temporary filling; the accident team put a temporary bandage on the wound**

temporo- ['tempərə, ˌ---] *prefix* referring to (i) the temple *temporo-, tinnings-;* (ii) the temporal lobe *temporo-, temporallobs-, tinninglobs-*

temporomandibular joint [ˌtempərəmæn'dɪbjʊlə ˌdʒɔɪnt] *subst.* joint between the jaw and the skull, in front of the ear *articulatio temporomandibularis*

temporär ⇨ **temporary**

tenaculum [tə'nækjʊləm] *subst.* surgical instrument shaped like a hook, used to pick up small pieces of tissue during an operation *tenaculum, klotång*

tenar- ⇨ **thenar**

tend [tend] *vb.* **to tend to do something** = to do something generally *or* as a normal process *bruka göra något;* **the prostate tends to enlarge as a man grows older**

tendency ['tendənsi] *subst.* being likely to do something *tendens, benägenhet, anlag;* **to have a tendency to something** = to be likely to have something *ha benägenhet (anlag) för något;* **there is a tendency to obesity in her family; the children of the area show a tendency to vitamin-deficiency diseases**

QUOTE premature babies have been shown to have a higher tendency to develop a squint during childhood
Nursing Times

tender ['tendə] *adj.* (skin *or* flesh) which is painful when touched *öm, ömmande;* **the bruise is still tender; her shoulders are still tender where she got sunburnt; a tender spot on the abdomen indicates that an organ is inflamed**

tenderness ['tendənəs] *subst.* feeling painful when touched *ömhet;* **tenderness when pressure is applied is a sign of inflammation**

tendineae ['tendɪniː] *subst. pl.* **chordae tendineae** = tiny fibrous ligaments in the heart which attach the edges of some of the valves to the walls of the ventricles *chordae tendineae*

tendinitis [ˌtendɪ'naɪtɪs] *subst.* inflammation of a tendon, especially after playing sport, and often associated with tenosynovitis *tendinit, seninflammation*

tendinous ['tendɪnəs] *adj.* referring to a tendon *sen-*

tend(o)- ⇨ **teno-**

tendo calcaneus [ˌtendəʊ kæl'keɪniəs] *or* **Achilles tendon** [əˌkɪliːz 'tendən] *subst.* tendon at the back of the ankle which connects the calf muscles to the heel and pulls the heel upwards when the calf muscles are tense *tendo calcaneus (Achillis), akillessenan*

tendon ['tendən] *subst.* strip of connective tissue which attaches a muscle to a bone *tendo, sena;* **tendon sheath** = tube of membrane which covers and protects a membrane *senskida*

tendonit ⇨ **tenonitis**

tendovaginitis [ˌtendəʊˌvædʒə'naɪtɪs] *subst.* inflammation of a tendon sheath, especially in the thumb *ten(d)ovaginit, senskideinflammation*
NOTE: for other terms referring to a tendon. see also words beginning with **teno-**

tenens ['tenəns] *see* LOCUM

tenesmus [tə'nezməs] *subst.* condition where the patient feels he needs to pass faeces, but is unable to do so and experiences pain *tenesm(er), smärtsam(ma) trängning(ar)*

tennis elbow [ˌtenɪs 'elbəʊ] *subst.* inflammation of the tendons of the extensor muscles in the hand which are attached to the bone near the elbow *tennisarmbåge*

teno- ['tenəʊ, ˌ--] *prefix* referring to a tendon *ten(o)-, tend(o)-, sen-*

tenonitis [ˌtenəʊ'naɪtɪs] *subst.* inflammation of a tendon *tenontit, tendonit, seninflammation*

Tenon's capsule ['tiːnɒns ˌkæpsjuːl] *subst.* tissue which lines the orbit of the eye *vagina bulbi, Tenons kapsel*

tenoplasty ['tenə(ʊ)plæsti] *subst.* surgical operation to repair a torn tendon *tenoplastik, tend(in)oplastik*

tenorrhaphy [tɪ'nɒrəfi] *subst.* surgical operation to stitch pieces of a torn tendon together *teno(r)rafi, sensutur, sensöm*

tenosynovitis [ˌtenəʊˌsaɪnəʊ'vaɪtɪs] *or* **peritendinitis** [ˌperiˌtendi'naɪtɪs] *subst.* painful inflammation of the tendon sheath and the tendon inside *ten(d)osynovit, peritendinit, senskideinflammation*

tenotomy [tə'nɒtəmi] *subst.* surgical operation to cut through a tendon *tenotomi*

tenovaginitis [ˌtenəʊˌvædʒə'naɪtɪs] *subst.* inflammation of the tendon sheath, especially in the thumb *ten(d)ovaginit, senskideinflammation*

tense [tens] *adj.* **(a)** *(of a muscle)* contracted *spänd, sammandragen* **(b)** nervous and worried *spänd;* **the patient was very tense while he waited for the report from the laboratory**

tension ['tenʃ(ə)n] *subst.* nervous stress *spänning;* **tension headache** = headache all over the head, caused by worry and stress *spänningshuvudvärk*

tensor ['tensə] *subst.* muscle which makes a joint stretch out *(musculus) tensor, sträckmuskel; compare* EXTENSOR, FLEXOR

tent [tent] *subst.* small shelter put over and round a patient's bed so that gas *or* vapour can be passed inside *tält;* **oxygen tent** = type of cover put over a patient's bed so that he can inhale oxygen *syrgastält*

tentorium cerebelli [ten'tɔːriəm ˌserə'beli] *subst.* part of the dura mater which separates the cerebellum from the cerebral hemispheres *tentorium cerebelli, lillhjärnstältet*

teori ⇨ **theory**

terapeut ⇨ **therapist**

terapeutisk ⇨ **therapeutic**

terapi ⇨ **therapy**

terat- ['terət, ˌ--] *or* **terato-** ['terətə(ʊ), ˌ---] *prefix* meaning congenitally abnormal *terat(o)-, missbildnings-*

teratogen ['terətədʒen] *subst.* substance (such as the German measles virus) which causes an abnormality to develop in an embryo *teratogen, missbildningsframkallande*

teratogenesis [ˌterətə'dʒenəsɪs] *subst.* development of abnormalities in an embryo and fetus *teratogenes, utveckling av missbildning hos foster*

teratology [ˌterə'tɒlədʒi] *subst.* study of abnormal development of embryos and fetuses *teratologi*

teratoma [ˌterə'təʊmə] *subst.* tumour which is formed of abnormal tissue, usually developing in an ovary or testis *teratom*

teres ['tɪəriːz] *subst.* one of two shoulder muscles running from the shoulder blade to the top of the humerus *musculus teres*

COMMENT: the larger of the two muscles, the teres major, makes the arm turn towards the inside, and the smaller, the teres minor, makes it turn towards the outside

term [tɜːm] *subst.* **(a)** length of time, especially the period from conception to childbirth *tid, period, graviditetsperiod;* **she was coming near the end of her term** = she was near the time when she would give birth *hon skulle snart föda* **(b)** part of a college *or* school year *termin;* **the anatomy exams are at the beginning of the third term**

termal ⇨ **thermal**

termanestesi ⇨ **thermal, thermoanaesthesia**

termin ⇨ **term**

terminal ['tɜːmɪn(ə)l] **1** *adj.* (i) referring to the last stage of a fatal illness *terminal, dödlig;* (ii) referring to the end *or* being at the end of something *slut-, änd-, som befinner sig i slutstadiet;* **the disease is in its terminal stages; he is suffering from terminal cancer; terminal branch** = end part of a neurone which is linked to a muscle ⇨ *illustration* NEURONE *nervändslut;* **terminal illness** = illness from which the patient will soon die *dödlig sjukdom* **2** *subst.* ending *or* part at the end of an electrode *or* nerve *ändpunkt, slut(punkt)*

terminale [ˌtɜːmɪ'neɪli] *see* FILUM

terminally ill ['tɜːmɪn(ə)li ˌɪl] *adj.* very ill and about to die *dödssjuk, sjuk i terminalstadiet;* **she was admitted to a hospice for terminally ill patients** *or* **for the terminally ill**

termination [ˌtɜːmɪ'neɪʃ(ə)n] *subst.* ending *slut, avslutning, avbrytande;* **termination of pregnancy** = abortion *avbrytande av havandeskap, abort*

term(o)- ⇨ **thermo-**

termofil ⇨ **thermophilic**

termografi ⇨ **thermography**

termogram ⇨ **thermogram**

termokaustik ⇨ **thermocautery**

termolys ⇨ **thermolysis**

termometer ⇨ **thermometer**

termoplegi ⇨ **heat**

termostat ⇨ **incubator**

termotaxis ⇨ **thermotaxis**

termoterapi ⇨ **therapy**

tertian fever ['tɜːʃ(ə)n ˌfiːvə] *subst.* type of malaria where the fever returns every two days *febris tertiana, varannandagsfeber, varannandagsfrossa; see also* QUARTAN

tertiary ['tɜːʃ(ə)ri] *adj.* third *or* coming after secondary and primary *tertiär, tredje (gradens), i tredje stadiet;* **tertiary bronchi** = air passages supplying a segment of a lung *bronchi segmentali, segmentbronkerna; see also* SYPHILIS

test [test] **1** *subst.* short examination to see if a sample is healthy *or* if part of the body is working well *test, prov, undersökning;* **he had an eye test this morning; laboratory tests showed that she was a meningitis carrier; tests are being carried out on swabs taken from the operating theatre; blood test** = test of a blood sample to find the chemical composition of a patient's blood *blodprov;* **the patient will have to have a blood test; the urine test was positive** = the examination of the urine sample showed the presence of an infection *urinprovet var positivt (visade ett positivt resultat)* **2** *vb.* to examine a sample of tissue to see if it is healthy *or* an organ to see if it is is working well *testa, prova, undersöka;* **they sent the urine sample away for testing; I must have my eyes tested**

COMMENT: the testes produce both spermatozoa and the sex hormone, testosterone. Spermatozoa are formed in the testes, and passed into the epididymis to be stored. From the epididymis they pass along the vas deferens through the prostate gland which secretes the seminal fluid, and are ejaculated through the penis

testa ⇨ **process, test**

testicle ['testɪkl] *or* **testis** ['testɪs] *subst.* one of two male sex glands in the scrotum *testis, testikel* NOTE: the plural of **testis** is **testes**

testicular [te'stɪkjʊlə] *adj.* referring to the testes *testikular, testikulär, testikel-, orki(o)-, orkid(o)-;* **testicular cancer comprises only 1% of all malignant neoplasms in the male; testicular hormone** = testosterone *testosteron* NOTE: for other terms referring to the testes see words beginning with **orchi-** = UROGENITAL SYSTEM (male)

testikel ⇨ **orchis, testicle**

testikel- ⇨ **orchi-, testicular**

testikelexcision ⇨ **orchidectomy**

testikelinflammation ⇨ **orchitis**

testikelsmärta ⇨ **orchidalgia**

testikulär ⇨ **testicular**

test meal ['test mi:l] *subst.* test to test the secretion of gastric juices *provfrukost, magsaftundersökning*

testosteron ⇨ **testicular, testosterone**

testosterone [te'stɒstərəʊn] *subst.* male sex hormone, secreted by the Leydig cells in the testes, which causes physical changes (such as the development of body hair and deep voice) to take place in males as they become sexually mature *testosteron*

test tube ['test tju:b] *subst.* small glass tube with a rounded bottom, used in laboratories to hold samples of liquids *provrör;* **test-tube baby** = baby which develops after the mother's ova have been removed from the ovaries, fertilized with a man's spermatozoa in a laboratory, and returned to the mother's womb to continue developing normally *provrörsbarn*

> COMMENT: this process of in vitro fertilization is carried out in cases where the mother is unable to conceive, though both she and the father are normally fertile

tetani ⇨ **tetany**

tetanic [te'tænɪk] *adj.* referring to tetanus *tetanus-, stelkramps-*

tetanus ['tet(ə)nəs] *subst.* **(a)** continuous contraction of a muscle, under repeated stimuli from a motor nerve *tonisk muskelkramp* **(b)** lockjaw *or* infection caused by **Clostridium tetani** in the soil, which affects the spinal cord and causes spasms in the muscles which occur first in the jaw *tetanus, stelkramp*

> COMMENT: people who are liable to infection with tetanus, such as farm workers, should be immunized against it, though booster injections are needed from time to time

tetanus- ⇨ **tetanic**

tetanusserum ⇨ **antitetanus serum (ATS)**

tetany ['tet(ə)ni] *subst.* spasms of the muscles in the feet and hands, caused by a reduction in the level of calcium in the blood *or* by lack of carbon dioxide *tetani; see* PARATHYROID HORMONE

tetracycline [ˌtetrə'saɪkli:n] *subst.* antibiotic used to treat a wide range of bacterial diseases *tetracyklin*

tetradactyly [ˌtetrə'dæktɪli] *subst.* congenital deformity where a child has only four fingers or toes *tetradaktyli, fyrfingrighet, fyrtåighet*

tetrajodtyronin ⇨ **thyroxine**

tetralogy of Fallot [te'trælədʒi əv fæˌləʊ] *or* **Fallot's tetralogy** [fæ'ləʊz teˌtrælədʒi] *subst.* disorder of the heart which makes a child's skin blue *Fallots tetrad (tetralogi); see also* WATERSTON'S OPERATION

> COMMENT: the condition is formed of four disorders occurring together: the artery leading to the lungs is narrow, the right ventricle is enlarged, there is a defect in the membrane between the ventricles, and the aorta is not correctly placed

tetraplegia [ˌtetrə'pli:dʒə] = QUADRIPLEGIA

textbook ['teks(t)bʊk] *subst.* book which is used by students *lärobok;* **a haematology textbook** *or* **a textbook on haematology; textbook case** = case which shows symptoms which are exactly like those described in a textbook *typfall, typiskt fall*

thalam- ['θæləm, ˌ--] *or* **thalamo-** ['θæləməʊ, ˌ---] *prefix* referring to the thalamus *thalam(o)-, thalamus-, talamus-*

thalamencephalon [ˌθæləmen'kef(ə)lɒn] *subst.* group of structures in the brain linked to the brain stem, formed of the epithalamus, hypothalamus, and thalamus *thalamencephalon, diencefalon, mellanhjärnan*

thalamencephalon ⇨ **diencephalon**

thalamic syndrome [θə'læmɪk ˌsɪndrəʊm] *subst.* condition where a patient is extremely sensitive to pain, caused by a disorder of the thalamus *talamussyndrom*

thalamocortical tract [ˌθæləməʊ'kɔ:tɪk(ə)l ˌtrækt] *subst.* tract containing nerve fibres, running from the thalamus to the sensory cortex *fasciculus thalamocorticalis, talamusstjälken, talamusstrålningen*

thalamotomy [ˌθæləˈmɒtəmi] *subst.* surgical operation to make an incision into the thalamus to treat intractable pain *avskärning av centrala smärtfibrer i hjärnan*

thalamus [ˈθæləməs] *subst.* one of two masses of grey matter situated beneath the cerebrum where impulses from the sensory neurones are transmitted to the cerebral cortex ⇨ *illustration* BRAIN *thalamus, talamus*
NOTE: plural is **thalami**

thalamus- ⇨ **thalam-**

thalassaemia [ˌθælæˈsiːmiə] *or* **Cooley's anaemia** [ˈkuːlɪz əˌniːmiə] *subst.* hereditary type of anaemia, found in Mediterranean countries, due to a defect in the production of haemoglobin *talass(an)emi, Cooleyanemi*

thaw [θɔː] *vb.* to bring something which is frozen back to normal temperature *tina (upp)*

theatre [ˈθɪətə] *subst.* **operating theatre** *or* *US* **operating room** = special room in a hospital where surgeons carry out operations *operationssal;* **theatre gown** = gown worn by a patient *or* by a surgeon *or* nurse in an operating theatre *operationsrock, operationsskjorta, steril rock;* **theatre nurse** = nurse who is specially trained to assist in operations *operationssköterska*

theca [ˈθiːkə] *subst.* tissue shaped like a sheath *theca, hölje*

thenar [ˈθiːnə] *adj.* (referring to) the palm of the hand *thenar-, tenar-, tumvalks-;* **thenar eminence** = the ball of the thumb *or* lump of flesh in the palm of the hand below the thumb *t(h)enar, tumvalken; compare* HYPOTHENAR

theory [ˈθɪəri] *subst.* argument which explains a scientific fact *teori, lära*

therapeutic [ˌθerəˈpjuːtɪk] *adj.* (treatment *or* drug) which is given in order to cure a disorder *or* disease *terapeutisk;* **therapeutic abortion** = abortion carried out because the health of the mother is in danger *abort pga att havandeskapet medför allvarlig fara för moderns liv eller hälsa*

therapeutics [ˌθerəˈpjuːtɪks] *subst.* study of various types of treatment and their effect on patients *läran om sjukdomars behandling*

therapist [ˈθerəpɪst] *subst.* person specially trained to give therapy *terapeut;* **an occupational therapist**

therapy [ˈθerəpi] *subst.* treatment of a patient to help cure a disease *or* disorder *terapi, behandling;* **aversion therapy** = treatment where the patient is cured of a type of behaviour by making him develop a great dislike for it *aversionsterapi;* **behaviour therapy** = psychiatric treatment where the patient learns to improve his condition *beteendeterapi;* **group therapy** = type of treatment where a group of people with the same disorder meet together with a therapist to discuss their condition and try to help each other *gruppterapi;* **heat therapy** *or* **thermotherapy** = using heat (from infrared lamps *or* hot water) to treat certain conditions such as arthritis and bad circulation *termoterapi, värmebehandling;* **light therapy** = treatment of a disorder by exposing the patient to light (sunlight, UV light, etc) *ljusterapi, ljusbehandling;* **occupational therapy** = work *or* hobbies used as a means of treatment, especially for handicapped *or* mentally ill patients *arbetsterapi;* **psychotherapy** = treatment of mental and personality disorders which does not involve drugs or surgery, but where a psychotherapist talks to the patient and encourages him to talk about his problems *psykoterapi;* **radiotherapy** = treating a disease by exposing the affected part to radioactive rays *radioterapi, strålbehandling;* **shock therapy** = method of treating some mental disorders by giving the patient an electric shock to induce convulsions and loss of consciousness *ECT, elektrokonvulsiv terapi (behandling), "chockbehandling", "elchock";* **speech therapy** = treatment to cure a speech disorder such as stammering *talterapi, logopedisk behandling*
NOTE: both therapy and therapist are used as suffixes: **psychotherapist, radiotherapy**

thermal [ˈθɜːm(ə)l] *adj.* referring to heat *termal, värme-;* **thermal anaesthesia** = loss of feeling of heat *termanestesi, värmeokänslighet*

thermo- [ˈθɜːmə(ʊ), ˌ--] *prefix* referring to (i) heat *term(o)-, värme-;* (ii) temperature *term(o)-, temperatur-*

thermoanaesthesia [ˌθɜːmə(ʊ)ˌænəsˈθiːziə] *subst.* condition where the patient cannot tell the difference between hot and cold *termanestesi, värmeokänslighet*

thermocautery [ˌθɜːmə(ʊ)ˈkɔːtəri] *subst.* removing dead tissue by heat *termokaustik*

thermocoagulation [ˌθɜːmə(ʊ)kəʊˌægjuˈleɪʃ(ə)n] *subst.* removing tissue and coagulating blood by heat *koagulation med hjälp av brännande instrument (diatermi)*

thermogram ['θɜːmə(ʊ)græm] *subst.* infrared photograph of part of the body *termogram*

thermography [θɜː'mɒgrəfi] *subst.* technique of photographing part of the body using infrared rays, which record the heat given off by the skin, and show variations in the blood circulating beneath the skin, used especially in screening for breast cancer *termografi*

thermolysis [θɜː'mɒləsɪs] *subst.* loss of body temperature (as by sweating) *termolys*

thermometer [θə'mɒmɪtə] *subst.* instrument for measuring temperature *termometer;* **clinical thermometer =** thermometer used in a hospital *or* by a doctor for taking a patient's body temperature *febertermometer;* **oral thermometer =** thermometer which is put into the mouth to take a patient's temperature *muntermometer;* **rectal thermometer =** thermometer which is inserted into the patient's rectum to take the temperature *rektaltermometer*

thermophilic [ˌθɜːmə(ʊ)'fɪlɪk] *adj.* (organism) which needs a high temperature to grow *termofil, värmeälskande*

thermoreceptor [ˌθɜːmə(ʊ)rɪ'septə] *subst.* sensory nerve which registers heat *värmereceptor*

thermotaxis [ˌθɜːmə(ʊ)'tæksɪs] *subst.* automatic regulation of the body's temperature *termotaxis*

thermotherapy [ˌθɜːmə(ʊ)'θerəpi] *subst.* heat treatment *or* using heat (as in hot water *or* infrared lamps) to treat conditions such as arthritis and bad circulation *termoterapi, värmebehandling*

thiamin ⇨ **aneurine**

thiamine ['θaɪ(ɪ)əmiːn] = VITAMIN B_1

thicken ['θɪk(ə)n] *vb.* to become thicker *tjockna, bli tjockare;* **the walls of the arteries thicken under deposits of fat**

Thiersch graft ['tɪəʃ ˌgrɑːft] = SPLIT-SKIN GRAFT

thigh [θaɪ] *subst.* top part of the leg from the knee to the groin *låret*

thighbone ['θaɪbəʊn] *or* **femur** ['fiːmə] *subst.* bone in the top part of the leg, which joins the acetabulum at the hip and the tibia at the knee *femur, lårbenet*
NOTE: for other terms referring to the thigh see words beginning with **femor-**

thin [θɪn] *adj.* **(a)** not fat *smal, mager;* **his arms are very thin; she's getting too thin - she should eat more; he became quite thin after his illness (b)** not thick *tunn;* **they cut a thin slice of tissue for examination under the microscope (c)** watery (blood) *tunnflytande, vattnig*

thirst [θɜːst] *subst.* feeling of wanting to drink *törst;* **he had a fever and a violent thirst**

thirsty ['θɜːsti] *adj.* wanting to drink *törstig;* **if the patient is thirsty, give her a glass of water**
NOTE: **thirsty - thirstier - thirstiest**

Thomas's splint ['tɒməs ˌsplɪnt] *subst.* type of splint used on a fractured femur, with a ring at the top round the thigh, and a bar under the foot at the bottom *Thomasskena*

thoracectomy [ˌθɔːrə'sektəmi] *subst.* surgical operation to remove one or more ribs *torakektomi*

thoracentesis [ˌθɔːrəsen'tiːsɪs] *subst.* operation where a hollow needle is inserted into the pleura to drain fluid *torakocentes, pleurocentes, pleurapunktion*

thoracic [θɔː'ræsɪk] *adj.* referring to the chest *or* thorax *thorakal, torakal, bröst-, bröstkorgs-;* **thoracic cavity =** chest cavity, containing the diaphragm, heart and lungs *cavum thoracis, brösthålan;* **thoracic duct =** one of the main terminal ducts in the lymphatic system, running from the abdomen to the left side of the neck *ductus thoracicus, stora bröstgången, stora lymfgången;* **thoracic inlet =** small opening at the top of the thorax *apertura thoracis superior, övre toraxaperturen (toraxöppningen);* **thoracic inlet syndrome** *or* **scalenus syndrome =** pain in an arm, caused when the scalenes press the brachial plexus against the vertebrae *scalenussyndrom;* **thoracic outlet =** large opening at the bottom of the thorax *apertura thoracis inferior, nedre toraxaperturen (toraxöppningen);* **thoracic vertebrae =** the twelve vertebrae in the spine behind the chest, to which the ribs are attached ⇨ *illustration* VERTEBRAL COLUMN *vertebrae thoracicae, bröstkotorna*

thorac(o)- ['θɔːrək(əʊ), ˌ---] *prefix* referring to the chest *thorac(o)-, torak(o)-, bröstkorgs-*

thoracocentesis [ˌθɔːrəkəʊsenˈtiːsɪs] *subst.* operation where a hollow needle is inserted into the pleura to drain fluid *pleurocentes, pleurapunktion, torakocentes*

thoracoplasty [ˈθɔːrəkəʊplæsti] *subst.* surgical operation to cut through the ribs to allow the lungs to collapse, formerly a treatment for pulmonary tuberculosis *toraxplastik, torakoplastik*

thoracoscope [ˈθɔːrəkəskəʊp] *subst.* surgical instrument, like a tube with a light at the end, used to examine the inside of the chest *torakoskop*

thoracoscopy [ˌθɔːrəˈkɒskəpi] *subst.* examination of the inside the chest, using a thoracoscope *torakoskopi*

thoracotomy [ˌθɔːrəˈkɒtəmi] *subst.* surgical operation to make a hole in the wall of the chest *torakotomi*

thorakal ⇨ **thoracic**

thorax [ˈθɔːræks] *or* **chest** [tʃest] *subst.* cavity in the top part of the body above the abdomen, containing the diaphragm, heart and lungs, all surrounded by the rib cage *thorax, torax, bröstkorgen*

thread [θred] *subst.* thin piece of cotton, etc. *tråd;* **the surgeon used strong thread to make the suture**

threadworm [ˈθredwɜːm] *or* **pinworm** [ˈpɪnwɜːm] *subst.* thin parasitic worm, **Enterobius** which infests the large intestine and causes itching round the anus *Enterobius vermicularis, springmask*

threonine [ˈθriːəniːn] *subst.* essential amino acid *treonin*

threshold [ˈθreʃ(h)əʊld] *subst.* (i) point below which a drug has no effect *tröskel(värde);* (ii) point at which a sensation is strong enough to be sensed by the sensory nerves *tröskel(värde);* **she has a low hearing threshold; pain threshold** = point at which a person cannot bear pain without crying *smärttröskel*

QUOTE if intracranial pressure rises above the treatment threshold, it is imperative first to validate the reading and then to eliminate any factors exacerbating the rise in pressure
British Journal of Hospital Medicine

thrill [θrɪl] *subst.* vibration which can be felt with the hands *fremitus, frémissement, skälvning*

thrive [θraɪv] *vb.* to do well *or* to live and grow strongly *(växa och) frodas, utvecklas;* **failure to thrive** = wasting disease of small children who have difficulty in absorbing nutrients *or* who are suffering from malnutrition *failure to thrive*

throat [θrəʊt] *subst.* (i) top part of the tube which goes down from the mouth to the stomach *svalget, strupen;* (ii) front part of the neck below the chin *halsen;* **if it is cold, wrap a scarf round your throat; a piece of meat got stuck in his throat; to clear the throat** = to give a little cough *klara strupen, harkla sig;* **sore throat** = condition where the mucous membrane in the pharynx is inflamed (sometimes because the person has been talking too much, but usually because of an infection) *ont i halsen, halsont*

COMMENT: the throat carries both food from the mouth and air from the nose and mouth. It divides into the oesophagus, which takes food to the stomach, and the trachea, which takes air into the lungs

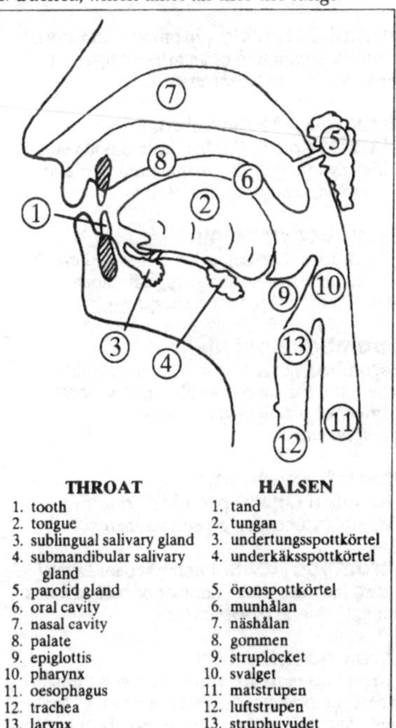

THROAT	HALSEN
1. tooth	1. tand
2. tongue	2. tungan
3. sublingual salivary gland	3. undertungsspottkörtel
4. submandibular salivary gland	4. underkäksspottkörtel
5. parotid gland	5. öronspottkörtel
6. oral cavity	6. munhålan
7. nasal cavity	7. näshålan
8. palate	8. gommen
9. epiglottis	9. struplocket
10. pharynx	10. svalget
11. oesophagus	11. matstrupen
12. trachea	12. luftstrupen
13. larynx	13. struphuvudet

throb [θrɒb] *vb.* to have a regular beat, like the heart *bulta, banka, dunka,* **his head was throbbing with pain**

throbbing ['θrɒbɪŋ] *adj.* (pain) which comes again and again like a heart beat *dunkande;* **she has a throbbing pain in her finger; he has a throbbing headache**

thrombectomy [θrɒm'bektəmi] *subst.* surgical operation to remove a blood clot *trombektomi*

thrombin ['θrɒmbɪn] *subst.* substance which converts fibrinogen to fibrin and so coagulates blood *trombin*

thrombo- ['θrɒmbəʊ, ˌ--] *prefix* referring to (i) blood clot *tromb(o)-, blodlever-;* (ii) thrombosis *tromb(o)-, blodpropps-*

thromboangiitis obliterans [ˌθrɒmbəʊˌændʒi'aɪtɪs əbˌlɪtərəns] *or* **Buerger's disease** ['bɜːgəz dɪˌziːz] *subst.* disease of the arteries, where the blood vessels in a limb (usually the leg) become narrow, causing gangrene *tromb(o)angiitis obliterans, endangiitis (endarteritis) obliterans, trombangit, Buergers sjukdom*

thromboarteritis [ˌθrɒmbəʊˌɑːtə'raɪtɪs] *subst.* inflammation of an artery caused by thrombosis *tromb(o)arterit*

thrombocyte ['θrɒmbəʊsaɪt] *or* **platelet** ['pleɪtlət] *subst.* little blood cell which encourages the coagulation of blood *trombocyt, blodplätt, blodplatta*

thrombocythaemia [ˌθrɒmbəʊsi'θiːmiə] *subst.* disease where the patient has an abnormally high number of platelets in his blood *trombocytemi*

thrombocytopenia [ˌθrɒmbəʊˌsaɪtə(ʊ)'piːniə] *subst.* condition where the patient has an abnormally low number of platelets in his blood *trombocytopeni*

thrombocytopenic [ˌθrɒmbəʊˌsaɪtə(ʊ)'penɪk] *adj.* referring to thrombocytopenia *trombo(cyto)penisk*

thrombocytosis [ˌθrɒmbəʊsaɪ'təʊsɪs] *subst.* increase in the number of platelets in a patient's blood *trombocytos*

thromboembolism [ˌθrɒmbəʊ'embəlɪz(ə)m] *subst.* condition where a blood clot forms in one part of the body and moves through the blood vessels to block another part *tromboemboli*

thromboendarterectomy [ˌθrɒmbəʊˌendɑːtə'rektəmi] *subst.* surgical operation to open an artery to remove a blood clot which is blocking it *trombendarterektomi, trombektomi*

thromboendarteritis [ˌθrɒmbəʊˌendɑːtə'raɪtɪs] *subst.* inflammation of the inside of an artery, caused by thrombosis *tromb(o)arterit*

thrombokinase [ˌθrɒmbəʊ'kaɪneɪz] *or* **thromboplastin** [ˌθrɒmbəʊ'plæstɪn] *subst.* substance which converts prothrombin into thrombin *trombokinas, tromboplastin, koagulationsfaktor III*

thrombolysis [θrɒm'bɒləsɪs] *subst.* breaking up of blood clots *trombolys, blodproppsupplösning*

thrombolytic [ˌθrɒmbəʊ'lɪtɪk] *adj.* (substance) which will break up blood clots *trombolytisk, blodproppsupplösande*

thrombophlebitis [ˌθrɒmbəʊflɪ'baɪtɪs] *subst.* blocking of a vein by a blood clot, sometimes causing inflammation *tromboflebit*

thromboplastin [ˌθrɒmbəʊ'plæstɪn] *or* **thrombokinase** [ˌθrɒmbəʊ'kaɪneɪz] *subst.* substance which converts prothrombin into thrombin *tromboplastin, trombokinas, koagulationsfaktor III*

thrombopoiesis [ˌθrɒmbəʊpɔɪ'iːsɪs] *subst.* process by which blood platelets are formed *trombocytbildning*

thrombosis [θrɒm'bəʊsɪs] *subst.* blood clotting *or* blocking of an artery *or* vein by a mass of coagulated blood *trombos, blodpropp;* **cerebral thrombosis** *or* **stroke** = condition where a blood clot enters and blocks a brain artery *cerebral trombos, blodpropp i hjärnan, stroke, slag(anfall);* **coronary thrombosis** = blood clot which blocks one of the coronary arteries, leading to a heart attack *koronarkärlstrombos;* **deep vein thrombosis** = blood clot in the deep veins of the leg or pelvis *djup ventrombos*

thrombus ['θrɒmbəs] *subst.* blood clot *or* mass of coagulated blood in an artery *or* vein *tromb, blodpropp*
NOTE: plural is **thrombi**

throw up [ˌθrəʊ 'ʌp] *vb.* to be sick *or* to vomit *kräkas, kasta upp, spy;* **she threw up all over the bathroom floor; he threw up his dinner**

thrush [θrʌʃ] *subst.* infection of the mouth (or sometimes the vagina) with the bacterium Candida albicans *moniliasis, muntorsk, torsk*

thumb [θʌm] *subst.* short thick finger, with only two phalanges, which is separated from the other four fingers on the hand *pollex, tummen;* **he hit his thumb with the hammer; the baby was sucking its thumb**

thumb-sucking ['θʌmsʌkɪŋ] *subst.* action of sucking a thumb (by a baby) *tumsugning;* **thumb-sucking tends to push the teeth forward**

thym- ['θaɪm, ˌ-] *prefix* referring to the thymus gland *tym(o)-, bräss-*

thymectomy [θaɪ'mektəmi] *subst.* surgical operation to remove the thymus gland *tymektomi*

-thymia ['θaɪmiə] *suffix* referring to a state of mind *-tymi*

thymic ['θaɪmɪk] *adj.* referring to the thymus gland *som avser el. hör till brässen*

thymitis [θaɪ'maɪtɪs] *subst.* inflammation of the thymus gland *tymit*

thymocyte ['θaɪməʊsaɪt] *subst.* lymphocyte formed in the thymus gland *tymocyt*

thymoma [θaɪ'məʊmə] *subst.* tumour in the thymus gland *tymom*

thymus (gland) ['θaɪməs (ˌglænd)] *subst.* endocrine gland in the front part of the top of the thorax, behind the breastbone *thymus, tymus, brässen, halsbrässen*

> COMMENT: the thymus gland produces lymphocytes and is responsible for developing the system of natural immunity in children. It grows less active as the person becomes an adult. Lymphocytes produced by the thymus are known as T-lymphocytes or T-cells

thyro- ['θaɪ(ə)rəʊ, ˌ---] *prefix* referring to the thyroid gland *thyre(o)-, tyre(o)-, tyr(o)-, sköldbrosks-, sköldkörtels-*

thyrocalcitonin [ˌθaɪ(ə)rəʊˌkælsi'təʊnɪn] *or* **calcitonin** [ˌkælsɪ'təʊnɪn] *subst.* hormone, produced by the thyroid gland, which is believed to regulate the level of calcium in the blood *tyrokalcitonin, kalcitonin*

thyrocele ['θaɪ(ə)rəʊsiː(ə)l] *subst.* swelling of the thyroid gland *sköldkörtelsvullnad*

thyroglobulin [ˌθaɪ(ə)rəʊ'glɒbjʊlɪn] *subst.* protein stored in the thyroid gland which is broken down into thyroxine *tyreoglobulin*

thyroglossal [ˌθaɪ(ə)rəʊ'glɒs(ə)l] *adj.* referring to the thyroid gland and the throat *som avser el. hör till både sköldkörteln och tungan;* **thyroglossal cyst** = cyst in the front of the neck *slags cysta på halsens framsida*

thyroid ['θaɪ(ə)rɔɪd] **1** *adj.* referring to the thyroid gland *tyreoid, sköld-, sköldkörtel-;* **thyroid cartilage** = large cartilage in the larynx, part of which forms the Adam's apple ⇨ *illustration* LUNGS *cartilago thyreoidea, sköldbrosket;* **thyroid extract** = substance extracted from thyroid glands of animals and used to treat hypothyroidism *sköldkörtelextrakt;* **thyroid hormone** = hormone produced by the thyroid gland *tyreoideahormon, sköldkörtelhormon* **2** *subst.* **thyroid (gland)** = endocrine gland in the neck below the larynx *glandula thyreoidea, tyreoidea, sköldkörteln*

> COMMENT: the thyroid gland is activated by the pituitary gland, and produces thyroxine, a hormone which regulates the body's metabolism. The thyroid gland needs a supply of iodine in order to produce thyroxine. If the thyroid gland malfunctions, it can result in hyperthyroidism (producing too much thyroxine) leading to goitre, or in hypothyroidism (producing too little thyroxine) which causes cretinism in children and myxoedema in adults

thyroidectomy [ˌθaɪ(ə)rɔɪ'dektəmi] *subst.* surgical operation to remove all *or* part of the thyroid gland *tyreoidektomi*

thyroiditis [ˌθaɪ(ə)rɔɪ'daɪtɪs] *subst.* inflammation of the thyroid gland *tyreoidit, sköldkörtelinflammation*

thyroid-stimulating hormone (TSH) [ˌθaɪ(ə)rɔɪd'stɪmjuleɪtɪŋ ˌhɔːməʊn (ˌtiːes'eɪtʃ)] *or* **thyrotrophin** [ˌθaɪ(ə)rəʊ'trəʊpɪn] *subst.* hormone secreted by the pituitary gland which stimulates the thyroid gland *tyreoideastimulerande hormon, TSH, tyreotropin*

thyrotomy [ˌθaɪ(ə)'rɒtəmi] *subst.* surgical opening made in the thyroid cartilage *or* the thyroid gland *tyreotomi*

thyrotoxic [ˌθaɪ(ə)rəʊ'tɒksɪk] *adj.* referring to severe hyperthyroidism *tyreotoxisk;* **thyrotoxic crisis** = sudden illness caused by hyperthyroidism *tyreotoxisk kris;* **thyrotoxic goitre** = goitre caused by thyrotoxicosis *tyreotoxikos, giftstruma*

thyrotoxicosis [ˌθaɪ(ə)rəʊˌtɒksɪ'kəʊsɪs] *or* **Graves' disease** ['greɪvz dɪˌziːz] *or* **exophthalmic goitre** [ˌeksɒf'θælmɪk ˌgɔɪtə] *or* **Basedow's disease** ['bæzɪdəʊz dɪˌziːz] *subst.* type of goitre, caused by hyperthyroidism, where the heart beats faster, the thyroid gland swells, the patient trembles and his eyes protrude *tyreotoxikos, giftstruma, Basedows sjukdom, Graves sjukdom*

thyrotrophin [ˌθaɪ(ə)rəʊ'trəʊfɪn] *or* **thyroid-stimulating hormone** [ˌθaɪ(ə)rɔɪd'stɪmjuleɪtɪŋ ˌhɔːməʊn] *subst.* hormone secreted by the pituitary gland which stimulates the thyroid gland *tyreotropin, tyreoideastimulerande hormon, TSH*

thyrotrophin-releasing hormone (TRH) [ˌθaɪ(ə)rəʊ'trəʊfɪnrɪˌliːsɪŋ 'hɔːməʊn (ˌtiːɑːr'eɪtʃ)] *subst.* hormone secreted by the hypothalamus, which makes the pituitary gland release thyrotrophin, which in turn stimulates the thyroid gland *tyreotropinfrigörande hormon, TRH, tyr(e)oliberin*

thyroxine [θaɪ(ə)'rɒksiːn] *subst.* hormone produced by the thyroid gland which regulates the body's metabolism and conversion of food into heat *tyr(e)oxin, tetrajodtyronin, T4;* synthetic thyroxine is used in treatment of hypothyroidism

TIA [ˌtiːaɪ'eɪ] = TRANSIENT ISCHAEMIC ATTACK

> QUOTE blood pressure control reduces the incidence of first stroke and aspirin appears to reduce the risk of stroke after TIAs by some 15%
> **British Journal of Hospital Medicine**

tiamin ⇨ **Vitamin B**

tibia ['tɪbiə] *or* **shin bone** ['ʃɪn bəʊn] *subst.* the larger of two long bones in the lower leg running from the knee to the ankle (the other, thinner, bone in the lower leg is the fibula) *tibia, skenbenet*

tibia- ⇨ **tibial, tibio-**

tibial ['tɪbiəl] *adj.* referring to the tibia *tibia-, skenbens-;* **tibial arteries** = two arteries which run down the front and back of the lower leg *arteriae tibiales, skenbensartärerna*

tibialis [ˌtɪbi'eɪlɪs] *subst.* one of two muscles in the lower leg running from the tibia to the foot *musculus tibialis*

tibio- ['tɪbiəʊ, ˌ--] *prefix* referring to the tibia *tibia-, skenbens-*

tibiofibular [ˌtɪbiəʊ'fɪbjʊlə] *adj.* referring to both the tibia and the fibula *som avser el. hör till både skenbenet och vadbenet*

tic [tɪk] *subst.* involuntary twitching of the muscles (usually in the face) *tic;* **tic douloureux** *or* **trigeminal neuralgia** = pain in the trigeminal nerve which sends intense pains shooting across the face *trigeminusneuralgi*

tick [tɪk] *subst.* tiny parasite which sucks blood from the skin *fästing;* **tick fever** = infectious disease transmitted by bites from ticks *fästingöverförd sjukdom*

tid ⇨ **stay, term**

t.i.d. [ˌtiːaɪ'diː] *or* **TID** [ˌtiːaɪ'diː] *abbreviation for the Latin phrase* "ter in die": three times a day (written on prescriptions) *ter in die, tre gånger dagligen*

"tiden ut" ⇨ **full term**

tie [taɪ] *vb.* to attach a thread with a knot *knyta, binda (fast);* **the surgeon quickly tied up the stitches; the nurse had tied the bandage too tight**
NOTE: **ties - tying - tied - has tied**

tight [taɪt] *adj.* which fits firmly *or* which is not loose *hård, åtsittande, fast;* **make sure the bandage is not too tight; the splint must be kept tight, or the bone may move; tight-fitting clothes can affect the circulation**
NOTE: **tight - tighter - tightest**

tightly ['taɪtli] *adv.* in a tight way *hårt, åtsittande, fast;* **she tied the bandage tightly round his arm**

tillbaka- ⇨ **retro-**

tillbakabildning ⇨ **involution**

tillbakablickande ⇨ **retrospection**

tillbakadragenhet ⇨ **withdrawal**

tillbakagång ⇨ **regress, regression, retrogression**

tillbakalöpande ⇨ **recurrent**

tillfriskna ⇨ **convalesce, get better, get well, recover, recuperate**

tillfrisknande ⇨ **convalescence, recovery, recuperation**

tillfällig ⇨ **provisional, temporary**

tillfällighet ⇨ **accident**

tillfälligt ⇨ **provisionally**

tillföra ⇨ **administer, supply**

tillförande lymfkärl ⇨ **vessel**

tillförsel ⇨ **supply**

tillgänglig ⇨ **available**

tillhandahålla ⇨ **provide, supply**

tillhandahållande ⇨ **provision**

tillräcklig ⇨ **adequate**

tillräknelig ⇨ **compos mentis**

tillsats ⇨ **additive; attachment**

tillslutningsfel ⇨ **malocclusion**

tillsnörd ⇨ **strangulated**

tillsnörning ⇨ **obstruction**

tillstyrka ⇨ **approve**

tillstånd ⇨ **condition, state, status**

tillstötande ⇨ **intercurrent disease**

tillsyn ⇨ **supervision**

tillsätta ⇨ **appoint**

tillta ⇨ **gain, rise**

tilltagande ⇨ **progressive, progressively**

tillträde ⇨ **admission**

tilltäppning ⇨ **obstruction, occlusion**

tillvänjning ⇨ **habituation, tolerance**

tillväxt ⇨ **growth, proliferation**

tillväxt- ⇨ **vegetative**

-tillväxt ⇨ **-trophy**

tillväxtfaktor ⇨ **factor**

tillväxthormon ⇨ **growth, somatotrophic hormone**

tillväxtperiod ⇨ **proliferative**

tillåta ⇨ **allow**

tillämpas ⇨ **apply**

timglasmage ⇨ **hourglass contraction**

timme ⇨ **hour**

tina (upp) ⇨ **thaw**

tincture ['tɪŋ(k)tʃə] *subst.* medicinal substance dissolved in alcohol *tinktur;* **tincture of iodine** = disinfectant made of iodine and alcohol *jodsprit*

tinea ['tɪniə] *or* **ringworm** ['rɪŋwɜ:m] *subst.* infection by a fungus, in which the infection spreads out in a circle from a central point *tinea, ringorm, revorm;* **tinea barbae** = ringworm in the beard *tinea barbae, skäggsvamp;* **tinea capitis** = ringworm on the scalp *revorm i hårbotten;* **tinea pedis** = athlete's foot *or* fungus infection between the toes *tinea pedis, fotsvamp*

tingle ['tɪŋg(ə)l] *vb.* to give a feeling like a slight electric shock *krypa, sticka;* **he had a tingling feeling in his fingers**

tinktur ⇨ **tincture**

tinning- ⇨ **temporal**

tinningbenet ⇨ **temporal bone**

tinningen ⇨ **temple**

tinninggropen ⇨ **temporal**

tinningloben ⇨ **temporal**

tinninglobs- ⇨ **temporo-**

tinnings- ⇨ **temporo-**

tinnitus [tɪ'naɪtəs] *subst.* ringing sound in the ears *tinnitus, öronringning, öronsusning*

> COMMENT: tinnitus can sound like bells, or buzzing, or a loud roaring sound. In some cases it is caused by wax blocking the auditory canal, but it is also associated with Ménière's disease and infections of the middle ear

tipped womb [ˌtɪpt 'wu:m] *US subst.* condition where the uterus slopes backwards away from its normal position *retroverterad livmoder, bakåtlutad livmoder*
NOTE: the UK English is **retroverted uterus**

tired ['ta(ɪ)əd] *adj.* feeling sleepy *or* feeling that a person needs to rest *trött;* **the patients are tired, and need to go to bed; there is something wrong with her - she's always tired**

tiredness ['taɪ(ɪ)ədnəs] *subst.* being tired *trötthet*

tired out [ˌtaɪ(ɪ)əd 'aʊt] *adj.* feeling extremely tired *or* feeling in need of a rest *utröttad, utmattad;* **she is tired out after the physiotherapy**

tissue ['tɪʃuː] *subst.* material made of cells, of which the parts of the body are formed *väv, vävnad;* **most of the body is made up of soft tissue, with the exception of the bones and cartilage; the main types of body tissue are connective, epithelial, muscular and nerve tissue; adipose tissue** = tissue where the cells contain fat *fettväv(nad), kroppsfett;* **connective tissue** = tissue which forms the main part of bones and cartilage, ligaments and tendons, in which a large amount of fibrous material surrounds the tissue cells *bindväv, stödjevävnad;* **elastic tissue** = connective tissue as in the walls of arteries, which contains elastic fibres *elastisk vävnad (bindväv);* **epithelial tissue** = tissue which forms the skin *epitel(vävnad);* **fibrous tissue** = strong white tissue which makes tendons and ligaments and also scar tissue *fibrös vävnad;* **lymphoid tissue** = tissue in the lymph nodes, the tonsils and the spleen, which forms lymphocytes and antibodies *lymfvävnad;* **muscle tissue** *or* **muscular tissue** = tissue which forms the muscles, and which can contract and expand *muskelvävnad;* **nerve tissue** = tissue which forms nerves, and which is able to transmit nerve impulses *nervvävnad;* **tissue culture** = live tissue grown in a culture in a laboratory *vävnadskultur;* **tissue typing** = identifying various elements in tissue from a donor and comparing them to those of the recipient to see if a transplant is likely to be rejected (the two most important factors are the ABO blood grouping and the HLA antigen system) *vävnadstypning*
NOTE: for other terms referring to tissue see words beginning with **hist-, histo-**

titer ▷ **titre**

titration [taɪ'treɪʃ(ə)n] *subst.* process of measuring the strength of a solution *titrering*

titre ['tiːtə] *subst.* measurement of the quantity of antibodies in a serum *titer, normalstyrka, normalkoncentration*

titrering ▷ **titration**

tjock ▷ **fat, fleshy, obese**

tjockna ▷ **thicken**

tjocktarmen ▷ **colon, large intestine**

tjocktarmsinflammation ▷ **colitis**

tjänst ▷ **duty, service**

tjänste- ▷ **official**

tjänstefel ▷ **malpractice, misconduct**

tjänstgöra ▷ **act, duty**

tjänst, i ▷ **take**

T-lymfocyt ▷ **lymphocyte, T-cell**

toalett ▷ **lavatory, toilet**

toalettpapper ▷ **toilet paper**

tobacco [tə'bækəʊ] *subst.* leaves of a plant which are dried and smoked, either in a pipe or as cigarettes or cigars *tobak*

> COMMENT: tobacco contains nicotine, which is an addictive stimulant. This is why it is difficult for a person who smokes a lot of cigarettes to give up the habit. Nicotine can enter the bloodstream and cause poisoning; tobacco smoking also causes cancer, especially of the lungs and throat

tobak ▷ **tobacco**

toco- ['təʊkə(ʊ), ˌ--] *prefix* referring to childbirth *toko-*

tocography [tɒ'kɒgrəfi] *subst.* recording of the contractions of the uterus during childbirth *tokografi*

Todd's paralysis ['tɒdz pəˌræləsɪs] *or* **Todd's palsy** ['tɒdz ˌpɔːlzi] *subst.* temporary paralysis of part of the body which has been the starting point of focal epilepsy *tillfällig förlamning pga fokal epilepsi*

toe [təʊ] *subst.* one of the five separate parts at the end of the foot (each toe is formed of three bones *or* phalanges, except the big toe, which only has two *dactylus, tå;* **big toe** *or* **great toe and little toe** = biggest and smallest of the five toes *hallux, stortån, digitus minimus, lilltån*

toenail ['təʊneɪl] *subst.* thin hard growth covering the end of a toe *tånagel*

tofi ▷ **urecchysis**

tofus ▷ **tophus**

toilet ['tɔɪlət] *subst.* **(a)** cleaning of the body *toalett;* **she was busy with her toilet (b)** lavatory *or* place or room where a person can pass urine or faeces *toalett*

toilet paper ['tɔɪlət peɪpə] *subst.* special paper for wiping the anus after defecating *toalettpapper*

toilet roll ['tɔɪlət rəʊl] *subst.* roll of toilet paper *rulle toalettpapper, toalettpappersrulle*

toilet training ['tɔɪlət treɪnɪŋ] *subst.* teaching a small child to pass urine *or* faeces in a toilet, and so no longer require nappies *potträning*

tokig ⇨ **mad**

toko- ⇨ **toco-**

tokografi ⇨ **tocography**

tolerance ['tɒl(ə)r(ə)ns] *subst.* ability of the body to tolerate a substance *or* an action *tolerans, tillvänjning;* **he has been taking the drug for so long that he has developed a tolerance to it; drug tolerance** = condition where a drug has been given to a patient for so long that his body no longer reacts to it, and the dosage has to be increased *läkemedelstolerans;* **glucose tolerance test** = test for diabetes mellitus, where the patient eats glucose and his blood and urine are tested regularly *glukosbelastning(sprov)*

> QUOTE 26 patients were selected from the outpatient department on grounds of disabling breathlessness, severely limiting exercise tolerance and the performance of activities of normal daily living
>
> **Lancet**

tolerans ⇨ **tolerance**

tolerate ['tɒləreɪt] *vb.* to accept *or* not to react to (a drug) *tolerera, tåla*

tolerera ⇨ **tolerate**

tolvfingertarm- ⇨ **duodenal, duoden-**

tolvfingertarmen ⇨ **duodenum**

tom ⇨ **empty**

tomo- ['təʊmə(ʊ), ˌ--, tə(ʊ)'mɒ] *prefix* meaning a cutting *or* section *tomo-*

tomografering ⇨ **tomography**

tomografi ⇨ **tomography**

tomogram ['təʊməgræm] *subst.* picture of part of the body taken by tomography *tomogram, skiktbild*

tomography [tə'mɒgrəfi] *subst.* scanning of a particular part of the body using X-rays *or* ultrasound *tomografi, tomografering, skiktröntgen;* **computerized axial tomography (CAT)** = X ray examination where a computer creates a picture of a section of the patient's body *datortomografi, DT, skiktröntgen, CT*

tomotocia [ˌtəʊmə'təʊsiə] *or* **Caesarean section** [sɪˌzeəriən 'sekʃ(ə)n] *subst.* surgical operation to deliver a baby by cutting through the mother's abdominal wall into the uterus *tomotoki, sectio caesarea, kejsarsnitt*

-tomy [təmi] *suffix* referring to a surgical operation *-tomi, -snitt*

ton ⇨ **sound**

tone [təʊn] *or* **tonus** ['təʊnəs] *subst.* state of a healthy muscle when it is not fully relaxed *tonus, muskeltonus, muskelspänning*

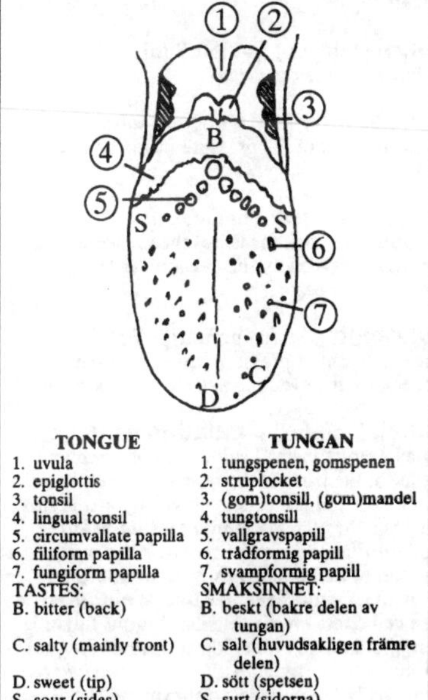

TONGUE	TUNGAN
1. uvula	1. tungspenen, gomspenen
2. epiglottis	2. struplocket
3. tonsil	3. (gom)tonsill, (gom)mandel
4. lingual tonsil	4. tungtonsill
5. circumvallate papilla	5. vallgravspapill
6. filiform papilla	6. trådformig papill
7. fungiform papilla	7. svampformig papill
TASTES:	SMAKSINNET:
B. bitter (back)	B. beskt (bakre delen av tungan)
C. salty (mainly front)	C. salt (huvudsakligen främre delen)
D. sweet (tip)	D. sött (spetsen)
S. sour (sides)	S. surt (sidorna)

tongue [tʌŋ] *or* **glossa** ['glɒsə] *subst.* long muscular organ inside the mouth which can move and is used for tasting, swallowing and speaking *lingua, glossa, tungan;* **the doctor told him to stick out his tongue and say "Ah"** NOTE: for other terms referring to the tongue, see **lingual** and words beginning with **gloss-**

COMMENT: the top surface of the tongue is covered with papillae, some of which contain buds. The tongue is also necessary for speaking certain sounds such as "l", "d", "n" and "th"

tonic ['tɒnɪk] **1** *adj.* (muscle) which is contracted *tonisk* **2** *subst.* substance which improves the patient's general health *or* which makes a tired person stronger *tonikum, stärkande medel;* **he is taking a course of iron tonic tablets; she asked the doctor to prescribe a tonic for her anaemia**

tonicity [tə(ʊ)'nɪsəti] *subst.* normal state of a muscle which is not fully relaxed *tonicitet, muskeltonus, muskelspänning*

tonikum ⇨ **tonic**

tonisk ⇨ **tonic**

tonisk muskelkramp ⇨ **myotonia, tetanus**

tono- ['təʊnə(ʊ), ˌ--, tə(ʊ)'nɒ] *prefix* referring to pressure *tono-*

tonography [ˌtə(ʊ)'nɒgrəfi] *subst.* measurement of the pressure inside an eyeball *mätning av ögontrycket*

tonometer [tə(ʊ)'nɒmɪtə] *subst.* instrument which measures the pressure inside an organ, especially the eye *tonometer, oftalmotonometer*

tonometry [ˌtə(ʊ)'nɒmɪtri] *subst.* measurement of pressure inside an organ, especially the eye *tonometri, oftalmotonometri*

tonsil ['tɒns(ə)l] *or* **palatine tonsil** ['pælətaɪn ˌtɒns(ə)l] *subst.* area of lymphoid tissue at the back of the throat in which lymph circulates and protects the body against germs entering through the mouth *tonsilla palatina, gomtonsill, gommandel, mandel;* **the doctor looked at her tonsils; they recommended that she should have her tonsils out; there are red spots on his tonsils; lingual tonsil** = lymphoid tissue on the top surface of the back of the tongue *"tungtonsillen", lymfvävnad i tungans bakre övre del;* **pharyngeal tonsil** *or* **adenoidal tissue** = lymphoid tissue at the back of the throat where the passages from the nose join the pharynx ⇨ *illustration* TONGUE *tonsilla pharyngea, farynxtonsillen, svalgtonsillen, svalgmandeln*

COMMENT: the tonsils are larger in children than in adults, and are more liable to infection. When infected, the tonsils become enlarged and can interfere with breathing

tonsillar ['tɒns(ə)lə] *adj.* referring to the tonsils *tonsillar, tonsillär*

tonsillectomy [ˌtɒnsə'lektəmi] *subst.* surgical operation to remove the tonsils *tonsillektomi*

tonsillinflammation ⇨ **gingivitis, ulceromembranous gingivitis**

tonsillitis [ˌtɒnsə'laɪtɪs] *subst.* inflammation of the tonsils *tonsillit, inflammation i halsmandlarna, halsfluss*

tonsillotom ⇨ **guillotine, tonsillotome**

tonsillotome [tɒn'sɪlətəʊm] *subst.* surgical instrument used in operations on the tonsils *tonsillotom, giljontinsax*

tonsillotomy [ˌtɒnsɪ'lɒtəmi] *subst.* surgical operation to make an incision into the tonsils *tonsillotomi*

tonsillär ⇨ **tonsillar**

tonus ['təʊnəs] *or* **tone** [təʊn] *subst.* state of a healthy muscle which is not fully relaxed *tonus, muskeltonus, muskelspänning*

tonåring ⇨ **adolescent**

tooth [tu:θ] *subst.* one of a set of bones in the mouth which are used to chew food *dens, tand;* **dental hygiene involves cleaning the teeth every day after breakfast; you will have to see the dentist if one of your teeth hurts; he had to have a tooth out** = he had to have a tooth taken out by the dentist *han måste dra ut en tand (få en tand utdragen);* **impacted tooth** = tooth which is pressed into the jawbone and so cannot grow normally *dens impactus, retinerad (inklämd) tand;* **milk teeth** *or* **deciduous teeth** = a child's first twenty teeth, which are gradually replaced by the permanent teeth *dentes decidui, mjölktänderna;* **permanent teeth** = adult's teeth, which replace a child's teeth during late childhood *permanenta tänderna; see also* HUTCHINSON'S TEETH NOTE: plural is **teeth.** For terms referring to teeth see words beginning with **dent-, odont-**

COMMENT: a tooth is formed of a soft core of pulp, covered with a layer of hard dentine. The top part of the tooth (the crown), which can be seen above the gum, is covered with hard shiny enamel which is very hard-wearing. The lower part of the tooth (the root), which attaches the tooth to the jaw, is covered with cement, also a hard substance, but which is slightly rough and holds the periodontal ligament which links the tooth to the jaw. The milk teeth in a child appear over the first two years of childhood and consist of incisors, canines and molars. The permanent teeth which replace them are formed of eight incisors, four canines, eight premolars and twelve molars, the last four molars (the third molars or wisdom teeth), are not always present, and do not appear much before the age of twenty. Permanent teeth start to appear about the age of 5 to 6. The order of eruption of the permanent teeth is: first molars, incisors, premolars, canines, second molars, wisdom teeth

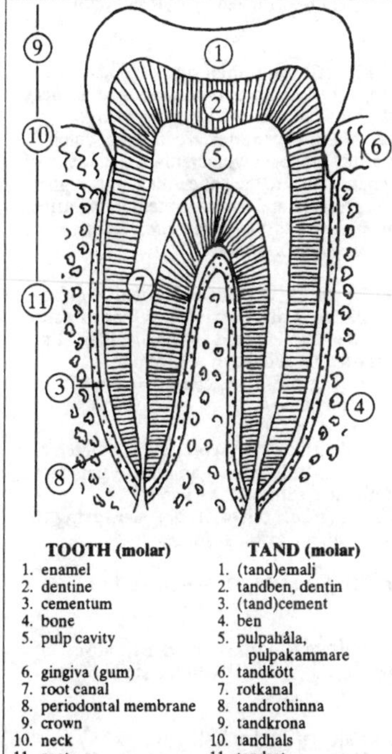

TOOTH (molar)	TAND (molar)
1. enamel	1. (tand)emalj
2. dentine	2. tandben, dentin
3. cementum	3. (tand)cement
4. bone	4. ben
5. pulp cavity	5. pulpahåla, pulpakammare
6. gingiva (gum)	6. tandkött
7. root canal	7. rotkanal
8. periodontal membrane	8. tandrothinna
9. crown	9. tandkrona
10. neck	10. tandhals
11. root	11. tandrot

toothache ['tu:θeɪk] *subst.* pain in a tooth *tandvärk;* **he went to the dentist because he had toothache** NOTE: no plural

toothbrush ['tu:θbrʌʃ] *subst.* small brush which is used to clean the teeth *tandborste*

toothpaste ['tu:θpeɪst] *subst.* soft cleaning material which is spread on a toothbrush and then used to brush the teeth *tandkräm;* **he always brushes his teeth with fluoride toothpaste**

topagnosis [ˌtəʊpəg'nəʊsɪs] *subst.* being unable to tell which part of your body has been touched, caused by a disorder of the brain *topagnosi*

tophus ['təʊfəs] *subst.* deposit of solid crystals in the skin, or in the joints, especially with gout *tophus (arthriticus), tofus, giktknöl* NOTE: plural is **tophi**

topical ['tɒpɪk(ə)l] *adj.* referring to one particular part of the body *topisk, lokal;* **topical drug** = drug which is applied to one part of the body only *läkemedel för lokal administrering (lokalbehandling)*

> QUOTE one of the most common routes of neonatal poisoning is percutaneous absorption following topical administration
> **Southern Medical Journal**

topically ['tɒpɪk(ə)li] *adv.* (applied) to one part of the body only *lokalt (administrerad);* **the drug is applied topically**

topisk ⇨ **topical**

topografi ⇨ **topography**

topografisk ⇨ **topographical**

topographical [ˌtɒpə'græfɪk(ə)l] *adj.* referring to topography *topografisk*

topography [tə'pɒgrəfi] *subst.* description of each particular part of the body *topografi, lägesbeskrivning*

topp ⇨ **head**

torakal ⇨ **thoracic**

torakektomi ⇨ **thoracectomy**

torak(o)- ⇨ **thorac(o)-**

torakocentes ⇨ **pleurocentesis, thoracentesis, thoracocentesis**

torakoplastik ⇨ **thoracoplasty**

torakoskop ⇨ **thoracoscope**

torakoskopi ⇨ **thoracoscopy**

torakotomi ⇨ **thoracotomy**

torax ⇨ **thorax**

toraxplastik ⇨ **thoracoplasty**

torgskräck ⇨ **agoraphobia**

tork ⇨ **swab, tampon**

torka ⇨ **dry, dryness**

torka (ut) ⇨ **dehydrate**

tormina ['tɔːmɪnə] *subst.* colic *or* pain in the intestine *tormina, buksmärtor, magknip*

torpor ['tɔːpə] *subst.* condition where a patient seems sleepy *or* slow to react *torpor, tröghet, slöhet*

torr ⇨ **dry**

torr- ⇨ **xero-**

torrdrunkning ⇨ **drowning**

torrhet ⇨ **dryness, kraurosis**

torris ⇨ **ice, snow**

torrögdhet ⇨ **xerophthalmia**

torsk ⇨ **candidiasis, perleche, thrush**

torskleverolja ⇨ **cod liver oil**

torso ['tɔːsəʊ] *subst.* main part of the body, not including the arms, legs and head *torso, bålen*

torticollis [ˌtɔːtɪ'kɒlɪs] *or* **wry neck** [ˌraɪ 'nek] *subst.* deformity of the neck, where the head is twisted to one side by contraction of the sternocleidomastoid muscle *torticollis, halsvred, nackspärr*

total ['təʊt(ə)l] *adj.* complete *or* covering the whole body *total, fullständig, hel;* **he has total paralysis of the lower part of the body**

totally ['təʊt(ə)li] *adv.* completely *totalt, fullständigt, helt;* **she is totally paralysed; he will never totally regain the use of his left hand**

touch [tʌtʃ] *subst.* one of the five senses, where sensations are felt by part of the skin, especially by the fingers and lips *känsel(sinnet), beröring(ssinnet)*

> COMMENT: touch is sensed by receptors in the skin which send impulses back to the brain. The touch receptors can tell the difference between hot and cold, hard and soft, wet and dry, and rough and smooth

tough [tʌf] *adj.* solid *or* which cannot break or tear easily *stark, seg;* **the meninges are covered by a layer of tough tissue, the dura mater**
NOTE: **tough - tougher - toughest**

tourniquet ['tɔːnɪkeɪ] *subst.* instrument *or* tight bandage wrapped round a limb to constrict an artery, so reducing the flow of blood and stopping bleeding from a wound *tourniquet, kompressor*

towel ['ta(ʊ)əl] *subst.* **(a)** piece of soft cloth which is used for drying *handduk, duk* **(b) sanitary towel** = wad of absorbent cotton placed over the vulva to absorb the menstrual flow *dambinda*

tox- ['tɒks, ˌ-, tɒk's] *or* **toxo-** ['tɒksə(ʊ), ˌ--, tɒk'sɒ] *prefix* meaning poison *tox(o)-, gift-*

toxaemia [tɒk'siːmiə] *subst.* blood poisoning *or* presence of poisonous substances in the blood *tox(ik)emi, blodförgiftning;* **toxaemia of pregnancy** = condition which can affect pregnant women towards the end of pregnancy, where the patient develops high blood pressure and passes protein in the urine *graviditetstoxikos, havandeskapstoxikos, havandeskapsförgiftning*

toxic ['tɒksɪk] *adj.* poisonous *toxisk, giftig;* **toxic goitre** *or* **thyrotoxicosis** = type of goitre where the thyroid gland swells, the patient's limbs tremble and the eyes protrude *tyreotoxikos, giftstruma, Basedows sjukdom, Graves sjukdom*

toxicity [tɒk'sɪsəti] *subst.* level to which a substance is poisonous *or* amount of poisonous material in a substance *toxicitet, giftighet(sgrad);* **scientists are measuring the toxicity of car exhaust fumes**

toxico- ['tɒksɪkə(ʊ), ˌ---, ˌtɒksɪ'kɒ] *prefix* meaning poison *toxiko-, gift-*

toxicologist [ˌtɒksɪ'kɒlədʒɪst] *subst.* scientist who specializes in the study of poisons *toxikolog*

toxicology [ˌtɒksɪ'kɒlədʒi] *subst.* scientific study of poisons and their effects on the human body *toxikologi*

toxicosis [ˌtɒksɪ'kəʊsɪs] *subst.* poisoning *toxiko(no)s, förgiftning*

toxikolog ⇨ **toxicologist**

toxikologi ⇨ **toxicology**

toxin ['tɒksɪn] *subst.* poisonous substance produced in the body by germs or microorganisms, and which, if injected into an animal, stimulates the production of antitoxins *toxin*

toxisk ⇨ **poisonous, toxic**

toxocariasis [ˌtɒksəkəˈraɪəsɪs] *or* **visceral larva migrans** [ˈvɪsərəl ˌlɑːvə ˈmaɪgrəns] *subst.* infestation of the intestine with worms from a dog or cat *tarminfektion med toxocara (slags spolmask)*

toxoid [ˈtɒksɔɪd] *subst.* toxin which has been treated and is no longer poisonous, but which can still provoke the formation of antibodies *toxoid, anatoxin*

> COMMENT: toxoids are used as vaccines, and are injected into a patient to give immunity against a disease

toxoid-antitoxin [ˌtɒksɔɪdˌæntɪˈtɒksɪn] *subst.* mixture of toxoid and antitoxin, used as a vaccine *blandning av toxoid och antitoxin*

toxoplasmosis [ˌtɒksə(ʊ)plæzˈməʊsɪs] *subst.* disease caused by the parasite **Toxoplasma** which is carried by animals *toxoplasmos;* **congenital toxoplasmosis** *or* **toxoplasma encephalitis** = condition of a baby which has been infected with toxoplasmosis by its mother while still in the womb *medfödd toxoplasmos*

> COMMENT: toxoplasmosis can cause encephalitis or hydrocephalus and can be fatal

trabecula [trəˈbekjʊlə] *subst.* thin strip of stiff tissue which divides an organ *or* bone tissue into sections *trabecula, bjälkliknande anatomisk bildning* NOTE: plural is **trabeculae**

trabeculectomy [trəˌbekjʊˈlektəmi] *or* **goniotomy** [ˌgəʊniˈɒtəmi] *subst.* surgical operation to treat glaucoma by cutting a channel through trabeculae to link with Schlemm's canal *goniotomi*

trace [treɪs] *subst.* very small amount *spår;* **there are traces of the drug in the blood sample; the doctor found traces of alcohol in the patient's urine; trace element** = element which is essential to the human body, but only in very small quantities *spårelement, spårämne*

> COMMENT: the trace elements are cobalt, chromium, copper, magnesium, manganese, molybdenum, selenium and zinc

tracer [ˈtreɪsə] *subst.* substance (often radioactive) injected into a substance in the body, so that doctors can follow its passage round the body *spårelement, spårämne*

trachea [trəˈkiːə] *or* **windpipe** [ˈwɪndpaɪp] *subst.* main air passage which runs from the larynx to the lungs, where it divides into the two main bronchi ⇨ *illustration* LUNGS, THROAT *trachea, trakea, luftstrupen*

> COMMENT: the trachea is about 10 centimetre long, and is formed of rings of cartilage and connective tissue

tracheal [trəˈkiːəl] *adj.* referring to the trachea *trakeal, luftstrups-;* **tracheal tugging** = feeling that something is pulling on the windpipe when the patient breathes in, a symptom of aneurysm *känsla av att ngt drar i luftstrupen vid inandning*

tracheitis [ˌtreɪkiˈaɪtɪs] *subst.* inflammation of the trachea due to an infection *trakeit, luftstrupskatarr*

trachelorrhaphy [ˌtreɪkiˈlɒrəfi] *subst.* surgical operation to repair tears in the cervix of the uterus *trakelorrafi*

tracheobronchitis [ˌtreikiəʊbrɒŋˈkaɪtɪs] *subst.* inflammation of both the trachea and the bronchi *trakeobronkit*

tracheostomy [ˌtrækɪˈɒstəmi] *or* **tracheotomy** [ˌtrækɪˈɒtəmi] *subst.* surgical operation to make a hole through the throat into the windpipe, so as to allow air to get to the lungs in cases where the trachea is blocked, as in pneumonia, poliomyelitis or diphtheria *trakeo(s)tomi, luftrörssnitt*

> COMMENT: after the operation, a tube is inserted into the hole to keep it open. The tube may be permanent if it is to bypass an obstruction, but can be removed if the condition improves

trachoma [trəˈkəʊmə] *subst.* contagious viral inflammation of the eyelids, common in tropical countries, which can cause blindness if the conjunctiva becomes scarred *trakom, egyptiska ögonsjukdomen*

tract [trækt] *subst.* (i) series of organs *or* tubes which allow something to pass from one part of the body to another *system, apparat, kanal;* (ii) series *or* bundle of nerve fibres connecting two areas of the nervous system and transmitting nervous impulses in one or in both directions *bana, nervbana, stråk;* **cerebrospinal tracts** = main motor pathways in the white columns of the spinal cord *fasciculi cerebrospinales, tractus corticospinales, pyramidbanorna;* **olfactory tract** = nerve tract which takes the olfactory nerve from the nose to the brain *tractus olfactorius;* **pyramidal tract** = tract in the brain and spinal cord carrying motor neurone fibres from the cerebral cortex *pyramidbana*; *see also* DIGESTIVE TRACT

> QUOTE GI fistulae are frequently associated with infection because the effluent contains bowel organisms which initially contaminate the fistula tract
>
> **Nursing Times**

traction ['trækʃ(ə)n] *subst.* pulling applied to straighten a broken or deformed limb *traktion, sträck;* **the patient was in traction for two weeks** NOTE: no plural

> COMMENT: a system of weights and pulleys is fixed over the patient's bed so that the limb can be pulled hard enough to counteract the tendency of the muscles to contract and pull it back to its original position. Traction can also be used for slipped discs and other dislocations. Other forms of traction include frames attached to the body

tractotomy [træk'tɒtəmi] *subst.* surgical operation to cut the nerve pathway taking sensations of pain to the brain, as treatment for intractable pain *traktotomi*

tragofoni ⇨ **aegophony**

tragus ['treɪgəs] *subst.* piece of cartilage in the outer ear which projects forward over the entrance to the auditory canal *tragus, örflik*

training ['treɪnɪŋ] *see* TOILET

trait [treɪ(t)] *subst.* characteristic which is particular to a person *karakteristiskt drag, egenskap;* **physical genetic trait =** characteristic of the body of a person (such as red hair *or* big feet) which is inherited *ärftlig fysisk egenskap*

trakea ⇨ **trachea, windpipe**

trakeal ⇨ **tracheal**

trakealtub ⇨ **endotracheal**

trakeit ⇨ **tracheitis**

trakelorrafi ⇨ **trachelorrhaphy**

trakeobronkit ⇨ **tracheobronchitis**

trakom ⇨ **ophthalmia, trachoma**

traktion ⇨ **traction**

traktotomi ⇨ **tractotomy**

trance [trɑːns] *subst.* condition where a person is in a dream, but not asleep, and seems not to be aware of what is happening round him *trans;* **he walked round the room in a trance; the hypnotist waved his hand and she went into** *or* **came out of a trance**

tranquillizer ['træŋkwəlaɪzə] *or* **tranquillizing drug** ['træŋkwəlaɪzɪŋ ˌdrʌg] *subst.* drug which calms a patient and helps him to stop worrying and to relieve anxiety *sedativ(um), lugnande medel;* **she's taking tranquillizers to calm her nerves; he's been on tranquillizers ever since he started his new job**

trans ⇨ **trance**

trans- [træn's] *prefix* meaning through *or* across *trans-*

trans- ⇨ **trans-**

transaminase [træn'sæmɪneɪz] *subst.* enzyme involved in the transamination of amino acids *transaminas, aminotransferas*

transamination [trænˌsæmɪ'neɪʃ(ə)n] *subst.* process by which amino acids are metabolized in the liver *transaminering*

transection [træn'sekʃ(ə)n] *subst.* (i) cutting across part of the body *tvärsnitt;* (ii) sample of tissue which has been taken by cutting across a part of the body *tvärsnitt*

transfer [træns'fɜː] *vb.* to pass from one place to another *överföra, flytta, transportera;* **the hospital records have been transferred to the computer; the patient was transferred to a special burns unit**

transference ['trænsf(ə)r(ə)ns] *subst. (in psychiatry)* condition where the patient transfers to the psychoanalyst the characteristics belonging to a strong character from his past (such as a parent), and reacts to the analyst as if he were that person *överföring*

transferrin [træns'fɜːrɪn] *or* **siderophilin** [ˌsaɪdə'rɒfəlɪn] *subst.* substance found in the blood, which carries iron in the bloodstream *transferrin*

transfusion [træns'fjuːʒ(ə)n] *subst.* transferring blood *or* saline fluids from a container into a patient's bloodstream *transfusion;* **blood transfusion =** transferring blood which has been given by another person into a patient's vein *blodtransfusion;* **exchange transfusion =** method of treating leukaemia *or* erythroblastosis where almost all the abnormal blood is removed from the body and replaced by normal blood *utbytestransfusion*

transient ['trænzɪənt] *adj.* which does not last long *övergående, kortvarig;* **transient**

ischaemic attack (TIA) = mild stroke caused by a short stoppage of blood supply *transitorisk ischemisk attack, TIA*

transillumination [ˌtrænsiˌluːmɪ'neɪʃ(ə)n] *subst.* examination of an organ by shining a bright light through it *transillumination, genomlysning*

transitional [træn'zɪʃ(ə)n] *adj.* which is in the process of developing into something *övergångs-;* **transitional epithelium** = type of epithelium found in the urethra *övergångsepitel*

translocation [ˌtrænsləʊ'keɪʃ(ə)n] *subst.* moving of part of a chromosome to a different chromosome pair which causes abnormal development of the fetus *translokation*

translumbar [træns'lʌmbə] *adj.* through the lumbar region *genom lumbalområdet (ländområdet)*

transmigration [ˌtrænzmaɪ'greɪʃ(ə)n] *subst.* movement of a cell through a membrane *cellvandring genom membran*

transmit [trænz'mɪt] *vb.* to pass (a message *or* a disease) *överföra, sprida, leda;* **impulses are transmitted along the neural pathways; the disease is transmitted by lice**

transmittorsubstans ⇨ **neurotransmitter**

transparent [træns'pær(ə)nt] *adj.* which can be seen through *genomskinlig;* **the cornea is a transparent tissue on the front of the eye**

transpiration ⇨ **perspiration, sweat, sudor**

transpirera ⇨ **perspire**

transplacental [ˌtrænsplə'sent(ə)l] *adj.* through the placenta *genom placenta (moderkakan)*

transplant 1 ['trænsplɑːnt] *subst.* (i) act of taking an organ (such as the heart *or* kidney) or tissue (such as skin) and grafting it into a patient to replace an organ *or* tissue which is diseased or not functioning properly *transplantation;* (ii) the organ or tissue which is grafted *transplantat, graft;* **she had a heart-lung transplant; the kidney transplant was rejected 2** [træns'plɑːnt] *vb.* to graft an organ *or* tissue onto a patient to replace an organ *or* tissue which is diseased or not functioning correctly *transplantera*

transplantat ⇨ **graft, transplant, transplantation**

transplantation [ˌtrænsplɑːn'teɪʃ(ə)n] *subst.* transplant *or* the act of transplanting *transplantat, transplantation*

> QUOTE unlike other transplant systems, bone marrow transplantation has the added complication of graft-versus-host disease
>
> **Hospital Update**

transplantation ⇨ **graft, implantation, transplant, transplantation**

transplantera ⇨ **graft, transplant**

transport [træns'pɔːt] *vb.* to carry to another place *transportera, forsla;* **arterial blood transports oxygen to the tissues**

> QUOTE insulin's primary metabolic function is to transport glucose into muscle and fat cells, so that it can be used for energy
>
> **Nursing 87**

transportera ⇨ **transfer, transport**

transportör ⇨ **carrier**

transposition [ˌtrænspə'zɪʃ(ə)n] *subst.* congenital condition where the aorta and pulmonary artery are placed on the opposite side of the body to their normal position *transposition, omkastning*

transrectal [træns'rekt(ə)l] *adj.* through the rectum *genom rektum (ändtarmen)*

transsexual [træn'sekʃu(ə)l] *subst. & adj.* (person) who feels a desire to be a member of the opposite sex *or* (behaviour) showing that a person wants to be a member of the opposite sex *transsexuell*

transsexualism [træn'sekʃu(ə)lɪz(ə)m] *subst.* sexual abnormality where a person wants to be a member of the opposite sex *transsexualism*

transudation [ˌtrænsju'deɪʃ(ə)n] *subst.* passing of a fluid from the body's cells outside the body *transudation*

transurethral [ˌtrænsju'riːər(ə)l] *adj.* through the urethra *transuretral;* **transurethral prostatectomy** *or* **transurethral resection (TUR)** = surgical operation to remove the prostate gland, where the operation is carried out through the urethra *transuretral prostatektomi (resektion), TUR*

transverse [trænz'vɜːs] *adj.* across *or* at right angles to an organ *tvär-;* **transverse arch** = arched structure across the sole of the foot *tvärgående fotvalvet, hålfoten;* **transverse colon** = second section of the colon, which crosses the body below the stomach ⇨ *illustration* DIGESTIVE SYSTEM *colon transversum, tvärgående delen av tjocktarmen;* **transverse fracture** = fracture where the bone is broken straight across *tvärfraktur;* **transverse presentation** = position of a baby in the womb, where the baby's side will appear first *tvärläge;* **transverse process** = part of a vertebra which protrudes at the side *processus transversus, tvärutskott*

transvesical prostatectomy [træns'vesɪk(ə)l ˌprɒstə'tektəmi] *subst.* operation to remove the prostate gland, where the operation is carried out through the bladder *transvesikal prostatektomi*

transvestite [trænz'vestaɪt] *subst.* person who dresses in the clothes of the opposite sex, as an expression of transsexualism *transvestit*

trapetsbenet ⇨ **trapezium**

trapetslika benet ⇨ **trapezius**

trapezium [trə'piːziəm] *subst.* one of the eight small carpal bones in the wrist *os trapezium, trapetsbenet*

trapezius [trə'piːziəs] *subst.* triangular muscle in the upper part of the back and the neck, which moves the shoulder blade and pulls the head back *musculus trapezius, trapetslika benet*

trapezoid (bone) ['træpɪzɔɪd (bəʊn)] *subst.* one of the eight small carpal bones in the wrist ⇨ *illustration* HAND *os trapezoideum, trapetslika benet*

trasigt nagelband ⇨ **hangnail**

trattbröst ⇨ **funnel chest**

trauma ['trɔːmə] *subst.* (i) wound *or* injury *trauma, skada, sår;* (ii) mental shock caused by a sudden happening which was not expected to take place *trauma, chock*

traumatic [trɔː'mætɪk] *adj.* referring to trauma *or* caused by an injury *traumatisk, chockartad;* **traumatic fever** = fever caused by an injury *sårfeber;* **traumatic shock** = state of general weakness caused by an injury and loss of blood *traumatisk chock*

traumatisk pneumotorax ⇨ **pneumothorax**

traumatology [ˌtrɔːmə'tɒlədʒi] *subst.* branch of surgery which deals with injuries received in accidents *traumatologi*

travel sickness ['træv(ə)l sɪknəs] *or* **motion sickness** ['məʊʃ(ə)n sɪknəs] *subst.* illness and nausea felt when travelling *kinetos, rörelsesjuka, åksjuka, ressjuka*

> COMMENT: the movement of liquid inside the labyrinth of the middle ear causes motion sickness, which is particularly noticeable in vehicles which are closed, such as planes, coaches, hovercraft

treat [triːt] *vb.* to look after a sick or injured person *or* to try to cure a sick person *behandla;* **after the accident the passengers were treated in hospital for cuts; she has been treated with a new antibiotic; she's being treated by a specialist for heart disease**

treatment ['triːtmənt] *subst.* way of looking after a sick *or* injured person *behandling, kur;* **this is a new treatment for heart disease; he is receiving** *or* **undergoing treatment for a slipped disc; she's in hospital for treatment to her back**

tredagarsfeber ⇨ **roseola**

tredje (gradens) ⇨ **tertiary**

tredje gradens brännskada ⇨ **burn**

tredje trimestern ⇨ **antepartum**

trefin ⇨ **trephine**

trehövdad muskel ⇨ **triceps**

trematode ['tremətəʊd] *subst.* fluke *or* parasitic flatworm *trematod, sugmask*

tremble ['tremb(ə)l] *vb.* to shake *or* shiver slightly *darra, skaka;* **his hands are trembling with cold; her body trembled with fever**

trembling ['tremblɪŋ] *subst.* making rapid small movements of a limb or muscles *darrning, skakning;* **trembling of the hands is a symptom of Parkinson's disease**

tremens ['triːmenz] *see* DELIRIUM

tremor ['tremə] *subst.* shaking *or* making slight movements of a limb *or* muscle *tremor, darrning, skakning;* **coarse tremor** = severe trembling *grov tremor;* **essential tremor** = involuntary slow trembling movement of the hands often seen in old people *essentiell tremor;* **intention tremor** = trembling of the hands when a person suffering from certain brain disease makes a voluntary movement to try to touch something *intentionstremor;* **physiological tremor** = normal small movements of limbs which take place when a person tries to remain still *fysiologisk tremor*

trench fever ['tren(t)ʃ ˌfiːvə] *subst.* fever caused by Rickettsia bacteria, similar to typhus but recurring every five days *slags rickettsios;* **trench foot** *or* **immersion foot** = condition caused by exposure to cold and damp, where the skin of the foot is red and blistered, and gangrene may set in *skyttegravsfot, köldskada efter långvarig vattenkontakt;* **trench mouth** *see* GINGIVITIS

Trendelenburg's position [tren'deləbɜːgz pəˌzɪʃ(ə)n] *subst.* position where the patient lies on a sloping bed, with the head lower than the feet, and the knees bent (used in surgical operations to the pelvis) *Trendelenburgs läge, bäckenhögläge;* **Trendelenburg's operation** = operation to tie a saphenous vein in the groin before removing varicose veins *Trendelenburgs operation;* **Trendelenburg's sign** = symptom of congenital dislocation of the hip, where the patient's pelvis is lower on the opposite side to the dislocation *Trendelenburgs tecken (symtom)*

treonin ⇨ **threonine**

trepan [trɪ'pæn] *vb. (formerly)* to cut a hole in the skull, as a treatment for some diseases of the head *trepanera*

trephine [trɪ'fiːn] *subst.* surgical instrument for making a round hole in the skull *or* for removing a round piece of tissue *trefin*

Treponema [ˌtrepə'niːmə] *subst.* spirochaete which causes disease such as syphilis or yaws *Treponema*

treponematosis [ˌtrepəniːmə'təʊsɪs] *subst.* yaws *or* infection by the bacterium **Treponema pertenue**

treslagspuls ⇨ **trigeminy**

TRH [ˌtiːɑːr'eɪtʃ] = THYROTROPHIN-RELEASING HORMONE

triad ['traɪæd] *subst.* three organs *or* symptoms which are linked together in a group *triad*

triangel ⇨ **triangle**

triangelformad ⇨ **triangular**

triangle ['traɪæŋg(ə)l] *subst.* flat shape which has three sides *triangel;* part of the body with three sides *triangel;* **rectal triangle** *or* **anal triangle** = posterior part of the perineum *bakre delen av bäckenbotten; see also* FEMORAL, SCARPA

triangular [traɪ'æŋgjʊlə] *adj.* with three sides *triangulär, triangelformad;* **triangular bandage** = bandages made of a triangular piece of cloth, used to make a sling for an arm *mitella;* **triangular muscle** = muscle in the shape of a triangle *triangelformad muskel*

triangulär ⇨ **triangular**

triceps ['traɪseps] *subst.* muscle formed of three parts, which are joined to form one tendon *trehövdad muskel;* **triceps brachii** = muscle in the back part of the upper arm which makes the forearm stretch out *musculus triceps brachii, armsträckaren*

trichiasis [trɪ'kaɪəsɪs] *subst.* painful condition where the eyelashes grow in towards the eye and scratch the eyeball *trichiasis*

trichinosis [ˌtrɪkɪ'nəʊsɪs] *or* **trichiniasis** [ˌtrɪkɪ'naɪəsɪs] *subst.* disease caused by infestation of the intestine by larvae of roundworms *or* nematodes, which pass round the body in the bloodstream and settle in muscles *trichinosis, trikinos;* the larvae enter the body from eating meat which has not been cooked, especially pork

trich(o)- ['trɪk(ə), ˌ--] *prefix* (i) referring to hair *trich(o)-, trik(o)-, hår-;* (ii) like hair *trich(o)-, trik(o)-, hårliknande*

Trichocephalus [ˌtrɪkə'sef(ə)ləs] *subst.* whipworm *or* parasitic worm in the intestine *Trichocephalus (dispar), Trichuris trichiura, slags trådmask, piskmask*

trichology [trɪ'kɒlədʒi] *subst.* study of hair and the diseases which affect it *läran om hår och deras sjukdomar*

Trichomonas [ˌtrɪkə'məʊnəs] *subst.* species of long thin parasite which infests the intestines *Trichomonas, trikomonas;* **Trichomonas vaginalis** = parasite which infests the vagina and causes an irritating discharge *Trichomonas vaginalis*

trichomoniasis [ˌtrɪkəʊmə'naɪəsɪs] *subst.* infestation of the intestine *or* vagina with Trichomonas *trikomonasinfektion*

trichomycosis [ˌtrɪkə(ʊ)maɪ'kəʊsɪs] *subst.* disease of the hair caused by a corynebacterium *trikomykos*

Trichophyton [traɪ'kɒfɪtɒn] *subst.* fungus which affects the skin, hair and nails *Trichophyton*

trichophytosis [ˌtrɪkə(ʊ)faɪ'təʊsɪs] *subst.* infection caused by Trichophyton *trikofytos*

trichosis [traɪ'kəʊsɪs] *subst.* abnormal condition of the hair *trikos, hårsjukdom*

trichotillomania [ˌtrɪkə(ʊ)ˌtɪləʊ'meɪniə] *subst.* condition where a person pulls his hair out compulsively *trikotillomani*

trichromatic [ˌtraɪkrə(ʊ)'mætɪk] *adj.* (vision) which is normal, where the person can tell the difference between the three primary colours *trikromatisk; compare* DICHROMATIC

trichrome stain ['traɪkrəʊm ˌsteɪn] *subst.* stain in three colours used in histology *trikromatisk färgning*

trichuriasis [ˌtrɪkju'raɪəsɪs] *subst.* infestation of the intestine with whipworms *trichuriasis, trikuriasis*

Trichuris [trɪ'kjʊərɪs] *subst.* whipworm *or* thin roundworm which infests the intestine *Trichuris (trichiura), piskmask*

tricuspid valve [traɪ'kʌspɪd ˌvælv] *subst.* inlet valve with three cusps between the right atrium and the right ventricle in the heart ⇨ *illustration* HEART *valva tricuspidalis (atrioventricularis dextra), trikuspidalklaffen, atrioventrikularklaffen*

trifocal lenses [traɪ'fəʊk(ə)l lenzɪz] *or* **trifocals** [traɪ'fəʊk(ə)lz] *subst pl.* type of glasses, where three lenses are combined in one piece of glass to give clear vision over different distances *trifokalglas; see also* BIFOCAL

trifokalglas ⇨ **trifocal lenses**

trigeminal [traɪ'dʒemɪn(ə)l] *adj.* in three parts *trigeminus-;* **trigeminal nerve** = fifth cranial nerve (formed of the ophthalmic nerve, the maxillary nerve, and the mandibular nerve) which controls the sensory nerves in the forehead, face and chin, and the muscles in the jaw *nervus trigeminus, 5:e kranialnerven;* **trigeminal neuralgia** *or* **tic douloureux** = pain in the trigeminal nerve, which sends intense pains shooting across the face *trigeminusneuralgi*

trigeminus- ⇨ **trigeminal**

trigeminusneuralgi ⇨ **trigeminal**

trigeminy [traɪ'dʒemɪni] *subst.* irregular heartbeat, where a normal beat is followed by two ectopic beats *pulsus trigeminus, treslagspuls*

trigger ['trɪgə] *vb.* to start something happening *starta, utlösa, sätta igång;* **it is not known what triggers the development of shingles**

> QUOTE the endocrine system releases hormones in response to a change in the concentration of trigger substances in the blood or other body fluids
> **Nursing 87**

trigger finger ['trɪgə ˌfɪŋgə] *subst.* condition where a finger can bend but is difficult to straighten, probably because of a nodule on the flexor tendon *Dupuytrens kontraktur*

triglycerid ⇨ **triglyceride**

triglyceride [traɪ'glɪsəraɪd] *subst.* substance (such as fat) which contains three fatty acids *triglycerid*

trigone ['traɪgəʊn] *subst.* triangular piece of the wall of the bladder, between the openings for the urethra and the two ureters *trigonum vesicae (urinariae), urinblåsetrekanten*

trigonitis [ˌtrɪgə'naɪtɪs] *subst.* inflammation of the bottom part of the wall of the bladder *trigonocystit*

trigonocephalic [traɪˌgɒnəsə'fælɪk] *adj.* (skull) which shows signs of trigonocephaly *som visar tecken på triangulär missbildning av skallen*

trigonocephaly [traɪˌgɒnə'sef(ə)li] *subst.* condition where the skull is deformed in the shape of a triangle, with points on either side of the face in front of the ears *triangulär missbildning av skallen*

trigonocystit ⇨ **trigonitis**

triiodothyronine [ˌtraɪaɪˌəʊdəʊ'θaɪrəniːn] *subst.* hormone synthesized in the body from thyroxine secreted by the thyroid gland *trijodtyronin, T3, liot(h)yronin*

trijodtyronin ⇨ **liothyronine, triiodothyronine**

trikinos ⇨ **trichinosis**

trik(o)- ⇨ **trich(o)-**

trikofytos ⇨ **trichophytosis**

trikomonas ⇨ **Trichomonas**

trikomonasinfektion ⇨ **trichomoniasis**

trikomykos ⇨ **trichomycosis**

trikos ⇨ **trichosis**

trikotillomani ⇨ **trichotillomania**

trikromatisk ⇨ **trichromatic**

trikuriasis ⇨ **trichuriasis**

trikuspidalklaffen ⇨ **tricuspid valve, valve**

trilling ⇨ **triplet**

trimester [traɪ'mestə] *subst.* one of the three 3-month periods of a pregnancy *trimester, tremånadersperiod under graviditeten*

trip [trɪp] **1** *subst.* **(a)** journey *resa;* **he finds it too difficult to make the trip to the outpatients department twice a week (b)** trance induced by drugs *tripp, narkotikarus;* **bad trip** = trance induced by drugs, where the patient becomes ill *dålig tripp, snedtändning* **2** *vb.* to fall down because of knocking the foot on something *snubbla, snava;* **he tripped over the piece of wood; she tripped up and fell down**

triphosphate [traɪ'fɒsfeɪt] *see* ADENOSINE TRIPHOSPHATE (ATP)

triplet ['trɪplət] *subst.* one of three babies born to a mother at the same time *trilling; see also* QUADRUPLET, QUINTUPLET, SEXTUPLET, TWIN

triploid ['trɪplɔɪd] *subst. & adj.* (cell, organ, etc.) having 3N chromosomes *or* three times the haploid number *triploid (kromosomuppsättning)*

tripp ⇨ **trip**

triquetral (bone) [traɪ'kwetr(ə)l (bəʊn)] *or* **triquetrum** [traɪ'kwetrəm] *subst.* one of the eight small carpal bones in the wrist ⇨ *illustration* HAND *os triquetrum*

trismus ['trɪzməs] *subst.* lockjaw *or* spasm in the lower jaw, which makes it difficult to open the mouth, a symptom of tetanus *trismus, munläsa, käkläsa*

trisomi ⇨ **trisomy**

trisomic [traɪ'səʊmɪk] *adj.* referring to Down's syndrome *som avser el. hör till trisomi*

trisomy ['traɪsəʊmi] *subst.* condition where a patient has three chromosomes instead of a pair *trisomi;* **trisomy 21** = DOWN'S SYNDROME

trissa ⇨ **pulley**

tritanopi ⇨ **tritanopia**

tritanopia [ˌtraɪtə'nəʊpiə] *subst.* rare form of colour blindness, a defect in vision where the patient cannot see blue *tritanopi, blåblindhet, violettblindhet; compare* DALTONISM, DEUTERANOPIA

troakar ⇨ **stilet, trocar**

trocar ['trəʊkɑː] *subst.* surgical instrument *or* pointed rod which slides inside a cannula to make a hole in tissue to drain off fluid *trokar, troakar*

trochanter [trə(ʊ)'kæntə] *subst.* two bony lumps on either side of the top end of the femur where muscles are attached *trochanter*

> COMMENT: the lump on the outer side is the greater trochanter, and that on the inner side is the lesser trochanter

trochlea ['trɒkliə] *subst.* any part of the body shaped like a pulley, especially (i) part of the lower end of the humerus, which articulates with the ulna *trochlea humeri;* (ii) curved bone in the frontal bone through which one of the eye muscles passes *trochlea musculi obliqui superioris bulbi*

trochlear ['trɒkliə] *adj.* referring to a ring in a bone *troklear, trokleär;* **trochlear nerve** = fourth cranial nerve, which controls the muscles of the eyeball *nervus trochlearis, 4:e kranialnerven*

trochoid joint ['trəʊkɔɪd ˌdʒɔɪnt] *or* **pivot joint** ['pɪvət ˌdʒɔɪnt] *subst.* joint where a bone can rotate freely about a central axis as in the neck, where the atlas articulates with the axis *articulatio trochoidea, rotationsled, vridled*

-trofi ⇨ **-trophy**

trofiskt sår ⇨ **ulcer**

trof(o)- ⇨ **troph(o)-**

trofoblast ⇨ **trophoblast**

trokar ⇨ **trocar**

troklear ⇨ **trochlear**

trokleär ⇨ **trochlear**

trolley ['trɒli] *subst.* wheeled table *or* cupboard, which can be pushed from place to place *bår(vagn), rullbord, rullvagn;* **she takes newspapers and books round the wards on a trolley; the patient was placed on a trolley to be taken to the operating theatre**
NOTE: the US English is **cart**

tromb ⇨ **blood, coagulum, thrombus**

trombangit ⇨ **thromboangiitis obliterans**

trombektomi ⇨ **thrombectomy, thromboendarterectomy**

trombendarterektomi ⇨ **thromboendarterectomy**

trombin ⇨ **thrombin**

tromb(o)- ⇨ **thrombo-**

trombocyt ⇨ **blood, thrombocyte**

trombocytbildning ⇨ **thrombopoiesis**

trombocytemi ⇨ **thrombocythaemia**

trombocytopeni ⇨ **thrombocytopenia**

trombocytos ⇨ **thrombocytosis**

tromboemboli ⇨ **thromboembolism**

tromboflebit ⇨ **thrombophlebitis**

trombokinas ⇨ **thrombokinase, thromboplastin**

trombolys ⇨ **thrombolysis**

trombolytisk ⇨ **thrombolytic**

tromboplastin ⇨ **thrombokinase, thromboplastin**

trombos ⇨ **thrombosis**

-trop ⇨ **-tropic**

troph(o)- ['trɒf(əʊ), ˌ--] *prefix* referring to food *or* nutrition *trof(o)-*

trophoblast ['trɒfə(ʊ)blæst] *subst.* tissue which forms the wall of a blastocyst *trofoblast*

-trophy [trəfi] *suffix* meaning (i) nourishment *-trofi, -näring;* (ii) development of an organ *-trofi, -tillväxt*

-tropic ['trɒpɪk] *suffix* meaning (i) turning towards *-trop;* (ii) which influences *-trop*

tropical ['trɒpɪk(ə)l] *adj.* referring to the tropics *tropisk, tropik-;* **the disease is carried by a tropical insect; tropical disease =** disease which is found in tropical countries, such as malaria, dengue, Lassa fever *tropisk sjukdom;* **tropical medicine =** branch of medicine which deals with tropical diseases *tropikmedicin;* **tropical ulcer** *or* **Naga sore =** large area of infection which forms round a wound, especially in tropical countries *slags infekterat sår (som uppstår i tropikerna)*

tropics [trɒpɪks] *or* **tropical countries** ['trɒpɪk(ə)l ˌkʌntriz] *subst pl.* hot areas of the world *or* countries near the equator *tropikerna;* **he lives in the tropics; disease which is endemic in tropical countries**

tropik- ⇨ **tropical**

tropikerna ⇨ **tropics**

tropikmedicin ⇨ **tropical**

tropisk ⇨ **tropical**

trouble ['trʌb(ə)l] *subst.* any type of illness *or* disorder *besvär, åkomma, sjukdom;* **he has had stomach trouble for the last few months; she is undergoing treatment for back trouble; his bladder is giving him some trouble; what seems to be the trouble?** = what are your symptoms *or* what are you suffering from? *hur står det till här då?, vad lider ni av (har ni) för besvär (åkomma)?*

Trousseau's sign [tru'səʊz ˌsaɪn] *subst.* spasm in the muscles in the forearm, causing the index and middle fingers to extend, when a tourniquet is applied to the upper arm, a sign of latent tetany, showing that the blood contains too little calcium *Trousseaus fenomen (tecken)*

trubbig ⇨ **blunt**

true [tru:] *adj.* correct *or* right *sann, äkta, egentlig;* **true ribs =** top seven pairs of ribs which are attached to the breastbone *costae verae, äkta revbenen*

trum- ⇨ **tympanic, tympan(o)-**

trumhinnan ⇨ **eardrum, tympanic**

trumhinne- ⇨ **tympanic, tympan(o)-**

trumhinneinflammation ⇨ **myringitis**

trumhinneparacentes ⇨ **tympanotomy**

trumhålan ⇨ **atrium, tympanic, tympanum**

trumpet ⇨ **tube**

trumpinnefingrar ⇨ **clubbing**

truncus ['trʌŋkəs] *subst.* main blood vessel in a fetus, which develops into the aorta and pulmonary artery *truncus (arteriosus), artärstammen*

trunk [trʌŋk] *subst.* main part of the body, without the head, arms and legs *bålen; see also* COELIAC

truss [trʌs] *subst.* belt worn round the waist, with pads to hold a hernia in place *bråckband*

tryck ⇨ **compression, pressure**

trycka ⇨ **press**

tryckfall ⇨ **drop**

tryckförband ⇨ **pack**

tryckminskning ⇨ **decompression**

tryckpunkt ⇨ **pulse**

tryckreceptor ⇨ **corpuscle**

trycksår ⇨ **bedsore, pressure, ulcer**

tryckvåg ⇨ **blast**

trypanocide ['trɪp(ə)nə(ʊ)saɪd] *subst.* drug which kills trypanosomes *trypanosomdödande medel*

Trypanosoma [ˌtrɪp(ə)nə(ʊ)'səʊmə] *or* **trypanosome** ['trɪp(ə)nə(ʊ)səʊm, trɪ'pænəsəʊm] *subst.* genus of parasite which causes sleeping sickness and Chagas' disease *Trypanosoma, trypanosom, borrkropp*

trypanosomiasis [ˌtrɪp(ə)nə(ʊ)sə(ʊ)'ma(ɪ)əsɪs] *subst.* disease, spread by insect bites, where trypanosomes infest the blood *trypanos(omiasis)*

COMMENT: symptoms are pains in the head, general lethargy and long periods of sleep. In Africa, sleeping sickness, and in South America, Chagas' disease, are both caused by trypanosomes

trypsin ['trɪpsɪn] *subst.* enzyme converted from trypsinogen by the duodenum and secreted into the digestive system where it absorbs protein *trypsin*

trypsinogen [trɪp'sɪnədʒ(ə)n] *subst.* enzyme secreted by the pancreas into the duodenum *trypsinogen*

tryptophan ['trɪptə(ʊ)fæn] *subst.* essential amino acid *tryptofan*

tråd ⇨ **fibre, suture, thread**

tråd- ⇨ **fibr-, fibrous, fil-**

trådformig ⇨ **filiform**

trådliknande ⇨ **filamentous**

trådmask ⇨ **nematode, roundworm**

trång ⇨ **narrow**

träna ⇨ **exercise**

tränga bort ⇨ **repress**

tränga in i ⇨ **penetrate**

trängande ⇨ **urgent**

träning ⇨ **exercise**

träningsvärk ⇨ **compression**

träsocker ⇨ **xylose**

träsprit ⇨ **methyl alcohol, wood**

trögflytande ⇨ **viscid, viscous**

tröghet ⇨ **inertia, obtusion, torpor, viscosity**

tröskel ⇨ **limit, threshold**

tröskel- ⇨ **liminal**

tröskelvärde ⇨ **threshold**

trösta ⇨ **comfort, reassure**

tröstnapp ⇨ **dummy, pacifier**

trött ⇨ **tired**

trötthet ⇨ **fatigue, tiredness**

tsetse fly ['tetsi flaɪ] *subst.* African insect which passes trypanosomes into the human bloodstream, causing sleeping sickness *tse-tsefluga*

TSH [ˌtiːes'eɪtʃ] = THYROID-STIMULATING HORMONE

tsutsugamushi disease [ˌtsuːtsəgə'muːʃi dɪˌziːz] *or* **scrub typhus** ['skrʌb taɪfəs] *subst.* form of typhus caused by the Rickettsia bacteria, passed to humans by mites (found in South East Asia) *tsutsugamushifeber*

tub ⇨ **hose, tube**

tub- ⇨ **tubular**

tubal ['tjuːb(ə)l] *adj.* referring to a tube *tubar(-), tubär, salping(o)-, äggledar-;* **tubal pregnancy** = the most common form of ectopic pregnancy, where the fetus develops in a Fallopian tube instead of the uterus *tubargraviditet*

tubar(-) ⇨ **tubal**

tubargraviditet ⇨ **tubal**

tubarplastik ⇨ **salpingostomy**

tube [tjuːb] *subst.* **(a)** long hollow passage in the body, like a pipe *tuba, rör, trumpet* **(b)** soft plastic pipe with a lid, which is filled with a paste *tub;* **a tube of eye ointment** *see also* EUSTACHIAN, FALLOPIAN

tuber ['tjuːbə] *subst.* swollen *or* raised area *tuber, knöl, utsprång, utväxt, svulst;* **tuber cinereum** = part of the brain to which the stalk of the pituitary gland is connected *den del av hjärnan som hypofysstjälken fäster vid*

tubercle ['tjuːbək(ə)l] *subst.* **(a)** small bony projection (as on a rib) *knöl, utskott* **(b)** small infected lump characteristic of tuberculosis, where tissue is destroyed and pus forms *tuberkel;* **primary tubercle** = first infected spot where tuberculosis starts to infect a lung *primär tuberkel, primärhärd, primärkomplex*

tubercular [tju'bɜːkjʊlə] *adj.* (i) which causes *or* refers to tuberculosis *tuberkulös, tb(c)-;* (ii) (patient) suffering from tuberculosis *tuberkulös, tb(c)-;* (iii) with small lumps, though not always due to tuberculosis *tuberös, knölig, knutformig*

tuberculid(e) [tju'bɜːbjʊlɪd] *subst.* skin wound caused by tuberculosis *tuberkulid*

tuberculin [tjʊ'bɜːkjʊlɪn] *subst.* substance which is derived from the culture of the tuberculosis bacillus and is used to test patients for the presence of tuberculosis *tuberkulin;* **tuberculin test** *or* **Mantoux test** = test to see if someone has tuberculosis, where the patient is given an intracutaneous injection of tuberculin and the reaction of the skin is noted *tuberkulinprov, Mantoux prov, pure protein derivative, PPD; see also* PATCH TEST

tuberculosis (TB) [tjuˌbɜːkju'ləʊsɪs (ˌtiː'biː)] *subst.* infectious disease caused by the tuberculosis bacillus, where infected lumps form in the tissue *tuberkulos, tb(c), TB(C);* **miliary tuberculosis** = form of tuberculosis which occurs as little nodes in many parts of the body, including the meninges of the brain and spinal cord *miliartuberkulos;* **post-primary tuberculosis** = reappearance of tuberculosis in a patient who has been infected before *postprimär (sekundär) tuberkulos;* **primary tuberculosis** = infection with tuberculosis for the first time *primär tuberkulos;* **pulmonary tuberculosis** = tuberculosis in the lungs, which makes the patient lose weight, cough blood and have a fever *lungtuberkulos*

COMMENT: tuberculosis can take many forms: the commonest form is infection of the lungs (pulmonary tuberculosis), but it can also attack the bones (Pott's disease), the skin (lupus), or the lymph nodes (scrofula). Tuberculosis is caught by breathing in germs or by eating contaminated food, especially unpasteurized milk; it can be passed from one person to another, and the carrier usually shows no signs of the disease. Tuberculosis can be cured by treatment with antibiotics, and can be prevented by inoculation with BCG vaccine. The tests for the presence of TB are the Mantoux test and Patch test; it can also be detected by X-ray screening

tuberculous [tju'bɜːkjʊləs] *adj.* referring to tuberculosis *tuberkulös, tb(c)-*

tuberkel ⇨ **tubercle**

tuberkelbacillen ⇨ **Koch's bacillus**

tuberkulid ⇨ **tuberculid(e)**

tuberkulin ⇨ **tuberculin**

tuberkulinprov ⇨ **tuberculin, purify**

tuberkulos ⇨ **tuberculosis (TB)**

tuberkulosmedel ⇨ **antituberculous drug**

tuberkulös ⇨ **tubercular, tuberculous**

tuberose ['tju:bərəʊz] *adj.* with lumps *or* nodules *tuberös, knölig, knutformig;* **tuberose sclerosis** *or* **epiloia** = hereditary disease of the brain, where a child is mentally retarded, suffers from epilepsy and many little tumours appear on the skin and on the brain *sclerosis tuberosis, tuberös skleros, epiloia*

tuberosity [ˌtju:bə'rɒsəti] *subst.* large lump on a bone *tuberositas, knölighet;* **deltoid tuberosity** = raised part of the humerus to which the deltoid muscle is attached *tuberositas deltoidea*

tuberous ['tju:b(ə)rəs] *adj.* with lumps *or* nodules *tuberös, knölig, knutformig*

tuberös ⇨ **tubercular, tuberose, tuberous**

tubgas ⇨ **tubular**

tubo- ['tju:bəʊ, ˌ--] *prefix* referring to a Fallopian tube *or* the auditory meatus *tubo-, salping(o)-, äggledar-, örontrumpets-*

tuboabdominal [ˌtju:bəʊæb'dɒmɪn(ə)l] *adj.* referring to a Fallopian tube and the abdomen *som avser el. hör till både äggledare och buk*

tubo-ovarian [ˌtju:bəʊəʊ'veəriən] *adj.* referring to a Fallopian tube and an ovary *tuboovarial*

tubotympanal [ˌtju:bəʊ'tɪmp(ə)n(ə)l] *adj.* referring to the Eustachian tube and the tympanum *som avser el. hör till både örontrumpeten och trumhålan*

tubular ['tju:bjʊlə] *adj.* (i) shaped like a tube *rörformig, tub-;* (ii) referring to a tubule *tubulär;* **tubular bandage** = bandage made of a tube of elastic cloth *(förband av) tubgas;* **tubular reabsorption** = process where some substances filtered into the kidney are reabsorbed into the bloodstream *tubulär resorption;* **tubular secretion** = secretion of substances by the tubules of a kidney into the urine *tubulär sekretion*

tubule ['tju:bju:l] *subst.* small tube in the body *tubulus, litet rör el. liten kanal i kroppen;* **renal tubule** = small tube in the kidney, part of the nephron **renal tubules** *tubuli renales, njurkanalerna*

tubulus ⇨ **tubule**

tubulus, proximala ⇨ **proximal**

tubulär ⇨ **tubular**

tubär ⇨ **salping-, tubal**

tudelad ⇨ **bicipital, bicornuate, bifid**

tudelning ⇨ **binary**

tuft [tʌft] *subst.* small group of hairs *or* of blood vessels *hårtott, hårtest, nystan;* **glomerular tuft** = group of blood vessels in the kidney which filters the blood *glomerulus, kärlnystan*

tugga ⇨ **chew, masticate; mouthful**

tugging ['tʌgɪŋ] *see* TRACHEAL

tuggmuskeln ⇨ **masseter (muscle)**

tuggning ⇨ **mastication**

tuggummi ⇨ **chewing gum**

tularaemia [ˌtu:lə'ri:miə] *or* **rabbit fever** ['ræbɪt ˌfi:və] *subst.* disease of rabbits, caused by the bacterium **Pasteurella** *or* **Brucella tularensis** , which can be passed to humans *tularemi, harpest*

COMMENT: in humans, the symptoms are headaches, fever and swollen lymph nodes

tulle gras ['tju:l ˌgrɑ:] *subst.* dressing made of open gauze covered with soft paraffin wax which prevents sticking *gasväv indränkt i paraffin*

tumefaction [ˌtju:mɪ'fækʃ(ə)n] *subst.* swelling of tissue caused by liquid which accumulates underneath *tumefaktion, tumescens, svullnad*

tumescence [tju:'mes(ə)ns] *subst.* swollen tissue where liquid has accumulated underneath *tumescens, tumefaktion, svullnad*

tumid ['tju:mɪd] *adj.* swollen *svullen, uppsvälld*

tummen ⇨ **thumb, pollex**

tummy ['tʌmi] *subst. informal* child's word for stomach *or* abdomen *magen;* **tummy ache** = child's expression for stomach pain *magont, ont i magen; see* GIPPY

tumoral ['tju:mər(ə)l] *or* **tumorous** ['tju:mərəs] *adj.* referring to a tumour *tumör-*

tumour ['tju:mə] *or US* **tumor** [tu:mər] *subst.* abnormal swelling *or* growth of new cells *tumör, svulst, svullnad;* **the X-ray showed a tumour in the breast; she died of a brain tumour; the doctors diagnosed a tumour in the liver; benign tumour** = tumour which is not cancerous, and which will not grow again *or* spread to other parts of the

body if is is removed surgically *benign (godartad) tumör;* **malignant tumour** = tumour which is cancerous and can grow again *or* spread into other parts of the body, even if removed surgically *malign (elakartad) tumör*
NOTE: for other terms referring to tumours, see words beginning with **onco-**

tumsugning ⇨ **thumb-sucking**

tumvalken ⇨ **ball, thenar**

tumvalks- ⇨ **thenar**

tumör ⇨ **neoplasm, tumor**

tumör- ⇨ **onco-, tumoral**

tumörframkallande ⇨ **oncogenic**

tung ⇨ **heavy**

tung- ⇨ **gloss-, lingual**

tungan ⇨ **tongue, glossa**

tungartären ⇨ **lingual**

tungbenet ⇨ **hyoid bone**

tungförlamning ⇨ **glossoplegia**

tung- och svalgnerven ⇨ **glossopharyngeal nerve**

tungspatel ⇨ **depressor**

tungspenen ⇨ **uvula**

tungt ⇨ **heavily**

tungvenen ⇨ **lingual**

tunica ['tju:nɪkə] *subst.* layer of tissue which covers an organ *tunica, hinna;* **tunica albuginea** = white fibrous membrane covering the testes and the ovaries *tunica albuginea;* **tunica vaginalis** = membrane covering the testes and epididymis *tunica vaginalis*

> COMMENT: the wall of a blood vessel is made up of several layers: the outer layer (tunica adventitia); the inner layer (tunica intima), and in between the central layer (tunica media)

tuning fork ['tju:nɪŋ ˌfɔ:k] *subst.* special metal fork which, if hit, gives out a perfect note, used in hearing tests, such as Rinne's test *stämgaffel*

tunn ⇨ **thin**

tunnelseende ⇨ **tunnel vision**

tunnel vision ['tʌn(ə)l ˌvɪʒ(ə)n] *subst.* field of vision which is restricted to the area directly in front of the eye *tunnelseende*

tunnflytande ⇨ **thin**

tunntarmen ⇨ **jejunum, small**

tuppkammen ⇨ **crista**

TUR [ˌti:ju:'ɑ:] = TRANSURETHRAL RESECTION

turbinal bones ['tɜ:bɪn(ə)l ˌbəʊnz] *or* **turbinate bones** ['tɜ:bɪnət bəʊnz] *or* **nasal conchae** ['neɪz(ə)l ˌkɒŋki:] *subst. pl.* three little bones which form the sides of the nasal cavity *conchae nasales, näsmusslorna*

turbinectomy [ˌtɜ:bɪ'nektəmi] *subst.* surgical operation to remove a turbinate bone *excision av näsmussla*

turbulent flow ['tɜ:bjʊlənt ˌfləʊ] *subst.* rushing *or* uneven flow of blood in a vessel *turbulent ström(ning), virvelström(ning)*

turcica ['tɜ:sɪkə] *see* SELLA

turgescence [tɜ:'dʒes(ə)ns] *subst.* swelling of tissue, when fluid accumulates underneath *svullnad*

turgid ['tɜ:dʒɪd] *adj.* swollen with blood *svullen*

turgor ['tɜ:gə] *subst.* being swollen *turgor, vätskefyllnad, svullnad*

turistdiarré ⇨ **gippy tummy, Montezuma's revenge**

turksadeln ⇨ **pituitary body**

turn [tɜ:n] **1** *subst. informal* slight illness *or* attack of dizziness *attack, anfall;* **she had one of her turns on the bus; he had a bad turn at the office and had to be taken to hospital 2** *vb.* **(a)** to move the head *or* body to face in another direction *vrida (på), vända (på);* **he turned to look at the camera; she has difficulty in turning her head (b)** to change into something different *ändra (sig), förvandlas;* **the solution is turned blue by the reagent; his hair has turned grey**

turn away [ˌtɜ:n ə'weɪ] *vb.* to send people away *avvisa;* **the casualty ward is closed, so we have had to turn the accident victims away**

Turner's syndrome ['tɜ:nəz ˌsɪndrəʊm] *subst.* congenital condition of females, where sexual development is retarded and no ovaries develop *Turners syndrom*

> COMMENT: the condition is caused by the absence of one of the pair of X chromosomes

turricephaly [ˌtʌrɪ'sef(ə)li] = OXYCEPHALY

tuss ⇨ **wad**

tussis ['tʌsɪs] *subst.* coughing *tussis, hosta*

tutor ['tju:tə] *subst.* teacher *or* person who teaches small groups of students *handledare;* **nurse tutor** = experienced nurse who teaches student nurses *vårdlärare*

tvilling ⇨ **gemellus, twin**

tvinga ⇨ **force**

tvinsot ⇨ **phthisis**

två- ⇨ **bi-**

tvådelad ⇨ **bicipital, bicornuate, bifid**

tvåfliktig ⇨ **bicuspid**

två gånger dagligen ⇨ **b.i.d.**

tvåkärnig ⇨ **binucleate**

tvångs- ⇨ **obsessional**

tvångsföreställning ⇨ **obsession**

tvångshandling ⇨ **obsession, obsessive**

tvångsmässig ⇨ **compulsive**

tvångstanke ⇨ **obsession**

tvåslagspuls ⇨ **bigeminy**

tvåspetsig ⇨ **bicuspid**

tvåäggs- ⇨ **binovular**

tvåäggstvillingar ⇨ **fraternal twins, twin**

tvär- ⇨ **transverse**

tvärfraktur ⇨ **transverse**

tvärgående ⇨ **oblique**

tvärläge ⇨ **lie, transverse**

tvärsnitt ⇨ **cross-section, transection**

tvärstrimmig ⇨ **striated**

tvärstrimmig muskel ⇨ **muscle**

tvärt ⇨ **sharply**

tvärutskott ⇨ **transverse**

tvätta ⇨ **bathe, clean**

tvätta sig ⇨ **scrub up**

tvättinrättning ⇨ **laundry**

tvätt(kläder) ⇨ **laundry**

tvättmedel ⇨ **detergent**

tvättsprit ⇨ **spirit**

tvättstuga ⇨ **laundry**

tweezers ['twi:zəz] *subst.* instrument shaped like small scissors, with ends which pinch, and do not cut, used to pull out or pick up small objects *pincett;* **she pulled out the splinter with her tweezers; he removed the swab with a pair of tweezers**

twenty-twenty vision [ˌtwenti'twenti ˌvɪʒ(ə)n] *subst.* perfect normal vision *normal syn*

twilight ['twaɪlaɪt] *subst.* time of day when the light is changing from daylight to night *skymning;* **twilight myopia** = condition of the eyes, where the patient has difficulty in seeing in dim light *slags närsynthet med besvär särskilt i dåligt ljus;* **twilight state** = condition (of epileptics and alcoholics) where the patient can do certain automatic actions, but is not conscious of what he is doing *tillstånd då automatiska handlingar kan utföras omedvetet;* **twilight sleep** = type of anaesthetic sleep, where the patient is semi-conscious but cannot feel any pain *halvslummer, ung. smärtlindring och sedering*

> COMMENT: twilight state is induced at childbirth, by introducing anaesthetics into the rectum

twin [twɪn] *subst.* one of two babies born to a mother at the same time *tvilling;* **fraternal** *or* **dizygotic twins** = twins who are not identical because they come from two different ova fertilized at the same time *dizygoter, tvåäggstvillingar;* **identical** *or* **monozygotic twins** = twins who are exactly the same in appearance because they developed from the same ovum *monozygoter, enäggstvillingar;*

see also QUADRUPLET, QUINTUPLET, SEXTUPLET, SIAMESE, TRIPLET

> COMMENT: twins are relatively frequent (about one birth in eighty) and are often found in the same family, where the tendency to have twins is passed through females

twinge [twɪn(d)ʒ] *subst.* sudden feeling of sharp pain *hugg, plötslig smärta;* **he sometimes has a twinge in his right shoulder; she complained of having twinges in the knee**

twist [twɪst] *vb.* to turn *or* bend a joint in a wrong way *vrida (ur led), vricka, stuka;* **he twisted his ankle** = he hurt it by bending it in an odd direction *han vrickade (stukade) foten*

twitch [twɪtʃ] *vb.* to make small movements of the muscles *rycka till, ha ryckningar;* **the side of his face was twitching**

twitching ['twɪtʃɪŋ] *subst.* small movements of the muscles in the face *or* hands *ryckning*

tydlig ⇨ **clear, distinct**

tydligt ⇨ **clearly**

tyflit ⇨ **typhlitis**

tyfoid ⇨ **typhoid fever**

tyfus ⇨ **typhus**

tyfus/paratyfusvaccin ⇨ **TAB vaccine**

tylosis [taɪ'ləʊsɪs] *subst.* development of a callus *tylos*

tymektomi ⇨ **thymectomy**

-tymi ⇨ **-thymia**

tymit ⇨ **thymitis**

tym(o)- ⇨ **thym-**

tymocyt ⇨ **thymocyte**

tymom ⇨ **thymoma**

tympanic [tɪm'pænɪk] *adj.* referring to the eardrum *tympan(o)-, trumhinne-, trum-;* **tympanic cavity** *or* **middle ear** = section of the ear between the eardrum and the inner ear, containing the three ossicles *cavum tympani, trumhålan, mellanörat;* **tympanic membrane** *or* **tympanum** *or* **eardrum** = membrane at the inner end of the external auditory meatus which vibrates with sound and passes the vibrations on to the ossicles in the middle ear *membrana tympani, myrinx, trumhinnan*

tympanites [ˌtɪmpə'naɪtiːz] *or* **meteorism** ['miːtiərɪz(ə)m] *subst.* expansion of the stomach with gas *meteorism, tympani(sm), väderspänning(ar)*

tympanitis [ˌtɪmpə'naɪtɪs] *or* **otitis** [ə(ʊ)'taɪtɪs] *subst.* middle ear infection *otitis media, inflammation i mellanörat, örsprång*

tympan(o)- ['tɪmpən(əʊ), ˌ---] *prefix* referring to the eardrum *tympan(o)-, trumhinne-, trum-*

tympan(o)- ⇨ **tympanic, tympan(o)-**

tympanoplastik ⇨ **myringoplasty, tympanoplasty**

tympanoplasty ['tɪmpənəʊˌplæsti] *or* **myringoplasty** [mɪ'rɪŋgəʊˌplæsti] *subst.* surgical operation to correct a defect in the eardrum *tympanoplastik, myringoplastik*

tympanotomi ⇨ **myringotomy, tympanotomy**

tympanotomy [ˌtɪmpə'nɒtəmi] *or* **myringotomy** [ˌmɪrɪŋ'gɒtəmi] *subst.* surgical operation to make an opening in the eardrum to allow fluid to escape *myringotomi, tympanotomi, paracentes, trumhinneparacentes*

tympanum ['tɪmpənəm] *subst.* **(a)** eardrum *or* membrane at the inner end of the external auditory meatus leading from the outer ear, which vibrates with sound and passes the vibrations on to the ossicles in the middle ear ⇨ *illustration* EAR *membrana tympani, myrinx, trumhinnan* **(b)** the tympanic cavity *or* section of the ear between the eardrum and the inner ear, containing the three ossicles *cavum tympani, trumhålan, mellanörat*

tymus ⇨ **thymus (gland)**

tyna av (bort) ⇨ **waste away**

tyngdlöshet ⇨ **weightlessness**

typfall ⇨ **textbook**

typhlitis [tɪ'flaɪtɪs] *subst.* inflammation of the caecum (large intestine) *tyflit, egentlig blindtarmsinflammation*

typhoid fever [ˌtaɪfɔɪd 'fiːvə] *subst.* infection of the intestine caused by **Salmonella typhi** in food and water *febris typhoides, tyfoid*

COMMENT: typhoid fever gives a fever, diarrhoea and the patient may pass blood in the faeces. It can be fatal if not treated; patients who have had the disease may become carriers, and the Widal test is used to detect the presence of typhoid fever in the blood

typhus ['taɪfəs] *subst.* one of several fevers caused by the Rickettsia bacterium, transmitted by fleas and lice *tyfus, fläcktyfus;* **endemic typhus** = fever transmitted by fleas from rats *endemisk tyfus;* **epidemic typhus** = fever with headaches, mental disturbance and a rash, caused by lice which come from other humans *epidemisk tyfus; see also* SCRUB TYPHUS

COMMENT: typhus victims have a fever, feel extremely weak and develop a dark rash on the skin. The test for typhus is Weil-Felix reaction

typical ['tɪpɪk(ə)l] *adj.* showing the usual symptoms of a condition *typisk, karakteristisk;* **his gait was typical of a patient suffering from Parkinson's disease**

typically ['tɪpɪk(ə)li] *adv.* in a typical way *typiskt, karakteristiskt;* **the anorexia patient is typically an adolescent or young woman, who is suffering from stress**

typisk ▷ **characteristic, distinctive, typical**

typiskt ▷ **typically**

tyramine ['taɪ(ə)rəmi:n] *subst.* enzyme found in cheese, beans, tinned fish, red wine and yeast extract, which can cause high blood pressure if found in excessive quantities in the brain *tyramin; see also* MONOAMINE OXIDASE

tyre(o)- ▷ **thyro-**

tyreoglobulin ▷ **thyroglobulin**

tyreoid ▷ **thyroid**

tyreoidea ▷ **thyroid**

tyreoideahormon ▷ **thyroid**

tyreoidektomi ▷ **thyroidectomy**

tyreoidit ▷ **thyroiditis**

tyreostatikum ▷ **depressant**

tyreotomi ▷ **thyrotomy**

tyreotoxikos ▷ **thyrotoxic, thyrotoxicosis, toxic**

tyreotoxisk ▷ **thyrotoxic**

tyreotropin ▷ **thyroid-stimulating hormone (TSH), thyrotrophin**

tyr(o)- ▷ **thyro-**

tyrokalcitonin ▷ **calcitonin, thyrocalcitonin**

tyrosine ['taɪ(ə)rə(ʊ)si:n] *subst.* amino acid in protein which is a component of thyroxine *tyrosin*

tyrosinosis [ˌtaɪ(ə)rə(ʊ)sɪ'nəʊsɪs] *subst.* condition caused by abnormal metabolism of tyrosine *tyrosinos*

tyst ▷ **quiescent, silent**

tystnad ▷ **silence**

tå ▷ **toe, dactyl, digit**

tå- ▷ **dactyl, digital**

tåla ▷ **resist, tolerate**

tåled ▷ **interphalangeal joint**

tålig ▷ **patient**

tåligt ▷ **patiently**

tålmodig ▷ **patient**

tålmodigt ▷ **patiently**

tånagel ▷ **toenail**

tång ▷ **algae, caliper, forceps**

tångförlossning ▷ **delivery**

tår ▷ **tear**

tår- ▷ **dacryo-, lacrimal**

tårapparaten ▷ **lacrimal**

tåras ▷ **water**

tårbenen ▷ **lacrimal**

tårflöde ▷ **lacrimation**

tårkanalen ▷ **nasolacrimal**

tårkarunkeln ▷ **lacrimal**

tårkörtel ▷ **lacrimal**

tårkörtelinflammation ▷ **dacryoadenitis**

tårproduktion ⇨ **lacrimation**

tårpunkterna ⇨ **lacrimal**

tårröret ⇨ **lacrimal**

tårsäcken ⇨ **lacrimal**

tårsäcksinflammation ⇨ **dacryocystitis**

tårvägskonkrement ⇨ **dacryolith**

tårvägssten ⇨ **dacryolith**

tåvalken ⇨ **ball**

täcka ⇨ **coat**

täckprov ⇨ **cover**

tält ⇨ **tent**

tämligen ⇨ **fairly**

täppa till ⇨ **block, obstruct**

täppt ⇨ **congested, stuffy, snuffles**

tärande sjukdom ⇨ **wasting**

tära (på) ⇨ **debilitate**

tärningsbenet ⇨ **cuboid bone**

tät ⇨ **dense**

tömma ⇨ **deplete, empty**

tömma (blåsan, tarmen) ⇨ **pass**

tömma (ut) ⇨ **discharge**

tömning ⇨ **aspiration, evacuation**

törst ⇨ **thirst**

törstig ⇨ **thirsty**

Uu

UKCC [ˌjuːkeɪsiːˈsiː] = UNITED KINGDOM CENTRAL COUNCIL

ulcer [ˈʌlsə] *subst.* open sore in the skin *or* in mucous membrane, which is inflamed and difficult to heal *ulcus, ulceration, sår;* **he is on a special diet because of his stomach ulcers; aphthous ulcer** = little ulcer in the mouth *aftöst sår;* **decubitus ulcer** *or* **bedsore** = inflamed patch of skin on a bony part of the body (usually found on the shoulder blades, buttocks, base of the back or heels), which develops into an ulcer, caused by pressure of the part of the body against the mattress *dekubitus, trycksår, liggsår;* **dendritic ulcer** = branching ulcer on the cornea, caused by herpesvirus *ceratitis dendritica (herpetica);* **duodenal ulcer** = ulcer in the duodenum *ulcus duodeni, sår i tolvfingertarmen;* **gastric ulcer** = ulcer in the stomach *ulcus ventriculi, magsår;* **peptic ulcer** = benign ulcer in the stomach or duodenum *ulcus pepticum, peptiskt magsår;* **trophic ulcer** = ulcer caused by lack of blood (such as a bedsore) *trofiskt sår;* **varicose ulcer** = ulcer in the leg as a result of bad circulation and varicose veins *ulcus varicosum, variköst sår, bensår; see also* RODENT

ulcerated [ˈʌlsəreɪtɪd] *adj.* covered with ulcers *ulcererad, ulcerös, sårig*

ulcerating [ˈʌlsereɪtɪŋ] *adj.* which is developing into an ulcer *som håller på att övergå till sår*

ulceration [ˌʌlsəˈreɪʃ(ə)n] *subst.* (i) condition where ulcers develop *ulceration, sårbildning;* (ii) the development of an ulcer *ulceration, sårbildning*

ulcerative [ˈʌls(ə)rətɪv] *adj.* referring to ulcers *or* characterized by ulcers *ulcererad, ulcerös, sårig, sår-;* **ulcerative colitis** = severe pain in the colon, with diarrhoea and ulcers in the rectum (the cause is not known) *colitis ulcerosa, ulcerös colit*

ulcererad ⇨ **ulcerated, ulcerative**

ulceromembranous gingivitis [ˌʌlsərəʊˈmembrənəs ˌdʒɪndʒɪˈvaɪtɪs] *subst.* inflammation of the gums, which can also affect the mucous membrane in the mouth *Vincents angina, tonsillinflammation*

ulcerous [ˈʌls(ə)rəs] *adj.* (i) referring to an ulcer *ulcerös, sårig, sår-;* (ii) like an ulcer *sårliknande*

ulcerös ⇨ **ulcerated, ulcerative, ulcerous**

ulcus ⇨ **ulcer**

ulitis [juˈlaɪtɪs] *subst.* inflammation of the gums *ulit, tandköttsinflammation*

ullhår ⇨ **lanugo**

ulna ['ʌlnə] *subst.* the longer and inner of the two bones in the forearm between the elbow and the wrist (the other, outer bone, is the radius) ⇨ *illustration* HAND *ulna, armbågsbenet*

ulnar ['ʌlnə] *adj.* referring to the ulna *ulnar, ulnaris-, armbågsbens-;* **ulnar artery** = artery which branches from the brachial artery at the elbow and runs down the inside of the forearm to join the radial artery in the palm of the hand *arteria ulnaris;* **ulnar nerve** = nerve which runs from the neck to the elbow and controls the muscles in the forearm and some of the fingers (and passes near the surface of the skin at the elbow, where it can easily be hit, giving the effect of the "funny bone") *nervus ulnaris;* **ulnar pulse** = secondary pulse in the wrist, taken near the inner edge of the forearm *ulnarispuls*

> QUOTE the whole joint becomes disorganised, causing ulnar deviation of the fingers resulting in the typical deformity of the rheumatoid arthritic hand
>
> **Nursing Times**

ulnaris- ⇨ **ulnar**

ulnarispuls ⇨ **ulnar**

ultra- ['ʌltrə, ˌ--] *prefix* meaning (i) further than *ultra-;* (ii) extremely *ultra-*

ultrafiltration [ˌʌltrəfɪl'treɪʃ(ə)n] *subst.* filtering of the blood where tiny particles are removed, as when the blood is filtered by the kidney *ultrafiltration, ultrafiltrering*

ultraljud ⇨ **ultrasound**

ultraljuds- ⇨ **ultrasonic**

ultraljudssond ⇨ **probe**

ultraljudsundersökning ⇨ **echography, ultrasonography**

ultramicroscopic [ˌʌltrəˌmaɪkrə'skɒpɪk] *adj.* so small that it cannot be seen using a normal microscope *ultramikroskopisk*

ultrasonic [ˌʌltrə'sɒnɪk] *adj.* referring to ultrasound *ultraljuds-*

ultrasonics [ˌʌltrə'sɒnɪks] *subst.* study of ultrasound and its use in medical treatments *läran om ultraljud*

ultrasonograph [ˌʌltrə'sɒnəgrɑːf] *subst.* machine which takes pictures of internal organs, using ultrasound *ultrasonograf*

ultrasonography [ˌʌltrəsə'nɒgrəfi] *subst.* passing ultrasound waves through the body and recording echoes which show details of internal organs *(ultra)sonografi, ultraljudsundersökning*

ultrasonotomography [ˌʌltrəˌsɒnətə'mɒgrəfi] *subst.* making pictures of organs which are placed at different depths inside the body, using ultrasound *ultraljudsundersökning med skiktbilder*

ultrasound ['ʌltrəsaʊnd] *or* **ultrasonic waves** [ˌʌltrə'sɒnɪk ˌweɪvz] *subst.* very high frequency sound wave *ultraljud;* **the nature of the tissue may be made clear on ultrasound examination; the ultrasound provides a picture of the ovary and the eggs inside it** NOTE: no plural for **ultrasound**

> COMMENT: the very high frequency waves of ultrasound can be used to detect and record organs *or* growths inside the body (in a similar way to the use of X-rays), by recording the differences in echoes sent back from different tissues. Ultrasound is used to treat some conditions such as internal bruising and can also destroy bacteria and calculi

ultraviolet rays (UV rays) [ˌʌltrə'va(ɪ)ələt ˌreɪz (ˌjuː'viː ˌreɪz)] *subst.* invisible rays of light, which have very short wavelengths and are beyond the violet end of the spectrum, and form the tanning and burning element in sunlight *ultravioletta strålar, UV-strålning, UV-ljus;* **ultraviolet lamp** = lamp which gives off ultraviolet rays which tan the skin, help the skin produce Vitamin D, and kill bacteria *ultraviolett lampa*

umbilical [ʌm'bɪlɪk(ə)l] *adj.* referring to the navel *umbilikal, omfal(o)-, navel-;* **umbilical circulation** = circulation of blood from the mother's bloodstream through the umbilical cord into the fetus *blodcirkulation i navelsträngen;* **umbilical hernia** *or* **exomphalos** = hernia which bulges at the navel, mainly in young children *hernia umbilicalis, omfalocele, navelbråck;* **umbilical region** = central part of the abdomen, lower than the epigastrium *navelområdet*

umbilical cord [ʌmˌbɪlɪk(ə)l 'kɔːd] *subst.* cord containing two arteries and one vein which links the fetus inside the womb to the placenta *chorda (funiculus) umbilicalis, navelsträngen*

> COMMENT: the arteries carry the blood and nutrients from the placenta to the fetus and the vein carries the waste from the fetus back to the placenta. When the baby is

born, the umbilical cord is cut and the end tied in a knot. After a few days, this drops off, leaving the navel marking the place where the cord was originally attached

umbilicated [ʌm'bɪlɪkeɪtɪd] *adj.* with a small depression, like a navel, in the centre *med en liten fördjupning i mitten*

umbilicus [ʌm'bɪlɪkəs] *or* **navel** ['neɪv(ə)l] *or* **omphalus** ['ɒmfələs] *subst.* scar with a depression in the middle of the abdomen where the umbilical cord was attached to the fetus *umbilicus, omphalus, naveln*

umbilikal ⇨ **umbilical**

umbo ['ʌmbəʊ] *subst.* projecting part in the middle of the outer side of the eardrum *umbo membranae tympani*

umbärande ⇨ **exposure**

un- [ʌn, 'ʌn, ˌ-] *prefix* meaning not *o-, inte*

unaided [ˌʌn'eɪdɪd] *adj.* without any help *ensam, utan hjälp, på egen hand;* **two days after the operation, he was able to walk unaided across the ward**

unblock [ˌʌn'blɒk] *vb.* to remove something which is blocking *sota, ta bort något som blockerar (täpper till);* **an operation to unblock an artery; if you swallow it will unblock your ears**

unboiled [ˌʌn'bɔɪld] *adj.* which has not been boiled *okokt;* **in some areas, it is dangerous to drink unboiled water**

unborn [ˌʌn'bɔːn] *adj.* not yet born *ofödd;* **a pregnant woman and her unborn child**

unciform bone ['ʌnsɪfɔːm ˌbəʊn] *or* **hamate bone** ['hemeɪt ˌbəʊn] *subst.* one of the eight small carpal bones in the wrist, shaped like a hook ⇨ *illustration* HAND *os hamatum, hakbenet*

uncinate ['ʌnsɪnət] *adj.* shaped like a hook *krokig;* **uncinate epilepsy** = type of temporal lobe epilepsy, where the patient has hallucinations of smell and taste *uncinatusanfall*

uncinatusanfall ⇨ **uncinate**

unconscious [ˌʌn'kɒnʃəs] **1** *adj.* not conscious *or* not aware of what is happening *medvetslös;* **he was found unconscious in the street; the nurses tried to revive the unconscious accident victims; she was unconscious for two days after the accident**

2 *subst. (in psychology)* **the unconscious** = the part of the mind which stores feelings *or* memories *or* desires, which the patient cannot consciously call up, but which influence his actions *det omedvetna, det undermedvetna; see also* SEMI-CONSCIOUS, SUBCONSCIOUS

unconsciousness [ʌn'kɒnʃəsnəs] *subst.* being unconscious (it may be the result of lack of oxygen or some other external cause such as a blow on the head) *medvetslöshet;* **he relapsed into unconsciousness, and never became conscious again**

uncontrollable [ˌʌnkən'trəʊləb(ə)l] *adj.* which cannot be controlled *okontrollerbar, omöjlig att kontrollera;* **she has an uncontrollable desire to drink alcohol; the uncontrollable spread of the disease through the population**

uncoordinated [ˌʌnkəʊ'ɔːdɪneɪtɪd] *adj.* not joined together *or* not working together *okoordinerad, inte samordnad;* **his finger movements are completely uncoordinated; the symptoms are uncoordinated movements of the arms and legs**

uncus ['ʌŋkəs] *subst.* projecting part of the cerebral hemisphere, shaped like a hook *uncus*

under- ['ʌndə, ˌ--] *prefix* meaning less than *or* not as strong as *under-, låg;* **underactivity** = less activity than usual *låg aktivitet;* **underhydration** = having too little water in the body *undervätskning;* **undernourished** = having too little food *undernärd;* **underproduction** = producing less than normal *underproduktion*

under- ⇨ **hyp-, hypo-, sub-, under-**

underarmen ⇨ **forearm**

underarmsbenen ⇨ **forearm**

underbegåvad ⇨ **feebleminded**

underbegåvning ⇨ **feeblemindedness**

underbett ⇨ **prognathism**

underbinda ⇨ **ligate**

underbindning ⇨ **ligation, ligature**

underburen ⇨ **premature**

underburenhet ⇨ **prematurity**

undergo (surgery) [ˌʌndə'gəʊ (ˌsɜːdʒ(ə)ri)] *vb.* to have (an operation) *undergå, genomgå, gå igenom;* **he underwent an appendicectomy; she will probably have to undergo another operation; there are six patients undergoing physiotherapy**

undergå ➪ **undergo (surgery)**

underhudsfettväv ➪ **panniculus**

underkäken ➪ **jaw, mandible**

underkäks- ➪ **mandibular**

underkäksgrenen ➪ **ramus**

underkäksspottkörteln ➪ **submandibular gland**

underlägsenhet ➪ **inferiority**

underläkare ➪ **houseman**

underlätta ➪ **aid, facilitate**

undermedveten ➪ **subconscious, subliminal**

undermedvetna, det ➪ **unconscious**

undernärd ➪ **under-**

undernäring ➪ **malnutrition**

underproduktion ➪ **under-**

underrätta ➪ **inform**

underskrift ➪ **signature**

understöd ➪ **welfare**

undersöka ➪ **examine, inquire, inspect, investigate, process, study, test**

undersökning ➪ **checkup, examination, exploration, inquiry, inspection, investigation, study, test**

undersökningsrum ➪ **surgery**

undertake [ˌʌndəˈteɪk] *vb.* to carry out (a surgical operation) *företa, utföra;* **replacement of the joint is mainly undertaken to relieve pain**

underteckna ➪ **sign**

undertrycka ➪ **suppress**

undertryckande ➪ **suppression**

undertungsspottkörteln ➪ **sublingual**

underutveckling ➪ **prematurity**

underviktig ➪ **underweight**

undervisa ➪ **teach**

undervisningsgrupp, klinisk ➪ **clinic**

undervisningssjukhus ➪ **hospital**

undervätskning ➪ **under-**

underweight [ˌʌndəˈweɪt] *adj.* too thin *or* not heavy enough *underviktig, under normalvikt;* **he is several pounds underweight for his age**

undescended testis [ˌʌndɪˌsendɪd ˈtestɪs] *subst.* condition where a testis has not descended into the scrotum *testiklar som inte har vandrat ner i pungen, kryptorkism*

undigested [ˌʌndɪˈdʒestɪd] *adj.* (food) which is not digested in the body *osmält*

undine [ˈʌndiːn] *subst.* glass container for a solution to bathe the eyes *undin*

undre ➪ **inferior**

undress [ʌnˈdres] *vb.* to take off all *or* most of your clothes *klä av (sig), ta av sig kläderna;* **the doctor asked the patient to undress** *or* **to get undressed**

undulant fever [ˌʌndjʊlənt ˈfiːvə] = BRUCELLOSIS

undvara ➪ **spare**

undvika ➪ **avoid**

unfertilized [ˌʌnˈfɜːtəlaɪzd] *adj.* which has not been fertilized *obefruktad;* **unfertilized ova are produced in the ovaries and can be fertilized by spermatozoa**

unfit [ˌʌnˈfɪt] *adj.* not fit *or* not healthy *i dålig kondition;* **she used to play a lot of tennis, but she became unfit during the winter**

ungdom ➪ **adolescent**

ungdoms- ➪ **juvenile**

ungdomstiden ➪ **adolescence**

ungual [ˈʌŋgwəl] *adj.* referring to the fingernails *or* toenails *nagel-*

unguent ['ʌŋgwənt] *subst.* ointment *or* smooth oily medicinal substance which can be spread on the skin to soothe irritations *unguentum, salva*

unguentum [ʌŋ'gwentəm] *subst. (in pharmacy)* ointment *unguentum, salva*

unguis ['ʌŋgwɪs] = NAIL

unhealthy [ʌn'helθi] *adj.* not healthy *or* which does not make someone healthy *ohälsosam, osund;* **the children have a very unhealthy diet; not taking any exercise is an unhealthy way of living; the office is an unhealthy place, and everyone always feels ill there**

unhygienic [ˌʌnhaɪ'dʒiːnɪk] *adj.* which is not hygienic *ohygienisk;* **the conditions in the hospital laundry have been criticized as unhygienic**

uni- ['juːni, ˌ--] *prefix* meaning one *uni-, en-*

unicellular ['juːni'seljʊlə] *adj.* (organism) formed of one cell *unicellulär, encellig*

uniform ['juːnɪfɔːm] *subst.* special clothes worn by a group of people, such as the nurses in a hospital *uniform;* **the nurses' uniform does not include a cap; he was wearing the uniform of the St John Ambulance Brigade**

unigravida [ˌjuni'grævɪdə] = PRIMIGRAVIDA

unilateral [ˌjuːni'læt(ə)r(ə)l] *adj.* affecting one side of the body only *unilateral, ensidig;* **unilateral oophorectomy** = surgical removal of one ovary *unilateral ooforektomi*

union ['juːniən] *subst.* joining together of two parts of a fractured bone *läkning, sammanväxning; see also* MALUNION
NOTE: opposite is **non-union**

uniovular twins [ˌjuːni'ɒvjulə ˌtwɪnz] *or* **monozygotic twins** [ˌmɒnəzaɪ'gɒtɪk ˌtwɪnz] *subst.* twins who are identical in appearance because they developed from a single ovum *monozygoter, enäggstvillingar*

unipara [ju'nɪpərə] = PRIMIPARA

unipolar [ˌjuːni'pəʊlə] *adj.* (neurone) with a single process *unipolar, unipolär, monopolar, monopolär, enpolig; compare with* BIPOLAR, MULTIPOLAR; **unipolar lead** = electric lead to a single electrode *unipolär avledning*

unit ['juːnɪt] *subst.* **(a)** single part (as of a series of numbers) *enhet;* **SI units** = international system of measurement for physical properties *SI-enheter;* **lumen is the SI unit of illumination (b)** specialized section of a hospital *avdelning;* **she is in the maternity unit; he was rushed to the intensive care unit; the burns unit was full after the plane accident**

> QUOTE the blood loss caused his haemoglobin to drop dangerously low, necessitating two units of RBCs and one unit of fresh frozen plasma
> **RN Magazine**

United Kingdom Central Council (for Nursing, Midwifery and Health Visiting) (UKCC) [juˌnaɪtɪd ˌkɪŋdəm ˌsentr(ə)l 'kaʊnsɪl (fɔː ˌnɜːsɪŋ ˌmɪd'wɪf(ə)ri ænd ˌhelθ 'vɪzɪtɪŋ) (ˌjuːkeɪsiː'siː)] *subst.* official body which regulates and registers nurses, midwives and health visitors

universalmedicin ⇨ **panacea**

unmedicated dressing [ˌʌn'medɪkeɪtɪd ˌdresɪŋ] *subst.* sterile dressing with no antiseptic or other medication on it *sterilt förband*

unpasteurized [ˌʌn'pæstʃəraɪzd] *adj.* which has not been pasteurized *opastöriserad;* **unpasteurized milk can carry bacilli**

unprofessional conduct [ˌʌnprəˌfeʃ(ə)n(ə)l 'kɒndʌkt] *subst.* action by a professional person (a doctor *or* nurse, etc.) which is considered wrong by the body which regulates the profession *ej lege artis*

> QUOTE refusing to care for someone with HIV-related disease may well result in disciplinary procedure for unprofessional misconduct
> **Nursing Times**

unqualified [ˌʌn'kwɒlɪfaɪd] *adj.* (person) who has no qualifications *or* who has no licence to practise *okvalificerad, outbildad, inte meriterad;* **the hospital is employing unqualified nursing staff**

unsaturated fat [ʌn'sætʃəreɪtɪd ˌfæt] *subst.* fat which does not have a large amount of hydrogen, and so can be broken down more easily *omättat fett; see also* FAT, SATURATED

unstable [ˌʌn'steɪb(ə)l] *adj.* not stable *or* which may change easily *instabil, labil;* **the patient was showing signs of an unstable mental condition; unstable angina** = angina which has suddenly become worse *instabil angina (pectoris)*

unsteady [ˌʌn'stedi] *adj.* likely to fall down when walking *ostadig, osäker;* **he is still very unsteady on his legs**

unsterilized [ˌʌn'sterəlaɪzd] *adj.* which has not been sterilized *osteril, inte steriliserad;* **he had to carry out the operation using unsterilized equipment**

unsuitable [ˌʌn'suːtəb(ə)l] *adj.* not suitable *olämplig, inte passande;* **radiotherapy is unsuitable in this case**

untreated [ˌʌn'triːtɪd] *adj.* which has not been treated *obehandlad;* **the disease is fatal if left untreated**

unwanted [ˌʌn'wɒntɪd] *adj.* which is not wanted *oönskad, ovälkommen;* **a cream to remove unwanted facial hair**

unwashed [ˌʌn'wɒʃt] *adj.* which has not been washed *otvättad, odiskad;* **dysentery can be caused by eating unwashed fruit**

unwell [ˌʌn'wel] *adj.* sick or not well *dålig, sjuk, krasslig;* **she felt unwell and had to go home**
NOTE: not used before a noun: **a sick woman** but **the woman was unwell**

uppblossande ⇨ **flare, flush**

uppblåsbar ⇨ **inflatable**

uppbyggnad ⇨ **structure**

uppegående ⇨ **ambulation, ambulatory**

uppenbara ⇨ **reveal**

upper ['ʌpə] *adj.* at the top *or* higher *övre, över-;* **the upper limbs** = the arms *armarna;* **upper arm** = part of the arm from the shoulder to the elbow *överarmen;* **he had a rash on his right upper arm; upper respiratory infection** = infection of the upper part of the respiratory system *övre luftvägsinfektion, ÖLI, "förkylning"; see also* NEURONE
NOTE: opposite is **lower**

uppfatta ⇨ **sense**

uppfattning ⇨ **opinion**

uppfinna ⇨ **invent**

uppfinning ⇨ **invention**

uppfostra ⇨ **bring up**

uppföljning ⇨ **follow-up**

uppförande ⇨ **performance**

uppgift ⇨ **duty, function**

uppgång ⇨ **gain**

upphetsad ⇨ **agitated, excited**

upphetsande ⇨ **excitatory**

upphetsning ⇨ **exaltation, excitation, excitement**

upphetta ⇨ **heat**

upphostning ⇨ **expectoration, phlegm, sputum**

upphov ⇨ **source**

upphöjning ⇨ **elevation, eminence**

uppiggande ⇨ **pep**

uppiggande medel ⇨ **analeptic**

uppkastning ⇨ **vomit, vomiting, vomitus**

uppkomma ⇨ **arise**

upplagra ⇨ **accumulate**

upplagring ⇨ **accumulation, cumulative**

uppleva ⇨ **experience**

upplevelse ⇨ **experience**

upplysa ⇨ **inform**

upplösa ⇨ **dissolve**

upplösas ⇨ **resolve**

upplösbar ⇨ **soluble**

upplösning ⇨ **decomposition, disintegration, lysis, maceration, resolution**

uppmjukning ⇨ **maceration, malacia**

uppmuntra ⇨ **encourage, reassure**

uppmärksam ⇨ **alert**

uppmärksamhet ⇨ **notice**

uppmärksamma ⇨ **notice**

uppochnedvänd ⇨ **upside down**

upprepa ⇨ **repeat, reproduce**

upprepa! ⇨ **re. mist., rep**

upprepade kräkningar ⇨ **cyclical**

upprymdhet ⇨ **elation**

upprätt ⇨ **erect, upright**

upprätthålla ⇨ **maintain**

upprättstående ⇨ **upright**

upprörd ⇨ **agitated**

uppskatta ⇨ **appreciate, evaluate**

uppslamning ⇨ **suspension**

uppstå ⇨ **arise, originate**

uppsugning ⇨ **absorption**

uppsvälld ⇨ **tumid**

upptag(ning) ⇨ **absorption**

upptagningsområde ⇨ **catchment area**

uppteckna ⇨ **record**

uppteckning ⇨ **record**

uppträda ⇨ **appear**

uppträdande ⇨ **behavior, manner**

upptäcka ⇨ **detect, discover**

upptäckare ⇨ **discoverer**

upptäckt ⇨ **detection, discovery**

uppvakningsavdelning ⇨ **day**

uppvakningsrum ⇨ **recovery**

uppväga ⇨ **compensate**

uppåtgående ⇨ **ascending**

uppåtstigande ⇨ **ascending**

upright ['ʌpraɪt] *adj. & adv.* in a vertical position *or* standing *upprätt(stående), rak(t);* **he became dizzy as soon as he stood upright**

upset ['ʌpset; ʌp'set] **1** *subst.* slight illness *rubbning, störning, besvär;* **stomach upset =** slight infection of the stomach *magbesvär, krångel med magen;* **she is in bed with a stomach upset 2** *adj.* slightly ill *dålig, störd, i olag;* **she is in bed with an upset stomach**

upside down [ˌʌpsaɪd 'daʊn] *adv.* with the top turned to the bottom *uppochnedvänd; US* **upside-down stomach =** DIAPHRAGMATIC HERNIA

uraemia [ju(ə)'riːmiə] *subst.* disorder caused by kidney failure, where urea is retained in the blood, and the patient develops nausea, convulsions and in severe cases goes into a coma *uremi*

uraemic [ju(ə)'riːmɪk] *adj.* referring to and suffering from uraemia *uremisk*

uran- ['jʊərən, ˌ--] *prefix* referring to the palate *uran(o)-, gom-*

uraniscorrhaphy [ˌjʊərənɪ'skɒrəfi] = PALATORRHAPHY

urataemia [ˌjʊərə'tiːmiə] *subst.* condition where urates are present in the blood, as in gout *uratemi*

urate ['jʊəreɪt] *subst.* salt of uric acid found in urine *urat*

uratemi ⇨ **urataemia**

uraturia [ˌjʊərə'tjʊəriə] *subst.* presence of excessive amounts of urates in the urine, as in gout *urat i urinen*

urdjur ⇨ **Protozoa**

urea [ju(ə)'riːə] *subst.* substance produced in the liver from excess amino acids, and excreted by the kidneys into the urine *urea, urinämne*

urease ['juərieɪz] *subst.* enzyme which converts urea into ammonia and carbon dioxide *ureas*

urecchysis [ju'rekɪsɪs] *subst.* condition where uric acid leaves the blood and enters connective tissue *tofi, podagra, giktknölar, inlagring av urater i bindväv*

uremi ⇨ **azotaemia, uraemia**

uremisk ⇨ **uraemic**

ures ⇨ **micturition, uresis, urination**

uresis [ju'riːsɪs] *subst.* passing urine *ures, miktion, urinering, urinavgång*

ureter ['jʊərɪtə] *subst.* one of two tubes which take urine from the kidneys to the urinary bladder ⇨ *illustration* KIDNEY *ureter, uretär, urinledare*

ureter ⇨ **urinary**

ureter- [ju'riːtə, -ˌ--, 'jʊərɪtə, ˌ---] *or* **uretero-** [ju'riːtərəʊ, -ˌ---] *prefix* referring to the ureters *ureter(o)-, uretär-, urinledar-*

ureteral [ju'riːt(ə)r(ə)l] *or* **ureteric** [ˌjʊərɪ'terɪk] *adj.* referring to the ureters *ureter(o)-, uretär-, urinledar-;* **ureteric calculus** = kidney stone in the ureter *uretärsten;* **ureteric catheter** = catheter passed through the ureter to the kidney, to inject an opaque solution into the kidney before taking an X-ray *uretärkateter; see also* IMPACTED

ureterectomy [ˌjʊərɪtə'rektəmi] *subst.* surgical removal of a ureter *ureterektomi*

ureteritis [ˌjʊərətə'raɪtɪs] *subst.* inflammation of a ureter *ureterit, urinledarinflammation*

ureterocele [ju'riːtərəʊˌsiː(ə)l] *subst.* swelling in a ureter caused by narrowing of the opening where the ureter enters the bladder *ureterocele, uretärbråck*

ureterocolostomy [juˌriːtərəʊkɒ'lɒstəmi] *subst.* surgical operation to implant the ureter into the sigmoid colon, so as to bypass the bladder *ureterokolostomi*

ureteroenterostomy [juˌriːtərəʊˌentə'rɒstəmi] *subst.* artificial tube placed between the ureter and the intestine *avledning av urin till tarmen*

ureterokolostomi ⇨ **ureterocolostomy**

ureterolith [ju'riːtərəʊlɪθ] *subst.* calculus *or* stone in a ureter *ureterolit, uretärsten, konkrement i urinledare*

ureterolithotomy [juˌriːtərəʊlɪ'θɒtəmi] *subst.* surgical removal of a stone from the ureter *ureterolitotomi*

ureteronephrectomy [juˌriːtərəʊnɪ'frektəmi] *or* **nephroureterectomy** [ˌnefrəʊjuˌriːtə'rektəmi] *subst.* surgical removal of a kidney and the ureter attached to it *nefroureterektomi*

ureteroplasty [ju'riːtərəʊˌplæsti] *subst.* surgical operation to repair a ureter *ureteroplastik, uretärplastik*

ureteropyelonephritis [juˌriːtərəʊˌpaɪələʊnɪ'fraɪtɪs] *subst.* inflammation of the ureter and the pelvis of the kidney to which it is attached *njurbäckeninflammation*

ureterosigmoidostomy [juˌriːtərəʊˌsɪgmɔɪ'dɒstəmi] = URETEROCOLOSTOMY

ureterostomy [ˌjʊərɪtə'rɒstəmi] *subst.* surgical operation to make an artificial opening for the ureter into the abdominal wall, so that urine can be passed directly out of the body *ureterostomi*

ureterotomy [ˌjʊərɪtə'rɒtəmi] *subst.* surgical operation to make an incision into the ureter mainly to remove a stone *ureterotomi*

ureterovaginal [juˌriːtərəʊ'vædʒɪn(ə)l] *adj.* referring to the ureter and the vagina *ureterovaginal*

urethr- [ju'riːθr, -ˌ-, jʊərɪ'θr] *or* **urethro-** [ju'riːθrəʊ, -ˌ--, jʊərɪ'θrɒ] *prefix* referring to the urethra *uretr(o)-, urinrörs-*

urethra [ju(ə)'riːθrə] *subst.* tube which takes urine from the bladder to be passed out of the body ⇨ *illustration* UROGENITAL SYSTEM *urethra, urinröret;* **penile urethra** = channel in the penis through which both urine and semen pass *pars spongiosa, mannens urinrör;* **prostatic urethra** = section of the urethra which passes through the prostate *pars prostatica, den del av urinröret som ligger i blåshalskörteln*

> COMMENT: in males, the urethra serves two purposes: the discharge of both urine and semen. The male urethra is about 20cm long; in women it is shorter, about 3cm. The urethra has sphincter muscles at either end which help control the flow of urine

urethral [ju(ə)'riːθr(ə)l] *adj.* referring to the urethra *uretral, urinrörs-;* **urethral catheter** = catheter passed up the urethra to allow urine to flow out of the body *urinkateter, tappningskateter;* **urethral stricture** = URETHROSTENOSIS

urethritis [ˌjʊərə'θraɪtɪs] *subst.* inflammation of the urethra *uretrit, urinrörsinflammation;* **specific urethritis** = inflammation of the urethra caused by gonorrhoea *gonorroisk uretrit; see also* NON-SPECIFIC URETHRITIS

urethrocele [ju'riːθrə(ʊ)ˌsiː(ə)l] *subst.* (i) swelling formed in a weak part of the wall of the urethra *uretrocele;* (ii) prolapse of the urethra in a woman *urinrörsprolaps (hos kvinna)*

urethrogram [ju'ri:ərə(ʊ)græm] *subst.* X-ray photograph of the urethra *uretrogram*

urethrography [ˌjʊərɪ'ərɒgrəfi] *subst.* X-ray examination of the urethra after an opaque substance has been introduced into it *uretrografi*

urethroplasty [ju'ri:ərə(ʊ)ˌplæsti] *subst.* surgical operation to repair a urethra *uretroplastik, urethraplastik*

urethrorrhaphy [ˌjʊərɪ'ərɒrəfi] *subst.* surgical operation to repair a torn urethra *uretro(r)rafi*

urethrorrhoea [juˌri:ərə(ʊ)'ri:ə] *subst.* discharge of fluid from the urethra, usually associated with urethritis *uretrorré, flytning från urinröret*

urethroscope [ju'ri:ərə(ʊ)skəʊp] *subst.* surgical instrument, used to examine the interior of a man's urethra *uretroskop*

urethroscopy [ˌjʊərɪ'ərɒskəpi] *subst.* examination of the inside of a man's urethra with a urethroscope *uretroskopi*

urethrostenosis [juˌri:ərə(ʊ)stə'nəʊsɪs] *or* **urethral stricture** [ju'ri:ər(ə)l ˌstrɪktʃə] *subst.* narrowing *or* blocking of the urethra by a growth *uretrostenos, uretrostriktur, urinrörsförträngning*

urethrostomy [ˌjʊərɪ'ərɒstəmi] *subst.* surgical operation to make an opening for a man's urethra between the scrotum and the anus *uretrostomi*

urethrotomy [ˌjʊərɪ'ərɒtəmi] *subst.* surgical operation to open a blocked *or* narrowed urethra *uretrotomi*

uretral ⇨ **urethral**

uretrit ⇨ **urethritis**

uretr(o)- ⇨ **urethr-**

uretrocele ⇨ **urethrocele**

uretrografi ⇨ **urethrography**

uretrogram ⇨ **urethrogram**

uretroplastik ⇨ **urethroplasty**

uretrorré ⇨ **urethrorrhoea**

uretroskop ⇨ **urethroscope**

uretroskopi ⇨ **urethroscopy**

uretrostenos ⇨ **urethrostenosis**

uretrostomi ⇨ **urethrostomy**

uretrostriktur ⇨ **urethrostenosis**

uretrotomi ⇨ **urethrotomy, Wheelhouse's operation**

uretär ⇨ **ureter, urinary**

uretär- ⇨ **ureter-, ureteral**

uretärbråck ⇨ **ureterocele**

uretärkateter ⇨ **ureteral**

uretärplastik ⇨ **ureteroplasty**

uretärsten ⇨ **ureteral, ureterolith**

urge [ɜ:dʒ] *subst.* strong need to do something *stark längtan, begär, drift;* **he was given drugs to reduce his sexual urge**

urgent ['ɜ:dʒ(ə)nt] *adj.* which has to be done quickly *brådskande, angelägen, viktig, trängande;* **he had an urgent message to go to the hospital; urgent cases are referred to the accident unit; she had an urgent operation for strangulated hernia**

urgently ['ɜ:dʒ(ə)ntli] *adv.* immediately *som kräver omedelbar åtgärd;* **the relief team urgently requires more medical supplies**

-uria ['jʊəriə] *suffix* meaning (i) a condition of the urine *-uri;* (ii) a disease characterized by a condition of the urine *-uri*

uric acid [ˌjʊərɪk 'æsɪd] *subst.* chemical compound which is formed from nitrogen in waste products from the body, and which also forms crystals in the joints of patients suffering from gout *urinsyra*

uricosuric (drug) [ˌjʊərɪkə(ʊ)'sjʊərɪk (ˌdrʌg)] *subst.* drug which increases the amount of uric acid excreted in the urine *medel som befrämjar utsöndringen av urinsyra*

uridrosis [ˌjʊərɪ'drəʊsɪs] *subst.* condition where excessive urea forms in the sweat *ur(h)idros, urinsvettning, urinhaltig svettning*

urikacidemi ⇨ **lithaemia**

urin ⇨ **urine, water**

urin- ['jʊərɪn, ˌ--] *or* **urino-** ['jʊərɪnə(ʊ),

,---] *prefix* referring to urine *urin-*

urin- ⇨ **urin-, urinary**

urinal ⇨ **urinary**

urinalysis [ˌjʊərɪˈnæləsɪs] *subst.* analysis of a patient's urine, to detect diseases such as diabetes mellitus *urinanalys*

urinanalys ⇨ **urinalysis**

urinary [ˈjʊərɪn(ə)ri] *adj.* referring to urine *urin-, urinal;* **urinary bladder** = sac where the urine collects from the kidneys through the ureters, before being passed out of the body through the urethra ⇨ *illustration* KIDNEY, UROGENITAL SYSTEM *vesica urinaria, urinblåsan;* **urinary catheter** = catheter passed up the urethra to allow urine to flow out of the bladder *urinkateter, tappningskateter;* **urinary duct** *or* **ureter** = one of two tubes which take urine from the kidneys to the bladder *ureter, uretär, urinledare;* **urinary obstruction** = blockage of the urethra which prevents urine being passed *urinstopp, urinstämma;* **urinary system** = system of organs and ducts which separates waste liquids from the blood and excretes them as urine (including the kidneys, urinary bladder, ureters and urethra) *njurarna och urinvägarna;* **urinary tract** = tubes down which the urine passes from the kidneys to the bladder and from the bladder out of the body *urinvägarna;* **urinary trouble** = disorder of the urinary tract *urinvägsbesvär, problem med urinvägarna*

urinate [ˈjʊərɪneɪt] *vb.* to pass urine from the body *urinera, kasta vatten;* **the patient has difficulty in urinating; he urinated twice this morning**

urination [ˌjʊərɪˈneɪʃ(ə)n] *or* **micturition** [ˌmɪktjʊˈrɪʃ(ə)n] *subst.* passing of urine out of the body *miktion, ures, urinering, urinavgång*

urinavgång ⇨ **micturition, uresis, urination**

urinblåsan ⇨ **urinary**

urinblåse- ⇨ **cyst-, cystic, vesical**

urinblåsebråck ⇨ **cystocele**

urinblåseneuralgi ⇨ **cystalgia**

urinblåsetrekanten ⇨ **trigone**

urindensitometer ⇨ **urinometer**

urindrivande (medel) ⇨ **diuretic**

urine [ˈjʊərɪn] *subst.* yellowish liquid, containing water and waste products (mainly salt and urea), which is excreted by the kidneys and passed out of the body through the ureters, bladder and urethra *urin*

urinera ⇨ **urinate**

urinering ⇨ **micturition, uresis, urination**

urinförande ⇨ **uriniferous**

uriniferous [ˌjʊərɪˈnɪf(ə)rəs] *adj.* which carries urine *urinförande;* **uriniferous tubule** *or* **renal tubule** = tiny tube which is part of a nephron **uriniferous (renal) tubules** *tubuli renales, njurkanalerna*

urinkateter ⇨ **urethral, urinary**

urinledar- ⇨ **ureter-, ureteral**

urinledare ⇨ **ureter, urinary**

urinledarinflammation ⇨ **ureteritis**

urinogenital [ˌjʊərɪnə(ʊ)ˈdʒenɪt(ə)l] *or* **urogenital** [ˌjʊərə(ʊ)ˈdʒenɪt(ə)l] *adj.* referring to the urinary and genital systems *urogenital*

urinometer [ˌjʊərɪˈnɒmɪtə] *subst.* instrument which measures the specific gravity of urine *urindensitometer*

urinretention ⇨ **ischuria, retention**

urinröret ⇨ **urethra**

urinrörs- ⇨ **urethr-, urethral**

urinrörsförträngning ⇨ **urethrostenosis**

urinrörsinflammation ⇨ **urethritis**

urinsten ⇨ **urolith**

urinstopp ⇨ **urinary**

urinstämma ⇨ **ischuria, retention, strangury, urinary**

urinsvettning ⇨ **uridrosis**

urinsyra ⇨ **uric acid**

urinutsöndring ⇨ **diuresis**

urinvägarna ⇨ **urinary, waterworks**

urinvägsbesvär ⇨ **urinary**

urinämne ⇨ **urea**

urkalkning ⇨ **decalcification, osteolysis, osteomalacia**

urladdning ⇨ **discharge**

urledvridning ⇨ **dislocation, luxation**

urnjuren ⇨ **mesonephros**

uroartrit ⇨ **Reiter's syndrome**

urobilin [ˌjʊərə(ʊ)ˈbaɪlɪn] *subst.* yellow pigment formed when urobilinogen comes into contact with air *urobilin, sterkobilin*

urobilin ⇨ **stercobilin**

urobilinogen [ˌjʊərə(ʊ)baɪˈlɪnədʒən] *subst.* colourless pigment formed when bilirubin is reduced to stercobilinogen in the intestines *urobilinogen, sterkobilinogen*

urobilinogen ⇨ **stercobilinogen**

urocele [ˈjʊərə(ʊ)siː(ə)l] *subst.* swelling in the scrotum which contains urine *urocele*

urochesia [ˌjʊərə(ʊ)ˈkiːziə] *subst.* passing of urine through the rectum, due to injury of the urinary system *fistelgång (efter skada) mellan urinvägar och tarm*

urochrome [ˈjʊərə(ʊ)krəʊm] *adj.* pigment which colours the urine yellow *urokrom*

urogenital [ˌjʊərə(ʊ)ˈdʒenɪt(ə)l] *adj.* referring to the urinary and genital systems *urogenital;* **urogenital diaphragm** = layer of fibrous tissue beneath the prostate gland, through which the urethra passes *diaphragma urogenitalis;* **urogenital system** = the whole of the urinary tract and reproductive system *urogenitalsystemet, urogenitala systemet*

urogenitalsystemet ⇨ **genitourinary, urogenital**

urografi ⇨ **pyelogram, pyelography, urography**

urography [ju(ə)ˈrɒgrəfi] *subst.* X-ray examination of part of the urinary system after injection of radio-opaque dye *intravenös pyelografi, urografi*

urokinase [ˌjʊərə(ʊ)ˈkaɪneɪz] *subst.* enzyme formed in the kidneys, which begins the process of breaking down blood clots *urokinas*

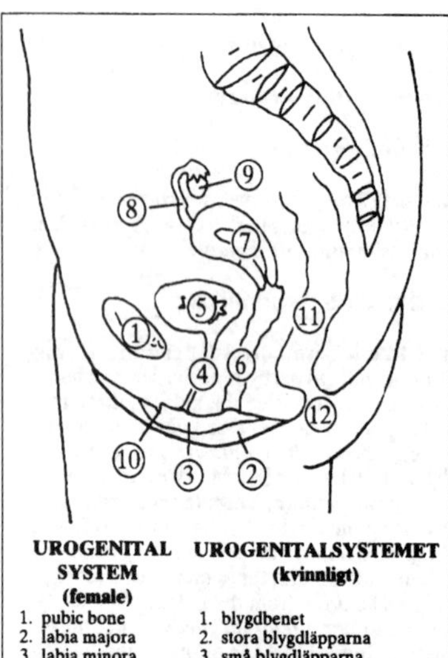

UROGENITAL SYSTEM (female)	**UROGENITALSYSTEMET (kvinnligt)**
1. pubic bone	1. blygdbenet
2. labia majora	2. stora blygdläpparna
3. labia minora	3. små blygdläpparna
4. urethra	4. urinröret
5. urinary bladder	5. urinblåsan
6. vagina	6. slidan
7. uterus	7. livmodern
8. Fallopian tube	8. äggledare
9. ovary	9. äggstock
10. clitoris	10. klitoris, kittlaren
11. rectum	11. ändtarmen
12. anus	12. analöppningen

urokrom ⇨ **urochrome**

urolith [ˈjʊərə(ʊ)lɪθ] *subst.* stone in the urinary system *urolit, urinsten*

urological [ˌjʊərəˈlɒdʒɪk(ə)l] *adj.* referring to urology *urologisk*

urologist [ju(ə)ˈrɒlədʒɪst] *subst.* doctor who specializes in urology *urolog*

urology [ju(ə)ˈrɒlədʒi] *subst.* scientific study of the urinary system and its diseases *urologi*

ursprung ⇨ **origin, source**

ursprunglig ⇨ **original, primary, primordial, radical**

urticaria [ˌɜːtɪˈkeəriə] *or* **hives** [haɪvz] *or* **nettlerash** [ˈnet(ə)læʃ] *subst.* allergic reaction (to injections *or* to certain foods) where the skin forms irritating reddish patches *urticaria, nässelfeber, nässelutslag*

urval ⇨ **selection**

urvals- ⇨ **selective**

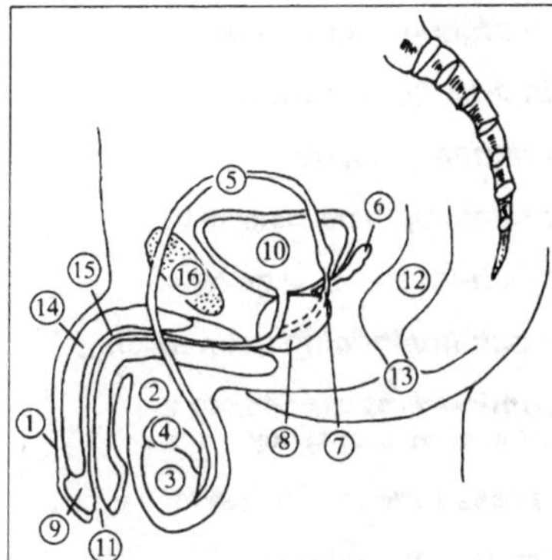

UROGENITAL SYSTEM (male)	UROGENITALSYSTEMET (manligt)
1. penis	1. penis, manslemmen
2. scrotum	2. pungen
3. testis	3. testikel
4. epididymis	4. bitestikel
5. ductus deferens	5. sädesledare
6. seminal vesicle	6. sädesblåsa
7. ejaculatory duct	7. utsprutningskanal
8. prostate gland	8. blåshalskörteln, prostata
9. glans	9. ollonet
10. urinary bladder	10. urinblåsan
11. urethra	11. urinröret
12. rectum	12. ändtarmen
13. anus	13. analöppningen
14. corpus cavernosum	14. corpus cavernosum, svällkropp
15. corpus spongiuosum	15. corpus spongiosum, svällkropp
16. pubic bone	16. blygdbenet

urägg ➪ **oogonium**

USP [ˌju:es'pi:] = UNITED STATES PHARMACOPOEIA

ut- ➪ **ex-, exo-**

utandning ➪ **exhalation, expiration**

utan remiss ➪ **informal**

utbildning ➪ **qualification**

utbredd ➪ **diffuse, prevalent**

utbredning ➪ **prevalence, proliferation, propagation**

utbrott ➪ **outbreak**

utbyte ➪ **exchange, replacement, substitution**

utbytestransfusion ➪ **replacement**

utdragning ➪ **extraction**

utdrivning ➪ **ejection**

utdrivningsskiftet ➪ **bearing down, lightening**

uter- ['ju:tə, ˌ--] *or* **utero-** ['ju:tərə(ʊ), ˌ---] *prefix* referring to the uterus *uter(o)-, hyster(o)-, metr(o)-, livmoder(s)-*

uterine ['ju:təraɪn] *adj.* referring to the uterus *uterin, uterus-, livmoder(s)-;* **the fertilized ovum becomes implanted in the uterine wall; uterine cavity** = the inside of the uterus *cavum uteri, livmodershålan;* **uterine fibroma** *or* **fibroid** = benign tumour in the muscle fibres of the uterus *uterusfibrom, fibromyom;* **uterine procidentia** *or* **uterine prolapse** = condition where part of the uterus has passed through the vagina (usually after childbirth) *hysteroptos, metroptos, prolapsus uteri, uterusprolaps, livmoderframfall*

> COMMENT: uterine prolapse has three stages of severity: in the first the cervix descends into the vagina, in the second the cervix is outside the vagina, but part of the uterus is still inside, and in the third stage, the whole uterus passes outside the vagina

uterine subinvolution = condition where the uterus does not go back to its normal size after childbirth *subinvolutio uteri;* **uterine tube** = FALLOPIAN TUBE *see also* INTRAUTERINE

uterocele ['ju:tərə(ʊ)ˌsi:(ə)l] *or* **hysterocele** ['hɪstərə(ʊ)ˌsi(ə)l] *subst.* hernia of the uterus *hysterocele, hernia uteri*

uterogestation [ˌjutərə(ʊ)dʒe'steɪʃ(ə)n] *subst.* normal pregnancy, where the fetus develops in the uterus *normal graviditet med fostret i livmodern*

uterography [ˌju:tə'rɒgrəfi] *subst.* X-ray examination of the uterus *hysterografi*

utero-ovarian [ˌju:tərəʊəʊ'veəriən] *adj.* referring to the uterus and the ovaries *som avse el. hör till både livmoder och äggstockar*

uterosalpingography [ˌju:tərə(ʊ)ˌsælpɪŋ'gɒgrəfi] = HYSTEROSALPINGOGRAPHY

uterovesical [ˌju:tərə(ʊ)'vesɪk(ə)l] *adj.* referring to the uterus and the bladder *uterovesikal*

uterus ['ju:t(ə)rəs] *or* **womb** [wu:m] *subst.* hollow organ in a woman's pelvic cavity, behind the bladder and in front of the rectum ➪ *illustration* UROGENITAL SYSTEM (female) *uterus, livmodern;* **double uterus** = condition where the uterus is divided into two sections by a membrane *uterus didelphys, dubbel livmoder; see also*

DIMETRIA NOTE: for other terms referring to the uterus, see words beginning with **hyster-, metr-**

COMMENT: the top of the uterus is joined to the Fallopian tubes which link it to the ovaries, and the lower end (or cervix uteri *or* neck of the uterus) opens into the vagina. When an ovum is fertilized it becomes implanted in the wall of the uterus and develops into an embryo inside it. If fertilization and pregnancy do not take place, the lining of the uterus (endometrium) is shed during menstruation. At childbirth, strong contractions of the wall of the uterus (myometrium) help push the baby out through the vagina.

uterus- ⇨ **uterine**

uterusfibrom ⇨ **fibroid, uterine**

uterusprolaps ⇨ **hysteroptosis, metroptosis, uterine**

utfällning ⇨ **precipitate, precipitation**

utföra ⇨ **effect, perform, undertake**

utförsgång ⇨ **duct, efferent**

utgjutning ⇨ **contusion, ecchymosis, effusion, haematoma, suffusion**

utgångspunkt ⇨ **basis**

utgöra ⇨ **form**

utklämning ⇨ **expression**

utlåtande ⇨ **opinion**

utländsk ⇨ **exotic, foreign**

utlänning ⇨ **foreigner**

utlösa ⇨ **provoke, trigger**

utmatta ⇨ **exhaust, fatigue**

utmattad ⇨ **tired out**

utmattning ⇨ **exhaustion, fatigue**

utmattning, fullständig ⇨ **prostration**

utmattningsfraktur ⇨ **stress**

utmärglad ⇨ **emaciated**

utmärgling ⇨ **emaciation**

utmärka ⇨ **characterize**

utnämna ⇨ **appoint**

utnämning ⇨ **appointment**

ut-och-invänd ⇨ **extroverted**

ut-och-invändning ⇨ **inversion**

utomkvedshavandeskap ⇨ **extrauterine pregnancy**

utpressande ⇨ **expression**

utreda ⇨ **investigate**

utredning ⇨ **inquiry, investigation**

utricle ['juːtrɪk(ə)l] *or* **utriculus** [ju'trɪkjʊləs] *subst.* **(a)** large sac inside the vestibule of the ear, which relates information about the upright position of the head to the brain *utriculus, säckliknande bildning i hinnlabyrinten* **(b) prostatic utricle** = sac branching off the urethra as it passes through the prostate gland *utriculus prostaticus*

utrota ⇨ **eradicate, stamp out**

utrotning ⇨ **eradication**

utrusta ⇨ **equip**

utrustning ⇨ **equipment**

utrymme ⇨ **space**

utrymning ⇨ **evacuation, evisceration**

utsatthet ⇨ **exposure**

utse ⇨ **select**

utseende ⇨ **appearance**

utsida ⇨ **surface**

utskalning ⇨ **enucleation**

utskott ⇨ **process, projection, prominence, spine, spur, tubercle**

utskrivning ⇨ **discharge**

utskärning ⇨ **excision**

utslag ⇨ **rash, spot**

utsliten ⇨ **worn out**

utsnitt ➪ **slice**

utsprång ➪ **process, projection, prominence, protuberance, tuber**

utspädd ➪ **dilute**

utspädning ➪ **dilution**

utspädningsmedel ➪ **diluent**

utspänd ➪ **patulous**

utspänd blåsa ➪ **distend**

utstryk ➪ **smear**

utsträckning ➪ **extension**

utstående ➪ **prominent, protrude**

utstående ögon ➪ **popeyes**

utstötning ➪ **ejection**

utsugning ➪ **aspiration**

utsöndra ➪ **discharge, eliminate, excrete, pass, secrete**

utsöndring ➪ **discharge, elimination, emission, excreta, excretion, exudate, exudation, secretion**

utsöndringsprodukt ➪ **waste**

utsöndring, tunn ➪ **gleet**

uttagning ➪ **selection**

uttalad ➪ **pronounced**

uttorkning ➪ **dehydration, xerosis**

uttryck ➪ **expression**

uttröttad ➪ **tired out, worn out**

uttänjning ➪ **distension**

uttömning ➪ **emission, excretion, exudate, exudation**

utveckling ➪ **development, progress, progression**

utvecklings- ➪ **developmental**

utvecklingsstörd ➪ **retarded**

utvecklingsstörd, psykiskt ➪ **subnormal**

utvidgad ➪ **cirsoid**

utvidgas ➪ **dilate**

utvidgning ➪ **dilatation, distension, ectasia, enlargement, expansion**

utvidgning(sfas) ➪ **diastole**

utvändig ➪ **outer**

utvärdera ➪ **evaluate**

utvärdering ➪ **evaluation**

utvärtes ➪ **external, externally**

utväxt ➪ **excrescence, growth, horn, tuber**

utåtbuktande ➪ **convex**

utåtledande ➪ **efferent**

utåtriktad ➪ **extrovert**

utåtskelning ➪ **divergent strabismus, exotropia, squint**

utåtvridning ➪ **eversion**

utöva ➪ **exert, practise**

UV [ˌjuːˈviː] = ULTRAVIOLET

uvea [ˈjuːviə] *subst.* layer of organs in the eye beneath the sclera, formed of the iris, the ciliary body and the choroid *uvea, ögats pigmentförande delar*

uveal [ˈjuːviəl] *adj.* referring to the uvea *uveal;* **uveal tract** = layer of organs in the eye beneath the sclera, containing the iris, the ciliary body and choroid *druvhinnan*

uveit ➪ **iridocyclitis, uveitis**

uveitis [ˌjuːviˈaɪtɪs] *subst.* inflammation of any part of the uvea *uveit*

uveoparotid fever [ˌjuːviəˌpærətɪd ˈfiːvə] *or* **syndrome** [ˈsɪndrəʊm] *subst.* inflammation of the uvea and of the parotid gland *samtidig inflammation i ögats druvhinna och öronspottkörteln*

UV-ljus ➪ **ultraviolet rays (UV rays)**

UV-strålning ➪ **ultraviolet rays (UV rays)**

uvula [ˈjuːvjʊlə] *subst.* piece of soft tissue which hangs down from the back of the the soft palate *uvula, tungspenen, gomspenen*

uvular ['ju:vjʊlə] *adj.* referring to the uvula *som avser el. hör till tungspenen*

uvulectomy [ˌju:vjʊ'lektəmi] *subst.* surgical removal of the uvula *uvulektomi, uvulotomi*

uvulektomi ➪ **uvulectomy**

uvulitis [ˌju:vjʊ'laɪtɪs] *subst.* inflammation of the uvula ➪ *illustration* TONGUE *uvulit*

uvulotomi ➪ **uvulectomy**

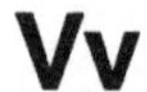

vaccinate ['væksɪneɪt] *vb.* to use a vaccine to give a person immunization against a specific disease *vaccinera, skyddsympa;* **she was vaccinated against smallpox as a child** NOTE: you vaccinate someone **against** a disease

vaccination [ˌvæksɪ'neɪʃ(ə)n] *subst.* action of vaccinating *vaccination, skyddsympning*

vaccination ➪ **inoculation**

vaccinationsterapi ➪ **vaccinotherapy**

vaccine ['væksi:n] *subst.* substance which contains the germs of a disease, used to inoculate or vaccinate *vaccin;* **the hospital is waiting for a new batch of vaccine to come from the laboratory; new vaccines are being developed all the time; MMR vaccine is given to control measles, mumps and rubella**

> COMMENT: a vaccine contains the germs of the disease, sometimes alive and sometimes dead, and this is injected into the patient so that his body will develop immunity to the disease. The vaccine contains antigens, and these provoke the body to produce antibodies, some of which remain in the bloodstream for a very long time and react against the same antigens if they enter the body naturally at a later date when the patient is exposed to the disease. Vaccination is mainly given against cholera, diphtheria, rabies, smallpox, tuberculosis, and typhoid

vaccinera ➪ **immunize, inoculate, vaccinate**

vaccinia [væk'sɪniə] = COWPOX

vaccinotherapy [ˌvæksɪnəʊ'θerəpi] *subst.* treatment of a disease with a vaccine *vaccinationsterapi* NOTE: Originally the words **vaccine** and **vaccination** applied only to smallpox immunization, but they are now used for immunization against any disease

vackla ➪ **stagger**

vacuole ['vækjuəʊl] *subst.* space in a fold of a cell membrane *vacuol, vakuol*

vacuum extractor [ˌvækjuəm ɪk'stræktə] *subst.* surgical instrument formed of a rubber suction cup which is used in vacuum extraction *or* pulling on the head of the baby during childbirth *sugklocka*

vadbenet ➪ **fibula**

vadbens- ➪ **peroneal**

vadd ➪ **wadding**

vaddtuss ➪ **wad**

vaden ➪ **calf**

vadmuskeln ➪ **peroneal**

vadmuskeln, stora ➪ **gastrocnemius**

vagal ['veɪg(ə)l] *adj.* referring to the vagus nerve *vagal;* **vagal tone** = action of the vagus nerve to slow the beat of the SA node *vagotoni*

vagel ➪ **hordeolum, stye**

vagel, kronisk ➪ **meibomian cyst**

vagina [və'dʒaɪnə] *subst.* passage in a woman's reproductive tract between the entrance to the uterus (the cervix) and the vulva, able to stretch enough to allow a baby to pass through during childbirth *vagina, slidan*

vaginal [və'dʒaɪn(ə)l] *adj.* referring to the vagina *vaginal, slid-;* **vaginal bleeding** = bleeding from the vagina *vaginal blödning;* **vaginal diaphragm** = contraceptive device, inserted into the woman's vagina and placed over the neck of the uterus *pessar, slidpessar;* **vaginal discharge** = flow of liquid from the vagina *vaginalfluor, flytning från slidan;* **vaginal douche** = (i) washing out of the vagina *slidsköljning;* (ii) the device used to wash out the vagina *sköljkanna; see also* DOUCHE; **vaginal examination** = checking the vagina for signs of disease or growth *vaginalundersökning;* **vaginal orifice** = opening leading from the vulva to the uterus

➪ *illustration* UROGENITAL SYSTEM (female) *ostium uteri, livmodermunnen*
NOTE: for other terms referring to the vagina see words beginning with **colp-**

vaginal- ➪ **colp-, vagin(o)-**

vaginalfluor ➪ **vaginal**

vaginalis [ˌvædʒɪ'neɪlɪs] *see* TRICHOMONAS, TUNICA

vaginalplastik ➪ **colpoplasty**

vaginalprolaps ➪ **colpoptosis**

vaginalsmear ➪ **Papanicolaou test**

vaginalsnitt ➪ **colpotomy**

vaginalundersökning ➪ **vaginal**

vaginalutstryk ➪ **Papanicolaou test**

vaginectomy [ˌvædʒɪ'nektəmi] *subst.* surgical operation to remove the vagina or part of it *vaginektomi*

vaginismus [ˌvædʒɪ'nɪzməs] *subst.* painful contraction of the vagina which prevents sexual intercourse *vaginism*

vaginitis [ˌvædʒɪ'naɪtɪs] *subst.* inflammation of the vagina which is mainly caused by the bacterium Trichomonas vaginalis or by a fungus Candida albicans *vaginit, kolpit, slidinflammation*

vagin(o)- [və'dʒaɪn(əʊ)] *prefix* referring to the vagina *vagin(o)-, vaginal-, colp(o)-, kolp(o)-, slid-*

vaginography [ˌvædʒɪ'nɒgrəfi] *subst.* X-ray examination of the vagina *röntgenundersökning av slidan*

vaginoplasty [və'dʒaɪnə(ʊ)ˌplæsti] *subst.* surgical operation to graft tissue on to the vagina *vaginoplastik*

vaginoscope ['vædʒɪnəʊskəʊp] *or* **colposcope** ['kɒlpəskəʊp] *subst.* surgical instrument inserted into the vagina to inspect the inside of it *kolposkop*

vaginotomi ➪ **colpotomy**

vagitorium ➪ **pessary**

vago- ['veɪgə(ʊ), ˌ--, və'gɒ, veɪ'gɒ] *prefix* referring to the vagus nerve *vago-, vagus-*

vagotomy [veɪ'gɒtəmi] *subst.* surgical operation to cut through the vagus nerve which controls the nerves in the stomach, as a treatment for peptic ulcers *vagotomi*

vagotoni ➪ **vagal**

vagus nerve ['veɪgəs ˌnɜːv] *subst.* tenth cranial nerve, which controls swallowing and the nerve fibres in the heart, stomach and lungs *(nervus) vagus, 10:e kranialnerven*

vaka ➪ **wakefulness**

vaken ➪ **alert, awake, wakeful**

vakenhet ➪ **wakefulness**

vakna (upp) ➪ **awake, wake**

vaktmästare ➪ **orderly, porter**

vakuol ➪ **vacuole**

vakuumextraktion ➪ **extraction**

valfri ➪ **elective**

valgus ['vælgəs] *subst.* type of deformity where the foot *or* hand bends away from the centre of the body *utåtvriden (sned) ställning;* **genu valgum** = knock knee *or* state where the knees touch and the feet are apart when a person is standing straight *genu valgum, kobenthet, X-benthet;* **hallux valgus** = condition of the foot, where the big toe turns towards the other toes and a bunion is formed *hallux valgus; compare* VARUS

valine ['veɪliːn] *subst.* essential amino acid *valin*

valk ➪ **callosity, callus**

vallate papillae ['væleɪt pəˌpiliː] *subst.* large papillae which form a line towards the back of the tongue and contain taste buds ➪ *illustration* TONGUE *papillae vallatae (circumvallatae)*

vallecula [və'lekjʊlə] *subst.* natural depression *or* fissure in an organ as between the hemispheres of the brain *vallecula*

vallgravspapiller ➪ **circumvallate papillae**

vallning ➪ **flush, hot**

value ['væljuː] *subst.* quantity shown as a number *värde;* **calorific value** = number of calories which a certain amount of a certain food contains *kalorivärde;* **energy value** = amount of energy produced by a certain amount of a certain food *energivärde*

valv ▷ **arc, arch, fornix**

valve [vælv] *subst.* flap, mainly in the heart *or* blood vessels *or* lymphatic vessels but also in other organs, which opens and closes to allow liquid to pass in one direction only *valva, valvel, klaff;* **aortic valve** = valve with three flaps at the opening into the aorta *valva aortae, aortaklaffen;* **bicuspid (mitral) valve** = valve in the heart which allows blood to flow from the left atrium to the left ventricle but not in the opposite direction *valvula mitralis (bicuspidalis), mitralisklaffen, bikuspidalklaffen;* **ileocaecal valve** = valve at the end of the ileum, which allows food to pass from the ileum into the caecum *valva ileocaecalis, ileocekalklaffen, Bauhins klaff;* **pulmonary valve** = valve at the opening of the pulmonary artery *valva trunci pulmonalis, pulmonalisklaff;* **semilunar valves** = two valves in the heart, the aortic valve and the pulmonary valve *valvulae semilunares, semilunarklaffarna, fickklaffarna;* **tricuspid valve** = inlet valve with three cusps between the right atrium and the right ventricle in the heart *valva tricuspidalis (atrioventricularis dextra), trikuspidalklaffen, atrioventrikularklaffen*

valvel ▷ **valve**

valvotomy [væl'vɒtəmi] *or* **valvulotomy** [ˌvælvju'lɒtəmi] *subst.* surgical operation to cut into a valve to make it open wider *valvotomi;* **mitral valvotomy** = surgical operation to detach the cusps of the mitral valve in mitral stenosis *slags operation vid mitralisstenos*

valvula ['vælvjʊlə] *subst.* small valve *valvula, liten valvel, liten klaff* NOTE: plural is **valvulae**

valvular ['vælvjʊlə] *adj.* referring to a valve *valvulär, klaff-;* **valvular disease of the heart (VDH)** = inflammation of the membrane which lines the valves of the heart *vitium organicum cordis, VOC, klaffel*

valvulitis [ˌvælvju'laɪtɪs] *subst.* inflammation of a valve in the heart *valvulit*

valvuloplasty ['vælvjʊləʊˌplæsti] *subst.* surgery to repair valves in the heart without opening the heart *slags plastik av hjärtklaff*

> QUOTE in percutaneous balloon valvuloplasty a catheter introduced through the femoral vein is placed across the aortic valve and into the left ventricle; the catheter is removed and a valve-dilating catheter bearing a 15mm balloon is placed across the valve
> **Journal of the American Medical Association**

valvulär ▷ **valvular**

van ▷ **experienced**

vana ▷ **experience, habit**

van den Bergh test [ˌvæn den 'bɜːgz ˌtest] *subst.* test of blood serum to see if a case of jaundice is caused by an obstruction in the liver or by haemolysis of red blood cells *Hijman van den Berghs reaktion*

vandrande njure ▷ **nephroptosis**

vandring ▷ **passage**

vanebildande ▷ **addictive, habit-forming**

vanföreställning ▷ **delusion**

vanlig ▷ **common**

vanligen ▷ **commonly, generally, normally**

vanpryda ▷ **disfigure**

vansinne ▷ **insanity**

vansinnig ▷ **insane, mad**

vanställa ▷ **disfigure**

vaporize ['veɪpəraɪz] *vb.* to turn a liquid into a vapour *vaporisera, förånga(s), avdunsta*

vaporizer ['veɪpəraɪzə] *subst.* device which warms a liquid to which medicinal oil has been added, so that it provides a vapour which a patient can inhale *evaporator, förgasare, sprej, spray*

vapour ['veɪpə] *subst.* substance in the form of gas *ånga, dimma;* medicinal oil in steam *förångad medicinsk olja*

Vaquez-Osler disease [væˌkeɪz'ɒslə dɪˌziːz] = POLYCYTHAEMIA VERA

var ▷ **ichor, matter, plastic, pus, sanies**

var- ▷ **py-, pyo-**

vara ['veərə] *subst. pl. see* VARUS

varaktig ▷ **perennial**

varannandagsfrossa ▷ **tertian fever**

varansamling ▷ **empyema**

vara sig ⇨ **fester, suppurate**

varbildande ⇨ **pyogenic**

varbildning ⇨ **pyosis, suppuration**

varflöde ⇨ **pyorrhoea**

varhärd ⇨ **abscess**

variation [ˌveərɪ'eɪʃ(ə)n] *subst.* change from one level to another *variation, växling;* **there is a noticeable variation in his pulse rate; the chart shows the variations in the patient's temperature over a twenty-four hour period**

varicectomy [ˌværi'sektəmi] *subst.* surgical operation to remove a vein *or* part of a vein *varicektomi, åderbråcksoperation*

varicella [ˌværi'selə] = CHICKENPOX

varicer ⇨ **varicose veins**

varices ['værɪsiːz] *see* VARIX

varicocele ['værɪkəʊsiː(ə)l] *subst.* swelling of a vein in the spermatic cord and which can be corrected by surgery *varikocele, pungåderbråck*

varicose veins [ˌværɪkəʊs 'veɪnz] *subst pl.* veins, usually in the legs, which become twisted and swollen *varicer, åderbråck;* **she wears special stockings to support her varicose veins; varicose eczema** = form of eczema which develops on the legs, caused by bad circulation *variköst eksem, hypostatiskt eksem;* **varicose ulcer** = ulcer in the leg as a result of varicose veins *ulcus varicosum, variköst sår, bensår*

varicosity [ˌværɪ'kɒsəti] *subst. (of veins)* being swollen and twisted *variköst tillstånd*

varicotomy [ˌværɪ'kɒtəmi] *subst.* surgical operation to make a cut into a varicose vein *varikotomi*

variera ⇨ **vary**

varig ⇨ **purulent, suppurating**

varigt sår ⇨ **sore**

varikocele ⇨ **varicocele**

varikotomi ⇨ **varicotomy**

variola [və'ra(ɪ)ələ] = SMALLPOX

varioloid ['veəriəlɔɪd] *subst.* type of mild smallpox which affects patients who have already had smallpox *or* have been vaccinated against it *variola mitigata*

varix ['veərɪks] *subst.* swollen blood vessel, especially a swollen vein in the leg *varix, åderbråck*
NOTE: plural is **varices**

varjedagsfrossa ⇨ **quotidian**

varm ⇨ **hot, warm**

varmblodig ⇨ **homoiothermic**

varning ⇨ **notice, warning**

varsam ⇨ **gentle**

varseblivning ⇨ **perception**

varsel ⇨ **notice**

varsko ⇨ **warn**

vartredjedagsfrossa ⇨ **quartan fever**

varumärke ⇨ **proprietary**

varus ['veərəs] *subst.* deformity where the foot or hand bends in towards the centre of the body *sned (inåtvänd) ställning;* **coxa vara** = deformity of the hip bone, making the legs bow *cox vara;* **genu varum** = bow legs *or* state where the ankles touch and the knees are apart when a person is standing straight *genu varum, hjulbenthet, O-benthet; compare* VALGUS
NOTE: plural is **vara**

varv ⇨ **layer**

vary ['veəri] *vb.* to change *or* to try different actions *variera, anpassa, ändra;* **the dosage varies according to the age of the patient; the patient was recommended to change to a more varied diet**

vas [væs] *subst.* tube in the body *vas, kärl, kanal;* **vasa vasorum** = tiny blood vessels in the walls of larger blood vessels *vasa vasorum*
NOTE: plural is **vasa**

vas- ['væs, ˌ-] *prefix* referring to (i) a blood vessel *vas(o)-, blodkärls-, kärl-;* (ii) the vas deferens *vas(o)-, sädesledar-*

vascular ['væskjʊlə] *adj.* referring to blood vessels *vaskulär, blodkärls-, kärl-;* **vascular lesion** = damage to a blood vessel *kärlskada;* **vascular system** = series of vessels such as veins, arteries and capillaries, carrying blood around the body *kärlsystemet*

vascularization [ˌvæskjʊlərarˈzeɪʃ(ə)n] *subst.* development of new blood vessels *vaskularisation, kärlbildning*

vasculitis [ˌvæskjuˈlartɪs] *subst.* inflammation of a blood vessel *vaskulit, kärlinflammation*

vas deferens [ˌvæs ˈdefərenz] *or* **ductus deferens** [ˌdʌktəs ˈdefərenz] *or* **sperm duct** [ˈspɜːm ˌdʌkt] *subst.* one of two tubes along which sperm passes from the epididymis to the prostate gland for ejaculation ⇨ *illustration* UROGENITAL SYSTEM (male) *(vas) ductus deferens, sädesledaren*
NOTE: plural is **vasa deferentia**

vasectomy [væˈsektəmi] *subst.* surgical operation to cut a vas deferens, to prevent sperm travelling from the epididymis up the duct *vasektomi, vasoresektion;* **bilateral vasectomy** = cutting of both the vasa deferentia which makes a man sterile *bilateral vasektomi (vasoresektion)*

COMMENT: bilateral vasectomy is a safe method of male contraception

vas efferens [ˌvæs ˈefərenz] *subst.* one of many tiny tubes which take the spermatozoa from the testis to the epididymis *vas efferens*
NOTE: plural is **vasa efferentia**

vasektomi ⇨ **vasectomy**

vaskularisation ⇨ **vascularization**

vaskulit ⇨ **vasculitis**

vaskulär ⇨ **vascular**

vaso- [ˈveɪzə(ʊ), ˌ--] *prefix* referring to (i) a blood vessel *vas(o)-, blodkärls-, kärl-;* (ii) the vas deferens *vas(o)-, sädesledar-*

vasoactive [ˌveɪzəʊˈæktɪv] *adj.* (agent) which has an effect on the blood vessels (especially one which constricts the arteries) *vasoaktiv*

vasoaktiv ⇨ **vasoactive**

vasoconstriction [ˈveɪzə(ʊ)kənˈstrɪkʃ(ə)n] *subst.* contraction of blood vessels which makes them narrower *vasokonstriktion, kärlsammandragning*

vasoconstrictor [ˌveɪzə(ʊ)kənˈstrɪktə] *subst.* chemical substance which makes blood vessels become narrower, so that blood pressure rises *vasokonstriktor, kärlsammandragande medel*

vasodilatation [ˌveɪzə(ʊ)daɪˈleɪteɪʃ(ə)n] *subst.* relaxation of blood vessels which makes them wider *vasodilatation, kärlutvidgning*

vasodilator [ˌveɪzə(ʊ)daɪˈleɪtə] *subst.* chemical substance which makes blood vessels become wider, so that blood flows more easily and blood pressure falls *vasodila(ta)tor, kärl(ut)vidgande medel;* **peripheral vasodilator** = chemical substance which acts to widen the blood vessels in the arms and legs, and so helps bad circulation as in Raynaud's disease *perifer vasodila(ta)tor, perifert verkande kärl(ut)vidgande medel*

vasokonstriktion ⇨ **vasoconstriction**

vasokonstriktor ⇨ **vasoconstrictor**

vasoligation [ˌveɪzə(ʊ)laɪˈgeɪʃ(ə)n] *subst.* surgical operation to tie the vasa deferentia to prevent infection entering the epididymis from the urinary system *vasoligatur*

vasomotion [ˌveɪzə(ʊ)ˈməʊʃ(ə)n] *subst.* vasoconstriction *or* vasodilatation *vasokonstriktion eller vasodilatation*

vasomotor [ˌveɪzə(ʊ)ˈməʊtə] *adj.* which makes blood vessels narrower *or* wider *vasomotorisk, vasomotor-;* **vasomotor centre** = nerve centre in the brain which changes the rate of heartbeat and the diameter of blood vessels and so regulates blood pressure *vasomotorcentrum;* **vasomotor nerve** = nerve in the wall of a blood vessel which affects the diameter of the vessel *vasomotorisk nerv*

vasomotorcentrum ⇨ **vasomotor**

vasomotorisk ⇨ **vasomotor**

vasopressin [ˌveɪzə(ʊ)ˈpresɪn] *or* **antidiuretic hormone (ADH)** [ˌæntɪˌdaɪju(ə)ˌretɪk ˈhɔːməʊn (ˌeɪdiːˈeɪtʃ)] *subst.* hormone secreted by the pituitary gland which acts on the kidneys to regulate the quantity of salt in body fluids and the amount of urine excreted by the kidneys *vasopressin, antidiuretiskt hormon, ADH*

vasopressor [ˌveɪzə(ʊ)ˈpresə] *subst.* substance which increases blood pressure by narrowing the blood vessels *vasopressor*

vasoresektion ⇨ **vasectomy**

vasospasm [ˈveɪzə(ʊ)spæz(ə)m] *or* **Raynaud's disease** [reɪˈnəʊz dɪˌziːz] *subst.* condition where the fingers become cold, white and numb *vasospasm,* *acrocyanosis chronica anaesthetica, Raynauds fenomen (sjukdom, symtom)*

vasovagal [ˌveɪzə(ʊ)'veɪg(ə)l] *adj.* referring to the vagus nerve and its effect on the heartbeat and blood circulation *vasovagal;* **vasovagal attack** = fainting fit (following a slowing down of the heartbeats caused by the vagus nerve) *vasovagalt synkope, vasovagal svimning*

vasovasostomy [ˌveɪzə(ʊ)və'sɒstəmi] *subst.* surgical operation to reverse a vasectomy *operation för att återställa fertilitet efter vasektomi*

vasovesiculitis [ˌveɪzə(ʊ)veˌsɪkju'laɪtɪs] *subst.* inflammation of the seminal vesicles and a vas deferens *vasovesikulit*

vass ➪ **sharp**

vastus intermedius [ˌvæstəs ˌɪntə'miːdiəs] *or* **vastus medialis** [ˌvæstəs ˌmiːdi'eɪlɪs] *or* **vastus lateralis** [ˌvæstəs ˌlætə'reɪlɪs] *subst.* three of the four parts of the quadriceps femoris *or* muscle of the thigh *musculus vastus intermedius (medialus, lateralis)*

vatten ➪ **water**

vatten- ➪ **aqueous, hydr-, hydro-**

vattenbehandling ➪ **hydrotherapy**

vattenbråck ➪ **hydrocele**

vattenhaltig ➪ **watery**

vattenkoppor ➪ **chickenpox**

vattenkräfta ➪ **noma**

vattenlösning ➪ **liquor**

vattenskalle ➪ **hydrocephalus**

vattensäng ➪ **water bed**

vattentät ➪ **waterproof**

vattkoppor ➪ **chickenpox**

vattnas ➪ **water**

vattnig ➪ **thin, watery**

vattuskräck ➪ **hydrophobia, rabies**

vax ➪ **wax**

v.b. ➪ **p.r.n.**

VD [ˌviː'diː] = VENEREAL DISEASE; **VD clinic** = clinic specializing in the diagnosis and treatment of venereal diseases *klinik för veneriska sjukdomar (könssjukdomar), könsklinik;* **he is attending a VD clinic; the treatment for VD takes several weeks**

VDH [ˌviːdiː'eɪtʃ] = VALVULAR DISEASE OF THE HEART

veck ➪ **convolution, flexure, fold, plica, plication, ruga**

veckad ➪ **plicate**

veckning ➪ **plication**

vectis ['vektɪs] *subst.* curved surgical instrument used in childbirth *kirurgiskt instrument som används vid förlossning*

vector ['vektə] *subst.* insect *or* animal which carries a disease and can pass it to humans *vektor, bärare;* **the tsetse fly is a vector of sleeping sickness**

vegan ['viːg(ə)n] *subst. & adj.* strict vegetarian *or* (person) who eats only vegetables and fruit, and does not eat milk, fish, eggs or any meat *vegan, strikt vegetarian*

vegetable ['vedʒtəb(ə)l] *subst.* plant grown for food, not usually sweet *grönsak;* **green vegetables are a source of dietary fibre**

vegetarian [ˌvedʒə'teəriən] *subst. & adj.* (person) who eats mainly vegetables, and eggs or cheese and sometimes fish, but no meat *vegetarian, vegetarisk;* **he is on a vegetarian diet**

vegetarian, strikt ➪ **vegan**

vegetarisk ➪ **vegetarian**

vegetation [ˌvedʒə'teɪʃ(ə)n] *subst.* growth on a membrane (as on the cusps of valves in the heart) *vegetation, (vävnads)tillväxt*

vegetative ['vedʒətətɪv] *adj.* (i) referring to growth of tissue *or* organs *vegetativ, växande, tillväxt-;* (ii) (state) after brain damage, where a person is alive and breathing but shows no responses *vegeterande*

vegeterande ➪ **vegetative**

vehicle ['viːɪk(ə)l] *subst.* liquid in which a dose of a drug is put *vehikel*

vein [veɪn] *subst.* blood vessel which takes deoxygenated blood containing waste carbon dioxide from the tissues back to the heart *ven,*

blodåder; **azygos vein** = vein which brings blood back to the heart from the abdomen *vena azygo, opariga venen;* **basilic vein** = vein in the arm, running from the hand along the forearm to the elbow *vena basilica;* **deep vein** = vein which is deep in tissue, near the bones *djup ven;* **hepatic vein** = vein which carries blood from the liver to the vena cava *vena hepatica, leverven;* **lingual vein** = vein which takes blood away from the tongue *vena lingualis, tungvenen;* **portal vein** = vein which takes blood from the stomach, pancreas, intestines and spleen to the liver *vena portae, portvenen, portådern;* **pulmonary vein** = vein which carries oxygenated blood from the lungs back to the left atrium of the heart (it is the only vein which carries oxygenated blood) *vena pulmonalis, pulmonalisven, lungven;* **superficial vein** = vein which is near the surface of the skin *ytlig ven*
NOTE: for other terms referring to the veins, see words beginning with **phleb-**

veka livet ⇨ **small of the back**

vektor ⇨ **carrier, vector**

ven ⇨ **vein**

ven- ⇨ **phleb-, venous**

vena cava [ˌviːnə 'keɪvə] *subst.* one of two large veins which take deoxygenated blood from all the other veins into the right atrium of the heart ⇨ *illustration* HEART, KIDNEY *vena cava, hålvenen* NOTE: plural is **venae cavae**

COMMENT: the superior vena cava brings blood from the head and the top part of the body, while the inferior vena cava brings blood from the abdomen and legs

vene- ['venɪ, ˌ--] *or* **veno-** [vɪ'nɒ, -ˌ-, 'viːnə(ʊ), ˌ--] *prefix* referring to veins *ven(e)-, veno-, fleb(o)-, blodåder-*

venene [və'niːn] *subst.* mixture of different venoms, used to produce antivenene *venin, (orm)gift*

venepuncture ['venɪˌpʌŋktʃə] *or* **venipuncture** ['venɪˌpʌŋktʃə] *subst.* puncturing a vein either to inject a drug *or* to take a blood sample *venpunktion*

venereal disease (VD) [vəˌnɪəriəl dɪˌziːz (ˌviː'diː)] *subst.* disease which is passed from one person to another during sexual intercourse *venerisk sjukdom, VS, könssjukdom, sexuellt överförd sjukdom, STD*

COMMENT: now usually called sexually transmitted diseases (STDs), the main types of venereal disease are syphilis, gonorrhoea, AIDS, non-specific urethritis, genital herpes and chancroid. The spread of sexually transmitted diseases can be limited by use of condoms. Other forms of contraceptive offer no protection against the spread of disease

venereology [vəˌnɪəri'ɒlədʒi] *subst.* scientific study of venereal diseases *venereologi*

venereum [və'nɪəriəm] *see* LYMPHOGRANULOMA

veneris ['venərɪs] *see* MONS

venerisk sjukdom ⇨ **sexually transmitted disease (STD), social, venereal disease (VD)**

venesection [ˌvenɪ'sekʃ(ə)n] = PHLEBOTOMY

venin ⇨ **venene**

ven, liten ⇨ **venule**

veno- ⇨ **vene-**

venoclysis [və'nɒkləsɪs] *subst.* introducing slowly a saline *or* other solution into a vein *infusion, infundering, långsam ingjutning*

venogram ['viːnə(ʊ)græm] = PHLEBOGRAM

venography [vɪ'nɒgrəfi] = PHLEBOGRAPHY

venol ⇨ **venule**

venom ['venəm] *subst.* poison in the bite of a snake *or* insect *gift*

COMMENT: depending on the source of the bite, venom can have a wide range of effects, from a light irritating spot after a mosquito sting, to death from a scorpion. Antivenene will counteract the effects of venom, but is only effective if the animal which gave the bite can be correctly identified

venomous ['venəməs] *adj.* (animal) which has poison in its bite *giftig;* **the cobra is a venomous snake; he was bitten by a venomous spider**

venosus [vɪ'nəʊsəs] *see* DUCTUS

venous ['viːnəs] *adj.* referring to the veins *venös, ven-, blodåder-;* **venous bleeding** = bleeding from a vein *venös blödning;* **venous**

blood = deoxygenated blood, from which most of the oxygen has been removed by the tissues and is darker than oxygenated arterial blood (it is carried by all the veins except for the pulmonary vein which carries oxygenated blood) *venöst (syrefattigt) blod;* **venous system** = system of veins which bring blood back to the heart from the tissues *vensystemet;* **venous thrombosis** = blocking of a vein by a blood clot *ventrombos, flebotrombos;* **venous ulcer** = ulcer in the leg, caused by varicose veins or by a blood clot *venöst sår;* **central venous pressure** = blood pressure in the right atrium, which can be measured by means of a catheter *centrala ventrycket, CVP*

QUOTE venous air embolism is a potentially fatal complication of percutaneous venous catheterization

Southern Medical Journal

QUOTE a pad was placed under the Achilles tendon to raise the legs, thus aiding venous return and preventing deep vein thrombosis

NATNews

venpunktion ⇨ **venepuncture**

vensten ⇨ **phlebolith**

vensystemet ⇨ **venous**

venter ⇨ **belly**

ventilation [ˌventɪ'leɪʃ(ə)n] *subst.* breathing air in or out of the lungs, so removing waste products from the blood in exchange for oxygen *ventilation, respiration, andning; see also* DEAD SPACE; **artificial ventilation** = breathing which is assisted *or* controlled by a machine *artificiell ventilation, konstgjord andning;* **mouth-to-mouth ventilation** = making a patient start to breathe again by blowing air through his mouth into his lungs *andning med hjälp av mun-mot-munmetoden*

ventilation ⇨ **respiration**

ventilator ['ventɪleɪtə] *or* **respirator** ['respəreɪtə] *subst.* machine which pumps air into and out of the lungs of a patient who has difficulty in breathing *ventilator, respirator;* **the newborn baby was put on a ventilator**

ventilatory failure ['ventɪleɪt(ə)ri ˌfeɪljə] *subst.* failure of the lungs to oxygenate the blood correctly *andningsinsufficiens*

ventilpneumotorax ⇨ **pneumothorax**

ventral ['ventr(ə)l] *adj.* referring to (i) the abdomen *ventral;* (ii) the front of the body *ventral*

NOTE: the opposite is **dorsal**

ventri- ⇨ **ventro-**

ventricle ['ventrɪk(ə)l] *subst.* cavity in an organ, especially in the heart or brain ⇨ *illustration* HEART *ventrikel, hjärtventrikel, kammare, hjärnventrikel, magsäcken*

COMMENT: there are two ventricles in the heart: the left ventricle takes oxygenated blood from the pulmonary vein through the left atrium, and pumps it into the aorta to circulate round the body; the right ventricle takes blood from the veins through the right atrium, and pumps it into the pulmonary artery to be passed to the lungs to be oxygenated. There are four ventricles in the brain, each containing cerebrospinal fluid. The two lateral ventricles in the cerebral hemispheres contain the choroid processes which produce cerebrospinal fluid. The third ventricle lies in the midline between the two thalami. The fourth ventricle is part of the central canal of the hindbrain

ventricular [ven'trɪkjʊlə] *adj.* referring to the ventricles *ventrikulär, ventrikel-, kammar-;* **ventricular fibrillation** = serious heart condition where the ventricular muscles flutter and the heart no longer beats *fibrillatio ventriculi cordis, ventrikelflimmer, kammarflimmer;* **ventricular folds** *or* **vocal cords** = two folds in the larynx which make sounds as air passes between them *stämbanden*

ventriculitis [venˌtrɪkju'laɪtɪs] *subst.* inflammation of the brain ventricles *inflammation i hjärnventriklarna*

ventricul(o)- [ven'trɪkjʊl(əʊ), -ˌ---] *prefix* referring to a ventricle in the brain *or* heart *ventrikul(o)-, ventrikel-*

ventriculoatriostomy [venˌtrɪkjʊləʊˌeɪtri'ɒstəmi] *subst.* operation to relieve pressure caused by excessive quantities of cerebrospinal fluid in the brain ventricles *slags shuntoperation (avlastning)*

ventriculogram [ven'trɪkjʊlə(ʊ)græm] *subst.* X-ray picture of the brain ventricles *ventrikulogram*

ventriculography [venˌtrɪkju'lɒgrəfi] *subst.* method of taking X-ray pictures of the ventricles of the brain after air has been introduced to replace the cerebrospinal fluid *ventrikulografi, pneumoencefalografi, encefalografi, luftskalle*

ventriculoscopy [ven,trıkju'lɒskəpi] *subst.* examination of the brain using an endoscope *slags undersökning av hjärnan*

ventriculostomy [ven,trıkju'lɒstəmi] *subst.* surgical operation to pass a hollow needle into a brain ventricle so as to reduce pressure *or* take a sample of fluid *slags shuntoperation (avlastning)*

ventrikel ⇨ **ventricle**

ventrikel- ⇨ **ventricular, ventricul(o)-**

ventrikelflimmer ⇨ **ventricular**

ventrikeln ⇨ **stomach**

ventrikelsond ⇨ **nasogastric, stomach**

ventrikul(o)- ⇨ **ventricul(o)-**

ventrikulografi ⇨ **encephalography, pneumoencephalography, ventriculography**

ventrikulogram ⇨ **ventriculogram**

ventrikulär ⇨ **ventricular**

ventro- ['ventrə(ʊ), ,--] *prefix* (i) meaning ventral *ventral;* (ii) referring to the abdomen *ventro-, ventri-, buk-*

ventrofixation [,ventrəʊfık'seıʃ(ə)n] *subst.* surgical operation to treat retroversion of the uterus by attaching the uterus to the wall of the abdomen *antefixation*

ventrombos ⇨ **phlebothrombosis, venous**

ventrosuspension [,ventrəʊsə'spenʃ(ə)n] *subst.* surgical operation to treat retroversion of the uterus *antefixation*

venula ⇨ **venule**

venule ['venju:l] *subst.* small vein, vessel leading from the tissue to a vein *venula, venol, liten ven*

venusberget ⇨ **mons pubis**

venös ⇨ **venous**

vera ['vıərə] *see* DECIDUA

verbigeration [vɜ:,bıdʒə'reıʃ(ə)n] *subst.* condition seen in mental patients, where the patient keeps saying the same words over and over again *verbigeration*

verka ⇨ **act, appear**

verkan ⇨ **action, effect, operation**

verklig ⇨ **actual**

verkligen ⇨ **actually**

verksam ⇨ **active, effective, efficient**

verksamhet ⇨ **activity**

verkställa ⇨ **effect**

verktyg ⇨ **instrument**

vermicide ['vɜ:mısaıd] *subst.* substance which will kill worms in the intestines *vermicid, maskdödande medel, maskmedel*

vermiform ['vɜ:mıfɔ:m] *adj.* shaped like a worm *vermiform, maskformig;* **vermiform appendix** = small tube attached to the caecum which serves no function, but can become infected, causing appendicitis *appendix vermiformis, blindtarmens maskformiga bihang, "blindtarmen"*

vermifuge ['vɜ:mıfju:dʒ] *subst. & adj.* substance which will make worms leave the intestine *maskfördrivande medel*

vermilion border [və,mıliən 'bɔ:də] *subst.* red edge of the lips *rubor labii, läppsömmen*

vermis ['vɜ:mıs] *subst.* central part of the cerebellum, which forms the top of the fourth ventricle *vermis (cerebelli), lillhjärnsmasken*

vermix ['vɜ:mıks] *subst.* vermiform appendix *appendix vermiformis, blindtarmens maskformiga bihang, "blindtarmen"*

vernix caseosa [,vɜ:nıks ,keısi'əʊsə] *subst.* oily substance which covers a baby's skin at birth *vernix caseosa, smegma embryonum (embryonale)*

verruca [və'ru:kə] *subst.* wart *or* small hard benign growth on the skin, caused by a virus *verruca, vårta*
NOTE: plural is **verrucae**

version ['vɜ:ʃ(ə)n] *subst.* turning the fetus in a womb so as to put it in a better position for birth *version, vändning, fostervändning;* **cephalic version** = turning a fetus in the womb so that the baby will be born head first *vändning till huvudläge;* **podalic version =** turning a fetus in the womb so that the baby will be born feet first *vändning på fot;* **spontaneous version =** movement of a fetus to take up another position in the the womb, caused by the contractions of the womb during childbirth *fostrets egna lägesändringar i livmodern*

vertebra ['vɜːtɪbrə] *subst.* one of twenty-four ring-shaped bones which link together to form the backbone *vertebra, kota, ryggkota* NOTE: plural is **vertebrae**

COMMENT: the top vertebra (the atlas) supports the skull; the first seven vertebrae in the neck are the cervical vertebrae; then follow the twelve thoracic or dorsal vertebrae which are behind the chest and five lumbar vertebrae in the lower part of the back. The sacrum and coccyx are formed of five sacral vertebrae and four coccygeal vertebrae which have fused together

vertebral ['vɜːtɪbr(ə)l] *adj.* referring to the vertebrae *vertebral(-), ryggkote-, kot-;* **vertebral arteries =** two arteries which go up the back of the neck into the brain *arteriae vertebrales, ryggkoteartärerna;* **vertebral canal =** channel formed of the holes in the centre of each vertebra, through which the spinal cord passes *canalis vertebralis, spinalkanalen, vertebralkanalen, ryggradskanalen;* **vertebral column =** backbone *or* series of bones and discs linked together to form a flexible column running from the base of the skull to the pelvis *columna spinalis (vertebralis), kotpelaren, ryggraden;* **vertebral disc** *or* **intervertebral disc =** thick piece of cartilage which lies between two vertebrae and acts as a cushion **vertebral discs** *disci intervertebrales, intervertebralbrosken;* **vertebral foramen =** hole in the centre of a vertebra which links with others to form the vertebral canal *foramen vertebrale, ryggkotehålet*
NOTE: the vertebrae are referred to by numbers and letters: **C6** = the sixth cervical vertebra; **T11** = the eleventh thoracic vertebra, and so on

vertebralkanalen ⇨ **spinal, vertebral**

vertex ['vɜːteks] *subst.* top of the skull *vertex, hjässan;* **vertex delivery =** normal birth of a baby, where the head appears first *huvudbjudning, kronbjudning, hjässbjudning*

vertigo ['vɜːtɪgəʊ] *subst.* **(a)** dizziness *or* giddiness *or* loss of balance where the patient feels that everything is rushing round him, caused by a malfunction of the sense of balance *vertigo, yrsel* **(b)** fear of heights *or* sensation of dizziness which is felt when high up (especially on a tall building) *vertigo, svindel;* **he won't sit near the window - he suffers from vertigo**

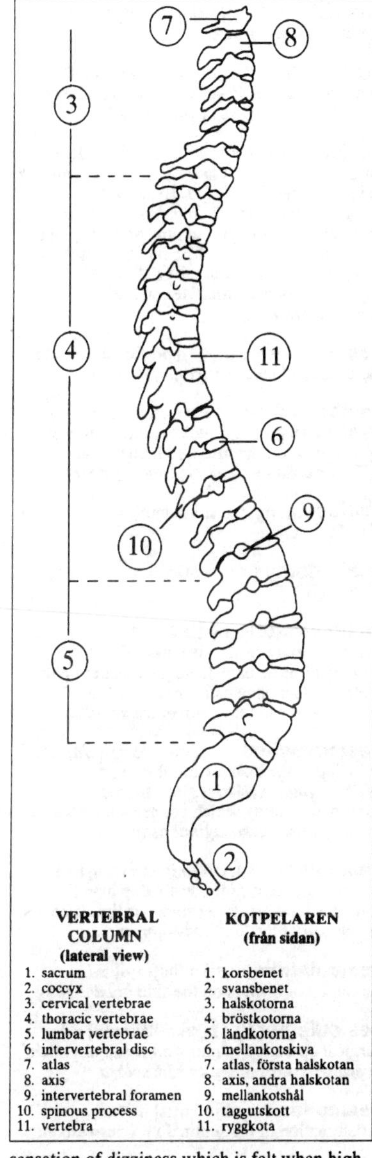

VERTEBRAL COLUMN (lateral view)

1. sacrum
2. coccyx
3. cervical vertebrae
4. thoracic vertebrae
5. lumbar vertebrae
6. intervertebral disc
7. atlas
8. axis
9. intervertebral foramen
10. spinous process
11. vertebra

KOTPELAREN (från sidan)

1. korsbenet
2. svansbenet
3. halskotorna
4. bröstkotorna
5. ländkotorna
6. mellankotskiva
7. atlas, första halskotan
8. axis, andra halskotan
9. mellankotshål
10. taggutskott
11. ryggkota

vesical ['vesɪk(ə)l] *adj.* referring to the bladder *vesikal, urinblåse-*

vesicant ['vesɪk(ə)nt] *or* **epispastic** [ˌepɪ'spæstɪk] *subst.* substance which makes the skin blister *blåsdragande medel*

vesicle ['vesɪk(ə)l] *subst.* **(a)** small blister on the skin (such as those caused by eczema) *liten vätskefylld hudblåsa* **(b)** sac which contains liquid *vesikel, liten blåsa;* **seminal vesicles** = two organs near the prostate gland which secrete seminal fluid into the vas deferens ⇨ *illustration* UROGENITAL SYSTEM (male) *vesiculae seminales, sädesblåsorna*

vesico- ['vesɪkə(ʊ), ˌ---] *prefix* referring to the urinary bladder *vesiko-, cyst-, blås-*

vesicofixation [ˌvesɪkəʊfɪk'seɪʃ(ə)n] *or* **cystopexy** ['sɪstəʊˌpeksi] *subst.* surgical operation to fix the urinary bladder in a different position *vesikofixation, cystopexi*

vesicostomy [ˌvesɪ'kɒstəmi] = CYSTOSTOMY

vesicotomy [ˌvesɪ'kɒtəmi] = CYSTOTOMY

vesicoureteric reflux [ˌvesɪkəʊˌjʊərə'terɪk ˌriːflʌks] *subst.* flowing of urine back from the bladder up the ureters, which may carry infection from the bladder to the kidneys *vesikouretär reflux*

vesicovaginal [ˌvesɪkəʊ'vædʒɪn(ə)l] *adj.* referring to the bladder and the vagina *vesikovaginal;* **vesicovaginal fistula** = abnormal opening which connects the bladder to the vagina *vesikovaginal fistel*

vesicular [və'sɪkjʊlə] *adj.* referring to a vesicle *vesikulär, blås-;* **vesicular breathing sound** = faint breathing sound as the air enters the alveoli of the lung *vesikulär andning*

vesiculation [vəˌsɪkju'leɪʃ(ə)n] *subst.* formation of blisters on the skin *blåsbildning*

vesiculectomy [vəˌsɪkju'lektəmi] *subst.* surgical operation to remove a seminal vesicle *operativt avlägsnande av sädesblåsa*

vesiculitis [vəˌsɪkju'laɪtɪs] *subst.* inflammation of the seminal vesicles *vesikulit*

vesiculography [vəˌsɪkju'lɒgrəfi] *subst.* X-ray examination of the seminal vesicles *vesikulografi*

vesiculopapular [vəˌsɪkjʊləʊ'pæpjʊlə] *adj.* (skin disorder) which has both blisters and papules *vesikulopapulär, med både blåsor och papler*

vesiculopustular [vəˌsɪkjʊləʊ'pʌstjʊlə] *adj.* (skin disorder) which has both blisters and pustules *vesikulopustulär, med både blåsor och pustler*

vesikal ⇨ **vesical**

vesikel ⇨ **vesicle**

vesiko- ⇨ **vesico-**

vesikocele ⇨ **cystocele**

vesikofixation ⇨ **vesicofixation**

vesikotomi ⇨ **cystotomy**

vesikovaginal ⇨ **vesicovaginal**

vesikulit ⇨ **vesiculitis**

vesikulografi ⇨ **vesiculography**

vesikulopapulär ⇨ **vesiculopapular**

vesikulopustulär ⇨ **vesiculopustular**

vesikulär ⇨ **vesicular**

vessel ['ves(ə)l] *subst.* tube in the body along which liquid flows, especially a blood vessel *kärl, blodkärl;* **afferent vessel** = tube which brings lymph to a gland *vas afferentia, tillförande lymfkärl;* **blood vessel** = any tube (artery *or* vein *or* capillary) which carries blood round the body *blodkärl;* **efferent vessel** = tube which drains lymph from a gland *vas efferentia, bortförande lymfkärl;* **lymphatic vessel** = tube which carries lymph round the body *vas lymphaticum, lymfkärl*
NOTE: for other terms referring to vessels, see words beginning with **vasc-**, **vaso-**

vestibular [ve'stɪbjʊlə] *adj.* referring to a vestibule, especially the vestibule of the inner ear *vestibular, vestibulär;* **vestibular folds** = folds in the larynx, above the vocal cords *plicae vestibulares, falska stämbanden;* **vestibular glands** = glands at the point where the vagina and vulva join, which secrete a lubricating liquid *glandulae vestibularis;* **greater vestibular gland** *or* **Bartholin's gland** = the more posterior of the vestibular glands *glandula vestibularis major, Bartholins körtel;* **lesser vestibular gland** = the more anterior of the vestibular glands *glandula vestibularis minor;* **vestibular nerve** = part of the auditory nerve which carries information about balance to the brain *nervus vestibuli,* *vestibularisnerven, gren av 8:e kranialnerven (hörsel- och balansnerven)*

vestibularisnerven ⇨ **vestibular**

vestibule ['vestɪbju:l] *subst.* cavity in the body at the entrance to an organ, especially (i) the first cavity in the inner ear *vestibulum labyrinthi ossei;* (ii) the space in the larynx above the vocal cords *vestibulum laryngis*

vestibuli [ve'stɪbjʊlaɪ] *see* FENESTRA

vestibulocochlear nerve [veˌstɪbjʊləʊ'kɒkliə ˌnɜ:v] *or* **acoustic nerve** [ə'ku:stɪk ˌnɜ:v] *or* **auditory nerve** ['ɔ:dɪt(ə)ri ˌnɜ:v] *subst.* eighth cranial nerve which governs hearing and balance *nervus vestibulo-cochlearis, hörsel- och balansnerven, 8:e kranialnerven*

vestibulär ⇨ **vestibular**

vestigial [ves'tɪdʒiəl] *adj.* which exists in a rudimentary form *rudimentär;* **the coccyx is a vestigial tail**

vetenskap ⇨ **science**

vetenskaplig ⇨ **scientific**

vetenskapsman ⇨ **scientist**

viability [ˌva(ɪ)ə'bɪləti] *subst.* being viable *viabilitet, livsduglighet;* **the viability of the fetus before the 22nd week is doubtful**

viable ['va(ɪ)əb(ə)l] *adj.* (fetus) which can survive if born *viabel, livsduglig;* **a fetus is viable by about the 28th week of pregnancy**

vibrate [vaɪ'breɪt] *vb.* to move rapidly and continuously *vibrera, darra, skaka*

vibration [vaɪ'breɪʃ(ə)n] *subst.* rapid and continuous movement *vibration, darrning, skakning;* **speech is formed by the vibrations of the vocal cords; sounds makes the eardrum vibrate, and the vibrations are sent to the brain as electric impulses; vibration white finger** = condition caused by using a chain saw *or* pneumatic drill, which affects the circulation in the fingers *slags vibrationsskada, vita fingrar pga vibration*

vibrator [vaɪ'breɪtə] *subst.* device to produce vibrations, which may be used for massages *vibrator, massageapparat*

vibrera ⇨ **vibrate**

Vibrio ['vɪbriəʊ] *subst.* genus of Gram-negative bacteria which are found in water and cause cholera *Vibrio*

vibrissae [vaɪ'brɪsi:] *subst. pl.* hairs in the nostrils *or* ears *vibrissae, näshår*

vicarious [vɪ'keəriəs] *adj.* (done by one organ *or* agent) in place of another *ställföreträdande, vikarierande;* **vicarious menstruation** = discharge of blood other than by the vagina during menstrual periods *vikarierande blödning*

victim ['vɪktɪm] *subst.* person who is injured in an accident *or* who has caught a disease *offer;* **the victims of the rail crash were taken to the local hospital; half the people eating the restaurant fell victim to salmonella poisoning; the health authority is planning a special hospital for AIDS victims**

Vidals prov ⇨ **Widal reaction**

vid behov ⇨ **p.r.n.**

vidga ⇨ **enlarge, widen**

vidgning ⇨ **enlargement**

vidmakthålla ⇨ **conserve**

vidöppen ⇨ **patulous**

vigour ['vɪgə] *see* HYBRID

vikande ⇨ **recessive**

vikarie ⇨ **locum (tenens)**

vikariera (för) ⇨ **cover**

vikarierande ⇨ **vicarious**

vikt ⇨ **weight**

viktig ⇨ **key, major, urgent**

viktigast ⇨ **primary**

viktlöshet ⇨ **weightlessness**

viktminskning ⇨ **loss**

viktökning ⇨ **weight**

vila ⇨ **rest**

vilande ⇨ **recumbent**

vilja ⇨ **volition, will**

viljeförlamning ⇨ **abulia**

viljekraft ⇨ **willpower**

viljestyrka ⇨ **willpower**

***viljesvaghet* ⇨ abulia**

villous ['vɪləs] *adj.* shaped like a villus *or* formed of villi *villös, luddig, luden*

villus ['vɪləs] *subst.* tiny projection like a finger on the surface of mucous membrane *villus;* **villi** *villi, ludd, fransar;* **arachnoid villi** = villi in the arachnoid membrane which absorb cerebrospinal fluid *spindelvävsliknande hjärnhinnans villi;* **chorionic villi** = tiny folds in the membrane covering the fertilized ovum *villi chorii, chorionvilli;* **intestinal villi** = projections on the walls of the intestine which help in the digestion of food *villi intestinales, tarmludd* NOTE: plural is **villi**

***vimmelkantig* ⇨ dazed, giddy**

Vincent's angina ['vɪnsents æn'dʒaɪnə] = ULCERATIVE GINGIVITIS

vinculum ['vɪŋkjʊləm] *subst.* thin connecting band of tissue *vinculum, band* NOTE: plural is **vincula**

***vindel* ⇨ gyrus**

***vindling* ⇨ convolution**

***vindögd* ⇨ cross-eyed, strabismal**

***vindögdhet* ⇨ squint, strabismus**

***vingla* ⇨ stagger**

***vinkel* ⇨ angle**

***vinkelled* ⇨ ginglymus, hinge joint**

violent ['va(ɪ)ələnt] *adj.* very strong *or* very severe *våldsam, häftig, stark, svår;* **he had a violent headache; her reaction to the injection was violent**

violently ['va(ɪ)ələntli] *adv.* in a strong way *våldsamt, häftigt, starkt;* **he reacted violently to the antihistamine**

violet ['va(ɪ)ələt] *subst.* dark blue colour at the end of the visible spectrum *violett; see also* CRYSTAL, GENTIAN

***violett* ⇨ violet**

***violettblindhet* ⇨ tritanopia**

viraemia [vaɪ'riːmiə] *subst.* virus in the blood *viremi*

viral ['vaɪ(ə)r(ə)l] *adj.* caused by a virus *or* referring to a virus *viral, virus-;* **he caught viral pneumonia on a plane**

***viremi* ⇨ viraemia**

virgin ['vɜːdʒɪn] *subst.* female who has not experienced sexual intercourse *virgo intacta, jungfru, oskuld*

virginity [və'dʒɪnəti] *subst.* condition of a woman who is a virgin *jungfrulighet, oskuld*

virile ['vɪraɪ(ə)l] *adj.* like a man *or* with strong male characteristics *viril, manlig, maskulin*

***virilisation* ⇨ virilization**

***virilisering* ⇨ virilization**

virilism ['vɪrɪlɪz(ə)m] *subst.* male characteristics (such as body hair *or* deep voice) in a woman *virilism, manhaftighet*

virilization [ˌvɪrɪlaɪ'zeɪʃ(ə)n] *subst.* development of male characteristics in a woman, caused by a hormone defect *or* therapy *virilisation, virilisering*

virology [ˌvaɪ(ə)'rɒlədʒi] *subst.* scientific study of viruses *virologi*

virulence ['vɪrʊləns] *subst.* (i) ability of a microbe to cause a disease *virulens;* (ii) violent effect (of a disease) *styrka, kraft, elakartad karaktär*

virulent ['vɪrʊlənt] *adj.* (i) (microbe) which can cause a disease *virulent, sjukdomsalstrande;* (ii) (disease) which has violent effects and develops rapidly *stark, kraftig, elakartad*

virus ['vaɪ(ə)rəs] *subst.* tiny germ cell which can only develop in other cells, and often destroys them *virus;* **scientists have isolated a new flu virus; shingles is caused by the same virus as chickenpox; infectious virus hepatitis** = hepatitis transmitted by a carrier through food or drink *hepatitis epidemica (infectiosa), infektiös virushepatit;* **virus pneumonia** = inflammation of the lungs caused by a virus *pneumonia virogenes, viruspneumoni*

> COMMENT: many common diseases such as measles or the common cold are caused by viruses; viral diseases cannot be treated with antibiotics

***virus-* ⇨ viral**

***viruspneumoni* ⇨ virus**

***virvelström(ning)* ⇨ turbulent flow**

visa ➪ **demonstrate, expose, guide, indicate, present, reveal**

visa sig ➪ **appear**

viscera ['vɪs(ə)rə] *subst pl.* internal organs (such as the heart, lungs, stomach, intestines) *viscera, inre organen;* **abdominal viscera** = the organs inside the abdomen *inälvorna*
NOTE: the singular (rarely used) is **viscus**

visceral ['vɪs(ə)r(ə)l] *adj.* referring to the internal organs *visceral;* **viscera larva migrans** = toxocariasis *or* infestation of the intestine with worms from a dog or cat *tarminfektion med toxocara (slags spolmask);* **visceral muscle** *or* **smooth muscle** = muscle in the wall of the intestine which makes the intestine contract *glatt muskel i tarmvägg;* **visceral pericardium** = inner layer of serous pericardium attached to the wall of the heart *epikardiet, hjärtsäckens inre blad;* **visceral peritoneum** = part of the peritoneum which covers the organs in the abdominal cavity *peritoneum viscerale, inälvsbukhinnan;* **visceral pleura** = inner pleura *or* membrane attached to the surface of a lung *pleura viscerale (pulmonalis), lungsäckens inre blad;* **visceral pouch** = PHARYNGEAL POUCH

visceromotor [ˌvɪsərə(ʊ)'məʊtə] *adj.* (reflex, etc) which controls the movement of viscera *som styr de inre organens rörelser*

visceroptosis [ˌvɪsərə(ʊ)'təʊsɪs] *subst.* movement of an internal organ downwards from its usual position *visceroptos*

visceroreceptor [ˌvɪsərə(ʊ)rɪ'septə] *subst.* receptor cell which reacts to stimuli from organs such as the stomach, heart and lungs *sinnescell som känner av inre organ*

viscid ['vɪsɪd] *adj.* sticky *or* slow-moving (liquid) *klibbig, seg, trögflytande*

viscosity [vɪ'skɒsəti] *subst.* state of a liquid which moves slowly *viskositet, klibbighet, tröghet*

viscous ['vɪskəs] *adj.* thick *or* slow-moving (liquid) *viskös, klibbig, trögflytande*

viscus ['vɪskəs] *see* VISCERA

visdomstand ➪ **wisdom tooth**

visible ['vɪzəb(ə)l] *adj.* which can be seen *synlig, märkbar;* **there were no visible symptoms of the disease**

vision ['vɪʒ(ə)n] *subst.* ability to see *or* eyesight *visus, syn(sinnet), synförmåga, seende;* **after the age of 60, many people's vision begins to fail; binocular vision** = ability to see with both eyes at the same time, which gives a stereoscopic effect and allows a person to judge distances *binokulärt seende;* **blurred vision** = condition where the patient does not see objects clearly *suddig (oskarp) syn;* **field of vision** = area which can be seen without moving the eye *synfält, synkrets;* **impaired vision** = eyesight which is not fully clear *nedsatt syn;* **monocular vision** = seeing with one eye only, so that the sense of distance is absent *monokulärt seende;* **partial vision** = being able to see only part of the total field of vision *begränsad syn(förmåga);* **stereoscopic vision** = being able to judge how far something is from you, because of seeing it with both eyes at the same time *stereoskopiskt (tredimensionellt) seende, stereoseende, djupseende;* **tunnel vision** = field of vision which is restricted to the area immediately in front of the eye *tunnelseende;* **twenty-twenty vision** = perfect normal vision *normal syn*

visit ['vɪzɪt] **1** *subst.* **(a)** short stay with someone (especially to comfort a patient) *besök;* **the patient is too weak to have any visits; he is allowed visits of ten minutes only (b)** short stay with a professional person *besök;* **they had a visit from the district nurse; she paid a visit to the chiropodist; on the patient's last visit to the physiotherapy unit, nurses noticed a great improvement in her walking 2** *vb.* to stay a short time with someone *besöka, hälsa på;* **I an going to visit my brother in hospital; she was visited by the health visitor; visiting times** = times of day when friends are allowed into a hospital to visit patients *besökstider*

visitor ['vɪzɪtə] *subst.* person who visits *besökare;* **visitors are allowed into the hospital on Sunday afternoons; how many visitors did you have this week?; health visitor** = registered nurse with qualifications in midwifery or obstetrics and preventive medicine, who visits mothers and babies, and sick people in their homes and advises on treatment *slags barnmorska (distriktssköterska) som gör hembesök*

viska ➪ **whisper**

viskning ➪ **whisper**

viskositet ➪ **viscosity**

viskös ➪ **viscous**

vismut ➪ **bismuth**

vismutsalter ➪ **bismuth**

vistas ➪ **stay**

vistelse ⇨ **stay**

visual ['vɪʒu(ə)l] *adj.* referring to sight *or* vision *visuell, syn-;* **visual acuity** = being able to see objects clearly *visus, synskärpa;* **visual axis** = the line between the object on which the eye focuses, and the fovea *synaxel;* **visual cortex** = part of the cerebral cortex which receives information about sight *syncentrum;* **visual field** = field of vision *or* area which can be seen without moving the eye *synfält, synkrets;* **visual purple** *or* **rhodopsin** = purple pigment in the rods of the retina which makes it possible to see in bad light *rodopsin, synpurpur*

visus ⇨ **acuity, vision, visual**

vit ⇨ **white, leuco-**

vitae ['vaɪti:] *see* ARBOR

vital ['vaɪt(ə)l] *adj.* most important for life *vital(-), livsnödvändig, livsviktig;* **if circulation is stopped, vital nerve cells begin to die in a few minutes; oxygen is vital to the human system; vital capacity** = largest amount of air which a person can exhale *vitalkapacitet;* **vital centre** = group of nerve cells in the brain which govern a particular function of the body (such as the five senses) *centrum för livsnödvändig funktion;* **vital organs** = the most important organs in the body, without which a human being cannot live (such as the heart, lungs, brain) *vitala organ;* **vital signs** = measurement of pulse, breathing and temperature *vitala tecken, värden på vitala funktioner;* **vital statistics** = official statistics relating to the population of a place (such as the percentage of live births per thousand, the incidence of a certain disease, the numbers of births and deaths) *vitalstatistik, befolkningsstatistik*

vitalkapacitet ⇨ **vital**

vitalstatistik ⇨ **vital**

vitamin ['vɪtəmɪn] *subst.* essential substance not synthesized in the body, but found in most foods, and needed for good health *vitamin;* **vitamin deficiency** = lack of necessary vitamins *vitaminbrist;* **he is suffering from Vitamin A deficiency; Vitamin C deficiency causes scurvy** *see also section on vitamins in the Supplement*

vitaminbrist ⇨ **vitamin**

vitelline sac [vɪˌtelaɪn 'sæk] *subst.* sac attached to an embryo, where the blood cells first form *äggulesäcken, gulesäcken*

vitellus [vɪ'teləs] *subst.* yolk of an egg (ovum) *vitellus, äggula, näringsgula*

vitiligo [ˌvɪti'laɪgəʊ] *or* **leucoderma** [ˌlu:kə(ʊ)'dɜ:mə] *subst.* condition where white patches appear on the skin *vitiligo, leukodermi*

vitium ⇨ **hole**

vitreous body [ˌvɪtriəs 'bɒdi] *or* **vitreous humour** [ˌvɪtriəs 'hju:mə] *subst.* transparent jelly which fills the main cavity behind the lens in the eye *corpus vitreum, glaskroppen*

vitro ['vi:triəʊ] *see* IN VITRO

Vitus ['vaɪtəs] *see* ST VITUS

vitögat ⇨ **white**

viviparous [vɪ'vɪp(ə)rəs] *adj.* (animal) which bears live young (such as humans, as opposed to birds and reptiles which lay eggs) *vivipar, som föder levande ungar*

vivisection [ˌvɪvɪ'sekʃ(ə)n] *subst.* dissecting a living animal as an experiment *vivisektion*

VOC ⇨ **valvular**

vocal ['vəʊk(ə)l] *adj.* referring to the voice *vokal, röst-, stäm-, tal-;* **vocal cords** *or* **vocal folds** *see* CORD; **vocal fremitus** = vibration of the chest as a patient speaks *or* coughs *fremitus vocalis (pectoralis), stämfremitus, pektoralfremitus;* **vocal ligament** = ligament in the centre of the vocal cords **vocal ligaments** *ligamenta vocalia, plica(e) vocalis(es), inlagrat i äkta stämbanden;* **vocal resonance** = sound heard by a doctor when he listens through a stethoscope while a patient is speaking *förstärkt talljud i stetoskop*

VOC congenitum ⇨ **congenital**

voice [vɔɪs] *subst.* sound made when a person speaks *or* sings *röst, stämma;* **the doctor has a quiet and comforting voice; I didn't recognize your voice over the phone; to lose one's voice** = not to be able to speak because of a throat infection *tappa (förlora) rösten;* **his voice has broken** = his voice has become deeper and adult, with the onset of puberty *han har kommit i målbrottet*

voice box ['vɔɪs ˌbɒks] *or* **larynx** ['lærɪŋ(k)s] *subst.* organ at the back of the throat which produces sounds *larynx, struphuvudet*

COMMENT: the voice box is a hollow organ containing the vocal cords, situated behind the Adam's apple

vokal ⇨ **vocal**

volar ['vəʊlə] *adj.* referring to the palm of the hand *or* sole of the foot *volar, handflate-, fotsule-*

volatile ['vɒlətaɪ(ə)l] *adj.* (liquid) which turns into gas at normal room temperature *flyktig;* **volatile oils** = concentrated oils from plants used in cosmetics and as antiseptics *flyktiga (eteriska) oljor*

volitantes [ˌvɒlɪ'tæntiːz] *see* MUSCAE

volition [və(ʊ)'lɪʃ(ə)n] *subst.* ability to use the will *vilja*

Volkmann's canal ['fɒlkmɑːnz kəˌnæl] *subst.* canal running across compact bone, carrying blood to the Haversian systems *Volkmanns (volkmannsk) kanal*

Volkmann's contracture ['fɒlkmɑːnz kən'træktʃə] *see* CONTRACTURE

volontär ⇨ **volunteer**

volsella [vɒl'selə] *or* **vulsella** [vʌl'selə] *subst.* type of forceps with hooks at the end of each arm *haktång*

volume ['vɒljuːm] *subst.* amount of a substance *volym, mängd;* **blood volume** = total amount of blood in the body *blodvolym;* **stroke volume** = amount of blood pumped out of a ventricle at each heartbeat *slagvolym*

voluntary ['vɒlənt(ə)ri] *adj.* not forced *or* (action) done because one wishes to do it *voluntär, frivillig;* **voluntary admission** = admitting a patient into a psychiatric hospital with the consent of the patient *frivillig inläggning;* **voluntary movement** = movement (such as walking *or* speaking) directed by the person's willpower, using voluntary muscles *frivillig rörelse;* **voluntary muscles** = muscles which are moved by the willpower of the person acting through the brain *skelettmuskel*

COMMENT: voluntary muscles work in pairs, where one contracts and pulls, while the other relaxes to allow the bone to move

volunteer [ˌvɒlən'tɪə] **1** *subst.* person who offers to do something freely *or* without being paid *volontär, frivillig;* **the hospital relies on volunteers to help with sports for handicapped children; they are asking for volunteers to test the new cold cure 2** *vb.* to offer to do something freely *frivilligt erbjuda (ge, lämna, åta sig);* **the research team volunteered to test the new drug on themselves**

volvulus ['vɒlvjʊləs] *subst.* condition where a loop of intestine is twisted and blocked, so cutting off its blood supply *volvulus, tarmvred*

volym ⇨ **capacity, volume**

vomer ['vəʊmə] *subst.* thin flat vertical bone in the septum of the nose *vomer, plogbenet*

vomering ⇨ **vomit, vomitus**

vomica ['vɒmɪkə] *subst.* **(a)** cavity in the lungs containing pus *vomica, kavern, abscesshåla* **(b)** vomiting pus from the throat or lungs *vomica, upphostning av var*

vomit ['vɒmɪt] **1** *subst.* vomitus *or* partly digested food which has been brought up into the mouth from the stomach *vomitus, vomering, kräkning, uppkastning;* **his bed was covered with vomit; she died after choking on her own vomit 2** *vb.* to bring up partly digested food from the stomach into the mouth *kräkas, kasta upp, spy;* **he had a fever, and then started to vomit; she vomited her breakfast**

vomiting ['vɒmɪtɪŋ] *or* **emesis** ['eməsɪs] *subst.* being sick *or* bringing up vomit into the mouth *emes, kräkning, uppkastning*

vomitus ['vɒmɪtəs] *subst.* vomit *vomitus, vomering, kräkning, uppkastning*

von Hippel-Lindau syndrome [vɒn ˌhɪpəl'lɪndaʊ ˌsɪndrəʊm] *subst.* disease in which angiomas of the brain are related to angiomas and cysts in other parts of the body *Hippel-Lindaus sjukdom*

von Recklinghausen's disease [vɒn 'reklɪŋhaʊzənz dɪˌziːz] *subst.* **(a)** = NEUROFIBROMATOSIS **(b)** osteitis fibrosa *or* weakness of the bones caused by excessive activity of the thyroid gland *osteodystrophia fibrosa (cystica) generalizata, von Recklinghausens sjukdom*

von Willebrand's disease [vɒn 'vɪlɪbrændz dɪˌziːz] *subst.* hereditary blood disease where the mucous membrane starts to bleed without any apparent reason *Willebrands sjukdom*

voyeurism [vwaɪ'ɜːrɪz(ə)m] *subst.* condition where a person experiences sexual pleasure by watching others having intercourse *voyeurism*

vredesutbrott ⇨ **temper**

vricka ⇨ **distort, twist, sprain**

vrickning ⇨ **distortion, twist, sprain**

vrida (på) ⇨ **turn**

vrida (ur led) ⇨ **twist**

vridled ⇨ **pivot**

vrist- ⇨ **tarsal, tars(o)-**

vristbenen ⇨ **tarsal**

vristen ⇨ **ankle, tarsus**

VS ⇨ **sexually transmitted disease (STD), social, venereal disease (VD)**

vu [vu:] *see* DEJA VU

vulgaris [vʌl'geərɪs] *see* ACNE, LUPUS

vulnerable ['vʌln(ə)rəb(ə)l] *adj.* likely to catch (a disease) because of being in a weakened state *vulnerabel, sårbar, känslig;* **premature babies are especially vulnerable to infection**

vulnus ⇨ **wound**

vulsella [vʌl'selə] = VOLSELLA

vulva ['vʌlvə] *subst.* a woman's external sexual organs, at the opening leading to the vagina *vulva, kvinnliga blygden; see also* KRAUROSIS

COMMENT: the vulva is formed of folds (the labia), surrounding the clitoris and the entrance to the vagina

vulvectomy [ˌvʌl'vektəmi] *subst.* surgical operation to remove the vulva *vulvektomi*

vulvitis [vʌl'vaɪtɪs] *subst.* inflammation of the vulva, causing intense irritation *vulvit*

vulv(o)- ['vʌlv(əʊ), ˌ--] *prefix* referring to the vulva *vulv(o)-*

vulvovaginitis [ˌvʌlvəʊˌvædʒɪ'naɪtɪs] *subst.* inflammation of the vulva and vagina *vulvovaginit*

NOTE: for other terms referring to the vulva see words beginning with **episio-**

vuxen ⇨ **adult, grown-up**

vådlig ⇨ **dangerous**

våg ⇨ **balance, scale**

vågrät ⇨ **horizontal**

våldsam ⇨ **violent**

våldsamt ⇨ **violently**

vålla ⇨ **provoke**

vård ⇨ **assistance, attention, care, nursing**

vårda ⇨ **attend, attend to, care for, look after, nurse, take care of**

vårdare ⇨ **carer**

vårdavdelning ⇨ **ward**

vårdcentral ⇨ **health**

vårdhem ⇨ **nursing**

vårdlärare ⇨ **tutor**

vårdplan ⇨ **care plan**

vårta ⇨ **verruca, wart**

vårtgården ⇨ **areola**

vårtliknande ⇨ **papillary**

vårtutskottet ⇨ **mastoid**

våt ⇨ **wet**

våtvarmt omslag ⇨ **stupe**

väcka ⇨ **awaken, elicit**

väcka (upp) ⇨ **awake, wake**

väderspänd ⇨ **flatulent**

väderspänning(ar) ⇨ **flatulence, gas, meteorism, wind**

väga ⇨ **weigh**

vägg ⇨ **paries, wall**

väggbukhinnan ⇨ **peritoneum**

vägglus ⇨ **bedbug**

väl ⇨ **welfare, well-being**

välbefinnande ⇨ **well-being**

välfärd ⇨ **welfare, well-being**

välja ⇨ **select**

vända (på) ⇨ **turn**

vändning ⇨ **version**

vändning på fot ⇨ **podalic version**

vändpunkt ⇨ **crisis**

vänlig ⇨ **gentle**

vänster ⇨ **left**

vänster- ⇨ **left-hand**

vänsterhänt ⇨ **left-handed**

vänsterhänthet ⇨ **left-handedness**

vänta ⇨ **wait**

väntelista ⇨ **wait**

väntetid ⇨ **wait**

väntrum ⇨ **wait**

värd ⇨ **host**

värddjur ⇨ **host**

värde ⇨ **reading, value**

värk ⇨ **ache, dolor, pain**

"värk" ⇨ **contraction**

värka ⇨ **ache, hurt**

värkande ⇨ **aching**

värkar ⇨ **contraction, labour, pain**

Världshälsoorganisationen ⇨ **World Health Organization (WHO)**

värme ⇨ **calor, heat**

värme- ⇨ **thermal, thermo-**

värmebehandling ⇨ **therapy**

värmekramp ⇨ **heat**

värmeokänslighet ⇨ **thermal, thermoanaesthesia**

värmereceptor ⇨ **thermoreceptor**

värmeslag ⇨ **exhaustion, heat**

värmeutslag ⇨ **heat, miliaria**

värmeälskande ⇨ **thermophilic**

värva ⇨ **recruit**

väsa ⇨ **wheeze**

väsande ⇨ **sibilant, wheezy**

väte ⇨ **hydrogen**

vätska ⇨ **fluid, humour, liquid, water**

vätska, applicera utvärtes ⇨ **paint**

vätskande sår ⇨ **sore**

vätskeersättning ⇨ **Hartmann's solution**

vätskefyllnad ⇨ **turgor**

vätskeprov, ta ⇨ **tap**

väv ⇨ **tissue**

vävnad ⇨ **tissue**

vävnads- ⇨ **histo-**

vävnadsdöd ⇨ **necrobiosis**

vävnadskompatibla ⇨ **histocompatible**

vävnadskultur ⇨ **tissue**

vävnadsskada ⇨ **damage**

vävnadstypning ⇨ **tissue**

vävnadsupplösning ⇨ **histolysis**

växa ⇨ **grow**

växande ⇨ **vegetative**

(växa och) frodas ⇨ **thrive**

växelvarm ⇨ **poikilothermic**

växelvård ⇨ **day**

växling ⇨ **variation**

växt ⇨ **growth, horn**

växtvärk ⇨ **growing pains**

Ww

wad [wɒd] *subst.* pad of material used to put on a wound *tuss, vaddtuss;* **the nurse put a wad of absorbant cotton over the sore**

wadding ['wɒdɪŋ] *subst.* material used to make a wad *vadd, cellstoff;* **put a layer of cotton wadding over the eye**

waist [weɪst] *subst.* narrow part of the body below the chest and above the buttocks *midjan, livet;* **he measures 85 centimetres around the waist**

wait [weɪt] *vb.* to stay somewhere until something happens *or* someone arrives *vänta, stanna;* **he has been waiting for his operation for six months; there are ten patients waiting to see Dr Smith; waiting list** = list of patients waiting for admission to hospital usually for treatment of non-urgent disorders *väntelista;* **hospital waiting lists are getting longer because of the shortage of nurses; waiting room** = room where patients wait at a doctor's *or* dentist's surgery *väntrum;* **please sit in the waiting room - the doctor will see you in ten minutes; waiting time** = period between the time when the name of a patient has been put on the waiting list and his admission into hospital *väntetid*

wake [weɪk] *vb.* (i) to interrupt someone's sleep *väcka (upp);* (ii) to stop sleeping *vakna (upp);* **the nurse woke the patient** *or* **the patients was woken by the nurse; the patient had to be woken to have his injection** NOTE: **wakes - waking - woke - has woken**

wakeful ['weɪkf(ə)l] *adj.* being wide awake *or* not wanting to sleep *vaken, sömnlös*

wakefulness ['weɪkf(ə)lnəs] *subst.* being wide awake *vakenhet, vaka, sömnlöshet*

wake up [ˌweɪk 'ʌp] *vb.* to stop sleeping *vakna (upp);* **the old man woke up in the middle of the night and started calling for the nurse**

Waldeyer's ring ['vɑːldaɪəz ˌrɪŋ] *subst.* ring of lymphoid tissue made by the tonsils *Waldeyers svalgring, lymfatiska svalgringen*

walk [wɔːk] *vb.* to go on foot *gå;* **the baby is learning to walk; he walked when he was only eleven months old; she can walk a few steps with a Zimmer**

wall [wɔːl] *subst.* side part of an organ *or* a passage in the body *vägg;* **an ulcer formed in the wall of the duodenum; the doctor made an incision in the abdominal wall; they removed a fibroma from the wall of the uterus** *or* **from the uterine wall**

wall eye ['wɔːl ˌaɪ] *subst.* eye which is very pale *or* eye which is squinting so strongly that only the white sclera is visible *färglöst öga, öga med ogenomskinlig vit hornhinna*

Wangensteen tube ['wæŋgənstiːn ˌtjuːb] *subst.* tube which is passed into the stomach to remove the stomach's contents by suction *slags ventrikelsond*

ward [wɔːd] *subst.* room or set of rooms in a hospital, with beds for the patients *sal, rum, avdelning, vårdavdelning;* **he is in Ward 8B; the children's ward is at the end of the corridor; ward sister** = senior nurse in charge of a ward *avdelningsföreståndare;* **accident ward** *or* **casualty ward** = ward for urgent accident victims *akutmottagning, olycksfallsavdelning;* **emergency ward** = ward for patients who require urgent attention *akutmottagning, olycksfallsavdelning;* **geriatric ward** = ward for the treatment of geriatric patients *geriatrisk avdelning;* **isolation ward** = special ward where patients suffering from dangerous infectious diseases can be kept isolated from other patients *isoleringsavdelning;* **medical ward** = ward for patients who are not undergoing surgery *medicinavdelning, medicinsk (vård)avdelning;* **surgical ward** = ward for patients who have undergone surgery *kirurgavdelning, kirurgisk (vård)avdelning*

warm [wɔːm] *adj.* quite hot *or* pleasantly hot *varm;* **the patients need to be kept warm in cold weather**
NOTE: **warm - warmer - warmest**

warn [wɔːn] *vb.* to tell someone that a danger is possible *(för)varna, varsko;* **the children were warned about the dangers of solvent abuse; the doctors warned her that her husband would not live more than a few weeks**

warning ['wɔːnɪŋ] *subst.* telling someone about a danger *varning, förvarning;* **there's a warning on the bottle of medicine, saying that it should be kept away from children; each packet of cigarettes has a government health warning printed on it; the health department has given out warnings about the danger of hypothermia**

wart [wɔːt] *or* **verruca** [vəˈruːkə] *subst.* small hard benign growth on the skin *verruca, vårta;* **common wart** = wart which appears mainly on the hands *verruca simplex (vulgaris), enkel (vanlig) vårta;* **plantar wart** = wart on the sole of the foot *verruca plantaris, fotvårta;* **venereal wart** = wart on the genitals or in the urogenital area *kondylom, venerisk vårta*

COMMENT: warts are caused by a virus, and usually occur on the hands, feet or face

Wassermann reaction (WR) [ˈwɒsəmæn rɪˌækʃ(ə)n (ˌdʌb(ə)ljuːˈɑː)] *or* **Wassermann test** [ˈwɒsəmæn ˌtest] *subst.* blood serum test to see if a patient has syphilis *Wassermanns reaktion, WR*

waste [weɪst] **1** *adj.* useless *or* which has no use *avfalls-, utsöndrings-;* **the veins take blood containing waste carbon dioxide back into the lungs; waste matter is excreted in the faeces or urine; waste product** = substance which is not needed in the body (and is excreted in urine *or* faeces) *avfallsprodukt, utsöndringsprodukt* **2** *vb.* to use more than is needed *slösa (bort);* **the hospital kitchens waste a lot of food**

waste away [ˌweɪst əˈweɪ] *vb.* to become thinner *or* to lose flesh *tyna av (bort), magra;* **when he caught the disease he simply wasted away**

wasting [ˈweɪstɪŋ] *subst.* condition where a person *or* a limb loses weight and becomes thin *borttynande, avmagring;* **wasting disease** = disease which causes severe loss of weight *or* reduction in size (of an organ) *tärande sjukdom*

water [ˈwɔːtə] **1** *subst.* **(a)** common liquid which forms rain, rivers, the sea etc., and which makes up a large part of the body *vatten, vätska;* **can I have a glass of water please? they suffered dehydration from lack of water; water balance** = state where the water lost by the body (in urine *or* perspiration, etc.) is balanced by water absorbed from food and drink *vätskebalans;* **water on the knee** = fluid in the knee joint under the kneecap, caused by a blow on the knee *vatten i knät (knäna)* **(b)** urine *urin;* **he passed a lot of water during the night; she noticed blood streaks in her water; the nurse asked him to give a sample of his water (c) the waters** = amniotic fluid *or* fluid in the amnion in which a fetus floats *liquor amni, amnionvattnet, amnionvätskan, fostervattnet* **2** *vb.* to fill with tears *or* saliva *vattnas, vattna sig, tåras;* **onions made his eyes water; her mouth watered when she saw the ice cream; watering eye** = eye which fills with tears because of an irritation *öga som vattnas (tåras)*

COMMENT: since the body is formed of about 50% water, a normal adult needs to drink about 2.5 litres (5 pints) of fluid each day. Water taken into the body is passed out again as urine or sweat

water bed [ˈwɔːtə ˌbed] *subst.* mattress made of a large sack filled with water, used to avoid bedsores developing *vattensäng*

waterbrash [ˈwɔːtəbræʃ] *subst.* condition caused by dyspepsia, where there is a burning feeling in the stomach and the mouth suddenly fills with acid saliva *halsbränna*

Waterhouse-Friderichsen syndrome [ˌwɔːtəhaʊsˌfriːdəˈrɪks(ə)n ˌsɪndrəʊm] *subst.* condition caused by blood poisoning with meningococci, where the tissues of the adrenal glands die and haemorrhage *Waterhouse-Friderichsens syndrom*

waterproof [ˈwɔːtəpruːf] *adj.* which will not let water through *vattentät, impregnerad;* **put a waterproof sheet on the baby's bed**

water sac [ˈwɔːtə sæk] *or* **bag of waters** [ˌbæg əv ˈwɔːtəz] = AMNION

Waterston's operation [ˈwɔːtəstənz ˌɒpəˌreɪʃ(ə)n] *subst.* surgical operation to treat Fallot's tetralogy, where the right pulmonary artery is joined to the ascending aorta *operation av Fallots tetrad*

waterworks [ˈwɔːtəwɜːks] *subst.* *(informal)* the urinary system *urinvägarna;* **there's nothing wrong with his waterworks**

watery [ˈwɔːtəri] *adj.* liquid, like water *vattnig, vattenhaltig;* **he passed some watery stools** NOTE: for other terms referring to water, see words beginning with **hydr-**

Watson knife [ˈwɒts(ə)n ˌnaɪf] *subst.* type of very sharp surgical knife for skin transplants *slags kniv som används vid hudtransplantation, "hyvel"*

wax [wæks] *subst.* **(a)** soft yellow substance produced by bees *or* made from petroleum *vax;* **hot wax treatment** = treatment for arthritis in which the joints are painted with hot liquid wax *behandling med varmt vax* **(b) ear wax** *or* **cerumen** = wax which forms in the ear *cerumen, öronvax*

WBC [ˌdʌb(ə)ljuːbiːˈsiː] = WHITE BLOOD CELL

weak [wi:k] *adj.* not strong *svag, klen, kraftlös, skröplig;* **after his illness he was very weak; she is too weak to dress herself; he is allowed to drink weak tea or coffee; weak pulse** = pulse which is not strong *or* which is not easy to feel *svag puls*
NOTE: **weak - weaker - weakest**

weaken ['wi:k(ə)n] *vb.* to make something *or* someone weak *försvaga;* to become weak *försvagas;* **he was weakened by the disease and could not resist further infection; the swelling is caused by a weakening of the wall of the artery**

weakness ['wi:knəs] *subst.* not being strong *svaghet, klenhet, kraftlöshet, skröplighet;* **the doctor noticed the weakness of the patient's pulse**

weal [wi:l] *or* **wheal** [wi:l] *subst.* small area of skin which swells because of a sharp blow *or* an insect bite *strimma, rand*

wean [wi:n] *vb.* (i) to make a baby start to eat solid food after having only had liquids to drink *börja vänja barn vid fast föda;* (ii) to make a baby start to drink from a bottle and start eating solid food after having been only breastfed *avvänja;* **the baby was breastfed for two months and then was gradually weaned onto the bottle**

wear [weə] *vb.* to become damaged through being used *nötas, slitas, bli nött (sliten);* **the cartilage of the knee was worn from too much exercise** NOTE: **wears - wearing - wore - has worn**

wear and tear [ˌweərən'teə] *subst.* normal use which affects an organ *slitage, förslitning, påfrestning(ar);* **a heart has to stand a lot of wear and tear; the wear and tear of a strenuous job has begun to affect his heart**

wear off [ˌweər'ɒf] *vb.* to disappear gradually *gå över (bort), minska, avta;* **the effect of the pain killer will wear off after a few hours; he started to open his eyes, as the anaesthetic wore off**

Weber-Christian disease [ˌwebə'krɪstʃ(ə)n dɪˌzi:z] *subst.* type of panniculitis where the liver and spleen become enlarged *Weber-Christians sjukdom*

Weber's test ['veɪbəz ˌtest] *subst.* test to see if both ears hear correctly, where a tuning fork is struck and the end placed on the head *Webers test (jfr Rinne)*

Wegener's granulomatosis ['vegənəz ˌgrænjʊləʊmə'təʊsɪs] *subst.* disease of connective tissue, where the nasal passages, lungs and kidneys are inflamed and ulcerated, with formation of granulomas; it is usually fatal *granulomatosis Wegener, Wegeners granulomatos*

weigh [weɪ] *vb.* (i) to measure how heavy something is *väga;* (ii) to have a certain weight *väga;* **the nurse weighed the baby on the scales; she weighed seven pounds (3.5 kilos) at birth; a woman weighs less than a man of similar height; the doctor asked him how much he weighed; I weigh 120 pounds** *or* **I weigh 54 kilos**

weight [weɪt] *subst.* **(a)** how heavy a person is *vikt;* **what's the patient's weight?; her weight is only 105 pounds** = she weighs only 105 pounds *hon väger bara 105 pund (c 48 kilo);* **to lose weight** = to get thinner *magra, gå ned i vikt;* **she's trying to lose weight before she goes on holiday; to put on weight** = to become fatter *öka (gå upp) i vikt;* **he's put on a lot of weight in the last few months; weight gain** *or* **gain in weight** = becoming fatter *or* heavier *viktökning;* **weight loss** = action of losing weight *or* of becoming thinner *viktminskning;* **weight loss can be a symptom of certain types of cancer (b)** something which is heavy *börda;* **don't lift heavy weights, you may hurt your back**

weightlessness ['weɪtləsnəs] *subst.* state where the body seems to weigh nothing (as experienced by astronauts) *viktlöshet, tyngdlöshet*

Weil-Felix reaction [ˌvaɪl'feɪlɪks rɪˌækʃ(ə)n] *or* **Weil-Felix test** [ˌvaɪl'feɪlɪks ˌtest] *subst.* test to see if the patient has typhus, where the patient's serum is tested for antibodies against Proteus vulgaris *Weil-Felix reaktion*

Weil's disease ['vaɪlz dɪˌzi:z] = LEPTOSPIROSIS

welder's flash [ˌweldəz 'flæʃ] *subst.* condition where the eye is badly damaged by very bright light *ögonskada efter exposition för starkt ljus, svetsblände*

welfare ['welfeə] *subst.* **(a)** good health *or* good living conditions *väl, välfärd;* **they look after the welfare of the old people in the town (b)** money paid by the government to people who need it *socialbidrag, understöd;* **he exists on welfare payments**

well [wel] *adj.* healthy *frisk, kry, bra;* **he's not a well man; you're looking very well after your holiday; he's quite well again after his flu; he's not very well, and has had to stay in bed; well-women clinic** = clinic which specializes in preventive medicine for women (such as screening) and giving advice on pregnancy, contraception and the menopause *slags klinik för gynekologisk och preventivmedelsrådgivning*

well-being [ˌwel'biːɪŋ] *subst.* being in good health *or* in good living conditions *väl, välfärd, välbefinnande;* **she is responsible for the well-being of the patients under her care**

wen [wen] *subst.* cyst which forms in a sebaceous gland *steatom, aterom, talg(körtel)cysta*

Wernicke's encephalopathy ['vɜːnɪkiːz enˌkefə'lɒpəθi] *subst.* condition caused by lack of vitamin B (often in alcoholics), where the patient is delirious, moves his eyes about rapidly (nystagmus), walks unsteadily and is subject to constant vomiting *Wernickes encefalopati*

Wertheim's operation ['vɜːthaɪmz ˌɒpəˌreɪʃ(ə)n] *subst.* type of hysterectomy *or* surgical operation to remove the womb, the lymph nodes which are next to it, and most of the vagina, the ovaries and the tubes, as treatment for cancer of the womb *Wertheims operation*

wet [wet] **1** *adj.* not dry *or* covered in liquid *våt, blöt, fuktig;* **he got wet waiting for the bus in the rain and caught a cold; the baby has nappy rash from wearing a wet nappy** NOTE: **wet - wetter - wettest 2** *vb.* to urinate (in bed) *kissa (på sig), väta (ner);* **he is eight years old and he still wets his bed every night; bedwetting** = passing urine in bed at night *sängvätning*

wet dressing [ˌwet 'dresɪŋ] *subst. see* COMPRESS

Wharton's duct ['wɔːt(ə)nz ˌdʌkt] *subst.* duct which takes saliva into the mouth from the salivary glands under the lower jaw *or* submandibular salivary glands *ductus submandibularis, Whartons gång*

Wharton's jelly ['wɔːt(ə)nz ˌdʒeli] *subst.* jelly-like tissue in the umbilical cord *Whartons sylta*

wheal [wiː(ə)l] = WEAL

wheel [wiː(ə)l] *vb.* to push along something which has wheels *rulla, köra, dra, skjuta;* **the orderly wheeled the trolley into the operating theatre**

wheelchair ['wiː(ə)ltʃeə] *subst.* chair with wheels in which an invalid can sit and move around *rullstol;* **he manages to get around in a wheelchair; she has been confined to a wheelchair since her accident**

Wheelhouse's operation ['wiː(ə)lhaʊsɪz ˌɒpəˌreɪʃ(ə)n] *or* **urethrotomy** [ˌjʊəri'θrɒtəmi] *subst.* surgical operation to relieve blockage of the urethra by making an incision into the urethra *uretrotomi*

wheeze [wiːz] **1** *subst.* whistling noise in the bronchi *väsande (rosslande, pipande) ljud;* **the doctor listened to his wheezes 2** *vb.* to make a whistling sound when breathing *väsa, rossla, pipa, andas med väsande (rosslande, pipande) ljud;* **when she has an attack of asthma, she wheezes and has difficulty in breathing**

wheezing ['wiːzɪŋ] *subst.* whistling noise in the bronchi when breathing *väsande (rosslande, pipande) ljud*

> COMMENT: wheezing is often found in asthmatic patients or associated with bronchitis

wheezy ['wiːzi] *adj.* making a whistling sound when breathing *väsande, rosslig, pipande, andfådd;* **he was quite wheezy when he stopped running**

whiplash injury ['wɪplæʃ ˌɪndʒ(ə)ri] *subst.* injury to the vertebrae in the neck, caused when the head jerks backwards, often occurring in a car crash *whiplash(skada), whiplashsyndrom, pisksnärtskada*

Whipple's disease ['wɪp(ə)lz dɪˌziːz] *subst.* disease where the patient has difficulty in absorbing nutrients and passes fat in the faeces, where the joints are inflamed and the lymph glands enlarged *intestinal lipodystrofi, Whipples sjukdom*

Whipple's operation ['wɪp(ə)lz ˌɒpəˌreɪʃ(ə)n] = PANCREATECTOMY

whipworm ['wɪpwɜːm] *or* **Trichocephalus** [ˌtrɪkəʊ'sef(ə)ləs] *or* **Trichuris** [trɪ'kjʊərɪs] *subst.* thin round parasitic worm which infests the caecum *Trichuris trichiura, piskmask*

whisper ['wɪspə] **1** *subst.* speaking very quietly *viskning;* **she has a sore throat and can only speak in a whisper 2** *vb.* to speak in a very quiet voice *viska;* **he whispered to the nurse that he wanted something to drink**

white [waɪt] **1** *adj. & subst.* of a colour like snow or milk *vit;* **white patches developed on his skin; her hair has turned quite white;**

white blood cell (WBC) *or* **leucocyte** = blood cell which contains a nucleus, is formed in bone marrow, and creates antibodies *leukocyt, vit blodkropp;* **white commissure** = part of the white matter in the spinal cord near the central canal *commisura (ventralis) alba, vit kommissur;* **white leg** *or* **milk leg** *or* **phlegmasia alba dolens** = condition which affects women after childbirth, where a leg becomes pale and inflamed *phlegmasia alba dolens;* **white matter** = nerve tissue in the central nervous system which contains more myelin than grey matter *substantia alba, vit substans*
NOTE: **white - whiter - whitest 2** *subst.* main part of the eye which is white *ögonvitan, vitögat;* **the whites of his eyes turned yellow when he developed jaundice** *see also* LEUCORRHOEA

whitlow ['wɪtləʊ] *or* **felon** ['felən] *subst.* inflammation caused by infection, near the nail in the fleshy part of the tip of a finger *panaritium, nagelböld, fulslag, infektion i fingerpulpan; see also* PARONYCHIA

WHO [ˌdʌb(ə)lju:eɪtʃ'əʊ] = WORLD HEALTH ORGANIZATION

whoop [wu:p, hu:p] *subst.* loud noise made when inhaling by a person suffering from whooping cough *kikning*

whooping cough ['hu:pɪŋ kɒf] *or* **pertussis** [pə'tʌsɪs] *subst.* infectious disease caused by **Bordetella pertussis** affecting the bronchial tubes, common in children, and sometimes very serious *pertussis, kikhosta*

> COMMENT: the patient coughs very badly and makes a characteristic "whoop" when he breathes in after a coughing fit. Whooping cough can lead to pneumonia, and is treated with antibiotics. Vaccination against whooping cough is given to infants

Widal reaction [vi:'dɑ:l rɪˌækʃ(ə)n] *or* **Widal test** [vi:'dɑ:l ˌtest] *subst.* test to detect typhoid fever *Vidals prov*

> COMMENT: a sample of the patient's blood is put into a solution containing typhoid bacilli *or* anti-typhoid serum is added to a sample of bacilli from the patient's faeces. If the bacilli agglutinate (i.e. form into groups) this indicates that the patient is suffering from typhoid fever

widen ['waɪd(ə)n] *vb.* to make wider *vidga;* **an operation to widen the blood vessels near the heart**

widespread ['waɪdspred] *adj.* affecting a large area of a country *or* a large number of people *allmän, allmänt utbredd (spridd);* **the government advised widespread immunization; glaucoma is widespread in the northern part of the country**

will [wɪl] *subst.* power of the mind to decide to do something *vilja*

Willebrands sjukdom ⇨ **von Willebrand's disease**

Willis ['wɪlɪs] *see* CIRCLE OF WILLIS

Willis fenomen ⇨ **paracusis**

willpower ['wɪlpa(ʊ)ə] *subst.* having a strong will *viljekraft, viljestyrka;* **the patient showed the willpower to start walking again unaided**

Wilm's tumour ['vɪlmz ˌtju:mə] = NEPHROBLASTOMA

Wilson's disease ['wɪls(ə)nz dɪˌzi:z] *or* **hepatolenticular degeneration** [ˌhepətəʊlen'tɪkjʊlə dɪˌdʒenəˌreɪʃ(ə)n] *subst.* hereditary disease where deposits accumulate in the liver and the brain, causing cirrhosis *degeneratio hepatolenticularis, Wilsons sjukdom*

wind [wɪnd] *subst.* (i) flatus *or* gas which forms in the digestive system *flatus, gaser, väder (i magen);* (ii) flatulence *or* accumulation of gas in the digestive system *flatulens, väderspänning(ar), gasfyllnad (i tarmen);* **the baby is suffering from wind; he has pains in the stomach caused by wind; to break wind** = to bring up gas from the stomach *or* to let gas escape from the anus *rapa, släppa sig (väder)*

windchill factor ['wɪn(d)tʃɪl ˌfæktə] *subst.* way of calculating the risk of exposure in cold weather by adding the speed of the wind to the number of degrees of temperature below zero *köldfaktor*

window ['wɪndəʊ] *subst.* small opening in the ear *fönster;* **oval window** *or* **fenestra ovalis** = oval-shaped opening between the middle ear and the inner ear, closed by a membrane and covered by the base of the stapes *fenestra ovalis (vestibuli), ovala fönstret;* **round window** *or* **fenestra rotunda** = round opening closed by a membrane, between the middle ear and the cochlea ⇨ *illustration* EAR *fenestra rotunda (cochleae), runda fönstret*

windpipe ['wɪn(d)paɪp] *or* **trachea** [trə'ki:ə] *subst.* main air passage from the nose and mouth to the lungs *trachea, trakea, luftstrupen*

wink [wɪŋk] *vb.* to close one eye and open it again rapidly *blinka*

wisdom tooth ['wɪzdəm tu:θ] *or* **third molar** [ˌθɜ:d 'məʊlə] *subst.* one of the four last molars in the back of the jaw (which only appear about the age of 20, and sometimes do not appear at all) *dens sapientiae, visdomstand*

witch hazel ['wɪtʃ ˌheɪz(ə)l] *or* **hamamelis** [ˌhæmə'mi:lɪs] *subst.* lotion made from the bark of a tree, used to check bleeding and harden inflamed tissue and bruises *medel berett av hamamelis virginia (häxhassel)*

withdraw [wɪð'drɔ:] *vb.* **(a)** to stop being interested in the world *or* to become isolated *dra sig tillbaka (undan, ur);* **the patient withdrew into himself and refused to eat (b)** to remove (a drug) *or* to stop (a treatment) *dra in (bort, undan), ta bort (ut);* **the doctor decided to withdraw the drug from the patient** NOTE: **withdrawing - withdrew - has withdrawn**

withdrawal [wɪð'drɔ:(ə)l] *subst.* (i) removing of interest *or* becoming isolated *tillbakadragenhet;* (ii) removal of a drug *or* treatment *abstinens, indragning, borttagande;* **withdrawal symptom** = unpleasant physical condition (vomiting *or* headaches *or* fever) which occurs when a patient stops taking an addictive drug *abstinenssymtom*

> QUOTE she was in the early stages of physical withdrawal from heroin and showed classic symptoms: sweating, fever, sleeplessness and anxiety
>
> **Nursing Times**

wolffska kroppen ⇨ **mesonephros**

woman ['wʊmən] *subst.* female adult person *kvinna;* **it is a common disease of women of 45 to 60 years of age; on average, women live longer than men; women's ward** *or* **women's hospital** = ward *or* hospital for female patients *kvinnosal, kvinnoavdelning, kvinnosjukhus; see also* WELL WOMEN CLINIC NOTE: plural is **women.** Note that for medical terms referring to women see words beginning with **gyn-**

womb [wu:m] *or* **uterus** ['ju:t(ə)rəs] *subst.* hollow organ in a woman's pelvic cavity in which a fertilized ovum develops into a fetus *uterus, livmodern*
NOTE: for other terms referring to the womb see words beginning with **hyster-, hystero-, metr-, metro-, utero-**

wood [wʊd] *subst.* material that comes from trees *trä;* **wood alcohol** = methyl alcohol, a poisonous alcohol used as fuel *metylalkohol, metanol, träsprit*

Wood's lamp ['wʊdz ˌlæmp] *subst.* lamp which allows a doctor to see fluorescence in the hair of a patient suffering from fungal infection *Woods lampa*

woolsorter's disease ['wʊlsɔ:təz dɪˌzi:z] *subst.* form of anthrax which affects the lungs *slags mjältbrand*

word [wɜ:d] *subst.* separate piece of language, in writing and speech, not joined to other separate pieces *ord;* **there are seven words in this sentence**

word blindness ['wɜ:d blaɪndnəs] *see* ALEXIA

World Health Organization (WHO) [ˌwɜld 'helθ ɔ:gənaɪˌzeɪʃ(ə)n (ˌdʌb(ə)lju:eɪtʃ'əʊ)] *subst.* organization (part of the United Nations Organization) which aims to improve health in the world by teaching *or* publishing information, etc. *Världshälsoorganisationen, WHO*

worm [wɜ:m] *subst.* long thin animal with no legs or backbone, which can infest the human body, especially the intestines *mask; compare* RINGWORM *see also* FLATWORM, HOOKWORM, ROUNDWORM, TAPEWORM, WHIPWORM

worn out [ˌwɔ:n 'aʊt] *adj.* very tired *uttröttad, utsliten;* **he came home worn out after working all day in the hospital; she was worn out by looking after all the children**

wound [wu:nd] **1** *subst.* damage to external tissue which allows blood to escape *vulnus, sår, skada;* **he had a knife wound in his leg; the doctors sutured the wound in his chest; contused wound** = wound caused by a blow, where the skin is bruised, torn and bleeding *vulnus contusum, kontusion(ssår), krossår;* **gunshot wound** = wound caused by a pellet *or* bullet from a gun *vulnus sclopetarium, skottskada, skottsår;* **incised wound** = wound with clear edges, caused by a sharp knife or razor *vulnus incisum, skärsår;* **lacerated wound** = wound where the skin is torn *vulnus laceratum, slitsår, rivsår;* **puncture wound** = wound made by a sharp point which makes a hole in the flesh *vulnus ictum (punctum), sticksår* **2** *vb.* to harm someone by making a hole in the tissue of the body *såra, skada;* **he was wounded three times in the head**

WR [ˌdʌb(ə)lju:'ɑ:] = WASSERMANN REACTION

wrinkle ['rɪŋk(ə)l] *subst.* fold in the skin *rynka, fåra;* **old people have wrinkles on the neck; she had a face lift to remove wrinkles**

wrinkled ['rɪŋk(ə)ld] *adj.* covered with wrinkles *rynkig*

wrist [rɪst] *subst.* joint between the hand and forearm *handled, handlov(e);* **he sprained his wrist and can't play tennis tomorrow; wrist drop** = paralysis of the wrist muscles, where the hand hangs limp, caused by damage to the radial nerve in the upper arm *dropphand, hänghand* NOTE: for other terms referring to the wrist see words beginning with **carp-** = HAND

COMMENT: the wrist is formed of eight small bones in the hand which articulate with the bones in the forearm. The joint allows the hand to rotate and move downwards and sideways. The joint is easily fractured or sprained

writer's cramp [ˌraɪtəz 'kræmp] *subst.* painful spasm of the muscles in the forearm and hand which comes from writing too much *skrivkramp*

wry neck ['raɪ ˌnek] *or* **wryneck** ['raɪˌnek] *or* **torticollis** [ˌtɔːti'kɒlɪs] *subst.* deformity of the neck, where the head is twisted to one side by contraction of the sternocleidomastoid muscle *torticollis, halsvred, nackspärr*

Wuchereria [ˌvʊkə'rɪəriə] *subst.* type of tiny nematode worm which infests the lymph system, causing elephantiasis *Wuchereria, slags trådmask*

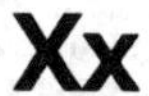

X ⇨ **oocyesis, pregnancy**

xantelasm ⇨ **xanthelasma**

xantemi ⇨ **carotenaemia**

xanth- ['zænθ, ˌ-, zæn'θ] *or* **xantho-** ['zænθə(ʊ), ˌ--] *prefix* meaning yellow *xant(o)-, gul-*

xanthaemia [zæn'θiːmiə] = CAROTENAEMIA

xanthelasma [ˌzænθə'læzmə] *subst.* formation of little yellow fatty tumours on the eyelids *xantelasm, xantom*

xanthochromia [ˌzænθə(ʊ)'krəʊmiə] *subst.* yellow colour of the skin as in jaundice *xantokromi, gulfärgning*

xanthoma [zæn'θəʊmə] *subst.* yellow fatty mass (often on the eyelids and hands), found in patients with a high level of cholesterol in the blood *xantom* NOTE: plural is **xanthomata**

xanthomatosis [ˌzænθə(ʊ)mə'təʊsɪs] *subst.* condition where several small masses of yellow fatty substance appear in the skin or some internal organs, caused by an excess of fat in the body *xantomatos*

xanthopsia [zæn'θɒpsiə] *subst.* disorder of the eyes, making everything appear yellow *xantopsi*

xanthosis [zæn'θəʊsɪs] *subst.* yellow colouring of the skin, caused by eating too much food containing carotene *xantos*

xantokromi ⇨ **xanthochromia**

xantom ⇨ **xanthelasma, xanthoma**

xantomatos ⇨ **xanthomatosis**

xantopsi ⇨ **xanthopsia**

xantos ⇨ **xanthosis**

X-bent ⇨ **knock-kneed**

X-benthet ⇨ **knock knee**

X chromosome ['eks ˌkrəʊməsəʊm] *subst.* sex chromosome *X-kromosom*

COMMENT: every person has a series of pairs of chromosomes, one of which is always an X chromosome; a normal female has one pair of XX chromosomes, while a male has one XY pair. Defective chromosomes affect sexual development: a person with an XO chromosome pair (i.e. one X chromosome alone) has Turner's syndrome; a person with an extra X chromosome (making an XXY set) has Klinefelter's syndrome. Haemophilia is a disorder linked to the X chromosome

xeno- ['zenə(ʊ), ˌ--] *prefix* meaning different *xeno-*

xenograft ['zenə(ʊ)grɑːft] *or* **heterograft** ['het(ə)rə(ʊ)grɑːft] *subst.* tissue taken from an individual of one species and grafted on an individual of another species *xenograft, xenotransplantat, heterotransplantat*
NOTE: the opposite is **homograft** *or* **allograft**

xenograft ▷ **heterograft**

xenotransplantat ▷ **heterograft, xenograft**

xero- ['zɪərə(ʊ), ˌ--] *prefix* meaning dry *xero-, torr-*

xeroderma [ˌzɪərə(ʊ)'dɜːmə] *subst.* skin disorder where dry scales form on the skin *xerodermi, xeroderma, hudtorrhet*

xerodermi ▷ **xeroderma**

xerophthalmia [ˌzɪərɒf'θælmiə] *subst.* condition of the eye, where the cornea and conjunctiva become dry because of lack of Vitamin A *xeroftalmi, torrögdhet*

xeroradiography [ˌzɪərəʊˌreɪdi'ɒgrəfi] *subst.* X-ray technique used in producing mammograms on selenium plates *slags mammografi*

xerosis [zɪ'rəʊsɪs] *subst.* abnormally dry condition (of skin *or* mucous membrane) *xeros, uttorkning*

xerostomia [ˌzɪərə(ʊ)'stəʊmiə] *subst.* dryness of the mouth, caused by lack of saliva *xerostomi, muntorrhet*

xiphisternal plane [ˌzɪfɪ'stɜːn(ə)l ˌpleɪn] *subst.* imaginary horizontal line across the middle of the chest at the point where the xiphoid process starts *tänkt horisontalplan genom processus xiphoideus (bröstbenets svärdsutskott)*

xiphisternum [ˌzɪfɪ'stɜːnəm] *or* **xiphoid process** ['zɪfɔɪd ˌprəʊses] *or* **xiphoid cartilage** ['zɪfɔɪd ˌkɑːt(ə)lɪdʒ] *or* **ensiform cartilage** ['ensɪfɔːm ˌkɑːt(ə)lɪdʒ] *subst.* bottom part of the breastbone *or* sternum, which in young people is formed of cartilage and becomes bone only by middle age *processus xiphoideus (ensiformis), svärdsutskottet*

X-kromosom ▷ **X chromosome**

X-ray ['eksreɪ] **1** *subst.* **(a)** ray with a very short wavelength, which is invisible, but can go through soft tissue and register as a photograph on a film *röntgen, röntgenstråle, röntgenstrålning;* **the X-ray examination showed the presence of a tumour in the colon; the X-ray department is closed for lunch (b)** photograph taken using X-rays *röntgenbild;* **the dentist took some X-rays of the patient's teeth; he pinned the X-rays to the light screen; all the staff had to have chest X-rays 2** *vb.* to take an X-ray photograph of a patient *röntga, röntgenfotografera;* **there are six patients waiting to be X-rayed**

> COMMENT: because X-rays go through soft tissue, it is sometimes necessary to make internal organs opaque so that they will show up on the film. In the case of stomach X-rays, patients take a barium meal before being photographed (contrast radiography); in other cases, such as kidney X-rays, radioactive substances are injected into the bloodstream or into the organ itself. X-rays are used not only in radiography for diagnosis but as a treatment in radiotherapy. Excessive exposure to X-rays, either as a patient being treated, or as a radiographer, can cause radiation sickness

xylose ['zaɪləʊz] *subst.* pentose which has not been metabolized *xylos, träsocker*

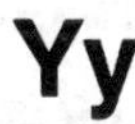

yawn [jɔːn] **1** *subst.* reflex action when tired *or* sleepy, where the mouth is opened wide and after a deep intake of air, the breath exhaled slowly *gäspning;* **his yawns made everyone feel sleepy 2** *vb.* to open the mouth wide and breathe in deeply and then breathe out slowly *gäspa*

> COMMENT: yawning can be caused by tiredness as the body prepares for sleep, but it can have other causes, such as a hot room, or even can be started by unconsciously imitating someone who is yawning near you

yaws [jɔːz] *or* **framboesia** [fræm'biːziə] *or* **pian** [piː'ɑːn] *subst pl.* tropical disease caused by the spirochaete Treponema pertenue *granuloma (papilloma) tropicum, yaws, framboesi*

> COMMENT: symptoms include fever with raspberry-like swellings on the skin, followed in later stages by bone deformation

Y chromosome ['waɪ ˌkrəʊməsəʊm] *subst.* male chromosome *Y-kromosom*

> COMMENT: the Y chromosome has male characteristics and does not form part of the female genetic structure. A normal male has an XY pair of chromosomes. See also the note at X CHROMOSOME

yeast [jiːst] *subst.* fungus which is used in the fermentation of alcohol and in making bread *jäst*

> COMMENT: yeast is a good source of Vitamin B, and can be taken in dried form in tablets

yellow [ˈjeləʊ] *adj. & subst.* of a colour like that of the sun or of gold *gul;* **his skin turned yellow when he had hepatitis; the whites of the eyes become yellow as a symptom of jaundice; yellow atrophy** = old name for severe damage to the liver *allvarlig leverskada;* **yellow fibres** *or* **elastic fibres** = fibres made of elastin, which can expand easily and are found in the skin and in the walls of arteries or the lungs *elastiska fibrer (trådar);* **yellow spot** *or* **macula lutea** = yellow patch on the retina of the eye around the fovea *macula lutea, gula fläcken*

yellow fever [ˌjeləʊ ˈfiːvə] *subst.* infectious disease, found especially in Africa and South America, caused by an arbovirus carried by the mosquito **Aedes aegypti** *febris flava, gula febern*

> COMMENT: the fever affects the liver and causes jaundice. There is no known cure for yellow fever and it can be fatal, but vaccination can prevent it

Yersinia pestis [jɜːˈsɪniə ˌpestɪs] *subst.* bacterium which causes plague *Yersinia pestis*

Y-kromosom ⇨ **Y chromosome**

ymnig ⇨ **profuse**

ympning ⇨ **inoculation**

yolk sac [ˈjəʊk ˌsæk] = VITELLINE SAC

yr ⇨ **dizzy, giddy**

yrke ⇨ **occupation, profession**

yrkes- ⇨ **occupational, professional**

yrkesdermatit ⇨ **occupational**

yrkesförening ⇨ **professional**

yrkeskår ⇨ **profession**

yrkessjukdom ⇨ **industrial, occupational**

yrkesutbildad ⇨ **skilled**

yrsel ⇨ **dizziness, giddiness, vertigo**

yta ⇨ **area, surface**

ytaktivt medel ⇨ **surfactant**

ytlig ⇨ **superficial**

ytspänningsnedsättande ⇨ **surfactant**

ytter- ⇨ **outer**

yttertemperatur ⇨ **temperature**

ytterörat ⇨ **ear**

yttre ⇨ **appearance; ect-, external, externally, extrinsic, lateral, outer, peripheral**

yttre kroppsbeskaffenhet ⇨ **habitus**

yttre respiration ⇨ **respiration**

yttring ⇨ **manifestation**

yuppie disease ⇨ **postviral**

Zz

Zadik's operation [ˈzeɪdɪks ˌɒpəˌreɪʃ(ə)n] *subst.* surgical operation to remove the whole of an ingrowing toenail *Königs operation*

Zimmer (frame) [ˈzɪmə (ˌfreɪm)] *subst.* trade mark for a metal frame used by patients who have difficulty in walking *slags gångstöd;* **she managed to walk some steps with a Zimmer**

zinc [zɪŋk] *subst.* white metallic trace element *zink, Zn* NOTE: chemical symbol is **Zn**

zinc ointment [ˈzɪŋk ˌɔɪntmənt] *subst.* soothing ointment made of zinc oxide and oil *zinkliniment, zinksalva*

zinc oxide [ˌzɪŋk ˈɒksaɪd] *subst.* compound of zinc and oxygen which forms a soft white soothing powder used in creams *zinkoxid*

zink ⇨ **zinc**

zinkliniment ⇨ **calamine (lotion), zinc ointment**

zinkoxid ⇨ **zinc oxide**

zinksalva ⇨ **zinc ointment**

Z line ['zed laɪn] *subst.* part of the pattern of muscle tissue, a dark line seen in the light I band *z-skiva*

Zollinger-Ellison syndrome [ˌzɒlɪndʒər'elɪs(ə)n ˌsɪndrəʊm] *subst.* condition where tumours are formed in the islet cells of the pancreas together with peptic ulcers *Zollinger-Ellisons syndrom*

zon ⇨ **zona, zone**

zona ['zəʊnə] *subst.* **(a)** = HERPES ZOSTER **(b)** zone *or* area *zon, område;* **zona pellucida** = membrane which forms around an ovum *zona pellucida*

zone [zəʊn] *subst.* area of the body *zon, område;* **erogenous zone** = part of the body which, if stimulated, produces sexual arousal (such as the penis *or* clitoris *or* nipples) *erogen (erotogen) zon*

zonula ['zɒnjʊlə] *or* **zonule** ['zɒnju:l] *subst.* small area of the body *zonula, liten zon;* **zonule of Zinn** = suspensory ligament of the lens of the eye *zonula Zinni (ciliaris), Zinns zonula*

zonulolysis [ˌzɒnju'lɒləsɪs] *subst.* removal of a zonule by dissolving it *borttagande av zonula genom upplösning*

zoonosis [ˌzəʊɒ'nəʊsɪs, zəʊ'ɒnəsɪs] *subst.* disease which a human can catch from an animal *zoonos*
NOTE: plural is **zoonoses**

zoster ['zɒstə] *see* HERPES ZOSTER

z-skiva ⇨ **intercalated, Z line**

zygoma [zaɪ'gəʊmə] *subst.* (i) zygomatic arch *arcus zygomaticus, okbågen, kindbågen;* (ii) zygomatic bone *or* cheek bone *os zygomaticum, okbenet, kindknotan*

zygomatic [ˌzaɪgə(ʊ)'mætɪk] *adj.* referring to the zygoma *zygomatisk, ok-, kind-;* **zygomatic arch** *or* **zygoma** = arch of bone in the temporal bone, running between the ear and the bottom of the eye socket *arcus zygomaticus, okbågen, kindbågen;* **zygomatic bone** *or* **cheekbone** *or* **malar bone** = bone which forms the prominent part of the cheek and the lower part of the orbit ⇨ *illustration* SKULL *os zygomaticum, okbenet, kindknotan*

zygomatisk ⇨ **zygomatic**

zygomycosis [ˌzaɪgə(ʊ)maɪ'kəʊsɪs] *subst.* disease caused by a fungus which infests the blood vessels in the lungs *slags svampsjukdom i lungornas kärl*

zygote ['zaɪgəʊt] *subst.* fertilized ovum *or* the first stage of development of an embryo *zygot, befruktad äggcell*

zym(o)- ['zaɪm(əʊ), ˌ--] *prefix* meaning (i) enzymes *zym(o)-;* (ii) fermentation *zym(o)-*

zymogen ['zaɪmədʒen] = PROENZYME

zymosis [zaɪ'məʊsɪs] *subst.* fermentation *or* process where carbohydrates are broken down by enzymes and produce alcohol *slags jäsning el. fermentering*

zymotic [zaɪ'mɒtɪk] *adj.* referring to zymosis

Åå

åderbråck ⇨ **varicose veins, varix**

åderbråcksoperation ⇨ **varicectomy**

åderförkalkning ⇨ **arteriosclerosis, artery, atherosclerosis**

åderförkalknings- ⇨ **atherosclerotic**

åderhinnan ⇨ **choroid**

åderlåtning ⇨ **blood, phlebotomy**

ådra sig ⇨ **catch, contract, get, pick up**

åkomma ⇨ **complaint, condition, trouble**

åksjuk ⇨ **carsick**

åksjuka ⇨ **carsickness, travel sickness**

ålder ⇨ **age**

ålderdom(en) ⇨ **age**

ålderdoms- ⇨ **senile**

ålderdomshem ⇨ **home**

ålderdomssvaghet ⇨ **infirmity, senility**

ålders- ⇨ **presby-, senile**

åldersgrupp ⇨ **group**

ålderssynthet ⇨ **presbyopia**

ålderstigen ⇨ **aged**

åldrande ⇨ **ageing, senescence, senescent**

åldrande, för tidigt ⇨ **presenility**

åldras ⇨ **age**

åldring ⇨ **elderly**

åldrings- ⇨ **geriatric**

åldringsbåge ⇨ **arcus**

ånga ⇨ **vapour**

ångest ⇨ **anxiety**

ångestneuros ⇨ **anxiety, neurosis**

åsikt ⇨ **opinion**

åstadkomma ⇨ **create, effect, get**

åter- ⇨ **retro-**

återanpassa ⇨ **rehabilitate**

återanpassning ⇨ **rehabilitation**

återbilda ⇨ **regenerate**

återbildning ⇨ **regeneration**

återblick ⇨ **retrospection**

återfall ⇨ **recrudescence, recurrence, relapse**

återfalla ⇨ **relapse**

återfallsfeber ⇨ **fever, recurrent**

återflöde ⇨ **reflux, regurgitation**

återfå ⇨ **recover, regain**

återgång ⇨ **regress, regression, retrogression**

återhämta sig ⇨ **pull through, recover**

återhämtning ⇨ **recovery, recuperation**

återkommande ⇨ **continual, palindromic, recurrent**

återkoppling ⇨ **feedback**

återomvandla ⇨ **reconvert**

återstående ⇨ **residual**

återställa ⇨ **restore**

återuppbygga ⇨ **rebuild**

återuppliva ⇨ **resuscitate, revive**

återupplivning ⇨ **resuscitation**

återuppsuga ⇨ **reabsorb**

återuppsugning ⇨ **reabsorption, resorption**

återuppta ⇨ **reabsorb**

återupptag ⇨ **reabsorption, resorption**

återuppträdande ⇨ **reappearance, re-emergence**

återuppvätskning ⇨ **rehydration**

återvinna ⇨ **regain**

åtfölja ⇨ **accompany**

åtsittande ⇨ **tight, tightly**

åtskild ⇨ **discrete**

åttatalsturer, förband med ⇨ **spica**

Ää

äcklad ⇨ **nauseous**

ägg ⇨ **egg, ovum**

ägg- ⇨ **oo-**

äggbildning ⇨ **oogenesis**

äggblåsa ⇨ **ovarian**

äggcell ▷ egg, ovum

äggcell, befruktad ▷ zygote

ägghinnan, yttersta ▷ decidua

äggledar- ▷ salping-, tubal, tubo-

äggledaren ▷ Fallopian tube

äggledarinflammation ▷ salpingitis

äggl ossning ▷ ovulation

äggstock ▷ oophoron, ovary

äggstocks- ▷ oopho-, ov-, ovarian

äggstockscysta ▷ ovarian

äggstocksinflammation ▷ oophoritis, ovaritis

äggula ▷ vitellus

äggulesäcken ▷ vitelline sac

"äggvita" ▷ globulinuria

äggviteämne ▷ protein

äkta ▷ true

äldre (person) ▷ elderly

ämbetsbrott ▷ misconduct

ämne ▷ material, matter, subject, substance

ämnesomsättning ▷ metabolism

ämnesomsättningsprodukt ▷ metabolite

änd- ▷ distal, telo-, terminal

ändamålsenlig ▷ efficient

ändamålsenligt ▷ efficiently

ändartär ▷ end

ändfalangerna ▷ distal

ändhjärnan ▷ telencephalon

ändkropp ▷ end

ändplatta ▷ end plate

ändpunkt ▷ terminal

ändra ▷ vary

ändtarmen ▷ rectum

ändtarms- ▷ proct-, rect-, rectal

ändtarmsbråck ▷ rectocele

ändtarmsinflammation ▷ proctitis

ändtarmsklåda ▷ pruritus

ändtarmsmynningen ▷ passage

ängslan ▷ anxiety, nervousness

ängslig ▷ anxious, nervous, nervy

änkestöt ▷ funny

ärftlig ▷ familial, hereditary

ärftlighet ▷ heredity

ärr ▷ scar, cicatrix, mark

ärrbråck ▷ incisional

ärrig ▷ pitted

ärrvävnad ▷ scar

ärtbenet ▷ pisiform (bone)

ärva ▷ inherit

äta ▷ eat, feed

ätbar ▷ edible

ätlig ▷ edible

ättiksyra ▷ acetic acid

äventyra ▷ endanger

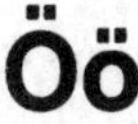

ödem ▷ dropsy, oedema

ödematös ▷ oedematous

ödem, utbrett ▷ anasarca

öga ▷ eye

öga, färglöst ▷ wall eye

ögats ringmuskel ⇨ orbicularis

ögon- ⇨ ocular, ophth-, ophthalmic

ögonbad ⇨ bath

ögonbank ⇨ corneal, eye bank

ögonbotten ⇨ fundus

ögonbryn ⇨ brow, eyebrow

ögonbrynsrynkaren ⇨ corrugator muscle

ögonfrans ⇨ cilium, eyelash

ögongloben ⇨ eyeball

ögonhålan ⇨ socket

ögonhåle- ⇨ orbital

ögonhår ⇨ cilium, eyelash

ögoninflammation ⇨ ophthalmia, ophthalmitis

ögon, insjunkna ⇨ enophthalmos

ögonkammaren ⇨ chamber

ögonkammarvatten ⇨ aqueous (humour)

ögonkarunkeln ⇨ caruncle

ögonkirurg ⇨ ophthalmic

ögonlocket ⇨ eyelid, blepharon, palpebra

ögonlocks- ⇨ blephar-, palpebral

ögonlock, sammanvuxna ⇨ ankyloblepharon

ögonlocksinflammation ⇨ blepharitis

ögonlockskramp ⇨ blepharospasm

ögonlocksrands- ⇨ tars(o)-

ögonläkare ⇨ oculist

ögonmuskelförlamning ⇨ ophthalmoplegia

ögonrörelsenerven ⇨ oculomotor

ögonskrofler ⇨ phlyctenule

ögonsmärtor ⇨ photalgia

ögonspecialist ⇨ oculist, ophthalmologist

ögonspegel ⇨ ophthalmoscope

ögonspegling ⇨ ophthalmoscopy

ögonspringefläck ⇨ pinguecula

ögonvatten ⇨ collyrium

ögonvinkeln ⇨ canthus

ögonvitan ⇨ albuginea, sclera, sclerotic, white

ögonvrån ⇨ canthus

öka ⇨ gain, raise

öka(s) ⇨ rise

ökenreumatism ⇨ coccidioidomycosis

ökning ⇨ gain, increase

ÖLI ⇨ respiratory, upper

öm ⇨ raw, sore, tender

ömhet ⇨ tenderness

ömmande ⇨ tender

ömtålig ⇨ delicate, susceptible

ömtålighet ⇨ susceptibility

önskad effekt ⇨ require

önske- ⇨ ideal

öppen ⇨ open, patent

öppen fraktur ⇨ compound fracture

öppenhet ⇨ patency

öppetstående ⇨ patent

öppnande ⇨ dehiscence

öppning ⇨ aditus, aperture, foramen, gap, inlet, lumen, opening, orifice, ostium, outlet, pore, stoma

öppningsskedet ⇨ engagement

örat ⇨ ear

örflik ⇨ tragus

örnnäsa ⇨ aquiline nose

öron- ⇨ aural, auricular, ot-, otic

öronblödning ⇨ otorrhagia

öronflytning ⇨ otorrhoea

öroninflammation ⇨ -itis, otitis

öronkirurgi ⇨ aural

öronmusslan ⇨ concha, helix

öronringning ⇨ tinnitus

öronsnäckan ⇨ cochlea

öronspecialist ⇨ otologist

öronspottkörtel ⇨ parotid

öronsten ⇨ otolith

öronsusning ⇨ tinnitus

örontrumpeten ⇨ Eustachian tube

örontrumpets- ⇨ salping-, tubo-

öronvax ⇨ earwax

öronvaxkörtlarna ⇨ ceruminous glands

örsnibb ⇨ lobe

örsprång ⇨ earache, middle ear, tympanitis

ört ⇨ herb

örtmedicin ⇨ herbal; herbalism

örtte ⇨ tea

östradiol ⇨ oestradiol

östriol ⇨ oestriol

östrogen ⇨ oestrogen, oestrogenic hormone

östron ⇨ oestrone

öva ⇨ exercise

över ⇨ above, all over

över- ⇨ epi-, hyper-, over-, senior, super-, upper

överallt ⇨ all over

överanstränga ⇨ exhaust

överansträngning ⇨ exhaustion, overexertion, overwork

överansträngning av ögonen ⇨ eyestrain

överarmen ⇨ brachium, upper

överarmsbenet ⇨ humerus

överbefruktning ⇨ superfecundation, superfetation

överburenhet ⇨ postmaturity

överburet barn ⇨ postmature baby

överdos ⇨ overdose, o.d.

överdosering ⇨ overdose

överdriva ⇨ overdo (things)

överensstämmelse ⇨ agreement

överfylld ⇨ engorged

överföra ⇨ transfer, transmit

överförbar sjukdom ⇨ communicable disease

överförd smärta ⇨ synalgia

överföring ⇨ conduction, passage, transference

övergående ⇨ transient

övergång ⇨ isthmus

övergångsepitel ⇨ transitional

övergångsålder ⇨ menopause

överhuden ⇨ cuticle, epidermis

överhudsavlossning ⇨ epidermolysis

överjaget ⇨ superego

överkompensera ⇨ overcompensate

överkäken ⇨ jaw, maxilla (bone)

överkäks- ⇨ maxillary

överkäkshålan ⇨ maxillary

överkänslig ⇨ hypersensitive

överkänslighet ⇨ hypersensitivity, intolerance, sensitization

överlappa ⇨ overlap

överledning ⇨ conduction

överleva ⇨ survive

överlevande ⇨ survivor

överlevnad ⇨ survival

överlägsenhet ⇨ superiority

överlägsenhetskomplex ⇨ superiority

överläkare ⇨ consultant, director

överordnad ⇨ senior

överproduktion ⇨ overproduction

överraskande ⇨ astonishing

överskott ⇨ excess

överskotts- ⇨ excessive

överskrida ⇨ exceed

överspänd ⇨ overwrought

överstiga ⇨ exceed

överstigande ⇨ excess

översvämma ⇨ flood, infest

översvämning ⇨ flood

översynthet ⇨ farsightedness

övertalig ⇨ supernumerary

övertrycks- ⇨ hyperbaric

övertrycksventilation ⇨ positive

övervaka ⇨ control, monitor, supervise

övervakning ⇨ monitoring, supervision

övervaknings-TV ⇨ cardiac

överviktig ⇨ obese, overweight

övervinna ⇨ get over, overcome

övervägande ⇨ predominant

överväxt ⇨ overgrowth

övning ⇨ exercise

övre ⇨ superior, upper

övre hjärnbihanget ⇨ pineal (body)

övre magmunnen ⇨ cardia

ANATOMICAL TERMS

The body is always described as if standing upright with the palms of the hands facing forward. There is only one central vertical plane, termed the *median* or *sagittal* plane, and this passes through the body from front to back. Planes parallel to this on either side are *parasagittal* or *paramedian* planes. Vertical planes at right angles to the median are called *coronal* planes. The term *horizontal* (or *transverse*) plane speaks for itself. Two specific horizontal planes are (a) the *transpyloric*, midway between the suprasternal notch and the symphysis pubis, and (b) the *transtubercular* or *intra-tubercular* plane, which passes through the tubercles of the iliac crests. Many other planes are named from the structures they pass through.

Views of the body from some different points are shown on the diagram; a view of the body from above is called the *superior aspect*, and that from below is the *inferior aspect*.

Cephalic means toward the head; *caudal* refers to positions (or in a direction) towards the tail. *Proximal* and *distal* refer to positions respectively closer to and further from the centre of the body in any direction, while *lateral* and *medial* relate more specifically to relative sideways positions, and also refer to movements. *Ventral* refers to the abdomen, front or anterior, while *dorsal* relates to the back of a part or organ. The hand has a *dorsal* and a *palmar* surface, and the foot a *dorsal* and a *plantar* surface.

Note that *flexion of the thigh* moves it forward while *flexion of the leg* moves it backwards; the movements of *extension* are similarly reversed. Movement and rotation of limbs can be *medial*, which is with the front moving towards the centre line, or *lateral*, which is in the opposite direction. Specific terms for limb movements are *adduction*, towards the centre line, and *abduction*, which is away from the centre line. Other specific terms are *supination* and *pronation* for the hand, and *inversion* and *eversion* for the foot.

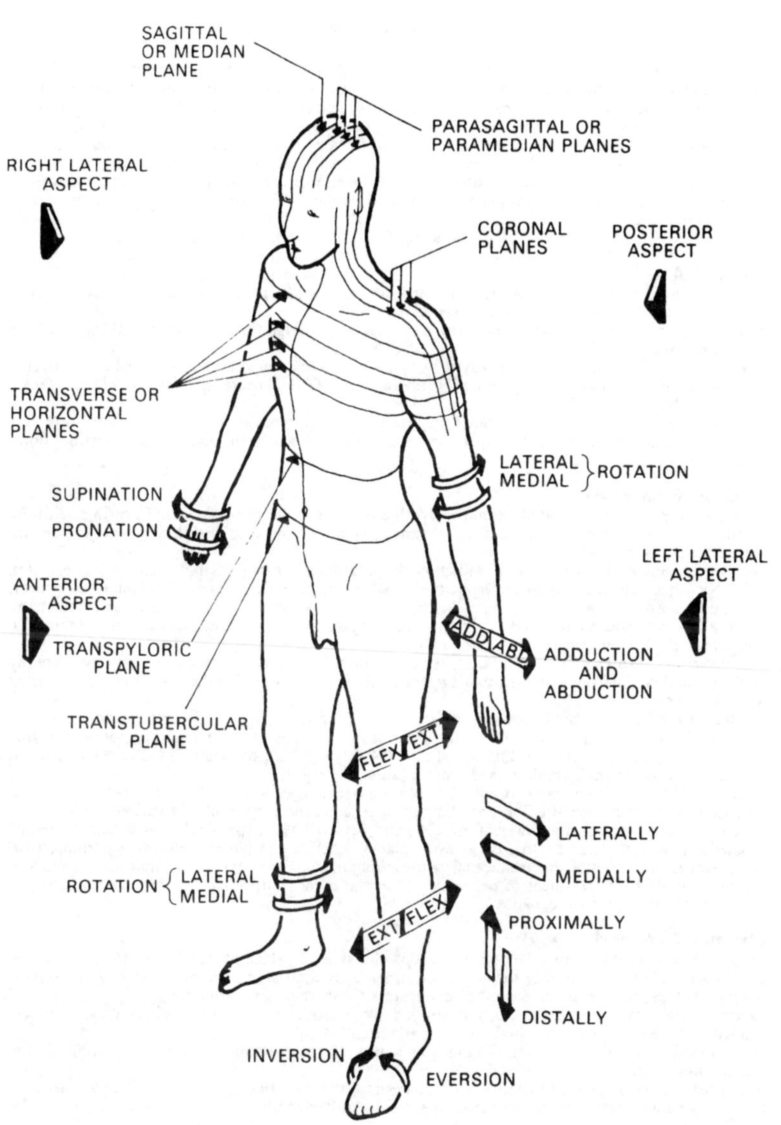
SAGITTAL
OR MEDIAN
PLANE
PARASAGITTAL OR
PARAMEDIAN PLANES
RIGHT LATERAL
ASPECT
CORONAL
PLANES
POSTERIOR
ASPECT
TRANSVERSE OR
HORIZONTAL
PLANES
LATERAL
MEDIAL
ROTATION
SUPINATION
PRONATION
LEFT LATERAL
ASPECT
ANTERIOR
ASPECT
ADD
ABD
TRANSPYLORIC
PLANE
ADDUCTION
AND
ABDUCTION
TRANSTUBERCULAR
PLANE
FLEX
EXT
LATERALLY
MEDIALLY
ROTATION
LATERAL
MEDIAL
EXT
FLEX
PROXIMALLY
DISTALLY
INVERSION
EVERSION

VITAMINS

Vitamins are substances which are required in tiny amounts in food. They promote the normal health and metabolism of the body, and can normally be obtained in a diet of natural foods. Although they are complex chemical substances, the structure and composition of most of them are known, most have been isolated, and some have been synthesized. As they are concerned with metabolism, it follows that absence or deficiency of certain vitamins can result in malnutrition and specific deficiency diseases. Almost all must be obtained preformed from external sources, the exceptions being vitamin A which is formed from its precursor carotene, vitamin D which is formed by the action of ultraviolet light on the skin, and vitamin K which is formed by the action of intestinal bacteria.

The following is a summary of the characteristics, actions, and sources of vitamins:

Vitamin A

This keeps mucous membranes healthy, is necessary for normal growth, formation of skin, glands and bone, and for properly functioning eyesight.

Sources. Liver, butter, margarine, milk, eggs, yellow and orange fruits, green vegetables, cod liver oil and halibut liver oil.

Characteristics. Fat soluble; not destroyed by normal cooking temperatures; is stored in the liver.

Recommended daily intake. Adults: 5000 IU (pregnancy: 6000IU; lactation: 8000IU); children: 2000–5000 IU; infants: 1500 IU.

Results of deficiency. Reduced resistance to infection; interference with normal growth; imperfect calcium metabolism and formation of bone, teeth, and cartilage; imbalance of the intestinal flora; night blindness.

Vitamin B complex

This is a large number of related vitamins: B_1 (thiamine); B_2 (riboflavine); niacin (nicotinic acid); B_6 (pyridoxine); biotin; pantothenic acid; B_{12} (cyanocobalamin); and folic acid. Many other factors are present in the B complex.

Sources. Thiamine (B_1): wheat germ, bread, pork, potatoes, liver, milk; Riboflavine (B_2): liver, eggs, milk; Nicotinic acid (niacin): yeast, liver, bread, wheat germ, milk, kidney; Pyridoxine (B_6): meat, fish, milk, yeast; Biotin: liver, yeast, milk, butter; Pantothenic acid: liver, yeast, eggs, and many other foods; Cyanocobalamin (B_{12}): liver, kidney, eggs, fish; Folic acid (also called vitamin B_c): green vegetables, liver, mushrooms, yeast.

Characteristics. Water soluble; not destroyed by normal cooking temperatures, but overcooking (and an alkaline environment) can damage them; B_1 can be stored by the body only in a limited way; B_2 is not stable to light.

Recommended daily intake. Thiamine: Adults: 1.0–1.6 mg (pregnancy: 1.3 mg; lactation: 1.7 mg); children: 0.7–1.8 mg; infants: 0.4–0.5 mg. Riboflavine: Adults: 1.4–2.5 mg (pregnancy: 2.0 mg; lactation: 2.5 mg); children: 1.0–2.0 mg; infants: 0.4–0.9 mg. Niacin: Adults: 17–21 mg (pregnancy: 15 mg; lactation: 15 mg); children: 8–21 mg; infants: 6–7 mg.

Results of deficiency. Generally, B complex vitamin deficiency results in loss of appetite, impaired digestion of starches, constipation and diarrhoea; severe deficiency results in various nervous disorders, loss of co-ordinating power of muscles, and beriberi. More specifically, B_2 deficiency results in cheilosis, weakness, and impaired growth; niacin deficiency results in pellagra, gastrointestinal disturbances, and mental disturbance. Cyanocobalamin deficiency results in anaemia (cyanocobalamin is used in the treatment of pernicious anaemia, sprue, nutritional anaemia, and macrocytic anaemias of infancy and pregnancy).

Vitamin C (Ascorbic acid)

This increases resistance to infection and keeps the skin in a healthy condition. It improves the circulation and the condition of the gums and other body tissues, and promotes healing of wounds.

Sources. Citrus fruits, rose-hip syrup, blackcurrants, fresh vegetables, tomatoes.

Characteristics. Water soluble; easily destroyed by overcooking; storage reduces efficacy unless canned or frozen; stored in the body only to a limited extent.

Recommended daily intake. Adults: 70 mg (pregnancy: 100 mg; lactation: 150 mg); children: 35–100 mg; infants: 30 mg.

Results of deficiency. Lowered vitality; joint tenderness; dental caries; lowered resistance to infection; fibrous tissue abnormalities. Severe deficiency results in haemorrhage, anaemia, and scurvy.

Vitamin D

This vitamin is essential for the proper utilization of calcium and phosphorus, and thus directly influences the structure of bones and teeth. It affects the blood chemistry.

Sources. Butter, egg yolk, fish liver oils and oily fish, yeast. As mentioned, the vitamin can be synthesized by the skin under the stimulus of sunlight or ultraviolet light.

Characteristics. Fat soluble; can be stored in the liver.

Recommended daily intake. The adult can generally synthesize sufficient of this vitamin, but deficiencies have occurred in dark-skinned individuals or elderly people who live in temperate areas where the sunlight they receive is insufficient. In pregnancy: 400 IU; lactation: 400 IU; children: 400 IU; infants: 400 IU.

Results of deficiency. Interference with calcium and phosphorous metabolism; weakness and irritability. Severe deficiency results in rickets in children and osteomalacia in adults.

Vitamin E

Little is known about the physiological activity of this vitamin, but animal experiments suggest that it is concerned with the reproductive cycle and fertility; it may also have an effect on the ageing process. It is present in most foods, particularly in green vegetables.

Vitamin K

This is responsible for the biosynthesis of prothrombin and for maintaining plasma prothrombin levels.

Sources. Green leafy vegetables, liver.

Characteristics. Fat soluble; not destroyed by cooking.

Recommended daily intake. Not known, but children should receive 1 microgram.

CALORIE REQUIREMENTS

The calorie requirements of the human body depend upon age and activity. Children need a greater energy input for their weight than adults, as they are building up their body tissues.

A 'calorie' is, in the context of dietetics, a 'kilocalorie' (kcal); it is a unit of energy, and is the amount of heat required to raise 1 000 g of water by 1° Celsius. The term kilojoule (kJ) is sometimes preferred; a kilocalorie is approximately 4.2 kilojoules.

The following is a list of approximate daily calorie requirements for varying ages and activities.

Children

Age (years)	*Daily kcal*	*(kJ)*
up to 1	800	3 360
1–2	1 200	5 040
2–3	1 400	5 880
3–5	1 600	6 720
5–7	1 800	7 560
7–9	2 100	8 820

Boys	*kcal*	*kJ*	*Girls*	*kcal*	*kJ*
9–12	2 500	10 500	9–12	2 300	9 660
12–15	2 800	11 760	12–15	2 300	9 660
15–18	3 000	12 600	15–18	2 300	9 660

Men

Age (years)	*Activity*	*kcal*	*kJ*
18–35	sedentary	2 700	11 340
	moderately active	3 000	12 600
	very active	3 600	15 120
35–65	sedentary	2 600	10 920
	moderately active	2 900	12 180
	very active	3 600	15 120
65–75	sedentary	2 300	9 660
over 75	sedentary	2 100	8 820

Women

Age (years)	*Activity*	*kcal*	*kJ*
18–35	moderately active	2 200	9 240
	very active	2 500	10 500
	pregnant	2 400	10 080
	lactating	2 700	11 340
35–65	moderately active	2 200	9 240
65–75	sedentary	2 050	8 610
over 75	sedentary	1 900	7 980

CALORIE CONTENT OF FOODS

Because the average portion of foods varies so much, both by custom and by personal preference, the following list shows the calorific value of various foods per 30 gram portion.

	per 30 gram portion	
	kcal	*kJ*
Meat (cooked)		
Bacon	160	672
Beef (roast)	108	454
(steak)	86	361
(corned)	66	277
Ham	125	525
Kidney	46	193
Liver (fried)	80	336
Lamb (chop)	36	151
(roast leg)	83	349
Luncheon meat	96	403
Pork (roast)	90	378
Sausages	90	378
Tripe	30	126
Veal (roast)	66	277
Poultry (cooked)		
Chicken (roast)	55	232
Duck (roast)	90	378
Turkey (roast)	56	236
Fish (cooked)		
Cod (steamed)	24	101
Haddock	28	118
Hake	30	126
Halibut	37	156
Herring	55	230
Kippers	57	239
Lemon sole	26	108
Mackerel	53	223
Plaice	26	108
Salmon (canned)	39	164
(fresh)	57	239
Sardines (canned)	83	350
Sole	25	105
Shellfish		
Crab	36	151
Lobster	34	143
Oysters	14	59
Prawns	30	126
Shrimps	32	134
Vegetables		
Beans (runner)	3	13
(broad)	12	50
(butter)	26	109
(haricot)	25	105
(French)	3	13
Beetroot	13	55
Broccoli	4	17
Brussels sprouts	5	21
Cabbage (raw)	7	29
(cooked)	2	8
Carrots (raw)	6	25
(cooked)	5	21
Cauliflower	3	13
Celery (raw)	3	13
Cucumber	3	13
Lettuce	3	13
Onions	4	17
Peas (raw)	18	76
(cooked)	28	118
Potatoes (new)	21	88

	per 30 gram portion	
	kcal	*kJ*
Vegetables		
(old)	23	97
(chips)	68	286
(crisps)	160	672
Spinach	7	29
Spring greens	3	13
Swedes	5	21
Tomatoes	4	17
Turnips	3	13
Watercress	4	17
Fruit		
Apples	13	55
Apricots (raw)	8	34
(dried)	52	218
Bananas	22	92
Blackcurrents	8	34
Grapes (black)	17	71
(white)	18	76
Grapefruit	6	25
Lemons	4	17
Melon	7	29
Oranges	10	42
Peaches	11	46
Pears	12	50
Plums	11	46
Prunes	46	193
Raisins	71	298
Raspberries	7	29
Rhubarb	1	4
Strawberries (raw)	5	21
Sultanas	72	302
Dairy Products		
Butter	225	945
Cheese (Cheddar)	118	496
(Cottage)	30	126
(Curd)	40	168
(Blue)	105	441
(Edam)	88	370
(Gruyere)	130	546
Cream (double)	130	546
(single)	62	260
Eggs	46	193
Margarine	225	946
Milk (whole fresh)	19	80
(skimmed)	10	42
(evaporated)	45	125
(condensed)	95	400
Oil (cooking)	250	1 050
Yoghurt (low fat)	15	63
Preserves and Sugar		
Chocolate (milk)	170	714
(plain)	156	655
Honey	95	399
Ice cream	56	235
Jam	74	311
Marmalade	75	315
Sugar (brown or white)	111	466
Syrup (golden)	90	378
Treacle	74	311
Cereals		
Bread (white, brown, or wholemeal)	70	294

Cereals	*per 30 gram portion* kcal	kJ
Cornflakes	105	441
Cornflour	100	420
Crispbread	100	420
Flour (white, wholemeal)	100	420
Macaroni (boiled)	30	126
Porridge (oatmeal)	14	59
Rice	35	147
Sago	100	420
Semolina	100	420
Spaghetti	106	445

Cereals	*per 30 gram portion* kcal	kJ
Tapioca	102	428
Nuts (shelled)		
Almonds	170	714
Brazils	182	764
Chestnuts	50	210
Coconut	180	756
Peanuts	170	714
Walnuts	154	647

INCUBATION PERIOD AND DURATION OF ISOLATION OF PATIENTS IN HOSPITAL

Disease	*Incubation period*	*Isolation of the infected person*
Chickenpox (Varicella)	10–21 days (14–15 days usually)	Until 6 days after the last crop of vesicles clear.
*Diphtheria	1–6 days	Until two consecutive negative swabs are obtained from the nose and throat
*Enteric group	3–23 days	Until three consecutive negative stools *off treatment* are obtained
*Infectious hepatitis (Hepatitis A)	15–40 days	7 days
*Measles (Morbilli)	12–14 days (8–11 days to catarrhal stage)	7 days from the date of appearance of the rash. (But the patient is infective even in the prodromal phase)
Meningococcal meningitis	2 days but frequently much more prolonged	3 days from commencement of antibacterial treatment
Mumps (Epidemic parotitis)	14–28 days (17–18 days usually)	9 days after appearance of the swelling
Paratyphoid fevers	About a week	Until the stools are negative
*Poliomyelitis	5–21 days (7–14 days is probably usual)	Until the stools are negative for poliovirus
Rubella	14–19 days (17–18 days usually)	7 days from onset of the rash
*Scarlet fever	2–5 days	For not less than 3 days following the start of chemotherapy
*Pertussis (whooping cough)	7–14 days to catarrhal stage A further 7–14 days to paroxysmal stage	For 3 weeks from the onset of paroxysmal cough, or until 14 days of chemotherapy
Tetanus	4 days to 3 weeks	None
Typhoid fever	Usually 1 to 3 weeks	Until cultures of faeces and urine are negative

* Notifiable disease in UK

SI Unit Conversions

The SI system (Système International d'Unités) has been introduced into many branches of science and technology. In medicine it has replaced older units of measurements (such as mg/100ml and mEq/l) but many textbooks still give both types of units.

The SI unit for chemical measurement of quantity where the molecular weight (MW) of the substance is known is the *mole*, or a fraction of a mole.

$$\text{Number of moles (mol)} = \frac{\text{weight (wt) in grams (g)}}{\text{MW}}$$

The normal subdivisions are millimoles (mmol, 10^{-3}), micromoles (μmol, 10^{-6}), nanomoles (nmol, 10^{-9}), and picomoles (pmol, 10^{-12})

The SI unit of volume is the cubic metre (m^3), but the *litre* (l) is now accepted as exactly equivalent to one cubic decimetre (dm^3), and in clinical medicine and biochemistry the *litre* is the unit of volume. Units of concentration are therefore millimoles per litre (mmol/l), micromoles per litre (μmol/l), nanomoles per litre (nmol/l) etc. There are, however, occasions where the molecular weight of a substance to be measured is not known, is uncertain or is of a mixed nature; in these instances the units will be grams or milligrams per litre (g/l, mg/l) (see 'Exceptions').
For results previously expressed as mEq/l (milliequivalents per litre):

$$\text{Number of equivalents} = \frac{\text{weight (wt) in grams (g)}}{\text{equivalent weight}}$$

$$= \frac{\text{wt in g} \times \text{valency}}{\text{MW}}$$

Thus, in the case of univalent ions such as sodium (Na) and potassium (K) the units will remain numerically the same, and a serum Na of 140 mEq/l becomes 140 mmol/l. For polyvalent ions such as calcium (Ca) or magnesium (Mg) (which are both divalent) the units are divided by the valency, and a serum Ca of 5.0 mEq/l becomes 2.5 mmol/l and an Mg of 2.0 mEq/l becomes 1.0 mmol/l.

For results previously expressed as mg/100ml, the method is to divide by the molecular weight (which converts from mg to mmol) and then to multiply by 10 (which converts from 100 ml to 1 litre). This conversion can therefore be made by dividing the old units by one tenth of the molecular weight. As an example, the molecular weight of glucose is 180 and of urea is 60. A glucose concentration of 180 mg/100 ml and a urea value of 60 mg/100 ml are both equivalent to 10 mmol/l.

Exceptions
For a variety of reasons there are exceptions to the above general notes.

Proteins. Body fluids contain a complex mixture of proteins of varying molecular weights. In these instances the litre is used, but the gram is retained. For example, total serum protein is measured in this manner, and a total serum protein of 7.0 g/100 ml becomes 70 g/l.

Units of pressure. In most cases these are measured in *Pascals* (Pa) (newtons per square metre), or *kilopascals* (kPa). Nevertheless, when blood pressure measurements are made with a mercury manometer, millimetres of mercury (mmHg) should be retained.

Enzyme units. The use of standard 'International Units' is still controversial. Results are expressed as *activities* rather than concentrations.

Some hormone concentrations are still expressed as 'International Units' or other special units.

Note that the expression '100 ml' should be shown as *decilitre* (dl).

There follows a list of some of the more important biochemical measurements and molecular weights, with approximate conversion factors to and from SI units.

CONVERSION FACTORS FOR SI UNITS

	MW	*From SI Units*	*To SI Units*
Amino-acid nitrogen	14.01		
plasma		mmol/l × 1.401 = mg/dl	mg/dl × 0.714 = mmol/l
urine		mmol/24 hr × 14.01 = mg/24 hr	mg/24 hr × 0.0714 = mmol/24 hr
Ammonium	17.03	μmol/l × 1.703 = μg/dl	μg/dl × 0.587 = μmol/l
Barbiturate	184.2	μmol/l × 0.0184 = mg/dl	mg/dl × 54.29 = μmol/l
Bilirubin	584.7	μmol/l × 0.0585 = mg/dl	mg/dl × 17.1 = μmol/l
Calcium	40.08		
plasma		mmol/l × 4.008 = mg/dl	mg/dl × 0.251 = mmol/l
urine		mmol/24 hr × 40.08 = mg/24 hr	mg/24 hr × 0.0251 = mmol/24 hr
Catecholamines (urine)	183.2	μmol/24 hr × 183 = μg/24 hr	μg/24 hr × 0.00546 = μmol/24 hr
Cholesterol	386.7	mmol/l × 38.7 = mg/dl	mg/dl × 0.0259 = mmol/l
Copper	63.54		
plasma		μmol/l × 6.35 = μg/dl	μg/dl × 0.157 = μmol/l
urine		μmol/24 hr × 63.5 = μg/24 hr	μg/24 hr × 0.0157 = μmol/24 hr
Cortisol (plasma)	362.5	nmol/l × 0.0362 = μg/dl	μg/dl × 27.62 = nmol/l
(urine)		nmol/24 hr × 0.362 = μg/24 hr	μg/24 hr × 2.76 = nmol/24 hr
Creatinine	113.1		
plasma		μmol/l × 0.0113 = mg/dl	mg/dl × 88.4 = μmol/l
urine		mmol/24 hr × 0.113 = g/24 hr	g/24 hr × 8.84 = mmol/24 hr
Ethanol (alcohol)	46.07	mmol/l × 4.607 = mg/dl	mg/dl × 0.217 = mmol/l
Fat (faecal)	284.5	mmol/24 hr × 0.284 = g/24 hr	g/24 hr × 3.52 = mmol/24 hr
Fibrinogen	Uncertain	g/l × 100 = mg/dl	mg/dl × 0.01 = g/l
Glucose	180.2		
blood or plasma		mmol/l × 18.02 = mg/dl	mg/dl × 0.0555 = mmol/l
urine		mmol/l × 0.018 = g/dl	g/dl × 55.5 = mmol/l
CSF		(as blood or plasma)	(as blood or plasma)
HMMA (or VMA) (urine)	198.2	μmol/24 hr × 0.198 = mg/24 hr	mg/24 hr × 5.05 = μmol/24 hr
Hydroxyproline (urine)	131.1	mmol/24 hr × 131.1 = mg/24 hr	mg/24 hr × 0.00763 = mmol/24 hr
Iron and TIBC	55.85	μmol/l × 5.59 = μg/dl	μg/dl × 0.179 = μmol/l

	MW	*From SI Units*	*To SI Units*
Lead	207.2		
blood		μmol/l × 20.7 = μg/dl	μg/dl × 0.0483 = μmol/l
urine		μmol/24 hr × 207 = μg/24 hr	μg/24 hr × 0.00483 = μmol/24 hr
Magnesium	24.31		
plasma		mmol/l × 2.43 = mg/dl	mg/dl × 0.411 = mmol/l
urine		mmol/24 hr × 24.3 = mg/24 hr	mg/24 hr × 0.0411 = mmol/24 hr
Oestriol (urine)	288.4	μmol/24 hr × 0.288 = mg/24 hr	mg/24 hr × 3.47 = μmol/24 hr
17-Oxosteroids (urine)	288.4	μmol/24 hr × 0.288 = mg/24 hr	mg/24 hr × 3.47 = μmol/24 hr
Phenylalanine	165.2	μmol/l × 0.0165 = mg/dl	mg/dl × 60.5 = μmol/l
Phosphate	30.97		
serum		mmol/l × 3.10 = mg/dl	mg/dl × 0.323 = mmol/l
urine		mmol/24 hr × 0.0310 = g/24 hr	g/24 hr × 32.3 = mmol/24 hr
Pregnanediol (urine)	320.5	μmol/24 hr × 0.320 = mg/24 hr	mg/24 hr × 3.12 = μmol/24 hr
Pregnanetriol (urine)	336.5	μmol/24 hr × 0.366 = mg/24 hr	mg/24 hr × 2.97 = μmol/24 hr
Protein	Uncertain	g/l × 0.1 = g/dl	g/dl × 10 = g/l
Serum Albumin	Uncertain	g/l × 0.1 = g/dl	g/dl × 10 = g/l
CSF Protein	Uncertain	g/l × 100 = mg/dl	mg/dl × 0.01 = g/l
Protein-bound Iodine	126.9	nmol/l × 0.0127 = μg/dl	μg/dl × 78.8 = nmol/l
Salicylate	138.1	mmol/l × 13.81 = mg/dl	mg/dl × 0.0724 = mmol/l
Thyroxine	776.9	nmol/l × 0.0777 = μg/dl	μg/dl × 12.87 = nmol/l
Triiodothyronine	651.01	nmol/l × 0.651 = ng/dl	ng/dl × 1.54 = nmol/l
Triglyceride	885.4	mmol/l × 88.5 = mg/dl	mg/dl × 0.0113 = mmol/l
Urate (uric acid)	168.1	mmol/l × 16.81 = mg/dl	mg/dl × 0.0595 = mmol/l
Urea	60.06	mmol/l × 6.01 = mg/dl	mg/dl × 0.166 = mmol/l
PO_2, PCO_2	—	kPa × 7.52 = mmHg	mmHg × 0.133 = kPa
Units of Energy	—	Joules (kJ) × 0.238 = calories	calories × 4.2 = Joules (kJ)

LIST OF EPONYMOUS TERMS

An eponym, in medicine, is a disease, procedure or anatomical structure that bears a person's name or the name of a place. It is usually the name of the person who discovered or first described it. The following is a list of the *eponymous* terms in this dictionary.

Addison's disease Described 1849. Thomas Addison (1793–1860), from Northumberland, founder of the science of endocrinology. His name is also applied to **Addison's anaemia** (pernicious anaemia) described in 1849.

Albee's operation Frederick Houdlett Albee (1876–1945), New York surgeon.

Alzheimer's disease Described 1906. Alois Alzheimer (1864–1915), Bavarian physician.

Apgar score Described 1952. Virginia Apgar (1909–1974), American anaesthesiologist.

Arnold-Chiari malformation Described 1894. Julius A. Arnold (1835–1915), Professor of Pathological Anatomy at Heidelberg; Hans von Chiari (1851–1916), Viennese pathologist who was Professor of Pathological Anatomy at Strasbourg and later at Prague.

Auerbach's plexus Described 1862. Leopold Auerbach (1828–1897), Professor of Neuropathology at Breslau.

Babinski reflex *or* **test** Described 1896. Joseph François Felix Babinski (1857–1932), French-born son of Polish refugees. A pupil of Charcot, he was head of the Neurological clinic at Hôpital de La Pitié, 1890–1927.

Baker's cyst Described 1877. William Morrant Baker (1838–1896), member of the staff at St Bartholomew's Hospital, London.

Bankart's operation First performed 1923. Arthur Sydney Blundell Bankart (1879–1951), first orthopaedic surgeon at the Middlesex Hospital.

Banti's syndrome Described 1882. Guido Banti (1852–1925), Florentine pathologist and physician.

Barlow's disease Described 1882. Sir Thomas Barlow (1845–1945), Physician at various London hospitals; also physician to Queen Victoria, King Edward VII, and King George V.

Barr body Described 1949. Murray Llewellyn Barr (born 1908), Head of the Department of Anatomy at the University of Western Ontario, Canada.

Basedow's disease Described 1840. Carl Adolphe Basedow (1799–1854), General practitioner in Mersburg, Germany.

Bazin's disease Described 1861. Pierre Antoine Ernest Bazin (1807–1878), Dermatologist at Hôpital St Louis, Paris, he was an expert in parasitology associated with skin conditions.

Beer's knife George Joseph Beer (1763–1821), German ophthalmologist.

Behçet's syndrome Described 1937. Halushi Behçet (1889–1948), Turkish dermatologist.

Bellocq's cannula Jean Jacques Bellocq (1732–1807), French surgeon.

Bell's mania Luther Vose Bell (1806–1862), American physician.

Bell's palsy Described 1821. Sir Charles Bell (1774–1842), Scottish surgeon. He ran anatomy schools, first in Edinburgh and then in London. Professor of Anatomy at the Royal Academy.

Bence Jones protein Described 1848. Henry Bence Jones (1814–1873), Physician at St George's Hospital, London.

Benedict's test Described 1915. Stanley Rossiter Benedict (1884–1936), Physiological chemist at Cornell University, New York.

Bennett's fracture Described 1886. Edward Halloran Bennett (1837–1907), Irish anatomist, later Professor of Surgery at Trinity College, Dublin.

Besnier's prurigo Ernest Besnier (1831–1909), French dermatologist.

Billroth's operations Described 1881. Christian Albert Theodore Billroth (1829–1894), Prussian surgeon; studied at Griefswald, Göttingen, and Berlin.

Binet's test Originally described 1914 but later modified at Stanford University, California. Alfred Binet (1857–1911), French psychologist and physiologist.

Bitot's spots Described 1863. Pierre A. Bitot (1822-1888), Bordeaux physician.

Blalock's operation Described 1945. Alfred Blalock (1899–1964), Emeritus Professor of Surgery at Johns Hopkins University, Baltimore.

Boeck's sarcoid Described 1899. Caesar Peter Moeller Boeck (1845–1917), Professor of Dermatology at Oslo.

Bonney's blue William Francis Victor Bonney, (1872–1953), London gynaecologist.

Bowman's capsule Described 1842. Sir William Paget Bowman (1816–1892), surgeon in Birmingham and later in London. A pioneer in work on the kidney and also in ophthalmology.

Braille Introduced 1829–1830. Louis Braille (1809–1852), blind Frenchman and teacher of the blind; he introduced the system which had originally been proposed by Charles Barbier in 1820.

Braun's splint *or* **frame** Heinrich Friedrich Wilhelm Braun (b. 1862), German surgeon.

Bright's disease Described 1836. Richard Bright (1789–1858), physician at Guy's Hospital, London.

Broadbent's sign Sir William Henry Broadbent (1835–1907) English physician.

Broca's area Described 1861. Pierre Paul Broca (1824–1880), Paris surgeon and anthropologist. A pioneer of neurosurgery, he also invented various instruments, described muscular dystrophy before Duchenne, and recognized rickets as a nutritional disorder before Virchow.

Brodie's abscess Described 1832. Sir Benjamin Collins Brodie (1783–1862), English surgeon

Brown-Séquard syndrome Described 1851. Charles Edouard Brown-Séquard (1817–1894), French physiologist.
Brunner's glands Described 1687. Johann Konrad Brunner (1653–1727), Swiss anatomist at Heidelberg, then at Strasbourg.
Budd-Chiari syndrome Described 1845. George Budd (1808–1882), Professor of Medicine at King's College Hospital, London. Hans von Chiari (1851–1916), Viennese pathologist, Professor of Pathological Anatomy at Strasbourg, then at Prague.
Buerger's disease Described 1908. Leo Buerger (1879–1943), New York physician of Viennese origins.
Burkitt's tumour Described 1958. Denis Parsons Burkitt (b. 1911), Formerly Senior Surgeon, Kampala, Uganda; later a member of the Medical Research Council (UK).
Caldwell-Luc operation Described 1893. George Walter Caldwell (1834–1918), American physician; Henry Luc (1855–1925), French laryngologist.
Celsius Described 1742. Anders Celsius (1701–1744), Swedish astronomer and scientist.
Chagas' disease Described 1909. Carlos Chagas (1879–1934), Brazilian scientist and physician.
Charcot's joints Described 1868. Jean-Martin Charcot (1825–1893), French neurologist.
Cheyne-Stokes respiration Described 1818 by Cheyne; 1854 by Stokes. John Cheyne (1777–1836), Scottish physician; William Stokes (1804–1878), Irish physician.
Christmas disease Named after Mr Christmas, the patient in whom the disease was first studied in detail.
Clutton's joints Described 1886. Henry Hugh Clutton (1850–1909), surgeon at St Thomas's Hospital, London.
Cooley's anaemia Described 1927. Thomas Benton Cooley (1871–1945), Professor of Paediatrics at Wayne College of Medicine, Detroit.
Coombs' test Robin Royston Amos Coombs (b. 1921), Quick Professor of Biology, and Fellow of Corpus Christi College, Cambridge.
Corti (organ of) Described 1851. Marquis Alfonso Corti (1822–1888), Italian anatomist and histologist.
Cowper's glands Described 1700. William Cowper (1666–1709), English surgeon.
Coxsackie virus Named after Coxsackie, New York, where the virus was first identified.
Credé's method Described 1860. Karl Sigmund Franz Credé (1819–1892), German gynaecologist.
Crohn's disease Described 1932. Burrill Bernard Crohn (b. 1884), New York physician.
Cushing's disease Described 1932. Harvey Williams Cushing (1869–1939), Boston, US, surgeon.
da Costa's syndrome Described 1871. Jacob Mendes da Costa (1833–1900), Philadelphia surgeon, who described this condition in soldiers in the American civil war.
Daltonism Described 1794. John Dalton (1766–1844), English chemist and physician. Founder of the atomic theory, he was himself colour-blind.
Denis Browne splint Described 1934. Sir Denis John Wolko Browne (1892–1967), Australian orthopaedic and general surgeon working in Britain.
Dercum's disease Described 1888. François Xavier Dercum (1856–1931), Professor of Neurology at Jefferson Medical College, Philadelphia.
Descemet's membrane Described 1785. Jean Descemet (1732–1810), French physician; Professor of Anatomy and Surgery in Paris.
Devic's disease Described 1894. Devic was a French physician who died in 1930.
Dick test Described 1924. George Frederick Dick (1881–1967), American physician who, in 1923 with Gladys Rowena Dick, identified streptococci as the cause of scarlet fever.
Dietl's crisis Joseph Dietl (1804–1878), Polish physician.
Döderlein's bacillus Albert Siegmund Gustav Döderlein (1860–1941), German obstetrician and gynaecologist.
Down's syndrome Described 1866. John Langdon Haydon Down (1828–1896), English physician.
Duchenne muscular dystrophy Described 1849. Guillaume Benjamin Arnaud Duchenne (1806–1875), French neurologist.
Ducrey's bacillus Described 1889. Augusto Ducrey (1860–1940), Professor of Dermatology in Pisa and then Rome.
Dupuytren's contracture Described 1831. Baron Guillaume Dupuytren (1775–1835), French surgeon.
Eisenmenger complex Described 1897. Victor Eisenmenger (1864–1932), German physician.
Epstein-Barr virus Michael Anthony Epstein, Bristol pathologist; Murray Llewellyn Barr (b. 1908), Canadian anatomist and cytologist.
Erb's palsy Described 1874. Wilhelm Erb (1840–1921), Professor of Medicine at Leipzig and later at Heidelberg.
Esmarch's bandage Described 1869. Johann Friedrich August von Esmarch (1823–1908), Professor of Surgery at Kiel.
Eustachian tube Described 1562, but actually named after Eustachio by Valsalva a century later. Bartolomeo Eustachio (1520–1574), Physician to the Pope and Professor of Anatomy in Rome.
Ewing's tumour Described 1922. James Ewing (1866–1943), Professor of Pathology at Cornell University, New York.
Fallopian tube Described 1561. Gabriele Fallopio (1523–1563), Italian man of medicine. He was Professor of Surgery and Anatomy at Padua, where he was also Professor of Botany.
Fallot's tetralogy Described 1888. Etienne-Louis Arthur Fallot (1850–1911), Professor of Hygiene and Legal Medicine at Marseilles.

Fanconi syndrome Described 1936. Guido Fanconi (b. 1892), Emeritus Professor of Paediatrics at the University of Zürich.
Fehling's solution Described 1848. Hermann Christian von Fehling (1812–1885), Professor of Chemistry at Stuttgart.
Felty's syndrome Described 1924. Augustus Roi Felty (1895–1963), Physician at Hartford Hospital, Connecticut.
Frei test Described 1925. Wilhelm Siegmund Frei (1885–1943), Professor of Dermatology at Berlin, he settled in New York.
Freiberg's disease Described 1914. Albert Henry Freiberg (1869–1940), Cincinnati surgeon.
Friedländer's bacillus Described 1882. (Now known as *Klebsiella pneumoniae*.) Carl Friedländer (1847–1887), pathologist at the Friederichshain Hospital, Berlin.
Friedreich's ataxia Described 1863. Nikolaus Friedreich (1825–1882), Professor of Pathological Anatomy at Würzburg, later Professor of Pathology and Therapy at Heidelberg.
Fröhlich's syndrome Described 1901. Alfred Fröhlich (1871–1953), Professor of Pharmacology at the University of Vienna.
Gallie's operation Described 1921. William Edward Gallie (1882–1959), Professor of Surgery at the University of Toronto, Canada.
Ganser's state Sigbert Joseph Maria Ganser (1853–1931), psychiatrist at Dresden and Munich.
Gasserian ganglion Johann Laurentius Gasser (1723–1765), Professor of Anatomy at Vienna. He left no writings, and the ganglion was given his name by Anton Hirsch, one of his students, in his thesis of 1765.
Gaucher's disease Described 1882. Philippe Charles Ernest Gaucher (1854–1918), French physician and dermatologist.
Geiger counter Described 1908. Hans Geiger (1882–1945), German physicist who worked with Rutherford at Manchester University.
Ghon's focus Described 1912. Anton Ghon (1866–1936), Professor of Pathological Anatomy at Prague.
Gilliam's operation David Tod Gilliam (1844–1923), Columbus, Ohio gynaecologist.
Girdlestone's operation Gathorne Robert Girdlestone (1881–1950), Nuffield Professor of Orthopaedics at Oxford.
Golgi apparatus Described 1898. Camillo Golgi (1843–1926), Professor of Histology and later Rector of the University of Pavia. In 1906 he shared the Nobel Prize with Santiago Ramon y Cajal for work on the nervous system.
Goodpasture's syndrome Described 1919. Ernest William Goodpasture (1886–1960), American pathologist.
Graefe's knife Friedrich Wilhelm Ernst Albrecht von Graefe (1828–1870), Professor of Ophthalmology in Berlin.
Gram stain Described 1884. Hans Christian Joachim Gram (1853–1938), Professor of Medicine in Copenhagen. He discovered the stain by accident while a student in Berlin.
Graves' disease Described 1835. Robert James Graves (1796–1853), Irish physician at the Meath Hospital, Dublin, where he was responsible for introducing clinical ward work for medical students.
Grawitz tumour Described 1883. Paul Albert Grawitz (1850–1932), Professor of Pathology at Griefswald.
Guillain-Barré syndrome Described 1916. Georges Guillain (1876–1961), Professor of Neurology at Paris; Jean Alexandre Barré (1880–1967), Professor of Neurology at Strasbourg.
Hand-Schüller-Christian disease Described 1893. (Described 1915 by Schüller and 1920 by Christian.) Alfred Hand Jr. (1868–1949), Philadelphia paediatrician; Artur Schüller (1874–1958), Vienna neurologist; Henry Asbury Christian (1876–1951), Harvard Professor of Medicine.
Hansen's bacillus (*Mycobacterium leprae*) Discovered 1873. Gerhard Henrik Armauer Hansen (1841–1912), Norwegian physician.
Harrison's sulcus Edward Harrison (1766–1838), Lincolnshire general practitioner. Also ascribed to Edwin Harrison (1779–1874), London physician.
Hartmann's solution Described 1932. Alexis Frank Hartmann (1898–1964), St Louis, Missouri paediatrician.
Hartnup disease Name of the family in whom this inherited disease was first recorded.
Hashimoto's disease Described 1912. Hakaru Hashimoto (1881–1934), Japanese surgeon.
Haversian canals Described 1689. Clopton Havers (1657–1702), English surgeon.
Heberden's nodes Described 1802. William Heberden (1710–1801), London physician.
Hegar's sign Alfred Hegar (1830–1914), Professor of Obstetrics and Gynaecology at Freiburg.
Henle (loop of) Described 1862. Friedrich Gustav Jakob Henle (1809–1885), Professor of Anatomy at Göttingen.
Henoch-Schönlein purpura Described 1832 by Schönlein and 1865 by Henoch. Eduard Heinrich Henoch (1820–1910), Professor of Paediatrics at Berlin; Johannes Lukas Schönlein (1793–1864), physician and pathologist at Würzburg, Zürich, and Berlin.
Hering-Breuer reflex Karl Ewald Konstantin Hering (1834–1918), physiologist in Vienna and Leipzig; Josef Breuer (1842–1925), Vienna psychiatrist.
Higginson's syringe Alfred Higginson (1808–1884), Liverpool surgeon.
Highmore (antrum of) Described 1651. Nathaniel Highmore (1613–1685), Dorset physician.
Hirschsprung's disease Described 1888. Harald Hirschsprung (1830–1916), Professor of Paediatrics in Copenhagen.

His (bundle of) Described 1893. Willhelm His Jr. (1863–1934), Professor of Anatomy successively at Leipzig, Basle, Göttingen, and Berlin.
Hodgkin's disease Described 1832. Thomas Hodgkin (1798–1866), London physician.
Homans' sign Described 1941. John Homans (1877–1954), Professor of Clinical Surgery at Harvard.
Horner's syndrome Described 1869. Johann Friedrich Horner (1831–1886), Professor of Ophthalmology at Zürich.
Horton's headache *or* **syndrome** Bayard Taylor Horton (b. 1895), Minnesota physician.
Huhner's test Max Huhner (1873–1947), New York urologist.
Huntington's chorea Described 1872. George Sumner Huntington (1850–1916), New York physician.
Hurler's syndrome Described 1920. Gertrud Hurler, Munich paediatrician.
Jacksonian epilepsy Described 1863. John Hughlings Jackson (1835–1911), English neurologist.
Jacquemier's sign Jean Marie Jacquemier (1806–1879), French obstetrician.
Kahn test Described 1922. Reuben Leon Kahn (b. 1887), Michigan serologist.
Kaposi's sarcoma Described 1872. Moritz Kohn Kaposi (1837–1902), Professor of Dermatology at Vienna.
Kayser-Fleischer rings Described 1902 by Kayser, 1903 by Fleischer. Bernhard Kayser (1869-1954), German ophthalmologist; Bruno Richard Fleischer (1848–1904), German physician.
Keller's operation Described 1904. William Lordan Keller (1874–1959), American surgeon.
Kernig's sign Described 1882. Vladimir Mikhailovich Kernig (1840–1917), St Petersburg neurologist.
Killian's operation Gustav Killian (1860–1921), Berlin laryngologist.
Kimmelstiel-Wilson disease Described 1936. Paul Kimmelstiel (1900-1970), Boston pathologist; Clifford Wilson (b. 1906), Emeritus Professor of Medicine, London University.
Kirschner wire Described 1909. Martin Kirschner (1879–1942), Professor of Surgery at Heidelberg.
Klebs-Loeffler bacillus (*Corynebacterium diphtheriae*) Theodor Albrecht Edwin Klebs (1834–1913), bacteriologist in Zürich and Chicago; Friedrich August Johannes Loeffler (1852–1915) Berlin bacteriologist.
Klinefelter's syndrome Described 1942. Harry Fitch Klinefelter Jr. (b. 1912), Associate Professor of Medicine, Johns Hopkins Medical School, Baltimore.
Klumpke's paralysis Described 1885. Auguste Klumpke (Madame Déjerine-Klumpke) (1859–1927), Paris neurologist, one of the first women doctors to qualify there in 1888.
Koch's bacillus (*Mycobacterium tuberculosis*) Described 1882. Robert Koch (1843–1910), Professor of Hygiene in Berlin, and later Director of the Institute for Infectious Diseases. (Nobel Prize 1905).
Köhler's disease Described 1908 and 1926. Alban Köhler (1874–1947), German radiologist.
Koplik's spots Described 1896. Henry Koplik (1858–1927), American paediatrician.
Korsakoff's syndrome *or* **psychosis** Described 1887. Sergei Sergeyevich Korsakoff (1854–1900), Russian psychiatrist.
Krause corpuscles Described 1860. Wilhelm Johann Friedrich Krause (1833–1910), Göttingen and Berlin anatomist.
Krebs cycle Sir Hans Adolf Krebs (b. 1900), British biochemist.
Krukenberg tumour Georg Peter Heinrich Krukenberg (1856–1899), Bonn gynaecologist.
Kuntscher nail Described 1940. Gerhard Kuntscher (1900–1972), Kiel surgeon.
Kupffer's cells Described 1876. Karl Wilhelm von Kupffer (1829–1902), German anatomist.
Kveim test Morten Ansgar Kveim (b. 1892), Oslo physician.
Laennec's cirrhosis Described 1819. René Théophile Hyacinthe Laennec (1781-1826), Professor of Medicine at the Collège de France, and inventor of the stethoscope.
Landry's paralysis Jean Baptiste Octave Landry (1826–1865), Paris physician.
Lange test Described 1912. Carl Friedrich August Lange (b. 1883), German physician.
Langerhans (islets of) Described 1869. Paul Langerhans (1847–1888), Professor of Pathological Anatomy at Freiburg.
Lassa fever Named after a village in northern Nigeria where the fever was first reported.
Lassar's paste Oskar Lassar (1849–1907), Berlin dermatologist.
Legge-Calvé-Perthes disease Described 1910 separately by all three workers. Arthur Thornton Legg (1874–1939), American orthopaedic surgeon; Jacques Calvé (1875–1954), French orthopaedic surgeon; Georg Clemens Perthes (1869–1927), Leipzig surgeon.
Lembert's suture Described 1826. Antoine Lembert (1802–1851), Paris surgeon.
Leydig cells Described 1850. Franz von Leydig (1821–1908), Professor of Histology successively at Würzburg, Tübingen, and Bonn.
Lieberkuhn's glands Described 1745. Johann Nathaniel Lieberkuhn (1711–1756), Berlin anatomist and physician.
Little's disease Described 1843. William John Little (1810–1894), Physician at the London Hospital.
Ludwig's angina Described 1836. Wilhelm Friedrich von Ludwig (1790–1865), Professor of Surgery and Midwifery at Tübingen, and Court Physician to King Frederick II.
Magendie (foramen of) Described 1828. François Magendie (1783–1855), Paris physician and physiologist.

Mallory-Weiss tears Described 1929. G. Kenneth Mallory (b. 1900), Professor of Pathology, Boston University.
Malpighian body Described 1666. Marcello Malpighi (1628–1694), Rome and Bologna anatomist and physiologist.
Mantoux test Described 1908. Charles Mantoux (1877–1947), Paris physician.
Marfan's syndrome Described 1896. Bernard Jean Antonin Marfan (1858-1942), Paris paediatrician.
McBurney's point Described 1899. Charles McBurney (1845–1913), New York surgeon.
Meckel's diverticulum Described 1809. Johann Friedrich Meckell (II) (1781–1833), Halle surgeon and anatomist.
Meissner's plexus Described 1853. Georg Meissner (1829–1905), German anatomist and physiologist.
Mendel's laws Described 1865. Gregor Johann Mendel (1822–1884), Austrian Augustinian monk and naturalist of Brno, whose work was rediscovered by de Vries in 1900.
Mendelson's syndrome Described 1954. Curtis L. Mendelson. Contemporary American obstetrician and gynaecologist.
Ménière's disease Described 1861. Prosper Ménière (1799–1862), Paris physician.
Merkel's disc Friedrich Siegmund Merkel (1845–1919), German anatomist.
Michel's clips Gaston Michel (1874–1937), Professor of Clinical Surgery at Nancy.
Milroy's disease Described 1892. William Forsyth Milroy (1855–1942), Professor of Clinical Medicine at Nebraska.
Mönckeberg's arteriosclerosis Described 1903. Johann Georg Mönckeberg (1877–1925), Bonn physician and pathologist.
Montgomery's glands William Fetherstone Montgomery (1797–1859), Dublin gynaecologist.
Mooren's ulcer Albert Mooren (1828–1899), ophthalmologist in Düsseldorf.
Moro reflex Ernst Moro (1874–1951), paediatrician in Heidelberg.
Müllerian duct Described 1825. Johannes Peter Müller (1801–1858), Professor of Anatomy at Bonn, later Professor of Anatomy and Physiology at Berlin.
Munchhausen's syndrome Described by Richard Asher in 1951 and named after Baron von Munchhausen, a 16th century traveller and inveterate liar.
Murphy's sign Described 1912. John Benjamin Murphy (1857–1916), Chicago surgeon.
Negri bodies Described 1903. Adelchi Negri (1876–1912), Professor of Bacteriology at Pavia.
Nissl bodies Described 1894. Franz Nissl (1860–1919), Heidelberg neuropathologist.
Ortolani's sign Described 1937. Marius Ortolani, contemporary Italian orthopaedic surgeon.
Osler's nodes Described 1885. Sir William Osler (1849–1919), Professor of Medicine successively in Montreal, Philadelphia, Baltimore, and Oxford.
Pacinian corpuscles Described 1835. Filippo Pacini (1812–1883), anatomist and physiologist in Pisa and Florence.
Paget's disease Described 1877. Sir James Paget (1814–1899), London surgeon.
Papanicolaou test Described 1933. George Nicolas Papanicolaou (1883–1962), Greek anatomist and physician who worked in USA.
Parkinson's disease Described 1817. James Parkinson (1755–1824), English physician.
Paschen body Enrique Paschen (1860–1936), Hamburg pathologist.
Pasteurization Louis Pasteur (1822–1895), Paris chemist and bacteriologist.
Paul-Bunnell reaction Described 1932. John Rodman Paul (b. 1893), New Haven physician; Walls Willard Bunnell (1902–1966), Connecticut physician.
Paul's tube Described 1891. Frank Thomas Paul (1851–1941), English surgeon.
Pel-Ebstein fever Described 1885. Pieter Klaases Pel (1852–1919), Professor of Medicine in Amsterdam; Wilhelm Ebstein (1836–1912), Professor of Medicine at Göttingen.
Pellegrini-Stieda disease Described 1905. Augusto Pellegrini, surgeon in Florence; Alfred Stieda (1869–1945), Professor of Surgery at Königsberg.
Peyer's patches Described 1677. Johann Conrad Peyer (1653–1712), Swiss anatomist.
Peyronie's disease Described 1743. François de la Peyronie (1678–1747), Surgeon to Louis XV in Paris.
Placido's disk A. Placido (fl. 1882), Portuguese oculist.
Plummer-Vinson syndrome Described 1912 by Plummer, 1919 by Vinson (also described in 1919 by Patterson and Brown Kelly, whose names are frequently associated with the syndrome). Henry Stanley Plummer (1874–1937), Minnesota physician; Porter Paisley Vinson (1890–1959), physician at the Mayo Clinic, Minnesota.
Politzer bag Described 1863. Adam Politzer (1835–1920), Professor of Otology in Vienna.
Pott's disease described 1779; **Pott's fracture**, described 1765. Sir Percivall Pott (1714–1788), London surgeon.
Poupart's ligament Described 1705. François Poupart (1616–1708), Paris surgeon and anatomist.
Purkinje cells described 1837; **Purkinje fibres,** described 1839. Johannes Evangelista Purkinje (1787–1869), Professor of Physiology at Breslau and later at Prague.
Queckenstedt's test Described 1916. Hans Heinrich Georg Queckenstedt (1876–1918), German physician.
Quick test Described 1935. Armand James Quick (b. 1894), Milwaukee physician and biochemist.
Ramstedt's operation Described 1912. Wilhelm Conrad Ramstedt (1867–1963), Münster surgeon.

Raynaud's disease Described 1862. Maurice Raynaud (1834–1881), Paris physician.
Reiter's syndrome Described 1916. Hans Conrad Reiter (1881–1969), German bacteriologist and hygienist.
Rinne's test Described 1855. Friedrich Heinrich Rinne (1819–1868), Otologist at Göttingen.
Roentgen Named after Wilhelm Konrad von Röntgen (1845–1923), physicist at Strasbourg, Geissen, Würzburg, and Munich, and then Director of the Physics Laboratory at Würzburg, where he discovered X-rays in 1895.
Romberg's sign Described 1846. Moritz Heinrich Romberg (1795–1873), Berlin physician and pioneer neurologist.
Rorschach test Described 1921. Hermann Rorschach (1884–1922), German-born psychiatrist who worked in Bern, Switzerland.
Roth spots Moritz Roth (1839–1914), Basle pathologist and physician.
Rothera's test Arthur Cecil Hamel Rothera (1880–1915), biochemist in Melbourne, Australia.
Rovsing's sign Described 1907. Nils Thorkild Rovsing (1862–1927), Professor of Surgery at Copenhagen.
Rubin's test Isador Clinton Rubin (b. 1883), New York gynaecologist.
Ruffini corpuscles Described 1893. Angelo Ruffini (1864–1929), histologist at Bologna.
Russell traction (Hamilton Russell traction). Described 1924. R. Hamilton Russell (1860–1933), Melbourne surgeon.
Ryle's tube Described 1921. John Alfred Ryle (1882–1950), physician at London, Cambridge, and Oxford.
Sabin vaccine Albert Bruce Sabin (b. 1906), New York bacteriologist.
Salk vaccine Jonas Edward Salk (b. 1914), virologist in Pittsburgh.
Sayre's jacket Lewis Albert Sayre (1820–1901), New York surgeon.
Scarpa's triangle Antonio Scarpa (1747–1832), Italian anatomist and surgeon.
Scheuermann's disease Described 1920. Holger Werfel Scheuermann (1877–1960), Danish orthopaedic surgeon and radiologist.
Schick test Described 1908. Bela Schick (1877–1967), paediatrician in Vienna and New York.
Schilling test Robert Frederick Schilling (b. 1919), Wisconsin physician.
Schlatter's disease Described 1903. Carl Schlatter (1864–1934), Professor of Surgery at Zürich.
Schlemm (canal of) Described 1830. Friedrich Schlemm (1795–1858), Professor of Anatomy at Berlin.
Schönlein-Henoch purpura See Henoch-Schönlein purpura.
Schwann cell Described 1839. Friedrich Theodor Schwann (1810–1882), German anatomist.
Schwartze's operation Hermann Schwartze (1837–1910), Halle otologist.
Sengstaken tube Robert William Sengstaken (b. 1923), New Jersey surgeon.
Sertoli cells Described 1865. Enrico Sertoli (1842–1910), Italian histologist, Professor of Experimental Physiology at Milan.
Simmonds' disease Described 1914. Morris Simmonds (1855–1925), German physician and pathologist.
Sippy diet Bertram Welton Sippy (1866–1924), physician in Chicago.
Skene's glands Described 1880. Alexander Johnston Chalmers Skene (1838–1900), Scottish-born New York gynaecologist.
Smith-Petersen nail Described 1931. Marius Nygaard Smith-Petersen (1886–1953), Norwegian-born Boston orthopaedic surgeon.
Snellen chart Described 1862. Hermann Snellen (1834–1908), Utrecht ophthalmologist.
Sonne dysentery Described 1915. Carl Olaf Sonne (1882–1948), Danish bacteriologist and physician.
Sprengel's deformity Described 1891. Otto Gerhard Karl Sprengel (1852–1915), German surgeon.
Stacke's operation Ludwig Stacke (1859–1918), German otologist.
Stein-Leventhal syndrome Described 1935. Irving F. Stein (b. 1887), American gynaecologist; Michael Leo Leventhal (b. 1901), American obstetrician and gynaecologist.
Steinmann's pin Described 1907. Fritz Steinmann (1872–1932), Berne surgeon.
Stellwag's sign Carl Stellwag von Carion (1823–1904), ophthalmologist in Vienna.
Stensen's duct Described 1661. Niels Stensen (1638–1686), Danish physician-priest, anatomist, physiologist and theologian.
Stevens-Johnson syndrome Described 1922. Albert Mason Stevens (1884–1945), Frank Chambliss Johnson (1894–1934), paediatricians in New York.
Still's disease Described 1896. Sir George Frederic Still (1868–1941), London paediatrician and Physician to the King.
Stokes-Adams syndrome William Stokes (1804–1878), Irish physician; Robert Adams (1791–1875), Irish surgeon.
Sudeck's atrophy Described 1900. Paul Hermann Martin Sudeck (1866–1938), Hamburg surgeon.
Sydenham's chorea Described 1686. Thomas Sydenham (1624–1689), English physician.
Syme's amputation Described 1842. James Syme (1799–1870), Edinburgh surgeon and teacher; one of the first to adopt antisepsis (Joseph Lister was his son-in-law) and also among the early users of anaesthesia.
Tay-Sachs disease Described 1881. Warren Tay (1843–1927), London ophthalmologist; Bernard Sachs (1858–1944), New York neurologist.

Tenon's capsule Jacques René Tenon (1724–1816), Paris surgeon.
Thiersch's graft Described 1874. Karl Thiersch (1822–1895), German surgeon.
Thomas's splint Described 1875. Hugh Owen Thomas (1834–1891), Liverpool surgeon and bone-setter.
Trendelenburg operation, position, sign Friedrich Trendelenburg (1844–1924), Leipzig surgeon.
Trousseau's signs Armand Trousseau (1801–1867), Paris physician.
Turner's syndrome Described 1938. Henry Hubert Turner (b. 1892) American endocrinologist; Clinical Professor of Medicine, Oklahoma University.
Vincent's angina Described 1898. Jean Hyacinthe Vincent (1862–1950), physician and bacteriologist in Paris.
von Recklinghausen's disease Described 1882. Friedrich Daniel von Recklinghausen (1833–1910), Professor of Pathology at Strasbourg.
von Willebrand's disease Described 1926. E. A. von Willebrand (1870–1949), Finnish physician.
Waldeyer's ring Described 1884. Heinrich Wilhelm Gottfried Waldeyer-Hartz (1836–1921), Berlin anatomist.
Wangensteen tube Described 1932. Owen Harding Wangensteen (1898–1980), Minneapolis surgeon.
Wassermann reaction/test Described 1906. August Paul von Wasserman (1866–1925), Berlin bacteriologist.
Waterhouse-Friderichsen syndrome Described 1911. Rupert Waterhouse (1873–1958), physician at Bath; described 1918 by Carl Friderichsen (b. 1886) Copenhagen physician.
Waterston's anastomosis David James Waterston (b. 1910), paediatric surgeon in London.
Weber-Christian disease Frederick Parkes Weber (1863–1962), London physician; Henry Asbury Christian (1876–1951), Boston physician.
Weber's test Friedrich Eugen Weber-Liel (1832–1891), German otologist.
Weil-Felix test, reaction Described 1916. Edmund Weil (1880–1922), Viennese physician and bacteriologist; Arthur Felix (1887–1956), London bacteriologist.
Weil's disease Described 1886. Adolf Weil (1848–1916), physician in Estonia who also practiced at Wiesbaden.
Wernicke's encephalopathy Described 1875. Karl Wernicke (1848–1904), Breslau psychiatrist and neurologist.
Wertheim's operation Described 1900. Ernst Wertheim (1864–1920), Vienna gynaecologist.
Wharton's duct; Wharton's jelly Thomas Wharton (1614–1673), English physician and anatomist at St Thomas's Hospital, London.
Wheelhouse's operation Claudius Galen Wheelhouse (1826–1909), Leeds surgeon.
Whipple's disease Described 1907. George Hoyt Whipple (1878–1976), American pathologist.
Widal reaction Described 1896. Georges Fernand Isidore Widal (1862–1929), Paris physician and teacher.
Willis, circle of Described 1664. Thomas Willis (1621–1675), English physician and anatomist.
Wilms' tumour Described 1899. Max Wilms (1867–1918), Professor of Surgery successively at Leipzig, Basle, and Heidelberg.
Wilson's disease Described 1912. Samuel Alexander Kinnier Wilson (1878–1937), London neurologist.
Wood's lamp Robert Williams Wood (1868–1945), Baltimore physicist.
Zollinger-Ellison syndrome Described 1955. Robert Milton Zollinger (b. 1903) Professor of Surgery at Ohio State University; Edwin H. Ellison (1918–1970), Associate Professor of Surgery at Ohio State University.